D1751448

Medicinal Plants
of
Brazil

MEDICINAL PLANTS of BRAZIL

Walter B. Mors,
Carlos Toledo Rizzini
and
Nuno Alvares Pereira

Edited by
Robert A. DeFilipps

Reference Publications, Inc.

This book is No. 6 in the series "Medicinal Plants of the World."

Published 2000

Copyright © 2000 by Reference Pulications.

Printed in the United States of America

Library of Congress Cataloguing-in-Publication Data

Mors, Walter B.
    Medicinal plants of Brazil / Walter B. Mors, Carlos Toledo Rizzini, Nuno Alvares Pereira ; edited by Robert A. DeFilipps.
    p. cm -- (Medicinal plants of the world ; 6)
    Includes bibliographical references and indexes.
    ISBN-0-917256-42-5 (hardcover : alk. paper)
    1. Medicinal plants - Brazil. 2. Materia medica, Vegetable- Brazil. I. Rizzini, Carlos Toledo. II. Pereira, Nuno Alvares. III. DeFilipps, Robert A. IV. Title. V. Series.

RS175.B7 M67 2000
615'.32'0981--dc21

                                                                    00-055859

Library of Congress Catalog Card Number: ISBN-0-917256-42-5
ISBN-0-917256-07-7 (v. 1) (West Africa)
ISBN-0-917256-12-3 (v. 2) (West Indies)
ISBN-0-917256-16-6 (v. 3) (North Africa)
ISBN-0-917256-20-4 (v. 4) (China, set)
ISBN-0-917256-39-5 (v. 5) (India, set)
ISBN-0-917256-42-5 (v. 6) (Brazil)

All rights reserved. No part of this work may be reproduced or utilized in any form or by any means, electronic or mechanical, or by any information storage and retrieval system without permission in writing from the publisher.

Reference Publications, Inc.
218 St. Clair River Drive, Box 344
Algonac, Michigan 48001-0344

Contents

Foreword: Some Historical and Modern Facets of
the Brazilian Medicinal Plant Heritage xxiii
    I. Brazil named for brazilwood
    II. Disease and remedy in the colonial era and today
    III. Curare
    IV. Indians
Introduction xli
General Bibliography xlvii

ACANTHACEAE
Ruellia geminiflora H.B.K. 1
Ruellia tuberosa L. 1

ADIANTACEAE
Adiantopsis chlorophylla (Sw.) Fée 1
Adiantum concinnum Humb. & Bonp. 1
Adiantum cuneatum Langsd. & Fisch. 1
Adiantum trapeziforme L. 1

AIZOACEAE
Sesuvium portulacastrum L. 2
Aizoaceae–References 2

ALISMATACEAE
Alisma palaefolium Kunth 2
Echinodorus grandiflorus
  (Cham. & Schl.) Mich. 2
Echinodorus macrophyllus (Kunth) Mich. 2
Echinodorus pubescens Mart. 2

AMARANTHACEAE
Achyranthes ficoidea Lam. 3
Achyranthes indica L. 3
Alternanthera achyrantha R. Br. 3
Alternanthera brasiliana (L.) O. Ktze. 3
Amaranthus blitum L. 3
Amaranthus spinosus L. 3
Amaranthus viridis L. 3
Chamissoa altissima H.B.K. 4
Chamissoa macrocarpa H.B.K. 4
Gomphrena leucocephala Mart. 4
Gomphrena macrocephala St.-Hil. 4
Gomphrena mollis Mart. 4
Gomphrena officinalis Mart. 4
Iresine polymorpha Mart. 4
Pfaffia glomerata (Spreng.) Peders. 4
Pfaffia jubata Mart. 5
Pfaffia paniculata (Mart.) Kuntze 5
Philoxerus portulacoides St.-Hil. 5
Amaranthaceae–References 5

AMARYLLIDACEAE
Bomarea salsilloides Roem. 6
Bomarea spectabilis Schrenk 6
Crinum scabrum Sims 6
Griffinia hyacinthina Ker.-Gawl. 6
Hippeastrum psittacinum Herb. 6
Hippeastrum puniceum (Lam.) Kuntze 6
Hippeastrum vittatum (L'Hérit.) Herb. 7
Hymenocallis tubiflora Salisb. 7
Amaryllidaceae–References 7

ANACARDIACEAE
Anacardium humile St.-Hil. 7
Anacardium nanum St.-Hil. 7
Anacardium occidentale L. 7
Astronium fraxinifolium Schott 8
Lithraea molleoides (Vell.) Engl. 8
Myracroduon urundeuva Fr. All. 9
Schinopsis brasiliensis Engl. 9
Schinus lentiscifolius March. 9
Schinus molle L. 9
Schinus terebinthifolius Raddi 9
Spondias macrocarpa Engl. 10
Spondias mombin L. 10
Anacardiaceae–References 10

ANNONACEAE
Annona ambotay Aubl. 11
Annona coriacea Mart. 11
Annona cornifolia St.-Hil. 12
Annona crassifolia Mart. 12
Annona dioica St.-Hil. 12
Annona foetida Mart. 12
Annona glabra L. 12
Annona marcgravii Mart. 12
Annona muricata L. 13
Annona reticulata L. 13
Annona spinescens Mart. 13
Annona squamosa L. 13
Bocagea alba St.-Hil. 13
Bocagea viridis St.-Hil. 14
Duguetia furfuracea (St.-Hil.)
  Benth. & Hook. 14

Duguetia riparia Hub. 14
Guatteria nigrescens Mart. 14
Guatteria ouregon (Aubl.) Dun. 14
Guatteria scandens Ducke 15
Rollinia exalbida (Vell.) Mart. 15
Rollinia orthopetala DC. 15
Rollinia salicifolia Schl. 15
Rollinia sylvatica (St.-Hil.) Mart. 15
Xylopia aromatica (Lam.) Mart. 15
Xylopia benthamiana Fries 16
Xylopia frutescens Aubl. 16
Xylopia sericea St.-Hil. 16
Annonaceae–References 16

APIACEAE
Apium sellowianum Wolf 18
Eryngium elegans Cham. & Schlecht 19
Eryngium foetidum L. 19
Eryngium pandanifolium
   Cham. & Schlecht. 19
Eryngium paniculatum Cav.
   & Domb. ex Delar. 19
Eryngium pristis Cham. & Schlecht. 19
Hydrocotyle bonariensis Lam. 19
Hydrocotyle leucocephala
   Cham. & Schlecht. 19
Apiaceae–References 19

APOCYNACEAE
Allamanda blanchetii M. Arg. 20
Allamanda cathartica L. 20
Allamanda doniana M. Arg. 20
Ambelania tenuifolia Aubl. 20
Anacampta riedellii (M. Arg.) Mgf. 21
Anisolobus cururu (Mart.) M. Arg. 21
Aspidosperma desmanthum M. Arg. 21
Aspidosperma discolor Benth. 21
Aspidosperma excelsum Benth. 21
Aspidosperma nigricans Handro 21
Aspidosperma nitidum Benth. 21
Aspidosperma polyneuron M. Arg. 21
Aspidosperma spp. 22
Couma macrocarpa B. Rodr. 23
Couma utilis (Mart.) M. Arg. 23
Dipladenia fragrans DC. 23
Dipladenia illustris M. Arg. 23
Dipladenia spp. 23
Echites macrocalyx M. Arg. 24
Echites peltata Vell. 24
Geissospermum laeve (Vell.) Baill. 24
Geissospermum sericeum Benth. & Hook. 24
Geissospermum spp. 24
Haemadyction gaudichaudii DC. 24
Hancornia speciosa Gomes 24
Himatanthus alba (L.) Woods. 24
Himatanthus drastica (Mart.) Woods. 24
Himatanthus fallax (M. Arg.) Woods. 25
Himatanthus lancifolia (M. Arg.) Woods. 26
Himatanthus phagedaenica
   (Mart.) Woods. 26
Himatanthus sucuuba (Spr.) Woods. 26
Macrosiphonia longiflora (Desf.) M. Arg. 26
Macrosiphonia velame (St.-Hil.) M. Arg. 26
Mandevilla velutina (Mart.
   ex Stadelm.) Woods. var. velutina 27
Mesechites sulphurea (Vell.) M. Arg. 27
Odontadenia speciosa Benth. 27
Parahancornia amapa (Hub.) Ducke 27
Peschiera affinis (M. Arg.) Miers 27
Peschiera laeta (Mart.) Miers 27
Plumeria alba L. 28
Rauwolfia bahiensis DC. 28
Rauwolfia blanchetii DC. 28
Rauwolfia ligustrina Willd. ex
   Roem. & Schult. 28
Secondatia floribunda DC. 28
Tabernaemontana citrifolia L. 28
Thevetia ahouai (L.) DC. 28
Vallesia cymbifolia Ortega 29
Zschokkea arborescens M. Arg. 29
Apocynaceae–References 29

AQUIFOLIACEAE
Ilex acrodonta Reiss. 31
Ilex brevicuspis Reiss. 31
Ilex paraguariensis St.-Hil. 31
Aquifoliaceae–References 33

ARACEAE
Anthurium affine Schott 33
Anthurium oxycarpum Poepp. 33
Caladium bicolor (Aiton) Vent. 34
Caladium bicolor (Aiton) Vent.
   var. poecile (Schott) Engler 35
Caladium sororium Schott 35
Dieffenbachia seguine (Jacq.) Schott 35
Dracontium asperum K. Koch 35
Dracontium polyphyllum L. 36
Monstera adansonii Schott 36
Monstera obliqua Miquel 36
Montrichardia linifera (Arruda) Schott ... 36
Philodendron bipinnatifidum Schott 36
Philodendron hederaceum (Jacq.)
   Schott var. hederaceum 36
Philodendron imbe Schott 36
Philodendron ochrostemon Schott 37
Philodendron pedatum (Hook.) Kunth 37
Philodendron selloum Koch 37

Philodendron speciosum Schott 37
Urospatha caudata (Poepp.
  & Endl.) Schott 37
Xanthosoma striatipes (Kunth
  & Bouché) Madison 37
Xanthosoma violaceum Schott 37
Araceae–References 38

ARECACEAE
Allagoptera campestris (Mart.) Kuntze ... 39
Astrocaryum aculeatissimum
  (Schott) Burret 39
Astrocaryum murumuru Mart. 39
Attalea oleifera Barb. Rodr. 39
Attalea spectabilis Mart. 39
Bactris insignis (Mart.) Baill. 39
Butia yatay (Mart.) Becc. 39
Cocos nucifera L. 40
Copernicia prunifera (Mill.) H. Moore ... 40
Desmoncus orthacanthos Mart. 40
Desmoncus polyacanthos Mart. 40
Elaeis guineensis Jacq. 40
Elaeis oleifera (H.B.K.) Cortez 40
Euterpe edulis Mart. 41
Euterpe oleracea Mart. 42
Jessenia bataua (Mart.) Burret 43
Leopoldinia major Wallace 43
Mauritia flexuosa L. f. 43
Mauritiella aculeata (Kunth) Burret 43
Oenocarpus distichus Mart. 43
Orbignya phalerata Mart. 43
Raphia taedigera (Mart.) Mart. 45
Scheelea phalerata (Mart.
  ex Spreng.) Burret 45
Syagrus comosa Mart. 45
Syagrus coronata (Mart.) Becc. 45
Syagrus oleracea (Mart.) Becc. 45
Syagrus pseudococos (Raddi) Glassman . 45
Syagrus romanzoffiana (Cham.) Glassman 45
Syagrus schizophylla (Mart.) Glassman .. 46
Arecaceae–References 46

ARISTOLOCHIACEAE
Aristolochia birostris Duch. 46
Aristolochia cordigera Willd. 46
Aristolochia cymbifera Mart. & Zucc. 46
Aristolochia elegans Mast. 48
Aristolochia esperanzae O. Kuntze 48
Aristolochia gigantea Mart. & Zucc. 48
Aristolochia triangularis Cham. 48
Aristolochia trilobata L. 48
Aristolochia spp. 49
Holostylis reniformis Duch. 50
Aristolochiaceae–References 50

ASCLEPIADACEAE
Araujia sericifera Brot. 50
Calotropis procera (Ait.) Ait. f.. 50
Marsdenia amylacea
  (Barb.-Rodr.) Malme 51
Asclepiadaceae–References 51

ASTERACEAE
Acanthospermum australe
  (Loefl.) O. Ktze. 52
Acanthospermum hispidum DC. 52
Achyrocline satureioides (Lam.) DC. 52
Acmella oleracea (L.) R.K. Jansen 52
Acmella repens (Walt.) L.C. Rich. 52
Ageratum conyzoides L. 53
Ambrosia artemisiifolia L. 53
Ayapana triplinerve (Vahl)
  King & H. Robinson 53
Baccharidastrum triplinerve (Less.) Cabr. 53
Baccharis articulata (Lam.) Pers. 54
Baccharis dentata (Vell.) G.M. Barroso .. 54
Baccharis dracunculifolia DC. 54
Baccharis lundii DC. 54
Baccharis notosergila Gris. 54
Baccharis ramosissima Gardn. 54
Baccharis trimera (Less.) DC. 54
Baccharis spp. 56
Bidens cynapiifolia H.B.K. 56
Bidens graveolens Mart. 56
Bidens pilosa L. 57
Blanchetia heterotricha DC. 57
Calea pinnatifida (R. Br.) Less. 57
Chaptalia nutans (L.) Polak. 57
Chionolaena latifolia (Benth.) Baker 57
Chromolaena hirsuta (Hook. & Arn.)
  King & H. Robinson 58
Chromolaena laevigata (Lam.)
  King & H. Robinson 58
Clibadium leiocarpum Mart. 58
Clibadium rotundifolium DC. 58
Clibadium surinamense L. 58
Conocliniopsis prasiifolia (DC.)
  King & H. Robinson 58
Conyza blakei (Cabr.) Cabr. 58
Cyrtocymura scorpioides
  (Lam.) H. Robinson 58
Eclipta prostrata (L.) L. 59
Egletes viscosa (L.) Less. 59
Elephantopus micropappus Less. 59
Elephantopus mollis H.B.K. 59
Erigeron tweediei Hook. & Arn. 60
Flaveria bidentis (L.) Ktze. 60
Galinsoga parviflora Cav. 60

CONTENTS: ASTERACEAE / BOMBACACEAE

Gochnatia polymorpha (Less.) Cabr. 60
Grindelia buphthalmoides DC. 60
Grindelia scorzonerifolia Hook. & Arn. ... 60
Heterothalamus alienus (Spr.) O. Ktze. ... 60
Heterothalamus psiadioides Less. 60
Ichthyothere terminalis (Spr.) S.F. Blake . 61
Isostigma megapotamicum (Spr.) Sherff .. 61
Jungia floribunda Less. 61
Lucilia nitens Less. 61
Melampodium divaricatum (Rich.) DC. .. 61
Mikania cordifolia (L. f.) Willd. 61
Mikania glomerata Spreng. 61
Mikania hirsutissima DC. 62
Mikania lindleyana DC. 62
Mikania officinalis Mart. 62
Mikania parviflora (Aubl.) Karst. 62
Mikania periplocifolia Hook. & Arn. 62
Mikania setigera Schultz-Bip. ex Baker .. 62
Noticastrum diffusum (Pers.) Cabr. 62
Parthenium hysterophorus L. 64
Piptocarpha rotundifolia (Less.) Bak. 64
Pluchea laxiflora Hook. & Arn. 64
Pluchea suaveolens (Vell.) O. Ktze. 64
Porophyllum ruderale (Jacq.) Cass. 64
Pterocaulon virgatum DC. 64
Raulinoreitzia tremula (Hook.
 & Arn.) King & H. Robinson 64
Senecio brasiliensis Less. 65
Silybum marianum Gaertn. 65
Solidago chilensis Meyen 65
Sphagneticola trilobata (L.) Pruski 65
Stomatanthes oblongifolius
 (Spr.) H. Robinson 65
Tagetes erecta L. 67
Tagetes minuta L. 67
Tanacetum vulgare L. 67
Trixis antimenorrhoea (Schrank) Mart. ... 67
Unxia camphorata L. f. 67
Vernonanthura brasiliana
 (L.) H. Robinson 67
Xanthium orientale L., X. spinosum L.
 and X. strumarium L. 67
Asteraceae–References 68

BALANOPHORACEAE
Helosis cayennensis (Swartz) Spreng. 73
Lophophytum mirabile Schott & Endl. ... 73
Scybalium fungiforme Schott & Endl. 74

BEGONIACEAE
Begonia acida Mart. 75
Begonia hirtella Link 76
Begonia luxurians Scheidw. 76

Begonia paulensis DC. 76

BERBERIDACEAE
Berberis laurina Thunb. 76
Berberis spinulosa St.-Hil. 76
References–Berberidaceae 76

BIGNONIACEAE
Adenocalymma alliacea (Lam.) Miers 78
Anemopaegma arvense (Vell.) Stapf 78
Anemopaegma spp. 78
Arrabidaea agnus-castus (Cham.) DC. 78
Arrabidaea chica (H.B.K.) Bur. 78
Arrabidaea foetida Bur. & K. Sch. 79
Bignonia exoleta Vell. 79
Cremastus sceptrum Bur. & K. Sch. 79
Crescentia cujete L. 80
Cybistax antisyphilitica (Mart.) Mart. 80
Cydista aequinoctialis Miers 80
Jacaranda brasiliana (Lam.) Pers. 80
Jacaranda caroba (Vell.) DC. 80
Jacaranda copaia (Aubl.) D. Don 80
Jacaranda cuspidifolia Mart. 81
Jacaranda micrantha Cham. 81
Jacaranda mimosifolia D. Don 81
Jacaranda subrhombea DC. 81
Jacaranda spp. 81
Macfadyena unguis-cati (L.) Gentry 81
Martinella obovata (H.B.K.)
 Bur. & K. Sch. 82
Pyrostegia ignea (Vell.) Pres. 82
Sparattosperma leucanthum
 (Vell.) K. Sch. 82
Tabebuia aurea (Manso) Moore 82
Tabebuia barbata (May) Sandw. 82
Tabebuia caraiba (Mart.) Bur. 82
Tabebuia chrysotricha (Mart.) Standl. 82
Tabebuia impetiginosa (Mart.) Standl. ... 83
Tabebuia ipe (Mart.) Standl. 83
Tabebuia leucoxylon (L.) DC. 83
Tabebuia serratifolia (Vahl) Nichol. 83
Tabebuia umbellata (Sond.) Sandw. 83
Tabebuia spp. 83
Tanaecium nocturnum (B. Rodr.)
 Bur. & K. Sch. 84
Tynanthus cognatus (Cham.) Miers 84
Zeyheria digitalis (Vell.) Hoehne 84
Bignoniaceae–References 84

BIXACEAE
Bixa orellana L. 85
Bixaceae–References 86

BOMBACACEAE
Ceiba pentandra (L.) Gaertn. 86

Chorisia crispiflora H.B.K. 86
Ochroma pyramidale (Cav.) Urb. 86
Bombacaceae–References 86
BORAGINACEAE
Auxemma oncocalyx (Fr. All.) Taub. 87
Cordia coffeoides Warm. 87
Cordia ecalyculata Vell. 87
Cordia grandiflora DC. 87
Cordia insignis Cham. 87
Cordia magnolifolia Cham. 87
Cordia monosperma (Jacq.)
   Roem. & Schult. 87
Cordia multispicata Cham. 88
Cordia obscura Cham. 88
Cordia salicifolia Cham. 88
Cordia umbraculifera DC. 88
Cordia verbenacea DC. 88
Heliotropium curassavicum L. 88
Heliotropium elongatum Willd. 88
Heliotropium indicum L. 89
Heliotropium lanceolatum Loefgr. 89
Patagonula americana L. 89
Tournefortia elegans Cham. 89
Tournefortia laevigata Lam. 89
Tournefortia paniculata Cham. 89
Tournefortia volubilis L. 90
Boraginaceae–References 90
BROMELIACEAE
Ananas comosus (L.) Merrill 90
Bromelia antiacantha Bertol. 91
Bromelia arenaria Ule 91
Bromelia pinguin L. 91
Tillandsia aeranthos (Loisel.) L.B. Smith 91
Tillandsia usneoides L. 91
Bromeliaceae–References 92
BUDDLEJACEAE
Buddleja brasiliensis Jacq. ex Spr. 93
Buddleja cambara Arech. 93
Buddleja stachioides Cham. 93
BURSERACEAE
Protium aracouchini (Aubl.) March. 93
Protium heptaphyllum (Aubl.) March. 93
Protium icicariba (DC.) March. 94
Protium schomburgkianum Engl. 94
Protium spp. 94
Burseraceae–References 95
CACTACEAE
Brasilopuntia brasiliensis (Willd.) Berg. . 95
Cereus jamacaru DC. 95
Cereus peruvianus (L.) Mill. 95
Hylocereus undatus (Haw.) Br. & Rose ... 95

Lepismium myosurus Pfeiff. 96
Melocactus melocactoides (Hoffm.) DC. 97
Notocactus ottonis (Lem.) Berg. 97
Opuntia vulgaris Mill. 97
Pereskia aculeata Mill. 97
Pereskia bleo H.B.K. 97
Rhipsalis macrocarpa Miq. 97
Cactaceae–References 97
CAESALPINIACEAE
Apuleia leiocarpa (Vog.) MacBride 98
Bauhinia candicans Benth. 99
Bauhinia forficata Link 99
Bauhinia guianensis Aubl. 99
Bauhinia langsdorffiana Bong. 99
Bauhinia radiata Vell. 99
Bauhinia rutilans Spr. ex Benth. 99
Caesalpinia bonduc (L.) Roxb. 99
Caesalpinia bracteosa Tul. 100
Caesalpinia echinata Lam. 100
Caesalpinia ferrea Mart. ex Tul. 100
Caesalpinia microphylla Mart. 100
Caesalpinia pyramidalis Tul. 100
Campsiandra comosa Benth.
   var. *laurifolia* (Benth.) Cowan 100
Cassia ferruginea (Schrad.)
   Schrad. ex DC. 100
Cassia grandis L. 101
Chamaecrista cathartica
   (Mart.) Ir. & Barn. 101
Chamaecrista fasciculata
   (Michx.) Greene 102
Chamaecrista mimosoides
   (L.) Ir. & Barn. 102
Copaifera cearensis Huber ex Ducke 102
Copaifera multijuga Hayne 102
Copaifera officinalis (Jacq.) L. 102
Hymenaea courbaril L. 103
Hymenaea spp. 104
Parkinsonia aculeata L. 104
Senna affinis (Benth.) Ir. & Barn. 104
Senna alata (L.) Roxb. 104
Senna bicapsularis (L.) Roxb. 104
Senna corymbosa (Lam.) Ir. & Barn. 104
Senna hirsuta (L.) Ir. & Barn.
   var. *puberula* Ir. & Barn. 105
Senna latifolia (Meyer) Ir. & Barn. 105
Senna leiophylla (Vog.) Ir. & Barn. 105
Senna macranthera (Collad.) Ir. & Barn.105
Senna multijuga Rich.
   var. *verrucosa* (Vog.) Ir. & Barn. 105
Senna oblongifolia (Vog.) Ir. & Barn. 105

Senna obtusifolia (L.) Ir. & Barn. 105
Senna occidentalis (L.) Link 105
Senna quinqueangulata
  (Rich.) Ir. & Barn. 106
Senna rugosa (G. Don) Ir. & Barn. 106
Senna septentrionalis (Viv.) Ir. & Barn. 106
Senna uniflora (P. Miller) Ir. & Barn. 106
Senna spp. 106
Swartzia chrysantha B. Rodr. 107
Swartzia panacoco
  (Aubl.) Cowan var. *panacoco* 107
Vouacapoua americana Aubl. 107
Caesalpiniaceae–References 108
CAMPANULACEAE
Centropogon cornutus (L.) Druce 109
Haynaldia exaltata (Pohl) Kanitz 109
Hippobroma longiflora (L.) G. Don 109
Campanulaceae–References 110
CANELLACEAE
Cinnamodendron axillare
  (Nees & Mart.) Endl. 110
CANNACEAE
Canna edulis Ker-Gawl. 110
Canna gigantea Desf. 110
Canna glauca L. 110
Canna indica L. 111
Canna lanuginosa Roscoe 111
Canna lutea Roscoe 111
Canna warszewiczii Dietr. 111
Cannaceae–Reference 111
CAPPARACEAE
Capparis cynophallophora L. 111
Capparis lineata Pers. 111
Capparis urens B. Rodr. 111
Cleome aculeata L. 112
Cleome gigantea L. 112
Cleome polygama L. 112
Cleome speciosa H.B.K. 112
Cleome spinosa Jacq. 112
Crataeva benthamii Eichl. 112
Crataeva tapia L. 112
Capparaceae–References 113
CARICACEAE
Carica papaya L. 113
Jacaratia spinosa (Aubl.) A. DC. 113
Caricaceae–References 114
CARYOCARACEAE
Caryocar brasiliense Camb. 114
Caryocar coriaceum Wittm. 114
Caryocar glabrum (Aubl.) Pers. 114
Caryocar villosum (Aubl.) Pers. 114

Caryocaraceae–References 115
CARYOPHYLLACEAE
Polycarpaea corymbosa (L.) Lam. 115
CELASTRACEAE
Maytenus boaria Mol. 115
Maytenus communis Reiss. 115
Maytenus gonoclada Mart. 115
Maytenus ilicifolia Mart. 115
Maytenus laevis Reiss. 115
Maytenus obtusifolia Mart. 116
Maytenus spp. 116
Celastraceae–References 117
CHENOPODIACEAE
Chenopodium ambrosioides L. 118
Chenopodium hircinum Schrad. 119
Chenopodiaceae–References 119
CHLORANTHACEAE
Hedyosmum brasiliense Mart. 119
CHRYSOBALANACEAE
Chrysobalanus icaco L. 119
Licania macrophylla Benth. 120
Chrysobalanaceae–References 120
CLADONIACEAE
Cladonia miniata Mey. 120
Cladonia pyxidata (L.) Ach. 120
Cladoniaceae–Reference 120
CLUSIACEAE
Calophyllum brasiliense Camb. 120
Caraipa densifolia Mart. 121
Caraipa excelsa Ducke 121
Caraipa grandifolia Mart. 121
Caraipa insidiosa B. Rodr. 121
Caraipa minor Huber 121
Clusia grandiflora Splitg. 121
Clusia panapanari Choisy 122
Clusia rosea Jacq. 122
Hypericum brasiliense Choisy 122
Hypericum connatum Lam. 122
Hypericum teretiusculum St.-Hil. 122
Kielmeyera coriacea Mart. 122
Kielmeyera petiolaris Mart. 122
Kielmeyera speciosa St.-Hil. 123
Mammea americana L. 123
Platonia insignis Mart. 123
Symphonia globulifera L. f. 123
Tovomita brasiliensis (Mart.) Walp. 123
Vismia acuminata (L.) Pers. 123
Vismia guianensis (Aubl.) Choisy 124
Vismia japurensis Reich. 124
Vismia latifolia (Aubl.) Choisy 124
Vismia reichardtiana (O. Ktze.) Ewan ... 124

Clusiaceae–References 124
COCHLOSPERMACEAE
Cochlospermum orinocense
  (H.B.K.) Steud. 125
Cochlospermum regium
  (Mart. & Schl.) Pilg. 125
COMBRETACEAE
Combretum leprosum Mart. 126
Conocarpus erecta L. 126
Terminalia argentea Mart. 126
Terminalia tanibouca Smith 126
Combretaceae–Reference 126
COMMELINACEAE
Commelina nudiflora L. 126
Commelina platyphylla Klotz. ex Seub. . 126
Commelina pohliana Seub. 127
Commelina robusta Kunth 128
Commelina sulcata Willd. 128
Commelina vestita Seub. 128
Commelina virginica L. 128
Dichorisandra affinis Mart. 128
Dichorisandra leucophthalmos Hook. ... 128
Dichorisandra spp. 128
Tradescantia diuretica Mart. 128
Tradescantia effusa Mart. 129
Tradescantia spathacea Sw. 129
Commelinaceae–References 129
CONNARACEAE
Connarus patrisii Planch. 129
Connarus suberosus Planch. 129
CONVOLVULACEAE
Calonyction aculeatum (L.) House 129
Cuscuta racemosa Mart. 130
Evolvulus alsinoides L. 130
Evolvulus holosericeus H.B.K. 130
Ipomoea acetosifolia (Vahl)
  Roem. & Schult. 130
Ipomoea pentaphylla Jacq. 130
Ipomoea pes-caprae (L.) R. Br. 130
Operculina alata (Ham.) Urb. 131
Operculina macrocarpa Urb. 131
Convolvulaceae–References 131
COSTACEAE
Costus cuspidatus (Nees & Mart.) Maas 132
Costus spicatus (Jacq.) Sw. 132
Costus spiralis (Jacq.) Roscoe 132
Costaceae–References 132
CRASSULACEAE
Kalanchoe brasiliensis Camb. 133
Kalanchoe pinnata (Lam.) Pers. 133
Crassulaceae–References 134

CUCURBITACEAE
Anisosperma passiflora Manso 135
Cayaponia cabocla (Vell.) Mart. 135
Cayaponia espelina (Manso) Cogn. 135
Cayaponia martiana (Cogn.) Cogn. 135
Cayaponia pilosa Cogn. 135
Cayaponia tayuya (Mart.) Cogn. 135
Cayaponia spp. 136
Cucurbita pepo L. 136
Fevillea trilobata L. 136
Fevillea uncipetala Kuhlm. 138
Gurania multiflora Cogn. 138
Gurania paulista Cogn. 138
Lagenaria siceraria (Molina) Standl. 138
Luffa operculata (L.) Cogn. 138
Melothria fluminensis Gardn. 139
Melothrianthus smilacifolius
  (Cogn.) M. Crovetto 139
Momordica charantia L. 139
Sicana odorifera Naud. 139
Sicyos polyacanthus Cogn. 139
Trianosperma diversifolia Cogn. 139
Trianosperma glandulosa Mart. 140
Wilbrandia ebracteata Cogn. 140
Wilbrandia verticillata (Vell.) Cogn. 140
Wilbrandia spp. 140
Cucurbitaceae–References 140
CYATHEACEAE
Cyathea armata (Sw.) Domin 141
Cyathea microdonta (Desv.) Domin 141
CYPERACEAE
Bulbostylis capillaris Clarke 142
Cyperus corymbosus Rottb. 142
Cyperus gracilescens Roem. & Schult. . 142
Cyperus ligularis L. 142
Cyperus rotundus L. 142
Cyperus sesquiflorus (Torrey)
  Mattf. & Kükent. 142
Hypolytrum laxum Schrad. 143
Kyllinga pungens Link 143
Mariscus flavus Vahl 143
Mariscus jacquinii H.B.K. 143
Remirea maritima Aubl. 143
Scleria pratensis L. 143
Cyperaceae–References 143
DENNSTAEDTIACEAE
Pteridium aquilinum (L.) Kuhn 144
Dennstaedtiaceae–References 144
DILLENIACEAE
Curatella americana L. 144
Davilla rugosa Poir. 145

CONTENTS: DILLENIACEAE / FABACEAE

Doliocarpus rolandri Gmel. 146
Tetracera aspera Willd. 146
Tetracera breyniana Schl. 146
Tetracera volubilis L. 146
Dilleniaceae–References 146
DIOSCOREACEAE
Dioscorea basiclavicaulis
 Rizz. & Mattos 146
Dioscorea glandulosa Klotz. 147
Dioscorea laxiflora Mart. 147
Dioscorea silvestris Vell. 147
Dioscoreaceae–Reference 147
DRYOPTERIDACEAE
Rumohra adiantiformis
 (G. Forst.) Ching 147
EBENACEAE
Diospyros paralea Steud. 147
EPHEDRACEAE
Ephedra americana Willd. 147
Ephedra triandra Tul. 148
EQUISETACEAE
Equisetum giganteum L. 148
Equisetaceae–Reference 148
ERIOCAULACEAE
Leiothrix flavescens (Bong.) Ruhl. 148
ERYTHROXYLACEAE
Erythroxylum anguifugum Mart. 148
Erythroxylum campestre St.-Hil. 149
Erythroxylum cataractarum Spruce 149
Erythroxylum coca Lam. 149
Erythroxylaceae–References 150
EUPHORBIACEAE
Croton cajucara Benth. 150
Croton floribundus Spreng. 150
Croton hemiargyreus M. Arg. 151
Croton salutaris Casar. 151
Croton sincorensis Mart. 151
Croton sonderianus M. Arg. 151
Croton triqueter Lam. 151
Croton urucurana Baill. 151
Croton zehntneri Pax & Hoffm. 151
Dalechampia ficifolia Lam. 152
Dalechampia scandens L. 152
Euphorbia caecorum Mart. 152
Euphorbia cotinoides Miq. 152
Euphorbia hirta L. 152
Euphorbia hyssopifolia L. 153
Euphorbia phosphorea Mart. 153
Euphorbia thymifolia L. 153
Euphorbia tirucalli L. 153
Hura crepitans L. 153

Jatropha curcas L. 154
Jatropha elliptica (Pohl) M. Arg. 154
Jatropha gossypiifolia L. 154
Jatropha multifida L. 154
Jatropha urens L. 155
Joannesia heveoides Ducke 155
Joannesia princeps Vell. 155
Julocroton humilis Diedr. 155
Julocroton stipularis M. Arg. 155
Mabea fistulifera Mart. 155
Maprounea brasiliensis L. 155
Omphalea diandra M. Arg. 156
Phyllanthus acutifolius Spreng. 156
Phyllanthus conami Sw. 156
Phyllanthus diffusus Klotz. 156
Phyllanthus niruri L. 156
Phyllanthus nobilis M. Arg. 157
Phyllanthus sellowianus M. Arg. 157
Phyllanthus tenellus Roxb. 157
Sapium hamatum Pax & Hoffm. 157
Sebastiania klotzschiana M. Arg. 157
Sebastiania macrocarpa M. Arg. 157
Tragia volubilis L. 158
Euphorbiaceae–References 158
FABACEAE
Abrus precatorius L. 160
Acosmium dasycarpum (Vog.) Yakovl. ... 161
Acosmium subelegans
 (Mohlenb.) Yakovl. 162
Andira inermis (Sw.) H.B.K. 162
Andira retusa (Poir.) H.B.K. 162
Andira vermifuga Mart. ex Benth. 162
Bowdichia nitida Spruce ex Benth. 163
Bowdichia virgilioides H.B.K. 163
Clitoria guianensis (Aubl.) Benth. 163
Crotalaria verrucosa L. 163
Dahlstedtia pinnata (Benth.) Malme 163
Dalbergia gracilis Benth. 163
Dalbergia subcymosa Ducke 164
Desmodium axillare (Sw.) DC. 164
Desmodium triflorum DC. 164
Dipteryx alata Vog. 165
Dipteryx odorata (Aubl.) Willd. 166
Erythrina corallodendron L. 166
Erythrina crista-galli L. 166
Erythrina falcata Benth. 166
Erythrina fusca Lour. 166
Erythrina velutina Willd. 166
Erythrina verna Vell. 168
Galactia neesii DC. 168
Galactia peduncularis (Benth.) Taub. 168
Geoffroea striata (Willd.) Morong 168

Indigofera suffruticosa Mill. 168
Machaerium ferox (Mart.) Ducke 168
Machaerium lunatum (L.) Ducke 168
Monopteryx uacu Spruce ex Benth. 169
Mucuna pruriens (L.) DC. 169
Myrocarpus frondosus Fr. All. 170
Myroxylon balsamum (L.) Harms 170
Periandra mediterranea (Vell.) Taub. 170
Psoralea glandulosa L. 170
Pterodon appariciοi Peders. 170
Pterodon pubescens Benth. 171
Sophora tomentosa L. 172
Sweetia fruticosa Spreng. 172
Torresea cearensis Fr. All. 172
Vatairea guianensis Aubl. 172
Vataireopsis araroba (Aguiar) Ducke 172
Fabaceae–References 173

FLACOURTIACEAE
Carpotroche brasiliensis (Raddi) Endl. .. 176
Carpotroche longifolia Benth. 176
Casearia adstringens Mart. 176
Casearia cambessedesii Eichl. 176
Casearia guyanensis (Aubl.) Urb. 177
Casearia inaequilatera Camb. 178
Casearia ovata Willd. 178
Casearia sylvestris Sw. 178
Laetia apetala Jacq. 178
Flacourtiaceae–References 178

GENTIANACEAE
Calolisianthus pendulus (Mart.) Gilg 179
Coutoubea ramosa Aubl. 179
Coutoubea spicata Aubl. 179
Curtia tenuifolia (Aubl.) Knobl. 180
Deianira nervosa Cham. & Schl. 180
Deianira pallescens Cham. & Schl. 180
Leiphaimos aphylla (Jacq.) Gilg 180
Microcolea quadrangularis
(Lam.) Gris. 180
Schultesia stenophylla Mart. 180
Tachia guianensis Aubl. 180
Zygostigma australe
(Cham. & Schl.) Gris. 181
Gentianaceae–References 181

GESNERIACEAE
Sinningia allagophylla (Mart.) Wiehl. ... 181

HELICONIACEAE
Heliconia angusta Vell. 181
Heliconia bihai L. 181

HIPPOCRATEACEAE
Hippocratea volubilis L. 183
Peritassa calypsoides
(Camb.) A.C. Sm. 183
Salacia impressifolia (Miers) A.C. Sm. .. 183
Tontelea brachypoda Miers 183
Hippocrateaceae–Reference 183

HUMIRIACEAE
Humiria balsamifera (Aubl.) St.-Hil. 183
Saccoglottis guianensis Benth. 185
Humiriaceae–Reference 185

HYPOXIDACEAE
Hypoxis decumbens L. 185

ICACINACEAE
Citronella congonha (Mart.) Howard 185
Citronella mucronata (R. & Pav.) Don .. 186

IRIDACEAE
Cipura paludosa Aubl. 186
Cypella herbertii Herb. 186
Eleutherine plicata Herb. 186
Nothoscordum striatum Kunth 186
Sisyrinchium vaginatum Spreng. 186
Trimezia juncifolia Benth. & Hook. 186
Trimezia lurida Salisb. 186

ISOETACEAE
Isoetes martii A. Braun 189

KRAMERIACEAE
Krameria argentea Mart. 191
Krameria spartioides Berg 191
Krameria tomentosa St.-Hil. 191
Krameriaceae–Reference 191

LAMIACEAE
Coleus barbatus Benth. 191
Cunila microcephala Benth. 192
Cunila spicata L. 192
Glechon ciliata Benth. 192
Glechon spathulata Benth. 192
Hyptis atrorubens Poit. 192
Hyptis crenata Pohl 192
Hyptis fasciculata Benth. 192
Hyptis incana Briq. 192
Hyptis multiflora Pohl 193
Hyptis mutabilis (Rich.) Briq. 193
Hyptis plectranthoides Benth. 193
Hyptis spicigera Lam. 193
Hyptis suaveolens Poit. 193
Hyptis umbrosa Salzm. 193
Keithia denudata Benth. 193
Leonotis nepetaefolia R. Br. 194
Leonurus sibiricus L. 194
Leucas martinicensis (Jacq.) R. Br. 194
Marsypianthes chamaedrys
(Vahl) O. Ktze. 194
Mentha crispa L. 194

Ocimum fluminensis Vell. 195
Ocimum micranthum Willd. 195
Peltodon longipes St.-Hil. 195
Peltodon radicans Pohl 195
Lamiaceae–References 195
LAURACEAE
Aiovea brasiliensis Meissn. 196
Aiovea meissneri Mez 197
Aniba canelilla (H.B.K.) Mez 197
Aniba permollis (Nees) Mez 197
Aniba puchury-minor (Mart.) Mez 197
Aniba rosaeodora Ducke 197
Cassytha filiformis L. 198
Cryptocarya guyanensis Meissn. 198
Cryptocarya mandioccana Meissn. 198
Cryptocarya minima Mez 198
Cryptocarya moschata Nees
  & Mart. ex Nees 198
Dicypellium caryophyllatum
  Nees & Mart. 198
Licaria camara (Schomb.) Kosterm. 198
Licaria canella (Meissn.) Kosterm. 199
Licaria puchury-major
  (Mart.) Kosterm. 199
Mezilaurus crassiramea (Meissn.)
  Taub. ex Mez 199
Nectandra canescens Nees 199
Nectandra globosa (Aubl.) Mez 199
Nectandra leucantha Nees 199
Nectandra leucothyrsus Meissn. 199
Nectandra pichurim (H.B.K.) Mez 200
Nectandra puberula Nees 200
Nectandra turbacensis Nees 200
Ocotea cujumary Mart. 200
Ocotea cymbarum H.B.K. 200
Ocotea guianensis Aubl. 201
Ocotea opifera Mart. 201
Ocotea pretiosa (Nees & Mart.)
  Benth. & Hook. 201
Ocotea pulchella Mart. 201
Ocotea rodiei (Schomb.) Mez 201
Ocotea spectabilis (Meissn.) Mez 201
Ocotea squarrosa Mart. ex Nees 203
Ocotea teleiandra (Messn.) Mez 203
Pleurothyrium cuneifolium Nees 203
Lauraceae–References 203
LECYTHIDACEAE
Bertholletia excelsa Humb. & Bonpl. 204
Cariniana legalis (Mart.) O. Ktze. 204
Gustavia hexapetala (Aubl.)
  J.E. Smith 205

Lecythis amara Aubl. 205
Lecythis pisonis Camb. 206
LEMNACEAE
Lemna minor L. 207
Lemnaceae–References 207
LILIACEAE
Cordyline dracaenoides Kunth 207
Herreria salsaparilha Mart. 207
Smilax campestris Gris. 208
Smilax longifolia Rich. 208
Smilax oblongifolia Pohl 208
Liliaceae–References 208
LOGANIACEAE
Potalia amara Aubl. 209
Spigelia anthelmia L. 209
Spigelia flemingiana Cham. & Schl. 209
Spigelia glabrata Mart. 209
Strychnos spp. 209
Strychnos pseudoquina St.-Hil. 209
Strychnos subcordata Spr. ex Benth. 209
Strychnos trinervis (Vell.) Mart. 210
Loganiaceae–References 211
LORANTHACEAE
Phoradendron crassifolium
  (Pohl) Eichl. 211
Phthirusa adunca (Meyer) Maguire 211
Struthanthus marginatus (Desf.) Bl. 213
LYTHRACEAE
Cuphea aperta Koehne 213
Cuphea balsamona Cham. 213
Cuphea carthagenensis
  (Jacq.) MacBride 213
Cuphea ingrata Cham. & Schl. 214
Cuphea melvilla Lindl. 214
Heimia salicifolia
  (H.B.K.) Link & Otto 214
Lafoensia densiflora Pohl 214
Lafoensia pacari St.-Hil. 215
Lythraceae–References 211
MAGNOLIACEAE
Talauma ovata St.-Hil. 216
Magnoliaceae–Reference 216
MALPIGHIACEAE
Banisteriopsis caapi (Spr.) Morton 217
Byrsonima chrysophylla H.B.K. 218
Byrsonima coccolobifolia H.B.K. 218
Byrsonima crassifolia H.B.K. 219
Byrsonima spicata Rich. 219
Byrsonima verbascifolia (L.) Rich. 220
Galphimia brasiliensis Juss. 220
Heteropteris aphrodisiaca O. Mach. 220

Heteropteris syringifolia Gris. 220
Malpighiaceae–References 220
MALVACEAE
Hibiscus bifurcatus Cav. 221
Hibiscus cannabinus L. 221
Hibiscus sabdariffa L. 221
Hibiscus tiliaceus L. 221
Modiolastrum pinnatipartitum
   (St.-Hil. & Naudin) Krapovickas 221
Sida acuta Burm. 221
Sida angustifolia Lam. 222
Sida carpinifolia (L. f.) K. Sch. 222
Sida macrodon DC. 222
Sida micrantha St.-Hil. 222
Sida rhombea L. 222
Sida rhombifolia L. 222
Urena lobata L. 223
Wissadula periplocifolia Presl. 223
Malvaceae–References 223
MARANTACEAE
Calathea grandiflora Lindl. 223
Ischnosiphon arouma Koern. 223
Maranta arundinacea L. 223
Stromanthe sanguinea Sond. 224
Thalia geniculata L. 224
MARCGRAVIACEAE
Marcgravia rectiflora Tr. & Planch. 224
MARTYNIACEAE
Craniolaria annua L. 224
Craniolaria integrifolia Cham. 224
Ibicella lutea (Lindl.) Van Eselt. 224
MELASTOMATACEAE
Bellucia grossularioides (L.) Tr. 225
Clidemia blepharoides DC. 225
Leandra lacunosa Cogn. 225
Macairea radula (Bonpl.) DC. 225
Miconia albicans (Sw.) Tr. 225
Mouriri apiranga Spruce 225
Mouriri guianensis Aubl. 225
Nepsera aquatica Naud. 226
Tibouchina aspera Aubl. 226
Tibouchina clavata (Pers.) Wurdack 226
Melastomataceae–References 226
MELIACEAE
Cabralea canjerana (Vell.) Mart. 227
Carapa guianensis Aubl. 227
Cedrela fissilis Vell. 227
Cedrela odorata L. 227
Guarea spiciflora Juss. 227
Guarea trichilioides L. 227
Guarea tuberculata Vell. 229

Trichilia barraensis DC. 229
Trichilia cathartica Mart. 229
Trichilia catigua Juss. 229
Trichilia catuaba (Silva) Rizz. 229
Trichilia hirta L. 229
Meliaceae–References 229
MENISPERMACEAE
Abuta candicans Rich. 231
Abuta concolor Poepp. & Endl. 231
Abuta rufescens Aubl. 231
Abuta selloana Eichl. 231
Chondodendron platyphyllum
   (Mart.) Miers 231
Cissampelos fasciculata Benth. 231
Cissampelos fluminensis Eichl. 233
Cissampelos glaberrima St.-Hil. 233
Cissampelos ovalifolia DC. 233
Cissampelos pareira L. 233
Cissampelos sympodialis Eichl. 233
Cocculus filipendula Mart. 234
Sciadotenia paraensis (Eichl.) Diels 234
Menispermaceae–References 234
MENYANTHACEAE
Nymphoides indica (L.) O. Ktze. 235
MIMOSACEAE
Acacia paniculata Willd. 236
Albizzia lebbeck (L.) Benth. 236
Anadenanthera colubrina
   (Vell.) Brenan 236
Anadenanthera falcata
   (Benth.) Brenan 236
Anadenanthera macrocarpa
   (Benth.) Brenan 236
Anadenanthera peregrina (L.) Speg. 236
Calliandra tweedii Benth. 237
Entada paranaguana B. Rodr. 237
Entada polyphylla Benth. 237
Entada polystachya (Jacq.) DC. 237
Inga alba (Sw.) Willd. 237
Inga lateriflora Miq. 237
Inga setigera DC. 237
Mimosa acutistipula Benth. 237
Mimosa bimucronata (DC.) O. Ktze. 238
Mimosa caesalpiniaefolia Benth. 238
Mimosa hostilis Benth. 238
Mimosa invisa Mart. 239
Mimosa malacocentra Mart. 239
Mimosa pudica L. 240
Mimosa velloziana Mart. 240
Mimosa verrucosa Benth. 240
Parapiptadenia rigida (Benth.) Brenan . 240

CONTENTS: MIMOSACEAE / OCHNACEAE

Parkia oppositifolia (Spruce) Benth. 240
Parkia pectinata Benth. 240
Parkia pendula Benth. ex Walp. 240
Pentaclethra macroloba
  (Willd.) O. Ktze. 242
Piptadenia polyptera Benth. 242
Pithecellobium avaremotemo Mart. 242
Pithecellobium cochleatum
  (Willd.) Mart. 242
Pithecellobium unguis-cati (L.) Benth. ... 242
Schrankia leptocarpa DC. 242
Stryphnodendron adstringens
  (Mart.) Cov. 242
Stryphnodendron coriaceum Benth. 243
Stryphnodendron polyphyllum Mart. 244
Mimosaceae–References 244

MONIMIACEAE
Mollinedia schottiana (Spr.) Perk. 245
Siparuna brasiliensis (Spr.) DC. 245
Siparuna camporum (Tul.) DC. 245
Siparuna cujabana (Mart.) DC. 245
Siparuna guianensis Aubl. 245
Siparuna laurifolia (H.B.K.) DC. 246
Monimiaceae–References 246

MORACEAE
Brosimum acutifolium Huber 246
Brosimum gaudichaudii Tréc. 246
Brosimum parinarioides Ducke 246
Brosimum potabile Ducke 246
Brosimum utile (H.B.K.) Pittier 246
Cecropia hololeuca Miq. 247
Cecropia leucocoma Miq. 247
Cecropia palmata Willd. 247
Clarisia racemosa Ruiz & Pav. 247
Coussapoa asperifolia Tréc. 247
Dorstenia asaroides Gardn. 247
Dorstenia brasiliensis Lam. 247
Dorstenia cayapia Vell. 248
Dorstenia reniformis Pohl 248
Ficus gomelleira Kunth & Bouché 248
Ficus insipida Willd. 248
Ficus maxima P. Mill. 248
Ficus trigona L. f. 249
Maclura brasiliensis Endl. 249
Maclura tinctoria (L.) D. Don 249
Maquira sclerophylla
  (Ducke) C. C. Berg 249
Naucleopsis amara Ducke 249
Sorocea bonplandii (Baill.) Burger 249
Moraceae–References 250

MYRISTICACEAE
Virola macrophylla
  (Spr. ex Benth.) Warb. 250
Virola oleifera (Schott) A.C. Smith 250
Virola sebifera Aubl. 250
Virola surinamensis (Rol.) Warb. 252
Myristicaceae–References 252

MYRSINACEAE
Cybianthus detergens Mart. 253

MYRTACEAE
Blepharocalyx salicifolius
  (H.B.K.) Berg 253
Calyptranthes aromatica St.-Hil. 253
Calyptranthes variabilis Berg 253
Campomanesia aurea Berg 253
Eugenia brasiliensis Lam. 253
Eugenia dysenterica DC. 253
Eugenia sulcata Spring 254
Eugenia supra-axillaris Spring 254
Eugenia uniflora L. 254
Marlierea tomentosa Camb. 255
Myrcia amazonica DC. 255
Myrcia lanceolata Camb. 255
Myrcia sphaerocarpa DC. 255
Myrcia tingens Berg 255
Pseudocaryophyllus sericeus Berg 255
Psidium arboreum Vell. 255
Psidium cattleyanum Sabine 255
Psidium cinereum Mart. 255
Psidium guajava L. 255
Myrtaceae–References 255

NYCTAGINACEAE
Andradea floribunda Fr. All. 257
Boerhavia coccinea Mill. 257
Boerhavia erecta L. 258
Boerhavia paniculata Rich. 258
Neea theifera Oersted 258
Pisonia aculeata L. 258
Pisonia alcalina Fr. All. 258
Pisonia cordifolia Mart. 258
Torrubia olfersiana
  (Link, Klotzsch & Otto) Standl. 258
Nyctaginaceae–References 259

NYMPHAEACEAE
Cabomba piauhyensis Gard. 259
Nymphaea ampla DC. 259
Nymphaea rudgeana G. Meyer 259
Victoria amazonica (Poepp.) Sower. 259

OCHNACEAE
Luxemburgia glazioviana Gilg 260
Luxemburgia polyandra St.-Hil. 261
Ouratea guianensis Aubl. 261
Ouratea hexasperma (St.-Hil.) Baill. 261
Ouratea jabotapita Engl. 261

Ouratea parviflora (DC.) Baill. 261
Sauvagesia erecta L. 262
Ochnaceae–References 262
OLACACEAE
Ptychopetalum olacoides Benth. 262
Ptychopetalum uncinatum Anselm. 262
Ximenia americana L. 263
Ximenia coriacea Engl. 236
Olacaceae–References 263
ONAGRACEAE
Ludwigia natans (H.B.K.) Ell. 264
Ludwigia peruviana (L.) Hara 264
Ludwigia repens (L.) Hara 264
Ludwigia suffruticosa (L.) Gomes 264
Oenothera catharinensis Camb. 264
OPILIACEAE
Agonandra brasiliensis Miers 265
Opiliaceae–References 266
ORCHIDACEAE
Cyrtopodium andersoni R. Br. 266
Cyrtopodium punctatum Lindl. 266
OXALIDACEAE
Oxalis amara St.-Hil. 266
Oxalis cordata St.-Hil. 266
Oxalis corniculata L. 266
Oxalis martiana Zucc. 267
PASSIFLORACEAE
Passiflora alata Dryand. 267
Passiflora amethystina Mikan 269
Passiflora caerulea L. 269
Passiflora coccinea Aubl. 269
Passiflora edulis Sims 269
Passiflora foetida L. 269
Passiflora gardneri Mast. 270
Passiflora laurifolia L. 270
Passiflora macrocarpa Mast. 270
Passiflora mucronata Lam. 270
Passiflora spp. 270
Passifloraceae–References 270
PHYTOLACCACEAE
Gallesia gorazema (Vell.) Moq. 271
Microtea debilis Sw. 271
Petiveria alliacea L. 271
Seguieria americana L. 272
Phytolaccaceae–References 272
PIPERACEAE
Ottonia corcovadensis Miq. 272
Ottonia jaborandi (Vell.) Kunth 272
Peperomia elongata Miq. 273
Peperomia hederacea Miq. 273
Peperomia pellucida H.B.K. 273

Peperomia rotundifolia H.B.K. 274
Peperomia transparens Miq. 274
Piper aduncum L. 274
Piper angustifolium R. & Pav. 274
Piper arboreum Aubl. 274
Piper callosum R. & Pav. 274
Piper cavalcantei Yunck. 275
Piper ceanothifolium H.B.K. 275
Piper colubrinum Link 275
Piper elongatum Vahl 275
Piper eucalyptifolium (Miq.) Rudge 275
Piper geniculatum Sw. 275
Piper gigantifolium Jacq. 275
Piper marginatum Jacq. 275
Piper mikanianum (Kunth) Steud. 276
Piper mollicomum Kunth 276
Piper parthenium Mart. 276
Piper reticulatum L. 276
Piper rohrii C. DC. 276
Piper tuberculatum Jacq. 276
Pothomorphe peltata L. 277
Pothomorphe umbellata (L.) Miq. 277
Piperaceae–References 277
PLANTAGINACEAE
Plantago brasiliensis Sims 278
Plantago guilleminiana Dcne. 278
Plantago myosurus Lam. 278
PLUMBAGINACEAE
Limonium brasiliense (Boiss.) O. Ktze. . 278
Plumbago scandens L. 279
Plumbaginaceae–References 279
POACEAE
Andropogon bicornis L. 279
Andropogon minarum Kunth 280
Aristida pallens Cav. 280
Avena quadridentata Doell 280
Chloris distichophylla (Nees) Lag. 280
Chloris polydactyla Sw. 280
Cymbopogon schoenanthus (L.) Spreng. 280
Elionurus bilinguis (Trin.) Hack. 281
Elionurus candidus (Trin.) Hack. 281
Gynerium parviflorum Nees 281
Hackelochloa granularis (L.) O. Ktze. .. 281
Imperata brasiliensis Trin. 281
Luziola peruviana Pers. 281
Melinis minutiflora Beauv. 281
Panicum brevifolium L. 282
Panicum megiston Schult. 282
Panicum petrosum Trin. 282
Panicum trichanthum Nees 282
Pappophorum mucronulatum Nees 282
Paspalum extenuatum Nees 282

Sacciolepis myuros (Lam.) Chase 282
Setaria scandens Schrad. 282
Poaceae–References 282
POLYGALACEAE
Bredemeyera floribunda Willd. 283
Polygala angulata DC. 283
Polygala comata Mart. 284
Polygala klotzschii Chodat 284
Polygala paniculata L. 284
Polygala spectabilis DC. 284
Polygala timoutou Aubl. 284
Polygalaceae–References 284
POLYGONACEAE
Coccoloba arborescens (Vell.) How. 285
Coccoloba laevis Casar. 285
Coccoloba marginata Benth. 285
Coccoloba mollis Casar. 285
Muehlenbeckia sagittifolia
  (Ort.) Meissn. 285
Polygonum acuminatum H.B.K. 286
Polygonum hydropiperoides Michx. 286
Polygonum punctatum Elliot 287
Polygonum spectabile Mart. 287
Rumex brasiliensis Link 287
Triplaris macrocalyx Casar. 287
Triplaris noli-tangere Wedd. 287
Triplaris weigeltiana (Reichb.) O. Ktze. 287
Polygonaceae–Reference 287
POLYPODIACEAE
Microgramma vaccinifolia
  (Langsd. & Fisch.) Copel. 288
Phlebodium aureum (L.) J.E. Smith 288
Phlebodium decumanum
  (Willd.) J. Smith 288
Polypodium brasiliense Poir. 288
PONTEDERIACEAE
Eichhornia crassipes Solms 288
Pontederia cordifolia Mart. 288
PORTULACACEAE
Portulaca grandiflora Hook. 288
Portulaca oleracea L. 289
Portulaca pilosa L. 289
Talinum racemosum (L.) Rohr. 289
Portulacaceae–References 289
PRIMULACEAE
Samolus valerandi L. 290
RANUNCULACEAE
Anemone decapetala L. 290
Clematis denticulata Vell. 290
Clematis dioica L. 290
Ranunculus apiifolius Pers. 290

Ranunculus bonariensis Poir. 291
RHABDODENDRACEAE
Rhabdodendron amazonicum
  (Spr. ex Benth.) Hub. 291
RHAMNACEAE
Ampelozizyphus amazonicus Ducke 291
Colletia paradoxa (Spr.) Escalante 291
Discaria americana Gill. & Hook. 291
Reisseckia smilacina (Sm.) Steud. 293
Scutia buxifolia Reiss. 293
Zizyphus joazeiro Mart. 293
Rhamnaceae–References 293
RHIZOPHORACEAE
Rhizophora mangle L. 294
ROSACEAE
Margyricarpus setosus Ruiz & Pav. 294
Prunus subcoriacea (Chod.
  & Hassl.) Hoehne 294
Rubus brasiliensis Mart. 294
RUBIACEAE
Alibertia edulis (Rich.) Rich. 294
Bathysa cuspidata Hook. 296
Borreria asclepiadea Cham. & Schl. 296
Borreria poaya (St.-Hil.) DC. 296
Borreria tenella Cham. & Schl. 296
Borreria verbenoides Cham. & Schl. 296
Borreria verticillata (L.) Meyer 296
Cephaelis ipecacuanha Rich. 296
Chiococca alba (L.) Hitch. 297
Coutarea hexandra (Jacq.) K. Sch. 297
Declieuxia aristolochia M. Arg. 297
Declieuxia cordigera Mart. & Zucc. 297
Diodia polymorpha Cham. & Schl. 297
Exostemma australe St.-Hil. 298
Genipa americana L. 298
Guettarda angelica Mart. 298
Guettarda argentea Lam. 298
Guettarda uruguayensis Cham. & Schl. 298
Ladenbergia hexandra Klotz. 299
Ladenbergia lambertiana Klotz. 299
Lipostoma campanuliflorum D. Don 299
Machaonia brasiliensis Cham. & Schl. . 299
Manettia ignita (Vell.) K. Sch. 299
Oldenlandia corymbosa L. 299
Rubiaceae–References 299
RUTACEAE
Cusparia febrifuga Humb. 300
Cusparia toxicaria Spr. ex Engl. 301
Esenbeckia febrifuga Juss. 301
Esenbeckia intermedia Mart. 301
Galipea dichotoma Sald. 301

Galipea multiflora Schult. 301
Hortia brasiliensis Vand. 301
Metrodorea pubescens St.-Hil. & Tul. ... 301
Monnieria trifolia Loefl. 302
Pilocarpus pinnatifolius Lem. 302
Raputia alba (Nees & Mart.) Engl. 302
Raputia aromatica Aubl. 302
Raputia magnifica Engl. 302
Zanthoxylum hyemale St.-Hil. 302
Zanthoxylum pterota H.B.K. 303
Zanthoxylum rhoifolium Lam. 303
Zanthoxylum tingoassuiba St.-Hil. 303
Rutaceae–References 303

SALVINIACEAE
Azolla caroliniana Willd. 304

SANTALACEAE
Acanthosyris spinescens
  (Mart. & Endl.) Gris. 304
Jodina rhombifolia Hook. & Arn. 304
Santalaceae–Reference 304

SAPINDACEAE
Cardiospermum grandiflorum Sw. 305
Cupania racemosa Radlk. 305
Dodonaea viscosa Jacq. 305
Magonia pubescens St.-Hil. 305
Matayba purgans Radlk. 306
Paullinia cupana Kunth 306
Sapindus saponaria L. 306
Talisia esculenta Radlk. 306
Sapindaceae–References 308

SAPOTACEAE
Bumelia sartorum Mart. 308
Dipholis nigra Gr. 309
Lucuma caimito Roem. & Schult. 309
Lucuma rivicoa Gaertn. 309
Manilkara bidentata (A. DC.) Chev. 309
Manilkara zapota (L.) Van Royen 309
Pouteria laurifolia Radlk. 309
Pouteria obtusifolia Baehni 310
Pouteria salicifolia Hook. & Arn. 310
Pradosia lactescens (Vell.) Radlk. 310
Sapotaceae–Reference 310

SCHIZAEACEAE
Anemia phyllitidis (L.) Sw. 310

SCROPHULARIACEAE
Angelonia integerrima Spreng. 310
Buchnera aquatica Aubl. 310
Buchnera virgata H.B.K. 310
Capraria biflora L. 311
Conobea aquatica Aubl. 311
Conobea scoparioides Benth. 311

Lindernia crustacea F. Muell. 311
Lindernia diffusa Wettst. 311
Scoparia dulcis L. 312
Tetralacrium veroniciforme Turcz. 312
Scrophulariaceae–References 312

SELAGINELLACEAE
Selaginella convoluta Spring 313
Selaginella erythropus Spring 313
Selaginella stellata Spring 313
Selaginellaceae–Reference 313

SIMAROUBACEAE
Marupa francoana Miers 313
Picramnia bahiensis Turcz. 313
Picramnia camboita Engl. 314
Picramnia ciliata Mart. 314
Picrolemma pseudocoffea Ducke 314
Quassia amara L. 314
Simaba ferruginea St.-Hil. 314
Simaba glandulifera Gardn. 314
Simaba salubris Engl. 315
Simarouba amara Aubl. 315
Simarouba versicolor St.-Hil. 315
Simaroubaceae–References 315

SOLANACEAE
Acnistus arborescens (L.) Schl. 316
Bassovia lucida Dunal 316
Brunfelsia uniflora (Pohl) D. Don 316
Cestrum amictum Schl. 317
Cestrum bracteatum Link & Otto 317
Cestrum calycinum Willd. 317
Cestrum parqui L'Herit. 317
Cestrum pseudoquina Mart. 317
Datura arborea L. 317
Datura insignis B. Rodr. 318
Datura stramonium L. 318
Datura suaveolens Humb. & Bonpl. 318
Nicandra physaloides (L.) Gaertn. 318
Physalis angulata L. 318
Physalis pubescens L. 318
Salpichroa origanifolia (Lam.) Thell. 319
Solanum aculeatissimum Jacq. 319
Solanum agrarium Sendt. 319
Solanum albidum Dun. 319
Solanum caavurana Vell. 319
Solanum cernuum Vell. 319
Solanum ciliatum Lam. 319
Solanum grandiflorum Ruiz & Pav. 320
Solanum insidiosum Mart. 320
Solanum juciri Mart. 321
Solanum lycocarpum St.-Hil. 321
Solanum mammosum L. 321

Solanum martii Sendt. 321
Solanum mauritianum Scop. 321
Solanum nigrum L. 321
Solanum paniculatum L. 321
Solanum pseudoquina St.-Hil. 322
Solanum variabile Mart. 322
Solanum verbascifolium L. 322
Solanum alkaloids, chemistry of 322
Solanaceae–References 322

STERCULIACEAE
Guazuma ulmifolia Lam.
   var. *tomentella* Schum. 323
Guazuma ulmifolia Lam. var. *ulmifolia* . 323
Helicteres ovata Lam. 324
Sterculia apetala (Jacq.) Karst.
   var. *elata* (Ducke) E. Taylor 324
Sterculia chicha St.-Hil. 325
Waltheria communis St.-Hil. 325
Waltheria indica L. 325
Waltheria viscosissima St.-Hil. 325

STYRACACEAE
Styrax ferrugineum Nees & Mart. 325
Styrax glabratum Schott 325

SYMPLOCACEAE
Symplocos parviflora Benth. 326
Symplocos platyphylla (Pohl) Benth. 326
Symplocos pubescens Klotzsch 326

THEACEAE
Laplacea fruticosa (Schr.) Kobuski 326
Ternstroemia brasiliensis Camb. 326
Theaceae–Reference 326

TILIACEAE
Luehea divaricata Mart. & Zucc. 326
Luehea rufescens St.-Hil. 327
Muntingia calabura L. 327
Triumfetta rhomboidea Jacq. 327
Triumfetta semitriloba Jacq. 327

TROPAEOLACEAE
Tropaeolum pentaphyllum Lam. 327

TURNERACEAE
Turnera diffusa Willd. 327
Turnera guianensis Aubl. 328
Turnera opifera Mart. 328
Turnera rupestris Aubl. 328
Turnera ulmifolia L. 328
Turneraceae–References 328

TYPHACEAE
Typha domingensis Pers. 328

ULMACEAE
Celtis brasiliensis Planch. 330
Celtis iguanaea Sarg. 330
Celtis morifolia Planch. 330
Celtis spinosissima Miq. 330
Ulmaceae–Reference 330

URTICACEAE
Boehmeria caudata Sw. 330
Laportea aestuans (L.) Chew 330
Parietaria boehmerioides Mart. 331
Pilea microphylla (L.) Liebm. 331
Urera aurantiaca Wedd. 331
Urera baccifera Gaud. 331
Urera caracasana Jacq. 331
Urera subpeltata Miq. 331
Urticaceae–References 331

VERBENACEAE
Aloysia triphylla (L'Her.) Britt. 332
Amasonia arborea H.B.K. 333
Avicennia germinans (L.) L. 334
Bouchea laetevirens Schauer 334
Bouchea pseudogervao (St.-Hil.) Cham. 334
Glandularia peruviana (L.) Small 334
Lantana brasiliensis Link 334
Lantana camara L. 334
Lantana lilacina Desf. 335
Lantana macrophylla Schauer 335
Lantana microphylla Cham. 335
Lippia alba (Mill.) N.E. Brown 335
Lippia gratissima (Gill. & Hook.)
   Troncoso 335
Stachytarpheta cayennensis
   (Rich.) Vahl 335
Stachytarpheta dichotoma Vahl 336
Stachytarpheta elatior Schrad. 336
Stachytarpheta jamaicensis (L.) Vahl 336
Verbena bonariensis L. 336
Verbena erinoides Lam. 336
Vitex agnus-castus L. 336
Vitex gardneriana Schauer 336
Vitex montevidensis Cham. 337
Verbenaceae–References 337

VIOLACEAE
Alsodeia flavescens (Aubl.) Spreng. 337
Anchietea pyrifolia (Mart.) G. Don 338
Corynostylis hybanthus
   (L.) Mart. & Zucc. 338
Hybanthus atropurpureus Taub. 338
Hybanthus ipecacuanha (L.) Baill. 339
Ionidium poaya St.-Hil. 339
Violaceae–References 339

VITACEAE
Cissus palmata Poir. 339

Cissus salutaris H.B.K. 339
Cissus sicyoides L. 339
Vitaceae–References 340
VOCHYSIACEAE
Callisthene major Mart. 340
Vochysia thyrsoidea Pohl 340
Vochysiaceae–Reference 340
WINTERACEAE
Drimys winteri Forst. 340
Winteraceae–References 341

XYRIDACEAE
Abolboda poarchon Seub. 342
Xyris laxifolia Mart. 342
Xyris pallida Mart. 342
ZINGIBERACEAE
Hedychium coronarium Koenig 342
Renealmia exaltata L. f. 342
Renealmia occidentalis Sweet 342
Zingiberaceae–References 343

Notes & Synonyms 344
Glossary 350
Editor's Acknowledgements 358
Illustration Credits 363
Indices:
    Medicinal 364
    Common Names 421
    Species 487

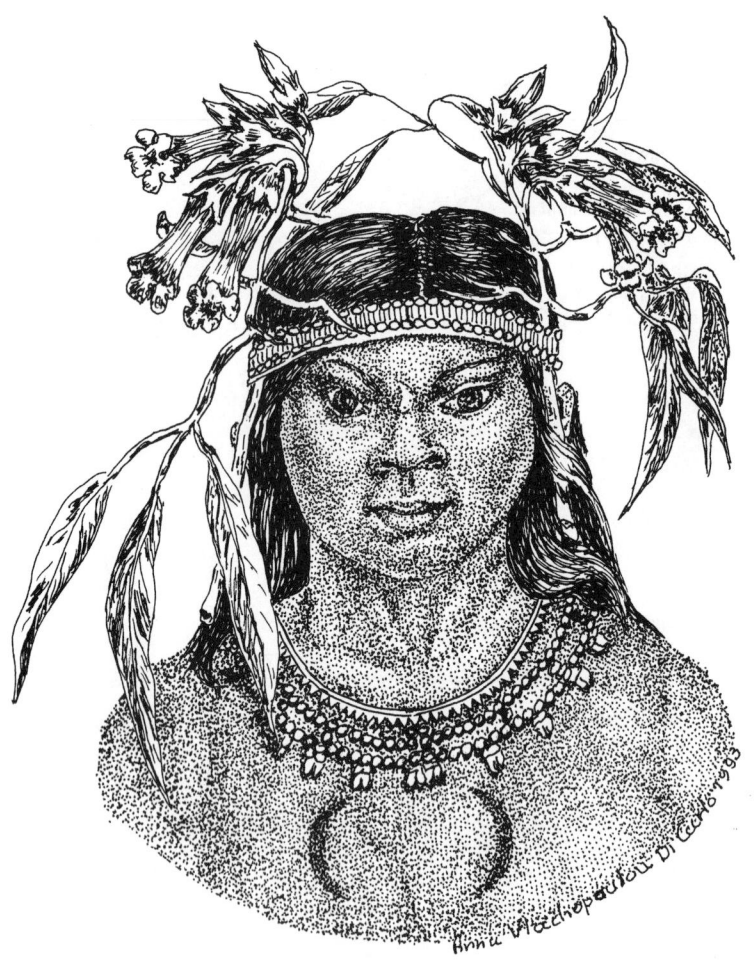

Brazilian Indian wearing flowering branches of Bignoniaceae.

FOREWORD

Some Historical and Modern Facets of the Brazilian Medicinal Plant Heritage

I. Brazil Named for Brazilwood

At an early age, Brazilians are taught that the Portuguese discoverers named the local dyewood tree "pau brazil," derived from the word "brasa" (then "braza"), meaning glow. In other words, "glowing red wood." From this, the official version suggests, the name of the country was derived.

However, many people accept a more historically accurate version of the source of the name, one that involves a fascinating interplay of botanical resources between the Old and New Worlds.

In the Middle Ages a thriving trade in bright crimson dyewood had developed between Europe and the wood source in India and Southeast Asia.[1] Extracts from the heartwood of an Asiatic shrubby tree, *Caesalpinia sappan* (a caesalpinoid legume), which the explorer Marco Polo had encountered, yielded the red dye sought for use in the European textile trade.[2] One of the plant's numerous Asian names was "brazilium"; it had been mentioned by rabbinical writers as early as the 12th century. This wood was also known in early Europe under the variant name "presillum," which was mentioned as such by Matthaeus Sylvaticus, an Italian medical writer who flourished in Salerno in 1317.[3] As "presilium," the Asiatic wood occurs in the first intelligible English-language description of America, namely *The Decades of the Newe Worlde or West India* (1555) by Richard Eden (1521–1576),[4] which is a translation of Decades I–III of Peter Martyr's 1516 *De Orbe Novo Decades*. In the *Decades*, Eden states that: "Presilium or brasyll, cometh from Darnasseri ... almost cc. leages from Calicut." So flourished the brazilwood (or, presillum) trade between Europe and the East.

---

[1] Cannon, J. & M. Cannon. 1994. DYE PLANTS AND DYEING. London: The Herbert Press. (Brazilwood, p. 36).

[2] Piergiovanni, P.M. 1991. *Capitolo dodicesimo. I coloranti del nuovo mondo e l'industria tessile europea: tra economia e tecnica*, pp. 233-249, in Orsini, L.C., Doria, Gio. & Giv. Doria, eds., 1492-1992. ANIMALI E PIANTE DALLE AMERICHE ALL'EUROPA. 323 pp. Genoa, Italy: Sagep Editrice.

[3] Pickering, C. 1879. CHRONOLOGICAL HISTORY OF PLANTS. 1222 pp. Boston: Little, Brown and Company.

[4] Eden, R. 1555. *The Decades of the Newe Worlde or West India*. 361 pp. London: Robert Toy.

Foreword

On April 23, 1500 Pedro Alvares Cabral, on a voyage to India sailing westward via the Atlantic, first sighted Brazil, which he claimed for Portugal and named "Santa Cruz." Friendly Amerindians, the Tupinambá cannibals, were encountered, and the Portuguese eventually learned that the land was neither a part of Asia nor an Asian island, both of which had been suspected (a mythical island named Brazil and source of abundant brazilwood was believed in as early as the 1300s). Cabral carried on with the voyage via Mozambique and in September 1500 reached India, where he loaded pepper and cinnamon at various ports, and finally returned to Lisbon in June 1501.

In various parts of the New World there occurs a native "brazilwood." Columbus had mentioned it as a Haitian plant, for example, in the account of his third voyage, and Spain exploited it in Haiti as early as 1501;[5] the plant was soon encountered in coastal Brazil. A different species from that of India, this Caribbean and Brazilian plant is the tree *Caesalpinia echinata*. It was referred to as the familiar "brazilwood" by New World explorers, who did not realize the botanical difference between *C. sappan* and *C. echinata,* although A. Thevet had struggled in 1558 to decide if the Old and New World kinds were the same.[6] This plant grew in extensive forests in northeastern South America, and the area itself soon came to be indicated on maps as "Brazil" or "Brasilia." Thus, Brazil was actually named for the major new source of brazilwood (dyewood), and the name replaced the original designation of "Santa Cruz" for the area.

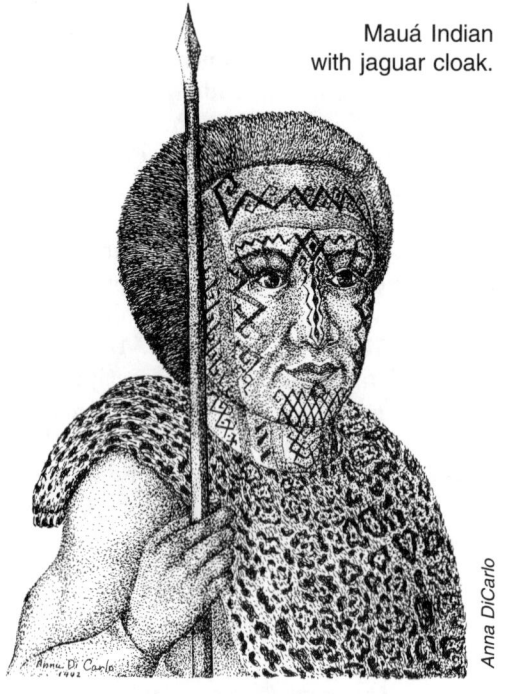

Mauá Indian with jaguar cloak.

Anna DiCarlo

As late as 1532, Brazil is labeled "Prisilia" (*cf.* "presi-

---

[5] *Cf.* Sauer, J.D. 1976. *Changing perception and exploitation of New World plants in Europe, 1492-1800,* pp. 813-832, in Chiappelli, F., et al., eds., First Images of America: The Impact of the New World on the Old. Vol. I. 515 pp. Berkeley, Los Angeles, London: University of California Press. *See also* Haiti discussion in Gerbi, A. 1985. Nature in the New World: From Christopher Columbus to Gonzalo Fernandez de Oviedo. 462 pp. Pittsburgh, Pennsylvania: University of Pittsburgh Press.

[6] *Cf.* Sauer, 1976.

lium") on a map attributed to Hans Holbein the Younger, printed in Basle, Switzerland by Johannes Hervagen.[7] The brazilwood tree, "Arbor Brasilia," is depicted in an herbal of the year 1583 published in Antwerp by Rembert Dodoens, entitled *Stirpium Historiae Pemptades* (History of Plants in Six Fifths or 30 Books).[8] Early maps of Brazil often included a cartouche-like drawing of Indians with axe in hand surrounded by the stumps of harvested brazilwood trees. Two such maps by Sebastião Lopes, made in 1558 and 1565, are reproduced in *Portugaliae Monumenta Cartographica*;[9] the originals are in The British Library (London) and The Newberry Library (Chicago, Illinois), respectively. Another 16th century map showing a brazilwood cutter is by Sebastian Cabot, and is conserved in the Bibliothèque Nationale, Paris; it is included in Gheerbrant.[10]

Additional early maps portraying the brazilwood harvest are reported

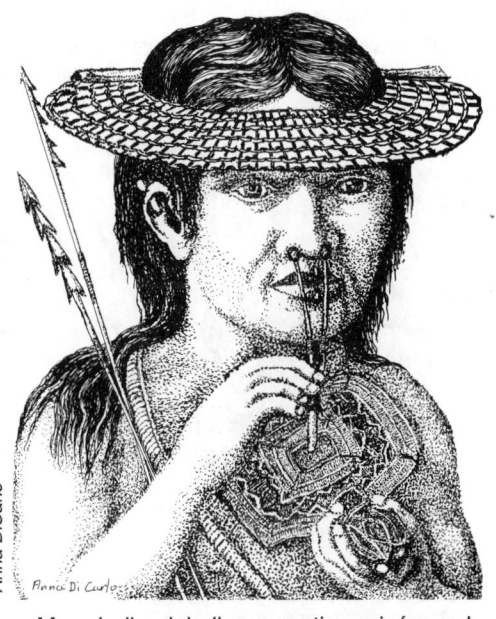

Mura Indian inhaling narcotic paricá powder.

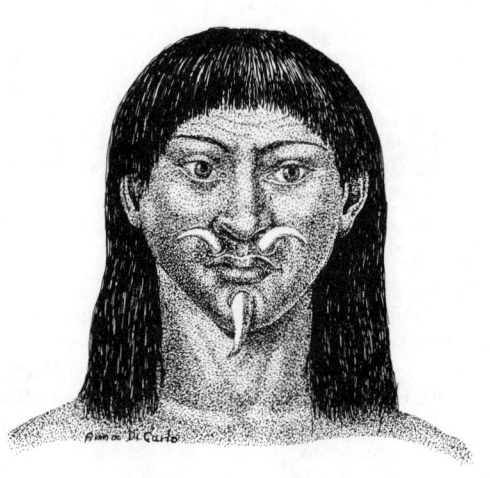

Mura Indian, state of Amazonas.

---

[7] Lehner, E. & J. Lehner. 1966. HOW THEY SAW THE NEW WORLD. 160 pp. New York: Tudor Publishing Company. (Hans Holbein the Younger, map p. 48).

[8] Dodoens, R. 1583. *Stirpium Historiae Pemptades Sex Sive Libri* XXX. 860 pp. Antwerp: Christophori Plantini.

[9] Cortesão, A. 1987. PORTUGALIAE MONUMENTA CARTOGRAPHICA. Vol. 4. Lisbon, Portugal: Imprensa Nacional – Casa da Moeda.

[10] Gheerbrant, A. 1992. THE AMAZON: PAST, PRESENT, AND FUTURE. 191 pp. New York: Harry N. Abrams, Inc. (Cabot map, p. 131).

Foreword

and/or reproduced by Sturtevant,[11] including maps in the 1519 *Miller Atlas;*[12] the 1547 atlas by Nicolas Vallard de Dieppe;[13] a 1553 map by Pierre Desceliers Presbetre;[14] and a 1556 map by Giovanni Battista Ramusio.[15] Tupinambá brazilwood cutters are illustrated in a book by André Thevet, an early Franciscan chaplain in Brazil, entitled *Les Singularitez de la France Antarctique, autrement nommée Amérique,*[16] which is shown in the more accessible publication *Amazonia Urgent*[17] by Ribeiro. The Ribeiro volume also includes a 16th century map of Brazil, from the Ajuda Library in Lisbon, showing brazilwood harvesters.[18]

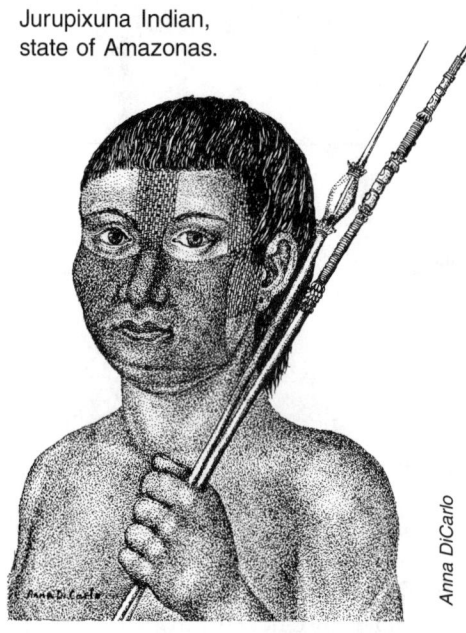

Jurupixuna Indian, state of Amazonas.

Anna DiCarlo

Exploitation of brazilwood began very early in the history of its namesake country. In 1501 Amerigo Vespucci carried large quantities of brazilwood to Portugal for the Portuguese crown. Then, as related by Wiznitzer, "In 1502 a consortium of New Christians [converted Jews] headed by Fernando de Noronha obtained from King Manuel I of Portugal a concession to colonize and exploit the newly discovered land. The main business of the group was to export brazilwood to Portu-

---

[11] Sturtevant, W.C. 1976. *First visual images of Native America,* pp. 417-454, in Chiappelli, F., et al., eds., FIRST IMAGES OF AMERICA: THE IMPACT OF THE NEW WORLD ON THE OLD. Vol. I. 515 pp. Berkeley, Los Angeles, London: University of California Press.

[12] Bibliothèque Nationale, Paris; also found in Belluzo, A.M. de Moraes. 1995. THE VOYAGER'S BRAZIL. Vol. I. Imagery of the New World. 156 pp.; Vol. II. A Place in the Universe. 168 pp.; Vol. III. The Construction of the Landscape. 192 pp. English edition translated by H.S. Gledhill. São Paulo: Metalivros, & Salvador, BA: Odebrecht Foundation.1: 2, 64–65, 68.

[13] Huntington Library, San Marino, California.

[14] Lost in Vienna in 1915.

[15] Library of Congress, Washington, DC.

[16] Paris, 1557. Thevet, A. 1557. *Les Singularitez de la France Antarctique, Autrement nommée Amérique.* 166 pp. Paris: S. Claude.

[17] Ribeiro, B.G. 1992. AMAZONIA URGENT: FIVE CENTURIES OF HISTORY AND ECOLOGY. 271 pp. "Reconquest of Brazil" Collection (Special Series), Vol. 13. Belo Horizonte, Brazil: Editora Itatiaia Limitada. p. 59.

[18] *Ibid,* p. 110.

gal for the purpose of dyeing textiles."[19] In the year 1519 alone, Noronha's monopoly felled 5,000 trunks of brazilwood and shipped them to Portugal; the monopoly scheme was discontinued in 1605. The French established a colony at Guanabara Bay (the site of present-day Rio de Janeiro) in the 1550s, and they also, despite being largely excluded from the equatorial New World by Spain and Portugal, employed Brazilian Tupinambá-Guarani, Tamoyo, Carijó and Potiguara Indians in the Atlantic coastal forests to harvest brazilwood which was sent to France for use in the wool and textile trade.[20]

Native Amerindians gradually came to be recognized in France, for approximately 50 Tupinambá Indians from the northern Brazilian coast had once been sent to Rouen (a major center of the French brazilwood trade since 1500). In October 1550 the Indians participated in a "Brazilian" festival and pageant which included a simulated habitat along the Seine river-bank and

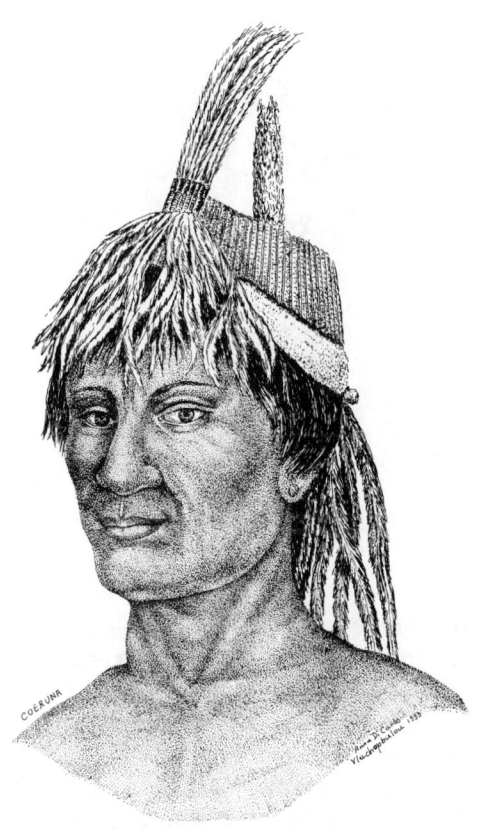

Coeruna Indian of Brazil.

---

[19] Wiznitzer, A.A. 1971. *Brazil: Colonial Period,* pp. 1322-1326, in ENCYCLOPEDIA JUDAICA. Vol. 4. Jerusalem: Keter Publishing House.

[20] Altman, I. 1992. *The contact of cultures in America* pp. 111-130, in Hebert, J.R., ed., 1492: AN ONGOING VOYAGE. 169 pp. Washington, DC: Library of Congress; Doggett, R., Hulvey, M. & J. Ainsworth. 1992. *The Catalogue,* pp. 34-79, in Doggett, R., ed., NEW WORLD OF WONDERS: EUROPEAN IMAGES OF THE AMERICAS, 1492-1700. 176 pp. Washington, DC: The Folger Shakespeare Library. [Distributed by University of Washington Press, Seattle & London]; Honour, H. 1975. THE NEW GOLDEN LAND: EUROPEAN IMAGES OF AMERICA FROM THE DISCOVERIES TO THE PRESENT TIME. 299 pp. New York: Pantheon Books; Nowell, C.E. 1949. *The French in sixteenth-century Brazil.* THE AMERICAS 5(4): 381-393; Dickason, O.P. 1984. THE MYTH OF THE SAVAGE: AND THE BEGINNINGS OF FRENCH COLONIALISM IN THE AMERICAS. 372 pp. Edmonton, Alberta, Canada: University of Alberta Press, pp. 183-193 for discussion of Tupinambá culture.

Foreword

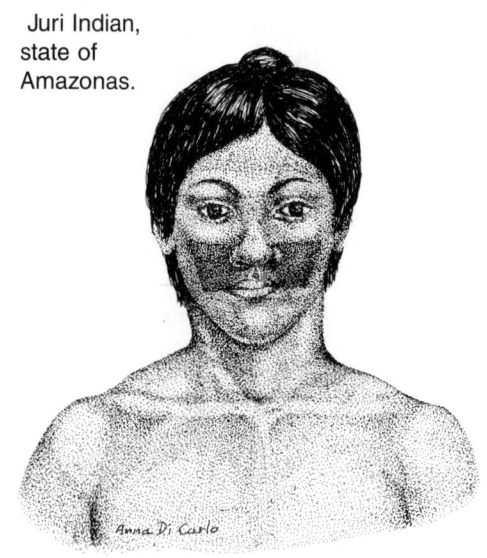

Juri Indian, state of Amazonas.

Anna DiCarlo

demonstrations of brazilwood harvesting, along with a mock battle between Tupinambá and Tabajara tribesmen.[21] The fete was held to celebrate the state visit of Henry II and Catherine de Medici to Rouen, and the artificial trees in the field in which the mock battle took place were painted red to signify brazilwood. A display of Tupinambá occurred again in 1613, since masquerades and carnivals of this nature were intended to help establish and reinforce France's perceived right to maintain settlements in the Portuguese New World.

As noted by Souza, "During a century and a half, the forests of Brazil were ravaged, until in 1652 a protest was raised against such abuse, which, however, was not repressed until 1751, when, by virtue of representations to the Crown, the first measures were adopted to limit the felling of hardwoods."[22] Today, brazilwood from Brazil is used largely for making violin bows and is shipped to Europe under the name of "pernambuco"; it is also a locally useful medicinal plant in that the wood is tonic and odontalgic. A different leguminous species, *Haematoxylon braziletto* from Central and South America, gradually became a replacement source for "brazilwood" imported to the North American dye industry.

By evidence of the above considerations, we may recognize the early and intimate connection between useful plant resources and the formative years of the Brazilian nation.

---

[21] *Cest la Deduction* (1551) cited in Moraes, R.B. de. 1958. Bibliographia Brasiliana. Vol. 1: 427 pp.; Vol. 2: 448 pp. Amsterdam & Rio de Janeiro: Colibris Editora 1: 151–154; *also* Belluzo, A.M. de Moraes. 1995. The Voyager's Brazil. Vol. I. Imagery of the New World. 156 pp.; Vol. II. A Place in the Universe. 168 pp.; Vol. III. The Construction of the Landscape. 192 pp. English edition translated by H.S. Gledhill. São Paulo: Metalivros & Salvador, BA: Odebrecht Foundation. 1: 26–35.

[22] Souza, P.F. 1945. *The Brazilian forests*, pp. 111-119, in Verdoorn, F., ed., Plants and Plant Science in Latin America. 381 pp. Waltham, Massachusetts: Chronica Botanica Company; *see also* Dean, W. 1995. With Broadax and Firebrand: The Destruction of the Brazilian Atlantic Forest. 482 pp. Berkeley, California: University of California Press.

II. Disease and Remedy in the Colonial Era and Today

The era in which Brazil was first explored corresponds to the Age of Herbals (the Age dates from 1470–1670) and of alchemists in Europe.[23] Meanwhile, in the New World, herbal medicine had developed among the sophisticated civilizations of the Aztec and Maya.[24] Medicinal plants were also utilized to a great extent by the lesser-advanced nomadic and sedentary Indian tribes of Brazil. In fact, one of the earliest phenomena noted about the Brazilian Indians was that they were able to treat or "doctor" themselves with plant preparations from the forest. Two examples of such relations include:[25] I. Ptolemy. 1508. *Ptolomaei Geographica*. In this book, Brazil is called *Terra de Santa Cruz*, and it is noted that the Indians "seldom fall sick and when they do they doctor themselves exclusively with roots and herbs"; II. Vespucci, Amerigo. 1510–1515. *Of the New Lands and of the People found by the Messengers of the King of Portugal named Emanuel*. The Indians live "many years more than other people for they have costly spices and roots, where they themself recover with, and heal them as they be sick."

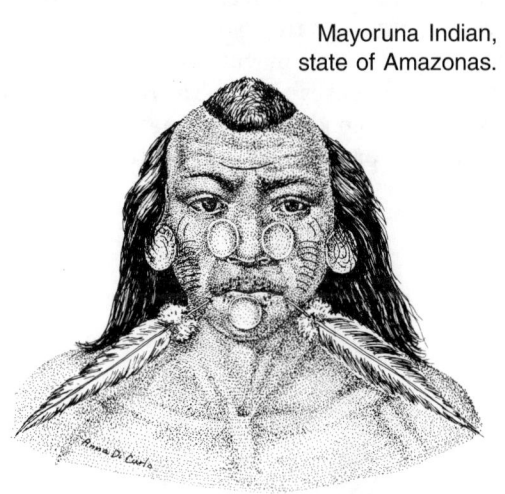

Mayoruna Indian, state of Amazonas.

Anna DiCarlo

As reported by Crosby, with regard to the original conditions which existed in the New World prior to the Discovery, "The Amerindians had at least *pinta* (a spirochaete-caused skin disease), yaws, venereal syphilis, hepatitis, encephalitis, polio, some varieties of tuberculosis (not those usually associated with pulmonary disease), and intestinal parasites, but they seem to have been without any experience with such Old World maladies as smallpox, measles, diphtheria, trachoma, whooping cough, chicken pox, bubonic plague, malaria, typhoid fever, cholera, yellow fe-

---

[23] Boorstin, D.J. 1983. THE DISCOVERERS. 745 pp. New York: Random House.

[24] King, S.R. 1992. Conservation and tropical medicinal plant research. *HerbalGram* 27: 28-35.

[25] Moraes, R.B. de. 1958. BIBLIOGRAPHIA BRASILIANA. Vol. 1: 427 pp.; Vol. 2: 448 pp. Amsterdam & Rio de Janeiro: Colibris Editora.

ver, dengue fever, scarlet fever, amebic dysentery, influenza, and a number of helminthic infestations."[26]

European colonists (Portuguese, etc.) in Brazil suffered from many discomforts and diseases in early times. This is evidenced by the writings of several observers, for example Alphonse Rendu, who in 1848 reported that the most common illnesses were intermittent fevers, syphilis, tuberculosis, stupor, buboes, goiters and leprosy.[27] Freyre reports that, in early Brazilian colonial times, "the diseases that affected children in those days were numerous: the "seven days sickness"; inflammation of the navel; mycosis; the itch in various forms; scurvy; measles; chicken pox; tapeworm — diseases that were combated with clysters, purgatives, leeches, cathartics, blood-lettings, emetics, mustard plasters."[28]

Another problem was presented by involuntary servitude. As explained by Symcox, "From the middle of the sixteenth century a profitable sugar economy began to develop in Brazil, necessitating the import of slaves from Elmina [a fort in the Gold Coast, now Ghana] and São Thomé in West Africa, and soon from Angola as well. Sugar from the Brazilian plantations was then shipped to Lisbon for distribution to the rest of Europe."[29]

Prior to the abolition of slavery in Brazil in 1888, Africans carried across the Atlantic Ocean several diseases that were prevalent in their West African homelands along the Gulf of Guinea. According to a 1934 lecture by Professor Octavio de Freitas, "the following were the maladies and afflictions brought to Brazil by the *"negros bichados"* (infected Negroes): *"bicho da Costa"* (a parasite), dysentery (*maculo*), buboes, bony

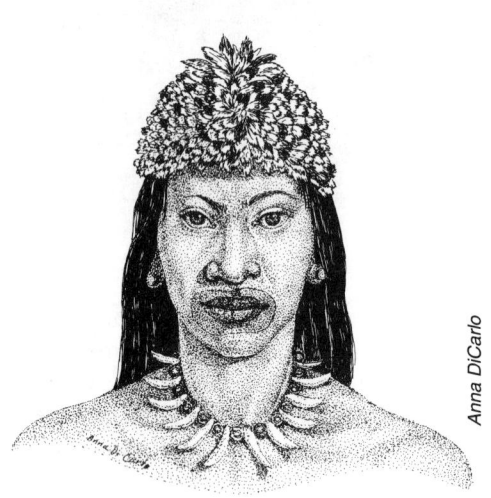

Mauhé Indian, state of Amazonas.

---

[26] Crosby, A.W. 1986. ECOLOGICAL IMPERIALISM: THE BIOLOGICAL EXPANSION OF EUROPE, 900–1900. 368 pp. Cambridge, London, New York: Cambridge University Press.

[27] Moraes, R.B. de. 1958.

[28] Freyre, G. 1956. THE MASTERS AND THE SLAVES. Ed. 2. 537 pp. New York: Alfred A. Knopf. [Translation by Samuel Putnam from original 1933 CASA GRANDE E SENZALA.]

[29] Symcox, G.W. 1976. *The battle of the Atlantic, 1500-1700*, pp. 265-277 in Chiappelli, F. et al., eds., FIRST IMAGES OF AMERICA: THE IMPACT OF THE NEW WORLD ON THE OLD. Vol. I. 515 pp. Berkeley, Los Angeles, London: University of California Press.

Right, Botocudos Indian, state of Amazonas.

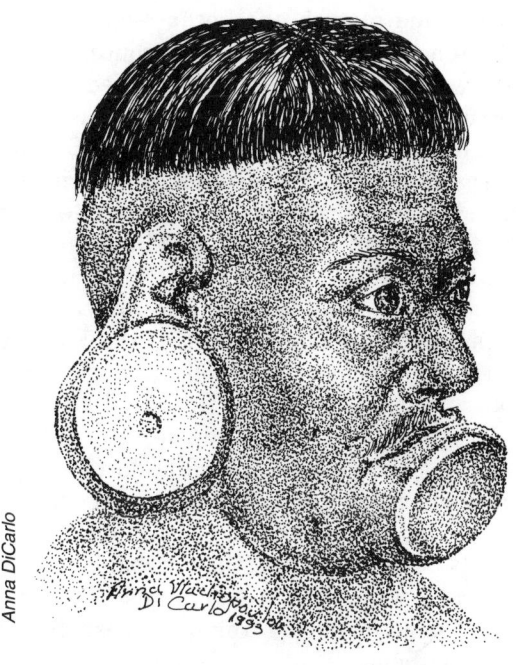

excrescences on the nose and cheek-bones (*gundu*), chills, thickening of the skin (*ainhum*), fleas, and nematode worms (*filarias*)."[30]

As noted by Grimé, the slaves introduced into Brazil the okra (*Abelmoschus esculentus*), a plant which in addition to the edible pod, was used by them as a softening cataplasm.[31] The slaves also were known to use gum arabic (*Acacia nilotica*) against goitre; this plant had previously been introduced from Africa to the New World.

Extended observations made in the year 1835 by José Martins da Cruz Jobim permit an overall view of the health of the non-European population: "the following maladies ... being prevalent among the workers and household slaves of Rio de Janeiro: syphilis; cardiac hypertrophy; rheumatism; bronchitis; affections of the respiratory passages; pneumonia; pleurisy; pericarditis; encephalic irritations and inflammations; tetanus; hepatitis; and erysipelas, commonly in the lower members and the scrotum, leading to hypertrophy and fibrolardaceous degeneration of the subcutaneous cellular tissue, extravasations in the various sonorous cavities, rarely in the joints but frequently in the abdomen, the pleura, the pericardium, the testicular membrane, and the cerebral ventricles, where it gave rise to paralysis. Still other affections were pulmonary tuberculosis, intermittent fevers, and ancylostomiasis. Worms, especially the tapeworm and lumbricoid roundworms, are to be found in great abundance."[32]

A typical Brazilian apothecary shop of the 1830s is depicted in a volume by Jean Baptiste Debret entitled *Viagem Pitoresca e Historica ao*

---

[30] As related by Freyre, G. (1956. THE MASTERS AND THE SLAVES).

[31] Grimé, W.E. 1979. ETHNO-BOTANY OF THE BLACK AMERICANS. 237 pp. Algonac, Michigan: Reference Publications, Inc.

[32] Freyre, 1956.

FOREWORD

Brasil.[33] Remedies, many of botanical derivation, for various ailments were stocked in such apothecary shops, as well as sought from doctors who often had rather primitive concepts for healing. In regard to the latter, we learn from sources recorded by Freyre, that colonial doctors prescribed "household remedies such as were common in Portugal and which from there were transmitted to Brazil: teas or infusions made of bedbugs ... for intestinal disorders; an ostrich's maw to dissolve gall-stones; ... the skin, bones, and flesh of toads, newts and crayfish."[34] Five toasted houseflies dissolved in a spoon of lukewarm water allegedly cured a case of urine suppression in a young girl of Rio de Janeiro.

It is understandable that, due to peculiar and unpleasant remedies such as the preceding examples, "the Portuguese colonizer in Brazil ... had the good sense not wholly to slight the native healers by having recourse always to officially approved medicine as practiced in Portugal. This despite the fact that the Jesuits had declared a war to the death upon the *"curandeiros,"* or tribal doctors. The priests themselves, however, even as they combated the mystic pharmacopoeia of the medicine-men, absorbed from the latter a knowledge of a number of plants and herbs. It is, indeed, altogether probable that the life of a patient in colonial Brazil was safer in the hands of the native practitioners than in those of some physician from overseas who was a stranger to the milieu and its pathology."[35]

During the period of Portuguese Enlightenment in the late 18th century, medical sciences flourished in Portugal, aided by contributions from Brazil. As noted by Simon, "There was a great interest in classical medicine as well as in the newly discovered drugs from the Orient as well as Brazil .... During the reign of King João V (1706–1750) the wealth of Brazilian diamond and gold mines allowed the King to build the convent-palaces of Mafra, patronize music, the sciences, arts, and literature, as well as send gifted students to study in northern Europe."[36]

Currently, as related by Walter B. Mors,[37] malaria, mainly of the *falciparum* variety, is the worst disease in Brazil. It is deadly, spreading fast, and is considered the main endemic disease at the moment, concentrated in the Amazon region and fast approaching one million new cases

---

[33] Debret, J.B. 1989. VIAGEM PITORESCA E HISTORICA AO BRASIL. 26 pp. + 139 plates. Belo Horizonte, Brazil: Editora Itatiaia Limitada. [Reprint. Original published Paris 1834] (Apothecary, plate 19.)

[34] Freyre, 1956.

[35] Freyre, 1956; *see also* Voeks, R.A. 1996. Tropical forest healers and habitat preference. *Economic Botany* 50(4): 381-400.

[36] Simon, W.J. 1983. SCIENTIFIC EXPEDITIONS IN THE PORTUGUESE OVERSEAS TERRITORIES (1783-1808). 193 pp. Lisboa, Portugal: Instituto de Investigacão Cientifica Tropical.

[37] Mors, W.B. 1995. *Pers. comm.*: Letter dated 22 January 1995; *see also* Milliken, W. 1997. Traditional anti-malarial medicine in Roraima, Brazil. *Economic Botany* 51 (3): 212-237.

annually. Secondarily, there is hepatitis B, mentioned in this publication under *Phyllanthus niruri* (Euphorbiaceae). In third place is leprosy, which is slowly coming back; it is mentioned under *Carpotroche brasiliensis* (Flacourtiaceae). Like malaria and hepatitis B, leprosy is also prevalent in Amazonia. Outside the Amazon region there are Chagas' disease which afflicts about five million Brazilians, and schistosomiasis (bilharzia) represented by about eight million cases. Schistosomiasis is mentioned herein under the leguminous *Pterodon pubescens* (Fabaceae).

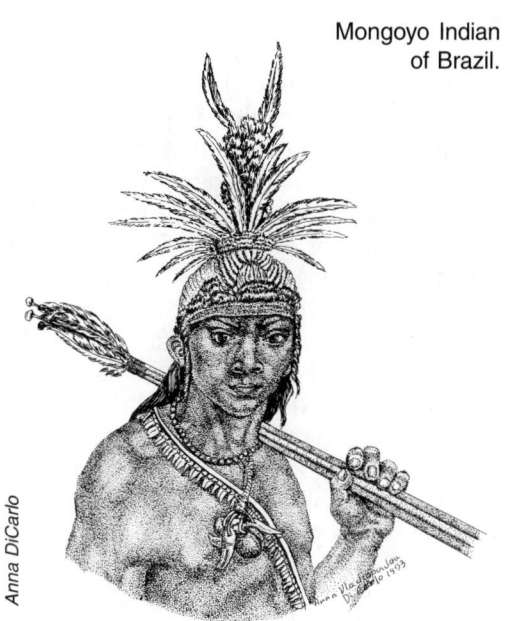

Mongoyo Indian of Brazil.

Anna DiCarlo

Also substantial, although far less so than the afflictions mentioned above, is the protozoan-caused skin disease known as leishmaniasis, wherein parasitic flagellates of the genus *Leishmania* are transmitted to humans through intermediate host (vector) sandflies. In Brazil, "uncontrolled deforestation is causing an increase ... in leishmaniasis, which is transmitted by phlebotomous insects commonly known by the name of "asa de palha" (straw wings),"[38] and in that connection the Leishmaniasis Research Laboratory of Minas Gerais has noted that "the insects that transmit leishmaniasis are currently in the process of adjusting to city life (in Belo Horizonte) after having been expelled from the jungle by indiscriminate deforestation." Fortunately, awareness of the ways human activities have an impact on the natural environment so as to cause the spread of disease is becoming more focused in modern societies.[39]

---

[38] Anonymous. 1990. *Deforestation linked to leishmaniasis.* JPRS REPORT: JPRS-TEN-90-006: 34 (27 June 1990). Washington, DC: Foreign Broadcast Information Service (FBIS), Joint Publication Research Service (JPRS). (Translation of broadcast on Brasilia Radio Nacional da Amazonia Network, 25 June 1990.)

[39] Garnett, G.P. & E.C. Holmes. 1996. *The ecology of emergent infectious disease.* BIOSCIENCE 46(2): 127-135; Garrett, L. 1995. THE COMING PLAGUE: NEWLY EMERGING DISEASES IN A WORLD OUT OF BALANCE. 750 pp. New York: Farrar, Straus; Grifo, F. & J. Rosenthal, 1997. BIODIVERSITY AND HUMAN HEALTH. 379 pp. Washington, DC & Covelo, California: Island Press; Morse, S.S., ed. 1993. EMERGING VIRUSES. 317 pp. New York & Oxford: Oxford University Press; Preston, R. 1994. THE HOT ZONE. 300 pp. New York: Random House.

FOREWORD

III. Curare

One of the interesting ethnotoxic gifts of the South American Indians for the advancement of Western medicine is the knowledge of skeletal muscle relaxants gained from the examination of curare, a hunting poison mixture used on the tips of darts and arrows by various tribes.[40]

The earliest accounts of curare were from Venezuela and the Guianas, referring to *Strychnos*-based mixtures, and later, in the 1820s, the famous explorer of Brazil, Karl von Martius found Menispermaceae-based (*Chondodendron*) curares being made along the Amazonian Rio Japurá. Researchers have learned that various neurological conditions such as convulsions and Parkinsonism are helped through use of "curarizing" agents, in addition to their use as a muscle relaxant. The compound d-tubocurarine, extracted from the bark of the liana *Chondodendron tomentosum*, has the most pronounced and useful curarizing effect.

As defined by Bisset, curare can have several different meanings: "1. To the anthropologist or ethnographer it stands for a group of dart (and arrow) poisons prepared by the Indians of tropical South America whose characteristic feature is to bring about paralysis; 2. To the pharmacolo-

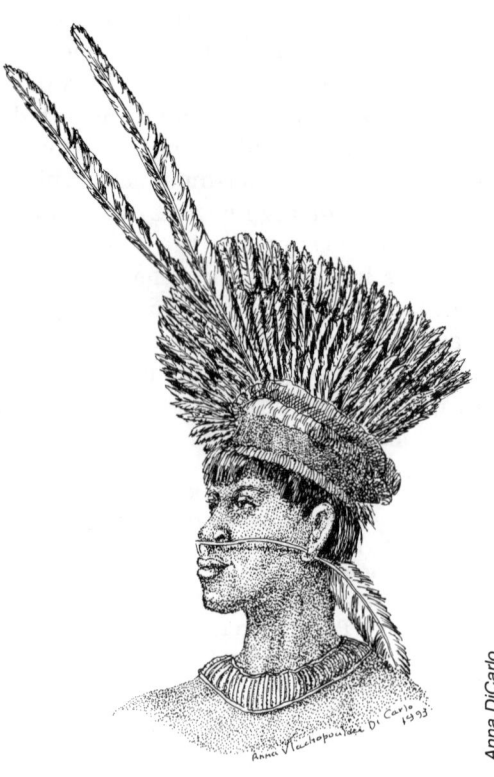

Indian of the Rio Xingu, Brazil.

Anna DiCarlo

[40] Bisset, N.G. 1995. *Arrow poisons and their role in the development of medicinal agents*, pp. 289-302, in Schultes, R.E. & S. von Reis, eds., ETHNOBOTANY: EVOLUTION OF A DISCIPLINE. 414 pp. Portland, Oregon: Dioscorides Press; Bovet, D., Bovet-Nitti, F. & G.B. Marini-Bettiolo, eds. 1959. CURARE AND CURARE-LIKE AGENTS. Amsterdam: Elsevier Publishing Co.; Joyce, C. 1994. EARTHLY GOODS: MEDICINE-HUNTING IN THE RAINFOREST. 304 pp. Boston, New York, Toronto, London: Little, Brown and Company. (Curare: Chapter 3. *The Arrow Poison and the Yam*, pp. 33-60); McIntyre, A.R. 1947. CURARE: ITS HISTORY, NATURE AND CLINICAL USE. 240 pp. Chicago, Illinois: University of Chicago Press; Smith, P. 1969. ARROWS OF MERCY. 244 pp. Toronto: Doubleday Canada Ltd.; Garden City, New York: Doubleday & Company, Inc.; Thomas, K.B. 1963. CURARE: ITS HISTORY AND USAGE. 144 pp. Philadelphia & Montreal: J.B. Lippincott Company.

gist curare is characterized by its action at the neuromuscular junction; this is to cause relaxation or paralysis of the musculature through blockade by a non-depolarizing, competitive mechanism, the effects of which are reversible by small doses of neostigmine; 3. To the anaesthetist curare often simply means the muscle-relaxant alkaloid (+)- tubocurarine."[41]

Within the boundaries of Brazil (although no curare-class is confined to Brazil), the Indians prepare four classes of curare, which have been arranged by Bisset, as follows: I. Curares based on Loganiaceae, e.g., in the states of Amapá, Pará, Amazonas, Roraima; II. Mixed Loganiaceae/ Menispermaceae curares, e.g., in the state of Amazonas; III. Curares based on Loganiaceae (savanna), e.g., in the states of Rondonia and Mato Grosso; IV. Loganiaceae and/or Menispermaceae-based arrow-tip curares, e.g., in the state of Amazonas.[42] The species employed in each of the above-mentioned classes are charted by Bisset.[43]

Curiously, as mentioned by Mors & Rizzini,[44] the convulsive properties of Old World species of *Strychnos* (Loganiaceae) have been known for a long time, with the Old World species often (but not exclusively) containing strychnine alkaloids in contrast to the New World species which have compounds that are related to strychnine, but are quaternary ammonium bases. Other examples given by Bisset are the arrowhead poisons made from *Strychnos usambarensis* by the Banyambo people of the Rwanda-Tanzania frontier, and the dart poison made from *Strychnos ignatii* by the Semai Senoi tribe of western Malaysia.[45]

It has recently been found that African species of *Strychnos* contain alkaloidal, quaternary ammonium curarizing compounds formerly thought to reside exclusively in the New World species,[46] and also that American species share with Old World plants such tetanizing tertiary bases as akagerine. The significant connections between the floras of South America and Africa as a whole have been discussed by Gentry.[47]

Based on various comparisons, Dr. Angenot[48] has suggested that the Brazilian *Strychnos* species should be further investigated for the follow-

---

[41] Bisset, N.G. 1988. *Curare — botany, chemistry, and pharmacology.* ACTA AMAZONICA 18(1-2) Suplemento: 255-290.

[42] *Ibid*, map p. 257.

[43] Bisset, 1988.

[44] Mors, W.B. & C.T. Rizzini. 1966. USEFUL PLANTS OF BRAZIL. 166 pp. San Francisco, London, Amsterdam: Holden-Day Inc.

[45] Bisset, 1988.

[46] Angenot, L. 1988. *Why further investigation of Brazilian Strychnos?* ACTA AMAZONICA 18(1-2) Suplemento: 241-254.

[47] Gentry, A.H. 1993. *Diversity and floristic composition of lowland tropical forest in Africa and South America*, pp. 500-547, in Goldblatt, P., ed., BIOLOGICAL RELATIONSHIPS BETWEEN AFRICA AND SOUTH AMERICA. 630 pp. New Haven & London: Yale University Press; Loganiaceae, p. 513.

[48] Angenot, 1988.

ing reasons: I. The lack of knowledge concerning the distribution of alkaloids among many species, and the fact that "the distribution of species in (the) southern part of the great Amazon Basin — particularly from the upper Rio Xingu and Rios Tapajós and Madeira — is poorly known and it is possible that new species may be found there." II. "There is little information available not only on the variation in composition of the alkaloidal mixture in the different parts of the plants (e.g., the leaves), but also on their biological activities too focused in the past on curarizing activity." III. Brazilian species may possibly contain new antimitotic alkaloids and antitumor drugs with properties similar to those which have been either long-known or recently discovered in African *Strychnos* species.

With regard to the Menispermaceae, some Brazilian menispermaceous curare ingredients have local medicinal uses, such as *Curarea tecunarum* used as a contraceptive in Amazonas; *Sciadotenia* cf. *pachnococca* used for toothache in Amazonas; *Sciadotenia paraensis* used as an abortifacient in Pará; *Abuta* cf. *grandifolia* as an abortifacient; *Abuta sandwithiana* for malaria in Mato Grosso, and as a female contraceptive in Rondonia; and *Cissampelos ovalifolia* tubers used in Pará to treat bite of the *Bothrops* snake "cobra jararaca."[49]

Concerning plants employed in curare which belong neither to the Menispermaceae nor Loganiaceae, one can only regret the lost knowledge once accumulated by the Juri tribe, a now-extinct people of western Amazonia, whom the early explorer Karl von Martius discovered using the admixture plant *Unonopsis (Guatteria) veneficiorum* (Annonaceae) as an ingredient in their curare. The *Unonopsis veneficiorum* has recently been shown to possibly contribute to the overall effect of the curare due to (-)- curine content, and therefore would be deserving of further research.[50] This (-)- form of curine also occurs in the menispermaceous curare species *Chondodendron platyphyllum, C. tomentosum* and *Curarea toxicoferum*.

IV. Indians

One thousand Indian tribes probably existed in Brazil in 1500 A.D.[51] Of 300 culturally distinct tribes identified in 1900, approximately one-third have disappeared for various reasons. The Brazilian government believes that there are still uncontacted Stone Age Indians in six locations in the state of Roraima; in 18 locations in Pará; four in Goias; eight each in Mato Grosso, Maranhão and Rondonia; and in 31 locations scattered throughout the state of Amazonas.[52]

---

[49] Bisset, 1988.

[50] *Ibid.*

[51] Ribeiro, 1992.

[52] Brooke, J. 1990. Conflicting pressures shape the future of Brazil Indians. *The New York Times,* February 25; Section E, page 5.

As previously noted, from the earliest times the Indians of Brazil were known to medicate themselves with plants from the local flora. The Amerindians of present times, such as the Kayapó, Tiriyo and Tenharins,[53] indeed know a great amount of information, although that is not to suggest that the various tribes know absolutely all potential medicinal plants.

The Brazilian scientist Dr. Otto R. Gottlieb has observed, concerning the extent of Indian medicinal knowledge, that "Not all medically useful Brazilian plants were discovered by indigenous populations. For example, various *Rauvolfia* species (Apocynaceae) with useful hypotensive alkaloids, never seem to have attained practical importance in indigenous medicine although they grow all over tropical South America ... Good examples of the relatively few plants used by traditional healers which also yielded useful drugs when subjected to chemical and pharmacological testing are *Cephaelis ipecacuanha* (Rubiaceae) with the emetic and expectorant emetine; *Chenopodium ambrosioides* (Chenopodiaceae) with the vermifugal ascaridole; *Dialyanthera otoba* (Myristicaceae) with the fungistatic or fungicidal otobain; possibly *Maytenus ilicifolia* (Celastraceae) with the antitumoral pristimerin; *Quassia amara* (Simaroubaceae) used against stomach disorders with quassin; *Carpotroche brasiliensis* (Flacourtiaceae) with esters of glycerol and hydnocarpic acid formerly used in the treatment of leprosy; *Stachytarpheta australis* (Verbenaceae) used as an antithermic and sudorific (sweat inducer) with ipoliimide, and *Calea pinnatifida* (Asteraceae) used as an amoebicide with a polyacetylene and a germacranolide."[54]

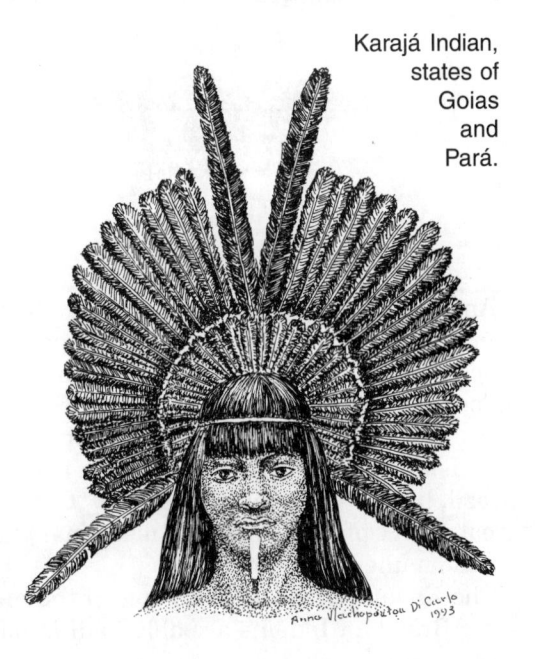

Karajá Indian, states of Goias and Pará.

Anna DiCarlo

---

[53] Souza Brito, A.R.M. & A.A. Souza Brito. 1996. *Medicinal plant research in Brazil: data from regional and national meetings,* pp. 386-401, in Balick, M.J., Elisabetsky, E. & S.A. Laird, eds., MEDICINAL RESOURCES OF THE TROPICAL FOREST: BIODIVERSITY AND ITS IMPORTANCE TO HUMAN HEALTH. 440 pp. New York: Columbia University Press.

[54] Gottlieb, O.R. 1985. *The chemical uses and chemical geography of Amazon plants,* pp. 218-238, in Prance, G.T. & T.E. Lovejoy, eds., AMAZONIA. KEY ENVIRONMENTS SERIES. 442 pp. Oxford & New York: Pergamon Press.

Bororo Indian, state of Mato Grosso.

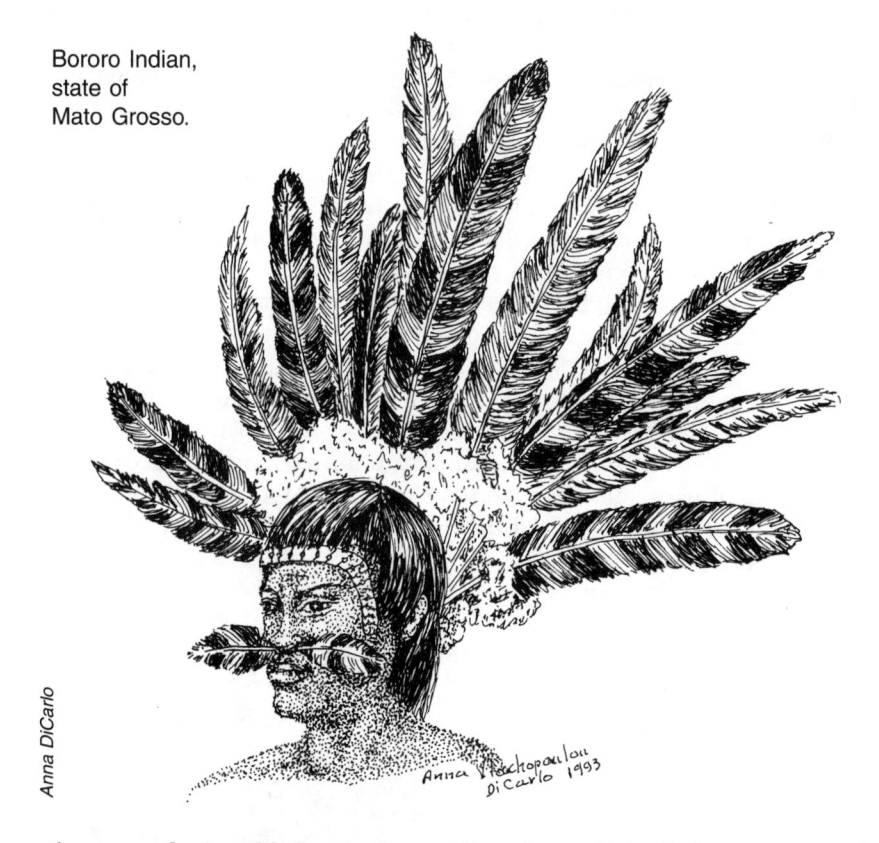

An example, in addition to *Rauvolfia*, of a medicinal plant apparently overlooked by the Indians, may be the genus *Alexa*, a papilionoid legume whose sap contains the drug castanospermine, a polyhydroxylated indolizidine alkaloid[55] which has potential in the treatment of HIV-1 AIDS (Acquired Immune Deficiency Syndrome). Species of *Alexa* occur on Maraca Island along the Rio Urancuera and other localities in Amazonian Brazil, but as reported by Macklin, "Curiously, the native Indians — a great source of information on medicinal plants — have no use for *Alexa*, and no name for the tree."[56]

The Kayapó tribe is an example of the highly refined degree to which some Brazilian Indians are able to differentiate between plant species,

---

[55] Nash, R.J., et al. 1988. *Castanospermine in Alexa species*. PHYTOCHEMISTRY 27(5): 1403-1404; Kaplan, M.A.C. 1995. *Amazonia versus Australia: Geographically distant, chemically close,* pp. 180-187, in Seidl, P.R., Gottlieb, O.R. & M.A.C. Kaplan, eds., CHEMISTRY OF THE AMAZON: BIODIVERSITY, NATURAL PRODUCTS, AND ENVIRONMENTAL ISSUES. 315 pp. American Chemical Society Symposium Series 588. Washington, DC: American Chemical Society.

[56] Macklin, D. 1989. *Last exit to the Amazon*. NEW SCIENTIST 122 (1666): 36-37.

and utilize them for various purposes. The most extensively studied Kayapó are in the state of Pará, where they practice a form of vegetation management by creating "islands" of domesticated and semi-domesticated indigenous, useful plants which they cultivate in isolated patches up to five acres in extent, within the surrounding savanna grasslands (campo). Among the various deliberately planted species are some which they use for medicine to treat headaches, fevers, body aches, diarrhea, dizziness, toothaches, and bleeding, as well as for contraceptives and abortifacients.[57]

The "Pau d'Arco," a group of 1,500 Kayapó Indians who succumbed to introduced diseases due to their lack of immunity, would certainly not have been expected to be familiar with the important immunostimulant properties (for allergies and weakened immune systems) of the pau d'arco trees (*Tabebuia* spp., Bignoniaceae) whose name they bore and wood their archers used for bows.[58] However, an elaboration of the wisdom of the Kayapó tribe (also known as the Mebengokre) of modern times would mention that they now employ preparations for treating scorpion stings, skin itches, black diarrhea, rheumatism and vitiligo (localized loss of skin pigment). More surprising, the Mebengokre, according to Posey, "classify over 150 types of diarrhoea/dysentery, each of which is treated with specific medicines";[59] see also Elisabetsky & Posey for 60 plant species used by the Kayapó to treat gastrointestinal disorders.[60] Similarly, the plant medicine of the Yanomami Indians of Brazil is derived from their knowledge of at least 198 species of plants and fungi used for treating various conditions or disorders.[61]

Dr. Robert A. DeFilipps, Editor
Smithsonian Institution
Washington, DC

---

[57] Posey, D.A. 1982. "The keepers of the forest." *Garden* 6(1): 18-24; Posey, D.A. 1984. "Keepers of the campo." *Garden* 8(6): 8-12; Posey, D.A. 1988. *Kayapó Indian natural resource management,* pp. 89-90, in Denslow, J.S. & C. Padoch, eds., People of the Tropical Rain Forest. 231 pp. Berkeley & Los Angeles: University of California Press; Posey, D.A., et al. 1987. *Introduction,* pp. 12-38, in Hamu, D.C., ed., Alternatives to Destruction: Science of the Mebengokre. 69 pp. Belem, Brazil: Museu Paraense Emilio Goeldi.

[58] Jones, K. 1995. PAU D'ARCO: IMMUNE POWER FROM THE RAIN FOREST. 152 pp. Rochester, Vermont: Healing Arts Press.

[59] Posey, D.A. 1989. "Alternatives to forest destruction: lessons from the Mebengokre Indians." *The Ecologist* 19(6): 241-244.

[60] Elisabetsky, E. & D.A. Posey. 1994. *Ethnopharmacological search for antiviral compounds: treatment of gastrointestinal disorders by Kayapó medical specialists,* pp. 77-94, in ETHNOBOTANY AND THE SEARCH FOR NEW DRUGS. 280 pp. Ciba Foundation Symposium 185. Chichester, England: John Wiley & Sons Ltd.

[61] Milliken, W. & B. Albert. 1996. "The use of medicinal plants by the Yanomami Indians of Brazil." *Economic Botany* 50(1): 10-25; Part II, *op. cit.* 51(3): 264-278 (1997).

Fig. 1: States of the Brazilian Federation.

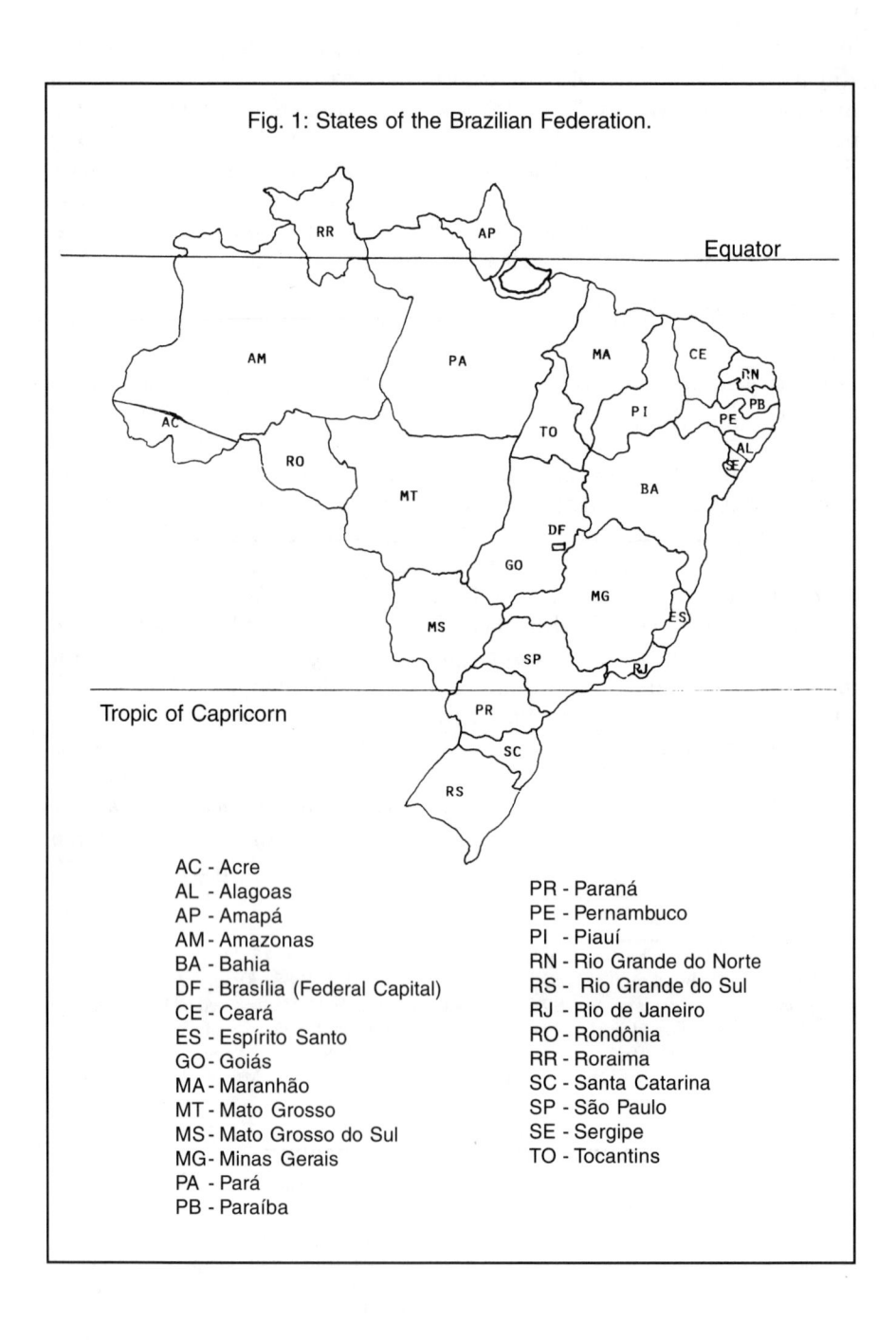

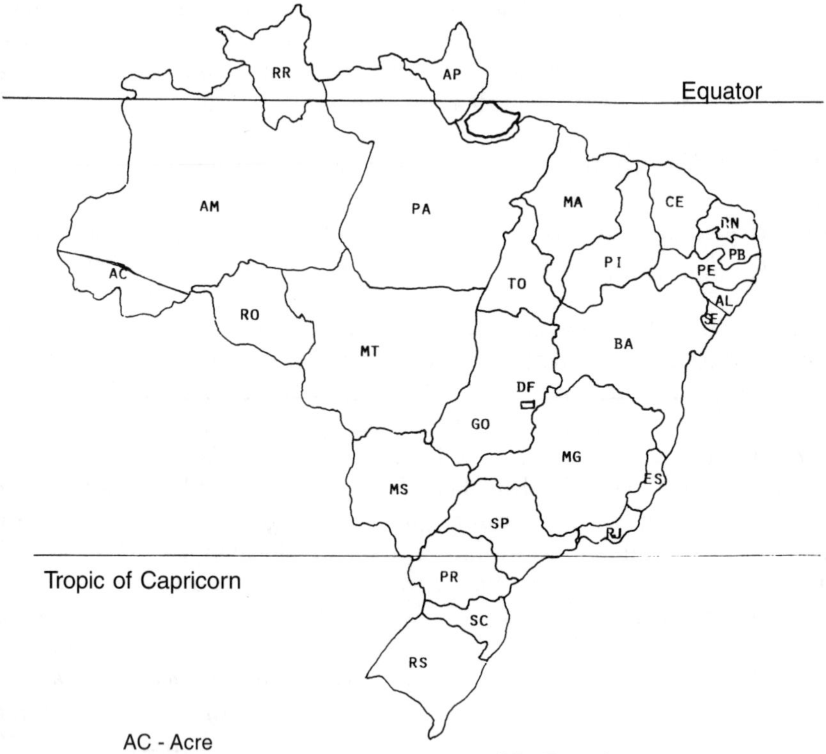

AC - Acre
AL - Alagoas
AP - Amapá
AM - Amazonas
BA - Bahia
DF - Brasília (Federal Capital)
CE - Ceará
ES - Espírito Santo
GO - Goiás
MA - Maranhão
MT - Mato Grosso
MS - Mato Grosso do Sul
MG - Minas Gerais
PA - Pará
PB - Paraíba
PR - Paraná
PE - Pernambuco
PI - Piauí
RN - Rio Grande do Norte
RS - Rio Grande do Sul
RJ - Rio de Janeiro
RO - Rondônia
RR - Roraima
SC - Santa Catarina
SP - São Paulo
SE - Sergipe
TO - Tocantins

INTRODUCTION

This book represents an overview of those plants which, since colonial times, have been gradually incorporated into the tradition of the Brazilian people as being of medicinal value. The first Europeans to settle in the country learned, of course, from the indigenous tribal populations. But in the course of four hundred years of depending on its natural wealth, the people of the country developed their own body of herbal knowledge, quite independent of the customs of the aboriginal Amerindians who today still live removed from, or merely brushed by, civilization.

The first person to record plants used for healing purposes in the newly settled Portuguese colony was Gabriel Soares de Sousa, who lived in Brazil during the second half of the 16th century. He released his writings, however, only after his return to Europe and published much later — in 1825 in Portugal and in 1851 in Brazil — under the title *"Tratado Descriptivo do Brazil."*

The next investigators were the Dutch physician Willem Pies (Gulielmus Piso) and the German botanist Georg Markgraf (Marcgrave). In the 17th century the Dutch secured a foothold in the Brazilian northeast, seizing the district of Pernambuco. Count Maurice of Nassau was nominated to govern this new possession, and proved himself an extremely able administrator during the seven years he remained at his post (1637–1644).

Piso embarked for Brazil upon Nassau's calling. His official position as physician notwithstanding, he dedicated himself exhaustively, with Nassau's encouragement, to the study of the natural resources used by the native population as medicines. He was joined somewhat later by Marcgrave and the collaboration of these two men led to the publication of the *"Historia Naturalis Brasiliae"* (1648), the most solid work on the natural sciences of colonial Brazil and, later, of *"De Indiae Utriusque re Naturali et Medica"* (1658), which covers both the East Indies and West Indies. Organized in fourteen books, the five dealing with Brazil were written by Piso. (Marcgrave died at an early age, in 1644.)

In *De Indiae*...we find the plants used for healing described in a most orderly fashion. They are, of course, named according to their native designations. But owing to the native names which have persisted to the present, and with the aid of the accompanying descriptions and illustrations, many, if not most of them, can be identified. To mention a few: the ipecacuanha, *Cephaelis ipecacuanha* Rich., emeto-cathartic; copaiva balsam, *Copaifera officinalis* (Jacq.) L., wound healing and antiseptic; japecanga or sarsaparilla, *Smilax longifolia* Rich., reputedly a powerful antiluetic; and jaborandi, *Pilocarpus pinnatifolius* Lem., with its salivation and sweat producing properties.

From that time on, the very same plants were repeatedly cited and described, and starting in the 18th century were given Latin scientific names. It is a most remarkable fact that plants held to be medicinal in those early times have conserved their reputation to this day. On the other hand, the huge store of Brazilian green medicine was enriched by additions from the newcomers. Europeans and Africans alike did not easily give up the plants to which they were accustomed in their homelands.

Portuguese settlers brought over angelica, *Angelica archangelica* L.; milk thistle, *Silybum marianum* Gaert.; rosemary, *Rosmarinus officinalis* L.; sweet sedge, *Acorus calamus* L.; and marsh mallow, *Althaea officinalis* L. They were the plants which came above deck. Below, in the holds of the slave ships, the captives brought their own herbs, among which we may note *Borreria verticillata* (L.) Meyer; *Kalanchoe pinnata* (Lam.) Pers.; *Vernonia condensata* Baker; and *Petiveria alliacea* L.

Jesuit priests in their missions reproduced their traditional theriacs (medicinal potions, often snakebite antidotes) using in part plants which they had introduced from Portugal, along with native substitutes which they found suitable. The most famous became the "Triaga Brasilica," produced in the 17th century in the Jesuit College in Bahia. At first maintained as a secret, its composition was made public in Rome, in 1766 (Pereira et al., 1996).

In the early search for surrogate plants in the Brazilian flora, which would tend to represent, and substitute for, the medicinal plants then known in Europe, some striking analogies were encountered. Old World species such as licorice, *Glycyrriza glabra* L.; nutmeg, *Myristica fragrans* Houtt.; and clove, *Eugenia caryophyllata* Thunb., found their New World counterparts in "Brazilian licorice," *Periandra mediterranea* (Vell.) Taub.; "Brazilian nutmeg," *Cryptocarya moschata* Nees & Mart.; and "Brazilian clove-bark," *Dicypellium caryophyllatum* Nees.

Two species from abroad, the European common rue, *Ruta graveolens* L. and the African cola nut, *Cola acuminata* Schott & Endl., became (and remain) elements in Afro-Brazilian religious rituals, the first under the Portuguese name "arruda," the latter under the Yoruba "obi."

Today, many of the medicinal plants treated in the present volume are common objects of commerce and can be found in specialized stores and open markets. Some of them are also exported. Examples are guaraná, *Paullinia cupana* H.B.K., as a general stimulant; and quebra-pedra, *Phyllanthus niruri* L., as a diuretic and for the elimination of kidney stones.

Thus came into being a fascinating blend which, developed through

INTRODUCTION

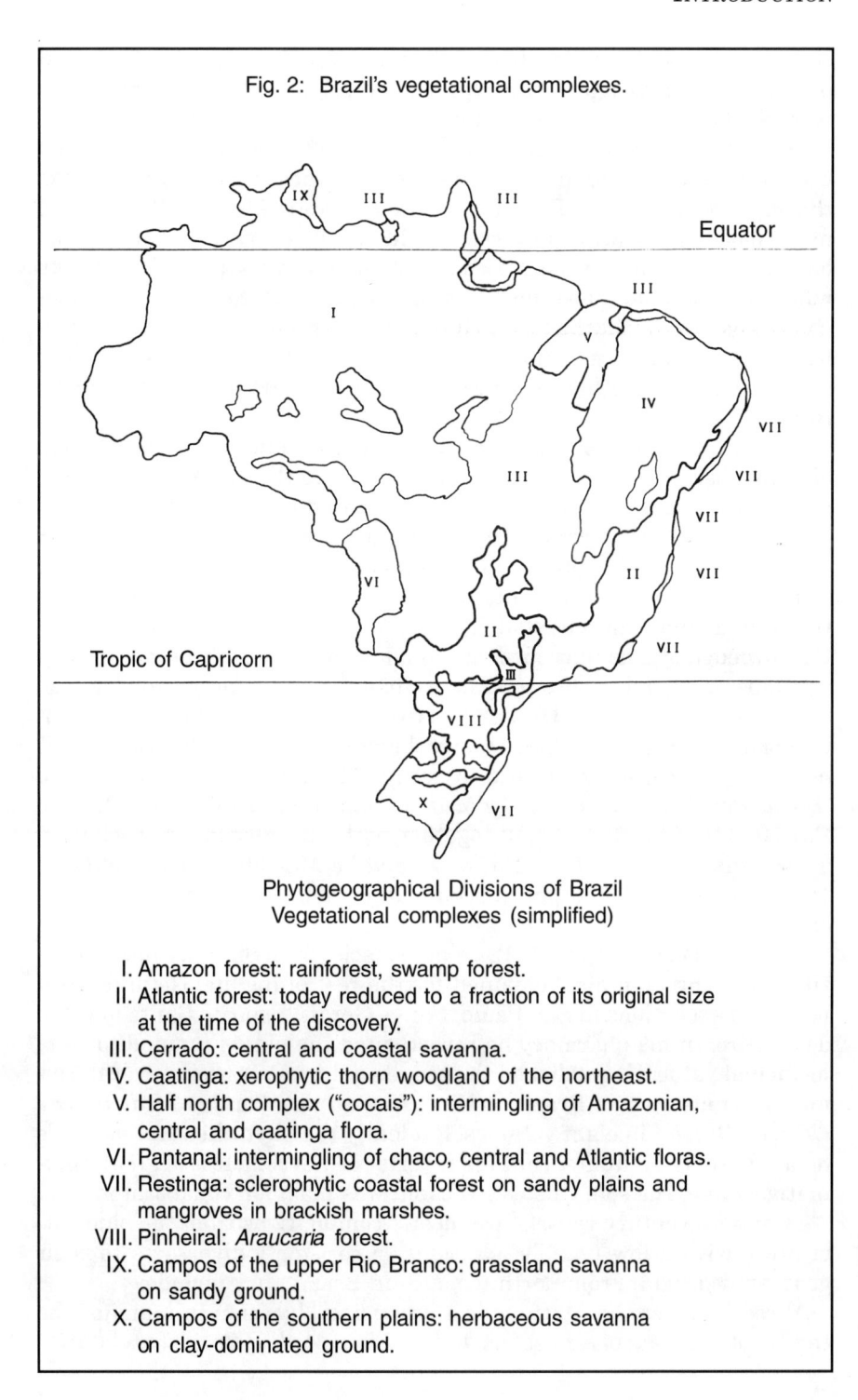

Fig. 2: Brazil's vegetational complexes.

Phytogeographical Divisions of Brazil
Vegetational complexes (simplified)

I. Amazon forest: rainforest, swamp forest.
II. Atlantic forest: today reduced to a fraction of its original size at the time of the discovery.
III. Cerrado: central and coastal savanna.
IV. Caatinga: xerophytic thorn woodland of the northeast.
V. Half north complex ("cocais"): intermingling of Amazonian, central and caatinga flora.
VI. Pantanal: intermingling of chaco, central and Atlantic floras.
VII. Restinga: sclerophytic coastal forest on sandy plains and mangroves in brackish marshes.
VIII. Pinheiral: *Araucaria* forest.
IX. Campos of the upper Rio Branco: grassland savanna on sandy ground.
X. Campos of the southern plains: herbaceous savanna on clay-dominated ground.

INTRODUCTION

centuries, has settled into what can be considered a Brazilian traditional pharmacopoeia. Original observations were later added by several renowned botanists when describing plants in their writings, including:

José Mariano da Conceição Velloso (1742–1811), a Franciscan friar who became best known for his work on the flora of the state of Rio de Janeiro, the "*Flora Fluminensis*"; Francisco Cysneiros Freire Allemão (1797–1874), naturalist at the National Museum of Rio de Janeiro and lecturer in the Faculty of Medicine; and Karl Friedrich Philipp von Martius (1794–1868), who became famous as editor and, in part, author of the "*Flora Brasiliensis*," a work which is fundamental to this day for botanical studies in Brazil. The observations of Martius on medicinal virtues of plants were brought together in "*Systema Materiae Medicae Vegetabilis Brasiliensis*" (1843).

Martius participated in the exploratory voyage undertaken by a group of naturalists who came to Brazil accompanying the Austrian archduchess Leopoldina, who was arriving to be married to the heir of the Portuguese throne, Dom Pedro de Alcântara, later the first Brazilian emperor under the name of Pedro I. Other famous botanists on this expedition were Heinrich Wilhelm Schott, Johann Emmanuel Pohl, Johann Christian Mikan and Giuseppe Raddi.

Knowledge of Brazilian medicinal plants was further systematized by a number of equally able scientists, among them Manuel Freire Allemão de Cysneiros (1834–1863), nephew of the older Freire Allemão and author of many articles published under the title "*Materia Medica Brasileira*" between 1862 and 1864; and Joaquim Monteiro Caminhoá, whose "*Elementos de Botânica Geral e Médica*" appeared in 1877. José Ricardo Pires de Almeida (1843– ?) put together, with the aid of many specialists, a huge dispensatory, "*Formulario Officinal e Magistral*" (four volumes, 1887), containing 6,000 pharmaceutical formulations from the practice of medicine in Brazil.

Theodoro Peckolt (1822–1912), a pharmacist from Silesia, came to Brazil as a young man and remained for the rest of his life. He undertook botanical excursions in São Paulo, Minas Gerais, Espírito Santo and Rio de Janeiro. In his pharmacy he investigated the plants reputed to be of medicinal value. He published the results of his analyses in several German journals and, in Brazil, in his "*História das Plantas Medicinais e Úteis do Brasil*," in eight volumes. Evidently the phytochemical methods he used are now outdated, but his reports are nevertheless of great informative value. His son, Gustavo Peckolt, was his main collaborator.

Twentieth century reports are mostly compilations from the older literature, with a few notable additions, surprisingly diverse as to their geographic origin. From north to south in Brazil, they include:

Alfredo Augusto da Matta was a practicing physician in Manaus, the capital of the state of Amazonas. In his "*Flora Medica Braziliense*" (1913) he included complete herbal formulations, describing their therapeutic applications and dosages.

Paul Le Cointe (1870–1956), French chemist and cartographer, lived most of his life in the state of Pará where, in the capital city of Belém, he organized a museum of Amazonian raw materials and a school for industrial chemists. His *"L'Amazonie Brésilienne"* was published in France in 1922 (two volumes) and a third volume, *"Árvores e Plantas Úteis,"* in Belém, in 1934. In his listing of plants of economic interest with their correct botanical identification, Le Cointe benefitted from the invaluable assistance of Adolpho Ducke (1876–1959), the foremost authority on Amazonian plants of our century.

Francisco Dias da Rocha (1869–1960), from the northeastern state of Ceará, published *"Botânica Médica Cearense"* in 1919, and a second edition in 1945 under the title *"Formulário Terapêutico de Plantas Medicinais Cearenses, Silvestres e Cultivadas."* This work was revised and updated in 1987 by Francisco José de Abreu Matos, again with the help of a knowledgeable botanist, Afrânio Fernandes.

Rodolpho Albino Dias da Silva (1889–1931) excelled in the pharmacognosy of Brazilian *materia medica*. With the inclusion of anatomical and microscopical descriptions of about one hundred plants, he was the sole author of the first *Brazilian Pharmacopoeia,* made official in 1929. Later editions tended to abandon the botanical data; but the first edition was never revoked and continues to be respected as a standard work in the field.

In São Paulo, Frederico Carlos Hoehne (1882–1959), as director of the Botanical Institute, started to update the *"Flora Brasiliensis"* with his *"Flora Brasilica,"* in collaboration with Brazilian botanists. Unfortunately, this work was interrupted after his death. Hoehne's knowledge and interest in medicinal plants is documented in *"Plantas e Substâncias Vegetais Tóxicas e Medicinais,"* published in 1939. The work was reprinted in 1979, but was soon sold out and, in spite of its relatively recent publication, is already a rarity.

The extreme south of the country is represented by Manuel Cypriano d'Avila who, in 1910, published *"Da Flora Medicinal do Rio Grande do Sul."* This was revised and updated by Lilly Charlotte Lutzenberger in 1985. Thus ends a general overview, summarizing the original contributions spanning several centuries.

As may be expected, second-hand compilations abound. Among these, the *Pio Corrêa* stands out as a masterpiece: Manoel Pio Corrêa (1874–1934), *"Dicionário das Plantas Úteis do Brasil e das Exóticas Cultivadas,"* six volumes, 1926–1975. True, it does not deal primarily with medicinal plants; rather, it is a dictionary of Brazilian economic botany. Nonethless, the important medicinals are all included, to the extent that it has become the first reference work to which everybody turns when looking for

Introduction

information on the subject. Credit must be given to Leonam de Azeredo Penna (1903–1979), who completed the work, of which only two volumes had come out in Pio Corrêa's lifetime.

This book obviously relies on the aforementioned publications. But it is not intended, nor was it designed from the beginning, as merely another all-embracing compilation. The plants cited here were chosen with much discernment and the botanical nomenclature was updated with extreme care. References to the chemical and pharmacological literature were added in order to give the reader information about the present state of scientific knowledge. Even this may soon be outdated, due to the dizzying pace at which plants with biodynamic properties are being investigated in our time.

The general area of distribution in Brazil, and often the extra-Brazilian area as well (geographical range, e.g., "Cosmopolitan" or "Eastern Brazil") of each species is indicated first, followed by a brief expression of its specific range within Brazilian political boundaries (e.g., "Rio de Janeiro" or "Minas Gerais") and the phytogeographic affiliation of the plant (e.g., "cerrado" or "caatinga"). For these purposes, two maps are included, one showing the states which make up the Brazilian federation (Fig. 1), the other outlining the characteristic vegetational complexes of the country (Fig. 2).

The authors wish to thank Mrs. Cecilia Rizzini and Ruth B. Toomey for the original botanical line drawings, and Mrs. Anna DiCarlo for the Amerindian illustrations. Thanks are also due to Graziella M. Barroso, Ida de Vattimo Gil, Haroldo C. de Lima, Pedro Carauta, Lúcia d'Avila Freire de Carvalho and Vera Lúcia Gomes Klein for information concerning a number of botanical names. Special thanks go to Dr. Robert A. DeFilipps for his excellent job of editing and for his patience in maintaining a sometimes exhausting correspondence. The authors also wish to express their recognition to the publishers for the careful and accomplished execution of the volume. Finally, thanks are also due to the Brazilian National Research Council, CNPq, for continued support during the course of many years.

W. B. M.
C. T. R.
N. A. P.

GENERAL BIBLIOGRAPHY

Almeida, E.R. de. 1993. *Plantas Medicinais Brasileiras: Conhecimentos Populares e Científicos*. São Paulo: Hemus Editoria Limitada. 341 pp.

✗ d'Avila, M.C. 1910. *Da Flora Medicinal do Rio Grande do Sul*. Porto Alegre. (Revised and updated 1985 by Lilly Charlotte Lutzenberger, Universidade Federal do Rio Grande do Sul).

Braga, R. 1953. *Plantas do Nordeste, Especialmente do Ceará*. Fortaleza: Imprensa Oficial. (Second edition: 1960; third edition: 1976, Mossoró).

Branch, L.C. and I.M.F. Silva. 1983. Folk medicine of "Alter do Chão," Pará, Brasil. *Acta Amazonica* 13: 737-797.

Caminhoá, J.M. 1877. *Elementos de Botanica Geral e Medica*. 6 vols. Rio de Janeiro: Typographia Nacional.

Corrêa, M. Pio. 1909. *Flora do Brazil. Algumas Plantas Úteis, suas Applicações e Distribuição Geographica*. Rio de Janeiro: Directoria Geral de Estatistica.

Corrêa, M. Pio. 1926-1975. *Dicionário das Plantas Úteis do Brasil e das Exóticas Cultivadas*. 6 vols. Ministério da Agricultura. (Completed by Leonam de Azeredo Penna.)

Costa, O. de A. 1963-1965. Bibliografia sobre Plantas Medicinais Brasileiras. *Anais da Faculdade Nacional de Farmácia* (Rio de Janeiro) 8: 175-328; 1966-1968, 9: 137-192, with additions on pp. 180-192.

Costa, O. de A. 1975. Plantas hipoglicemiantes brasileiras. *Leandra* (Rio de Janeiro) 5: 95-106.

Dias da Rocha, F. 1945. *Formulário Terapêutico de Plantas Medicinais Cearenses, Nativas e Cultivadas*. Fortaleza. (Updated revision: Abreu Matos, F.J. de. 1987. O Formulário Fitoterápico do Professor Dias da Rocha. *Coleção Mossoroense*, vol. 365. Mossoró).

Di Stasi, L.C., E.M.G. Santos, C.M. dos Santos, and C.A. Hiruma. 1989. *Plantas Medicinais na Amazonia*. 194 pp. São Paulo: Editora UNESP. (59 species from Municipio de Humaitá).

Elisabetsky, E. and P. Shanley. 1994. Ethnopharmacology in the Brazilian Amazon. *Pharmac. Ther.* 64: 201-214.

Hoehne, F.C. 1920. *O que vendem os Hervanarios da Cidade de São Paulo*. Serviço Sanitario do Estado de São Paulo.

Hoehne, F.C. 1920. *Vegetaes Anthelminticos ou Enumeração dos Vegetaes Empregados na Medicína Popular como Vermifugos*. São Paulo: Weiszflog Irmãos.

Hoehne, F.C. 1939. *Plantas e Substâncias Vegetais Tóxicas e Medicinais*. Departamento de Botânica do Estado de São Paulo. (Second edition, 1979.)

Le Cointe, P. 1934. *A Amazônia Brasileira. III. Árvores e Plantas Úteis*. Belém: Livraria Clássica. (Second edition: 1942, Companhia Editora Nacional, Rio de Janeiro, Coleção Brasiliana.)

GENERAL BIBLIOGRAPHY

Lemos, F. de. 1912. *Flora Medica de Minas Geraes*. 21 pp. VII Congresso Brasileiro de Medicina e Cirurgia, Rio de Janeiro.

Martius, K.F.P. von. 1843. *Systema Materiae Medicae Vegetabilis Brasiliensis*. Leipzig: F. Fleischer.

Martius, K.F.P. von. 1862-1863. *Materia Medica Brasileira*. (Several articles in *Gazeta Medica do Rio de Janeiro*; facsimile edition in Falcão, L.C. 1976. *Brasiliensia Documenta*, vol. 10, Rio de Janeiro.)

Martius, K.F.P. von. 1884. *Natureza, Doenças, Medicina e Remedios dos Indios Brasileiros*. (Republished 1939 by Companhia Editora Nacional, Rio de Janeiro, Série Brasiliana, vol. 154.)

Martius, K.F.P. von, A.W. Eichler and I. Urban. 1840-1906. *Flora Brasiliensis*. 40 vols. Leipzig.

da Matta, A.A. 1913. *Flora Medica Braziliense*. Manaus: Imprensa Official.

Mors, W.B. and C.T. Rizzini. 1966. *Useful Plants of Brazil*. 166 pp. San Francisco, California: Holden Day Inc.

Peckolt, T. and G. Peckolt. 1888-1914. *Historia das Plantas Medicinaes e Uteis do Brazil*. 8 vols. Rio de Janeiro: Typographia Laemmert.

Pereira, N.A. 1982. *A Contribuição de Manuel Freire Alemão de Cysneiros para o Conhecimento de nossos Fitoterápicos*. 88 pp. Thesis, Universidade Federal do Rio de Janeiro.

Pereira, N.A., R.J.S. Jaccoud and W.B. Mors. 1996. Triaga Brasilica: renewed interest in a seventeenth-century panacea. *Toxicon* 34(5): 511-516.

Pires de Almeida, J.R. 1897. *Formulario Officinal e Magistral Internacional*. 4 vols. Rio de Janeiro and São Paulo.

Plotkin, M.J. and M.J. Balick. 1984. Medicinal uses of South American palms. *Journal of Ethnopharmacology* 10: 157-179.

Rizzini, C.T. and W.B. Mors. 1976. *Botânica Econômica Brasileira*. Editora Pedagógica e Universitária and Editora Universidade de São Paulo. Second revised and updated edition, Ambito Cultural Edições Ltda., Rio de Janeiro, 1995.

Silva, M.C. da. 1979. *Inventário de Plantas Medicinais do Estado da Bahia*. 1206 pp. Salvador, Bahia: Subsecretaria de Ciência e Tecnologia, Governo do Estado da Bahia.

Simões, C.M.O., L.A. Mentz, E.P. Schenkel, B.E. Irgang & J.R. Stehmann. 1986. *Plantas da Medicina Popular no Rio Grande do Sul*. 173 pp. Porto Alegre: Editora da Universidade Federal do Rio Grande do Sul.

van den Berg, M.E. 1982. *Plantas Medicinais da Amazônia: Contribuição ao seu Conhecimento Sistemático*. 223 pp. Belém: Conselho Nacional de Desenvolvimento Científico e Tecnológico, Museu Paraense Emilio Goeldi, Programa Trópico Úmido. (Second printing: 1993.)

ACANTHACEAE

Ruellia geminiflora H.B.K.
AREA: Throughout Brazil.
NAME: Ipecacuanha-de-flor-roxa (Marajó).
USE: Root is vomitive.

Ruellia tuberosa L.
AREA: South America, including Venezuela and Colombia.
NAME: Falsa-ipeca.
USES: Root is purgative and emetic, used as a substitute for true ipecac. Leaves are sudorific and febrifuge; mixed with castor oil and given to relieve those skin eruptions in children which are believed to be a consequence of teething.

ADIANTACEAE

Adiantopsis chlorophylla (Sw.) Fée
AREA: Minas Gerais and Rio de Janeiro to Santa Catarina, forest.
NAME: Avenca-da-terra.
USE: Expectorant.

Adiantum concinnum Humb. & Bonp.
AREA: Amazonia, on rocks in forest.
NAME: Culantrilho.
USES: Infusion as a pectoral, depurative and emmenagogue.

Adiantum cuneatum Langsd. & Fisch.
AREA: Rio de Janeiro to Mato Grosso and Rio Grande do Sul.
NAMES: Avenca-de-folha-miúda, avencão, capilário.
USE: Bechic.

Adiantum trapeziforme L.
AREA: Rio de Janeiro to Mato Grosso and Santa Catarina.
NAMES: Avenca-dos-córregos, avencão, avenca-paulista.
USES: Emollient, diaphoretic, pectoral, also against baldness.

AIZOACEAE

Sesuvium portulacastrum L.
AREA: Bahia to Rio Grande do Sul, on the beach sands; cosmopolitan.
NAMES: Beldroega-da-praia, beldroega-miúda, bredo-da-praia.

USES: Leaves are edible, emollient and used against scurvy.
CHEM.: The plant is a rich source of phytoecdysones. Two flavonol glycosides and the respective aglycon have been identified (Ref: AIZO 1,2,3).

Aizoaceae – References

AIZO 1. Banerji, A., G.J. Chintalwar, N.K. Joshi & M.S. Chadha. 1971. Isolation of ecdysterone from Indian plants. *Phytochemistry 10*: 2225-2226.

AIZO 2. Banerji, A. & G.J. Chintalwar. 1971. Phytoecdysones and a new flavonol glycoside from *Sesuvium portulacastrum*. *Indian J. Chem. 9*: 1029-1030.

AIZO 3. Khajuria, R.K., K.A. Suri, O.P. Suri & C.K. Atal. 1982. 3,5,4'- Trihydroxy-6,7-dimethoxyflavone-3-glucoside from *Sesuvium portulacastrum*. *Phytochemistry 21*: 1179-1180.

ALISMATACEAE

Alisma palaefolium Kunth
AREA: Bahia, in swamps.
NAMES: Erva-do-pântano, erva-do-brejo.
USES: Juice is said to be active against snake bites.

Echinodorus grandiflorus (Cham. & Schl.) Mich.
AREA: Ceará to Rio Grande do Sul and Mato Grosso, in marshes.
NAMES: Aguapé, chá-da-campanha, congonha-do-brejo, erva-do-brejo, erva-do-pântano.
USES: Rhizome in poultices for hernia. Above-ground parts are used as a depurative, tonic, diuretic and cure for syphilis, skin diseases and liver ailments; said to arrest the progress of arteriosclerosis.

Echinodorus macrophyllus (Kunth) Mich.
AREA: Minas Gerais to Rio Grande do Sul, in swampy terrain.
NAMES: Chá-da-campanha, chapéu-de-couro, erva-do-brejo, erva-do-pântano.
USES: Rhizome prescribed against hydrophobia. Aerial parts are astringent, used as a tea-laxative and for arthritis, rheumatism, syphilis, dermatoses and liver ailments; in gargles for sore throat; in baths for chronic ulcers.

Echinodorus pubescens Mart.
AREA: Bahia to São Paulo.
NAME: Chá-mineiro.
USES: Same as *E. grandiflorus*.

AMARANTHACEAE

Achyranthes ficoidea Lam.
AREA: Guianas to Rio de Janeiro; on sandy beaches near the sea.
NAME: Corrente.
USE: Leaf infusion is employed as a diuretic.

Achyranthes indica L.
AREA: Amazonia.
NAME: Carrapicho.
USES: In baths, recommended for excessive menstrual flow.

Alternanthera achyrantha R. Br.
AREA: Rio de Janeiro to Rio Grande do Sul; cosmopolitan.
NAMES: Erva-de-pinto, periquito.
USES: Leaf infusion is diuretic, digestive, depurative, good for liver and bladder ailments, syphilis and certain dermatoses.

Alternanthera brasiliana (L.) O. Ktze.
AREA: Throughout Brazil, mainly in the littoral.
NAMES: Caaponga, ervanço, infalível, perpétua-da-mata, perpétua-do-brasil.
USE: Flowers used as a bechic.

Amaranthus blitum L.
AREA: Common in Brazil; cosmopolitan.
NAMES: Bredo, bredo-macho, bredo-malabar, bredo-rabaça, caruru-de-porco, caruru-miúdo, caruru-verdadeiro.
USE: Galactagogue.

Amaranthus spinosus L.
AREA: Common in Brazil; cosmopolitan.
NAMES: Bredo-de-espinho, bredo-branco, bredo-vermelho, bredo-de-santo-antonio, caruru, caruru-de-espinho, crista-de-galo.
USES: Leaves and roots are emollient, antiblennorrhagic. Leaves diuretic, laxative, used against hydropsy and bladder catarrh, also against snake-bite.
CHEM.: Leaves contain spinasterol and a saponin derived from oleanolic acid (Ref: AMAR 1).

Amaranthus viridis L.
AREA: Common in Brazil; cosmopolitan.
NAMES: Bredo, caruru, caruru-bravo, caruru-de-soldado, caruru-miúdo, caruru-verde.
USES: Leaves are mucilaginous, emollient, diuretic, resolvent, indicated

in cases of dropsy and bladder catarrh; also in gonorrhoea and to aid lactation.

Chamissoa altissima H.B.K.
AREA: Widely dispersed in Brazil.
NAME: Fumo-bravo.
USE: Root used as a diuretic.

Chamissoa macrocarpa H.B.K.
AREA: Pará to Rio de Janeiro.
NAMES: Fumo-bravo, fumo-bravo-do-ceará.
USES: Roots are diuretic, useful for dissolving kidney stones and to ease bladder catarrh; infusion of the fresh leaves used in enemas to mitigate malarial fever.

Gomphrena leucocephala Mart.
AREA: Maranhão to Alagoas.
NAMES: Corango, corongo, paratudo.
USES: Antipoison, antithermic, antidiarrhoeic, antidyspeptic.

Gomphrena macrocephala St.-Hil.
AREA: Minas Gerais and São Paulo; campos.
NAME: Paratudo-do-campo.
USES: Rootstock indicated as a panacea without specification. Flower-heads for dysmenorrhoea.

Gomphrena mollis Mart.
AREA: Alagoas to Paraná.
NAMES: Erva-mole, erva-mole-falsa.
USES: Roots are tonic and carminative.

Gomphrena officinalis Mart.
AREA: Goiás and Minas Gerais to São Paulo and Mato Grosso; cerrados.
NAMES: Panacéia, paratudo, perpétua-do-mato, paratudinho, raiz-do-padre, salerma.
USES: Rootstock for a bitter tonic, aromatic, excitant, febrifuge, panacea.

Iresine polymorpha Mart.
AREA: Ceará to Minas Gerais, ruderal.
NAME: Bredinho.
USES: Leaves are emollient, diuretic.

Pfaffia glomerata (Spreng.) Peders.
AREA: Amazonia.
NAME: Corrente.
USES: Leaves macerated in copaiva balsam (*Copaifera*) or andiroba oil

(*Carapa*) are locally applied to treat hemorrhoids and diarrhoea; also in the form of an enema. The juice has the same uses.

Pfaffia jubata Mart.
AREA: Campos of central and southern Brazil.
NAMES: Marcela, marcela-do-campo, marcela-do-cerrado.
USES: Stomach disorders; antipyretic, tonic, antiophidic.

Pfaffia paniculata (Mart.) Kuntze
AREA: Goiás, São Paulo, Paraná.
NAMES: Carango, paratudo.
USES: Roots for an antidiabetic, tonic, aphrodisiac; considered a substitute for the Asiatic and American ginseng, *Panax ginseng* C.A. Meyer and *Panax quinquefolius* L., respectively (Araliaceae). Thus, they are reputed to increase organic defenses against disease and prevent precocious aging.
CHEM. & PHARM.: The roots contain a mixture of stigmasterol and sitosterol and their glycosides, as well as allantoin, pfaffic acid and three nortriterpene glucuronosides named pfaffosides. Growth inhibition of cultured tumor cells by these compounds has been investigated (Ref: AMAR 2,3,4).

The roots of *Pfaffia iresinoides* Spreng., a species encountered in the same geographical area, have been introduced into commerce under the name of "Brazilian ginseng." They were shown to produce a high concentration of triterpenoid saponins as well as ecdysteroids (a type of insect moulting hormone) (Ref: AMAR 5,6).

Philoxerus portulacoides St.-Hil.
AREA: Sandy beaches from Ceará to Rio Grande do Sul.
NAMES: Bredo-da-praia, capetiraguá, pirixi.
USES: Leaf infusion for treating leucorrhoea.

Amaranthaceae – References
AMAR 1. Banerji, N. 1979. Chemical constituents of *Amaranthus spinosus. Indian J. Chem. 17 (b)*: 180-181.
AMAR 2. Oliveira, F., G. Akisue & M. Akisue. 1980. Contribuição para o estudo farmacognóstico do "ginseng brasileiro," *Pfaffia paniculata* (Mart.) Kuntze. *An. Farm. Quím. S. Paulo 20*: 261-277.
AMAR 3. Takemoto, T., N. Nishimoto, S. Nakai, N. Takagi, S. Hayashi, S. Odashima & Y. Wada. 1983. Pfaffic acid, a novel nortriterpene from *Pfaffia paniculata* Kuntze. *Tetrahedron Lett. 24*: 1057-1060.
AMAR 4. Nishimoto, N., S. Nakai, N. Takagi, S. Hayashi, T. Takemoto, S. Odashima, H. Kizu & Y. Wada. 1984. Pfaffosides and nortriterpenoid saponins from *Pfaffia paniculata. Phytochemistry 23*: 139-142.
AMAR 5. Nishimoto, N., Y. Shiobara, M. Fujino, S. Inoue, T. Takemoto, F. Oliveira, G. Akisue, M.K. Akisue, G. Hashimoto, O. Tanaka, R. Kasai & R. Matsuura. 1987. Ecdysteroids from *Pfaffia iresinoides* and reassignment of some ^{13}C NMR chemical shifts. *Phytochemistry 26*: 2505-2507.

AMAR 6. Nishimoto, N., Y. Shiobara, S. Inoue, M. Fujino, T. Takemoto, C.L. Yeoh, F. de Oliveira, G. Akisue, M.K. Akisue & G. Hashimoto. 1988. Three ecdysteroid glycosides from *Pfaffia iresinoides*. *Phytochemistry* 27: 1665-1668.

AMARYLLIDACEAE

Bomarea salsilloides Roem.
AREA: Pará to Rio de Janeiro.
NAMES: Cará-de-caboclo, jaraugaúba.
USES: Root considered diuretic and diaphoretic.

Bomarea spectabilis Schrenk
AREA: Mainly Rio de Janeiro and Mato Grosso.
NAME: Cará-do-mato.
USES: Bulb as a diuretic; also for bladder catarrh.

Crinum scabrum Sims
AREA: Brazilian littoral and surroundings.
NAMES: Cebola-brava, lírio rajado.
USES: Bulb is strongly diuretic; for dropsy.
CHEM.: Contains the alkaloid lycorine (Ref: AMARY 1).

Griffinia hyacinthina Ker.-Gawl.
AREA: Rio de Janeiro.
NAMES: Cebola-brava, cebola-do-mato.
USES: Bulb is purgative, diuretic; bruised bulbs are mixed with cassava flour in poultices and placed on boils.

Hippeastrum psittacinum Herb.
AREA: Minas Gerais to Rio Grande do Sul.
NAME: Açucena-do-campo.
USES: Juice of roots is said to be excitant and laxative.

Hippeastrum puniceum (Lam.) Kuntze
AREA: Amazonia.
NAMES: Açucena, cebola berrante.
USES: Juice of bulb is excitant, purgative, emetic.

Hippeastrum vittatum (L'Hérit.) Herb.
AREA: Central and southern Brazil.
NAMES: Açucena-do-jardim, cebola-barrão, cebola-cecem, cebola-do-mato.
USES: Bulb for an emetic, cathartic, antiasthmatic and for other pectoral problems.
CHEM.: Contains the phenanthridine alkaloid hippagine or pancracine (Ref: AMARY 2).

Hymenocallis tubiflora Salisb.
AREA: Guianas and Pará, in flooded areas.
NAMES: Açucena-d'água, cebola-branca, cebola-brava, cila, cila-da-terra.
USES: Bulbs are sour, used for an excitant, emetic, expectorant, diuretic; useful against bronchitis and hydropsy. Leaves, both fresh or bruised, are bound to boils.

For non-alkaloidal components in the family Amaryllidaceae, see Ref: AMARY 3.

Amaryllidaceae – References

AMARY 1. Reichert, B. 1938. Das Vorkommen des Alkaloids Lycorin in *Crinum scabrum*. Arch. Pharm. 276: 328-329.

AMARY 2. Ali, A.A., M.K. Mesbah & A.W. Frahm. 1984. Phytochemical investigation of *Hippeastrum vittatum*. Part IV: Stereochemistry of pancracine, the first 5,11-methanomorphanthridine alkaloid from *Hippeastrum* — structure of "hippagine." *Planta Medica 50*: 188-189.

AMARY 3. Piozzi, F., M.L. Marino, C. Fuganti & A. DiMartino. 1969. Occurrence of nonbasic metabolites in Amaryllidaceae. *Phytochemistry 8*: 1745-1748.

ANACARDIACEAE

Anacardium humile St.-Hil.
AREA: Throughout the cerrado of central Brazil.
NAMES: Cajueiro-do-campo, cajueiro-anão, cajuí.
USES: Oil from pericarp is vesicant, used for dermal afflictions; juice of pseudofruit is antisyphilitic.

Anacardium nanum St.-Hil.
AREA, NAMES, USES: Same as for *Anacardium humile* St.-Hil.

Anacardium occidentale L.
AREA: The entire Brazilian littoral; native to certain coastal forests (matas de restinga); extensively cultivated.
NAME: Cajueiro.
USES: Roots are purgative. Bark is astringent, a tonic stimulant, antidiabetic; gargle for sore throat and aphthae. Gum exuding from trunk is depurative and expectorant. Leaf-juice recommended against scurvy, aphthae, intestinal colics. Flowers for a tonic and aphrodisiac. Nuts used for impotence and debility from chronic diseases; oil of the shell is highly vesicant (therefore to be used with extreme care), and applied to inflammatory disorders, dermatoses, including leprosy, as well as to expel worms; active against ulcers, corns, warts; juice of the pseudofruit ("cashew apple") is said to be excitant, diaphoretic, diuretic, depurative, antisyphilitic, antidyspeptic and anticatarrhal.

ANACARDIACEAE

Anacardium occidentale

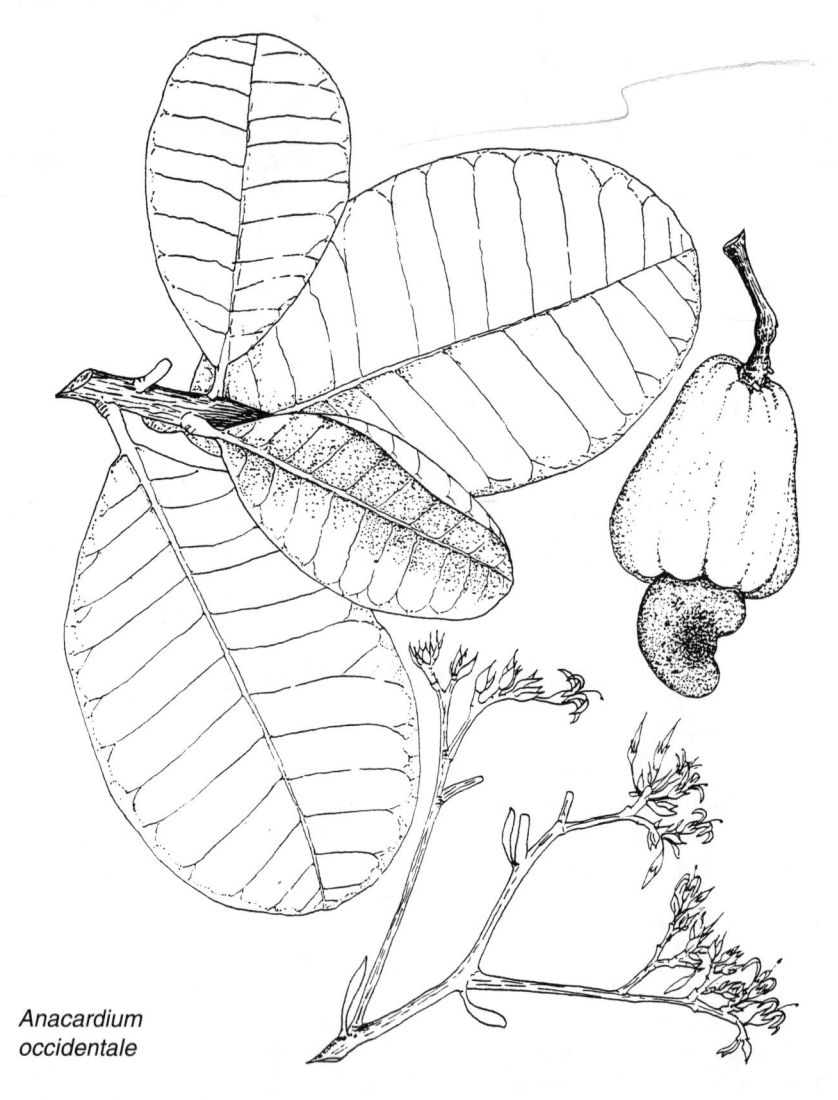

CHEM. & PHARM.: Pseudofruit is rich in vitamin C. Volatile flavor components have been identified (Ref: ANAC 1). Oil of the shells commercially known as "cashew nut shell liquid," used in the manufacture of varnishes; main phenolic components are anacardic acid and cardol, with antibacterial, anthelmintic and molluscicidal properties (Ref: ANAC 2,3,4,5,6,7). Flavonoids and their glycosides identified in leaves (Ref: ANAC 8,9). Hypoglycemic action of inner bark has been confirmed (Ref: ANAC 10,11). Tannins from bark show anti-inflammatory activity (Ref: ANAC 12). The essential oil of the leaves acts as a depressant on the central nervous system (Ref: ANAC 13). It is made up almost exclusively of alpha-pinene (Ref: ANAC 14).

ANACARDIACEAE

Astronium fraxinifolium Schott
AREA: Pará to Paraná and Mato Grosso, in dry forests and cerrados.
NAMES: Generally known as gonçalo-alves; other names, local and less important, are: aroeira, aroeira-do-campo, aroeira-preta, aroeira-vermelha, aratanha, batão, chibatã, cubatã-vermelho, gomável, guarabu, jujuíra, ubatã.
USES: Bark is astringent, pectoral, recommended for pulmonary tuberculosis including cases with hemoptyses. The small nuts yield a caustic oil, prescribed to remove corns and alleviate toothache.

Lithraea molleoides (Vell.) Engl.
AREA: Minas Gerais to Rio Grande do Sul.
NAMES: Aroeira-branca, aroeira-brava, aroeirinha.
USES: Bark is employed as an astringent, tonic, vulnerary, emmenagogue, diuretic, antileucorrhoeic, antidysenteric; useful against inflammations, tumors; resin to treat rheumatism and bubos; internally, purgative, bechic, for blennorrhagia and orchitis. Leaflets are considered a remedy for gonorrhoea, muscle spasms, hemorrhages, ophthalmia.

Myracroduon urundeuva Fr. All.
AREA: From Ceará to Paraguay, in dry forests, cerrados and caatingas.
NAMES: Aroeira, aroeira-do-sertão, aroeira-preta, urundeúva.
USES: Bark and resin are balsamic, hemostatic, used for pulmonary complaints, kidney troubles, hemoptyses, metrorrhagia, for post-natal vaginal washes, for stomach ulceer and colitis; resin is tonic. An excellent pharmacognostic monograph has been published (Ref: ANAC 15).
PHARM.: Both aqueous and alcoholic extracts of the bark strongly inhibit gastric ulceration induced in rats (Ref: ANAC 16).

Schinopsis brasiliensis Engl.
AREA: Northeastern Brazil, caatinga.
NAMES: Baraúna, braúna.
USE: Tea from sprouts helps to arrest hysteria.

Schinus lentiscifolius March.
AREA: Rio Grande do Sul.
NAMES: Aroeira-do-campo, caroba.
USES: Leaves for a depurative, antirheumatic.

Schinus molle L.
AREA: São Paulo to Rio Grande do Sul.
NAMES: Aroeira, aroeira-folha-de-salsa, aroeirinha, aroeira-mansa.
USES: Actions are the same as those of *Lithraea molleoides*; in addition, the bark, when heated, oozes out a kind of resin which is applied to adenitis; internally it is purgative; an infusion of the leaves is stimulant, sudorific, antirheumatic.

ANACARDIACEAE

CHEM.: Several mono- and sesquiterpenes have been identified in the essential oil of this plant (Ref: ANAC 17,24). The fruits contain triterpenoid acids (Ref: ANAC 18).

PHARM.: It is a general belief that both *Schinus molle* and *Lithraea molleoides* expel into the air a volatile irritant which causes a skin rash similar to urticaria, affecting persons who remain for some time under or close to these trees. It has been verified that their gum-resin in fact gives rise to contact dermatitis (Ref: ANAC 19).

Schinus terebinthifolius Raddi

AREA: Sands of the littoral, from Bahia to Rio de Janeiro.

NAMES: Aroeira-mansa, aroeira-vermelha, cambuí, fruta-de-sabiá.

USES: Gum-resin externally applied for cornea diseases, tumors, leprosy; bark is depurative, antifebrile, antineuralgic, used for hemoptyses and afflictions of the uterus.

CHEM.: Triterpenoid acids are present in the leaf, fruit and bark (Ref: ANAC 20,21,22). Pentagalloylglucose in crude drug (Ref: ANAC 23). Essential oil is predominantly gamma-terpinene (Ref: ANAC 14).

Spondias macrocarpa Engl.

AREA: Amazonia.

NAME: Taperebá-açu.

USES: Same as for *S. mombin* L.

Spondias mombin L.

AREA: Amazonia to Minas Gerais and Mato Grosso, forest and pantanal; much cultivated.

NAMES: Cajá-mirim, cajazeira, taperibá, cajá, taperebá, acaíba.

USES: Bark for an emetic, antidiarrhoeic, good for gonorrhoea and piles. Leaves useful for constipation, gastralgia, ophthalmia, laryngitis. Decoction of the bark and shoots reduces swelling of feet caused by erysipelas; bark is antispasmodic, emetic, astringent, tonic. Flower decoction is recommended for ophthalmia and laryngitis; also cardioactive and for children's diarrhoea; maceration is stomachic. Fruit pulp used for cystitis and urethritis; pit of fruit in a decoction for leucorrhoea.

CHEM. & PHARM.: Two ellagitannins from leaves and stems active against Coxsackie and Herpes simplex virus have been described (Ref: ANAC 25).

Anacardiaceae – References

ANAC 1. MacLeod, A.J. & N.G. Troconis. 1982. Volatile flavor components of cashew "apple" (*Anacardium occidentale*). *Phytochemistry* 21: 1517-1530.

ANAC 2. Eichbaum, F.W., H. Hauptmann & H. Rothschild. 1945. Preparação e ação biológica do ácido anacárdico e de alguns derivados. *An. Assoc. Quím. Brasil* 4: 83-94.

ANAC 3. Eichbaum, F.W. 1946. Biological properties of anacardic acid (0-pentadecadienyl-salicylic acid) and related compounds. *Mem. Inst. Butantan* 19: 69-134.

ANACARDIACEAE

ANAC 4. Leão, A.T. & F.W. Eichbaum. 1947. Ação vermicida do óleo de caju (*Anacardium occidentale*) e derivados. Experiências em cães. *Mem. Inst. Butantan* 20: 13-30.

ANAC 5. Eichbaum, F.W., D. Koch-Weser & A.T. Leão. 1950. Activity of cashew nutshell oil in human ancylostomiasis. *Am. J. Digestive Diseases* 17: 370-371.

ANAC 6. Pereira, J.P. & C.P. de Souza. 1974. Preliminary studies of *Anacardium occidentale* as a molluscicide. *Ciência e Cultura* 26: 1054-1057.

ANAC 7. Sullivan, J.T., C.S. Richards, H.A. Lloyd & G. Krishna. 1982. Anacardic acid: molluscicide in cashew nut shell liquid. *Planta Medica* 44: 175-177.

ANAC 8. Rahman, W., K. Ishratullah, H. Wagner, O. Seligman, V.M. Chari & B.G. Osterdahl. 1987. Prunin-6"-0-coumarate, a new acylated flavanone glycoside from *Anacardium occidentale*. *Phytochemistry* 17: 1064-1065.

ANAC 9. Subramanian, S.S., K.J. Joseph & A.G.R. Nair. 1969. Polyphenols of *Anacardium occidentale*. *Phytochemistry* 8: 673.

ANAC 10. Aguiar, F.J.C. & L.J.C. Lins. 1958. Hypoglycemic action of inner bark (bast) of cashew tree (*Anacardium occidentale*). II. Comparative studies on adrenalectomized rats. *An. Fac. Med. Univ. Recife* 18: 263-268.

ANAC 11. Teodósio, N.R. 1960. Contribuição experimental ao estudo fisiológico da hipoglicemia (atuação do fator hipoglicemiante do *Anacardium occidentale* L.). University of Recife. 146 pp.

ANAC 12. Mota, M.L.R., G. Thomas & J.M. Barbosa Filho. 1985. Anti-inflammatory actions of tannins isolated from the bark of *Anacardium occidentale* L. *J. Ethnopharmacol.* 13: 289-300.

ANAC 13. Garg, S.C. & H.L. Kasera. 1984. Neuropharmacological studies of the essential oil of *Anacardium occidentale*. *Fitoterapia* 55: 131-136.

ANAC 14. Craveiro, A.A., A.G. Fernandes, C.H.S. Andrade, F.J.A. Matos, J.W. Alencar & M.I.L. Machado. 1981. *Oleos Essenciais de Plantas do Nordeste*. Federal University of Ceará. 209 pp.

ANAC 15. Viana, G.S.B., F.J. Abreu-Matos, M.A.M. Bandeira &V.S.N. Rao. Aroeira-do-sertão (*Myracroduon urundeuva* Fr. All.) estudo botânico, farmacognóstico químico e farmacológico. Monograph published by the Federal University of Ceará, Fortaleza.

ANAC 16. Rao, V.S., G.S.B. Viana, A.M.S. Menezes & M.G.T. Gadelha. 1987. Studies on the antiulcerogenic activity of *Astronium urundeuva* Engl. aqueous extract. *Braz. J. Med. Biol. Res.* 20: 803-805.

ANAC 17. Terhune, S.J., J.W. Hogg & B.M. Lawrence. 1974. β-Spathulene: a new sesquiterpene in *Schinus molle* oil. *Phytochemistry* 13: 865-866.

ANAC 18. Pozzo-Balbi, T., L. Nobile, G. Scapini & M. Cini. 1978. The triterpenoid acids of *Schinus molle*. *Phytochemistry* 13: 2107-2110.

ANAC 19. Lloyd, H.A., T.M. Jaouni, S.L. Evans & J.F. Morton. 1977. Terpenes of *Schinus terebinthifolius*. *Phytochemistry* 16: 1301-1302.

ANAC 20. Kaistha, K.K. & L.B. Kier. 1962. Structural studies on terebinthone from *Schinus terebinthifolius*. *J. Pharm. Sci.* 51: 245-248, 1136-1139.

ANAC 21. Campello, J.P. & A.J. Marsaioli. 1974. Triterpenes of *Schinus terebinthifolius*. *Phytochemistry* 13: 659-660.

ANAC 22. Campello, J.P. & A.J. Marsaioli. 1975. Terebinthifolic acid and bauerenone: new triterpenoid ketones from *Schinus terebinthifolius*. *Phytochemistry* 14: 2300-2302.

ANAC 23. Hayashi, T., K. Nagayama, M. Arisawa, M. Shimizu, S. Suzuki, M. Yoshizaki, N. Morita, E. Ferro, I. Basualdo & L.H. Berganza. 1989. Pentagalloylglucose, a xanthine oxidase inhibitor from a Paraguayan crude drug, 'Mell-i' (*Schinus terebinthifolius*). *J. Nat. Prod.* 52: 210-211.

ANAC 24. Bernard, R.A. and R. Wrolstad. 1963. The essential oil of *Schinus molle*; the terpene hydrocarbon fraction. *J. Food Sci.* 28: 59-63.

ANAC 25. Corthout, J., Peiters, L.A., Claeys, M., Van den Berghe, D.A. & A.J. Vlietinck. 1991. Antiviral ellagitannins from *Spondias mombin*. *Phytochemistry* 30: 1129-1130.

ANNONACEAE

Annona ambotay Aubl.
AREA: Amazonia.
NAME: Envirataia.
USES: Fumes of burning wood are employed against stings. Decoction of leaves and bark applied externally to fortify women after labor.
CHEM.: Azanthracene alkaloid identified in wood (Ref: ANNO 1).

Annona coriacea Mart.
AREA: Ceará to São Paulo and Mato Grosso, in the cerrados and, to a lesser extent, in the campos.
NAMES: Araticum-do-campo, araticum-do-tabuleiro, cabeça-de-negro, marolo, marolinho.
USE: Seeds employed for dysentery.
CHEM.: Diterpenes isolated from underground organs (Ref: ANNO 2,3,4,5,6).

Annona cornifolia St.-Hil.
AREA: Bahia to São Paulo and Mato Grosso.
NAMES: Araticum-das-catingas, araticum-do-campo, araticum-do-pará, araticum-mirim, enfira-bobó, envireira.
USE: Fruit-flesh is applied to sloughing ulcers.

Annona crassifolia Mart.
AREA: Same as *A. coriacea*: cerrado.
NAMES: Araticum, araticum-do-cerrado, araticum-panã, cabeça-de-negro, marolo.
USES: Flesh of the berries is said to be laxative (if at all, certainly in very large doses!). Seeds used against snakebite.
CHEM.: Several alkaloids have been identified from the leaves, with analgesic, spasmolytic and limited antibacterial activity (Ref: ANNO 7).

Annona dioica St.-Hil.
AREA: São Paulo to Paraná; forest.
NAMES: Araticum-do-campo, araticum-grande.
USES: Leaves externally applied as antirheumatic. Fruit is resolvent.

Annona foetida Mart.
AREA: Bahia, forest.
NAME: Araticum-da-caatinga.
USES: Bark and leaves used externally for an antirheumatic; decoction for malaria. Fruit to clean ulcers.

Annona glabra L.
AREA: Amazonia to Santa Catarina, in swampy sites.
NAMES: Araticum, araticum-bravo, araticum-cortiça, araticum-da-água, araticum-do-brejo, araticum-do-mangue, corticeira.
USES: Leaves are anthelmintic and antirheumatic.

Annona marcgravii Mart.
AREA: Ceará to Minas Gerais.
NAMES: Araticum, araticum-cagão, araticum-de-paca, araticum-pana, araticum-ponhé.
USES: Unripe berries are prescribed for aphthae; mature fruits for reducing inflammation.

Annona muricata L.
AREA: Widely cultivated all over Brazil.
NAMES: Araticum-de-comer, araticum-do-grande, ata, graviola, pinha.
USES: Young shoots, leaves and flowers for cough and other chest problems. Contused leaves are strongly aromatic, indicated in cases of spasms and diarrhoea; same in decoction. Seeds are astringent, emetic. Root bark is calmative, antispasmodic, antidiabetic.
CHEM.: Free L(-)proline and GABA (gamma-aminobutyric acid) in fruit pulp (Ref: ANNO 8). Alkaloids in leaves and stem (Ref: ANNO 9).

Annona reticulata L.
AREA: Widely cultivated all over Brazil.
NAMES: Araticum, ata, condessa, fruta-de-condessa, miloló, pinha.
USES: Unripe fruits are astringent, antidysenteric. Seeds for a febrifuge, antidiarrhoeic. Leaves as a resolvent for abscesses; reported to be narcotic.
CHEM.: An unusual bistetrahydrofuran compound has been described from the bark (Ref: ANNO 10).

Annona spinescens Mart.
AREA: Bahia, in marshy places.
NAMES: Araticum-de-espinho, araticum-do-brejo, araticum-do-rio.
USES: Bark and leaves are antirheumatic. Fruit-pulp for abscesses and ulcers. Ground seeds used to heal pityriasis of children.

Annona squamosa L.
AREA: Widely cultivated throughout Brazil.
NAMES: Ata, fruta-de-conde, pinha.
USES: Leaves are sudorific, carminative, stomachic, antirheumatic, antidyspeptic; bruised and placed upon the head, they induce sleep in cases of insomnia and alleviate migraine; applied to wounds and ulcers, they repel worms and insects. Unripe berries are astringent and

laxative; they, as well as the seeds, are insecticidal.

CHEM. & PHARM.: Free amino acids were identified in the fruit pulp, among them, most abundant, L(+)citrulline, L(+)arginine, L(+)ornithine and GABA (gamma-aminobutyric acid) (Ref: ANNO 8). Aporphine alkaloids in bark (Ref. ANNO 11). Post-coital antifertility activity of seeds has been studied (Ref: ANNO 12). A cytotoxic bis-tetrahydrofuran derivative is present (Ref: ANNO 13). The essential oil from the bark contains aromadendrene as the predominant constituent (Ref: ANNO 26). A complete analysis of the leaf and fruit oils exists (Ref: 27).

Bocagea alba St.-Hil.
AREA: Rio de Janeiro.
NAME: Araticum.
USE: Seed infusion employed as a vermifuge.

Bocagea viridis St.-Hil.
AREA: Minas Gerais and Rio de Janeiro, forest.
NAME: Araticum.
USE: Same as for *B. alba*.

Duguetia furfuracea (St.-Hil.) Benth. & Hook.
AREA: Cerrados of central Brazil.
NAMES: Araticum-do-campo, araticum-grande.
USES: Ground seeds suspended in water are active against head lice.

Duguetia riparia Hub.
AREA: Amazonia.
NAMES: Envirataí, embirataia, invirataí.
USES: Roots useful for expelling worms; in baths for rheumatism. Bark antirheumatic.
CHEM.: Three aporphine alkaloids have been isolated from an unidentified Brazilian *Duguetia* species (Ref: ANNO 14).

Guatteria nigrescens Mart.
AREA: Rio de Janeiro and São Paulo.
NAME: Pindaíba-preta.
USES: Excitant, aromatic.

Guatteria ouregon (Aubl.) Dun.
AREA: Amazonia, forest.
NAMES: Ouregon, envira.
USES: Leaves and fruits are excitant for the nervous system. Seed infusion for dyspepsia, gastralgia, colics of uterus and bowels.
CHEM.: Fourteen isoquinoline alkaloids have been identified in leaves and bark (Ref: ANNO 15).

ANNONACEAE

Guatteria scandens Ducke
AREA: Pará, forest.
NAME: Cipó-ira.
USE: Stems are aromatic.
CHEM.: Aporphine-type alkaloids are present in leaves and bark (Ref: ANNO 16).

Rollinia exalbida (Vell.) Mart.
AREA: Rio de Janeiro to Rio Grande do Sul, forest.
NAMES: Araticum-alvadio, embira, fruta-de-conde pequena.
USES: From the astringent bark oozes a gum which is used as an antidiarrhoeic. Fruits are purgative if swallowed in large amounts.
CHEM.: The composition of the epicuticular wax of the leaves has been investigated (Ref: ANNO 17). Leaves contain a furofuran lignan (Ref: ANNO 18).

Rollinia orthopetala DC.
AREA: Amazonia, much cultivated.
NAME: Biribá.
USES: Bark is employed against enterocolitis. Fruits are analeptic, antiscorbutic. Seeds are dried and ground for intestinal infections.

Rollinia salicifolia Schl.
AREA: Rio de Janeiro to Rio Grande do Sul, forest.
NAMES: Araticum-folha-de-salgueiro, araticum-de-santa-catarina, embira-vermelha.
USES: Bark for an astringent, tonic.

Rollinia sylvatica (St.-Hil.) Mart.
AREA: Pernambuco to Mato Grosso and Rio Grande do Sul, forest.
NAMES: Araticum-da-mata, araticum-do-mato, araticum-do-morro, araticu-grande.
USES: Leaves used as a bechic, febrifuge, antispasmodic, antidysenteric; also for aphthae and sore throat.

Xylopia aromatica (Lam.) Mart.
AREA: Throughout Brazil, cerrado.
NAMES: Embira, envira, envireira, esfola-bainha, jejerecu, pachinhos, pacovi, pimenta-de-árvore, pimenta-de-bugre, pimenta-de-folha-grande, pimenta-de-gentio, pimenta-de-macaco, pimenta-de-negro, pimenta-do-campo, pimenta-do-sertão, pimenta-dos-negros, pimenta-da-costa.
USES: Seeds are aromatic, reminiscent of black pepper (*Piper nigrum*), used as condiment, carminative, eupeptic, aphrodisiac.
CHEM.: The essential oil of the fruits contains alpha- and beta-pinene,

myrcene, limonene, ocimene, citronellol and carvone (Ref: ANNO 19). Non-volatile constituents include diterpenes (Ref: ANNO 20).

Xylopia benthamiana Fries
AREA: Amazonia.
NAMES: Embiriba, embiriba-pacovi, envira-amarela.
USES: Fruits used as a tea, for gastralgia.

Xylopia frutescens Aubl.
AREA: Amazonia, forest.
NAMES: Coagerucu, jererecu, envira, pindaíba, pimenta-de-macaco, pimenta-do-mato, pimenta-do-sertão, pacovi, pimenta-de-gentio.
USES: Bark is aromatic. Seeds are aromatic, carminative, eupeptic, bladder stimulant, antirheumatic, prescribed for consumption, weakness accompanied by lumbar aches; said to be active against snake bites; to treat caries, catarrhal afflictions of the mucous membranes and urinary tract; seeds also useful for leucorrhoea and stomach colics; besides, considered aphrodisiac and tonic in some localities.
CHEM.: Rich in alkaloids (Ref: ANNO 21,22).

Xylopia sericea St.-Hil.
AREA: Amazonia, Goiás to São Paulo, forest.
NAMES: Pindaíba-vermelha.
USES: Seeds are aromatic, carminative, somewhat similar to black pepper; capsules employed to treat piles; supposed to have vasoconstricting properties.
CHEM.: Several diterpenes have been detected in the fruit (Ref: ANNO 23,24).

For a general account of the chemistry of Annonaceae, including the occurrence of diterpenes, flavonoids and alkaloids, see Ref: ANNO 25.

Annonaceae – References
ANNO 1. Oliveira, A.B., G.G. de Oliveira, F. Carazza & J.G.S. Maia. 1987. Geovanine, a new azanthracene alkaloid from *Annona ambotay* Aubl. *Phytochemistry 26*: 2650-2651.
ANNO 2. Ferrari, M., F. Pelizzoni & G. Ferrari. 1971. New terpenoids with clerodane skeleton. *Phytochemistry 10*: 3267-3269.
ANNO 3. Mussini, P., F. Orsini, F. Pelizzoni & G. Ferrari. 1973. Constituents of *Annona coriacea*. The structure of a new diterpenoid. *J. Chem. Soc. Perkin Trans.* I: 2551-2557.
ANNO 4. Mussini, P., F. Orsini, F. Pelizzoni, B.L. Buckwalter & E. Wenkert. 1973. The C-13 configuration of annonalide. *Tetrahedron Lett.*: 4849-4851.
ANNO 5. Orsini, F., F. Pelizzoni, A.T. McPhail, K.D. Onan & E. Wenkert. 1977. The structure of annonalide. *Tetrahedron Lett.*: 1085-1088.
ANNO 6. Onan, K.D. & A. T. McPhail. 1978. Crystal and molecular structure of annonalide, a 9 H-pimaradienic diterpenoid from *Annona coriacea*. *J. Chem. Res.* (S) 1978(I): 15.
ANNO 7. Hocquemiller, R., A. Cavé, H. Jacquemin, A. Touché & P. Forgacs. 1982. Alcaloïdes de Annonacées. XXXVI: alcaloïdes de l'*Annona crassifolia* Mart. *Plantes Méd. Phytothér. 16*: 4-6.

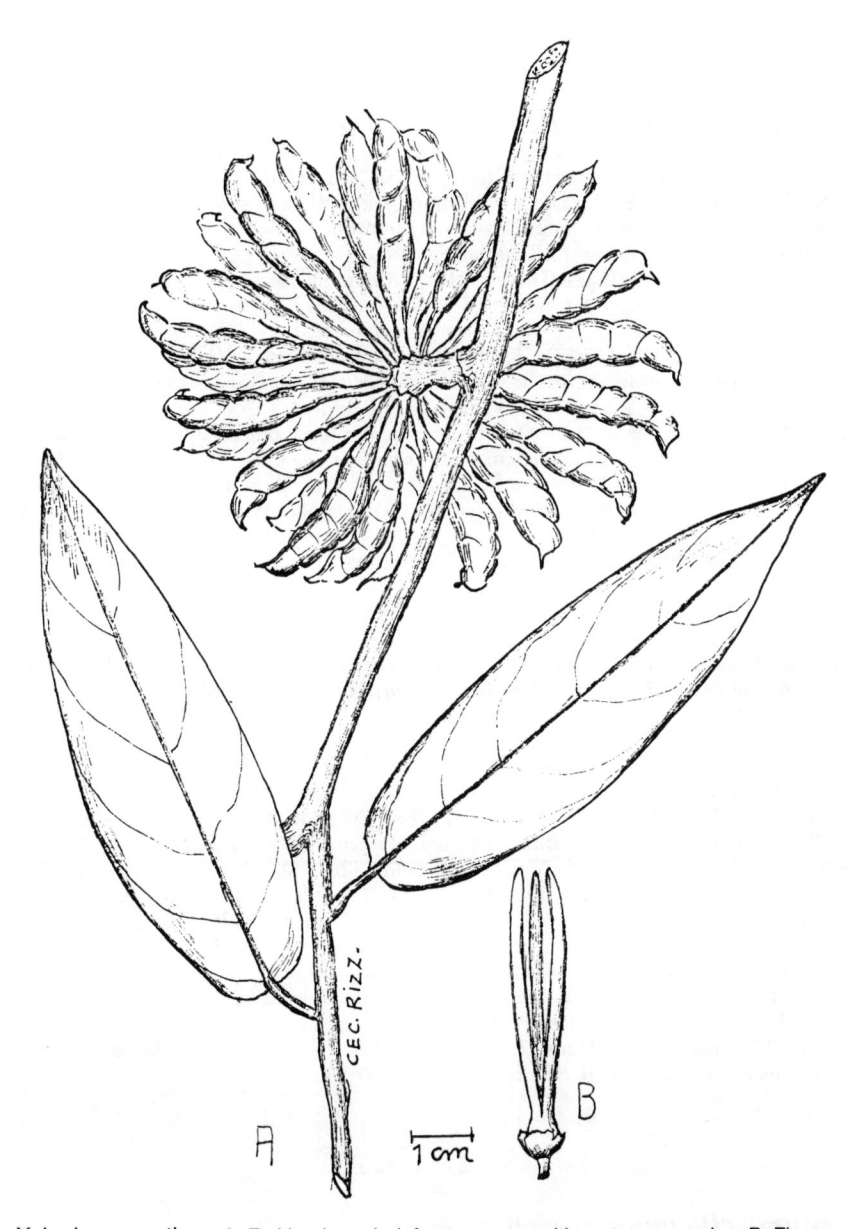

Xylopia aromatica: A. Fruiting branch; infructescence with mature capsules. B. Flower

ANNO 8. Ventura, M.M. & I.H. Lima. 1961. Ornithine cycle amino acids and other free amino acids in fruits of *Annona squamosa* and *A. muricata*. *Phyton* (Buenos Aires) *17*: 39-47.

ANNO 9. Leboeuf, M., C. Legneut, A. Cavé, J.F. Deconcluis & P. Forgacs. 1980. Anomurine et anomuricine, deux nouveaux alcaloïdes isoquinoleiques de l'*Annona muricata*. *Planta Medica 39*: 204-205.

ANNO 10. Etse, J.T. & P.G. Waterman. 1986. Chemistry in the Annonaceae. XXII. 14-Hydroxy-25-deoxyrollinicin from stem bark of *Annona reticulata. J. Nat. Prod. 49*: 684-686.
ANNO 11. Bhakuni, D.S., S. Thewari & M.M. Dhar. 1972. Aporphine alkaloids of *Annona squamosa. Phytochemistry 11*: 1819-1822.
ANNO 12. Mishra, A., J.U.V. Dogra, J.N. Singh & O.P. Iha. 1979. Post-coital antifertility activity of *Annona squamosa* and *Ipomoea fistulosa. Planta Medica 35*: 283-285.
ANNO 13. Fujimoto, Y., T. Eguchi, K. Kakinuma, N. Ikekawa, M. Sahai & Y.K. Gupta. 1988. Squamocin, a new cytotoxic bis-tetrahydrofuran containing acetogenin from *Annona squamosa. Chem. Pharm. Bull. 36*: 4802-4806.
ANNO 14. Casagrande, C. & G. Ferrari. 1970. Aporphine alkaloids. I. Alkaloids of Brazilian *Duguetia. Farmaco, Ed. Sci. 25*: 442-448.
ANNO 15. Leboeuf, J., D. Cortes, R. Hocquemiller & T.A. Cavé. 1983. Alcaloïdes des Annonacées. XLVII: Alcaloïdes de *Guatteria ouregon. Planta Medica 48*: 234-245.
ANNO 16. Hocquemiller, R., S. Razamifazy, A. Cavé & C. Moretti. 1983. Alcaloïdes des Annonacées. XXXVII. Alcaloïdes du *Guatteria scandens. J. Nat. Prod. 46*: 335-341.
ANNO 17. Salatino, M.L. 1983. Constituents of the unsaponifiable fraction of the foliar epicuticular wax and the systematics of the Annonaceae. *Rev. Bras. Bot. 6*: 23-28.
ANNO 18. Mesquita, L.M., J.F. Roque, L.M.B. Quintana, M. de Q. Paulo & J.M. Barbosa Filho. 1988. Lignans from *Rollinia* species (Annonaceae). *Biochem. Syst. Ecol. 16*: 379-380.
ANNO 19. Silva, J.B. & A.B. Rocha. 1981. Oleorresina do fruto de *Xylopia aromatica* (Lam.) Mart. *Rev. Ciênc. Farm.* (S. Paulo) *3*: 33-40.
ANNO 20. Moraes, M.P.L. & N.F. Roque. 1988. Diterpenes from the fruits of *Xylopia aromatica. Phytochemistry 27*: 3205-3208.
ANNO 21. Leboeuf, M., A. Cavé, J. Provost, P. Forgacs & H. Jacquemin. 1982. Alcaloïdes desAnnonacées. XLIII. Alcaloïdes du *Xylopia frutescens* Aubl. *Plantes Méd. Phytothér. 16*: 253-259.
ANNO 22. Silva, E.A. 1983. Isolamento e identificação de alguns constituintes químicos e estudos farmacológicos preliminares de *Xylopia frutescens* Aubl. (Annonaceae). Thesis, Federal University of Paraiba.
ANNO 23. Matos, M.E., F.J.A. Matos & R. Braz Filho. 1984. Constituintes químicios de *Xylopia sericea* St.-Hil. vel affinis. *Ciência e Cultura 36* (No. 7, Supl.): 528.
ANNO 24. Matos, M.E., F.J.A. Matos & R. Braz Filho. 1985. Constituintes químicios de *Xylopia sericea* St.-Hil. vel affinis. *Ciência e Cultura 37* (No. 7, Supl.): 521.
ANNO 25. Leboeuf, M., A. Cavé, P.K. Bhaumic, B. Mukherjee & R. Mukherjee. 1982. The phytochemistry of the Annonaceae. *Phytochemistry 21*: 2783-2813.
ANNO 26. Craveiro, A.A., A.G. Fernandes, C.H. Sousa Andrade, F.J.A. Matos, J.W. Alencar & M.I.L. Machado. 1981. Óleos essenciais de plantas do Nordeste. 209 pp. Published by the Federal University of Ceará, Fortaleza.
ANNO 27. Pelissier, Y., C. Marion, A. Dezeuze & J.M. Bessière. 1993. Volatile components of *Annona squamosa* L. *J. Essent. Oil Res. 5*: 557-560.

APIACEAE

Apium sellowianum Wolf
AREA: Rio Grande do Sul, in marshy sites.
NAMES: Aipo, aipo-bravo.
USES: Herb is used externally for skin injuries and burns, internally, as a diuretic and to remove dermal afflictions.
CHEM.: Leaves and twigs contain furocoumarins (Ref: APIA l).

PHARM.: The species has been proved toxic against the European corn borer (Ref: APIA 2).

Eryngium elegans Cham. & Schlecht.
AREA: South Brazil, campos.
NAMES: Caraguatá, caraguatá-elegante, gravatá-falso.
USES: Roots are diuretic.

Eryngium foetidum L.
AREA: Neotropical, Pará to Rio de Janeiro.
NAMES: Coentro-bravo, coentro-da-colônia, coentro-de-caboclo.
USES: Indicated for dropsy, spasms, sexual impotence, urine retention, as emmenagogue and abortifacient. Used as a condiment.
CHEM.: Dodecene aldehyde is the major component of the essential oil (Ref: APIA 3).

Eryngium pandanifolium Cham. & Schlecht.
AREA: Southern Brazil, in swampy terrain.
NAMES: Caraguatá, caraguatá-branco, caraguatá-do-banhado.
USE: Roots are diuretic.

Eryngium paniculatum Cav. & Domb. ex Delar.
AREA: Goiás to Rio Grande do Sul and Mato Grosso, along streams and lagoons.
NAMES: Caraguatá-falso, croatá-falso.
USES: Plant is diuretic.

Eryngium pristis Cham. & Schlecht.
AREA: Minas Gerais to Rio Grando do Sul, mainly in wasteland.
NAMES: Caraguatá, língua-de-araçari, língua-de-tucano.
USES: Plant is bitter, diuretic, active against aphthae and ulcers of the mouth and throat.
CHEM.: Leaves and rhizome contain caffeic acid, steroids and catechic tannins (Ref: APIA 4).

Hydrocotyle bonariensis Lam.
AREA: Common herb all over South America; in Brazil, frequent as a ruderal.
NAMES: Acariçoba, erva-capitão.
USES: Plant juice is employed to remove freckles. Rhizome is diuretic, vomitive, aperient, antirheumatic, useful for liver and kidney ailments. Leaves are considered toxic.
CHEM.: The essential oil has been analyzed, showing the presence of isothiocyanates (Ref: APIA 5).

Hydrocotyle leucocephala Cham. & Schlecht.
AREA: Bahia to Rio Grande do Sul.
NAMES: Acariçoba, cicuta-falsa, erva-capitão, erva-capitão-miúda, orelha-de-onça-rasteira.
USES: Same as for *Hydrocotyle bonariensis*.

Apiaceae – References

APIA 1. Silva, M. 1977. Some constituents of *Apium australe* Thouars. *Rev. Latinoam. Quím.* 8: 140-142.
APIA 2. Freedman, B. 1979. A bio-assay for plant-derivated pest control agents using the European corn borer. *J. Econ. Entomol.* 72: 541-545.
APIA 3. Koolhaas, D.R. 1932. Das aetherische Oel aus *Eryngium foetidum* L. Ueber das Vorkommen vom Dodecen-(2)-al-1. *Rec. Trav. Chim. Pays-Bas* 51: 460-468.
APIA 4. Wexel, M.D.B. 1977. *Contribuição à Análise Fitoquímica em* Eryngium horridum *Malme e* E. pristis *Cham. et Schlecht*. Thesis, Federal University of Rio Grande do Sul.
APIA 5. Salgues, R. 1963. Analysis of the essential oil of *Hydrocotyle bonariensis*. *Qual. Plant. Mat. Veget.* 9: 230-256.

APOCYNACEAE

Allamanda blanchetii M. Arg.
AREA: Bahia, caatinga.
NAME: Alamanda-de-jacobina.
USES: Latex is emetocathartic.
CHEM.: Contains the iridoid lactones plumericine and isoplumericine (Ref: APOC 1) and the coumarins umckalin and its methyl ether (Ref: APOC 2).

Allamanda cathartica L.
AREA: Widespread in Brazil, much cultivated in gardens.
NAMES: Alamanda, dedal-de-dama, orélia, quatro-patacas, santa-maria, alamanda-de-flor-grande.
USES: Latex is rubbed on skin against scabies. Leaf infusion is emetic, purgative, helminthicide.
CHEM.: Contains the iridoid lactones plumericine, isoplumericine (Ref: APOC 3) and allamandine (Ref: APOC 4).
PHARM.: Antileukemic properties of allamandine have been demonstrated (Ref: APOC 4).

Allamanda doniana M. Arg.
AREA: Maranhão to Bahia.
NAMES: Acapociba, itabocaba.
USES: Bark is vomitive, purgative, toxic.

Ambelania tenuifolia Aubl.
AREA: Amazonia, forest.

APOCYNACEAE

NAMES: Molongó, pepino-do-mato.
USE: Fruits are antitussive.

Anacampta riedellii (M. Arg.) Mgf.
AREA: Amazonia.
NAME: Pacaratepê, paqueretê.
USE: Latex is indicated for snakebite.

Anisolobus cururu (Mart.) M. Arg.
AREA: Amazonia.
NAMES: Cipó-cururu, cumapé, cururu.
USES: Root is emetic. Latex is used as a resolvent for abscesses. Bark infusion is purgative, useful for dyspepsy, splenitis, hepatitis.

Aspidosperma desmanthum M. Arg.
AREA: Amazonia, forest.
NAMES: Araracanga, araraúba-da-terra-firme.
USES: Leaves are antipyretic.

Aspidosperma discolor Benth.
AREA: Eastern Brazil, Atlantic forest.
NAMES: Cabo-de-machado, peroba, quina-de-rego.
USES: Bark is extremely bitter, reputedly antimalarial.

Aspidosperma excelsum Benth.
AREA: Amazonia, forest.
NAME: Carapanaúba.
USES: Bark is carminative, stomachic, recommended for bronchitis.
CHEM. & PHARM.: Alkaloids from bark are antimicrobial (Ref: APOC 5).

Aspidosperma nigricans Handro
AREA: Bahia and Minas Gerais, forest.
NAME: Pereiro-amarelo.
USE: Bark is reportedly carcinostatic.

Aspidosperma nitidum Benth.
AREA: Pará, forest.
NAMES: Carapanaúba, pau-de-remo, sapopema.
USES: Bark is antifebrile, reputed antimalarial.
PHARM.: The bark extract has been found inactive against *Plasmodium lophurae* (Ref: APOC 6).

Aspidosperma polyneuron M. Arg.
AREA: Bahia to Paraná, in forest.
NAMES: Peroba-amargosa, peroba-rosa, sobro.
USES: Bark is bitter, astringent, antipyretic.

APOCYNACEAE

Aspidosperma spp.

Much work was done on the chemistry of *Aspidosperma* alkaloids in the 1960s. More than 100 alkaloids were isolated and had their structures determined. The majority are indole and dihydroindole bases, subdivided into a series of structural groups. For complete reviews see Ref: APOC 8,9.

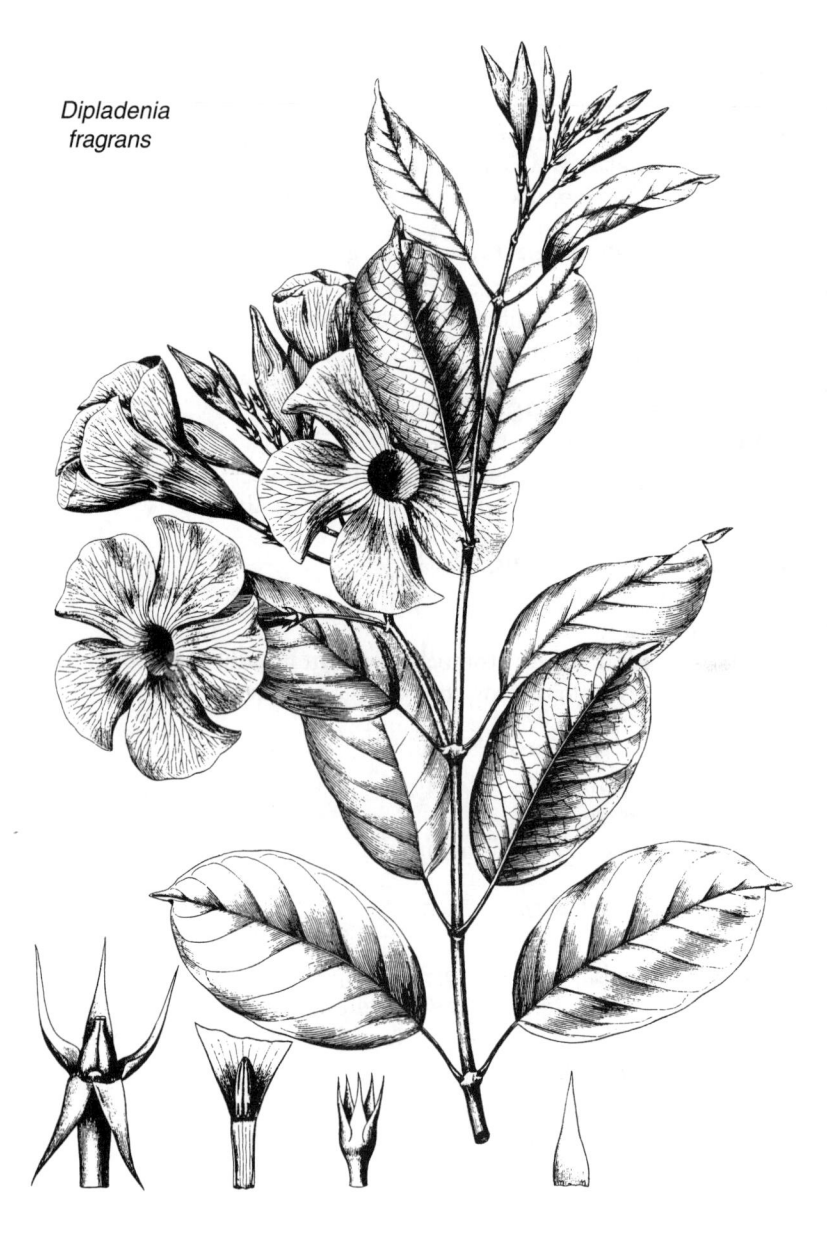

Dipladenia fragrans

Couma macrocarpa B. Rodr.
AREA: Amazonia, forest.
NAMES: Sorva, sorveira, sorva-da-mata.
USE: Latex is useful for amebiasis.

Couma utilis (Mart.) M. Arg.
AREA: Amazonia, forest.
NAMES: Sorva-do-pará, cumã, cumaí, sorva, sorva-pequena, sorveira, sorvinha.
USE: Latex is prescribed to expel intestinal worms.

Dipladenia fragrans DC.
AREA: Bahia to Minas Gerais and Rio de Janeiro, campo.
NAMES: Alamanda-cheirosa, rosa-do-campo.
USES: Flowers are antispasmodic, though toxic.

Dipladenia illustris M. Arg.
AREA: Widespread in Brazilian campos, from Bahia to Mato Grosso and São Paulo.
NAMES: Erva-venenosa, flor-de-babado, jalapa-vermelha, purga-do-campo, quina-de-camamu, rosa-do-campo, rosa-infalível.
USES: Leaves are poisonous, drastic in weak doses. Juice of roots is taken against snakebite.

Dipladenia spp.
Other *Dipladenia* species native to the campos and used for the same purposes as *D. illustris* are: *D. amabilis* Hort., *D. atropurpurea* (Lindl.) DC., *D. atroviolacea* (Lem.) DC., *D. gentianoides* M. Arg., *D. riedelii* M. Arg., *D. spigeliifolia* M. Arg., and *D. splendens* (Hook.) DC.

Echites macrocalyx M. Arg.
AREA: Bahia to Minas Gerais and São Paulo.
NAME: Folha-santa.
USES: Fresh leaves which are worked into fat and applied externally are said to be a resolvent for orchitis.

Echites peltata Vell.
AREA: Goiás to São Paulo and Rio de Janeiro, forest.
NAMES: Capa-homem, cipó-capador, cipó-de-paina, cipó-santo, erva-santa, joão-da-costa, paina-de-penas.
USES: Stem and leaves used for orchitis as well as inflammations in general; also indicated for chronic ulcers.

Geissospermum laeve (Vell.) Baill.
AREA: Bahia to Rio de Janeiro, forest.

Apocynaceae

NAMES: Canudo-amargoso, camará-de-bilro, pau-forquilha, pau-pereira, pereiro, pinguaciba.
USES: Bark is exceedingly bitter; infusion of bark used for fever, malaria, hypertension, and as tonic and stomachic.

Geissospermum sericeum Benth. & Hook.
AREA: Amazonia, forest.
NAMES: Acarirana, quinarana, acariquara-branca, pereira.
USE: Bark is taken as a febrifuge.

Geissospermum spp.

A complete summary of the chemistry and pharmacology of *Geissospermum* species is found in Ref: APOC 10. For more recent work on the indole and indoline bases see Ref: APOC 11,12,13. Among the isolated alkaloids some show antagonistic activity. Thus, geissoschizoline has curare-like action, while flavopereirine has anticholiesterase activity (Ref: APOC 14,15).

Haemadyction gaudichaudii DC.
AREA: Amazonia to Rio de Janeiro, forest.
NAME: Cipó-de-carneiro.
USES: Recommended for arresting hemorrhages of the lungs and, principally, of the womb.

Hancornia speciosa Gomes
AREA: Dry regions of northeast and central Brazil and part of the littoral.
NAMES: Mangabeira, mangabinha-do-norte.
USES: Tea from bark and leaves used against liver ailments; externally applied for cleaning skin eruptions. Decoction of the roots used against rheumatism.

Himatanthus alba (L.) Woods.
AREA: Amazonia, forest.
NAMES: Jasmim-de-caiena, jasmim-de-leite, jasmim-do-pará, pau-de-leite.
USES: Root bark is a strong purgative; latex used in poultices in cases of joint wrench and hernia; also used to cure snakebite. Latex is caustic, useful for removing warts. Flowers are pectoral.

Himatanthus drastica (Mart.) Woods.
AREA: Pará to Minas Gerais, in forests.
NAMES: Janaúba, jasmim-manga, raivosa, sabeú-una, sucuuba, tiborna.
USES: Bark is tonic, febrifuge in low doses; for hernia and sloughing ulcers.

APOCYNACEAE

Flowering branches

Hancornia speciosa
[above]

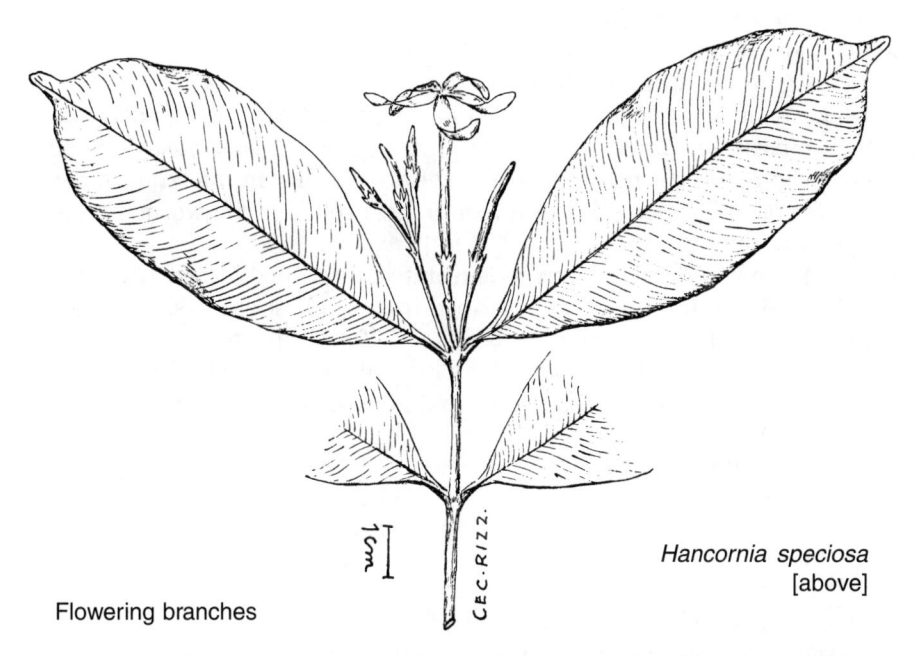

Parahancornia amapa
[below]

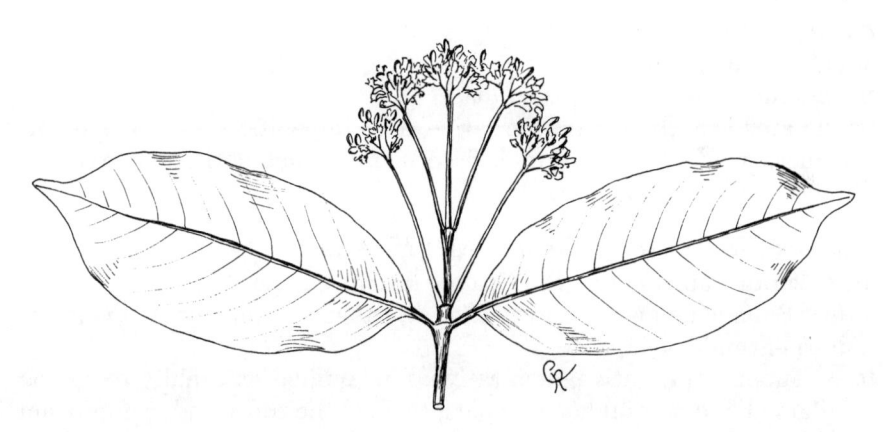

Himatanthus fallax (M. Arg.) Woods.
AREA: Amazonia to Alagoas, forest.
NAMES: Sucuuba, tiborna-traiçoeira.
USES: Formerly employed for venereal disease, though poisonous.

APOCYNACEAE

Himatanthus lancifolia (M. Arg.) Woods.
AREA: Espírito Santo to Rio Grande do Sul.
NAMES: Agoniada, quina-mole, tapuoca.
USES: Latex is anthelmintic. Bark employed as antiasthmatic, antisyphilitic, purgative, emmenagogue, against chlorosis, hypertrophy of lymphatic ganglia, dermatoses, said to induce fertility in infertile women. Leaves used in a decoction as a vermifuge, useful for ringworm, herpes, hysteria, pian (yaws).
CHEM.: A compound, agoniadin, was isolated from the bark in 1870 (Ref: APOC 16). Plumierid, later described from another species, was found to be identical with agoniadin (Ref: APOC 17). Although the latter name has priority, the designation plumierid prevailed in the literature. Its structure was elucidated as an iridoid glucoside (Ref: APOC 18).

Himatanthus phagedaenica (Mart.) Woods.
AREA: Amazonia, forest.
NAMES: Jasmim-mango-falso, sabiá-una, sucuuba, sucuíba, tiborna.
USES: Latex used for expelling intestinal worms; considered remedy for herpes, crustose ulcers, psoriasis, warts.
PHARM.: Pharmacological tests demonstrated spasmodic action of the wood extract on smooth muscle preparations of guinea pig ileum. (Ref: APOC 19).

Himatanthus sucuuba (Spr.) Woods.
AREA: Amazonia, forest.
NAMES: Janaguba, sucuba, sucuuba.
USES: Latex is anthelmintic, purgative, used in poultices as an emollient, vulnerary, antiarthritic. Bark is febrifuge, antirheumatic, used for treating cancer and bone fracture.

Macrosiphonia longiflora (Desf.) M. Arg.
AREA: Santa Catarina and Rio Grande do Sul, campo.
NAMES: Babado-de-nossa-senhora, flor-de-babado, velame-branco, velame-do-rio-grande-do-sul.
USES: Tuber is purgative, depurative, but applied externally to soothe inflamed and painful hemorrhoids; resin of the tuber and leaf infusion is highly esteemed in veterinary medicine for curing septic wounds in cattle.

Macrosiphonia velame (St.-Hil.) M. Arg.
AREA: Minas Gerais and Goiás to Rio Grande do Sul.
NAMES: Flor-de-babado, velame-branco, velame-do-rio-grande-do-sul.
USES: Depurative and antisyphilitic; for treating septic wounds in cattle.
CHEM.: Leaves contain free ursolic acid (triterpene) up to 4%, small amount

of an ursolic acid glucoside, and monopotassium salt of tartaric acid (Ref: APOC 20).

Mandevilla velutina (Mart. ex Stadelm.) Woods. var. ***velutina***
AREA: Minas Gerais, Rio de Janeiro, and Paraná, campos.
NAME: Jalapa.
USES: Tuber employed in tea or tincture as an anti-inflammatory and antiophidic.
PHARM.: The popular claim to anti-snakebite activity has been scientifically verified, the extract of the tubers being the first known naturally occurring bradykinin antagonist (Ref: APOC 21).

Mesechites sulphurea (Vell.) M. Arg.
AREA: Goiás and Rio de Janeiro to São Paulo.
NAMES: Cipó-de-leite, maquiné-do-mato.
USES: Latex is drastic purgative, poisonous.

Odontadenia speciosa Benth.
AREA: Amazonia, forest.
NAME: Cipó-cururu.
USES: Wood infusion useful in cases of dyspepsia and to improve appetite.

Parahancornia amapa (Hub.) Ducke
AREA: Pará, forest.
NAME: Amapá.
USES: Bark is tonic, antisyphilitic. Latex in large doses is an emetocathartic, diuretic; in moderate doses useful for asthma and bronchitis; externally resolving and wound healing.

Peschiera affinis (M. Arg.) Miers
AREA: Minas Gerais, Rio de Janeiro, São Paulo.
NAME: Leiteira.
USES: Bark is a tonic, vulnerary, antihemorrhoidal in local baths.
CHEM.: Indole alkaloids are present in bark and root bark (Ref: APOC 7,22,23).
PHARM.: Antitumor properties (Ref: APOC 24). Other pharmacological activity reported in isolated organ preparations (Ref: APOC 25).

Peschiera laeta (Mart.) Miers
AREA: Amazonia to São Paulo and Mato Grosso, forest.
NAMES: Esperta, café-do-mato, grão-de-galo, jasmin-de-cachorro, jasmim-de-leite, pau-de-colher.
USES: Bark is tonic, vulnerary, antihemorrhoidal in local baths; sap, bark and flowers are cardioactive.
CHEM.: Contains bisindole alkaloids (Ref: APOC 27).

APOCYNACEAE

PHARM.: Bark extract spasmolytic (Ref: APOC 26).

Plumeria alba L.
AREA: Amazonia, forest.
NAMES: Jasmim-de-caiena, jasmim-de-leita, jasmim-do-pará, pau-de-leite.
USES: Root-bark is a strong purgative. Latex used in poultices in cases of joint wrench and hernia; also to cure snakebite; latex is caustic, useful for removing warts. Flowers are pectoral.

Rauwolfia bahiensis DC.
AREA: Piauí to Bahia, forest.
NAMES: Casca-de-anta-brava, puçá.
USE: Plant is considered tonic.
CHEM.: Reserpine, reserpiline and rescinnamine have been identified by paper chromatography (Ref: APOC 28).

Rauwolfia blanchetii DC.
AREA: Bahia, forest.
NAME: Canudo-de-purga.
USES: Root-bark is emetocathartic. Bruised fruits are employed against ringworm and scabies.

Rauwolfia ligustrina Willd. ex Roem. & Schult.
AREA: Alagoas to Espírito Santo.
NAME: Pau-de-leite.
USES: Root is emetic, drastic.
CHEM.: Twenty-one *Rauwolfia* alkaloids were identified in this species by different authors (Ref: APOC 28,29,30).

Secondatia floribunda DC.
AREA: Ceará, cerrado.
NAME: Catuaba-cipó.
USES: Stem-bark is indicated as an aphrodisiac.

Tabernaemontana citrifolia L.
AREA: Amazonia.
NAMES: Jasmim-da-mata, paratucu.
USES: Bark is tonic, antipyretic. Leaves are febrifuge, purgative.

Thevetia ahouai (L.) DC.
AREA: Amazonia to Ceará, but widespread in cultivation.
NAMES: Agaí, auaí, cascaveleira, chapéu-de-napoleão, jorro-jorro, tinguí-de-leite.
USES: Leaves are emetic, cathartic, antiodontalgic, used for washing chronic ulcers. Bark is bitter, febrifuge, purgative, vomitive, but its use

is dangerous. Latex is useful for alleviating toothache. Fruit kernel applied in poultice is said to neutralize snake poison, specifically that of rattlesnakes.

CHEM. & PHARM.: Seeds contain the cardioactive glycosides thevetine, neriifoline, thevebioside, peruvoside and ruvoside (Ref: APOC 31,32,33,34,35). For an individual description of these compounds see Ref: APOC 36.

Vallesia cymbifolia Ortega
AREA: Amazonia.
NAME: Dumiringama.
USE: Juice of fruit is recommended for eye inflammation.

Zschokkea arborescens M. Arg.
AREA: Pará, forest.
NAMES: Comaí, cumaí, guajaraí, molongó, pau-de-colher, sorvinha, tucujá.
USES: Latex used for treating herpes and sloughing ulcers. Extract of bark prescribed for liver disorders.

Apocynaceae – References

APOC 1. Moraes e Souza, M.A., M.S.B. Cavalcanti, G.M. Maciel, M.C.M. Araújo & F.F. de Mello. 1980/81. Isolamento e caracterização dos constituintes ativos de *Allamanda blanchetii* A.D.C. *Rev. Inst. Antibióticos* 20: 29-34.

APOC 2. Bhattacharyya, J. & M.S. Q. de Moraes. 1986. 5,6-Dimethoxy-7-hydroxycoumarin (umckalin) from *Allamanda blanchetii*: isolation and 13C-NMR characteristics. *J. Nat. Prod.* 49: 354-355.

APOC 3. Pai, B.R., P.S. Subramanian & U.K. Ramdas. 1970. Isolation of plumericin and isoplumericin from *Allamanda cathartica*. *Indian J. Chem.* 8: 851.

APOC 4. Kupchan, S.M., A.L. Desserine, B.T. Blaylock & R.F. Bryan. 1974. Isolation and structural elucidation of allamandine, an antileukemic iridoid lactone from *Allamanda cathartica*. *J. Org. Chem.* 39: 2477-2482.

APOC 5. Verpoorte, R., E. Kos-Kuyck, A. Tjin a Tsoi, C.L.M. Ruigrok, G. de Jong & A.B. Svendsen. 1983. Medicinal plants of Suriname. III. Antimicrobially active alkaloids from *Aspidosperma excelsum*. *Planta Medica* 48: 283-289.

APOC 6. Becker, E.R. 1949. Report on thirty-five drugs and three plant materials tested against *Plasmodium lophurae* in White Peking duck. *Iowa State Coll. J. Sci.* 23: 189-194.

APOC 7. Wolter Filho, W., C.H.S. Andrada, R. Braz Filho & F.J.A. Matos. 1985. Alcalóïdes de *Peschiera affinis* (Muell. Arg.) Miers (Apocynaceae). *Acta Amazonica* 15 (1/2): 193-197.

APOC 8. Gilbert, B. 1965. The alkaloids of *Aspidosperma*, *Diplorrhynchus*, *Kopsia*, *Ochrosia*, *Pleiocarpa*, and related genera. *In*: R.H.F. Manske, THE ALKALOIDS, vol. 8: 335-513. Academic Press, New York and London.

APOC 9. Gilbert, B. 1968. The alkaloids of *Aspidosperma*, *Ochrosia*, *Pleiocarpa*, *Melodinus* and related genera. *In*: R.H.F. Manske, THE ALKALOIDS, vol. 11: 205-306. Academic Press, New York and London.

APOC 10. Henry, T.A. 1949. THE PLANT ALKALOIDS, 4th Ed. The Blakiston Co., Philadelphia, PA.

APOC 11. Rapoport, H., T.P. Onak, N.A. Hughes & M.G. Reinecke. 1958. Alkaloids of *Geissospermum vellosii*. *J. Am. Chem. Soc.* 80: 1601-1604.

Apocynaceae

APOC 12. Rapoport, H., R.J. Windgassen, N.A. Hughes & T.P. Onak. 1959. The structure of geissoschizine. *J. Am. Chem. Soc. 81*: 3166-3167.

APOC 13. Rapoport, H., & R.E. Moore. 1962. Alkaloids of *Geissospermum vellosii*. Isolation and structure determination of vellosimine, vellosiminol, and geissolosimine. *J. Org. Chem. 27*: 2981-2985.

APOC 14. Aurousseau, M. 1961. Étude pharmacodynamique de la geissospermine, l'alcaloïde principale du *Geissospermum laeve*. *Ann. Pharm. Franç. 19*: 104-116, 175, 515.

APOC 15. Buffolo, E., G. Rosa & J. Ribeiro do Valle. 1962. Ação anticolinesterásica de flavopereirina. *Ciência e Cultura 14*: 232.

APOC 16. Peckolt, T. 1870. Agoniadin. *Arch. Pharm.* (2) *142*: 40.

APOC 17. Schmid, H., H. Bickel & T.M. Meijer. 1952. Zur Kenntnis des Plumierids. *Helv. Chim. Acta 35*: 415-417.

APOC 18. Halpern, B. & H. Schmid. 1958. Zur Kenntnis des Plumierids. *Helv. Chim. Acta 41*: 1109-1154.

APOC 19. Vanderlei, M.F. & A.R.M. Souza Brito. 1989. Ações espasmogênicas do extrato etanólico bruto de *Himatanthus phagedaenica* (Mart.) Woodson, em íleo isolado de cobaia. *Rev. Bras. Farm. 70*: 15-18.

APOC 20. Lobato, J.E. 1980. Contribuição para o estudo fitoquímico do velame, *Macrosyphonia velame* (St.-Hil.) M.Arg. — Glucosidação do ácido ursólico. Thesis, Federal University of Rio de Janeiro.

APOC 21. Calixto, J.B., M.G. Pizzolatti & R.A. Yunes. 1988. The competitive antagonistic effect of compounds from *Mandevilla velutina* on kinin-induced contractions of the uterus and guinea-pig ileum *in vitro*. *Brit. J. Pharmacol. 94*: 1133-1142.

APOC 22. Cava, M.P., S.K. Talapatra, J.A. Weisbach, B. Douglas, R.F. Raffauf & O. Ribeiro. 1964. Structures of affinine and affinisine, alkaloids of *Peschiera affinis (Tabernaemontana affinis)*. *Chem. and Ind.*: 1193-4.

APOC 23. Matos, F.J.A., R. Braz Filho, O.R. Gottlieb, F.W. L. Machado & M.I.L.M. Madruga. 1976. 20-epiheyneanine, an iboga alkaloid from *Peschiera affinis*. *Phytochemistry 15*: 551-553.

APOC 24. Fonteles, M.C., M.C. Sampaio, J.H. Cardoso, M.E. Pereira & F.J.A. Matos. 1969. Verificação da atividade antitumoral de vegetais do nordeste brasileiro. *Ciência e Cultura 21*: 508.

APOC 25. Fonteles, M.C., D. Ferram, F.J.A. Matos & R.P. Ahlquist. 1974. Pharmacological activity of the major alkaloid from *Peschiera affinis*. *Planta Medica 25*: 175-182.

APOC 26. Barros, G.S.G., F.F.A. Matos, J.E.V. Vieira, M.P. Souza & M.C. Medeiros. 1970. Pharmacological screening of some Brazilian plants. *J. Farm. Pharmacol. 22*: 116-122.

APOC 27. Mattos, S.M.P., N.R.S. Brito & R.J.S. Jaccoud. 1979. Contribução ao estudo farmacognóstico da *Peschiera laeta* Mart. *Rev. Bras. Farm. 60*: 85-90.

APOC 28. Korzun, B.P., A.F. St. André & P.R. Ulschager. 1957. Paper chromatographic evaluation of *Rauwolfia* species. *J. Am. Pharm. Assoc. Sci. Ed. 46*: 720-723.

APOC 29. Cardoso, H.T. & I.A.A. Venâncio. 1956. Identifição da reserpina na *Rauwolfia ternifolia* H.B.K. *Rev. Bras. Biol. 16*: 231-234.

APOC 30. Müller, J.M. 1957. Über die Alkaloide von *Rauwolfia ligustrina* R.& S.; Raugustin, ein neues reserpinähnliches Alkaloid. *Experientia 13*: 479-481.

APOC 31. Chen, K.K. & A.L. Chen. 1934. The constituents of be-still nuts, *Thevetia neriifolia*. *J. Biol. Chem. 105*: 231-240.

APOC 32. Helfenberger, H. & T. Reichstein. 1948. Thevetin. I. *Helv. Chim. Acta 31*: 1470-1482.

APOC 33. Vohra, M.M., J.D. Kohli & N.N. De. 1961. Pharmacological studies on ruvoside — another new digitaloid from *Thevetia neriifolia* Juss. *Arch. Internat. Pharmacodyn. Thérapie 133*: 265-274.

APOC 34. Bisset, N.G., J. Euw, M. Frèrejacque, S. Rangaswami, O. Schindler & T. Reichstein. 1962. Die Cardenolide von *Thevetia peruviana*. *Helv. Chim. Acta 45*: 938-943.

APOC 35. Frèrejacque, M. & M. Durgeat. 1971. Structure de la thévéfoline. *Compt. Rend. Acad. Sci., Série D, 272*: 2620-2621.

APOC 36. Chen, K.K. & F.G. Henderson. 1962. Cardiac activity of apocynaceous glycosides and aglycones. *Arch. Internat. Pharmacodyn. Thérapie 140*: 8-19.

AQUIFOLIACEAE

Ilex acrodonta Reiss.
AREA: Rio de Janeiro and Minas Gerais, forest.
NAME: Pau-de-azeite.
USES: Bark is tonic, astringent.

Ilex brevicuspis Reiss.
AREA: Very common in Paraná and Santa Catarina, forest; rare in São Paulo.
NAMES: Caúna, caúna-da-serra, congonha, erva-mate, orelha-de-mico, voandeira.
USE: Used frequently in the adulteration of mate (erva-mate, *Ilex paraguariensis*).

Ilex paraguariensis St.-Hil.
AREA: Rio Grande do Sul, Paraná, Santa Catarina and Mato Grosso do Sul; particularly frequent in Rio Grande do Sul; widely cultivated.
NAMES: Mate,* erva-mate, chá-mate, congonha.
USES: The tea from the leaves is highly appreciated, mainly in southern Brazil and even more so in Argentina and Paraguay. The dried, sometimes slightly burned or toasted, leaves are an important article of commerce and can also regularly be found in open markets. The tea is tonic, stimulant, diuretic, reduces fatigue, improves appetite, and aids the gastric functions. It has recently become popular in Germany as a refreshing and stimulating beverage and slimming remedy. The leaves are sometimes applied in poultices to anthrax and ulcers. For a review see Ref: AQUI 1.
CHEM.: The leaves contain varying amounts of caffeine (1-1.5%) and a little theobromine (ca. 0.1%); concentrations are much lower in the infusion. Contains also choline, chlorogenic acid and inositol (Ref: AQUI 2,3), besides flavonoids and triterpenes (Ref: AQUI 4), and triterpenoid saponins (Ref: AQUI 5,6,7). Free and protein-bound amino acids (Ref: AQUI 8), free sugars (Ref: AQUI 9). Peroxidase (Ref: AQUI 10) and polyphenol-oxydase (Ref: AQUI 11) have been determined.
Leaf anatomy of this species, including its varieties and forms, has been

---

* The name *mate*, pronounced mah-tay, is often spelled "maté" in the international literature.

AQUIFOLIACEAE

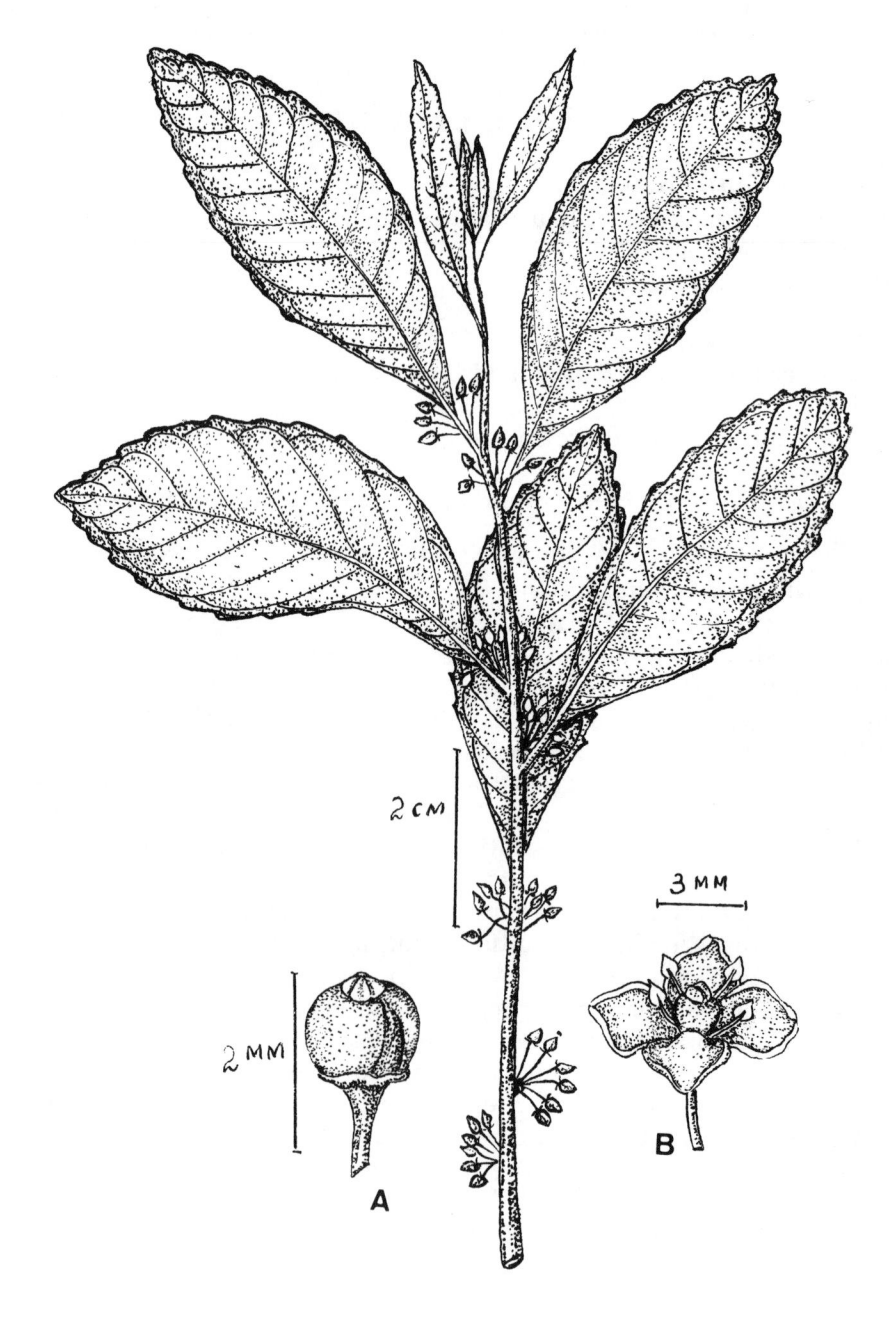

Ilex paraguariensis

described in detail as an aid to distinguish genuine mate from its adulterants (Ref: AQUI 12). The more commonly encountered admixtures have been similarly described (Ref: AQUI 13) and have also been chemically studied.

Aquifoliaceae – References

AQUI 1. Porter, R.H. 1950. Maté — South American or Paraguay tea. *Econ. Bot. 4*: 37-51.
AQUI 2. Badin, P., V. Deulofeu & O.L. Galmarini. 1962. Chlorogenic and chlorogenic-like acids in mate (*Ilex paraguariensis* St.Hil.). *Chem. & Ind.*: 257-258.
AQUI 3. Garcia Paula, R.D. 1968. *Novos Estudos Sobre o Mate*. Instituto Nacional de Tecnologia, Rio de Janeiro. 46 pp.
AQUI 4. Ohem, N. & J. Hölzl. 1988. Some new investigations on *Ilex paraguariensis*. Flavonoids and triterpenes. *Planta Medica 54*: 576.
AQUI 5. Gosmann, G., E.P. Schenkel & O. Seligman. 1989. A new saponin from mate, *Ilex paraguariensis* St.-Hil. (erva-mate). *J. Nat. Prod. 52*: 1367-1370.
AQUI 6. Gosmann, G., D. Guillaume, A.T.C. Taketa & E.P. Schenkel. 1995. Triterpenoid saponins from *Ilex paraguariensis. J. Nat. Prod. 58*: 438-441.
AQUI 7. Kraemer, K.H., A.T.C. Taketa, E.P. Schenkel, G. Gosmann & D. Guillaume. 1996. Matesaponin 5, a highly polar saponin from *Ilex paraguariensis. Phytochemistry 42*: 1119-1122.
AQUI 8. Cascon, S.C. 1955. Os amino-ácidos do mate. *Bol. Inst. Quím. Agrícola* (Rio de Janeiro) *38*: 7-15.
AQUI 9. Chlamtac, E.B. 1955. Açúcares do mate. *Bol. Inst. Quím. Agrícola* (Rio de Janeiro) *38*: 17-24.
AQUI 10. Panek, A.D. 1955. Peroxidase do mate. *Bol. Inst. Quím. Agrícola* (Rio de Janeiro) *39*: 7-12.
AQUI 11. Chlamtac, E.B. 1955. Enzimas do mate: polifenol-oxidase. *Bol. Inst. Quím. Agrícola* (Rio de Janeiro) *39*: 13-17.
AQUI 12. Gurgel, L. 1931. Primeira contribuição para o estudo do mate. Histologia e anatomia de algumas variedades de *Ilex paraguariensis* St. Hil. *Memória do Instituto de Química* (Ministério da Agricultura, Rio de Janeiro). no.3, 91 pp. + 15 pp. illustr.
AQUI 13. Gurgel, L. 1937. Segunda contribuição para o estudo do mate. Histologia e anatomia de alumas espécies de *Ilex*. *Memória do Instituto de Química* (Ministério da Agricultura, Rio de Janeiro), no.4, 95 pp. + 11 pp. illustr.

ARACEAE

Anthurium affine Schott
AREA: Extreme northwestern Brazil, extending into Colombia.
NAMES: Babosa-de-árvore, babosa-do-mato, zangatempo.
USE: Juice used against baldness.

Anthurium oxycarpum Poepp.
AREA: Amazonia.
NAMES: Folha-cheirosa, ieuri-cumajé.
USES: The dry leaves smell of vanilla, and are used to scent tobacco; infusion said to be aphrodisiac.

ARACEAE

Caladium bicolor

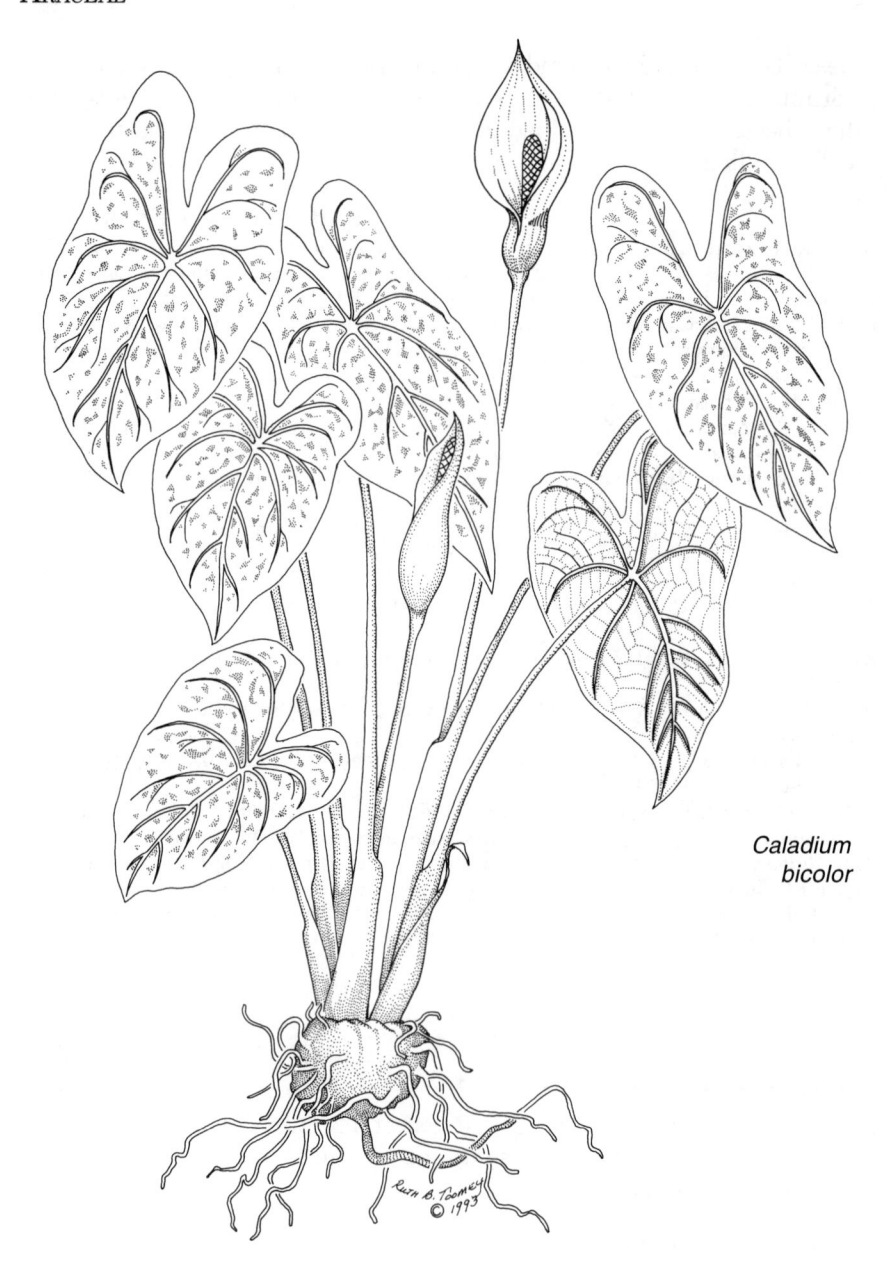

Caladium bicolor (Aiton) Vent.
AREA: Known only in cultivation.
NAMES: Ará, caládio, mangará, tajá, tinhorão.
USES: Fresh tubers are emetic, purgative. Leaves used as vulnerary, purgative, vermicide.

ARACEAE

Caladium bicolor (Aiton) Vent. var. *poecile* (Schott) Engler
AREA: Ceará.
NAME: Mão-aberta.
USES: Leaves heated and coated with olive oil are used to hasten the maturation of tumors.

Caladium sororium Schott
AREA: Amazonia, forest.
NAME: Aninga-da-água.
USES: Leaves employed in the treatment of skin ulcers.

Dieffenbachia seguine (Jacq.) Schott
AREA: Amazonia, forest; much cultivated as an ornamental.
NAMES: Aninga-uba, aninga-para, bananeira-d'água, cana-de-imbé, comigo-ninguém-pode.
USES: Root tincture against gout and genital pruritus. Leaf decoction in gargles for angina, in lotion for edematous inflammation. Stem extract in baths for dropsy; reportedly added to curare in arrow poison; stem juice to relieve snakebite and scorpion sting.
CHEM. & PHARM.: The stem juice, if placed in the mouth, is extremely dangerous, giving rise to a violent sensation of burning and producing severe edema of the glottis. The stems superficially resemble sugar-cane and are thus sometimes inadvertently chewed, mainly by children. As a result, speech is impaired (the plant is known as "dumb cane" in English-speaking countries) and death can be caused by asphyxia. Much has been speculated with regard to the causes of these effects.

It is now understood that they derive from a joint action of mechanical and chemical factors. The stem parenchyma contains raphides of calcium oxalate crystals which, when the stem is crushed, disintegrate into millions of minute needles. These penetrate into the mucous membranes of the mouth and throat, accompanied by a toxic material, which is responsible for producing the edema (Ref: ARAC 1,2,3). This material is a mixture of long carbon chain substances, possibly fatty acids, the exact chemical structure of which has not yet been ascertained (Ref: ARAC 4). Claims to a sterilizing effect of *D. seguine* extracts on humans are unsubstantiated.

Dracontium asperum K. Koch
AREA: Amazonia, forest.
NAMES: Erva-jararaca, jararaca, jararaca-taia, jararaca-tajá, milho-de-cobra, tajá-de-cobra.
USES: Powdered, dry rhizome used against snakebite, scabies, asthma, amenorrhoea, chlorosis, whooping cough; juice of the rhizome used to treat sores caused by blow-fly. Root-juice and petiole for snakebite. Whole plant decoction in baths for gout.

ARACEAE

Dracontium polyphyllum L.
AREA: Amazonia, forest.
NAMES: Erva-de-santa-maria, jararaca, jararaca-mirim, jiraraca.
USES: Plant is toxic, caustic, antispasmodic, antiasthmatic. Root decoction for cleansing ulcers of long standing.

Monstera adansonii Schott
AREA: Common in forests.
NAMES: Dragão-fedorento, folha-furada, folha-rota, imbê, imbê-furado, imbê-são-pedro, timbó-manso.
USES: Root infusion used against hydropsy and arthritis. Fresh leaves employed as a vesicatory, rubefacient and for chronic orchitis, otitis, erysipelas, eczema, dandruff, ulcers in general, post-partum lymphoadenitis; emollient and soothing in baths for rheumatism.

Monstera obliqua Miquel
AREA: Amazonia, forest.
NAME: Folha-rota.
USES: Though poisonous, considered to be of value for anasarca and gout.

Montrichardia linifera (Arruda) Schott
AREA: Piauí to Rio de Janeiro, in river mouths.
NAMES: Aninga, aninga-açu.
USES: Roots are diuretic, but toxic. Leaves for rheumatism and ulcers.

Philodendron bipinnatifidum Schott
AREA: Espírito Santo and Goiás, to Mato Grosso and Santa Catarina, in marshy campos, restinga and coppices.
NAMES: Banana-do-brejo, banana-imbê, cipó-gimbé, cipó-imbé or -imbê, folha-da-fonte, guimbê.
USES: Leaves and stem produce a caustic juice used for orchitis, rheumatism and ulcers. Root powder is drastic. Seeds said to destroy intestinal parasites.

Philodendron hederaceum (Jacq.) Schott var. **hederaceum**
AREA: Pará, Pernambuco and Rio de Janeiro.
NAMES: Folha-da-fonte, guimberana.
USES: Leaves are antirheumatic, antialgesic, indicated for inflamed nerves and joints. At night flowers send forth a strong odor of cloves.

Philodendron imbe Schott
AREA: Espirito Santo to São Paulo, forest.
NAMES: Cipó-de-imbê, cipó-imbê, cumba, imbé, tracuá.
USES: Powdered roots are drastic, useful for dropsy. Leaves are a purga-

tive diuretic, astringent, for erysipelas, rheumatism, orchitis, though use deserves care.

Philodendron ochrostemon Schott
AREA: Minas Gerais and Rio de Janeiro to São Paulo and Santa Catarina, forest.
NAMES: Cipó-de-imbê, imbê-miúdo.
USES: Same uses as *Philodendron imbe*, but perhaps less active.

Philodendron pedatum (Hook.) Kunth
AREA: Amazonia, forest.
NAMES: Folha-de-uruba, guembé.
USES: Leaf decoction used against rheumatism; leaves heated and coated with olive oil are calmative for pain and inflammations applied locally in cases of neuralgia and arthritis.

Philodendron selloum Koch
AREA: Alagoas to São Paulo, forest.
NAMES: Cipó-de-imbê, fruto de imbé, guambé, imbé-de-comer.
USES: Root is drastic. Seeds used as a vermifuge. Fruits are edible.

Philodendron speciosum Schott
AREA: Espírito Santo, Minas Gerais and Rio de Janeiro, forest.
NAME: Aninga.
USES: Stem juice is caustic, resolvent and used for rheumatic pains. Roots and seeds are recommended as anthelmintic.

Urospatha caudata (Poepp. & Endl.) Schott
AREA: Amazonia, forest.
NAME: Apê.
USES: Juice of the rhizome is caustic, prescribed for ringworm.

Xanthosoma striatipes (Kunth & Bouché) Madison
AREA: Amazonia to São Paulo, forest.
NAMES: Banana-do-brejo, cana-do-brejo.
USES: Fresh tubers employed for treating throat disorders. Leaf-juice used for the same purpose, but must be diluted with water.

Xanthosoma violaceum Schott
AREA: Cultivated throughout Brazil, sometimes disseminated or escaped from cultivation.
NAMES: Mangará, mangarito-grande, mangarito-roxo, taiá-açu, taioba, taioba-verdadeira, taiarana.
USES: Contused leaves are used in cataplasms on boils.

Philodendron pedatum

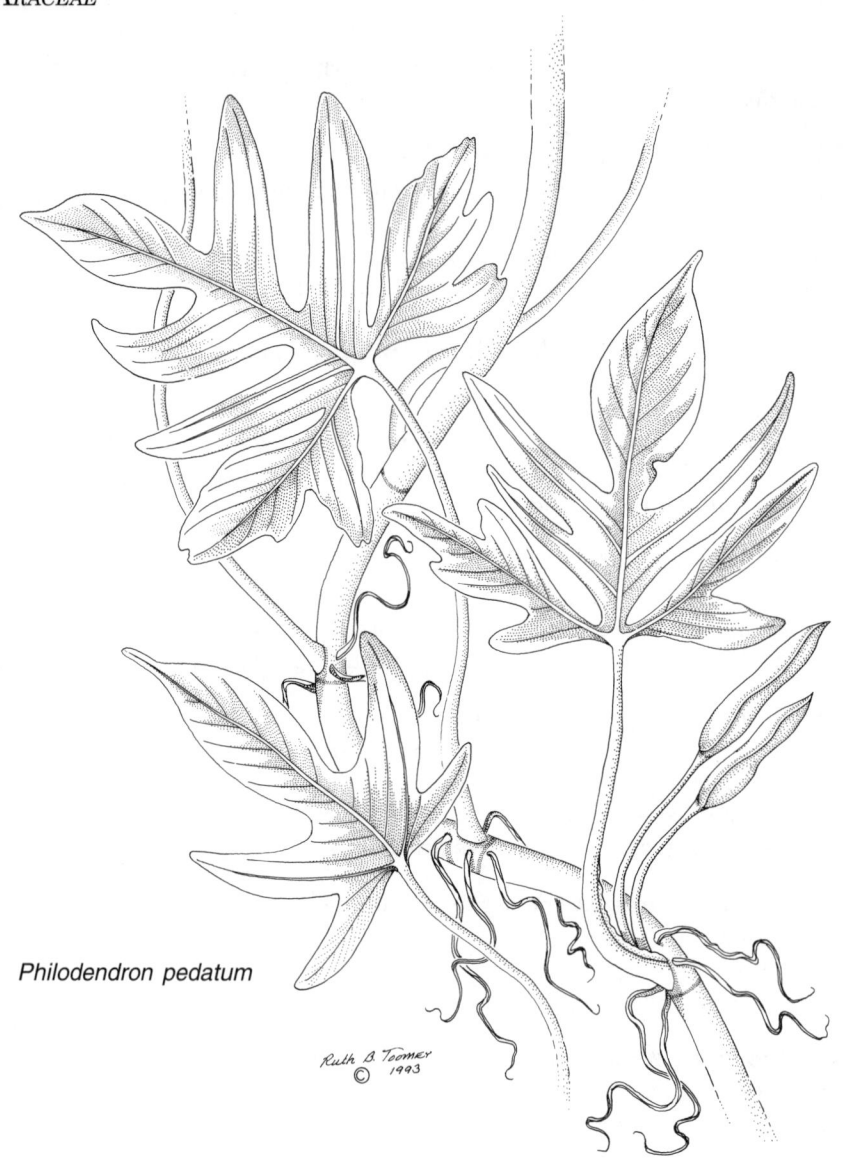

Araceae – References

ARAC 1. Rizzini, C.T. & P. Occhioni. 1957. Ação tóxica das *Dieffenbachia picta* e *D. seguine*. *Rodriguesia 20*: 5-19 + 3.

ARAC 2. Occhioni, P. & C.T. Rizzini. 1958. Ação tóxica de duas sp. de *Dieffenbachia*. *Rev. Bras. Med. 15*: 10-27.

ARAC 3. Arditti, J. & E. Rodriguez. 1982. *Dieffenbachia*: uses, abuses and toxic constituents. A review. *J. Ethnopharmacol. 5*: 293-302.

ARAC 4. Carneiro, C.M.T.S., L. de J. Neves, E. de F.R. Pereira & N.A. Pereira. 1989. Mecanismo tóxico de comigo-ninguém-pode, *Dieffenbachia picta* Schott, Araceae. *Rev. Bras. Farm. 70*: 11-13.

ARECACEAE*

Allagoptera campestris (Mart.) Kuntze
AREA: Central Brazil, campo and cerrado.
NAMES: Ariri, buri-do-campo, coco-de-vassoura, coqueiro-pissandó, emburi, guriri-do-campo, imburi, pissandu.
USES: Juice of the unripe nuts is used to treat infections. Mesocarp is bitter, antipyretic.

Astrocaryum aculeatissimum (Schott) Burret
AREA: Bahia to Santa Catarina, forest and restinga.
NAMES: Airi, brejaúva, coco-de-airi.
USES: Liquid endosperm of the unripe nut (known as água-de-airi) is considered laxative and useful for jaundice. Oil from ripe endosperm said to be taenifuge.

Astrocaryum murumuru Mart.
AREA: Amazonia, forest.
NAME: Murumuru.
USES: Mesocarp of fruit is aromatic and edible, used as a mild aphrodisiac.

Attalea oleifera Barb. Rodr.
AREA: Alagoas to Paraiba.
NAMES: Pindoba, palmeira.
USES: Kernel oil is active against chigoes (*Tunga penetrans*) and erysipelas.

Attalea spectabilis Mart.
AREA: Amazonia and Mato Grosso, forest.
NAMES: Carúa-piranga, uauaçu.
USES: Kernel used in liniments against rheumatism; ground and mixed with sugar and water it makes a refreshing and febrifuge emulsion.

Bactris insignis (Mart.) Baill.
AREA: Amazonia and Mato Grosso, forest.
NAMES: Ceriba, chonta, palmeira-real, piriguáo.
USES: Oil from kernel used to relieve rheumatic pains.

Butia yatay (Mart.) Becc.
AREA: Rio Grande do Sul (perhaps), campo.
NAMES: Butiá, coqueiro-jataí.
USE: Kernel is anthelmintic.

---

* For a review of the medicinal uses of Brazilian palms, see Ref: AREC 1.

ARECACEAE

Cocos nucifera L.
AREA: Along the entire Brazilian coast; much cultivated.
NAME: Coqueiro-da-bahia.
USES: Liquid endosperm (água de coco) reputed as a vermicide and taenifuge, considered efficient against beriberi, jaundice, gastrointestinal ailments, chest diseases, eye inflammations and vomiting during pregnancy. Young roots are said to be alexipharmic, antidysenteric, antidiarrhoeic, antiblennorrhagic and antipyretic; also applied to strengthen the gums. Sap obtained from stem or peduncles (vinho de coco), when newly extracted, has healing properties against piles, hemorrhage and fever in cases of smallpox.

Copernicia prunifera (Mill.) H. Moore
AREA: Northeast, in ancient dry riverbeds.
NAMES: Carnaúba, carnaubeira.
USES: Decoction of the roots is depurative and indicated as a specific medicine for syphilis; also for arthritis, rheumatism, dermal afflictions and to induce diuresis. The well-known carnauba wax, obtained from the leaves, has many industrial applications and is used medicinally to prepare ointments and cataplasms.

Desmoncus orthacanthos Mart.
AREA: Most of Brazil, including Atlantic Rainforest.
NAMES: Atitara, jacitara, jequitá, palmeira-do-brejo, urubamba, urum.
USES: Root decoction is drastic; excellent for curing dartre, eczema and certain dermatoses.

Desmoncus polyacanthos Mart.
AREA: On coastal sands, restinga.
NAMES: Crumbamba, jacitara, rutim, umbamba.
USE: Roots are depurative.

Elaeis guineensis Jacq.
AREA: Naturalized from Africa, much cultivated and subspontaneous, from Amazonia to Bahia.
NAME: Dendezeiro.
USES: Oil from pulp is emollient and used to treat suppuration, whitlow and swelling of the legs due to erysipelas and infestation by *Filaria*.

Elaeis oleifera (H.B.K.) Cortez
AREA: Amazonia, forest.
NAMES: Caiauá, caiauê, caiaué, dendezeiro-do-pará.
USES: Pulp oil is used for rheumatism, to invigorate hair, to combat dandruff and to repel insects. Hairs from the leaf axils are reputedly hemostatic.

ARECACEAE

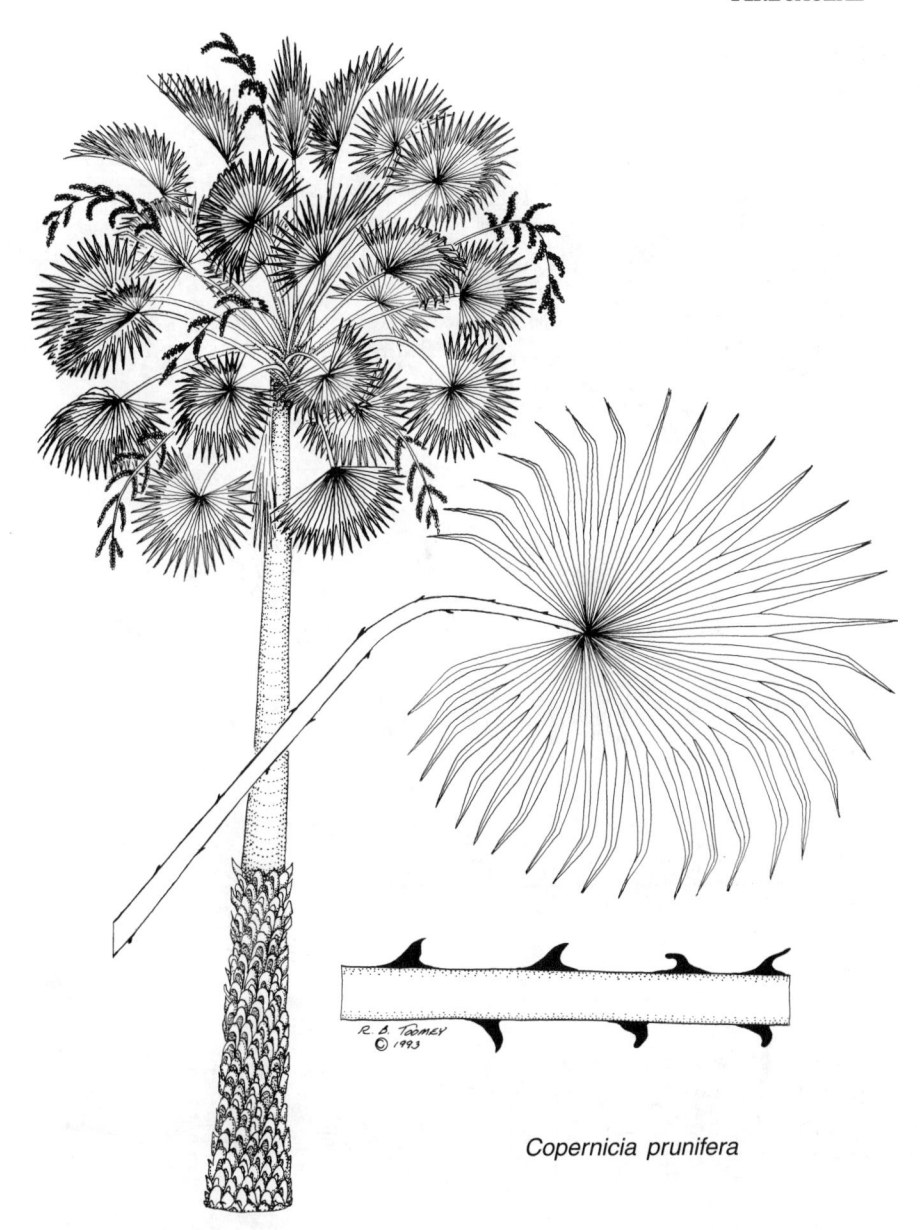

Copernicia prunifera

Euterpe edulis Mart.
AREA: Bahia to Rio Grande do Sul, very widespread in eastern Brazil forest.
NAMES: Iuçara, jiçara, juçara, palmito, palmito-doce, palmito-juçara.
USES: Juice squeezed from the young stem is put on wounds to stop bleeding.

ARECACEAE

Euterpe oleracea

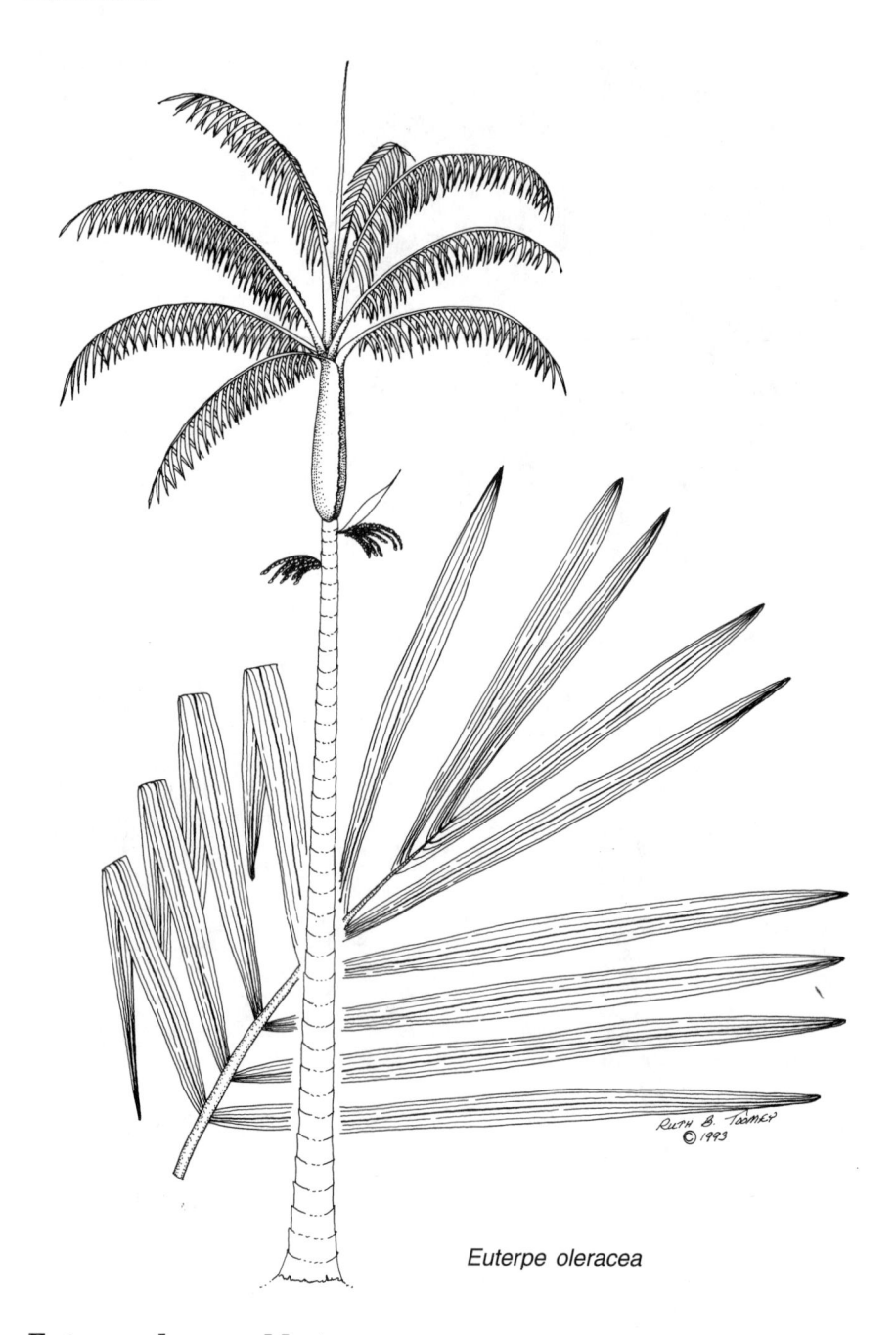

Euterpe oleracea Mart.
AREA: Amazonia, forest.
NAMES: Açaí, açaizeiro, juçara, palmiteiro, piriá.

USES: Fruit oil is antidiarrhoeic. Tea from roots is taken for jaundice and "to strengthen the blood." The grated rind, steeped in water, is recommended to wash ulcers. Tea from seeds is antifebrile.

Jessenia bataua (Mart.) Burret
AREA: Amazonia, forest.
NAME: Patauá.
USES: Kernel oil is employed to treat tuberculosis; also a purgative.

Leopoldinia major Wallace
AREA: Amazonia, forest.
NAMES: Iará-açu, jará-açu.
USES: The ash from the burned drupes is used against curare poisoning by applying it directly to the injury.

Mauritia flexuosa L. f.
AREA: Amazonia and central Brazil, in swampy sites known as buritizal or vereda.
NAMES: Buriti, miriti.
USES: Leaves in baths are emollient. The juice from the young stems is considered tonic.

Mauritiella aculeata (Kunth) Burret
AREA: Amazonia, forest.
NAMES: Buritirana, caraná, caranaí, canaiá.
USES: Fruits macerated in water yield a refreshing drink with tonic properties.

Oenocarpus distichus Mart.
AREA: Amazonia, forest.
NAMES: Cacaba, bacabá, bacaba-de-azeite, bacaba-de-óleo.
USES: Oil from fruit mesocarp is emollient.

Orbignya phalerata Mart.
AREA: Amazonia to Piaui and Mato Grosso.
NAMES: Aguaçu, auaçu, babaçu (formerly spelled 'babassu'), baguaçu, coconaiá, coco-pindo-ba.
USES: The oil from the kernels is industrially extracted on a huge scale, for use mainly in the food industry (Ref: AREC 2,3). The starchy powder from the mesocarp is used as a general anti-inflammatory, for menstrual colic, for treating gastric and duodenal ulcers, obesity, nervous exhaustion, anemia, varicose veins, as well as in certain carcinomatous conditions.
PHARM.: The ethanolic extract from the fruits failed to produce significant antitumor activity against transplantable Walker's sarcoma in rats.

ARECACEAE

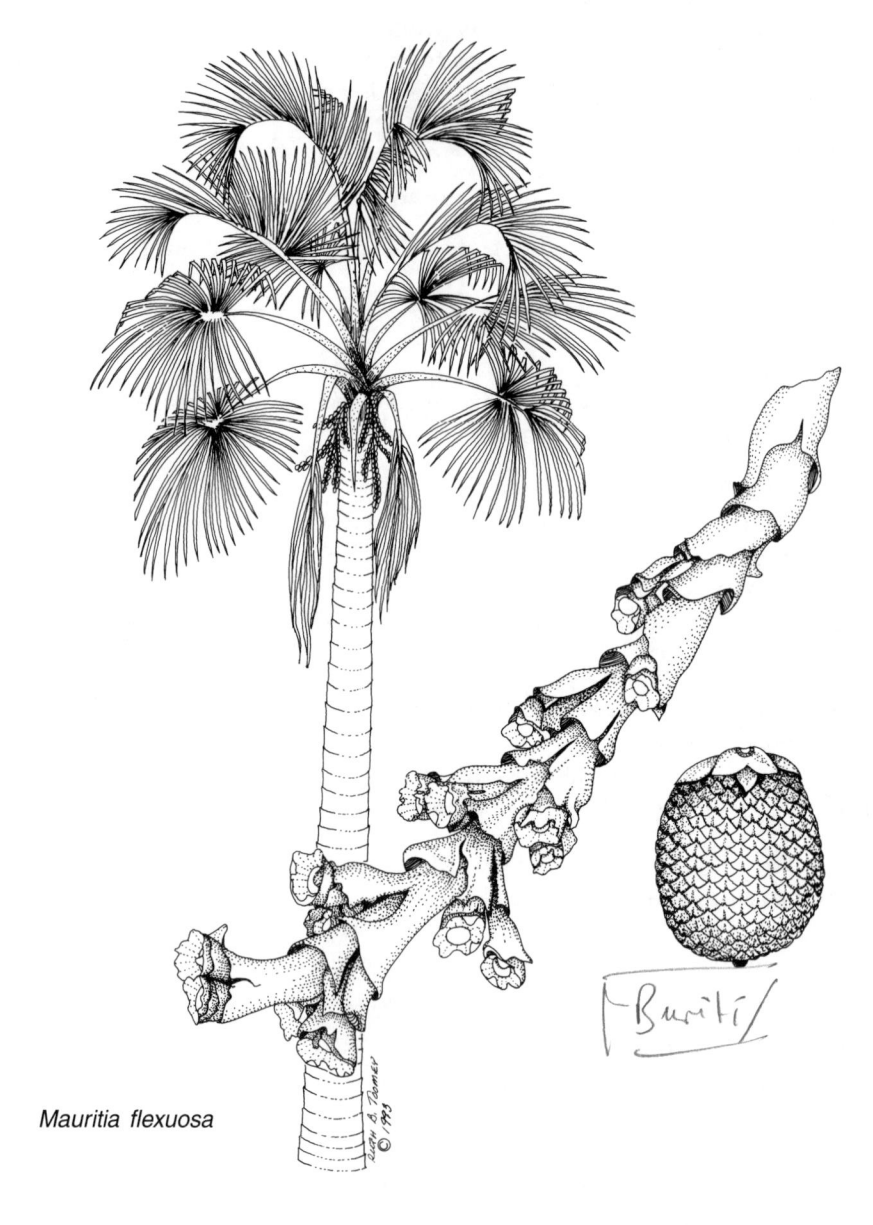

Mauritia flexuosa

However, the same extract demonstrated potent anti-inflammatory activity against carrageenan-induced paw edema in rats, by both oral and intraperitoneal administration (Ref: AREC 4).

Taxonomy of the species complex to which *O. phalerata* belongs is discussed in Ref: AREC 2; see also Notes and Synonyms.

Arecaceae

Raphia taedigera (Mart.) Mart.
AREA: Amazonia, forest.
NAME: Jupati.
USES: Oil from the pulp is used in rubs for gout, rheumatism and paralysis.

Scheelea phalerata (Mart. ex Spreng.) Burret
AREA: Mato Grosso.
NAMES: Acurí, anacuri, coqueiro-naiá, guacurí, naiá, rucurí, bacuri, uacurí.
USES: Liquid endosperm from immature drupes is prescribed for ophthalmia. Kernel oil prescribed for treating baldness.

Syagrus comosa Mart.
AREA: Piauí to Minas Gerais, and west to Bolivia, campo, cerrado and stretches of forest; also in Mato Grosso.
NAMES: Babão, coqueiro-catolé, catolé, guariroba, guariroba-do-campo, palmito amargoso.
USES: Terminal bud is bitter, stomachic. Pulp of the fruit is mucilaginous, diuretic. Roasted kernels are used to check diarrhoea.

Syagrus coronata (Mart.) Becc.
AREA: Pernambuco to northern Minas Gerais.
NAMES: Aricurí, licuri, licurizeiro, urucuri.
USES: Kernel oil is useful to treat wounds caused by sting rays.

Syagrus oleracea (Mart.) Becc.
AREA: Ceará to São Paulo and Mato Grosso.
NAMES: Catolé, coco-babão, coqueiro-amargoso, coco-de-quaresma, coco-guariroba, guariroba, pati, pati-amargosa.
USES: Terminal bud is bitter, tonic, carminative, stomachic; also used to control hysteric symptoms. Fermented mesocarp yields a diuretic beverage (aluá). Oil from kernels serves to invigorate the hair.

Syagrus pseudococos (Raddi) Glassman
AREA: Espirito Santo, Rio de Janeiro and São Paulo, forest.
NAMES: Coco-amargoso, coco-verde, guariroba, palmito-amargoso, pati-amargoso.
USES: Bitter terminal bud, when soaked in water, is prescribed for aiding indigestion.

Syagrus romanzoffiana (Cham.) Glassman
AREA: Bahia to Ri Grande do Sul, littoral and seasonal forest.
NAMES: Baba-de-boi, coco-de-cachorro, coco-de-sapo, coqueiro-de-santacatarina, coqueiro-juvena, jerivá, pindó.
USES: Fruits macerated in wine or made into syrup are reputedly an effective pectoral.

Syagrus schizophylla (Mart.) Glassman
AREA: Pernambuco to northern Espirito Santo, in coastal forest only.
NAMES: Alicurí, aricuri, arirí, urucuri.
USES: Juice of unripe nuts is used to treat ophthalmia.

Arecaceae – References

AREC 1. Plotkin, M.J. & M.J. Balick. 1984. Medicinal uses of South American palms. *J. Ethnopharmacol.* 10: 157-179.

AREC 2. Anderson, A.B. & M.J. Balick. 1988. Taxonomy of the babassu complex (*Orbignya* spp.: Palmae). *Syst. Bot.* 13(1): 32-50.

AREC 3. Anderson, A.B., Overal, W.L. & A. Henderson. 1988. Pollination ecology of a forest-dominant palm (*Orbignya phalerata* Mart.) in northern Brazil. *Biotropica* 20(3): 192-205.

AREC 4. Maia, M.B.S. & V.S. Rao. 1989. Avaliação experimental da atividade antineoplásica e antiinflamatória de *Orbignya phalerata* Mart. (babaçu). *Rev. Bras. Farm.* 70: 21-22.

ARISTOLOCHIACEAE

Most of the *Aristolochia* species so far investigated contain, mainly in the roots, organic nitro-compounds, the aristolochic acids and aristolactams (Ref: ARIS 1,2). Aristolochic acids were shown to be carcinogenic (Ref: ARIS 3) and pharmaceutical preparations containing these compounds, formerly available in Germany, have since been withdrawn from the market. All *Aristolochia* species in Brazil are considered alexipharmic against snake poison. This information will not be repeated under every species name.

Aristolochia birostris Duch.
AREA: Piauí to Bahia, forest.
NAMES: Capivara, jarrinha, mil-homens.
USES: Roots are prescribed especially against rattlesnake poison. Leaves are diaphoretic, anticatarrhal.
CHEM.: Volatile sesquiterpenoids in leaves (Ref: ARIS 4). In contrast to the Old World species, where monoterpenoids predominate in the composition of the essential oils, Brazilian *Aristolochia* species show a preponderance of the sesquiterpenic fraction (Ref: ARIS 4).

Aristolochia cordigera Willd.
AREA: Pará, forest.
NAMES: Angelicó, cipó-do-coração, guaco-bravo.
USES: Roots are emmenagogue, excitant, indicated for typhoid fever and malaria. Leaves are sudorific, used for colds and bronchial asthma.

Aristolochia cymbifera Mart. & Zucc.
AREA: Bahia to Rio Grande do Sul, in forest and coppice.
NAMES: Ambaia-caá, ambaia-embo, caçaú, caçaui, capa-homem, cipó-mata-

ARISTOLOCHIACEAE

Aristolochia cymbifera

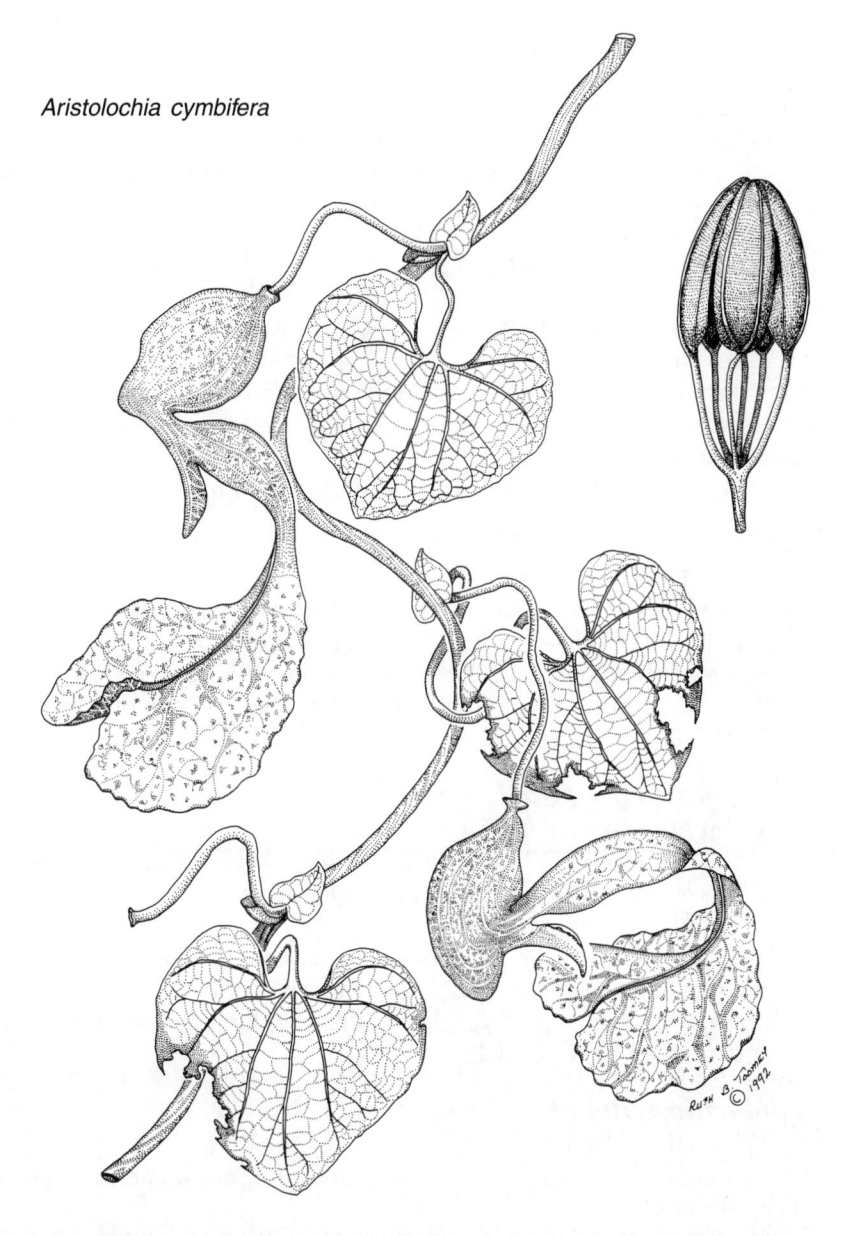

cobras, cipó-paratudo, coifa-do-diabo, jarrinha, jarra-do-diabo, milhome, milhomens, papo-de-galo, papo-de-peru, raiz-de-josé-domingues, touca-do-diabo, umbu-caá.
USES: Given for fever, dyspepsy, heavy diarrhoea, asthma, gout, dropsy, chlorosis, migraine, convulsions, palpitations, flatulence, prurigo, eczema; externally used for sloughing ulcers, arthralgia, dandruff, orchitis.

Aristolochiaceae

CHEM.: Diterpenes in roots and stems (Ref: ARIS 5). Volatile sesquiterpenoids in leaves (Ref: ARIS 4).

Aristolochia elegans Mast.
AREA: Minas Gerais, Rio de Janeiro, São Paulo.
NAMES: Cipó-milhomens, caçaú, jarrinha-pintada, milhome-de-babado, jarrinha, pao-de-peru.
USES: Against snakebite.
CHEM.: Diterpenoids (Ref: ARIS 5).

Aristolochia esperanzae O. Kuntze
AREA: Mato Grosso.
NAMES: Jarrinha, mil-homens, papo-de-peru-do-miudo.
USES: Used as an abortive and against amenorrhoea, malaria, facial neuralgia and scabies.
CHEM.: Lignans and diterpenes in stems (Ref: ARIS 5,6).

Aristolochia gigantea Mart. & Zucc.
AREA: Minas Gerais, São Paulo, Paraná.
NAMES: Milhomens, jarrinha-monstro, milhome, papo-de-peru, papo-de-peru-de-babado, papo-de-peru-do-grande, urubu-caá.
USES: Same as the other *Aristolochia* species in general.
CHEM.: Volatile sesquiterpenoids in leaves (Ref: ARIS 4). Alkaloids in leaves (Ref: ARIS 7). Antimicrobial properties (Ref: ARIS 4,8).

Aristolochia triangularis Cham.
AREA: Mainly Rio Grande do Sul.
NAMES: Caçaú, cipó-mil-homens, mil-homens-do-rio-grande-do-sul, jarrinha-concha, jarrinha-triangular, cipó-jarrinha.
USES: Internally for hysteria, poisoning, dropsy, cystitis, malaria, intestinal worms; externally for skin disease, ulcers; in baths against orchitis, as an emmenagogue, stimulant, tonic, and diuretic.
CHEM.: Sesquiterpenes and diterpenes, steroids, lignans and neolignans in roots and stems (Ref: ARIS 9).

Aristolochia trilobata L.
AREA: Amazonia to Bahia, forest.
NAMES: Angelicó, calunga, capa-homem, jarrinha, mil-homens, papo-de-peru, umbu-caá.
USES: Roots are bitter, tonic, excitant, stimulant, stomachic, antiseptic, sudorific, diuretic, antifebrile, abortive, antidiarrhoeic, and antihysteric. Leaves are recommended for gastralgia, chronic ulcers, dandruff and orchitis.

ARISTOLOCHIACEAE

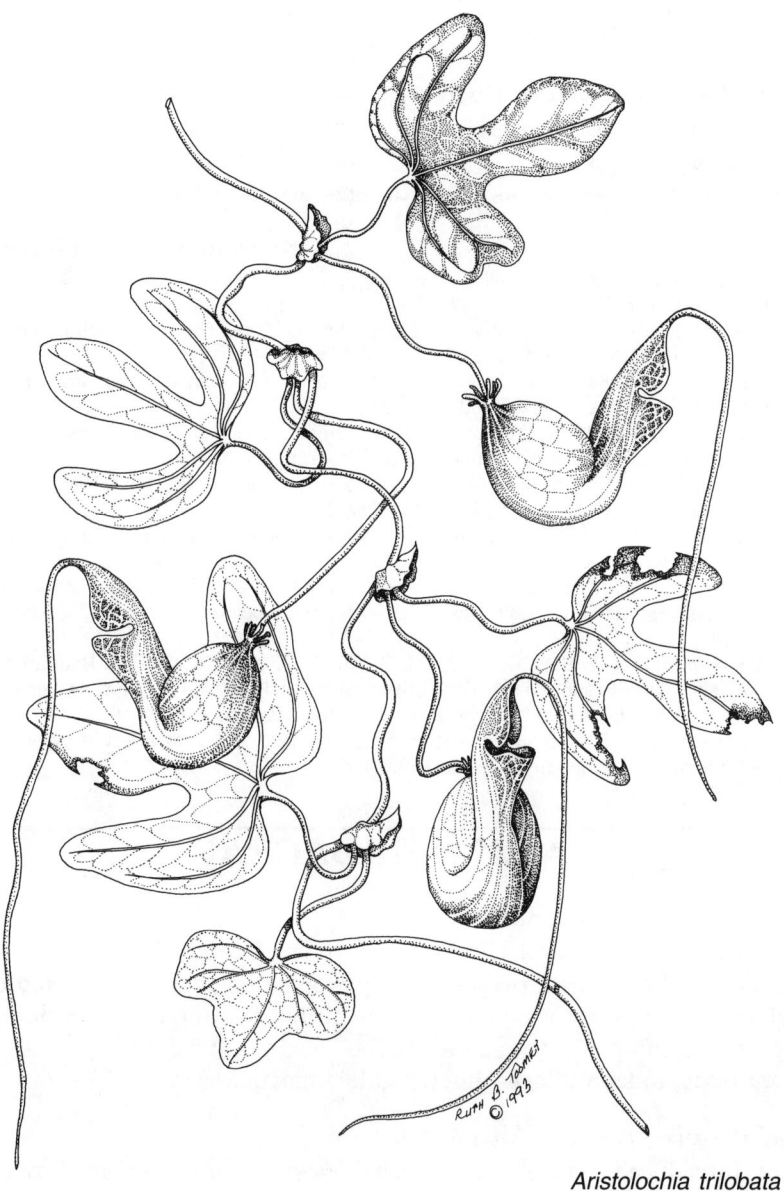

Aristolochia trilobata

Aristolochia spp.
The following additional *Aristolochia* species, among others less referred to, are frequently pointed out by the people as medicinal: *A. allemanii* Hoehne (Ceará), *A. amazonica* Ule (Amazonia), *A. arcuata* Mast. (Minas Gerais to Rio de Janeiro and Mato Grosso), *A. barbata* Jacq. (Amazonia),

A. *burchellii* Mast. (São Paulo), *A. maxima* Jacq. (Amazonia to São Paulo) and *A. sipho* L'Her. (introduced from the United States).

Holostylis reniformis Duch.
AREA: Goiás and Mato Grosso.
NAME: Flor-de-sapo.
USES: The same as those ascribed to other *Aristolochia* species.

Aristolochiaceae – References
ARIS 1. Pailer, M. 1960. Natürlich vorkommende Nitroverbindungen. *In*: L. Zechmeister, ed., *Progr. Chem. Org. Nat. Prod. 18*: 55-82.
ARIS 2. Mix, D.B., H. Guinaudeau & M. Shamma. 1982. The aristolochic acids and aristolactams. *J. Nat. Prod. 45*: 657-666.
ARIS 3. Mengs, U. 1983. On the histopathogenesis of rat forestomach carcinoma caused by aristolochic acid. *Arch. Toxicol. 52*: 209-220.
ARIS 4. Leitão, G.G. 1989. Química e farmacologia de espécies brasileiras do gênero *Aristolochia*. Thesis, Federal University of Rio de Janeiro.
ARIS 5. Lopes, L.M.X., V.S. Bolzani & L.M.V. Trevisan. 1987. Clerodane diterpenes from *Aristolochia* species. *Phytochemistry 26*: 2781-2784.
ARIS 6. Lopes, L.M.X. & V.S. Bolzani. 1988. Lignans and diterpenes of three *Aristolochia* species. *Phytochemistry 27*: 2265-2268.
ARIS 7. Cortes, D., H. Dadoun, R.L.R. Paiva & A.B. Oliveira. 1987. Nouveaux alcaloïdes bis-benzylisoquinoleiques isolés des feuilles de *Aristolochia gigantea*. *J. Nat. Prod. 50*: 910-914.
ARIS 8. Nunan, E.A., L.M.M. Campos, R.L.R. Paiva, S.T. de Oliveira, H.A. Dadoun & A.B. de Oliveira. 1985. Estudo da atividade antimicrobiana de extrato de folhas de *Aristolochia gigantea* Mart. et Zucc. *Rev. Farm. Bioquím.* (Belo Horizonte) *6*: 33-40.
ARIS 9. Rücker, G., B. Langmann & N.S. Siqueira. 1981. Inhaltsstoffe von *Aristolochia triangularis*. *Planta Medica 41*: 143-149.

ASCLEPIADACEAE

Araujia sericifera Brot.
AREA: Rio de Janeiro and Minas Gerais to Rio Grande do Sul.
NAMES: Angélica-de-rama, cipó-de-parque, cipó-de-rama, cipó-de-sapo, cipó-de-seda, cipó-ramo, cipó-seda, cipozinho-do-campo, paina-de-seda, paina-do-campo, seda-vegetal, timbó.
USES: Toxic; in small doses emetic; galactagogue.

Calotropis procera (Ait.) Ait. f.
AREA: Introduced from tropical Africa, now subspontaneous in Brazil as a ruderal plant, mostly from the Northeast to Minas Gerais.
NAMES: Ciúme, flor-de-seda, hortênsia.
USES: Decoction of the leaves used for rheumatism and as a tranquilizer. The latex is a powerful depilatory and also used as an odontalgic. The root-bark is considered tonic and stimulant.
CHEM. & PHARM.: The latex contains cardioactive glycosides, calotropin be-

ing the major one (Ref: ASCL 1). However, the chemical as well as the pharmacological studies with respect to these constituents (Ref: ASCL 2,3) have all been performed on Old World material (India, tropical Africa), whereas in the plants grown in Brazil the cardioactive components seem to be absent (Ref: ASCL 4,5). The latex is strongly proteolytic (Ref: ASCL 6). Anti-inflammatory and analgesic activity of the root extract has been reported (Ref: ASCL 7).

Marsdenia amylacea (Barb.-Rodr.) Malme
AREA: Amazonia (Marajó Island).
NAMES: Cumacaá, cumaná, cumacá, camucá.
USES: The tuberous root has a destructive effect on recently formed tissue, finding popular use in the removal of pterygium. Its starch is considered useful in the treatment of wounds and ulcers, including those caused by tegumentary leishmaniasis. Tea from the leaves is laxative.

Asclepiadaceae – References

ASCL 1. Crout, D.H.G., C.H. Hassal & T.L. Jones. 1964. Cardenolides. Part IV. Uscharidin, calotropin, and calotoxin. *J. Chem. Soc.*: 2187-2194.

ASCL 2. Chen, K.K., C.I. Bliss & E.B. Robbins. 1942. The digitalis-like principles of *Calotropis* compared with other cardiac substances. *J. Pharmacol. Exp. Therap.* 74: 223-234.

ASCL 3. Patel, M.B. & M. Rowson. 1964. Investigations of certain Nigerian medicinal plants. Part I. Preliminary pharmacological and phytochemical screenings for cardiac activity. *Planta Medica* 12: 34-42.

ASCL 4. Matos, F.J. de A. (Ceará) & N.A. Pereira (Rio de Janeiro), independent unpublished observations (personal communications).

ASCL 5. Canella, C.F.C., C.H. Tokarnia & J. Döbereiner. 1966. Experimentos com plantas tidas como tóxicas realizados em bovinos do nordeste do Brasil, com resultados negativos. *Pesquisa Agropecuária Brasileira* 1: 345-352.

ASCL 6. Atal, C.K. & P.D. Sethi. 1962. Proteolytic activity of some Indian plants. II. Isolation, properties and kinetic studies of calotropin. *Planta Medica* 10: 77-90.

ASCL 7. Basu, A. & A.K. Nag Chaudhuri. 1991. Preliminary studies on the anti-inflammatory and analgesic activities of *Calotropis procera* root extract. *J. Ethnopharmacol.* 31: 319-324.

ASTERACEAE

Acanthospermum australe (Loefl.) O. Ktze.
AREA: Widespread in Brazil, ruderal; prefers sandy tracts in the coastal region.
NAMES: Amor-de-negro, carrapicho-rasteiro, erva-mijona, erva-mineira, espinho-de-agulha, espinho-decarneiro, mata-pasto, picão-da-praia, poejo-da-praia.
USES: Leaves are mucilaginous, bitter, tonic, diaphoretic, anti-blennorrhagic, antidiarrhoeic, antimalarial; also used for erysipelas, anemia and diseases of the urinary system.

Asteraceae

CHEM.: Aerial parts contain numerous sesquiterpene and diterpene lactones (Ref: ASTE 1,2,3).
PHARM.: Flavonoid with lens aldolase inhibiting activity has been isolated (Ref: ASTE 4). Crude extracts tested in mice infected with *Plasmodium berghei* and tested *in vitro* against *P. falciparum* were shown to be partly active (Ref: ASTE 5).

Acanthospermum hispidum DC.
AREA: In all of Brazil, ruderal, but most frequent on sandy littoral.
NAMES: Amor-de-negro, carrapicho, maroto, retirante.
USES: Roots are indicated for cough, bronchitis, diarrhoea and liver disorders. Leaves are bitter, mucilaginous, pectoral, tonic, antifebrile, sudorific. Mixed with erva-tostão (*Boerhavia hirsuta*, Nyctaginaceae) and recommended as an aphrodisiac.
CHEM.: Roots contain one polyacetylene and four monoterpenes (Ref: ASTE 6). Sesquiterpene lactones have been described from the aerial parts (Ref: ASTE 1,6).

Achyrocline satureioides (Lam.) DC.
AREA: Common from Minas Gerais to Rio Grande do Sul.
NAMES: Macela, macela-do-campo, marcela, marcela-da-mata.
USES: Aerial parts furnish a tea which is aromatic, bitter, stomachic, antidysenteric, useful for indigestion and gastritis.
CHEM.: Plant contains essential oil with alpha- and beta-pinene (Ref: ASTE 7), flavonoids and other phenolics (Ref: ASTE 8,9,10) and one kawa-type pyrone (Ref: ASTE 11).
PHARM.: Anti-inflammatory and antispasmodic activity have been demonstrated (Ref: ASTE 12,13,14). Also contains polysaccharides with immune-stimulating action (Ref: ASTE 15,16).

Acmella oleracea (L.) R.K. Jansen
AREA: Amazonia to southern Brazil.
NAME: Agrião-do-pará.
USES: The same as for *A. repens*.
CHEM.: The substance responsible for the numbing effect of these plants is an isobutyl amide, spilanthol (Ref: ASTE 105).
PHARM.: The action of spilanthol on the electrical acitivity of the isolated rabbit heart has been studied. The compound could be used to generate arrhythmias in cardiologic research (Ref: ASTE 106,107). Intraperitoneal injection of the hexane extract in rats induced convulsions, suggesting a tool for new models of epilepsy (Ref: ASTE 108).

Acmella repens (Walt.) L.C. Rich.
AREA: Amazonia to Rio de Janeiro, in moist places.
NAMES: Abecedária, agrião-bravo, agrião-do-Brasil, agrião-do-pará, botão-

de-ouro, jambu, mambu-açu, mastruço, pimenta d'água.
USES: Employed for mouth and throat ailments, vesical lithiasis and pulmonary tuberculosis. Leaves and flowers when chewed have a numbing effect on the mucous membranes of the mouth and are thus used against toothache. Also used as a stimulant and appetizer. In Pará the herb is an obligatory condiment in some regional dishes.

Ageratum conyzoides L.
AREA: Ruderal throughout Brazil; cosmopolitan.
NAMES: Catinga-de-barrão, catinga-de-bode, erva-de-são-joão, maria-preta, mentrasto.
USES: Plant is aromatic, bitter, antirheumatic, antidiarrhoeic, febrifuge, carminative, tonic, utilized for curing colds; also against intestinal and uterine colics, amenorrhoea, gonorrhoea, bladder catarrh and for the healing of wounds.
CHEM.: The essential oil from the leaves has been studied, containing chromene derivatives among other compounds (Ref: ASTE 17,18,19). Flavonoids are also present (Ref: ASTE 20,21,22). Ageratochromene is one of the "precocenes," later found in other *Ageratum* species (Ref: ASTE 23). Pyrrolizidine alkaloids have been isolated (Ref: ASTE 24).
PHARM.: The precocenes are compounds which induce early larval stages of insects to develop into precocious adultoids (Ref: ASTE 25). The leaves have also been shown to exhibit antibacterial activity against *Staphylococcus aureus*, *in vitro* (Ref: ASTE 26).

Ambrosia artemisiifolia L.
AREA: Amazonas to Rio Grande do Sul, ruderal.
NAME: Ambrosia.
USES: Leaves with flowering summits are aromatic, tonic, employed against leucorrhoea, fever, intestinal worms. Fumigations induce menstruation.

Ayapana triplinerve (Vahl) King & H. Robinson
AREA: Amazonia.
NAMES: Aiapana, iapana, japana, japana-branca.
USES: The expressed juice and infusion of the whole plant are tonic, stimulant, astringent; antidysenteric and sudorific; for cough and inflamed throat. Externally for curing gingivitis and aphthae. Leaf juice is a cicatrizant and highly reputed against snakebite.
CHEM.: Two coumarins were isolated and shown to have pronounced haemostatic action (Ref: ASTE 82,83).

Baccharidastrum triplinerve (Less.) Cabr.
AREA: Minas Gerais and Mato Grosso to Rio Grande do Sul.
NAMES: Erva-de-santo-antônio, erva-santa.

Asteraceae

USES: Contused leaves hasten the healing of chronic skin ulcers.

Baccharis articulata (Lam.) Pers.
AREA: São Paulo to Rio Grande do Sul, campo.
NAMES: Carqueja-doce, carquejinha, carqueja-do-morro, carqueja-miúda.
USES: Bitter, digestive, tonic, antipyretic, diuretic, useful for dyspepsy, weakness, anemia, cholera morbus. Replaces wormwood (*Artemisia absinthium*, "losna" in Brazil) in veterinary medicine, in the treatment of cattle diarrhoea.
CHEM.: Diterpenes are found in the whole plant (Ref: ASTE 27) and in flowers (Ref: ASTE 28). The essential oil has been analyzed in comparison with that of *B. trimera* (Ref: ASTE 29).

Baccharis dentata (Vell.) G.M. Barroso
AREA: Goiás to São Paulo, campo.
NAMES: Alecrim-do-campo, alecrim-do-mato.
USES: Anticatarrhal and antirheumatic.

Baccharis dracunculifolia DC.
AREA: Central Brazil, Ceará and Marajó, campo.
NAMES: Alecrim-do-campo, vassoura, vassourinha.
USES: Tonic, eupeptic, febrifuge and antidyspeptic.
PHARM.: Slight toxic effects have been reported in cattle (Ref: ASTE 30).

Baccharis lundii DC.
AREA: Bahia to Rio Grande do Sul, on the banks of rivers and lakes.
NAME: Carqueja.
USES: Prescribed to wash and cure ulcers.

Baccharis notosergila Gris.
AREA: Rio Grande do Sul.
NAME: Carqueja.
USES: Flowering tips are used for diarrhoea and liver congestion; in baths for alleviating leprosy and muscular rheumatism.
PHARM.: Antimicrobial activity has been verified (Ref: ASTE 31).

Baccharis ramosissima Gardn.
AREA: Campos and cerrados of central and southern Brazil.
NAME: Alecrim-do-campo.
USES: Fumes from burning shrub repel and kill mosquitos.
CHEM.: Diterpenes have been described (Ref: ASTE 32).

Baccharis trimera (Less.) DC.
AREA: Throughout Brazil.
NAMES: Cacália-amarga, carqueja, carqueja-amargosa, vassoura.

ASTERACEAE

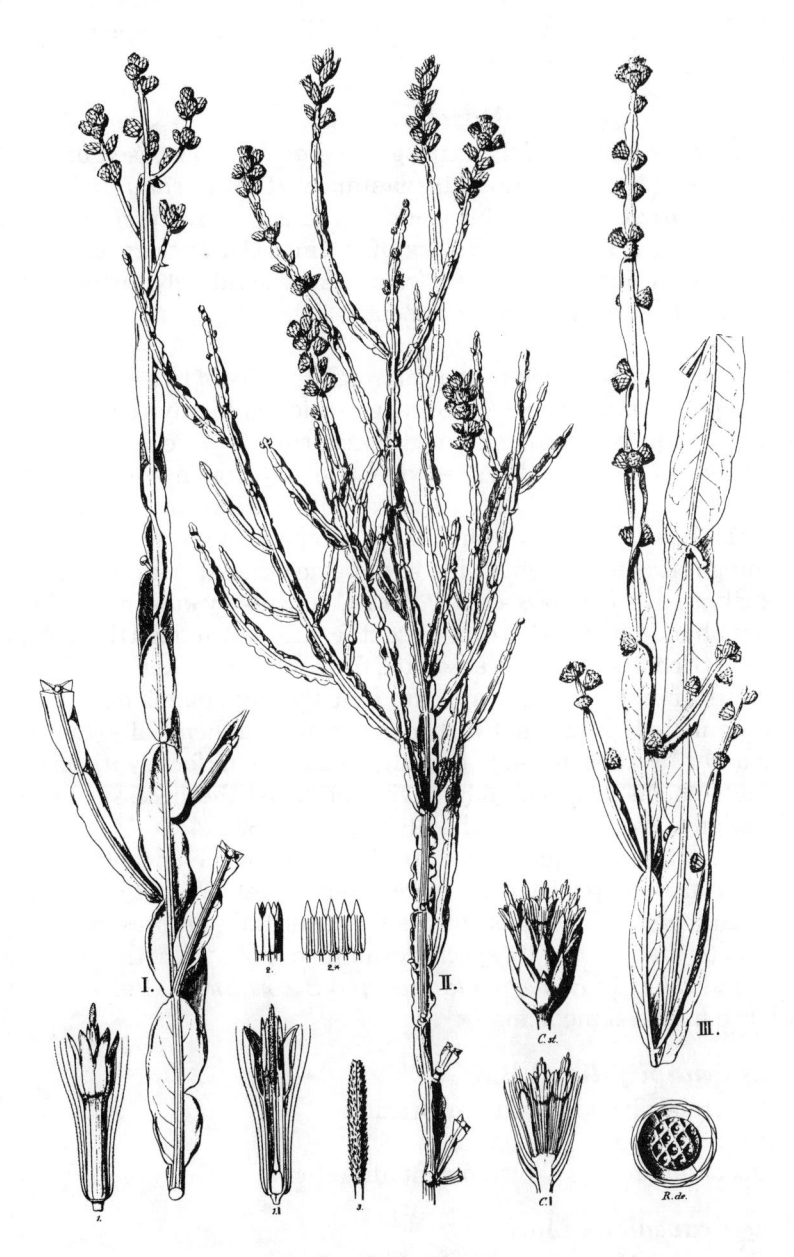

Baccharis trimera

USES: Tonic, stomachic, antirheumatic, antipyretic, anthelmintic; recommended for liver ailments, diabetes, leprosy and bleeding ulcers. The

ASTERACEAE

plant is being extensively used in the form of health teas, for slimming.
CHEM.: The plant is extremely rich in terpenoids, both volatile (Ref: ASTE 29,33,34,35,36) and non-volatile (Ref: ASTE 37,38,39). Flavonoids are also present (Ref: ASTE 40).

Baccharis spp.

Several other species of the large genus *Baccharis* are used under the general name of carqueja, as, for instance: *B. gaudichaudii* DC. (Rio Grande do Sul), *B. ochracea* Spr. (southern Brazil), *B. stenocephala* Baker (São Paulo) and *B. tarchonanthoides* DC. (Minas Gerais to Paraná). Popular uses are in majority derived from their exceedingly bitter taste, a quality which always suggests eupeptic, digestive, tonic and febrifuge properties.

Attention must be called to the very high toxicity of two species of this genus. From *B. megapotamica* Spreng., which is highly toxic to cattle, four macrocyclic compounds named baccharinoids were isolated. These were shown to be trichothecenes, a type of mycotoxin which until the 1970s had been observed only as metabolites of certain soil fungi (Ref: ASTE 41). It was suggested that these compounds are in fact plant-altered fungal products (Ref: ASTE 41,42). The other species notorious for its toxicity to livestock is *B. coridifolia* DC., popularly known as mio-mio. It occurs abundantly in pastures in southern Brazil and northern Argentina. Nine trichothecenes were isolated from this plant (Ref: ASTE 43,44). In this instance, however, it appears that the mycotoxins are absorbed and accumulated by the plant without being altered chemically (Ref: ASTE 44). Another hypothesis holds that the toxins are in fact synthesized by the plants themselves, possibly having acquired the necessary genetic information by transfer from the fungus (Ref: ASTE 45).

It appears that the question as to the origin of the trichothecenes in *Baccharis* has not yet been answered conclusively. With respect to the use of a number of *Baccharis* species for medicinal purposes, it is important to note that, among 21 species examined, toxic trichothecenes have been found solely in *B. megapotamica* and *B. coridifolia* (Ref: ASTE 46), which are not used medicinally.

Bidens cynapiifolia H.B.K.
AREA: Pantropical; widespread in Brazil.
NAMES: Carrapicho-de-agulha.
USES: Roots and leaves are resolvent, diuretic.

Bidens graveolens Mart.
AREA: Goiás and Minas Gerais, campo.
NAME: Picão.
USES: Plant is sour, antiscorbutic; bruised and applied to sloughing ulcers.

CHEM.: Acetylenic compounds have been identified (Ref: ASTE 47).

Bidens pilosa L.
AREA: Throughout Brazil as ruderal; cosmopolitan.
NAMES: Carrapicho, carrapicho-de-agulha, carrapicho-de-duas-pontas, cuambu, erva-picão, fura-capa, goambu, macela-do-campo, picão, picão-do-campo, picão-preto, piolho-de-padre.
USES: Bitter, mucilaginous, stimulant, antiscorbutic, antiodontalgic, sialagogue, antidysenteric, antidiabetic, antileucorrhoeic, anthelmintic, vulnerary; juice taken against jaundice; tea for sore throat, respiratory problems and hepatitis; also for stopping excessive milk production after childbirth and to aid healing of malignant sores.
CHEM. & PHARM.: Polyacetylenes and thiophene derivatives were identified (Ref: ASTE 48,49). Phenylheptatriyne was shown to have antibiotic and cytotoxic properties through photosensitization (Ref: ASTE 50,51). The compounds also proved to be antiparasitic (Ref: ASTE 52,53).

Blanchetia heterotricha DC.
AREA: Bahia.
NAMES: Erva-preá, maria-preta.
USES: Diaphoretic, antifebrile, emollient and vulnerary.

Calea pinnatifida (R. Br.) Less.
AREA: Rio de Janeiro to Rio Grande do Sul, forest.
NAMES: Aruca, erva-de-lagarto, guaçatonga, jasmim-do-mato, mata-paca, pau-de-lagarto.
USES: Bitter and astringent; flowering summits and leaves are used against amoebae; also used to combat stomach troubles and to treat bruises and cuts.
CHEM.: Sesquiterpene lactones and other compounds have been identified (Ref: ASTE 54).

Chaptalia nutans (L.) Polak.
AREA: Ruderal in eastern and southern Brazil.
NAMES: Costa-branca, lingua-de-vaca.
USES: Roots and leaves employed against jaundice and gastric ailments; externally applied for dressing ulcers. The heated leaves are placed on the forehead against headache; decoction for cleaning sores. Internally, the plant serves as a tonic, stimulant and bechic. Root tea for pulmonary diseases, skin problems, syphilis and gonorrhoea.
CHEM.: The plant is strongly cyanogenic (Ref: ASTE 55).

Chionolaena latifolia (Benth.) Baker
AREA: Minas Gerais, campo; Rio de Janeiro.
NAME: Arnica-do-campo.

ASTERACEAE

USES: Indicated as a substitute for the European arnica.

Chromolaena hirsuta (Hook. & Arn.) King & H. Robinson
AREA: São Paulo to Rio Grande do Sul, sandy or stony campos.
NAMES: Charrua, erva-de-charrua.
USES: Leaf infusion applied externally for suppurated eyes, ophthalmia, and in gargles for throat disorders.

Chromolaena laevigata (Lam.) King & H. Robinson
AREA: Minas Gerais to Rio Grande do Sul, cerrado and campo.
NAMES: Camará, cambará.
USES: Leaves employed for curing malignant ulcers.
CHEM.: The essential oil contains a furanoid sesquiterpene (Ref: ASTE 81).

Clibadium leiocarpum Mart.
AREA: Amazonia.
NAME: Barbasco.
USES: A narcotic herb.

Clibadium rotundifolium DC.
AREA: Southern Brazil.
NAME: Limpa-viola.
USES: Leaves and flowers for erysipelas.

Clibadium surinamense L.
AREA: Amazonia.
NAMES: Conabi, conambi.
USES: Bitter tonic, used for anemia and chlorosis. Leaves used for erysipelas and applied as a wash for skin diseases in general.
The plant is a powerful fish poison.
CHEM.: Contains acetylenic constituents (tetrahydropyranes), as do many other species of the genus (Ref: ASTE 56).

Conocliniopsis prasiifolia (DC.) King & H. Robinson
AREA: Pará to Bahia.
NAMES: Maria-preta, maria-preta-verdadeira.
USES: Excitant, emollient and against snakebite.

Conyza blakei (Cabr.) Cabr.
AREA: Along the seacoast.
NAMES: Erva-lanceta.
USES: Stimulant and emmenagogue.

Cyrtocymura scorpioides (Lam.) H. Robinson
AREA: Throughout Brazil as a ruderal.

NAMES: Assa-peixe, erva-preá.
USES: As decoctions in baths or as lotion for healing erysipelas and rheumatism.
CHEM. & PHARM.: Contains strongly tumor inhibiting sesquiterpene lactones (Ref: ASTE 113).

Eclipta prostrata (L.) L.
AREA: Brazil, ruderal.
NAMES: Agrião-do-brejo, erva-botão, erva-de-botão, surucuina.
USES: Antiasthmatic, pectoral, antiophidic; used against hair loss.
CHEM.: A thiophene derivative, flavonoids, steroids and triterpenoids have been identified (Ref: ASTE 57,58,59,60,61).
PHARM.: Hepato-protective activity has been verified, coumestans being the main active constituents (Ref: ASTE 62). Anti-snake venom activity has been confirmed, with wedelolactone (a coumestan), sitosterol and stigmasterol as the main active compounds (Ref: ASTE 63,64).

Egletes viscosa (L.) Less.
AREA: From Paraiba to Minas Gerais, campos and caatinga.
NAMES: Losna-do-mato, macela-da-terra, macela-do-sertão.
USES: Bitter, stomachic, antidiarrhoeic, emmenagogue.
CHEM. & PHARM.: Diterpene and flavonoids have been isolated (Ref: ASTE 65,66,70). The spasmolytic action of the flower extract and its constituents on cardiac and skeletal muscle has been studied (Ref: ASTE 67,68). Ternatin, a flavonoid isolated from the plant, showed strong anti-inflammatory activity (Ref: ASTE 69). The same compound (isolated from other sources) revealed antiviral properties (Ref: ASTE 71).

Elephantopus micropappus Less.
AREA: Minas Gerais and São Paulo, campo.
NAME: Suçuaiá.
USES: Leaves are diaphoretic and febrifuge.

Elephantopus mollis H.B.K.
AREA: Cosmopolitan, ruderal in Brazil.
NAMES: Erva-colégio, erva-de-colégio, erva-grossa, fumo-bravo, fumo-da-mata, lingua-de-vaca, pé-de-elefante, suçuaiá, suaçucaá, tapirapecu.
USES: Roots are tonic, diuretic, emmenagogue, antipyretic; also for herpes and to eliminate kidney stones. Leaves emollient, resolvent, sudorific, antitussive, antisyphilitic, antirheumatic and against snakebite; also reputedly useful for gastralgia, common cold and itches.
CHEM.: Flavonoids (Ref: ASTE 72) and triterpenes (Ref: ASTE 73) have been isolated. The plant is particularly rich in sesquiterpene lactones, some of which were shown to have cytotoxic and antitumor properties (Ref: ASTE 74,75,76,77,78,79,80).

ASTERACEAE

Erigeron tweediei Hook. & Arn.
AREA: Minas Gerais to Rio Grande do Sul, in swampy terrain.
NAME: Mal-me-quer-do-pântano.
USE: Vulnerary.

Flaveria bidentis (L.) Ktze.
AREA: Rio Grande do Sul, along humid river banks.
NAME: Contra-erva-do-Peru.
USES: Vermifuge and alexipharmic.

Galinsoga parviflora Cav.
AREA: Neotropical; ruderal in Brazil.
NAMES: Fazendaeiro, picão-branco.
USES: Vulnerary, aromatic, excitant.

Gochnatia polymorpha (Less.) Cabr.
AREA: Bahia to Rio Grande do Sul and Mato Grosso.
NAMES: Cambará-de-folha-grande, cambará-do-mato.
USES: Leaves for bronchopulmonary diseases.

Grindelia buphthalmoides DC.
AREA: Rio Grande do Sul.
NAMES: Girassol-do-mato, malmequer.
USES: Excitant, stomachic, emmenagogue.

Grindelia scorzonerifolia Hook. & Arn.
AREA: Rio Grande do Sul.
NAME: Malmequer.
USES: Digestive stimulant, emmenagogue, vulnerary.

Heterothalamus alienus (Spr.) O. Ktze.
AREA: Rio de Janeiro to Rio Grande do Sul.
NAMES: Alecrim-do-campo, arnica-da-serra.
USES: Aromatic, excitant, febrifuge, restorative. As such, it is used as a substitute for the European arnica and rosemary.

Heterothalamus psiadioides Less.
AREA: Southern Brazil.
NAMES: Alecrim-do-campo, coralina, erva-formiga.
USES: Antipyretic, anti-inflammatory and used against snakebite.
CHEM.: The flavone pinostrobin and flavonol galangin were isolated from the leaves and flowering summits. The essential oil contains monoterpenes and coumarins (Ref: ASTE 84).

Ichthyothere terminalis (Spr.) S.F. Blake
AREA: Amazonia, forest.
NAMES: Conabi, cunabi, cunambi.
USES: Juice applied on ulcers. Plant is a powerful fish poison. Ingested in the form of bait, it makes the fish jump out of the water.
CHEM.: The active constituent is an acetylenic compound, ichthyothereol (Ref: ASTE 85).

Isostigma megapotamicum (Spr.) Sherff
AREA: Minas Gerais to Mato Grosso and Rio Grande do Sul, campo.
NAME: Cravo-do-campo.
USES: Tuberous root is purgative.

Jungia floribunda Less.
AREA: Minas Gerais and Rio de Janeiro to Rio Grande do Sul, campo.
NAME: Arnica.
USE: Useful for dressing wounds.

Lucilia nitens Less.
AREA: São Paulo, Parana, Santa Catarina.
NAME: Vira-vira.
USE: To check children's diarrhoea.

Melampodium divaricatum (Rich.) DC.
AREA: Minas Gerais and São Paulo, campo.
NAME: Picão-da-praia.
USES: Aromatic, diaphoretic, diuretic, bitter; for leucorrhoea.

Mikania cordifolia (L. f.) Willd.
AREA: Throughout Brazil, particularly near beaches and on flooded tracts.
NAMES: Coração-de-Jesus, erva-de-cobra, erva-de-sapo, guaco, uaco.
USES: Aerial parts used against rheumatism and snakebite. Fresh flowers taken for intestinal troubles, menstrual colics and hysteria.
CHEM.: Eight sesquiterpenes (Ref: ASTE 86), quercetin glucoside, linalool glucoside and 3,5-dicaffeoylquinic acid (Ref: ASTE 87) have been isolated.

Mikania glomerata Spreng.
AREA: Southern campos.
NAME: Guaco.
USES: Bechic, expectorant, bronchodilating, bactericide, analgesic, antifebrile, anti-inflammatory and used against snakebite.
PHARM.: Relaxing effect on the tracheo-bronchic musculature has been demonstrated (Ref: ASTE 88).

ASTERACEAE

Mikania hirsutissima DC.
AREA: Bahia to São Paulo.
NAMES: Cipó-cabeludo, erva-dutra, guaco.
USES: Indicated for albuminuria, chronic diarrhoea, paralyses, rheumatism, nephritis, excess uric acid and intercostal neuralgia.
CHEM.: Flavonols and one triterpene acid have been isolated (Ref: ASTE 89).

Mikania lindleyana DC.
AREA: Amazonia.
NAME: Sucuriju.
USES: Leaves are antiphlogistic, rubefacient, prescribed for several dermatoses, chronic ulcers and hepatitis.

Mikania officinalis Mart.
AREA: Throughout Brazil.
NAMES: Coração-de-Jesus, guaco-da-serra.
USES: Aromatic, bitter, antipyretic, tonic, antidyspeptic, alexipharmic to snake poison, for oedema in the lower limbs and abdominal troubles.
CHEM.: Diterpenes have been identified (Ref: ASTE 90).

Mikania parviflora (Aubl.) Karst.
AREA: Native to Amazonia, but naturalized in various parts of the country.
NAMES: Cipó-catinga, guaco.
USES: Plant decoction recommended for malarial fevers, coughs, whooping cough, rheumatism, gout, syphilis, hydrophobia, cholera morbus, snakebite, scorpion sting and intestinal worms; externally applied for cleaning wounds and ulcers.

Mikania periplocifolia Hook. & Arn.
AREA: Throughout Brazil, in moist locations.
NAMES: Falso-guaco, guaco, guaco-de-quintal, guaco-verdadeiro.
USES: For afflictions of the respiratory tract.

Mikania setigera Schultz-Bip. ex Baker
AREA: Southern Brazil.
NAMES: Cipó-cabeludo, guaco.
USES: Strong diuretic and antialbuminuric, recommended especially for nephritis.

Noticastrum diffusum (Pers.) Cabr.
AREA: Rio Grande do Sul and Santa Catarina.
NAME: Mal-me-quer.
USE: Stimulant of the digestive tract.

ASTERACEAE

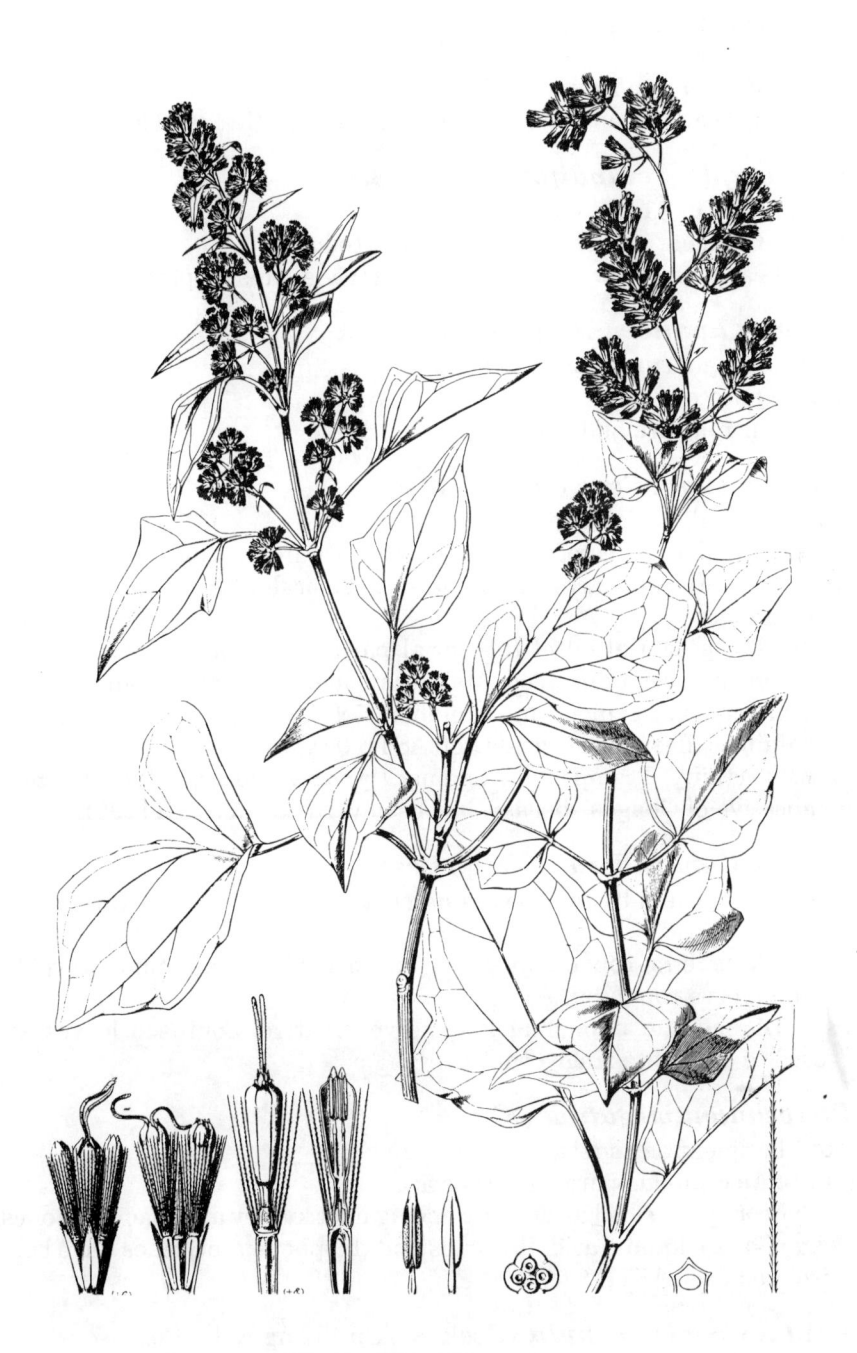

Mikania glomerata

ASTERACEAE

Parthenium hysterophorus L.
AREA: Southern Brazil, ruderal.
NAME: Vilanova.
USES: Emollient and resolvent.
CHEM.: A sesquiterpene lactone has been isolated (Ref: ASTE 91).

Piptocarpha rotundifolia (Less.) Bak.
AREA: Bahia to São Paulo, cerrado.
NAMES: Candeia, infalível, macieira, paratudo.
USES: Leaves and flowers reputedly effective against syphilis.

Pluchea laxiflora Hook. & Arn.
AREA: São Paulo and Rio de Janeiro.
NAME: Quitoco.
USES: Carminative and calmative.

Pluchea suaveolens (Vell.) O. Ktze.
AREA: Throughout Brazil, ruderal.
NAMES: Caculucage, estoraque, mandecravo, quitoco, tabacarana.
USES: Aromatic, stomachic, carminative, pectoral; also abortifacient and vermifuge.
CHEM.: The essential oil of the aerial parts of the plant, including the flowers, has been analyzed. Main components are alpha-pinene, camphene, cineol, p-cymene and camphor (Ref: ASTE 92,93). The plant also contains caffeoylquinic acid (Ref: ASTE 94).
PHARM.: Activity of components against *Trypanosoma cruzi*, the protozoan causative of Chagas' disease, has been verified (Ref: ASTE 95).

Porophyllum ruderale (Jacq.) Cass.
AREA: As indicated by the species name, the plant is ruderal throughout Brazil.
NAMES: Avoadeira, couve-cravinho, couve-de-vedado, couvinha, cravo-de-urubu, erva-couvinha.
USES: Diaphoretic, emmenagogue, nerve sedative. Contused leaves are used to eliminate ringworm.

Pterocaulon virgatum DC.
AREA: Frequent as ruderal.
NAMES: Alecrim-das-paredes, barbasco.
USES: Roots prescribed as diuretic and against kidney and bladder stones.
CHEM.: Caffeoylquinic acid, flavonols and thiophene acetylenes have been isolated (Ref: ASTE 94,96).

Raulinoreitzia tremula (Hook. & Arn.) King & H. Robinson
AREA: Piauí to Paranà and Mato Grosso, campos.

NAMES: Chilca, perna-de-saracura, vassoura-de-ferro.
USES: Astringent, tonic, stomachic.

Senecio brasiliensis Less.
AREA: From Minas Gerais and Mato Grosso southward, commonly as a ruderal.
NAMES: Erva-lanceta, flor-das-almas, maria-mole, tasneirinha.
USES: Dry leaves applied to wounds for healing. The plant is cited as toxic to cattle (Ref: ASTE 97).
CHEM.: The species of this genus contain typical alkaloids generally known as *Senecio* alkaloids. They are cyclic diesters of pyrrolizidines, having also been described in the present species (Ref: ASTE 98,99,100,101).

Silybum marianum Gaertn.
AREA: Widespread in southern Brazil: introduced from Europe and Asia.
NAMES: Cardo-asnal, cardo-santo.
USES: Seed tincture is antispasmodic, used for urinary, biliary and uterine disorders. Also as antifebrile and for persistent coughs.
CHEM. & PHARM.: Silymarin, a mixture of three flavonolignans isolated from the seeds, has been recognized as a powerful hepatoprotective agent (Ref: ASTE 102).

Solidago chilensis Meyen
AREA: Widespread as a ruderal, particularly in southern Brazil.
NAMES: Arnica, arnica-silvestre, erva-lanceta, espiga-de-ouro, macela-miúda, rabo-de-rojão, sapê-macho (English: goldenrod).
USES: Bitter, stomachic, vulnerary; for sprains and bruises as a substitute for the genuine arnica (*Arnica montana* L.). In veterinary medicine, the dry flowers are burnt to treat glanders.
CHEM.: Quercitrin, a flavonoid glucoside, in the aerial parts (Ref: ASTE 103); diterpenes in the roots (Ref: ASTE 104).

Sphagneticola trilobata (L.) Pruski
AREA: Throughout Brazil, much cultivated in gardens.
NAME: Agrião.
USES: The entire plant, mixed with honey, in the form of a syrup, is prescribed for flu, grippe and cough.
CHEM. & PHARM.: Sesquiterpenes and diterpenes have been isolated (Ref: ASTE 114,115). One secokaurene lactone showed antibiotic activity (Ref: ASTE 115).

Stomatanthes oblongifolius (Spr.) H. Robinson
AREA: Rio Grande do Sul, campos.
NAME: Erva-de-lagarto.
USES: Leaves prescribed for bronchopulmonary diseases and slight cases of hysteria.

ASTERACEAE

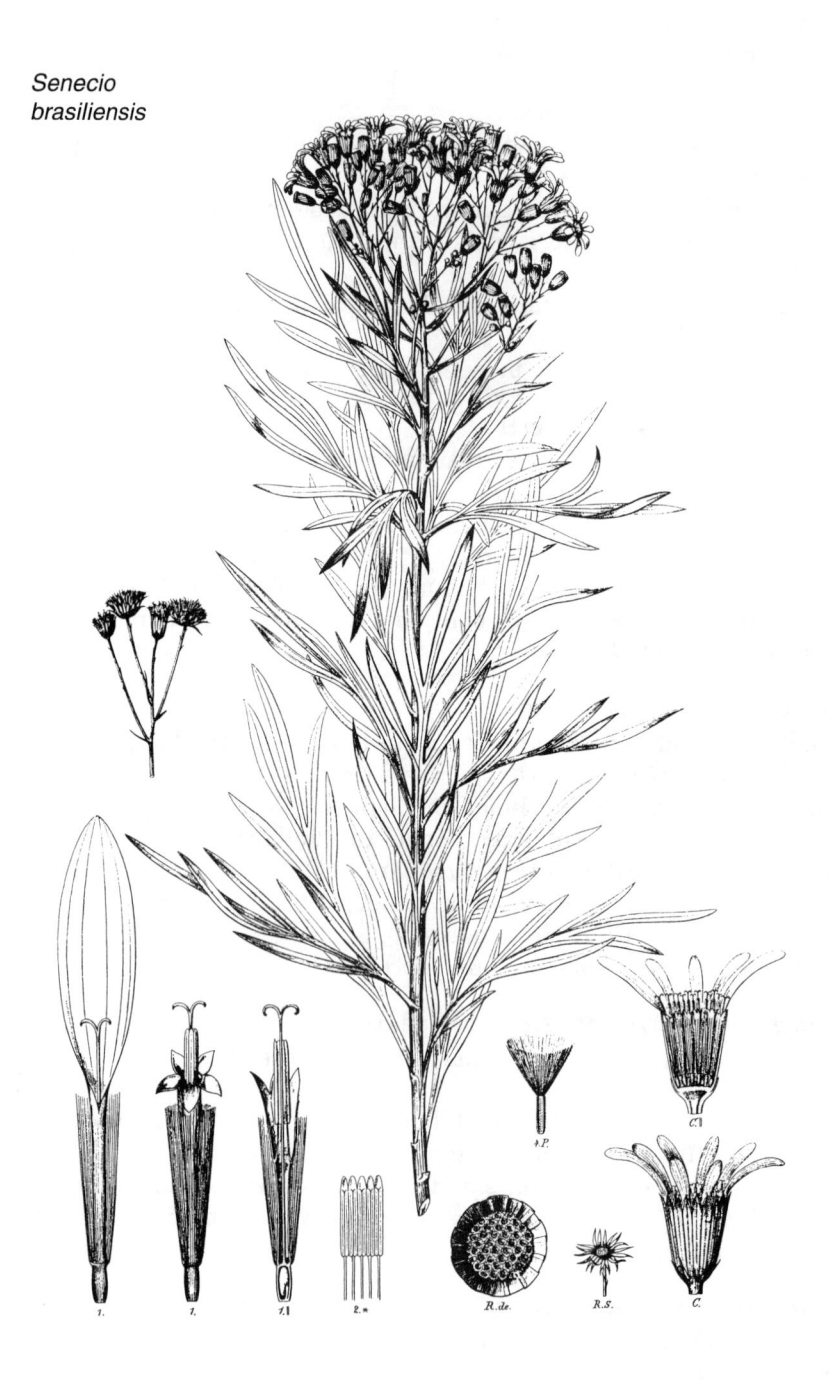

*Senecio
brasiliensis*

ASTERACEAE

Tagetes erecta L.
AREA: Naturalized in Brazil, ruderal.
NAME: Cravo-de-defunto.
USES: Infusion of the flowers used as a pectoral and sedative; also for rheumatic pain, colds, bronchitis and cough. Roots and seeds are considered laxative.
CHEM.: The roots contain acetylenic compounds (Ref: ASTE 109). Flavonoid glycocides were found in leaves and flower heads (Ref: ASTE 110). A review has been published in Hungarian (Ref: ASTE 111).

Tagetes minuta L.
AREA: Common in Brazil, mainly as a ruderal.
NAMES: Coari-bravo, cravo-de-defunto, cravo-de-defunto-miúdo.
USES: Aromatic, excitant, diuretic; for rheumatism, intestinal colics and dyspepsy. Also for expelling intestinal parasites and for stimulating menstrual flow.

Tanacetum vulgare L.
AREA: Introduced from Europe, very widespread, ruderal.
NAMES: Catinga-de-mulata, tasneira (English: tansy).
USES: Aromatic, bitter, tonic, stimulant, anthelmintic, abortifacient, emmenagogue. Leaves insectifuge.
CHEM.: Essential oil contains thujone (Ref: ASTE 112).

Trixis antimenorrhoea (Schrank) Mart.
AREA: Very widespread, particularly as second growth.
NAMES: Celidônia, erva-andorinha, erva-de-mulher, solidônia.
USES: Roots and leaves used to treat inflamed eyes and to stop uterine hemorrhage.

Unxia camphorata L. f.
AREA: Amazonia.
NAME: São-joão-caá.
USES: Leaf tea for kidney ailments and leucorrhoea.

Vernonanthura brasiliana (L.) H. Robinson
AREA: Pará to Espirito Santo, mainly as second growth.
NAMES: Assa-peixe, erva-preá, matias, pau-de-moquem, tramanhem.
USES: Aromatic, stimulant. Infusion of twigs used as antiophthalmic and antiphlogistic.

Xanthium orientale L., *X. spinosum* L. and *X. strumarium* L.
AREA: Cosmopolitan; ruderal.

ASTERACEAE

NAMES: Abroco, amor-de-negro, carrapicho-de-carneiro, carrapicho-grande, espinho-de-carneiro (English: cocklebur).
USES: Emollient, resolutive, indicated for scrophula and sores. Fruits are febrifuge; roots for bladder afflictions, liver ailments and dysentery.
CHEM. & PHARM.: A compound isolated from the seeds of *X. strumarium* exhibited potent hypoglycemic activity in the rat (Ref: ASTE 116). The responsible agent was identified as carboxyatractyloside, a complex diterpenoid glycoside (Ref: ASTE 117).

Asteraceae – References

ASTE 1. Herz, W. & P.S. Kalyanaraman. 1975. Acanthospermal A and acanthospermal B, two new melampolides from *Acanthospermum* species. *J. Org. Chem.* 40: 3486-3491.

ASTE 2. Bohlmann, F., J. Jakupovic, A.K. Dhar, R.M. King & H. Robinson. 1981. Two sesquiterpene and three diterpene lactones from *Acanthospermum australe*. *Phytochemistry* 20: 1081-1083.

ASTE 3. Bohlmann, F., H.G. Schmeda-Hirschmann & J. Jakupovic. 1984. Neue Melampolide aus *Acanthospermum australe*. *Planta Medica* 50: 37-39.

ASTE 4. Shimizu, M., S. Horie, M. Arisawa, T. Hayashi, S. Suzuki, M. Yoshizaki, M. Kawasaki, S. Terashima, H. Tsuji, S. Wada, H. Ueno, N. Morita, L.H. Berganza, E. Ferro & I. Basualdo. 1987. Chemical and pharmaceutical studies on medicinal plants in Paraguay. I. Isolation and identification of lens aldolase reductase inhibitor from "tapecue," *Acanthospermum australe*. *Chem. Pharm. Bull.* 35: 1234-1237.

ASTE 5. Carvalho, L.H., M.G.L. Brandão, D. Santos-Filho, J.C.C. Lopes & A.U. Krettli. 1991. Antimalarial activity of crude extracts from Brazilian plants studied "in vivo" in *Plasmodium berghei*-infected mice and "in vitro" against *Plasmodium falciparum* in culture. *Braz. J. Med. Biol. Res.* 24: 1113-1123.

ASTE 6. Bohlmann, F., J. Jakupovic, C. Zdero, R.M. King & H. Robinson. 1979. Neue Melampolide und *cic*, *cis*-Germacranolide aus Vertretern der Subtribus Melampodiinae. *Phytochemistry* 18: 625-630.

ASTE 7. Bauer, L., G.A.A. Brasil e Silva, N.C.S. Siqueira, C.T.M. Bacha & B.M.S. Sant' Ana. 1979. Contribuição à análise dos óleos essenciais de *Eupatorium ligulifolium* H.A. e *Achyrocline satureioides* DC. do Rio Grande do Sul. *Rev. Bras. Farm.* 60: 97-100.

ASTE 8. Hänsel, R. & O. Ohlendorf. 1971. Ein neues im Ring B unsubstituiertes Flavon aus *Achyrocline satureioides*. *Arch. Pharm.* 304: 893-896.

ASTE 9. Ferraro, G.E., C. Norbedo & J.D. Coussio. 1981. Polyphenols from *Achyrocline satureioides*. *Phytochemistry* 20: 2053-2054.

ASTE 10. Broussalis, A.M., G.E. Ferraro, A. Gurni & J.D. Coussio. 1988. Phenolic constituents of four *Achyrocline* species. *Biochem. Syst. Ecol.* 16: 401-402.

ASTE 11. Kaloga, M., R. Hänsel & E.-M. Cybulski. 1983. Isolierung eines Kawapyrons aus *Achyrocline satureioides*. *Planta Medica* 48: 103-104.

ASTE 12. Langeloh, A. & E.P. Schenkel. 1981/82. Atividade antiespasmódica do extrato alcoólico de marcela (*Achyrocline satureioides* DC., Compositae) sobre a musculatura lisa genital de ratos. *Oreades* (Belo Horizonte) 8 (14/15): 454-458.

ASTE 13. Simões, C.M.O. 1988. Antiinflammatory action of *Achyrocline satureioides* (Lam.) DC. extracts applied topically. *Fitoterapia* 59: 419-421.

ASTE 14. Simões, C.M.O., E.P. Schenkel, L. Bauer & A. Langeloh. 1988. Pharmacological investigations of *Achyrocline satureioides* (Lam.) DC., Compositae. *J. Ethnopharmacol.* 22: 281-283.

ASTE 15. Wagner, H., A. Proksch, I. Riess-Maurer, A. Vollmar, S. Odenthal, H. Stuppner, K. Jurcic, M. Le Turdue & J.N. Fang. 1985. Immunostimulierend wirkende Polysaccharide (Heteroglykane) aus höheren Pflanzen. *Arzneimittelforsch./Drug Res.* 35 (II): 1069-1075.

ASTE 16. Puhlmann, J., U. Knaus, L. Tubaro, W. Schäffer & H. Wagner. 1992. Immunologically active metallic ion-containing polysaccharides of *Achyrocline satureiodes*. *Phytochemistry 31*: 2617-2621.

ASTE 17. Kasturi, T.R. & T. Manithomas. 1967. Essential oil of *Ageratum conyzoides*. Isolation and structure of two new constituents. *Tetrahedron Lett.*: 2573-2575.

ASTE 18. von Rudloff, E. & V.K. Sood. 1969. Chemical composition of the leaf oil of *Ageratum conyzoides* L. *Perf. Essent. Oil Record*: 303-304.

ASTE 19. Ekundayo, O., I. Laakso & R. Hiltunen. 1988. Essential oil of *Ageratum conyzoides*. *Planta Medica 54*: 55-57.

ASTE 20. Nair, A.G.R., J.P. Kotiyal & S.S. Subramanian. 1977. Chemical constituents of the leaves of *Ageratum conyzoides*. *Indian J. Pharm. 39*: 108-109.

ASTE 21. Adegosan, E.K. & A.L. Okunada. 1979. A new flavone from *Ageratum conyzoides*. *Phytochemistry 18*: 1863-1864.

ASTE 22. Vyas, A.V. & N.B. Mulchandani. 1986. Polyoxygenated flavones from *Ageratum conyzoides*. *Phytochemistry 25*: 2625-2627.

ASTE 23. Alertsen, A.R. 1955. Ageratochromene, a heterocyclic compound from the essential oils of some *Ageratum* species. *Acta Chem. Scand. 9*: 1725-1726.

ASTE 24. Wiedenfeld, H. & E. Röder. 1991. Pyrrolizidine alkaloids from *Ageratum conyzoides*. *Planta Medica 57*: 578-579.

ASTE 25. Bowers, W.S., T. Ohta, J.S. Cleere & P.A. Marsella. 1976. Discovery of insect anti-juvenile hormones in plants. *Science 193*: 543-547.

ASTE 26. Durodola, J.I. 1977. Antibacterial property of crude extract from a herbal wound healing remedy — *Ageratum conyzoides* L. *Planta Medica 32*: 388-390.

ASTE 27. Stapel, G., H.G. Men Ben & G. Snatzke. 1980. Isolierung und Strukturaufklärung von zwei Diterpenen aus *Baccharis articulata*. *Planta Medica 39*: 366-374.

ASTE 28. Gianello, J.C. & O.S. Giordano. 1982. Barticulicidiol, nuevo diterpeno furanico isolado del *Baccharis articulata* (Lam.) Persoon. *Rev. Latinoam. Quím. 13*: 76-78.

ASTE 29. Siqueira, N.C.S., G.A.A.B. Silva, C.B. Alice & M. Nitschke. 1985. Análise comparativa dos óleos essenciais de *Baccharis articulata* (Lam.) Pers. e *Baccharis trimera* (Less.) DC. (Compositae), espécies espontâneas do Rio Grande do Sul. *Rev. Bras. Farm. 66*: 36-39.

ASTE 30. Tokarnia, C.H. & J. Döbereiner, unpublished; cit. in ASTE 44.

ASTE 31. Palacios, P., G. Gutkind, R.V.D. Rondina, R. de Torres & J.D. Coussio. 1983. Genus *Baccharis*. II. Antimicrobial activity of *B. crispa* and *B. notosergila*. *Planta Medica 49*: 128.

ASTE 32. Bohlmann, F., W. Kramp, M. Grenz, H. Robinson & R.M. King. 1981. Diterpenes from *Baccharis* species. *Phytochemistry 20*: 1907-1913.

ASTE 33. Naves, Y.R. 1959. Études sur les matières végétales volatiles. CLIX. Sur l'huile essentielle de Carquéja de l'État de Santa Catarina (Brésil). *Bull. Soc. Chim. France 26*: 1871-1879.

ASTE 34. Naves, Y.R. 1959. Études sur les matières végétales volatiles. CLXI. Présence de lédol dans l'huile essencielle de carquéja. *Helv. Chim. Acta 42*: 1996-1998.

ASTE 35. Dolejs, L., V. Herout & F. Sorm. 1961. On Terpenes. CXX. Sesquiterpenic compounds of *Baccharis genistelloides* Pers. Structure of palustrol. *Coll. Czech. Chem. Comm. 26*: 811-817.

ASTE 36. Santos Filho, D., S.J. Sarti, W. Vichnewski, M.S. Bulhões & H.F. Leitão Filho. 1980. Atividade moluscicida em *Biomphalaria glabrata*, de uma lactona diterpênica e de uma flavona isoladas de *Baccharis trimera* (Less.) A.P. De Candolle. *Rev. Fac. Farm. Odont. Ribeirão Preto 17*: 43-47.

ASTE 37. Herz, W., A.-M. Pilotti, A.-C. Söderholm, I.K. Shuhama & W. Vichnewski. 1977. New *ent*-clerodane diterpenoids from *Baccharis trimera*. *J. Org. Chem. 42*: 3913-3917.

ASTE 38. Bohlmann, F. & C. Zdero. 1969. Über neue Terpenderivate aus *Baccharis trimera*. *Tetrahedron Lett.*: 2419-2421.

ASTE 39. Daily, H., H. Wagner & O. Seligmann. 1984. Hispidolin and stigmasta-7, 22-dien-3-ol from *Baccharis genistelloides*. *Fitoterapia 55*: 236-238.

ASTERACEAE

ASTE 40. Soicke, H. & E. Leng-Peschlow. 1987. Characterization of flavonoids from *Baccharis trimera* and their antihepatotoxic properties. *Planta Medica 53*: 37-39.

ASTE 41. Kupchan, S.M., D.R. Streelman, B.B. Jarvis, R.G. Dailey Jr. & A.T. Sneden. 1977. Isolation of potent new antileukemic trichothecenes from *Baccharis megapotamica*. *J. Org. Chem. 42*: 4221-4225.

ASTE 42. Jarvis, B.B., J.O. Midiwo, D. Tuthill & G.A. Bean. 1981. Interaction between the antibiotic trichothecenes and the higher plant *Baccharis megapotamica*. *Science 214*: 460-462.

ASTE 43. Habermehl, G.G., L. Busam & M. Spraul. 1984. Miotoxin D und iso miotoxin D, zwei neue macrocyclische Trichothecene aus *Baccharis coridifolia* DC. *Justus Liebigs Ann., Chem. 75*: 1746-1754.

ASTE 44. Habermehl, G.G., L. Busam, P. Heydel, D. Mebs, C.H. Tokarnia, J. Döbereiner & M. Spraul. 1985. Macrocyclic trichothecenes: cause of livestock poisoning by the Brazilian plant *Baccharis coridifolia*. *Toxicon 23*: 731-745.

ASTE 45. Jarvis, B.B., J.O. Midiwo, G.A. Bean, M.B. Aboul-Nasr & C.S. Barros. 1988. The mystery of trichothecene antibiotics in *Baccharis* species. *J. Nat. Prod. 51*: 736-744.

ASTE 46. Jarvis, B.B., N. Mokhtari-Rejali, E.P. Schenkel, C.S. Barros & N. I. Matzenbacher. 1991. Trichothecene mycotoxins from Brazilian *Baccharis* species. *Phytochemistry 30*: 789-797.

ASTE 47. Bohlmann, F., M. Ahmed, R.M. King & H. Robinson. 1983. Acetylenic compounds from *Bidens graveolens*. *Phytochemistry 22*: 1281-1283.

ASTE 48. Bohlmann, F., H. Bornowski & K.-M. Kleine. 1964. Über neue Polyyne aus dem Tribus Heliantheae. *Chem. Ber. 97*: 2135-2138.

ASTE 49. Alvarez, L., S. Marquina, M.L. Villareal, D. Alonso, E. Aranda & G. Delgado. 1996. Bioactive polyacetylenes from *Bidens pilosa*. *Planta Medica 62*: 355-357.

ASTE 50. Wat, C.-K., R.K. Biswas, E.A. Graham, L. Bohm & G.H.N. Towers. 1978. UV-mediated antibiotic activity of phenylheptatriyne in *Bidens pilosa*. *Planta Medica 33*: 309-310.

ASTE 51. Wat, C.-K., R.K. Biswas, E.A. Graham, L.Bohm, G.H.N. Towers & E.R. Waygood. 1979. Ultraviolet-mediated cytotoxic activity of phenylheptatriene from *Bidens pilosa* L. *J. Nat. Prod. 42*: 103-111.

ASTE 52. Graham, K., E.A. Graham & G.H. Towers. 1980. Cercaricidal activity of phenylheptatriyne and alpha-terthienyl, naturally occurring compounds in species of Asteraceae (Compositae). *Can. J. Zool.* (Vancouver) *58*: 1955-1958.

ASTE 53. N'Dounga, L.M., G. Balansard, A. Baradjamian, P.T. Davis & M. Gasquet. 1983. Contribution à l'étude de *Bidens pilosa* L. Identification et activité antiparasitaire de la phénil-1-heptatriyne 1,3,5. *Plantes Méd. Phytothér. 17*: 64-75.

ASTE 54. Ferreira, Z.S., N.F. Roque, O.R. Gottlieb, F. Oliveira & H.E. Gottlieb. 1980. Structural clarification of germacranolides from *Calea* species. *Phytochemistry 19*: 1481-1484.

ASTE 55. Fikenscher, L.H. & R. Hegnauer. 1977. Cyanogenese bei den Cormophyten. 12. *Chaptalia nutans*, eine stark cyanogene Pflanze Brasiliens. *Planta Medica 31*: 266-267.

ASTE 56. Czerson, H., F. Bohlmann, F. Stuessy & H. Fischer. 1979. Sesquiterpenoid and acetylenic constituents of seven *Clibadium* species. *Phytochemistry 18*: 257-260.

ASTE 57. Govindachari, T.R., K. Nagarajan & B.R. Pai. 1956. Wedelolactone from *Eclipta alba*. *J. Sci. Ind. Research* (India) *15B*: 664-665.

ASTE 58. Krishnaswamy, N.R., T.R. Seshadri & B.R. Sharma. 1966. The structure of a new polythienyl from *Eclipta alba*. *Tetrahedron Lett.* 4227-4230.

ASTE 59. Bhargava, K.K., N.R. Krishnaswamy & T.R. Seshadri. 1972. Demethylwedelolactone glucoside from *Eclipta alba* leaves. *Indian J. Chem. 10*: 810-811.

ASTE 60. Sarg, T.M., N.A. Abdel Salam, M. El-Domiaty & S.M. Khafagy. 1981. The steroid, triterpenoid and flavonoid constituents of *Eclipta alba* (L.) Hassk. (Compositae) grown in Egypt. *Sci. Pharm. 49*: 262-264.

ASTE 61. Halim, A.F., S.I. Balboa, & A.T. Kalil. 1982. Phenolics and other constituents from *Eclipta alba*. *Planta Medica 45*: 163.

ASTE 62. Wagner, H., B. Geyer, Y. Kiso, H. Hikino & G.S. Rao. 1986. Coumestans as the main active principles of the liver drugs *Eclipta alba* and *Wedelia calendulacea*. *Planta Medica* 52: 370-374.

ASTE 63. Mors, W.B., M.C. Nascimento, J.P. Parente, M.H. da Silva, P.A. Melo & G. Suarez-Kurtz. 1989. Neutralization of lethal and myotoxic activities of South American rattlesnake venom by extracts and constituents of the plant *Eclipta prostrata* (Asteraceae). *Toxicon* 27: 1003-1009.

ASTE 64. Melo, P.A., W.B. Mors, M.C. Nascimento & G. Suarez-Kurtz. 1990. Antagonism of the myotoxic and hemorrhagic effects of crotalide venoms by *Eclipta prostrata* extracts and constituents. *Eur. J. Pharmacol.* 183: 572.

ASTE 65. Lima, M.A.S. & E.R. Silveira. 1989. Diterpenos de macela-da-terra: 12-acetoxihautriwaicolactona. *12th Brazilian Chemical Congress, São Paulo*. Abstracts of papers: J.5.10.

ASTE 66. Silveira, E.R., M.A. Sousa Lima & L.M.B. Macedo. 1989. Contribuição ao conhecimento quimico de plantas do nordeste: *Egletes viscosa* Less. *Ciência e Cultura* (São Paulo) 41 (Supl.): 511.

ASTE 67. Simões, E.R.B., E.A. Torres da Silva, E.R. Silveira, M.S. Lima & G.S.B.Viana. 1989. Pharmacological effects of active principles of *Egletes viscosa* Less. *Brazilian-Sino Symposium on Chemistry and Pharamacology of Natural Products* (Rio de Janeiro). Abstracts of papers: 111.

ASTE 68. Simões, E.R.B., E.R. Silveira, M.S. Lima & G.S.B. Viana. 1990. Efeitos de *Egletes viscosa* Less. sobre musculatura cardiaca e esquelética. *11th Symposium of Medicinal Plants of Brazil* (João Pessoa). Abstracts of papers: 4.53.

ASTE 69. Souza, M.F., J.C.R.Silva, V.S.N. Rao & E.R. Silveira. 1992. Atividade antiinflamatoria da ternatina, um flavonóide isolado da *Egletes viscosa* Less. *12th Symposium on Medicinal Plants of Brazil* (Curitiba). Abstracts of papers: 17.

ASTE 70. Machado, M.I.L., F.J.A. Matos, J.W. Alencar, A.A. Craveiro & A.C.S. de Brito. 1992. Diterpeno labdânico das folhas de *Egletes viscosa* Less., a macela do nordeste do Brasil. *12th Symposium on Medicinal Plants of Brazil*. Abstracts of papers: 121.

ASTE 71. Simões, C.M.O., M. Amoros, L. Girre, J. Gleye & M.-T. Fauvel. 1990. Antiviral activity of ternatin and meliternatin, 3-methoxyflavones from species of Rutaceae. *J. Nat. Prod.* 53: 989-992.

ASTE 72. Ghamin, A., A. Zaman & R.R. Kidwai. 1963. Chemical examination of *Elephantopus scaber*. *Indian J. Chem.* 1: 320-321.

ASTE 73. Sim, K. & H.T. Lee. 1969. Constituents of *Elephantopus scaber* (Compositae). *Phytochemistry* 8: 933-934.

ASTE 74. Govindachari, T.R., N. Viswanathan & H. Fuehrer. 1972. Isodeoxyelephantopin, a new germacranediolide from *Elephantopus scaber*. *Indian J. Chem.* 10: 272-273.

ASTE 75. Lee, K.H., H. Furukawa, M. Kozuka, H.C. Huang, P.A. Luhan & A.T. McPhail. 1973. Molephantin, a novel cytotoxic germacranolide from *Elephantopus mollis*. *J. Chem. Soc. Chem. Commun.* 14: 476-477.

ASTE 76. McPhail, A.T., K.D. Onan, K.H. Lee, T. Ibuka, M. Kozuka, T. Shingu & H. C. Huang. 1974. Structure and stereochemistry of the epoxide of phantomolin, a novel cytotoxic esquiterpene lactone from *Elephantopus mollis*. *Tetrahedron Lett.* 32: 2739-2741.

ASTE 77. Lee, K.H., T. Ibuka, H.C. Huang & D.L. Harris. 1975. Antitumor agents, XIV. Molephantin, a new potent antitumor sesquiterpene lactone from *Elephantopus mollis*. *J. Pharm. Sci.* 64: 1077-1078.

ASTE 78. Lee, K.H., T. Ibuka, H. Furokawa, M. Kozuka, R.Y. Wu, I.A. Hall & H.C. Huang. 1980. Antitumor agents. XXXVIII. Isolation and structural elucidation of novel germacranolides and triterpenes from *Elephantopus mollis*. *J. Pharm. Sci.* 69: 1050-1056.

ASTE 79. Silva, L.B., W.H.M.W. Herath, R.C. Jennings, M. Mahendran & G.E. Wannigama. 1982. A new sesquiterpene lactone from *Elephantopus scaber*. *Phytochemistry* 21: 1173-1175.

ASTERACEAE

ASTE 80. Banerjee, S., G. Schmeda-Hirschmann, V. Castro, A. Schuster, J. Jakupovic & F. Bohlmann. 1986. Further sesquiterpene lactones from *Elephantopus mollis* and *Centratherum punctatum*. *Planta Medica* 52: 29-32.

ASTE 81. Oliveira, A.B., G.G. Oliveira, F. Carazza, R. Braz Filho, C.T.M. Bacha, L. Bauer, G.A.A.B. Silva & N.C.S. Siqueira. 1978. Laevigatin, a sesquiterpenoid from *Eupatorium laevigatum* Lam. *Tetrahedron Lett.* 30: 2653-2654.

ASTE 82. Bose, P.K. & B.B. Sarkar. 1937. Haemostatic agents. Part I. Experiments with ayapanin and ayapin. *Nature* 139: 515.

ASTE 83. Bose, P.K. & P.B. Sen. 1941. Haemostatic agents. Part I. Experiments with ayapanin and ayapin. *Annals Biochem. Expt. Med.* (India) 1: 311-316.

ASTE 84. Kerber, V.A., O.G. Miguel & E.A. Moreira. 1993. Flavonoids from *Heterothalamus psiadioides*. *Fitoterapia* 64: 185.

ASTE 85. Cascon, S.C., W.B. Mors, B.M. Tursch, T.T. Aplin & L.J. Durham. 1965. Ichthyothereol and its acetate, the active polyacetylene constituents of *Ichthyothere terminalis* (Spreng.) Malme, a fish poison from the lower Amazon. *J. Am. Chem. Soc.* 87: 5237-5241.

ASTE 86. Gutierrez, A.B., J.C. Oberti, V.E. Sosa & W. Herz. 1987. Melampolides from *Mikania cordifolia*. *Phytochemistry* 26: 2315-2320.

ASTE 87. D'Agostino, M., F. de Simone, F. Zollo & C. Pizza. 1991. Constituents of *Mikania cordifolia*. *Fitoterapia* 62: 461.

ASTE 88. Portela, B.A.N., V.C. Gerhardt, S.M.G. Oliveira, R.C.M.M. Almeida & R. Soares de Moura. 1989. Efeito do extrato alcoólico do guaco, *Mikania glomerata*, no músculo traqueobrônquico da cobaia e do homem. *4th Annual Meeting of the Federation of Brazilian Societies of Experimental Biology* (Caxambu). Abstracts of papers: 86.

ASTE 89. Muradian, J., M. Motidome, P.C. Ferreira & R. Braz Filho. 1977. Flavonols and (-) kaur-16-en-19-oic acid from *Mikania hirsutissima*. *Rev. Latinoam. Quím.* 8: 88-89.

ASTE 90. Bohlmann, F., A. Adler, A. Schuster, R.K. Gupta, R.M. King & H. Robinson. 1981. Diterpenes from *Mikania* species. *Phytochemistry* 20: 1899-1902.

ASTE 91. Herz, W. & H. Watanabe. 1959. Parthenin, a new guaianolide. *J. Am. Chem. Soc.* 81: 6088-6089.

ASTE 92. Fester, G.A., E.A. Martinuzzi, J.A. Retamar & A.I.A. Ricciardi. 1961. Aceites esenciales de la República Argentina. *Acad. Nacional de Ciências* (Córdoba, Argentina): 51-52.

ASTE 93. Talenti, E.C.J., R. Manzi, F.A. Tedone, E. Arigoli & R.A. Yunes. 1969. Estudio metodologico de la *Pluchea sagittalis* (Lam.) Cabr. *Rev. Fac. Ingenieria Quimica* (Santiago del Estero, Argentina) 38: 251-267.

ASTE 94. Martino, V.S., S.L. Debenedetti & J.D. Cousso. 1979. Caffeoylquinic acids from *Pterocaulon virgatum* and *Pluchea sagittalis*. *Phytochemistry* 18: 2052.

ASTE 95. Zani, C.L., T.M.A. Alves, A.B. Oliveira, S.M.F. Murta, I.P. Ceravolo & A.J. Romanha. 1994. Trypanocidal components of *Pluchea quitoc* L. *Phytotherapy Research* 8: 375-377.

ASTE 96. Bohlmann, F., W.-R. Abraham, R.M. King & H. Robinson. 1981. Thiophene acetylenes and flavonols from *Pterocaulon virgatum*. *Phytochemistry* 20: 825-827.

ASTE 97. Habermehl, G.G., W. Martz, C.H. Tokarnia, J. Döbereiner & M.C. Mendez. 1988. Livestock poisoning in South America by species of the *Senecio* plants. *Toxicon* 26: 275-286.

ASTE 98. Adams, R. & M. Gianturco. 1956. *Senecio* alkaloids: The alkaloids of *Senecio brasiliensis*, *fremonti* and *ambrosioides*. *J. Am. Chem. Soc.* 78: 5315-5317.

ASTE 99. Motidome, M. & P. Carvalho Ferreira. 1966. Alcalóides do *Senecio brasiliensis* Less. *Rev. Fac. Farm. Bioquímica* (Univ. São Paulo) 4: 13-44.

ASTE 100. Motidome, M. & P. Carvalho Ferreira. 1966. Alcalóides do gênero *Senecio*. *Rev. Fac. Farm. Bioquímica* (Univ. São Paulo) 4: 175-179.

ASTE 101. Hirschmann, G.S., E.A. Ferraro, L. Franco, L. Recalde & C. Theoduloz. 1987. Pyrrolizidine alkaloids from *Senecio brasiliensis* populations. *J. Nat. Prod.* 50: 770-772.

ASTE 102. Hikino, H., Y. Kiso, H. Wagner & M. Fiebig. 1984. Antihepatotoxic actions of flavonolignans from *Silybum marianum* fruits. *Planta Medica* 3: 248-250.

ASTE 103. Torres, L.M.B., M.K. Akisue & N.F. Roque. 1987. Quercitrina em *Solidago microglossa* DC., a arnica-do-brasil. *Rev. Farm. Bioquímica* (Univ. São Paulo) *23*: 33-40.
ASTE 104. Torres, L.M.B., M.K. Akisue & N. F. Roque. 1989. Diterpenes from the roots of *Solidago microglossa* DC. *Rev. Latinoam. Quím. 20*: 94-97.
ASTE 105. Jacobson, M. 1957. The structure of spilanthol. *Chem. & Ind.*: 50-51.
ASTE 106. Herdy, G.V.H. & A. Paes de Carvalho. 1984. Ação do espilantol (extraído do jambu) sobre a atividade elétrica do coração do coelho. Eletrocardiograma experimental. *Arq. Bras. Cardiol. 43*: 315-320.
ASTE 107. Herdy, G.V.H. & A. Paes de Carvalho. 1984. Ação do espilantol (extraido do jambu) sobre o potencial de ação. Registros elétricos em tira atrial. *Arq. Bras. Cardiol. 43*: 423-428.
ASTE 108. Moreira, V.M.T.S., J.G.S. Maia, J.M. Souza, Z.A. Bortolotto & E.A. Cavalheiro. 1989. Characterization of convulsions induced by a hexane extract of *Spilanthes acmella* var. *oleracea* in rats. *Braz. J. Med. Biol. Res. 22*: 65-67.
ASTE 109. Bohlmann, F., M. Grenz, M. Wotschokowsky & E. Berger. 1967. Über neue Thiophenacetylenverbindungen. *Chem. Ber. 100*: 2518-2522.
ASTE 110. El-Emary, N.A. & A.A. Ali. 1983. Revised phytochemical study of *Tagetes erecta*. *Fitoterapia 54*: 9-12.
ASTE 111. Szabo, L.G. & E. Papp. 1975. Chemical and pharmacological revision of *Tagetes*. (Hungarian). *Gyogyszereszet 19*: 281-285 [*Chem. Abstr. 83*: 190324 t].
ASTE 112. Wallach, O. 1904. Zur Kenntnis der Terpene und der ätherische Öle. 70. Verbindungen der Thujonreihe. *Ann. Chem. 336*: 247-280.
ASTE 113. Jakupovic, J., R.N. Baruah, T.V. Cahu Thi, F. Bohlmann, J.D. Msonthi & G. Schmeda-Hirschmann. 1985. New vernolepin derivatives from *Vernonia glabra* and glaucolides from *Vernonia scorpioides*. *Planta Medica 51*: 378-380.
ASTE 114. Bohlmann, F., J. Ziesche, R.M. King & H. Robinson. 1981. Eudesmanolides and diterpenes from *Wedelia trilobata* and an ent-kaurenic acid derivative from *Aspilia parvifolia*. *Phytochemistry 20*: 751-756.
ASTE 115. Roque, N.F., T.L. Gianella, A.M. Giesbrecht & R.C.S.B.C. Barbosa. 1987. Kaurene diterpenes from *Wedelia paludosa*. *Rev. Latinoam. Quim. 18*: 110-111.
ASTE 116. Kupiecki, F.P., C.D. Ogzewalla & F.M. Schell. 1974. Isolation and characterization of a hypoglycemic agent from *Xanthium strumarium*. *J. Pharm. Sci. 63*: 1166-1167.
ASTE 117. Craig Jr., J.C., M.L. Mole, S. Billets & F. El-Feraly. 1976. Isolation and identification of the hypoglycemic agent, carboxyatractylate, from *Xanthium strumarium*. *Phytochemistry 15*: 1178.

BALANOPHORACEAE

Helosis cayennensis (Swartz) Spreng.

AREA: Amazonia to São Paulo and Mato Grosso, forest.

NAME: Espiga-de-sangue.

USES: Peduncles are astringent, used for stopping hemorrhages, especially hemop-tyses. Dried roots, reduced to powder, used for serious diarrhoea.

Lophophytum mirabile Schott & Endl.

AREA: Maranhão to Santa Catarina, inside the forest on the roots of trees.

NAMES: Batata-de-escamas, boa-noite, espiga-da-terra, milho-de-cobra, pinha-de-raiz.

USES: Tuber employed in baths for rachitism; powdered, for jaundice and epilepsy. Decoction of both the pollen and spadix is said to be aphrodisiac.

BALANOPHORACEAE

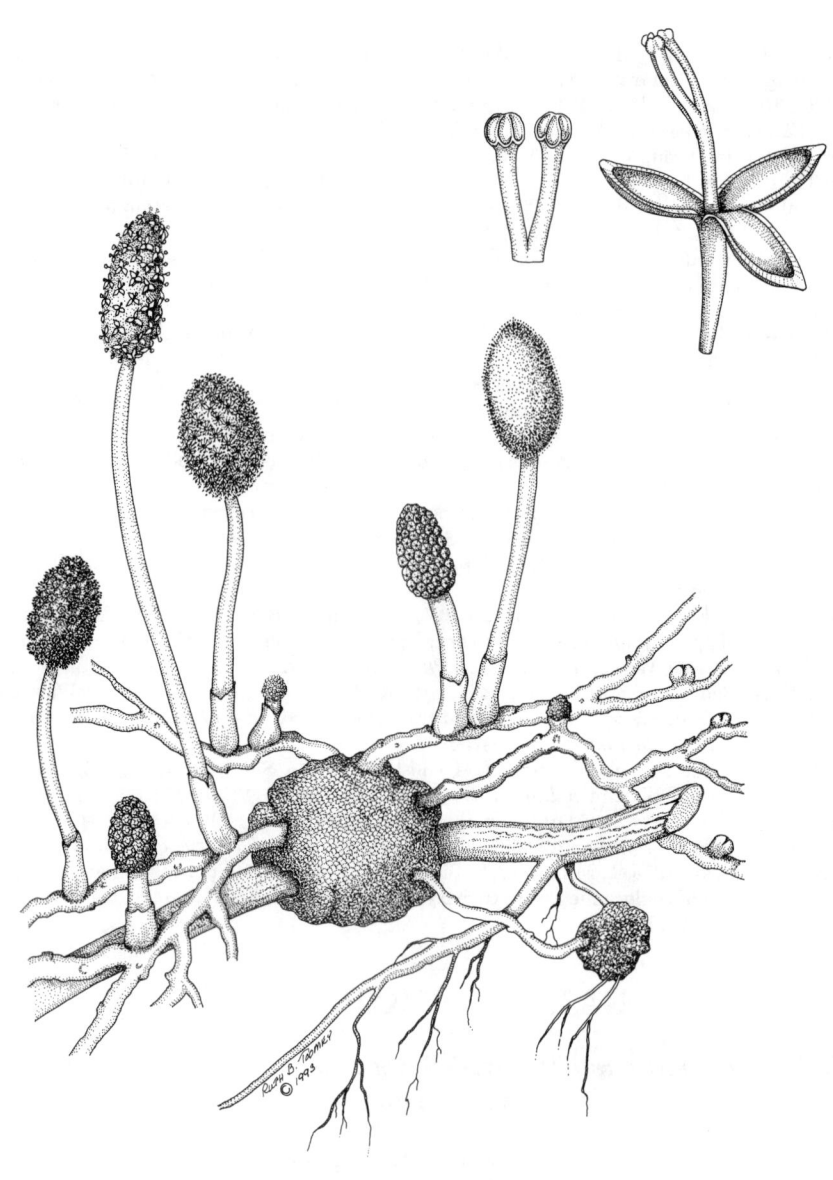

Helosis cayennensis

Scybalium fungiforme Schott & Endl.
AREA: Minas Gerais, Rio de Janeiro and São Paulo, forest.
NAMES: Cogumelo-de-caboclo, cogumelo-de-sangue, esponja-de-raiz, fel-da-terra.
USES: Peduncle and especially pollen is considered aphrodisiac.

BEGONIACEAE

Begonia acida Mart.
AREA: Bahia, forest.
NAMES: Azedinha, azedinha-do-brejo, azeda-de-ourives, erva-azeda, erva-de-sapo, erva-de-saracura.
USES: Prescribed to treat scurvy.

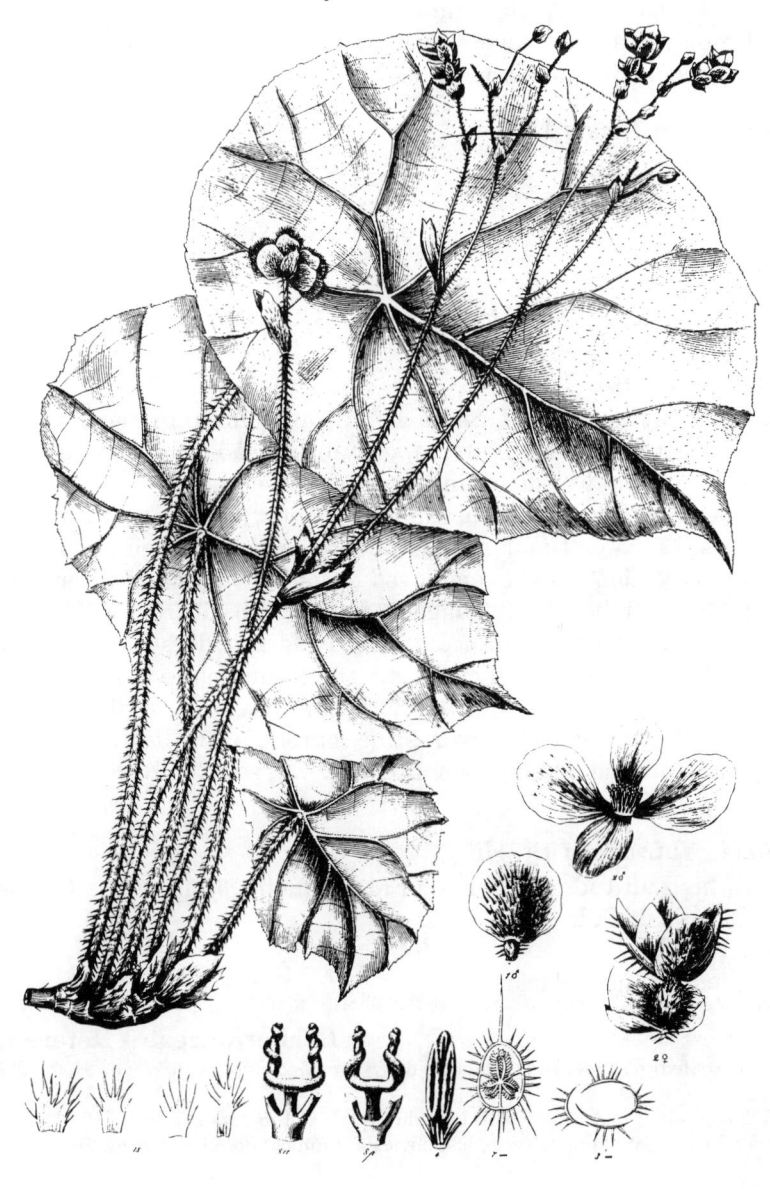

Begonia paulensis

BEGONIACEAE / BERBERIDACEAE

Begonia hirtella Link
AREA: Amazonia to São Paulo, forest.
NAMES: Erva-de-sapo, erva-de-saracura.
USES: Diuretic, antithermic, for diarrhoea and aphthae.

Begonia luxurians Scheidw.
AREA: Rio de Janeiro and Minas Gerais, forest.
NAMES: Begônia, coração-de-estudante.
USES: Employed against fevers, dysentery, hemorrhage; more frequently used for tonsillitis and stomatitis.

Begonia paulensis DC.
AREA: São Paulo, forest.
NAME: Azeda-de-são-paulo.
USES: Antipyretic, antiophthalmic (i.e., as an eyewash).

BERBERIDACEAE

Berberis laurina Thunb.
AREA: Minas Gerais to Rio Grande do Sul, on mountain ridges.
NAMES: Berberiz, berberiz-da-terra, espinho-de-são-joão, quina-cruzeiro, raiz-de-são-joão, uva-de-espinho, uva-espim-do-brasil.
USES: Leaves are astringent, used in gargles for mouth and throat troubles; as tea, antimalarial. Fruits are astringent, useful for scurvy; decoction of fruits employed to soothe burns and eczema.
CHEM.: The root has been suggested as a substitute for *Hydrastis canadensis* rhizome (Ranunculaceae). In fact, it does contain the two main alkaloids of that official drug, the isoquinoline bases berberine and hydrastine (Ref: BERB 1). Berberine has been verified in up to 2.5% yield (Ref: BERB 2). Hydrastine content is low (Ref: BERB 3). For these and additional alkaloids in *B. laurina*, see Ref: BERB 4,5.

Berberis spinulosa St.-Hil.
AREA: In high altitudes in Serra da Mantiqueira, from Minas Gerais to Rio Grande do Sul.
NAME: Berberiz.
USE: Tea as an antimalarial.

Berberidaceae – References

BERB 1. Stellfeld, C. 1934. Um sucedâneo do *Hydrastis canadensis*. *Tribuna Farm.* 2: 142-143.
BERB 2. Gurgel, L., O.A. Costa & R. Dias da Silva. 1934. *Berberis laurina* (Billb.) Thunb., Berberidácea. Estudo anatômico, histológico e químico. *Bol. Assoc. Bras. Farm.* 15: 11-20.

BERBERIDACEAE

Berberis laurina

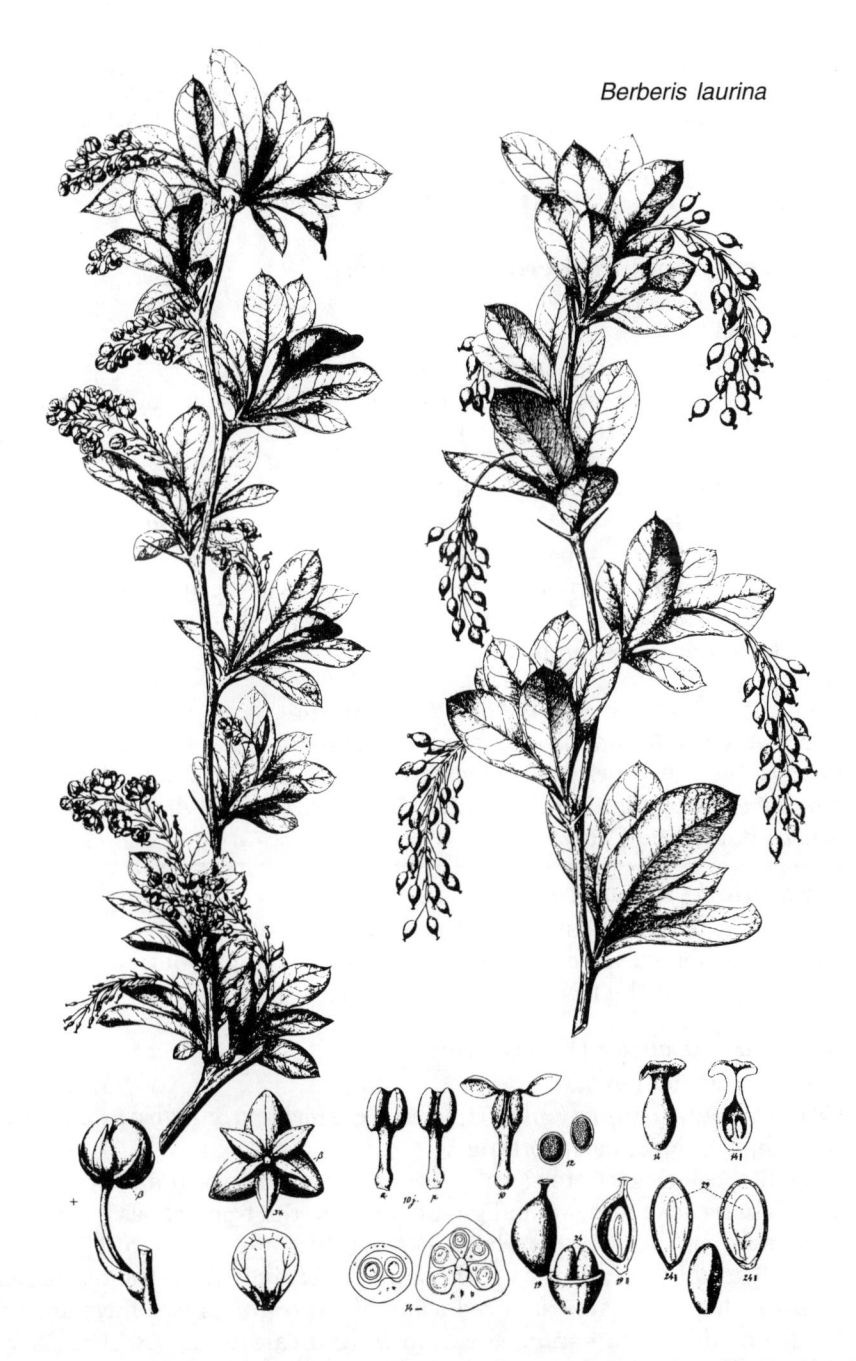

BERB 3. Janot, M.M. & R. Goutarel. 1941. Une falsification ou possible succédane du rhizome de l'*Hydrastis canadensis* L.: la racine de *Berberis laurina* Billb. ou racine de St. Jean. *Bull. Sci. Pharmacol.* 48: 215-224.

BERB 4. Liberalli, C.H. & C.A. Sharovski. 1958. Os alcalóides de *Berberis laurina* (Billb.) Thunb. (Raiz de São João). *An. Fac. Farm. Odont. Univ. São Paulo 15*: 135-158.

BERB 5. Falco, M.R., J.X. deVries, A.G. Bovetto, Z. Macció, S. Rebuffo & I.R.C. Bick. 1968. Two new alkaloids from *Berberis laurina* Billb. *Tetrahedron Lett.*: 1953-1959.

BIGNONIACEAE

Adenocalymma alliacea (Lam.) Miers
AREA: Pará, forest.
NAME: Cipó-d'alho.
USES: Infusion of leaves used against colds and fevers.
CHEM.: The pronounced garlic odor is due to the presence of a number of organic sulfides (Ref: BIGN 1).

Anemopaegma arvense (Vell.) Stapf
AREA: Minas Gerais to São Paulo and Mato Grosso, cerrado.
NAMES: Catuaba, catuaba-verdadeira.
USES: Roots for an aphrodisiac. The most famous of the aphrodisiac plants used in Brazil. Roots are taken in infusion in sugar cane brandy. Also pectoral and antisyphilitic.

Anemopaegma spp.
Other *Anemopaegma* species indicated as aphrodisiacs under the name of catuaba, but much less important, are: *A. album* Mart. (Bahia), *A. glaucum* Mart. (Piauí to Bahia and Minas Gerais) and *A. scabriusculum* Mart. (Bahia and Ceará).

Arrabidaea agnus-castus (Cham.) DC.
AREA: Alagoas to São Paulo, dry and humid forests.
NAMES: Cipó-camarão, cipó-de-rego, cipó-rego, cipó-três-quinas.
USES: Applied in the treatment of gonorrhoea.

Arrabidaea chica (H.B.K.) Bur.
AREA: Amazonia, forest.
NAMES: Carajuru, cajiru, chica, cipó-cruz, coapiranga, guagiru, guarajuru-piranga, oajuru, pariri piranga.
USES: Red coloring matter locally used against ringworm and other skin afflictions; also to clean malignant wounds. Tea from leaves for intestinal spasms, bleeding diarrhoea, enterocolitis and anaemia.
CHEM.: The coloring matter of this plant is obtained from the fermented leaves. It precipitates as a red solid which contains two flavonoids of quinonoid structure, named carajurin and carajurone (Ref: BIGN 2). The dye, once used in cosmetics, had a small export market in the 19th century, under the name of "chica red."

BIGNONIACEAE

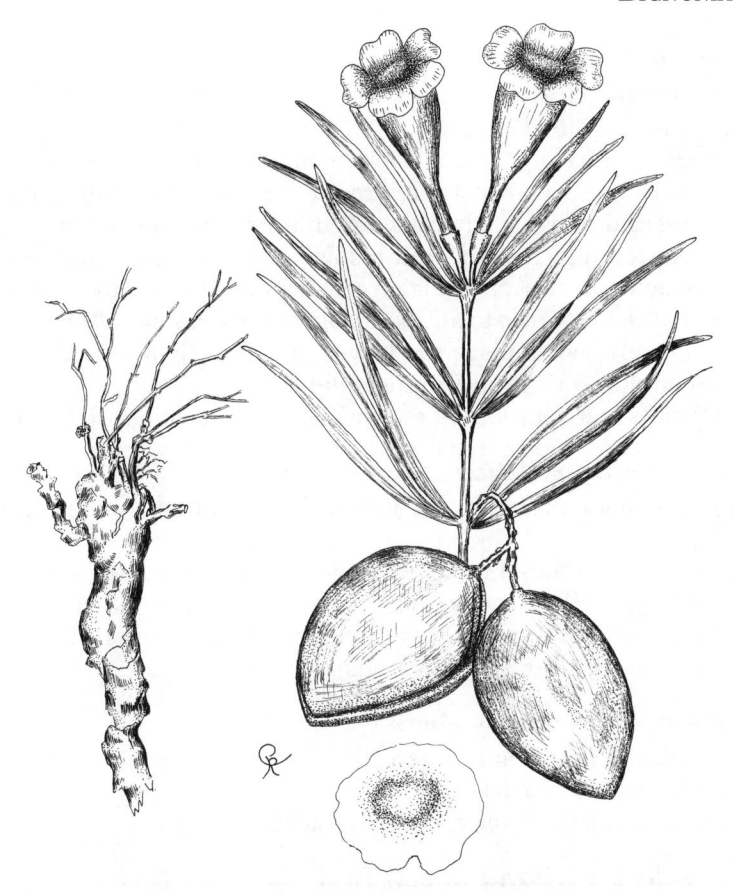

Anemopaegma arvense : A. Flowering and fruiting branch;
B. Thick root with leafless aerial portion; C. Seed.

Arrabidaea foetida Bur. & K. Sch.
AREA: Amazonia, forest.
NAME: Timborana.
USES: Roots are macerated in water, and taken internally against ant and scorpion stings.

Bignonia exoleta Vell.
AREA: Amazonia to Santa Catarina, forest.
NAMES: Andirá-poampé, batata-miúda, batata-de-caboclo.
USE: Antirheumatic.

Cremastus sceptrum Bur. & K. Sch.
AREA: Bahia, Goiás and Minas Gerais, campos.
NAMES: Caroba-do-campo, erva-cigana, erva-de-cigana, parreirinha.
USES: Depurative, antisyphilitic.

BIGNONIACEAE

Crescentia cujete L.
AREA: Amazonia, forest.
NAMES: Cuieira, coité, cuieté.
USES: Bark extract or decoction for membranous enteritis and dropsy. Flesh of the unripe fruit for hydrocele; incorporation into syrup with sugar results in a remedy considered antipyretic, purgative, expectorant, for treating chlorosis and respiratory afflictions; pulp in a poultice is emollient, anticephalalgic, recommended for erysipelas and other dermal afflictions; also to aid expulsion of the placenta after childbirth. It is also advised to place the leaves on the belly of women in labor. Leaves are diuretic if taken internally.
PHARM.: Fruits were shown to have antimicrobial activity (Ref: BIGN 3).

Cybistax antisyphilitica (Mart.) Mart.
AREA: Throughout Brazil, in forest and cerrado, from Amazonia to Rio Grande do Sul.
NAMES: Caroba-de-flor-verde, caroba-do-campo, carobinha-verde, cinco-chagas, cinco-folhas, ipê-de-flor-verde, ipê-verde, ipê-da-várzea.
USES: Bark and sprouts are strong depurative and antisyphilitic; used also in cases of anuria and hydropsy.

Cydista aequinoctialis Miers
AREA: Amazonia to Maranhão, forest.
NAMES: Cipó-de-cesto, cipó-de-corda.
USES: Bark is antidysenteric, bechic, resolvent.

Jacaranda brasiliana (Lam.) Pers.
AREA: Bahia to Rio Grande do Sul.
NAMES: Barbatimão, caroba, jacarandá, jacarandá-preto.
USES: Bark is prescribed for urinary problems; in decoction used for washing wounds and ulcers. Internally, leaf tea is taken for syphilis and skin diseases. Fruits are bechic.

Jacaranda caroba (Vell.) DC.
AREA: Goiás to São Paulo and Mato Grosso, campos.
NAMES: Caroba, caroba-do-campo, caroba-do-carrasco, caroba-miúda, carobinha, camboatá, camboatá-pequeno.
USES: Bark is bitter, astringent, diuretic and antisyphilitic. Leaves are tonic, used against syphilis and various dermatoses.

Jacaranda copaia (Aubl.) D. Don
AREA: Amazonia, forest.
NAMES: Caraúba, caroba-do-mato, carobuçu, marupá, marupá-falso, parapará, simaruba-copaia, simaruba-falsa.
USES: Root induces sweating. Bark is emetic, cathartic, good for syphilitic

lesions, itches and chronic urethritis. Leaves employed externally for dermal afflictions, including syphilis; in gargles for syphilitic lesions of the throat.

Jacaranda cuspidifolia Mart.
AREA: Minas Gerais to Mato Grosso.
NAMES: Caroba, mulher-pobre.
USE: Bark and leaves are antithermic.

Jacaranda micrantha Cham.
AREA: Rio Grande do Sul.
NAMES: Caroba, carobão.
USES: Depurative, antisyphilitic.
CHEM. & PHARM.: A quinol derivative with bacteriostatic properties, the ethyl ester of 1-hydroxy-4-oxo-2, 5-cyclohexadiene-6-acetic acid, has been isolated (Ref: BIGN 4).

Jacaranda mimosifolia D. Don
AREA: Southern Brazil; much used as a shade tree.
NAMES: Caroba-guaçu, jacarandá-caroba, jacarandá-mimoso, palissandra.
USE: Bark is antisyphilitic.

Jacaranda subrhombea DC.
AREA: Minas Gerais and Rio de Janeiro to Rio Grande do Sul.
NAMES: Carobinha-do-campo, caroba-preta, caroba-roxa.
USES: Bark is strongly sudorific. Leaves used for arthritic gout, blennorrhagia, bladder afflictions, ulcers and eczema.

Jacaranda spp.

The following *Jacaranda* species, also known as caroba and prized as antisyphilitic and depurative, are used by the people in different regions of the country: *J. clausseniana* Casar. (Goiás to São Paulo and Mato Grosso), *J. decurrens* Cham. (Minas Gerais to Paraná and Mato Grosso), *J. elegans* Mart. (Ceará), *J. heterophylla* Bur. & Pet. (Pernambuco), *J. oxyphylla* Cham. (Ceará to Paraná), *J. paucifoliata* Mart. (Bahia to Minas Gerais), *J. puberula* Cham. (Rio de Janeiro to Rio Grande do Sul), *J. rufa* Manso (Gioás to São Paulo), *J. semiserrata* Cham. (Minas Gerais to Rio de Janeiro) and *J. tomentosa* R.Br. (littoral).

Macfadyena unguis-cati (L.) Gentry
AREA: Almost all of Brazil, forest.
NAMES: Cipó-de-gato, erva-de-morcego, erva-de-são-domingos, mão-de-calango, unha-de-gato.
USES: Leaves useful for snakebite, diarrhoea, fever, rheumatism, intestinal inflammations; for inducing diuresis. Aqueous extract for venereal diseases and malaria.

CHEM.: Two glycosides were isolated from the roots, both with quinovic acid as aglycon. The sugar moieties were identified as fucose and glucose, respectively (Ref: BIGN 5).

Martinella obovata (H.B.K.) Bur. & K. Sch.
AREA: Amazonia.
NAMES: Gapuí, gapuí-cipó.
USES: Once reputedly useful in baths as a remedy for syphilitic lesions. Roots steeped in water for an eyewash.

Pyrostegia ignea (Vell.) Pres.
AREA: Ceará to Rio Grande do Sul; very frequent in waste land.
NAMES: Belas, cipó-bela-flor, cipó-de-fogo, cipó-de-lagarto, cipó-de-lagartixa, cipó-de-são-joão, marqueza-de-belas.
USES: Leaves are tonic and employed against diarrhoea.

Sparattosperma leucanthum (Vell.) K. Sch.
AREA: Goiás to Rio de Janeiro.
NAMES: Caroba-branca, caroba-de-flor-branca, cinco-chagas, cinco-folhas, ipê-batata, ipês-boia, ipê-branco.
USES: Bark is bitter, astringent, indicated for ulcers in the throat, stomatitis, syphilitic lesions, rheumatism, bladder stones; also said to be depurative in cases of chronic, prolonged diseases. Leaves are bitter, depurative, diuretic, recommended for biliar calculi.
CHEM.: A bitter compound has been isolated as a major constituent of the fruit, identified as pinocembrin 7-ß-neohesperidoside (Ref: BIGN 6).

Tabebuia aurea (Manso) Moore
AREA: São Paulo and Mato Grosso, forest.
NAMES: Paratudo, pau-d'arco.
USE: Leaves are purgative.

Tabebuia barbata (May) Sandw.
AREA: Amazonia.
NAME: Pau-d'arco-da-beira.
USE: Leaf tea is drunk to treat leucorrhoea.

Tabebuia caraiba (Mart.) Bur.
AREA: Cerrado and limestone forest in central Brazil.
NAMES: Caraíba, carobeira, caraúba-do-campo.
USE: Antisyphilitic.

Tabebuia chrysotricha (Mart.) Standl.
AREA: Southern Brazil, often planted along roadsides.
NAMES: Ipê, ipê-amarelo, ipê-do-brejo, ipê-tabaco, pau-d'arco-amarelo.

USE: Bark used against syphilis.

Tabebuia impetiginosa (Mart.) Standl.
AREA: Bahia to Rio de Janeiro, forest.
NAMES: Ipê-roxo, pau-d'arco-roxo, ipê-contra-sarna.
USES: Bark is bitter; used as an infusion or salve applied for scabies, ringworm and cancer.

Tabebuia ipe (Mart.) Standl.
AREA: Amazonia to Rio Grande do Sul, forest.
NAMES: Ipê-mirim, ipê-preto, ipê-rosa, ipê-roxo, ipê-tabaco, ipeúva, peúva, peúva-roxa.
USES: Bark in a decoction is astringent, mucilaginous, reputed for healing syphilitic ulcers. Leaves prescribed for the same purpose and also for gonorrhoea.
PHARM.: Anti-inflammatory activity of extracts has been demonstrated (Ref: BIGN 7).

Tabebuia leucoxylon (L.) DC.
AREA: Amazonia, forest.
NAMES: Ipê-açu, ipê-caboclo, ipê-tabaco, ébano-amarelo, pereira-das-ilhas, pau-d'arco, uruparaíba.
USES: Bark for a tonic, febrifuge. Juice of the leaves taken as an antidote against the effect of poisonous (hydrocyanic acid containing) cassava.

Tabebuia serratifolia (Vahl) Nichol.
AREA: Throughout Brazil, forest.
NAMES: Ipê, ipê-amarelo, ipê-do-campo, ipeúva, pau-d'arco, piúva, piúva-do-charco, tamurá-tuira.
USES: Antirheumatic, antisyphilitic and against leishmaniasis.

Tabebuia umbellata (Sond.) Sandw.
AREA: Minas Gerais and São Paulo, in swamps and on river banks.
NAMES: Ipê-amarelo, ipê-do-brejo.
USES: Bark is astringent, used for mouth and throat disorders.

Tabebuia spp.

The heartwood of a number of *Tabebuia* species contains a high proportion (sometimes over 5%) of the prenylnaphthoquinone lapachol (Ref: BIGN 8). Cytostatic properties of lapachol against a number of tumors has been reported (Ref: BIGN 9,10,11). The compound was approved by the Cancer Chemotherapy National Service Center (U.S.A.) for human clinical trials, but did not achieve final approval as a therapeutic agent. The inner bark (liber) of some *Tabebuia* species (especially that of *T. impetiginosa*) has gained a high popular reputation as an anticancer remedy, in the form of a tea. The drug is even being exported under the name of "Tahebo bark." Its claimed medicinal properties can possibly be explained, at least in part, by the presence of several furanonaphthoquinones with immunomodulating activity on human granulocytes and lymphocytes (Ref: BIGN 12,13,14,15,16,17).

Tanaecium nocturnum (B. Rodr.) Bur. & K. Sch.
AREA: Amazonia, forest.
NAMES: Cipó-corimbó, cipó-curimbo, cipó-paré, corimbó, corimbó-da-mata.
USES: Bark used to relieve upset stomach. The Kayapó Indians of the state of Pará make use of the toxic properties of this vine to kill wild or escaped bees for the extraction of honey. The grated bark also kills ants, caterpillars and other insects (Ref: BIGN 18). The Paumari Indians use the bark for preparing a hallucinogenic snuff (Ref: BIGN 21).
CHEM.: The whole plant is rich in cyanogenetic glycosides, releasing hydrocyanic acid and benzaldehyde on hydrolysis (Ref: BIGN 19,20).

Tynanthus cognatus (Cham.) Miers
AREA: Bahia to Minas Gerais and Rio de Janeiro, forest.
NAME: Cipó-cravo.
USES: Bark of the root and stem smells of cloves; highly esteemed as an aphrodisiac. *T. elegans* (Cham.) Miers (Minas Gerais and Rio de Janeiro to Santa Catarina) and *T. fasciculatus* (Vell.) Miers (Minas Gerais and São Paulo) have the same vernacular name, properties and uses.
CHEM.: Coumarins, phenylpropanoids and steroids were described from *T. fasciculatus* (REF: BIGN 22,23).

Zeyheria digitalis (Vell.) Hoehne
AREA: Piauí to São Paulo and Mato Grosso, always in cerrados.
USES: Bark of the roots useful for dermatoses; bark of the stem for syphilis.

Bignoniaceae – References
BIGN 1. Zoghbi, M.G.B., L.S. Ramos, J.G.S. Maia, M.L. Silva & A.I.R. Luz. 1984. Volatile sulfides of the Amazonian garlic bush. *J. Agric. Food Chem.* 32: 1009-1010.
BIGN 2. Chapman, E., A.G. Perkin & R. Robinson. 1927. The colouring matter of carajura. *J. Chem. Soc.* (London): 3015-3041.
BIGN 3. Verpoorte, R., A. Tjin a Tsot, H. van Doorne & A.B. Svendson. 1982. Medicinal plants of Suriname. I. Antimicrobial activity of some medicinal plants. *J. Ethnopharmacol.* 5: 221-226.
BIGN 4. Silva, M.G.M. 1980. *Jacaranda micrantha* Cham.: Isolamento e identificação de l-hidroxi-4-oxo-2, 5-ciclohexadien-6-acetato de etila. Ensaios antineoplásicos, antibacterianos e antifúngicos. Thesis, Federal University of Rio Grande do Sul.
BIGN 5. Ferrari, F., I.K. de Cornelio, F. Delle Monache & G.B. Marini-Bettòlo. 1981. Quinovic acid glycosides from roots of *Macfadyena unguis-cati*. *Planta Medica* 43: 24-27.
BIGN 6. Kutney, J.P., W.D.C. Warnock & B. Gilbert. 1970. Pinocembrin 6-â-neohesperidoside, a flavanone glycoside from *Sparattosperma vernicosum*. *Phytochemistry* 9: 1877-1878.

BIGN 7. Oga, S. & T. Sekino. 1969. Toxidez e atividade antiinflamatória de *tabebuia avellanedae*. *Rev. Fac. Farm. Bioquím. Univ. S. Paulo* 7: 47-53.
BIGN 8. Thomson, R.H. 1971. *Naturally Occurring Quinones*. Academic Press. London and New York.
BIGN 9. Rao, K.V., T.J. McBride & J.J. Oleson. 1968. Recognition and evaluation of lapachol as an antitumor agent. *Cancer Research* 28: 1952-1954.
BIGN 10. Hadler, H.I. & T.L. Moreau. 1969. Induction of ATP energized mitochondrial volume changes by the combination of the two antitumor agents showdomycin and lapachol. *J. Antibiotics* 22: 513-520.
BIGN 11. Lima, O.G., J.S.B. Coelho, I.L. d'Albuquerque, J.F. Mello, D.G. Martins, A.L. Lacerda & M.A. de M. e Souza. 1971. Substâncias antimicrobianas em plantas superiores. XXXV. Atividade antimicrobiana e antitumoral de lawsona em comparação com o lapachol. *Rev. Inst. Antibióticos* (Federal University of Pernambuco) *11*: 21-26.
BIGN 12. Driscoll, J.S., G.F. Hazard Jr., H.B. Wood & A. Goldin. 1974. Structure-antitumor activity relations among quinone derivatives. *Cancer Chemother. Rep.* 4 (2): 1-27.
BIGN 13. Casinovi, C.G., G.B. Marini-Bettòlo, O. Gonçalves de Lima. 1963. Sui chinoni isolati del legno di *Tabebuia avellanedae* Lor. ex Griseb. *Radiconti dell'Istituto Superiore di Sanitá* (Roma) *26*: 1-10.
BIGN 14. Girard, M., D. Kindack, B.A. Dawson, J.-C. Ethier, D.V.C. Awang & A.H. Gentry. 1988. Naphthoquinone constituents of *Tabebuia* spp. *J. Nat. Prod.* 51: 1023-1024.
BIGN 15. Kreher, B., H. Lotter, G.A. Cordell & H. Wagner. 1988. New furanonaphthoquinones and other constituents of *Tabebuia avellanedae* and their immunomodulating activities *in vitro*. *Planta Medica* 54: 562-563.
BIGN 16. Wagner, H., B. Kreher & K. Jurcic. 1988. In vitro stimulation of human granulocytes and lymphocytes by pico- and femtogram quantities of cytostic agents. *Arzneimittel-Forschung/Drug Research* 38: 273-275.
BIGN 17. Oliveira, A.B. , D.S. Raslan, M.C.M. Miraglia, A.A.L. Mesquita, C.L. Zani, D.T. Ferreira & J.G.S. Maia. 1990. Estrutura química e atividade biológica de naftoquinonas de Bignoniáceas brasileiras. *Química Nova* (São Paulo) *13*: 302-307.
BIGN 18. Kerr, W.E. & D.A. Posey. 1991. "Kangàrà Kanê," *Tanaecium nocturnum* (Bignoniaceae), um cipó usado pelos índios Kayapó como insecticida natural. *Boletim do Museu Paraense Emílio Goeldi, ser. Bot.* (Belém) 7: 23-26.
BIGN 19. Machado, O. & P. Occhioni. 1943. Contribuição ao estudo das plantas cianogênicas do Brasil. *Rodriguesia* (Rio de Janeiro) 7 (16): 35-44 + 9.
BIGN 20. Gottlieb, O.R., M. Koketsu, M.T. Magalhães, J.G. Maia, P.H. Mendes, A.I. da Rocha, M.L. Silva & V.C. Wilberg. 1981. Oleos essenciais da Amazônia. VII. *Acta Amazonica* (Manaus) *11*: 143-148.
BIGN 21. Prance, G.T., D.G. Campbell & B.W. Nelson. 1977. The ethnobotany of the Paumari Indians. *Econ. Bot.* 31: 129-139.
BIGN 22. Vilegas, W., J.H.Y. Vilegas, G.L. Pozetti & R.M.S. Moreno. 1992. The chemistry of cipó-cravo, *Tynanthus fasciculatus*. *Rev. Latinoam. Quim.* 23: 65-66.
BIGN 23. Vilegas, J.H.Y., W. Vilegas, G.L. Pozetti & G. Llabres. 1993. Constituents of *Tynanthus fasciculatus*. *Fitoterapia* 64: 476.

BIXACEAE

Bixa orellana L.   A G R O T K C

AREA: Amazonia. Extensively cultivated for coloring matter and condiment.
NAMES: Açafroa, açafroeira-da-terra, urucu, urucum.
USES: Roots for a digestive, diuretic. Fresh shoots steeped in water as an eyewash for inflamed eyes. Leaf decoction used to lessen vomiting dur-

ing pregnancy. Seed paste indicated as an aphrodisiac and as protection against insect stings; in syrup for pharyngitis and bronchitis. Coloring matter is said to be an antidote against the effect of hydrocyanic acid found in poisonous cassava. The seeds are also recommended in cases of intestinal catarrh, measles and as an emmenagogue.

CHEM.: The red dye from the seed arils, internationally known as annatto, contains a mixture of stereoisomers of bixin, a C-24 diapocarotenoid (Ref: BIXA 1,2). The oil extracted from the leaves is a rich source of a great number of terpenes (Ref: BIXA 3).

Bixaceae – References

BIXA 1. Kuhn, R. & L. Ekman. 1929. Über Konjugierte Doppelbindungen. XI. Über das Bixin und seine Abbau zum Bixan. *Helv. Chim. Acta 12*: 904-915.

BIXA 2. Barber, M.S., A. Hardisson, L.M. Jackman & B.C.L. Weedon. 1961. Studies in nuclear magnetic resonance. IV. Stereochemistry of the bixins. *J. Chem. Soc.*: 1625-1630.

BIXA 3. Lawrence, B.M. & J.W. Hogg. 1973. Ishwarane in *Bixa orellana* leaf oil. *Phytochemistry 12*: 2995.

BOMBACACEAE

Ceiba pentandra (L.) Gaertn.
AREA: Amazonia, forest.
NAMES: Árvore-de-lã, árvore-de-seda, barriguda-de-espinho, paina-lisa, sumaúma, sumaumeira, sumaumeira-da-várzea.
USES: Root bark used for wounds. Sap for conjunctivitis.
CHEM.: A methylglucuronoxylan has been identified in the seeds (Ref: BOMB 2). Composition of seed oil has been studied (Ref: BOMB 3).

Chorisia crispiflora H.B.K.
AREA: Rio de Janeiro to Santa Catarina, along the littoral.
NAMES: Barriguda, paineira.
USE: Bark resin used for hernia.
CHEM.: The leaves contain 0.15% of rhoifolin, a glycoside of the flavone apigenin (Ref: BOMB 1).

Ochroma pyramidale (Cav.) Urb.
AREA: Amazonia, forest.
NAMES: Balsa, pau-de-balsa, topa.
USE: Root bark for an emetic.

Bombacaceae – References

BOMB 1. Coussio, J.D. 1964. Isolation of rhoifolin from *Chorisia* species. *Experientia 20*: 562.

BOMB 2. Currie, A.L. & T.E. Timell. 1959. Constitution of a methylglucuronoxylan from kapok (*Ceiba pentandra*). *Can. J. Chem. 37*: 922-959.

BOMB 3. Griffing, E.P. & C.I. Alsberg. 1931. Composition of kapok seed. *Ind. Eng. Chem.* **23**: 908-909.

BORAGINACEAE

Auxemma oncocalyx (Fr. All.) Taub.
AREA: Northeastern Brazil, caatinga.
NAME: Pau-branco.
USES: Bark used for healing wounds and ulcers.

Cordia coffeoides Warm.
AREA: Rio de Janeiro and Minas Gerais.
NAMES: Café-do-mato, laranjeira-do-mato, limão-do-mato.
USES: Leaves are diaphoretic, depurative, antirheumatic; said to be active against yellow fever.

Cordia ecalyculata Vell.
AREA: Minas Gerais to Rio Grande do Sul; central Brazil and Acre.
NAMES: Chá-de-bugre, porangaba, cafezinho, café-do-mato, chá-de-frade, louro-salgueiro, louro-mole.
USES: Tea is diuretic and used for slimming; for treating cough; wound healing.
CHEM.: Contains allantoin and allantoic acid (Ref: BORA 1).

Cordia grandiflora DC.
AREA: Pernambuco to São Paulo.
NAMES: Acoara-muru, grão-de-galo, grão-de-porco.
USES: Fruits used in preparing a mucilaginous syrup for bronchitis.

Cordia insignis Cham.
AREA: Minas Gerais.
NAMES: Caraíba, grão-de-galo.
USE: Emollient.

Cordia magnolifolia Cham.
AREA: Rio de Janeiro.
NAMES: Acoara-muru, grão-de-galo, jaguara-muru.
USES: Drupes (fruits) are bechic.

Cordia monosperma (Jacq.) Roem. & Schult.
AREA: Southern Brazil.
NAMES: Baleeira, erva-baleeira.
USES: Drupes are slightly laxative.

BORAGINACEAE

Cordia multispicata Cham.
AREA: Amazonia.
NAMES: Canaru-caá, caru-caá.
USES: Leaves in infusion are appreciated as tonic; also for grippe, bronchitis and prolonged cough.

Cordia obscura Cham.
AREA: Minas Gerais and São Paulo.
NAMES: Capitão-do-campo, jurutê.
USE: Leaf tea used for slimming.

Cordia salicifolia Cham.
AREA: Amazonia to Rio Grande do Sul.
NAMES: Café-do-mato, chá-de-bugre, bugrinho, chá-de-negro-mina, laranjeira-do-mato, porangaba.
USES: Leaves are tonic and used for slimming.

Cordia umbraculifera DC.
AREA: Amazonia.
NAMES: Árvore-de-umbela, pará-pará.
USES: Smoke from the burning bark is used in fumigations to disinfect dwellings.

Cordia verbenacea DC.
AREA: Southeastern coast of Brazil.
NAMES: Erva-baleeira, catinga-preta, maria-rezadeira, maria-preta.
USES: Leaves for wound healing, anti-inflammatory, against ulcers; used by fishermen to cure wounds inflicted by fish.
CHEM. & PHARM.: Leaf extract strongly anti-inflammatory, with low toxicity (Ref: BORA 2,3,4). Two flavonoids (Ref: BORA 5) and two new triterpenes (Ref: BORA 6) have been identified. The active compound responsible for the anti-inflammatory properties is artemetin, 5-hydroxy-3,6,7,3',4'-pentamethoxyflavone. Its industrialization has been studied by a pharmaceutical laboratory in São Paulo (Ref: BORA 7).

Heliotropium curassavicum L.
AREA: Littoral, from Bahia to Rio Grande do Sul.
NAME: Crista-de-galo.
USES: Pectoral, mucilaginous.
CHEM.: Contains pyrrolizidine alkaloids (Ref: BORA 8,9,11).

Heliotropium elongatum Willd.
AREA: Ceará to Bahia.
NAMES: Aguaraquinhá, crista-de-galo, erva-ferro, fedegoso-do-mato.
USES: Herb is resolvent, antiasthmatic, diuretic; recommended for an-

thrax, syphilitic ulcers, liver diseases and bladder problems. Flowers as a pectoral and for colds.

Heliotropium indicum L.
AREA: Almost throughout Brazil.
NAMES: Borragem-brava, crista-de-galo, fedegoso.
USES: Roots, leaves and flowers are resolvent, diuretic, pectoral. Plant juice indicated for skin diseases. Leaves applied to boils, ulcers, wounds and insect stings.
CHEM.: Contains pyrrolizidine alkaloids (Ref: BORA 9,10,11).

Heliotropium lanceolatum Loefgr.
AREA: Northeastern Brazil.
NAME: Sete-sangrias.
USES: Root decoction is tonic, emmenagogue, antipyretic and diuretic.
Plants of the genus *Heliotropium* are rich in ester-alkaloids of the pyrrolizidine type. Some have interesting pharmacological properties, such as ganglion blocking and antineoplastic activity. All of them, however, are strongly hepatotoxic, making the use of these plants for medicinal purposes extremely dangerous (Ref: BORA 9,10).

Patagonula americana L.
AREA: Southern Brazil.
NAMES: Guajuvira, guaraiúva, guaiuvira, garapuvira, ipê-branco, pau-d'arco.
USES: Leaves are vulnerary and useful for suppurations, malignant wounds and syphilitic lesions. Tea is emollient.
CHEM.: Two terpenoid quinone pigments of the cordiachrome type, found mainly in a number of *Cordia* species (Ref: BORA 12), were identified in the wood of this plant (Ref: BORA 13), aside from a highly methoxylated cinnamaldehyde (Ref: BORA 14).

Tournefortia elegans Cham.
AREA: Minas Gerais.
NAME: Caruru-de-veado.
USES: Leaves are mucilaginous, used in poultices and hot baths for rheumatism.

Tournefortia laevigata Lam.
AREA: Amazonia.
NAME: Erva-de-lagarto.
USES: Leaf and root decoction for hydropsy and syphilis.

Tournefortia paniculata Cham.
AREA: Minas Gerais.

NAME: Marmelinho.
USE: Diuretic.

Tournefortia volubilis L.
AREA: Eastern Brazil, mainly Rio de Janeiro.
NAME: Chá-mineiro-verdadeiro.
USES: Leaf tea is aromatic, used as substitute for India tea (*Thea sinensis*).

Boraginaceae – References

BORA 1. Saito, M.L. & F. Oliveria. 1986. Morfodiagnose e identificação cromatográfica em camada delgada de chá-de-bugre — *Cordia ecalyculata* Vell. *Rev. Bras. Farm.* **67**: 1-16.

BORA 2. Sertié, J.A.A., A.C. Basile, S. Panizza, A.K. Matida & R. Zelnik. 1988. Pharmacological assay of *Cordia verbenacea*: Part I. Anti-inflammatory activity and toxicity of the crude extract of the leaves. *Planta Medica* **54**: 7-10.

BORA 3. Sertié, J.A.A., A.C. Basile, S. Panizza, A.K. Matida & R. Zelnik. 1990. Pharmacological assay of *Cordia verbenacea*. Part II. Anti-inflammatory activity and sub-acute toxicity of artemetin. *Planta Medica* **56**: 36-40.

BORA 4. Sertié, J.A.A., A.C. Basile, S. Panizza, T.T. Oshiro, C.P. Azzolini & S.C. Penna. 1991. Pharmacological assay of *Cordia verbenacea*. Part III. Oral and topical antiinflammatory activity and gastrotoxicity of a crude leaf extract. *J. Ethnopharmacol.* **31**: 239-247.

BORA 5. Lins, A.P., N.A. Alvarenga, O.R. Gottlieb & F. Oliveira. 1980. Flavonóis de *Cordia verbenacea*. *Ciência e Cultura* **32** (7): 457.

BORA 6. Van de Velde, V., D. Lavie, R. Zelnik, A.K. Matida & S. Panizza. 1982. Cordialin A and B, two new triterpenes from *Cordia verbenacea* DC. *J. Chem. Soc. Perkin Trans. 1*: 2697-2700.

BORA 7. Anon. 1989. Dose completa. *Rev. Bras. Tecnologia* **19**: 44-45.

BORA 8. Rajagopalan, T.R. & V. Batra. 1977. Alkaloidal constituents of *Heliotropium curassavicum*. *Indian J. Chem.* **15B**: 494.

BORA 9. Smith, L.W. & C.C.J. Culvenor. 1981. Plant sources of hepatotoxic pyrrolizidine alkaloids. *J. Nat. Prod.* **44**: 129-152.

BORA 10. Pandey, V.B., J.P. Singh, Y.V. Rao & S.B. Acharya. 1982. Isolation and pharmacological action of heliotrine, the major alkaloid of *Heliotropium indicum*. *Planta Medica* **45**: 229-233.

BORA 11. Catalfamo, J.L., W.B. Martin Jr. & H. Birecka. 1982. Accumulation of alkaloids and their necines in *Heliotropium curassavicum*, *H. spathulatum* and *H. indicum*. *Phytochemistry* **21**: 2669-2675.

BORA 12. Moir, M. & R.H. Thompson. 1973. Naturally occurring quinones. Part XXII. Terpenoid quinones in *Cordia* spp. *J. Chem. Soc. Perkin Trans. 1*: 1352-1357.

BORA 13. Moir, M. & R.H. Thompson. 1973. Naturally occurring quinones. Part XXIII. Cordiachromes from *Patagonula americana*. *J. Chem. Soc. Perkin Trans. 1*: 1556-1561.

BORA 14. Moir, M. & R.H. Thompson. 1973. New cinnamaldehyde from *Patagonula americana*. *Phytochemistry* **12**: 2501-2503.

BROMELIACEAE

Ananas comosus (L.) Merrill
AREA: Throughout Brazil, both native and extensively cultivated.
NAMES: Abacaxi, ananás.
USES: The juice of the syncarp is highly appreciated as a digestive, due to

its enzyme content; useful for dyspepsy, sore throat and bronchitis; also anti-inflammatory. Unripe fruit reputedly is vermifuge and abortifacient.

CHEM. & PHARM.: Syncarp and stem contain the plant protease bromelin or bomelain (Ref: BROM 1). The anthelmintic action is due to the digestion of the keratin carapace of worms (Ref: BROM 2). Also used as a meat tenderizer.

Bromelia antiacantha Bertol.

AREA: Minas Gerais to Rio Grande do Sul and Mato Grosso; in littoral, cerrados and dry forests.

NAMES: Carauatá, gravatá, gravatá-da-praia, gravatá-do-mato, gravatá-de-raposa, maná-de-raposa, banana-do-mato.

USES: Berries are sour, purgative, vermifuge, diuretic, even abortive. The flesh serves in a syrup recommended for asthma, bronchitis and ancylostomiasis. Also for kidney stones, jaundice and dropsy.

CHEM.: The plant has been cited as a possible source of bromelin (Ref: BROM 3).

Bromelia arenaria Ule

AREA: Bahia, caatinga.

USES: Juice of the berries is used for cleaning malignant sores, whose tissue it destroys; also against aphthae and afflictions of the mucous membranes.

Bromelia pinguin L.

AREA: Amazonia, forest.

NAMES: Caraguatá, caroatá, carauá.

USES: Fruit anthelmintic, diuretic, abortive; juice diluted with water to cure aphthae.

CHEM.: Contains protease with properties identical to those of bromelin (Ref: BROM 4,5).

Tillandsia aeranthos (Loisel.) L.B. Smith

AREA: Rio Grande do Sul.

NAME: Cravo-do-mato.

USES: Plant is diuretic; decoctions prescribed for blennorrhagia.

Tillandsia usneoides L.

AREA: Throughout Brazil, with the exception of Amazonia.

NAMES: Barba-de-velho, barba-de-pau.

USES: Recommended for rheumatism, hemorrhoids, hernia and enlarged liver.

CHEM.: Flavonols (Ref: BROM 6,7) and triterpenes (Ref: BROM 8) identified.

Tillandsia aeranthos

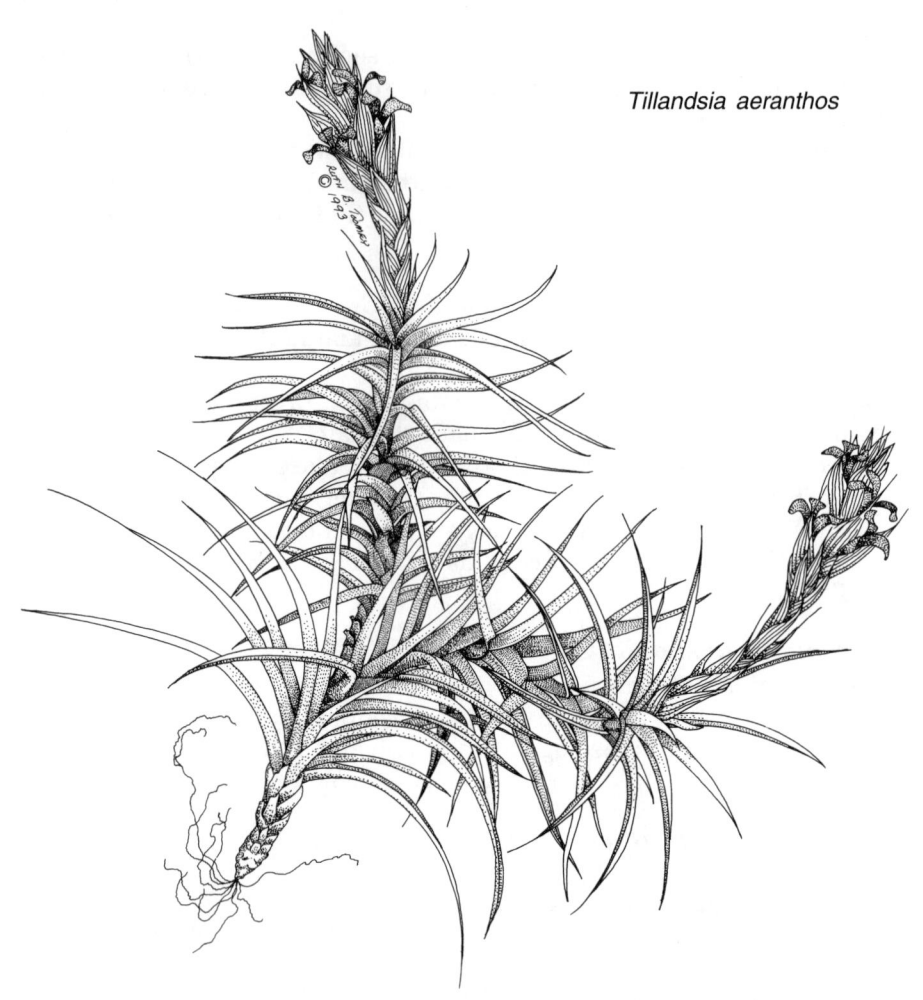

PHARM.: Extracts show weak antibiotic activity (Ref: BROM 6,9). Estrogenic activity has also been reported (Ref: BROM 10).

Bromeliaceae – References

BROM 1. Bells, A.K., R.R. Thompson & M.W. Kies. 1941. Bromelin. Properties and commercial production. *Ind. Eng. Chem. 33*: 950-953.

BROM 2. Asenjo, C.F. 1940. A preliminary study of the anthelmintic activity *in vitro* of fresh pineapple juice. *J. Am. Pharm. Assoc. 29*: 8-10.

BROM 3. Nakamura, S. 1972. *Alguns Estudos sobre Obtenção de Enzimas Proteolíticas em Bromelia antiacantha* Bertol. Thesis, University of São Paulo.

BROM 4. Asenjo, C.F. & M.C.C. Fernandez. 1942. New protease from *Bromelia pinguin* L. *Science 95*: 48-49.

BROM 5. Asenjo, C.F. & M.C.C. Fernandez. 1945. Uses, preparation and properties of pinguinain, the protein splitting enzyme of the maya fruit. *J. Agric. Univ. Puerto Rico 229*: 35-46.

BROM 6. Webber, M.G., W.M. Lauter & P.A. Fook. 1952. A preliminary phytochemical study of *Tillandsia usneoides* (Spanish moss). *J. Am. Pharm. Assoc. 41*: 230-235.

BROM 7. Lewis, D.S. & T.J. Mabry. 1977. 3,6,3',5'-tetramethoxy-5,7,4'-trihydroxyflavone from *Tillandsia usneoides*. *Phytochemistry 16*: 1114-1115.
BROM 8. Djerassi, C. & R. McCrindle. 1962. Terpenoids. LI. The isolation of some new cyclopropane-containing triterpenes from Spanish moss. *J. Chem. Soc.* (London): 4034-4039.
BROM 9. Wald, J.T. 1945. The antibiotic action of *Tillandsia usneoides* (Spanish moss). *Proc. Soc. Exptl. Biol. Med. 59*: 40-41.
BROM 10. Feurt, S.D. & L.E. Fox. 1952. The pharmacological activity of substances extracted from Spanish moss, *Tillandsia usneoides*. *J. Am. Pharm. Assoc. 41*: 453-454.

BUDDLEJACEAE

Buddleja brasiliensis Jacq. ex Spr.
AREA: Amazonia to Rio Grande do Sul.
NAMES: Barbasco, barbasco-do-brasil, calças-de-velho, calção-de-velho, tinguí-da-praia, verbasco, vassoura.
USES: Bark is bitter, applied for lung afflictions. Root infusion for snakebite. Leaves and flowers are soothing, sudorific, bechic, emollient, antiarthritic; also for piles, contusions, hemoptyses, bronchitis and asthma.

Buddleja cambara Arech.
AREA: Rio Grande do Sul, in marshy sites.
NAME: Cambará.
USES: Pectoral. In veterinary practice, a decoction is employed for washing inflamed eyes of mules; in baths to treat bruises.

Buddleja stachioides Cham.
AREA: Minas Gerais to Rio Grande do Sul.
NAMES: Vassoura, vassourinha, tupeiçaba.
USES: Anticatarrhal, antiarthritic, antihemorrhoidal.

BURSERACEAE

Protium aracouchini (Aubl.) March.
AREA: Amazonia, forest.
NAME: Aracuchini.
USE: Resin vulnerary.

Protium heptaphyllum (Aubl.) March.
AREA: Widespread throughout Brazil, in forest and cerrado.
NAMES: Almecegueira, breu, breu-branco, breu-jauaricica, jauaricica.
USES: Bark and leaves are used to treat gangrenous ulcers and inflammations in general; hemostatic.

BURSERACEAE

Protium icicariba (DC.) March.
AREA: Amazonia to São Paulo, forest and restinga.
NAMES: Almecegueira, breu-branco, guapoí, mescla.
USES: Root-bark is astringent, depurative, antisyphilitic. Leaves and bark used for cleaning sloughing ulcers and to expel chiggers (*Pulex penetrans*). Resinous exudate of the tree is known as almecega or Brazilian elemi, employed externally as stimulant, soothing, hemostatic, antigonorrhoeic, antirheumatic, as well as to soothe toothache.

Protium schomburgkianum Engl.
AREA: Amazonia, forest.
NAME: Aruru.
USE: Resin employed to treat blennorrhagia.

Protium spp.

Several other *Protium* species are also used, but are less important in popular medicine: *P. brasiliense* Engl. (plate below), *P. cordatum* Hub., *P. elegans* Engl., *P. insigne* Engl., *P. sagotianum* March., *P. spruceanum* (Benth.) Engl., and *P. unifoliolatum* Engl., found mostly in Amazonian territory.

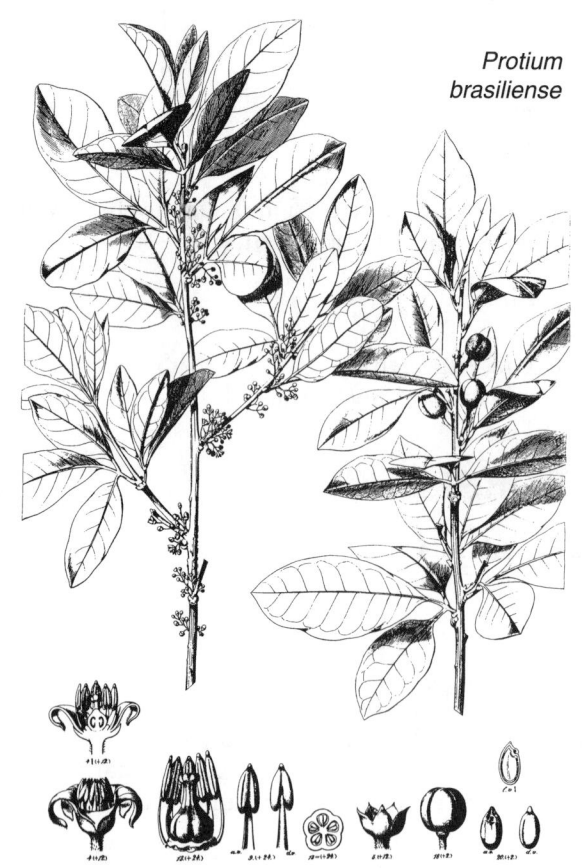

All *Protium* species secrete from incisions in the trunk a greenish-white or light grey oleoresin of pleasant odor, which hardens on exposure to the air. This is rich in triterpenes, mainly of the oleanane, ursane and euphane series, being analogous to frankincense or olibanum of India and Africa, which are obtained

Protium brasiliense

from trees of the same family (Ref: BURS 1). A coumarinolignoid has been described from the Amazonian *P. opacum* Swart., a species which, however, is not listed as medicinal (Ref: BURS 2).

Burseraceae – References

BURS 1. Parnet, R. 1972. Phytochimie des Burseracées. *Lloydia 35*: 280-287.
BURS 2. Zoghbi, M.G.B., N.F. Roque & O.R. Gottlieb. 1981. Propacin, a coumarinolignoid from *Protium opacum*. *Phytochemistry 20*: 180.

CACTACEAE

Brasilopuntia brasiliensis (Willd.) Berg.
AREA: Dispersed throughout Brazil, mainly along the littoral.
NAMES: Figueira, jumbeba, jurumbeba, palmatória-grande, urumbeba.
USES: Unripe berries are emollient; ripe berries used for tuberculosis; in poultices, for relieving pains of sciatica. Juice of roots and cladodes used as a febrifuge.

Cereus jamacaru DC.
AREA: Widely disseminated in the northeastern caatinga of Brazil.
NAMES: Cardieiro, facheiro, jamacaru, mandacaru, mandacaru-de-boi.
USES: Juice used for treating scurvy, lung and skin diseases; externally applied on ulcers.
CHEM.: Contains alkaloids (Ref: CACT 1).

Cereus peruvianus (L.) Mill.
AREA: Mainly Rio Grande do Sul and Mato Grosso.
NAMES: Mandacaru, urumbeva, tuna.
USES: Antiscorbutic and bechic. Juice of plant used mainly for treatment of burns; in cataplasms it hastens healing of wounds and chronic ulcers. Also used against snakebite.
CHEM.: Presence of alkaloids has been reported (Ref: CACT 2). Nonbasic components described in the juice (Ref: CACT 3) and in epicuticular wax (Ref: CACT 4).

Hylocereus undatus (Haw.) Br. & Rose
AREA: Mainly along the southern coast of Brazil.
NAMES: Cardo-ananás, cardo-limão, pitacaiá, urumbeba.
USES: Poultices made from the stem are sedative and emollient on ulcers and abscesses. Decoction is a cooling remedy for fevers in general. The juice, worked into syrup, is used in cases of pulmonary afflictions. Tincture of the flowers is diuretic and cardioactive. Fruit juice is used against scurvy. Plant juice is anthelmintic and also used to treat heart problems.

CACTACEAE

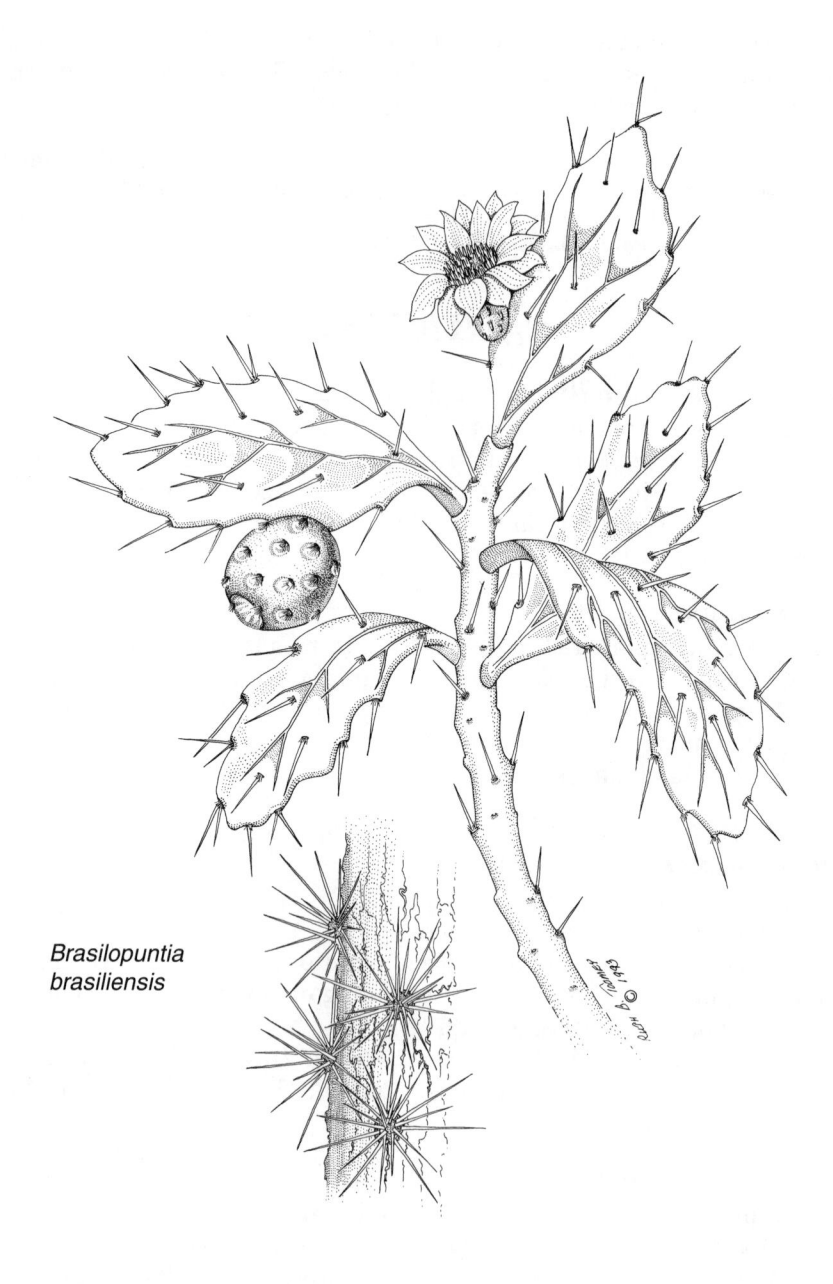

Brasilopuntia brasiliensis

Lepismium myosurus Pfeiff.
AREA: In and around Rio Grande do Sul.
NAME: Rabo-de-rato.
USE: Plant used for a sedative.

Melocactus melocactoides (Hoffm.) DC.
AREA: Paraíba to Rio de Janeiro, on sandy beaches.
NAMES: Cabeça-de-frade, cardo-melão, coroa-de-frade.
USE: Antiscorbutic.

Notocactus ottonis (Lem.) Berg.
AREA: Campos in Rio Grande do Sul.
NAME: Cardo-melão.
USE: Fruit used as a diuretic.

Opuntia vulgaris Mill.
AREA: Bahia to Rio Grande do Sul, in littoral and inland.
NAMES: Arumbeva, palma-santa, palmatória, urumbeva.
USE: Sedative.
CHEM.: Flavonoids are present in flowers; mucilage and pectin in fruits (Ref: CACT 5). Triterpenes present in whole plant (Ref: CACT 6).

Pereskia aculeata Mill.
AREA: Bahia to Rio Grande do Sul, restinga.
NAMES: Groselha-da-américa, ora-pro-nobis.
USES: Leaves are emollient. Fruit is expectorant and antisyphilitic.

Pereskia bleo H.B.K.
AREA: Subspontaneous in all of Brazil, ruderal.
NAMES: Cacto-rosa, jumbeba, jurubeba, ora-pro-nobis, rosa-curandeira, rosa-mole, sem-vergonha.
USES: Berries are bechic, antisyphilitic. Leaves used as an emollient.

Rhipsalis macrocarpa Miq.
AREA: Rio de Janeiro, forest.
NAME: Rabo-de-jacaré.
USES: Fruit is diuretic and sedative.

A review of the composition of the mucilages of Cactaceae has been published (Ref: CACT 7).

Cactaceae – References
CACT 1. Bruhn, J.G. & J.-E. Lindgren. 1976. Cactaceae alkaloids. XXIII. Alkaloids of *Pachycereus pecten-aboriginum* and *Cereus jamacaru*. *Lloydia 39*: 175-177.
CACT 2. Hefter, A. 1898. Über Cacteenalkaloïde. III. Mitteilung. *Ber. Deut. Chem. Ges. 31*: 1193-1199.
CACT 3. Kringstad, R. 1980. Cerheptaric acid, a new lactone-forming acid isolated from *Cereus peruvianus* (L.) Mill. *Carbohydrate Res. 80*: 285-289.
CACT 4. Hughes, J., G. Ramos & P. Moyna. 1980. Main components in *Cereus peruvianus* epicuticular wax. *J. Nat. Prod. 43*: 564-566.
CACT 5. Paris, R. 1951. Un flavonoïde des fleurs de l'*Opuntia vulgaris*. *Compt. Rend. 233*: 90-92.

Bauhinia forficata

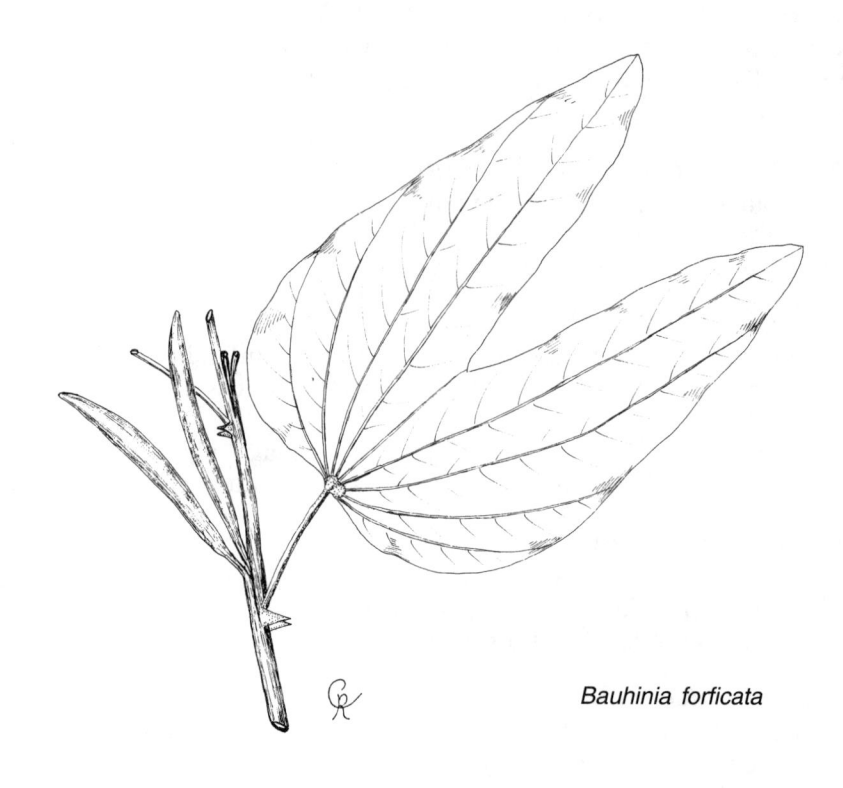

CACT 6. Chatterjee, A., S. Mukhopadhyay & K. Chattopadhyay. 1976. Lewis acid catalyzed rearrangement of triterpenes. *Tetrahedron 32*: 3051-3053.
CACT 7. Mindt, L. 1975. Cactaceae mucilage composition. *J. Sci. Food Agric. 26*: 993-1000.

CAESALPINIACEAE

Apuleia leiocarpa (Vog.) MacBride
AREA: Ceará to Rio de Janeiro, forest.
NAMES: Garapa, gema-de-ovo, grapiá, grapiapunha, jatobá, jitaí, jutaí.
USES: Bark reputedly is antisyphilitic.
CHEM.: Flavonoids identified in bark (Ref: CAES 1).
PHARM.: Aqueous extracts of wood and bark, administered orally to mice, showed anti-inflammatory and analgesic activity (Ref: CAES 2). The same extracts inhibited cutaneous vascular permeability caused by various agents and protected against the snake venom of *Bothrops jararaca* (Ref: CAES 3).

Bauhinia candicans Benth.
AREA: Rio Grande do Sul, forest.
NAMES: Pata-de-boi, pata-de-vaca, unha-de-boi, unha-de-vaca.
USES: Leaves are reputedly antidiabetic and hypocholesteremic.
CHEM.: Sterols, flavonoids, pinitol, choline and trigonellin isolated from leaves and flowers (Ref: CAES 4).

Bauhinia forficata Link
AREA: Minas Gerais, Rio de Janeiro and São Paulo, forest.
NAMES: Mororó, pata-de-vaca, unha-de-vaca.
USES: Leaves used as an anti-diabetic and for cystitis.
PHARM.: The highly reputed hypoglycemic action is still controversial. Early studies which confirmed this action (Ref: CAES 5) have recently been refuted (Ref: CAES 6).

Bauhinia guianensis Aubl.
AREA: Amazonia
NAME: Escada-de-jabuti.
USES: Roots considered active against amoebiasis and dysentery.

Bauhinia langsdorffiana Bong.
AREA: Throughout the Brazilian coastal region.
NAMES: Cipó-escada, unha-de-boi.
USES: Leaves are mucilaginous and astringent, used in gargles, poultices and clysters.

Bauhinia radiata Vell.
AREA: Ceará to Rio de Janeiro, mainly in the coastal forest.
NAME: Cipó-escada.
USES: A syrup is prepared from the stem, prescribed against coughs, bronchitis and whooping cough.

Bauhinia rutilans Spr. ex Benth.
AREA: Amazonia.
NAME: Escada-de-jabuti.
USES: Bark is antirheumatic and antiluetic (antisyphilitic).

Caesalpinia bonduc (L.) Roxb.
AREA: Amazonia to São Paulo, littoral.
NAMES: Arriózes, inimbó, inimboja, juquirirana, olho-de-gato, silva-da-praia.
USES: Young leaves used to expel worms in children; seeds are vomitive and employed in the treatment of snakebite.
CHEM.: The kernels contain a group of furanoditerpenes designated as caesalpins (Ref: CAES 7).

CAESALPINIACEAE

Caesalpinia bracteosa Tul.
AREA: Northeastern states of Brazil, in caatinga.
NAMES: Catingueira, pau-amarante.
USE: Flowers are bechic.

Caesalpinia echinata Lam.
AREA: Pernambuco to Rio de Janeiro, in both coastal and inland forest. This is the well-known "Brazil wood," which was almost extinct due to overexploitation in colonial times. Nowadays it is frequently replanted.
NAMES: Ibirapitanga, pau-brasil, pau-pernambuco.
USES: Wood is tonic and odontalgic.
CHEM.: The red dye for which the wood used to be procured owes its color to the substance brazilein, the aerial oxidation product of brazilin, which is colorless. An excellent review of the subject exists (Ref: CAES 8).

Caesalpinia ferrea Mart. ex Tul.
AREA: Piauí to Rio de Janeiro, forest and caatinga.
NAMES: Ibita-obi, jucá, muira-itá, pau-ferro.
USES: Roots are antipyretic and antidiarrhoeic. Decoction of wood is anticatarrhal and vulnerary. Root and stem bark are antidiabetic. Infusion of bast used for treating sores and for chronic cough and asthma.

Caesalpinia microphylla Mart.
AREA: Bahia.
NAMES: Catinga-de-porco, catingueiro-da-folha-miúda, catingueiro-de-porco, erva-de-rato, pau-de-rato.
USES: An aqueous extract of bast, leaves and flowers is drunk as an effective remedy to aid digestion.

Caesalpinia pyramidalis Tul.
AREA: Piauí do Bahia, caatinga.
NAMES: Catingueira, pau-de-rato.
USES: Bark and flowers are used against catarrhal infections and diarrhoea.

Campsiandra comosa Benth. var. *laurifolia* (Benth.) Cowan
AREA: Amazonia, forest.
NAMES: Acapu-do-igapó, acapurana, caacapoc, cumandá.
USES: Alcoholic extract or aqueous decoction is tonic and excitant, recommended for malarial fever and to clean sores.

Cassia ferruginea (Schrad.) Schrad. ex DC.
AREA: Ceará to Paraná, forest.
NAME: Canafístula.
USE: Seed pulp is laxative.

CAESALPINIACEAE

Caesalpinia echinata

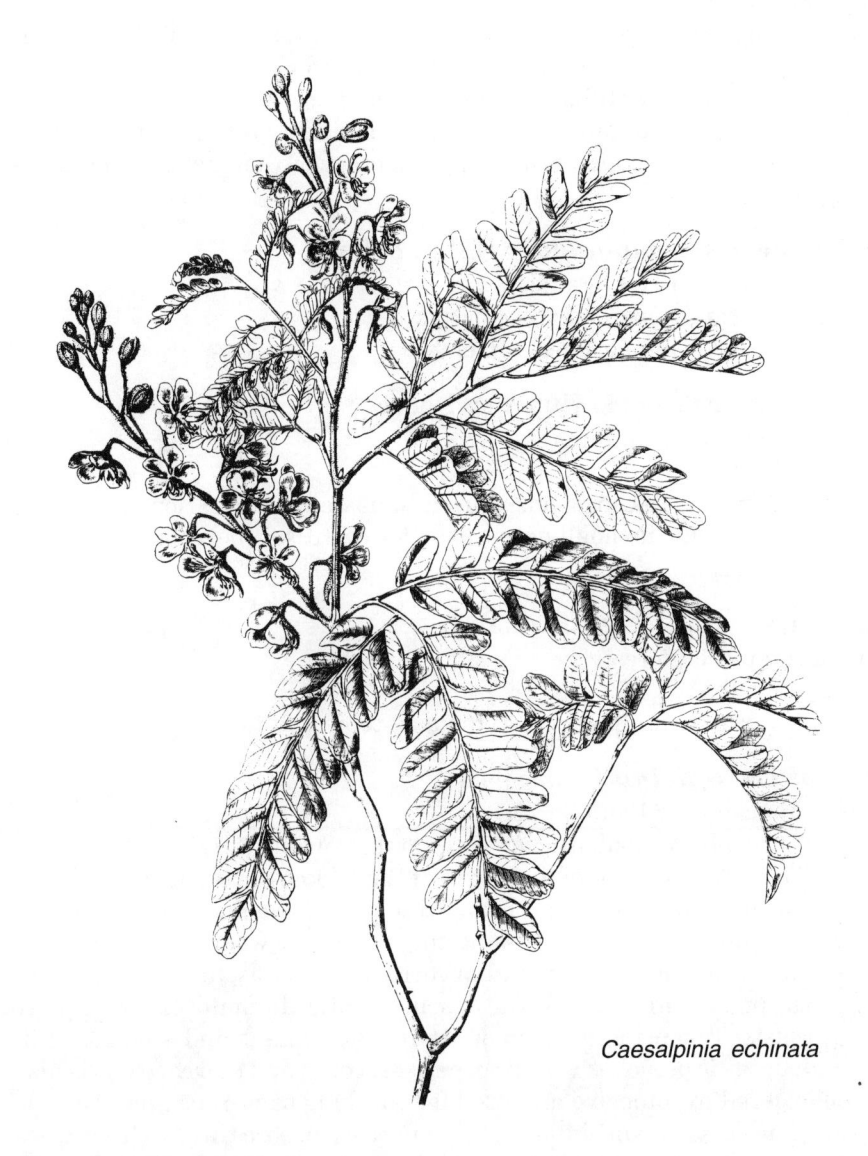

Cassia grandis L.
AREA: Amazonia, but extensively cultivated in other regions.
USES: Pulp of pods is laxative and also used for certain skin diseases.

Chamaecrista cathartica (Mart.) Ir. & Barn.
AREA: Minas Gerais and Rio de Janeiro to São Paulo.
NAME: Sene-do-campo.
USES: Laxative, like the genuine senna (cf. CHEM. under *Senna* spp.).

CAESALPINIACEAE

Chamaecrista fasciculata (Michx.) Greene
AREA: Rio de Janeiro to Rio Grande do Sul, preferably in littoral, but reaching as far as the interior of Minas Gerais and Goiás.
NAMES: Cássia-das-antilhas, fedegoso-dormideira.
USES: Leaves are purgative, serving as substitute for the genuine senna leaves (cf. CHEM. under *Senna* spp.); moreover, they have hypnotic effects.

Chamaecrista mimosoides (L.) Ir. & Barn.
AREA: Amazonia to São Paulo.
NAMES: Cássia-de-empingem, sensitiva.
USES: In a medicine for liver ailments.

Copaifera cearensis Huber ex Ducke
AREA: Ceará, on mountains.
NAME: Pau-d'óleo.
USES: Oil from trunk incisions is used to hasten cicatrization of wounds; emollient, tonic in small doses, used for cystitis, gonorrhoea and rheumatic pain.

Copaifera multijuga Hayne
AREA: Amazonia, forest.
NAME: Copaíba.
USES: Oil from trunk is added to tea as a tonic and to lower fever.

Copaifera officinalis (Jacq.) L.
AREA: Amazonia to Piauí, forest.
NAMES: Copaíba-verdadeira, copaíva, jatobá-mirim, pau-de-óleo.
USES: This species is the main source of the oil known as copaíba balsam, which oozes from incisions on the trunk. It is balsamic, wound healing, used as an antitetaic in dressing the navel of newborns, urinary antiseptic, antiblennorrhagic, antileucorrhoeic; also useful for vesical catarrh, pneumonia, bronchitis, dysentery and dermatoses, principally psoriasis. Taken in small amounts it is stimulant and stomachic; in high doses it provokes vomiting, nausea, colics and diarrhoea. It is also considered hypotensive and used for checking cancerous growths. It is much used as an anti-inflammatory in cases of sore throat. Other trees furnishing copaíba balsam are *C. langsdorffii* Desf. (central Brazil, cerrado) and *C. reticulata* Ducke (Amazon forest).
CHEM.: Copaíba oil or oleoresin, or 'balsam' as it is called, is made up of a mixture of sesquiterpenes (Ref: CAES 9,10) and diterpenes (Ref: CAES 11). Coumarins have been identified in seeds (Ref: CAES 12); and the use of the oleoresin as fuel oil has been suggested (Ref: CAES 13).
PHARM.: The reputed anti-inflammatory activity has been confirmed (Ref: CAES 14,15).

CAESALPINIACEAE

Hymenaea courbaril

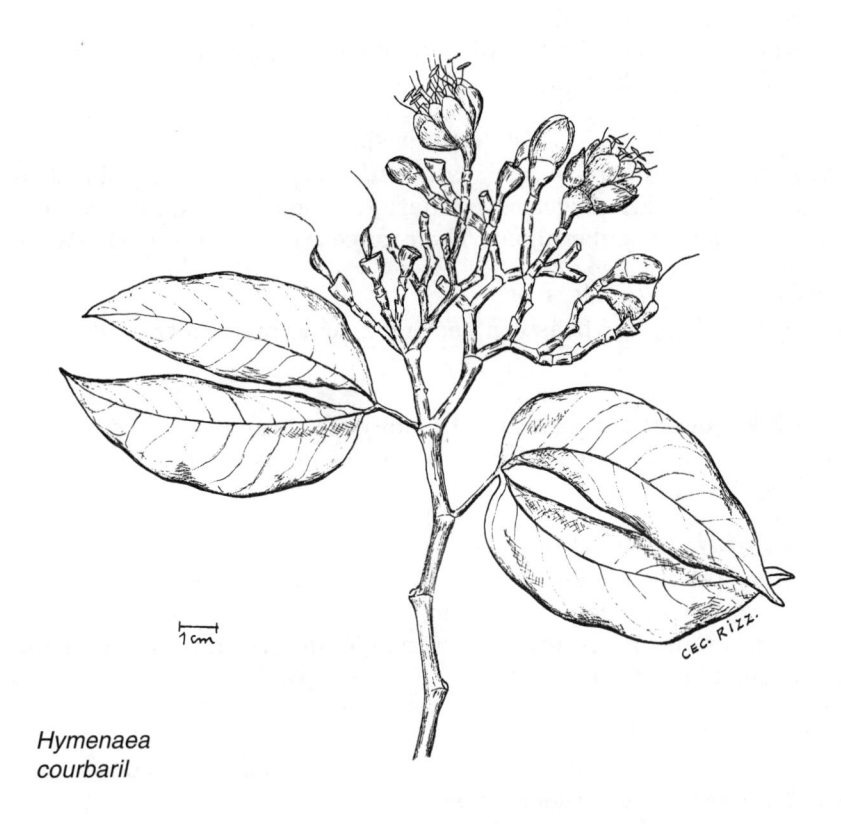

Hymenaea courbaril L.

AREA: Amazonia to Bahia and Mato Grosso, forest.

NAMES: Jataí, jatobá, jutaí, jutaí-açu.

USES: The tree spontaneously yields a resin which collects at the base of the trunk, where it appears in large, irregular masses. It is hard, translucent and brittle, light yellow to brown in color. The Brazilian name for this resin is jutaicica, whereas internationally it is known as 'Brazilian copal.' It is tonic, balsamic, bechic, stomachic and vermifuge in popular usage. The sap which flows from bore-holes in the trunk is considered fortifying, wound healing and used for treating chronic cystitis, urine retention, anemia, prostatitis, blennorrhagia and chronic bronchitis. The bark is astringent and pectoral. In baths it is used against skin diseases. The seeds within the pods are covered by a sweetish pulp which is edible and has a mild laxative action.

CHEM.: A diterpene acid, named copalic acid (Ref: CAES 16), and a mixture of sesquiterpenes of the bisabolene type (Ref: CAES 17) have been identified as constituents of the resin. Sesqui- and diterpenes have also been found in leaves (Ref: CAES 18), bark (Ref: CAES 19) and trunk resin (Ref: CAES 20,21,22).

Hymenaea spp.

Other *Hymenaea* species, such as *H. stilbocarpa* Hayne (dry forest in central Brazil) and *H. stigonocarpa* Mart. (cerrado), have similar properties and the same popular names. Their range is from Goiás to São Paulo.

Parkinsonia aculeata L.

AREA: Neotropical; northeastern caatinga; sometimes cultivated along streets.
NAMES: Rosa-da-turquia, turco.
USES: Bark, flowers and seeds used to lower fever and restore strength. Leaves are antipyretic, sudorific, antimalarial and recommended for epilepsy.

Senna affinis (Benth.) Ir. & Barn.

AREA: Minas Gerais, Rio de Janeiro and São Paulo.
NAMES: Cabo-verde, fedegoso-legítimo.
USES: Root-bark is tonic, diuretic, indicated for dropsy and liver ailments. Leaves and bracts are purgative.

Senna alata (L.) Roxb.

AREA: Cosmopolitan, common in Brazil from Amazonia to Rio de Janeiro and Mato Grosso as a ruderal plant.
NAMES: Dartrial, fedegoso, maria-preta, marigeriona-grande, matapasto.
USES: Root infusion is drastic, emmenagogue, for liver obstruction, antirheumatic, diuretic, febrifuge. Young leaves are purgative, used as substitute for genuine senna (cf. CHEM. under *Senna* spp.). Flowers, eaten raw, are used to remedy hemorrhoids.
CHEM.: Leaves contain rhein and its corresponding anthrone (Ref: CAES 24). Roots are also rich in anthraquinone pigments (Ref: CAES 25).

Senna bicapsularis (L.) Roxb.

AREA: Throughout Brazil.
NAMES: Caquera, são-joão.
USES: Leaves are purgative.

Senna corymbosa (Lam.) Ir. & Barn.

AREA: Minas Gerais to Rio Grande do Sul, mostly along creeks.
NAMES: Canafístula-da-mata, fedegoso, fedegoso-de-folha-torta, mangerioba.
USES: Leaves, bracts and seed pulp are laxative. Seeds are roasted, powdered and mixed with coffee grounds to make a laxative beverage.

CAESALPINIACEAE

Senna hirsuta (L.) Ir. & Barn. var. ***puberula*** Ir. & Barn.
AREA: Amazonia to Paraná and Mato Grosso.
NAMES: Fedegoso-do-mato, paramarioba.
USES: Roots used for a tonic. Plant infusion is recommended for kidney disorders; also for ulcers and fissures of the nipples during breast feeding. Febrifuge and antiluetic.

Senna latifolia (Meyer) Ir. & Barn.
AREA: Pará, forest.
NAMES: Fedegoso, lava-pratos.
USES: Leaves employed to clean sores. Roots are resolvent.

Senna leiophylla (Vog.) Ir. & Barn.
AREA: Southern Brazil.
NAME: Fedegoso.
USES: Infusion taken against common cold.

Senna macranthera (Collad.) Ir. & Barn.
AREA: Minas Gerais to São Paulo, forest.
NAMES: Aleluia, cabo-verde, ipê-falso, manduirana, pau-fava.
USES: Reputedly as an antisyphilitic.

Senna multijuga Rich. var. ***verrucosa*** (Vog.) Ir. & Barn.
AREA: Bahia to São Paulo, forest.
NAMES: Aleluia, canudo-de-pito, cássia-murici, murici-amarelo.
USES: Tonic and astringent.
CHEM.: Extraction of softwood yielded stearic acid, sitostenone and sitosterol. Sitosterol and pinitol were isolated from the petals (Ref: CAES 26).

Senna oblongifolia (Vog.) Ir. & Barn.
AREA: Minas Gerais and Rio de Janeiro, forest.
NAME: Fedegoso.
USE: Leaves are purgative.

Senna obtusifolia (L.) Ir. & Barn.
AREA: Neotropical; throughout Brazil.
NAME: Mata-pasto.
USES: Bitter, appetizer, antipyretic, purgative.

Senna occidentalis (L.) Link
AREA: Tropical cosmopolitan; widespread in Brazil as ruderal.
NAMES: Fedegoso, lava-prato, maioba, magerioba, mamangá, matapasto, pajamarioba, paramarioba.
USES: Root is bitter, antidote to poisons; diuretic, tonic, abortifacient,

CAESALPINIACEAE

malarial, for treating liver ailments and amygdalitis; juice for dressing burns; leaves used for skin diseases, hepatitis, dropsy, appetite stimulant, diaphoretic, antifebrile; tonic is diuretic, emmenagogue, purgative, vermifuge, also for treating yellow fever.

CHEM.: Pigments described from all parts of the plant (Ref: CAES 27,28,29,30,31).

PHARM.: Seeds showed antibiotic activity against bacteria and fungi (Ref: CAES 32).

Senna quinqueangulata (Rich.) Ir. & Barn.
AREA: Amazonia to São Paulo.
NAME: Fedegoso-grande.
USES: Same as for *S. occidentalis* (L.) Link.

Senna rugosa (G. Don) Ir. & Barn.
AREA: Piauí to São Paulo and Mato Grosso; frequent in cerrado.
NAMES: Alcaçuz-bravo, amendoeirana, boi-gordo.
USES: Roots used in a decoction against snake bites. Leaves are purgative.

Senna septentrionalis (Viv.) Ir. & Barn.
AREA: Amazonia to Paraná, forest.
NAME: Canudo-de-pito.
USES: Leaves are purgative; decoction of leaves used to wash scalp and kill skin parasites.

Senna uniflora (P. Miller) Ir. & Barn.
AREA: Amazonia to Bahia.
NAMES: Caquera, fedegoso-do-pará, matapasto.
USES: Root is tonic, febrifuge, diuretic. Leaves are emmenagogue, diaphoretic, laxative, alexipharmic. Bracts used as substitute for the genuine senna (cf. CHEM. under *Senna* spp.). Roasted seeds used as a coffee substitute, tonic.

Senna spp.

All species of *Senna* here considered have been previously treated as members of the genus *Cassia* and appear as such in most of the literature.

CHEM.: The leaves of all *Senna* species are rich in anthraquinone pigments and their reduction products, the corresponding athrones. These compounds are responsible for their laxative properties, acknowledged through the universal use of "senna" teas in normalizing the intestinal function and also account for their usefulness in treating afflictions of the skin (Ref: CAES 23).

The genuine senna of commerce, a purgative (cathartic) drug, is ob-

Senna rugosa

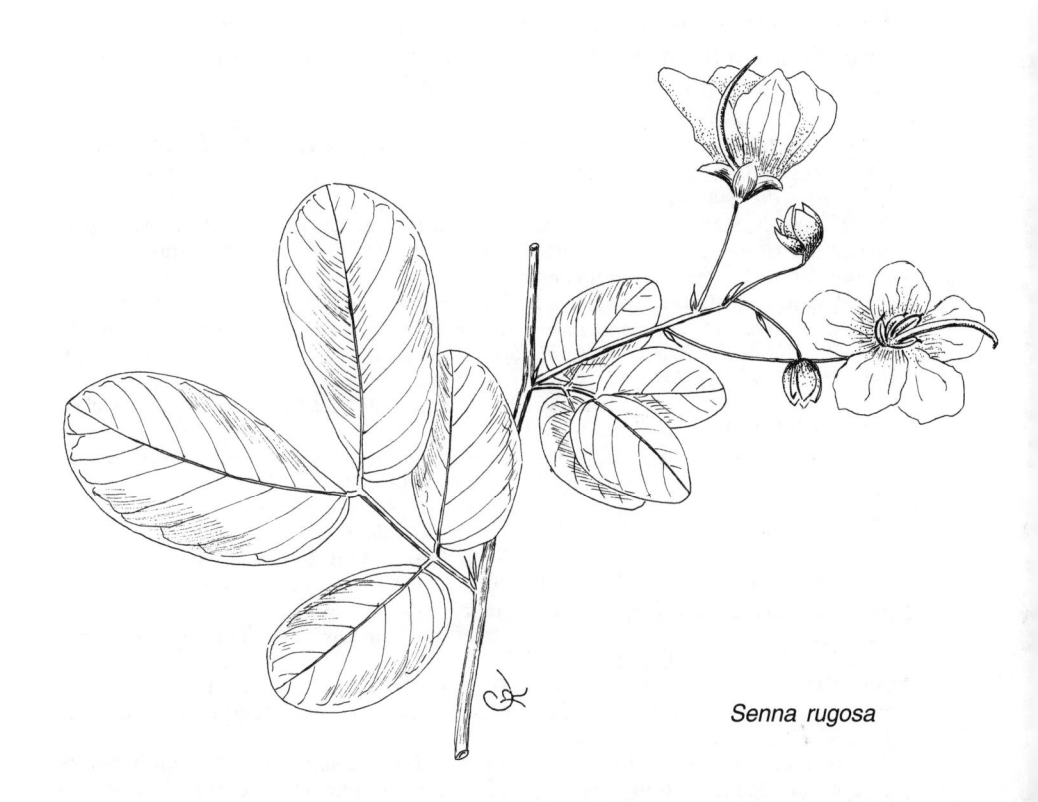

tained from several Old World species of *Senna*, including *S. alexandrina* Miller and *S. italica* Miller.

Swartzia chrysantha B. Rodr.
AREA: Amazonia, in igapós or terra firme.
NAME: Coquidá.
USES: Bark is considered effective against intestinal disorders and amenorrhoea.

Swartzia panacoco (Aubl.) Cowan var. **panacoco**
AREA: Amazonia, forest.
NAMES: Pau-ferro, pau-santo.
USE: Bark is sudorific.

Vouacapoua americana Aubl.
AREA: Amazonia, forest.

CAESALPINIACEAE

NAME: Acapu.
USES: Bark and wood are astringent, used to clean sloughing ulcers.
CHEM.: The main constituent of the wood extractive is the methyl ester of the diterpene vouacapenic acid (Ref: CAES 33,34).

Caesalpiniaceae – References

CAES 1. Braz Filho, R. & O.R. Gottlieb. 1971. The flavones of *Apuleia leiocarpa*. *Phytochemistry* 10: 2433-2450.

CAES 2. Ruppelt, B.M., E.F.R. Perreira, L.C. Gonçalves & N.A. Pereira. 1990. Abordagem farmacológica de plantas recomendadas na medicina folclórica como antiofídicas. I. Atividades analgésica e antiinflamatória. *Rev. Bras. Farm.* 71: 54-56.

CAES 3. Ruppelt, B.M., L.C. Gonçalves & N.A. Pereira. 1990. Abordagem farmacológica de plantas recomendadas na medicina folclórica como antiofídicas. II. Bloqueio da atividade na permeabilidade capilar e na letalidade do veneno de jararaca (*Bothrops jararaca*). *Rev. Bras. Farm.* 71: 57-58.

CAES 4. Iribarren, A.M. & A.B. Pomilio. 1983. Components of *Bauhinia candicans*. *J. Nat. Prod.* 46: 752-753.

CAES 5. Juliani, C. 1941. Ação hipoglicemiante da *Bauhinia forficata* Link. Novos estudos clínicos e experimentais. *Jornal dos Clínicos* (Rio de Janeiro) 3: 1-17.

CAES 6. Russo, E.M.K., A.A.J. Reichelt, J.R. de Sá, R.P. Furlanetto, R.C.S. Moisés, T.S. Kasamatsu & A.R. Chacra. 1990. Clinical trial of *Myrcia uniflora* and *Bauhinia forficata* leaf extracts in normal and diabetic patients. *Braz. J. Med. Biol. Res.* 23: 11-20.

CAES 7. Pascoe, K.O., B.A. Burke & W.R. Chan. 1986. Caesalpin F, a new furanoditerpene from *Caesalpinia bonducella*. *J. Nat. Prod.* 49: 913-915.

CAES 8. Robinson, R. 1958. Chemistry of brazilin and hematoxilin. *Bull. Soc. Chim. France* (5ᵉ série Memoires) 25: 125-134.

CAES 9. Wenninger, J.A., R.L. Yates & M. Dolinsky. 1967. Sesquiterpene hydrocarbons of commercial copaiba and American cedarwood oils. *J. Amer. Oil Chemists Soc. 50*: 1304-1312.

CAES 10. Delle Monache, G., I.L. d'Albuquerque, F. Delle Monache, G.B. Marini-Bettolo & G.M. Nano. 1971. á-Multijugenol, a new sesquiterpenic alcohol with caryophyllene carbon skeleton. *Tetrahedron Lett.*: 659-660.

CAES 11. Mahajan, J.R. & G. A.L. Ferreira. 1971. New diterpenoids from copaiba oil. *An. Acad. Bras. Ciênc. 43*: 611-613.

CAES 12. Mors, W.B. & H.J. Monteiro. 1959. Duas cumarinas nas sementes da *Copaifera langsdorffii*. *An. Assoc. Bras. Quím.* 18: 179-181.

CAES 13. Calvin, M. 1987. Fuel oils from euphorbs and other plants. *Bot. J. Linn. Soc.* (London) 94: 97-110.

CAES 14. Fernandes, R.M. 1986. *Contribuição para o conhecimento do efeito antiinflamatório e analgésico do bálsamo de copaíba e alguns de seus constituintes químicos*. Thesis, Federal University of Rio de Janeiro.

CAES 15. Basile, A.C., J.A.A. Sertié, P.C.D. Freitas & A.C. Zanini. 1988. Anti-inflammatory activity of oleoresin from Brazilian *Copaifera*. *J. Ethnopharmacol.* 22: 101-109.

CAES 16. Nakano, T. & C. Djerassi. 1961. Terpenoids. XLVI. Copalic acid. *J. Org. Chem.* 26: 167-173.

CAES 17. Harrison, I.T. & T. Nakano. 1962. Os sesquiterpenos da resina de jutaicica. *An. Assoc. Bras. Quím. 21*: 23-29.

CAES 18. Martin, S.S., J.H. Langenheim & E. Zavarin. 1972. Sesquiterpenes in leaf pocket resin of *Hymenaea courbaril*. *Phytochemistry 11*: 3049-3051.

CAES 19. Marsaioli, A.J., H. Freitas Leitão Filho & J.P. Campelo. 1975. Diterpenes in the bark of *Hymenaea courbaril*. *Phytochemistry 14*: 1882-1883.

CAES 20. Martin, S.S. & J.H. Langenheim. 1970. Studies of resins from *Hymenaea* and *Trachylobium* (Abstract). *Am. J. Bot. 57*: 765.

CAES 21. Martin, S.S., J.H. Langenheim & A. Cunningham. 1971. Resin acids in *Hymenaea* (Leguminosae). *Am. J. Bot. 58*: 479-480.

CAES 22. Cunningham, A., S.S. Martin & J. H. Langenheim. 1974. Labd-13-en-8-ol-15-oic acid in the trunk resin of Amazonian *Hymenaea courbaril*. *Phytochemistry 13*: 294-295.

CAES 23. Anton, R. & P.L. Duquenois. 1968. L'emploi des *Cassia* dans les pays tropicaux et subtropicaux examinés d'après quelques uns des constituants chimiques de ces plantes médicinales. *Plantes Méd. Phytothér. 2*: 255-268.

CAES 24. Hauptmann, H. & L.L. Nazario. 1950. Some constituents of leaves of *Cassia alata* L. *J. Am. Chem. Soc. 72*: 1492-1495.

CAES 25. Tiwari, R.D. & O.P. Yadava. 1971. Structural study of the quinone pigments from the roots of *Cassia alata*. *Planta Medica 19*: 299-305.

CAES 26. Oliveira, A.B., M.L.M. Fernandes, V.T. Shaat, I.A. Vasconcelos & O.R. Gottlieb. 1977. Constituents of *Cassia* species. *Rev. Latinoamer. Quím. 8*: 80-81.

CAES 27. Anton, R. & P.L. Duquenois. 1968. Étude chimique de *Cassia occidentalis*. *Ann. Pharm. Franç. 26*: 673-680.

CAES 28. Lal, J. & P.C. Gupta. 1973. Physcion and phytosterol from the roots of *Cassia occidentalis*. *Phytochemistry 12*: 1186.

CAES 29. Lal, J. & P.C. Gupta. 1974. Two new anthraquinones from the seeds of *Cassia occidentalis*. *Experientia 30*: 850-851.

CAES 30. Niranjan, M.G.S. & P.C. Gupta. 1973. Chemical constituents of the flowers of *Cassia occidentalis*. *Planta Medica 23*: 298-300.

CAES 31. Tiwari, R.D. & J. Singh. 1977. Anthraquinone pigments from *Cassia occidentalis*. *Planta Medica 32*: 375-377.

CAES 32. Gaind, K.N., R.D. Budhiraja & R.N. Kaul. 1966. Antibiotic activity of *Cassia occidentalis* L. *Indian J. Pharm. 28*: 248-250.

CAES 33. King, F.E., D.H. Godson & T.J. King. 1955. The chemistry of extractives from hardwoods. XXII. The structure of diterpenes from *Vouacapoua* species. *J. Chem. Soc.*: 1117-1125.

CAES 34. King, F.E. & T. J. King. 1953. The chemistry of extractives from hardwoods. XV. The constitution of methyl vinhaticoate. *J. Chem. Soc.*: 4158-4168.

CAMPANULACEAE

Centropogon cornutus (L.) Druce
AREA: Frequent all over Brazil, except for the extreme south.
NAMES: Bico-de-papagaio, crista-de-peru, ganha-saia.
USES: Leaf decoction used for toothache.

Haynaldia exaltata (Pohl) Kanitz
AREA: Minas Gerais, Rio de Janeiro and São Paulo, in swampy environment.
NAME: Arrebenta-cavalos.
USE: Latex is poisonous, but in small doses used for cardiac trouble.

Hippobroma longiflora (L.) G. Don
AREA: In moist places of the littoral, from Amazonia to São Paulo.
NAMES: Arrebenta-boi, cega-olho, jasmim-da-itália, jasmim-de-cachorro.
USES: Though toxic, recommended for syphilis and asthma.

CHEM. & PHARM.: Chemistry and pharmacology have not been studied in depth, but agree with the presence of *Lobelia*-type alkaloids (Ref: CAMP 1,2).

Campanulaceae – References

CAMP 1. Sanchez, G.C. 1945. Farmacologia de la *Isotoma longiflora*. *Rev. Med. Experimental* (Lima, Peru) *4*: 284-318.

CAMP 2. Borio, E.B.L. & Y. Kawase. 1966. Alacalóides da *Isotoma longiflora* Presl (Campanulaceae). *Ciência e Cultura 18* (Supl.): 184.

CANELLACEAE

Cinnamodendron axillare (Nees & Mart.) Endl.
AREA: Minas Gerais, Rio de Janeiro and São Paulo, forest.
NAMES: Canela-branca, erva-moura-do-sertão, paratudo-aromatico, pau-pimenta, casca-paratudo.
USES: Bark is aromatic, pungent, excitant, tonic, stomachic, antithermic, used for scurvy and tonsillitis.

CANNACEAE

Canna edulis Ker-Gawl.
AREA: Southern Brazil, also cultivated.
NAMES: Araruta-bastarda, araruta-de-porco, beri, biru-manso, meru.
USES: Rhizome is diuretic, effective against cystitis and gonorrhoea.
CHEM.: Chelidonic acid identified in roots (Ref: CANN 1).

Canna gigantea Desf.
AREA: Amazonia, forest.
NAMES: Bananeira-brava, caeté-açu, caeté-do-mato, erva-dos-feridos.
USES: Rhizome is diuretic, sudorific, used for treatment of injuries. Leaf juice is antirheumatic. Fruits are antiodontalgic. Stem indicated for pharyngitis.

Canna glauca L.
AREA: Amazonia, Bahia and Mato Grosso.
NAMES: Albará, bananeira-do-mato, bananeirinha, caeté-imbiri, coquilho, erva-dos-feridos, imbiri, maracá.
USES: Fresh rhizomes in a decoction are diuretic, diaphoretic, antiblennorrhagic, antirheumatic, useful for urethritis and bladder catarrh. In poultices to soften tumors. Plant juice in gargles to soothe salivation induced by the medical use of mercury compounds. Seeds bruised to relieve earache. Tea of the whole plant as diuretic.

Canna indica L.
AREA: Highly esteemed in gardens. Ruderal (subspontaneous) in many places.
NAMES: Bananeirinha-da-índia, cana, cana-da-índia.
USES: Leaf decoction used for washing malignant ulcers; in baths for rheumatism. Rhizome infusion is sudorific and excitant; tincture used as tonic.

Canna lanuginosa Roscoe
AREA: Amazonas to Alagoas, forest.
NAMES: Café-do-mato, pacuarana, panduarana.
USE: Leaves used for treatment of piles.

Canna lutea Roscoe
AREA: Amazonia, forest.
NAMES: Bananeirinha-de-flor-amarela, muru.
USES: Rhizome is diaphoretic and diuretic.

Canna warszewiczii Dietr.
AREA: Minas Gerais to Rio Grande do Sul, forest.
NAMES: Bananeirinha-roxa, caeté-de-talo-roxo, caeté-mirim, caeté-roxo.
USES: Rhizome is diuretic, antigonorrhoeic. Leaves are emollient.

Cannaceae – Reference

CANN 1. Ramstad, E. 1945. Distribution of chelidonic acid in drugs. *Pharm. Acta Helv.* 20: 145-154.

CAPPARACEAE

Capparis cynophallophora L.
AREA: Along the littoral, in restinga.
NAME: Sapo-taia.
USES: Root-bark for a hydragogue, diuretic, appetizer.

Capparis lineata Pers.
AREA: Amazonia.
NAME: Cipotaí.
USES: Tincture rubbed on body for leucorrhoea. Roots steeped in water to rub on body against sluggishness.

Capparis urens B. Rodr.
AREA: Amazonia, forest.
NAME: Cipotaí.
USES: Ground roots mixed with water are used as sinapisms, for instance

CAPPARACEAE

against rheumatic pains. Plant juice mixed with almond oil against suppurated otitis.

Cleome aculeata L.
AREA: Northeastern Brazil.
NAME: Muçambê-fedorento.
USE: Leaves used as a revulsive.

Cleome gigantea L.
AREA: Dispersed throughout Brazil.
NAMES: Catinga-de-negro, catinga-de-tatu, muçambê-catinga.
USES: Useful for rheumatism and paralysis.

Cleome polygama L.
AREA: Goiás.
NAMES: Bredo-fedorento, pimenta-de-macaco, muçambê-de-três-folhas.
USES: Aromatic, excitant, against scurvy; externally used as a vulnerary.

Cleome speciosa H.B.K.
AREA: Amazonia.
NAME: Catinga-de-negro.
USES: Excitant, diuretic, appetizer.

Cleome spinosa Jacq.
AREA: Amazonia to São Paulo.
NAMES: Muçambê, muçambê-de-espinhos, sete-marias.
USES: Plant used as an excitant for the stomach. Used for gonorrhoea and leucorrhoea. Externally as a vulnerary and for relieving orchitis. Leaf juice for purulent otitis. Contused leaves on the skin are rubefacient. Root infusion for treating bronchitis and asthma.

Crataeva benthamii Eichl.
AREA: Amazonia, on flooded river banks.
NAMES: Catauari, catauré, catoré, trapiá.
USES: Roots and flowers are tonic, stomachic. Leaf juice applied externally against rheumatism. Stem bark against snakebite.
CHEM.: Stem bark contains lupeol (Ref: CAPP 1).

Crataeva tapia L.
AREA: Pará to São Paulo, littoral.
NAMES: Pau-d'alho, tapiá, trapiá.
USES: Bark is a bitter tonic, febrifuge. In poultices for whitlow.
CHEM.: Stem bark contains ß-amyrin, lupeol and betulinic acid (Ref: CAPP 2).
PHARM.: Cardiorespiratory and oxytocic activity (Ref: CAPP 3,4).

The presence of thioglucosides is a common characteristic of all species of Capparaceae. These so-called glucosinolates liberate glucose, sulfate and isothiocyanate on hydrolysis. One of them, glucocapparin, is predominant in 38 species investigated, *Cleome spinosa* being one of them. For comprehensive reviews see Ref: CAPP 5,6.

Capparaceae – References

CAPP 1. Aynilian, G.H., N.R. Farnsworth & G.J. Persinos. 1972. Isolation of lupeol from *Crataeva benthamii*. *Phytochemistry* 11: 2885-2886.
CAPP 2. Souza, M.P., F.J.A. Matos, J.W. Alencar & P.A. Rouquayrol. 1970. Triterpenóides de plantas do nordeste brasileiro — *Byrsonima sericea* L., *Crataeva tapia* L., *Curatella americana* L. *Rev. Bras. Farm.* 51: 67-70.
CAPP 3. Barros, G.S.G., F.J.A. Matos, J.E.V. Vieira, M.P. Souza & M.C. Medeiros. 1970. Pharmacological screening of some Brazilian plants. *J. Farm. Pharmacol.* 22: 116-122.
CAPP 4. Vieira, J.E.V., F.J.A. Matos, G.S.G. Barros, M.P. Souza, M.C. Medeiros & M.J. Medeiros. 1968. Abordagem farmacológica de plantas do nordeste brasileiro. II. *Rev. Bras. Farm.* 49: 67-75.
CAPP 5. Kjaer, A. & H. Thomsen. 1963. Isothiocyanate producing glucosides in species of Capparidaceae. *Phytochemistry* 2: 29-32.
CAPP 6. Ahmed, Z.F., A.M. Rizk, F.M. Hammouda & M.M. Seif El-Nasr. 1972. Naturally occurring glucosinolates with special reference to those of the family Capparidaceae. *Planta Medica* 21: 35-60.

CARICACEAE

Carica papaya L.

AREA: Cultivated, sometimes spontaneous.
NAMES: Mamoeiro (plant), mamão (fruit); papaya, pawpaw.
USES: Latex, bruised seeds and roots for expelling intestinal worms. The latex destroys corns and warts. Fruit eupeptic. Flower infusion for an emmenagogue, antipyretic, pectoral. Leaves are stomachic, sedative and calmative, but toxic in higher doses.
CHEM. & PHARM.: Latex from bark and unripe fruit is source of the proteolytic enzyme papain. The antibacterial and anthelmintic properties of latex and fruit are due to the action of this enzyme (Ref: CARI 1); those of the seeds are due to the presence of benzyliso-thiocyanate (Ref: CARI 2,3). The leaves contain an alkaloid, carpaine. In small doses this slows down the heart and thus reduces blood pressure. Higher doses produce vasoconstriction. In addition, carpaine has a spasmolytic action on smooth muscle, besides being strongly amoebicidal (Ref: CARI 4).

Jacaratia spinosa (Aubl.) A. DC.

AREA: Amazonia to Rio Grande do Sul and Mato Grosso, forest.
NAMES: Barrigudo, jacaratiá, diamburu, mamão-de-veado, mamão-do-mato, mamão-rana, mamoiero bravo, mamuí.

USES: Fruit is a strong anthelmintic; hydragogue to a certain extent; anti-inflammatory for infections of the gut.
CHEM. & PHARM.: Latex from bark and fruit is strongly proteolytic (Ref: CARI 5).

Caricaceae – References

CARI 1. Emeruwa, A.C. 1982. Antibacterial substance from *Carica papaya* fruit extract. *J. Nat. Prod. 45*: 123-127.
CARI 2. Ettlinger, M.G. & J.E. Hodgkins. 1956. The mustard oil of papaya seed. *J. Org. Chem. 21*: 204.
CARI 3. El Tayeb, O., M. Kucera, V.O. Marquis & H. Kucerova. 1974. Contribution to the knowledge of Nigerian medicinal plants. III. Study on *Carica papaya* seeds as a source of reliable antibiotic, the benzylisothiocyanate. *Planta Medica 26*: 79-89.
CARI 4. Burdick, E.M. 1971. Carpaine, an alkaloid of *Carica papaya*. Its chemistry and pharmacology. *Econ. Botany 25*: 363-365.
CARI 5. Peckolt, T. 1903. Heil- und Nutzpflanzen Brasiliens. Caricaceae. *Ber. Deut. Pharm. Ges. 13*: 339-374.

CARYOCARACEAE

Caryocar brasiliense Camb.
AREA: Central Brazil, cerrado.
NAMES: Pequi, pequiá, piqui.
USES: Fruits and seed oil used against common cold and bronchitis, the seed oil mixed with honey. Bark infusion is febrifuge and diuretic.
CHEM.: Leaves contain triterpenes, sterols and ellagic acid (Ref: CARY 1).

Caryocar coriaceum Wittm.
AREA: Piauí to Goiás, cerrado.
NAMES: Pequi, pequiá, piqui.
USES: Oil from fruit flesh and seed kernel is used for bronchopulmonary infections; also to treat cuts and boils in animals.

Caryocar glabrum (Aubl.) Pers.
AREA: Amazonia, forest.
NAMES: Cabeleira, pequi-da-areia, pequiarana, pequiarana-vermelha, pequiarana-da-terra-firme.
USES: Ash from the burned bark is employed as antidysenteric.

Caryocar villosum (Aubl.) Pers.
AREA: Amazonia, forest.
NAMES: Amêndoa-de-espinho, grão-de-cavalo, pequi, pequiá-verdadeiro, petiá, piqui, piquiá.
USES: Leaves and bark induce sweating.
CHEM.: Fatty oil from pulp and kernels has been described (Ref: CARY 2).

Caryocaraceae – References

CARY 1. Oliveira, M.M., B. Gilbert & W.B. Mors. 1968. Triterpenes in *Caryocar brasiliense*. *An. Acad. Brasil. Ci.* 40: 451-452.
CARY 2. Cerqueira, P.O. 1943. Óleo de pequiá. *Revista Alimentar* (Rio de Janeiro) 7: 16-17.

CARYOPHYLLACEAE

Polycarpaea corymbosa (L.) Lam.
AREA: Disseminated throughout Brazil.
NAME: Sete-sangrias.
USE: Tea from plant used to fortify blood.

CELASTRACEAE

Maytenus boaria Mol.
AREA: Rio de Janeiro and Rio Grande do Sul.
NAME: Boaria.
USES: Decoction of leaves is antimalarial, febrifuge, drastic; used externally to wash wounds and ulcers.
CHEM. & PHARM.: See below, under *Maytenus obtusifolia*.

Maytenus communis Reiss.
AREA: Rio de Janeiro and São Paulo.
NAMES: Congonha-brava, congonha-grande.
USES: Dried leaves are made into a tea against fevers; decoction is vulnerary.

Maytenus gonoclada Mart.
AREA: São Paulo to Rio Grande do Sul.
USES: Leaves are tonic, stimulant.

Maytenus ilicifolia Mart.
AREA: Minas Gerais to Rio Grande do Sul, forest and high caatinga.
NAMES: Cancerosa, espinheira-santa, espinho-de-deus, erva-cancerosa, salvavidas, sombra-de-touro.
USES: Leaf decoction employed for hyperacidity and gastric ulcers, also depurative and general tonic as well as anti-febrile, externally used to clean wounds and ulcers of the skin. Used extensively; found in the drug market.
CHEM. & PHARM.: See below, under *Maytenus* spp.

Maytenus laevis Reiss.
AREA: Amazonia, forest.
NAMES: Chuchuhuasca, chuchuguacha.

USES: Bark is stimulant, anti-rheumatic.
CHEM. & PHARM.: See below, under *Maytenus* spp.

Maytenus obtusifolia Mart.

AREA: Piauí to Rio de Janeiro, mostly in coastal woody vegetation (caatinga).
NAMES: Carne-de-anta, carrancudo, congonha-brava-de-folha-miúda, lenha-branca, limãozinho.
USES: Leaf decoction is diuretic, used against stomachache and in the treatment of malignant ulcers.
CHEM. & PHARM.: See below, under *Maytenus* spp.

Maytenus spp.

CHEM. & PHARM.: Early chemical analyses on the leaves of *M. ilicifolia* were performed in 1962, leading to the isolation of several trivial compounds: ß-amyrin, chlorogenic acid tannins (Ref: CELA 1). The presence of caffeine was also claimed, but was later disproved (Ref: CELA 2). Antimicrobial and anticancer activity of extracts of *Maytenus* species were observed as far back as 1969 (Ref: CELA 3). Clinical experiments in humans were performed in 1971 (Ref: CELA 4).

The effects were at that time attributed to several substances — maytenin, pristimerin, tingenone — isolated from the plants by a research group in Pernambuco (Ref: CELA 5) and in Rome (Ref: CELA 6). The compound called maytenin was found to be identical to tingenone (Ref: CELA 7,8). These substances received the collective designation of "celastroids." They are pentacyclic triterpenes containing a stabilized quinone-methide moiety in the molecule which confers on them an orange color. Shortly afterwards, "maytansoids" were discovered — nitrogen containing ansa-macrolides — which are strongly tumor inhibiting (Ref: CELA 9,10). All these findings were summarized in two reviews published, respectively, in 1974 (Ref: CELA 11) and 1978 (Ref: CELA 12).

Additional pharmacological studies showed also a strong antiulcerogenic effect (Ref: CELA 13). Freeze-dried aqueous infusions of the leaves, administered both orally and intraperitoneally, showed a protective effect against various experimental models of gastric ulcers in laboratory animals (Ref: CELA 14). Toxicological trials, both preclinical and clinical, revealed total absence of undesirable side-effects (Ref: CELA 15).

Most of these studies were performed on extracts and compounds isolated from *M. ilicifolia*, the species of the highest reputation. Of the above-mentioned species, individual results were also published on *M. boaria* (Ref: CELA 16,17), *M. obtusifolia* (Ref: CELA 17) and *M. laevis* (Ref: CELA 18).

Maytenus ilicifolia

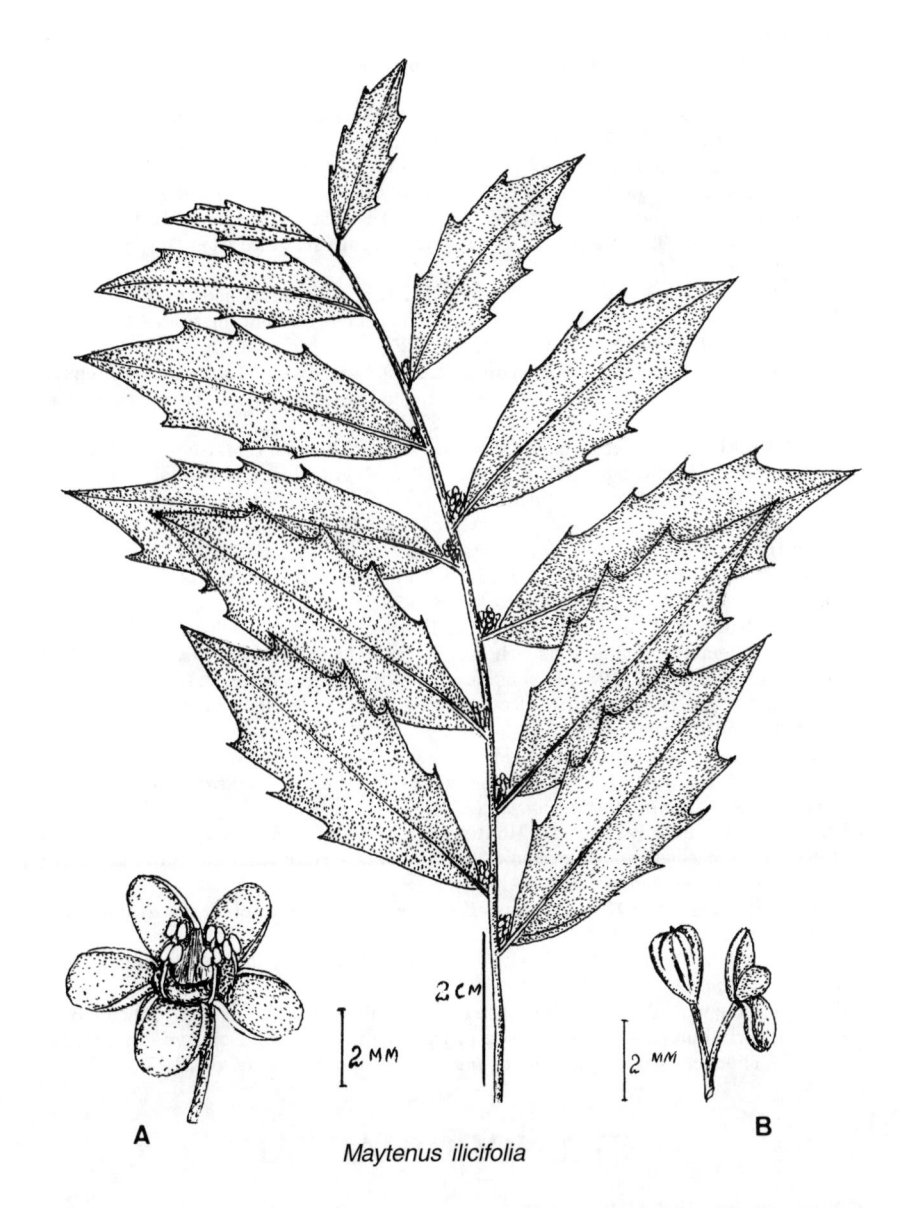

Celastraceae – References

CELA 1. Vaz Pereira, M. 1962. Princípio ativo e outros constitutintes básicos de *Maytenus ilicifolia*. *Rev. Bras. Quím.* (São Paulo) *54*: 416-417.

CELA 2. Bernardi, H.H. & M. Wasicky. 1963. A alegada ocorrencia de cafeina em *Maytenus ilicifolia*. *Tribuna Farmaceutica* (Curitiba) *31*: 38-39.

CELA 3. Gonçalves de Lima, O., I.L. d'Albuquerque, J.S.B. Coelho, D.G. Martins, A.L. Lacerda & G.M. Maciel. 1969. Substancias antimicrobianas de plantas superiores. XXXI. Maitenina novo antimicrobiano com ação antineoplásica, isolado de celastrácea de Pernambuco. *Rev. Inst. Antibiot.* (Recife) *9*. (1/2): 17-25.

CELA 4. Santana, C.F., J.J. Asfora & C.T. Cotias. 1971. Primeiras observações sobre o emprego da maitenina em pacientes cancerosos. *Rev. Inst. Antibiot.* (Recife) *11* (2): 37-49.

CELA 5. Gonçalves de Lima, O., J.S.B. Coelho, E. Weigert, I.L. d'Albuquerque, D.A. Lima & M. Moraes e Souza. 1971. Substâncias antimicrobianas de plantas superiores. XXXVI. Sobre a presença de maitenina e pristimerina na parte cortical das raizes de *Maytenus ilicifolia* procedente do Brasil meridional. *Rev. Inst. Antibiot.* (Recife) *11* (1): 35-38.

CELA 6. Delle Monache, F., G.-B. Marini-Bettòlo, O. Gonçalves de Lima, I.L. d'Albuquerque & J.S.B. Coelho. 1972. Maitenin, a new antitumoral substance from *Maytenus* species. *Gazz. Chim. Ital. 102*: 317-320.

CELA 7. Brown, P.M., M. Moir, R.H. Thomson, T.J. King, V. Krishnamoorthy & T.R. Seshadri. 1973. Tingenone and hydroxytingenone, triterpenoid quinone methides from *Euonymus tingens*. *J. Chem. Soc. Perkin I*: 2721-2725.

CELA 8. Delle Monache, F., G.-B. Marini-Bettòlo, O. Gonçalves de Lima, I.L. d'Albuquerque & J.S.B. Coelho. 1973. The structure of tingenone, a quinonoid triterpene related to pristimerin. *J. Chem. Soc. Perkin I*: 2725-2727.

CELA 9. Kupchan, S.M., Y. Komoda, W.A. Court, G.J. Thomas, R.M. Smith, A. Karim, C.J. Gilmore, R.C. Haltiwanger & R.F. Bryan. 1972. Maytansine, a novel antileukemic ansa macrolide from *Maytenus ovatus*. *J. Am. Chem. Soc. 94*: 1354-1356.

CELA 10. Remillard, S., L.I. Rebhun, G.A. Howe & S.M. Kupchan. 1975. Antimitotic activity of the potent tumor inhibitor maytansine. *Science 189*: 1002-1005.

CELA 11. Marini-Bettòlo, G.-B. 1974. La Chimie des principes actifs de Celastraceae-Hippocrateaceae. *Plant. Méd. Phytothér. 8*: 3-14.

CELA 12. Brüning, R. & H. Wagner. 1978. Übersicht über die Celastreen-Inhaltsstoffe: Chemie, Chemotaxonomie, Biosynthese, Pharmakologie. *Phytochemistry 17*: 1821-1858.

CELA 13. Carlini, E.L.A. 1988. ESTUDO DE AÇÃO ANTIÚLCERA GÁSTRICA DE PLANTAS BRASILEIRAS: MAYTENUS ILICIFOLIA (ESPINHEIRA-SANTA) E OUTRAS. Central de Medicamentos (CEME), Ministry of Health, Brasília. 87 pp.

CELA 14. Souza-Formigoni, M.L.O., M.G.M. Oliveira, M.G. Monteiro, N.G. Silveira-Filho, S. Braz & E.A. Carlini. 1991. Antiulcerogenic effects of two *Maytenus* species in laboratory animals. *J. Ethnopharmacol. 34*: 21-27.

CELA 15. Oliveira, M.G.M., M.G. Monteiro, C. Macaúbas, V.P. Barbosa & E.A. Carlini. 1991. Pharmacologic and toxicologic effects of two *Maytenus* species in laboratory animals. *J. Ethnopharmacol. 34*: 29-41.

CELA 16. Bahkuni, S. 1973. Anti-cancer agents from Chilean plants. *Maytenus boaria*. *Rev. Latinoam. Quím. 4*: 166-170.

CELA 17. De Luca, C. 1978. Triterpenoid quinones of *Maytenus obtusifolia* and *M. boaria*. *Rev. Latinoam. Quím. 9*: 208-209.

CELA 18. Gonzalez, J.G., G. delle Monache, F. delle Monache & G.-B. Marini-Bettòlo. 1982. Chuchuhuasca — A drug used in folk medicine in the Amazonian and Andean areas. A chemical study of *Maytenus laevis*. *J. Ethnopharmacol. 5*: 73-77.

CHENOPODIACEAE

Chenopodium ambrosioides L.

AREA: Cosmopolitan, ruderal in Brazil.

NAMES: Ambrósia, ambrósia-do-méxico, anserina-vermífuga, erva-de-santa-maria, mastruço, mastruz, quenopódio.

USES: Herb is an important vermicide; also emmenagogue, abortifacient, carminative, stomachic and sudorific; useful for cough and angina; said to be employed to ease the expulsion of a dead foetus.

CHEM.: The essential oil contains the active anthelmintic compound ascaridole, besides limonene, myrcene, beta-pinene and other minor monoterpenes (Ref: CHEN 1).

Chenopodium hircinum Schrad.
AREA: Rio de Janeiro, Minas Gerais, São Paulo and all southern Brazil.
NAMES: Caperiçoba-branc, quinôa.
USE: Substitute for *C. ambrosioides* as an anthelmintic.
CHEM.: Composition of the essential oil is similar to that of *C. ambrosioides*, except for an additional high camphor content (Ref: CHEN 2).

Chenopodiaceae – References
CHEN 1. Bauer, L. & G.A. de Assis Brasil e Silva. 1973. Os óleos essenciais de *Chenopodium ambrosioides* e *Schinus terebinthifolius* no Rio Grande do Sul. *Rev. Bras. Farm. 54*: 240-242.

CHEN 2. Pereira, N.A., G.A. de Assis Brasil e Silva, N.C. S. de Siqueira, L. Bauer, B.M.S. Sant'Ana, C.T.M. Bacha & C.B. Alice. 1982. Composição do óleo essencial de *Chenopodium hircinum* Schrad. *Rev. Bras. Farm. 63*: 141-143.

CHLORANTHACEAE

Hedyosmum brasiliense Mart.
AREA: Minas Gerais to São Paulo, forest.
NAMES: Chá-de-bugre, chá-de-soldado, erva-almíscar, erva-de-soldado, hortelã-do-brejo.
USES: Leaves are aromatic, analeptic, febrifuge, stomachic, refreshing. Recommended against migraine, athlete's foot and diseases of the ovaries. Tea from the leaves, served cold, is taken as a refreshing and stimulating beverage. Infusion in wine is said to be tonic and aphrodisiac.

CHRYSOBALANACEAE

Chrysobalanus icaco L.
AREA: From Pará southward, along the littoral, on sandy beaches.
NAMES: Abajeru (former spelling "abagerú"), ariu, guajeru, guajuru.
USES: Bark is antidiabetic. Root, bark and flowers are astringent, indicated for chronic diarrhoea, blennorrhagia, leucorrhoea and bladder catarrh.
PHARM.: The tea from the leaves produces hypoglycemia in mice and protects from a lethal dose of alloxane. It inhibits the intestinal absorption of glucose in anaesthetized rats and controls blood sugar level in humans suffering from type II diabetes (Ref: CHRY 1,2).

CHRYSOBALANACEAE / CLUSIACEAE

Licania macrophylla Benth.
AREA: Flooded forest of the lower Amazon.
NAME: Anauerá.
USES: Bark decoction against amoebae.

Chrysobalanaceae – References

CHRY 1. Presta, G.A. 1986. *Interferência do chá de abagerú* (Chrysobalanus icaco *L.) na glicemia de jejum de camundongos e indivíduos com Diabetes mellitus — Tipo II.* Thesis, Federal University of Rio de Janeiro.

CHRY 2. Presta, G.A. & N.A. Pereira. 1987. Atividade de abagerú, *Chrysobalanus icaco* Lin. (Chrysobalanaceae) em modelos experimentais para o estudo de plantas hipoglicemiantes. *Rev. Bras. Farm. 68:* 91-101.

CLADONIACEAE

Cladonia miniata Mey.
AREA: On high mountain plateaus, mainly in the Organ Mountains and Itatiaia, Rio de Janeiro, also in Minas Gerais and São Paulo.
NAME: Canduá.
USES: This lichen was formerly used for dying baskets and clothes in red. Medicinally, used for treating aphthae in children.
CHEM.: Rhodocladonic acid, *d*-usnic acid and several triterpenes have been described (Ref: CLAD 1).

Cladonia pyxidata (L.) Ach.
AREA: On sandy terrain of the restinga, Rio de Janeiro.
NAMES: Canduá, candeiá.
USES: This lichen is indicated for broncho-pulmonary afflictions.

Cladoniaceae – Reference

CLAD 1. Godoy, R.L.O. 1981. *Constituintes Quimicos do Liquen* Cladonia miniata *Meyer.* Thesis, Federal University of Rio de Janeiro.

CLUSIACEAE

Calophyllum brasiliense Camb.
AREA: Almost throughout Brazil, forest, restinga and cerrado.
NAMES: Guanandi, guanandi-cedro, guandi, guandi-carvalho, jacareúba, landim, olandi, uá-iandi.
USES: The gum-resin which exudes from the bark, known as "bálsamo-de-jacareúba" or "bálsamo-de-landim," is aromatic, bitter and astringent. Reputed as antirheumatic, it is also used for maturing tumors and treating old ulcers. In veterinary medicine it is used to strengthen the tendons of animals. Bark and leaves are considered antidiabetic.

CHEM.: Typical constituents of the wood are xanthones (Ref: CLUS 1,2,3).
PHARM.: No hypoglycemic action could be demonstrated in rats (Ref: CLUS 4).

Caraipa densifolia Mart.
AREA: Amazonia, forest and cerrado.
NAMES: Macucu; tamacoari, tamacuari or tamaquari; tamaquaré-brando, tamaquaré-do-cerrado.
USES: Resin and bark decoction are employed against scabies and other dermatoses.
CHEM.: Xanthones (Ref: CLUS 5) and one coumaroyltriterpene (Ref: CLUS 6) have been described.

Caraipa excelsa Ducke
AREA: Amazonia, forest.
NAME: Tamaquaré.
USES: Balsam is used for the removal of spots and shingles from skin.

Caraipa grandifolia Mart.
AREA: Amazonia, forest.
NAME: Tamaquaré-grande.
USES: Oleo-resin is prescribed against ringworm, scabies, herpes and stains on the skin; also for rheumatism, liver troubles, pruritus and intestinal worms.
CHEM.: Xanthones have been described from wood (Ref: CLUS 7).

Caraipa insidiosa B. Rodr.
AREA: Amazonia, forest.
NAMES: Inhambuquiçaua, tamacoaré, tamaquaré.
USES: Oleo-resin and bark decoction used in baths against skin diseases. The same applications are ascribed to *C. silvatica* B. Rodr. (Amazonia).

Caraipa minor Huber
AREA: Amazonia, forest.
NAMES: Baratinha, tamaquaré-miudo, tamaquari-miudo.
USES: Depurative, antirheumatic, antiherpetic.

Clusia grandiflora Splitg.
AREA: Amazonia, forest.
NAMES: Apuí, cebola-grande-da-mata, guapuí.
USES: Reddish-yellow exudate from flowers is mixed with cacao butter for healing cracks in the nipples of nursing mothers. The closely related *C. insignis* Mart. (Amazonia) is used in the same way.

CLUSIACEAE

Clusia panapanari Choisy
AREA: Amazonia, forest.
NAME: Panapanari.
USES: Latex is employed as a stomachic and febrifuge.

Clusia rosea Jacq.
AREA: Amazonia, forest.
NAMES: Cebola-brava, cupaí, matapau.
USES: Latex which flows from the punctured trunk is bitter, balsamic and drastic, used to treat injuries in cattle. Bark is astringent, used for rheumatism. Leaf infusion is pectoral. Latex from fruits is resolvent, used topically to treat sprains and fractures.

Hypericum brasiliense Choisy
AREA: Minas Gerais to Rio Grande do Sul, campo.
NAMES: Alecrim-bravo, milfacadas, milfuradas, orelha-de-gato.
USES: Aromatic, astringent, excitant, vulnerary, antispasmodic and antiophidic.

Hypericum connatum Lam.
AREA: Southern states of Brazil.
NAME: Orelha-de-gato.
USES: Decoction is used as a gargle against aphthae, stomatitis and tonsillitis.

Hypericum teretiusculum St.-Hil.
AREA: São Paulo and Paraná, campo.
NAME: Arruda-do-campo.
USES: Aromatic, stimulant and emmenagogue.

Kielmeyera coriacea Mart.
AREA: Piauí to São Paulo and Mato Grosso, cerrado.
NAMES: Folha-santa, pau-de-são-josé, pau-santo.
USES: Latex and resin are tonic and emollient. Leaves in baths are resolvent.
CHEM.: Xanthones, characteristic components of Clusiaceae in general, have been isolated (Ref: CLUS 9,10).

Kielmeyera petiolaris Mart.
AREA: Goiàs to São Paulo, cerrado and forest.
NAME: Pau-santo.
USE: Emollient.
CHEM.: Xanthones have been isolated (Ref: CLUS 11).
   Kielmeyera rosea Mart. (Goiás to Minas Gerais) is used for the same purpose.

CLUSIACEAE

Kielmeyera speciosa St.-Hil.
AREA: Bahia to São Paulo, cerrado.
NAMES: Boizinho, folha-santa, malva-do-campo, pau-de-cortiça, pau-santo, pinhão.
USES: Latex and resin are tonic, emollient, prescribed for toothache. Leaves are also indicated as emollient.
CHEM.: Xanthones have been isolated (Ref: CLUS 12).
  For additional information on xanthones in various Clusiaceae, see Ref: CLUS 13,14,15.

Mammea americana L.
AREA: Amazonia, spontaneous and cultivated.
NAMES: Abricó, abricó-do-pará.
USES: Bark of trunk and fruit together with seeds are given to combat internal and external parasites, to alleviate insect stings and for treating various dermal afflictions. Gum-resin is antiparasitic. Bark decoction is resolvent and vulnerary. Water distilled from the flowers is a stimulant and is drunk for easing digestion.
CHEM. & PHARM.: The seeds contain a number of coumarins of complicated structure, having insecticidal properties (Ref: CLUS 16,17, 18,19).

Platonia insignis Mart.
AREA: Amazonia to Piauí, forest and cultivated.
NAME: Bacuri.
USES: Bark and seed oil for healing dermatoses.

Symphonia globulifera L. f.
AREA: Almost throughout Brazil, preferably in swampy forests.
NAMES: Guanandi, landim, oanani, pau-breu, uanani.
USES: Bark is used for treating enlarged glands, biliary obstruction, rheumatism and bone ailments.

Tovomita brasiliensis (Mart.) Walp.
AREA: Amazonia, forest.
NAMES: Manguerana, paxiubarana-miúda.
USES: Infusion of flowers against diarrhoea. Oil from fruits in rubs against rheumatism.
CHEM.: Xanthones, betulinic acid and sitosterol have been described in the wood (Ref: CLUS 20,21).

Vismia acuminata (L.) Pers.
AREA: Amazonia, forest.
NAMES: Caparosa, lacre.
USE: Latex is purgative.

CLUSIACEAE

Vismia guianensis (Aubl.) Choisy
AREA: Amazonia, forest.
NAMES: Caá-opiá, caopiá, lacre, lacre-branco, pau-de-lacre.
USES: Gum-resin is resolvent, cathartic, indicated for skin diseases. Bark and leaves are antipyretic and antirheumatic.
CHEM.: The reddish gum-resin and fruits of *Vismia* species owe their color to a number of anthrace derivatives, such as anthraquinones and several partially hydrogenated anthracene derivatives for which the term "anthranoids" has been suggested (Ref: CLUS 22).

Vismia japurensis Reich.
AREA: Amazonia, forest.
NAMES: Lacrão, pau-de-lacre.
USES: Bark is antithermic, useful for diverse dermatoses.
CHEM.: Anthraquinones have been described (Ref: CLUS 23).

Vismia latifolia (Aubl.) Choisy
AREA: Amazonia to Bahia, forest.
NAMES: Lacre, pau-de-lacre, pau-de-sangue.
USES: Bark employed for a tonic, febrifuge and against ringworm.

Vismia reichardtiana (O. Ktze.) Ewan
AREA: Maranhão.
NAME: Lacre.
USES: Gum-resin exudate is used against skin diseases.
CHEM.: An anthraquinone of unusual structure has been described (Ref: CLUS 24).

Clusiaceae – References

CLUS 1. King, F.E., T.J. King & L. C. Manning. 1953. The chemistry of extractives from hardwoods. Part XIV. The constitution of jacareubin, a pyranoxanthone from *Calophyllum brasiliense*. *J. Chem. Soc.*: 3932-3937.

CLUS 2. Pereira, M.O.S., O.R. Gottlieb & M.T. Magalhães. 1966. A química de Gutíferas brasileiras. IX. Constituintes xantônicos do *Calophyllum brasiliense*. *An. Acad. Bras. Ci. 38*: 425-427.

CLUS 3. Pereira, M.O.S., O.R. Gottlieb & M.T. Magalhães. 1967. Novas xantonas do *Calophyllum brasiliense*. *An. Acad. Bras. Ci. 39*: 255-256.

CLUS 4. Ramoa, A.S.S. & P.C.A. Rodrigues. 1977. Efeito da infusão de *Calophyllum brasiliense* na glicemia de ratos. *Rev. Bras. Biol. 37*: 147-149.

CLUS 5. Lima, R.A., O.R. Gottlieb & A.A.L. Mesquita. 1972. Xanthones from *Caraipa densiflora*. *Phytochemistry 11*: 2307-2309.

CLUS 6. Gunasekera, S.P., G.A. Cordell & N.R. Farnsworth. 1983. 3 -Hydroxy-28-p-coumaroyl-lup-20(29)-en-27-oic acid from *Caraipa densiflora*. *J. Nat. Prod. 46*: 118-122.

CLUS 7. Lima, R.A. & O.R. Gottlieb. 1970. A química de Gutíferas brasileiras. XXV. Os constituintes da *Caraipa grandifolia*. *An. Acad. Bras. Ci. 42*(Supl.): 137.

CLUS 8. Rocha, L.M., 1991. Estudo Químico e Farmacológico de *Hypericum brasiliense*. Thesis, Federal University of Rio de Janeiro.

CLUS 9. Gottlieb, O.R., M.T. Magalhães, M. Camey, A.A.L. Mesquita & D.B. Corrêa. 1966. The chemistry of Brazilian Guttiferae. V. 2,3,4- and 1,3,5-trioxygenated xanthones from *Kielmeyera* species. *Tetrahedron* 22: 1777-1784.

CLUS 10. Lopes, J.L.C., B. Gilbert & S. Bonini. 1977. Osajaxanthone from *Kielmeyera coriacea*. *Phytochemistry* 16: 1101.

CLUS 11. Gottlieb, O.R., M.T. Magalhães & G.M. Stefani. 1966. 1,2,8-trioxygenated xanthones from *Kielmeyera petiolaris*. *Tetrahedron* 22: 1785.

CLUS 12. Gottlieb, O.R., A.A. Lins Mesquita, G.G. Oliveira & M.T. Melo. 1970. Xanthones from *Kielmeyera speciosa*. *Phytochemistry* 9: 2537-2544.

CLUS 13. Gottlieb, O.R., M.T. Magalhães, M. Ottoni, A.A. Lins Mesquita, D. Barros Corrêa & G.G. Oliveira. 1968. The chemistry of Brazilian Guttiferae. XII. Isoprenylated xanthones from *Kielmeyera* and *Calophyllum* species. *Tetrahedron* 24: 1601-1610.

CLUS 14. Rezende, C.M.A.M. & O.R. Gottlieb. 1973. Xanthones as systematic markers. *Biochem. Syst.* 1: 111-118.

CLUS 15. Castelão Jr., J.F., O.R. Gottlieb, R. Alves de Lima, A.A. Lins Mesquita, H.E. Gottlieb & E. Wenkert. 1977. Xanthonolignoids from *Kielmeyera* and *Caraipa* species. - ^{13}C NMR spectroscopy of xanthones. *Phytochemistry* 16: 735-740.

CLUS 16. Djerassi, C., E.J. Eisenbraum, B. Gilbert, A.J. Lemin, S.P. Marfey & M.P. Morris. 1958. Naturally occurring oxygen heterocyclics. II Characterization of an insecticidal principle from *Mammea americana*. *J. Am. Chem. Soc.* 80: 3686-3691.

CLUS 17. Djerassi, C., E.J. Eisenbraum, R.A. Finnegan & B. Gilbert. 1959. Naturally occurring oxygen heterocyclics. V. Mammein. *Tetrahedron Lett.*: 10-14.

CLUS 18. Djerassi, C., E.J. Eisenbraum, R.A. Finnegan & B. Gilbert. 1960. Naturally occurring oxygen heterocyclics. VII. Structure of mammein. *J. Org. Chem.* 25: 2164-2169.

CLUS 19. Finnegan, R.A. & W.H. Mueller. 1965. Constituents of *Mammea americana* L. IV. The structure of mammeigin. *J. Org. Chem.* 30: 2342-2344.

CLUS 20. Gabriel, S.J., O.R. Gottlieb, R. Alves de Lima & A.A. Lins Mesquita. 1977. The chemistry of Brazilian Guttiferae. XXXVI. Constituents of Amazonian species. *Acta Amazonica* 7: 289-291.

CLUS 21. Braz Filho, R., C.A.S. Miranda, O.R. Gottlieb & M.T. Magalhães. 1982. Constituintes químicos de *Tomovita brasiliensis*. *Acta Amazonica* 12: 901-804.

CLUS 22. Marini-Bettòlo, G.-B., F. Delle Monache & M.M. McQuahe. 1978. Biogenetic correlations of anthranoids in *Vismia* genus. *Acad. Nazionale dei Lincei, Rend. Sc. Fis., Mat. e Nat.* 65: 303-306.

CLUS 23. Miraglia, M.C.M., A.A.L. Mesquita, M.J.C. Varejão, O.R. Gottlieb, & H.E. Gottlieb. 1981. Anthraquinones from *Vismia* species. *Phytochemistry* 20: 2041-2042.

CLUS 24. Gonçalves, M.L.S. & W.B. Mors. 1981. Vismiaquinone, a Δ^1-isopentenyl substituted anthraquinone from *Vismia reichardtiana*. *Phytochemistry* 20: 1947-1950.

COCHLOSPERMACEAE

Cochlospermum orinocense (H.B.K.) Steud.

AREA: Amazonia, forest.

NAMES: Algodão-bravo, botuto, periquiteira-da-mata, periquiteira-grande-da-terra-firme, pacoté.

USES: Bark applied to contusions.

Cochlospermum regium (Mart. & Schl.) Pilg.

AREA: Cerrados of central Brazil; Bahia to São Paulo.

NAMES: Algodoeiro-do-campo, algodão-bravo, butuá-de-corvo, periquiteira, periquiteira-do-campo.

USES: Bark as a resolvent, for contusions and abscesses; antirheumatic. Roots recommended for enteritis.

COMBRETACEAE

Combretum leprosum Mart.
AREA: Northeastern caatinga.
NAME: Mofumbo.
USES: Bast and leaves are hemostatic, sudorific, calmative.
PHARM.: The tree inhibits the growth of other vegetation beneath its coppice; an extract of the leaves froths abundantly and inhibits the germination of bean seeds (Ref: COMB 1).

Conocarpus erecta L.
AREA: Neotropical; in Brazil near mangroves and salt lagoons.
NAMES: Jenipapinho, mangue, mangue-de-botão.
USES: Leaves are astringent, antibacterial, antidiabetic, antipyretic, antisyphilitic.

Terminalia argentea Mart.
AREA: Maranhão to São Paulo, cerrado.
NAMES: Capitão-do-campo, caxapora-do-gentio.
USES: Gum-resin from bark is purgative.

Terminalia tanibouca Smith
AREA: Amazonia.
NAMES: Cinzeiro, cuia-rana, tanibouca.
USES: Bark is tanniferous, used against diarrhoea and for washing ulcers.

Combretaceae – Reference
COMB 1. Tavares, S. & C.T. Rizzini. Personal communications.

COMMELINACEAE

Commelina nudiflora L.
AREA: Ruderal throughout Brazil.
NAMES: Capim-gomoso, didi-da-porteira, grama-da-terra, maria-mole, marianinha, trapoeraba, trapoeraba-azul, trapoeraba-rana.
USES: Diuretic, antigonorrhoeic, antirheumatic, antihydropic; also used to treat amygdalitis, skin eruptions, warts, tinea, leprosy, piles.

Commelina platyphylla Klotz. ex Seub.
AREA: Disseminated throughout Brazil.

COMMELINACEAE

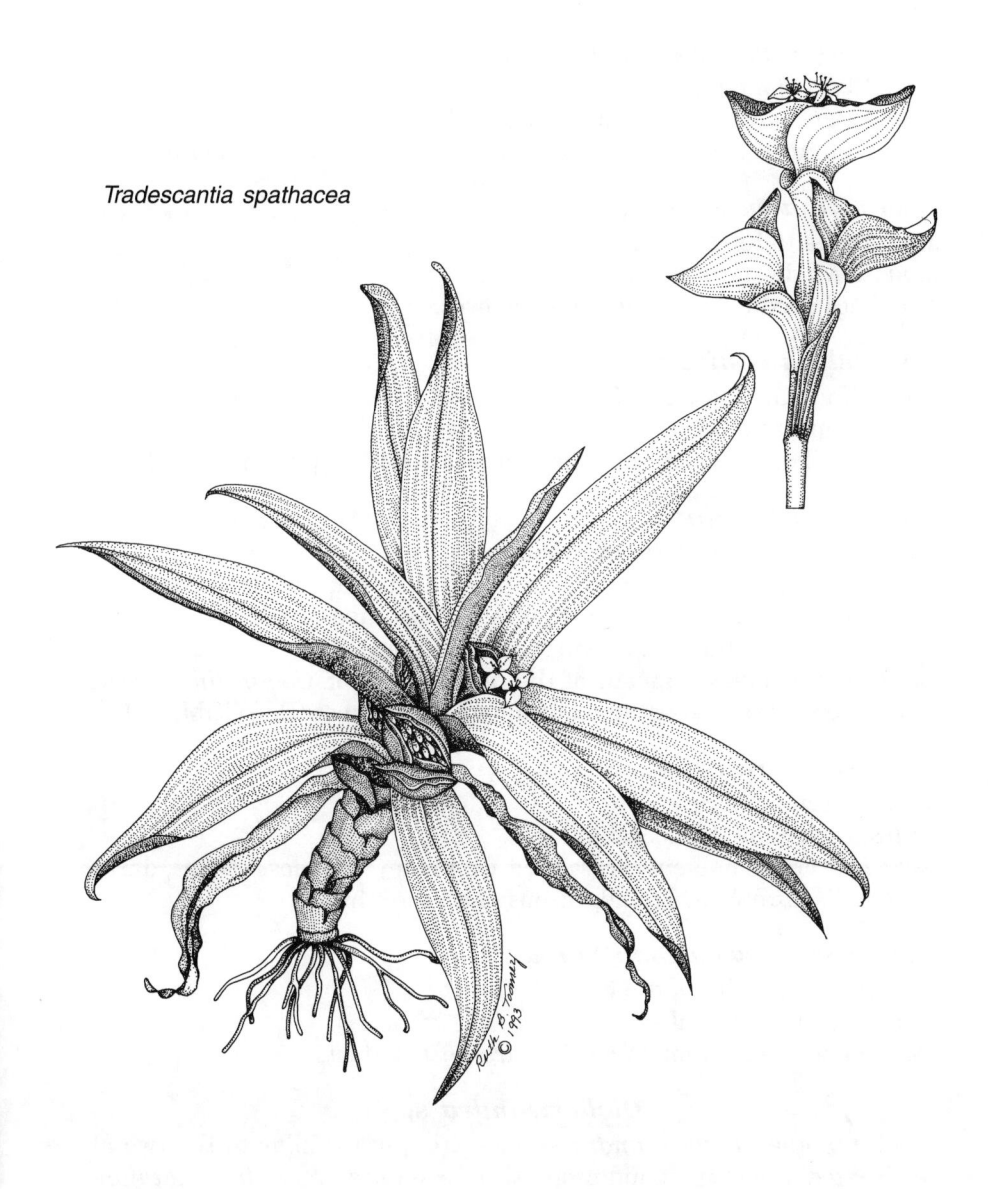

Tradescantia spathacea

NAME: Trapoeraba.
USES: Emollient, diuretic.

Commelina pohliana Seub.
AREA: Pernambuco to São Paulo, in shady places.
NAMES: Didi-da-porteira, trapoeraba-azul.
USES: Plant decoction used against dartre (skin disease) and dandruff.

COMMELINACEAE

Commelina robusta Kunth
AREA: Rio de Janeiro, on river banks.
NAMES: Batata-ovo, manobi-açu, trapoeraba-açu.
USES: Plant used in a decoction against dysentery; infusion for ophthalmia.

Commelina sulcata Willd.
AREA: Bahia to Rio Grande do Sul.
NAME: Erva-de-santa-luzia.
USE: Juice used for washing inflamed eyes.

Commelina vestita Seub.
AREA: Minas Gerais to São Paulo.
NAME: Trapoeraba-azul.
USES: Emollient, diuretic, antirheumatic; also for dropsy and sore throat.

Commelina virginica L.
AREA: Neotropical; ruderal in Brazil.
NAMES: Andacá, erva-mijona, erva-de-santa-luzia, flor-das-lavadeiras, maria-mole, marianinha, trapoeraba, trapoeraba-azul.
USES: Emollient, diuretic, for curing sore throat.
CHEM.: The complex pigment of the blue flowers of *Commelina* species has been extensively studied by Japanese workers (Ref: COMM 1).

Dichorisandra affinis Mart.
AREA: Amazonia, forest.
NAMES: Disciplina, trapoeraba.
USES: Diuretic, emollient, prescribed for kidney troubles, ascites, dartre (skin disease), hemorrhoids, dropsy and sore throat.

Dichorisandra leucophthalmos Hook.
AREA: Rio de Janeiro and São Paulo, forest.
NAME: Trapoeraba-azul.
USES: Same as given for *Dichorisandra affinis* Mart.

Dichorisandra spp.
Several other *Dichorisandra* species are quite similar to the two already cited, in features and properties. Examples are: *D. luschnathiana* Kunth, *D. picta* Hook., *D. thyrsiflora* Mikan and *D. villosula* Mart., all of which occur in the undergrowth of the Brazilian rainforest.

Tradescantia diuretica Mart.
AREA: Minas Gerais, Rio de Janeiro and Mato Grosso.
NAMES: Trapoeraba, trapoeraba-verdadeira.
USES: Strongly diuretic, more so than the preceding species; also useful for piles, dropsy or anasarca.

Tradescantia effusa Mart.
AREA: Throughout Brazil.
NAME: Trapoerba-branca.
USES: Emollient, diuretic, indicated for rheumatism, hydropsy, sore throat.

Tradescantia spathacea Sw.
AREA: Ruderal in Brazil, escaped from cultivation, e.g., in Rio de Janeiro. The species grows both in soil and as an epiphyte on trees.
NAMES: Cordobá, trapoeraba-açu, uru-de-pobre.
USES: Entire plant is used for an emollient, pectoral and diuretic.
CHEM.: Pigmented leaves contain a disaccharide glycoside of cyanidin (Ref: COMM 2).

There are numerous other *Tradescantia* species, all morphologically very similar and reputedly having the same medicinal purposes.

Commelinaceae – References

COMM 1. Goto, T., T. Hoshino & S. Takase. 1979. A proposed structure of commelinin, a sky-blue anthocyanin complex obtained from the flower petals of *Commelina*. *Tetrahedron Lett.*: 2905-2908.

COMM 2. Robinson, G.M. & R. Robinson. 1932. A survey of anthocyanine. II. *Biochem. J.* 26: 1647-1664.

CONNARACEAE

Connarus patrisii Planch.
AREA: Amazonia and Goiás.
NAME: Árvore-dos-feiticeiros.
USES: Seeds recommended to help recover strength after illnesses.

Connarus suberosus Planch.
AREA: Minas Gerais to Paraná, cerrado.
NAMES: Araruta-do-campo, cabelo-de-negro, pau-ferro.
USES: Bark used for curing diarrhoea.

CONVOLVULACEAE

Calonyction aculeatum (L.) House
AREA: Frequent in cultivation and escaped in eastern and southern Brazil.
NAMES: Boa-noite, dama-da-noite.
USES: In baths, to relieve rheumatic ailments; internally taken as drastic purgative.

CONVOLVULACEAE

Cuscuta racemosa Mart.
AREA: Widely dispersed parasite, devoid of chlorophyll; often found in cities, on fences, shrubs and trees.
NAMES: Cipó-chumbo, fios-de-ovos.
USES: Astringent, emollient, anti-inflammatory, stomachic, anticatarrhal, purgative, depurative, diuretic, antiblennorrhagic; also useful for throat infections, liver colics, bleeding diarrhoea, hemoptysis and for the treatment of a variety of wounds and sores.

There are more than a score of *Cuscuta* species in Brazil, all of them reputed to have similar properties. Some are very frequent, such as *C. umbellata* H.B.K. Morphologically very similar, they are difficult to distinguish, except by the specialists.

Evolvulus alsinoides L.
AREA: Tropical cosmopolitan; prefers sandy tracts.
NAME: Corre-corre.
USES: Bitter, tonic, antipyretic, used for upset stomach.
CHEM.: Triacontane and sitosterol identified (Ref: CONV 1).

Evolvulus holosericeus H.B.K.
AREA: Neotropical; sandy campos, e.g., in Minas Gerais.
NAME: Erva-galega.
USES: Against syphilitic manifestations.

Ipomoea acetosifolia (Vahl) Roem. & Schult.
AREA: On sandy beaches along the Brazilian coast.
NAMES: Campainha-branca, cipó-da-praia, salsa-da-praia.
USES: Latex is purgative. Bruised leaves placed on inflamed spots of the skin to provoke suppuration. Decoction is antihydropic, emollient, vulnerary. Roots are a mild laxative. Roots and seeds are diuretic, emmenagogue and used for the removal of obstructions.

Ipomoea pentaphylla Jacq.
AREA: Amazonia.
NAMES: Batatão-roxo, campainha-dos-tintureiros.
USE: Flowers in baths for conjunctivitis.

Ipomoea pes-caprae (L.) R. Br.
AREA: On beaches, all along the littoral.
NAMES: Batata-da-praia, batata-do-mar, cipó-da-praia, pé-de-cabra, salsa-da-praia.
USES: Decoction is emollient, vulnerary, employed in rubbings for rheumatism and against certain tumors. Roots are slightly purgative, diuretic. Contused leaves are used for maturing inflamed areas in the form of abscesses.

CHEM. & PHARM.: Summary analyses are found in the older literature (Ref: CONV 2,3). Extracts were shown to be spasmolytic and effective against dermatitis caused by venomous jellyfish (Ref: CONV 4). One acyclic diterpene (E-phytol) and one partially degraded sesquiterpene (â-damascenone) were found to be partially responsible for these actions (Ref: CONV 5). Crude extracts and several isolated compounds showed an inhibiting effect on prostaglandin synthesis *in vitro* (Ref: CONV 6).

A number of *Ipomoea* species have tuberous, fleshy roots with strong purgative action. In analogy to the *Operculina* species (see below) they are generally designated as "jalapa." Commonly cited are the following: *I. batatoides* Meissn. (Amazonia), *I. capparoides* Choisy (Amazonia to Rio de Janeiro), *I. echioides* Choisy (Ceará, Minas Gerais and Mato Grosso), *I. gigantea* Choisy (Goiás and Mato Grosso), *I. longicuspis* Meissn. (Amazonia), *I. silvana* Choisy (São Paulo and Paraná, used for purging horses) and *I. sinuata* Ortega (Paraná and São Paulo).

Operculina alata (Ham.) Urb.

AREA: From Amazonia southward, to Goiás and Rio de Janeiro.
NAMES: Batata-de-purga, batatão (Amazonia), jalapa.
USES: The starchy, fleshy tubers are strongly drastic. Both the sliced tubers and the roasted seeds are used in infusions against constipation, dropsy, syphilis, amenorrhoea and believed to prevent diseases of the digestive tract. The gum of the tubers is given to children to prevent diarrhoea and skin eruptions as consequences of teething. The drug is also used in the treatment of congestive respiratory conditions and cerebral palsy. The resin is widely industrialized in the form of laxative pills.

Operculina macrocarpa Urb.

AREA: On sandy soils, from Maranhão southward as far as São Paulo.
NAMES: Batata-de-purga, jalapa.
USES: Same as for *Operculina alata*.
CHEM.: The drastic resins of the Convolvulaceae have highly complex chemical structures. For an excellent review see Ref: CONV 7. More recent studies are presented in Ref: CONV 8.

Convolvulaceae – References

CONV 1. Mehta, C.R. & N.B. Shah. 1958. Chemical examination of *Evolvulus alsinoides*. *Sci. and Cult.* (Calcutta) 24: 180-181.
CONV 2. Christensen, B.V. & J.A. Reese. 1938. Study of the leaves of *Ipomoea pes-caprae*. *J. Am. Pharm. Assoc.* 27: 195-199.
CONV 3. Cwalina, G.E. & G.L. Jenkins. 1938. A phytochemical study of *Ipomoea pes-caprae*. *J. Am. Pharm. Assoc.* 27: 585-595.
CONV 4. Pongprayoon, U,. L. Bohlin & S. Wasuwat. 1991. Neutralization of toxic effects of different crude jellyfish venoms by an extract of *Ipomoea pes-caprae* (L.) R.Br. *J. Ethnopharmacol.* 35: 65-69.

CONV 5. Pongprayoon, U., P. Baeckström, U. Jacobsson, M. Lindström & L. Bohlin. 1992. Antispasmodic activity of â-demascenone and E-phytol isolated from *Ipomoea pes-caprae*. *Planta Medica 58*: 19-21.

CONV 6. Pongprayoon, U., P. Baeckström, U. Jacobsson, M. Lindström & L. Bohlin. 1991. Compounds inhibiting prostaglandin synthesis isolated from *Ipomoea pes-caprae*. *Planta Medica 57*: 515-518.

CONV 7. Wagner, H. 1973. The chemistry of resin glucosides of the Convolvulaceae family. *Nobel 25*: 235-240.

CONV 8. Ono, M., T. Kawasaki & K. Miyahara. 1989. Resin Glycosides. V. Identification and characterization of the component organic and glycosidic acids of the ether-soluble crude resin glycosides ("Jalapin") from Rhizoma jalapae brasiliensis (Roots of *Ipomoea operculata*). *Chem. Pharm. Bull. 37*: 3209-3213.

COSTACEAE

Costus cuspidatus (Nees & Mart.) Maas
AREA: Pará, Bahia and Rio de Janeiro; forest.
NAMES: Cana-da-terra, cana-do-mato, cana-do-rio, ubacaiá.
USES: Juice from shoots is febrifuge, antisyphilitic and used for bladder ailments.

Costus spicatus (Jacq.) Sw.
AREA: Amazonia, Pernambuco and Rio de Janeiro, forest; neotropical.
NAMES: Caatinga, cana-branca, cana-de-macaco, cana-do-brejo, canarana, jacuacanga, paco-caatinga, pacová, periná, pobre-velha, ubacaia.
USES: Shoots are tonic, diuretic, depurative, diaphoretic, emmenagogue; the expressed juice is used against fever, nephritis, urethritis, bladder lithiasis, gonorrhoea, leucorrhoea, and to calm coughs; in poultices to treat tumors.

Costus spiralis (Jacq.) Roscoe
AREA: Pará to São Paulo, forest.
NAMES: The same as for *Costus spicatus*.
USES: The juice expressed from the aerial parts is recommended for arteriosclerosis and as a calmative for nerves and the heart; also used for cleaning syphilitic sores. Fresh, contused leaves are used as a resolvent for tumors.
CHEM.: Diosgenin, which used to be an important raw material for the synthesis of steroidal hormones, has been detected in several *Costus* species, including those cited above (Ref: COST 1,2).

Costaceae is sometimes included in the family Zingiberaceae.

Costaceae – References
COST 1. Wilhuhn, G. & G. Pretzsch. 1985. Diosgenin und Sterine aus *Costus spiralis*. *Planta Medica 51*: 185-187.

COST 2. Lambert, N., J.-C. Baccou & Y. Sauvaire. 1988. Screening for diosgenin in rhizomes from three *Costus* species (*C. deistellii, C. igneus, C. lucanusianus*). *Planta Medica* 54: 366-367.

CRASSULACEAE

Kalanchoe brasiliensis Camb.
AREA: Bahia to São Paulo, along littoral.
NAMES: Coirama, coirama-branca, erva-da-costa, folha-da-costa, folha-da-fortuna, folha-grossa, orelha-de-monge, saião.
USES: Useful for treating insect stings and to hasten cicatrization. Fresh leaves roasted and applied to lessen cephalalgia; their infusion for lymphangitis and bubo and erysipelas of the legs. Leaf juice said to be efficient to remove corns and in treating athlete's foot and burns.

Kalanchoe pinnata (Lam.) Pers.
AREA: Grown in gardens and very common as a ruderal.
NAMES: Coirama, folha-da-costa, folha-da-fortuna, pirarucu, são-raimumdo, daião.
USES: Leaves for a sedative, bechic, emollient, antiphlogistic; indicated for amygdalitis and glaucoma.
CHEM. & PHARM.: Tissues of the Crassulaceae contain exceptionally high concentrations of isocitric and malic acids. The concentration of the latter oscillates greatly during the 24 hours of the day, accumulating during the night and being metabolized during the day (Ref: CRAS 1,2). The plants also produce high concentrations of seduheptulose, a rare seven-carbon sugar (Ref: CRAS 3). Other constituents shown to be present in *K. pinnata* are flavonoid glycosides (Ref: CRAS 4) and other phenolics (Ref: CRAS 5), alkanes, triterpenes and sterols (Ref: CRAS 6,7,8). Among the latter, a cytotoxic sterol has been reported (Ref: CRAS 9,10). Anti-inflammatory activity has been demonstrated (Ref: CRAS 11,12) and an antiallergic compound has been isolated (Ref: CRAS 13). An immunosuppressive effect of extracts of *K. pinnata* has been verified *in vivo* in mice and *in vitro* in the form of an inhibitory action on human lymphocyte proliferation (Ref: CRAS 14,15). In *K. brasiliensis* this effect was shown to be due, in part, to the presence of the flavonoid glycosides identified as patuletin acetylrhamnosides (Ref: CRAS 16).

Reports as to a reputed beneficial effect in cases of gastric ulcers are controversial. One study attests to the anti-ulcer activity of *K. pinnata* (Ref: CRAS 17), whereas other experiments yielded negative results for *K. pinnata* and inconclusive for *Sedum* sp. (Ref: CRAS 18). (These latter studies established the efficacy of extracts of *Maytenus ilicifolia*,

CRASSULACEAE

Celastraceae, *q.v.*). A review of the chemistry and biological properties of *Kalanchoe* species has been published (Ref: CRAS 19).

Crassulaceae – References

CRAS 1. Bruisma, J. 1958. Studies in the Crassulacean acid metabolism. *Acta Bot. Neerl.* 7: 531- 538.
CRAS 2. Soderstrom, T.R. 1962. Isocitric acid content of Crassulacean plants and a few succulent species from other families. *Am. J. Bot. 49*: 850-851.
CRAS 3. Nordal, A. & R. Klevstarnd. 1951. Constituents of Crassulacean plants (II). Paper chromatographic investigation of the free sugars. *Acta Chem. Scand. 5*: 898-900.
CRAS 4. Gaind, K.N. & R.L. Gupta. 1971. Flavonoid glycosides from *Kalanchoe pinnata*. *Planta Medica 20*: 368-373.
CRAS 5. Gaind, K.N. & R.L. Gupta. 1973. Phenolic compounds from the leaves of *Kalanchoe pinnata*. *Planta Medica 23*: 149-153.
CRAS 6. Gaind, K.N. & R.L. Gupta. 1972. Alkanes, alkanols, triterpenes and sterols of *Kalanchoe pinnata*. *Phytochemistry 11*: 1500-1502.
CRAS 7. Gaind, K.N. & R.L. Gupta. 1974. Identification of waxes from the leaves of *Kalanchoe pinnata*. *Planta Medica 23*: 193-196.
CRAS 8. Siddiqui, S., S. Faizi, B.S. Siddiqui & N. Sultana. 1989. Triterpenoids and phenanthrenes from leaves of *Bryophyllum pinnatum*. *Phytochemistry 28*: 2433-2438.
CRAS 9. Yamagishi, T., X.-Z. Yan, R.-Y. Wu, D.R. McPhail, A.T. McPhail & K.-H. Lee. 1988. Structure and stereochemistry of bryophyllin-A, a novel potent cytotoxic bufadienolide from *Bryophyllum pinnatum*. *Chem. Pharm. Bull.* (Japan) *36*: 1615-1617.
CRAS 10. Yamagishi, T., M. Haruna, X.-Z. Yan, J.-J. Chan & K.H. Lee. 1989. Antitumor agents. 110. Bryophyllin B, a novel potent cytotoxic bufadienolide from *Bryophyllum pinnatum*. *J. Nat. Prod. 52*: 1071-1079.
CRAS 11. Pal, S. & A.K.N. Chaudhuri. 1990. Anti-inflammatory action of *Bryophyllum pinnatum*. *Fitoterapia 61*: 527-533.
CRAS 12. Pal, S. & A.K.N. Chaudhuri. 1992. Further studies on the anti-inflammatory profile of the methanolic fraction of the fresh leaf extracts of *Bryophyllum pinnatum*. *Fitoterapia 63*: 451-459.
CRAS 13. Ishikawa, M., M. Ogura & T. Iijima. 1986. Antiallergic flavone glycoside from *Kalanchoe pinnatum*. *Chem. Abstr. 105*: 178423q.
CRAS 14. Rossi-Bergmann, B., S.S. Costa, M.B.S. Borges, S.A. da Silva, G.R. Noleto, M.L.M. Souza & V.L.G. Moraes. 1994. Immunosuppressive effect of the aqueous extract of *Kalanchoe pinnata* in mice. *Phytotherapy Res. 8*: 399-402.
CRAS 15. Moraes, V.L.G., L.F.M. Santos, S.B. Castro, L.H. Loureiro, O.A. Lima, M.L.M. Souza, L.M.K. Yien, B. Rossi-Bergmann & S.S. Costa. 1994. Inhibition of lymphocyte activation by extracts and fractions of *Kalanchoe, Alternanthera, Paullinia* and *Mikania* species. *Phytomedicine 1*: 199-204.
CRAS 16. Costa, S.S., A. Jossang, B. Bodo, M.L.M. Souza & V.L.G. Moraes. 1994. Patuletin acetylrhamnosides from *Kalanchoe brasiliensis* as inhibitors of human lymphocyte proliferative activity. *J. Nat. Prod. 57*: 1503-1510.
CRAS 17. Pal, S. & A.K.N. Chaidhuri. 1991. Studies on the anti-ulcer activity of *Bryophyllum pinnatum* leaf extract in experimental animals. *J. Ethnopharmacol. 33*: 97-102.
CRAS 18. Macaubas, C.I.P., M.G.M. Oliveira, M.L.O.S. Formigoni, N.G. Silveria Filho & E.A. Carlini. 1988. Estudo da eventual ação antiúlcera gástrica do bálsamo (*Sedum* sp.), folha-da-fortuna (*Bryophyllum calycinum*), couve (*Brassica oleracea*) e da espinheira santa (*Maytenus ilicifolia*) em ratos. In: E.A. Carlini (ed.): Estudo de ação antiúlcera gástrica de plantas brasileiras (*Maytenus ilicifolia* "espinheira-santa" e outras). Central de Medicamentos (CEME), Ministry of Health, Brasília. 1988. 87 pp. (pp. 5-20).
CRAS 19. Costa, S.S., A. Jossang & B. Bodo. 1995. Propriétés biologiques et phytochimie des *Kalanchoe*. In: Boiteau, P. & L. Allorge-Boiteau, Kalanchoe de Madagascar. Éditions Karthala (Paris) 1955, pp. 219-235.

CUCURBITACEAE

Anisosperma passiflora Manso
AREA: Amazonia to São Paulo.
NAMES: Andiroba, castanha-de-bugre, castanha-de-jatobá, castanha-mineira.
USES: Seeds prescribed for jaundice, gastrointestinal troubles; oil from seeds is bitter, purgative, antidyspeptic, recommended for liver ailments. Used in veterinary medicine against colics in cattle.

Cayaponia cabocla (Vell.) Mart.
AREA: Bahia to Paraná, capoeira.
NAMES: Anapinta, abobreira-do-mato, capitão-do-mato, purga-de-caboclo, purga-de-caiapó, purga-de-gentio.
USES: Roots for a purgative. Seeds drastic, used against ascites and malignant fevers.

Cayaponia espelina (Manso) Cogn.
AREA: Very frequent in cerrado from Ceará to Mato Grosso and São Paulo.
NAMES: Carijó, disciplina, fel-de-gentio, purga-de-carijó.
USES: Roots are tonic, diuretic, anti-asthmatic, antisyphilitic, antidysenteric, purgative, alexipharmic mainly against plant poisons; also indicated for epilepsy, pulmonary catarrh, bronchitis, whooping cough and hemorrhage.

Cayaponia martiana (Cogn.) Cogn.
AREA: Rio de Janeiro to Rio Grande do Sul, commonly ruderal.
NAMES: Abobrinha, abobrinha-do-mato, purga-de-caboclo, purga-de-gentio, taiyiá, taiuiá-de-pimenta, taiuiá-grande.
USES: Roots are purgative, emetic, antisyphilitic, depurative, antirabies.

Cayaponia pilosa Cogn.
AREA: Minas Gerais to São Paulo.
NAMES: Abobrinha-do-mato, fruta-de-gentio, purga-de-caboclo, purga-de-caiapó, purga-de-gentio, purga-do-mato.
USES: Roots and berries are bitter, drastic, emmenagogue, antisyphilitic, indicated for dropsy and ascites. In veterinary medicine the seeds are employed as a violent purgative for cattle.

Cayaponia tayuya (Mart.) Cogn.
AREA: Widely disseminated, from Amazonia to the extreme south.
NAMES: Anapinta, abobrinha-do-mato, azougue-do-brasil, cabeça-de-negro, guardião, raiz-de-bugre, taiuiá, tomba.
USES: Highly esteemed as a depurative. Entire plant is bitter, emetocathartic, antisyphilitic, antirabies, and also recommended for

dermatoses, boils, eczema, rheumatism, epilepsy, amenorrhoea and dilated stomach.

Cayaponia spp.

Several other *Cayaponia* species reputedly have the same properties, such as *C. cordifolia* Cogn. (Minas Gerais to São Paulo), *C. pedata* Cogn. (Rio de Janeiro and São Paulo) and *C. triangularis* Cogn. (Amazonia); in general they are known by the same vernacular names as those given above.

All species of the genus *Cayaponia* so far investigated contain in their roots cucurbitacins, highly oxygenated triterpenes of bitter taste and some toxicity (Ref: CUCU 1). The crude drug which is commercialized under the name 'taiuiá' is supposed to be represented by the roots of *Cayaponia tayuya*, official according to the BRAZILIAN PHARMACOPOEIA (1st edition, 1929). A careful survey, however, has shown that almost any species of *Cayaponia* is marketed under the same label. Even material from another genus, *Wilbrandia ebracteata*, has frequently been found among the roots of commerce (Ref: CUCU 2). Besides cucurbitacins, flavone glycosides were characterized (Ref: CUCU 3) and anti-inflammatory activity has been verified (Ref: CUCU 4).

Cucurbita pepo L.

AREA: Cultivated and often escaped from cultivation.
NAMES: Abóbora, gerimum (English: pumpkin).
USES: Seeds are vermicidal (taenifuge); fresh and peeled, they are given especially to children, in association with coconut milk.
CHEM. & PHARM.: The active compound is cucurbitin (3-amino-pyrrolidine-3-carboxylic acid), a water-soluble, non-proteinogenic amino acid (Ref: CUCU 5). Besides being taenifuge, the substance inhibits the growth of immature worms of *Schistosoma japonicum*, in vivo (Ref: CUCU 6).

Fevillea trilobata L.

AREA: Amazonia to Paraná, forest and capoeira.
NAMES: Cipó-de-jaboti, cipó-escada, fava-de-santo-inácio-falsa, guapeva, nhandiroba, noz-de-serpente.
USES: Roots are purgative, prescribed for eruptive diseases. Seeds are febrifuge, tonic, stomachic, emetic, emmenagogue, useful for jaundice and liver troubles. Oil from seeds is applied externally against rheumatic pains, erysipelas, ringworm, snake bites (here also the juice of the leaves). Also used as an antidote against the toxic action of bitter cassava.
CHEM.: The glyceride constituents of the seed oil contain conjugated unsaturated fatty acids (Ref: CUCU 7).

CUCURBITACEAE

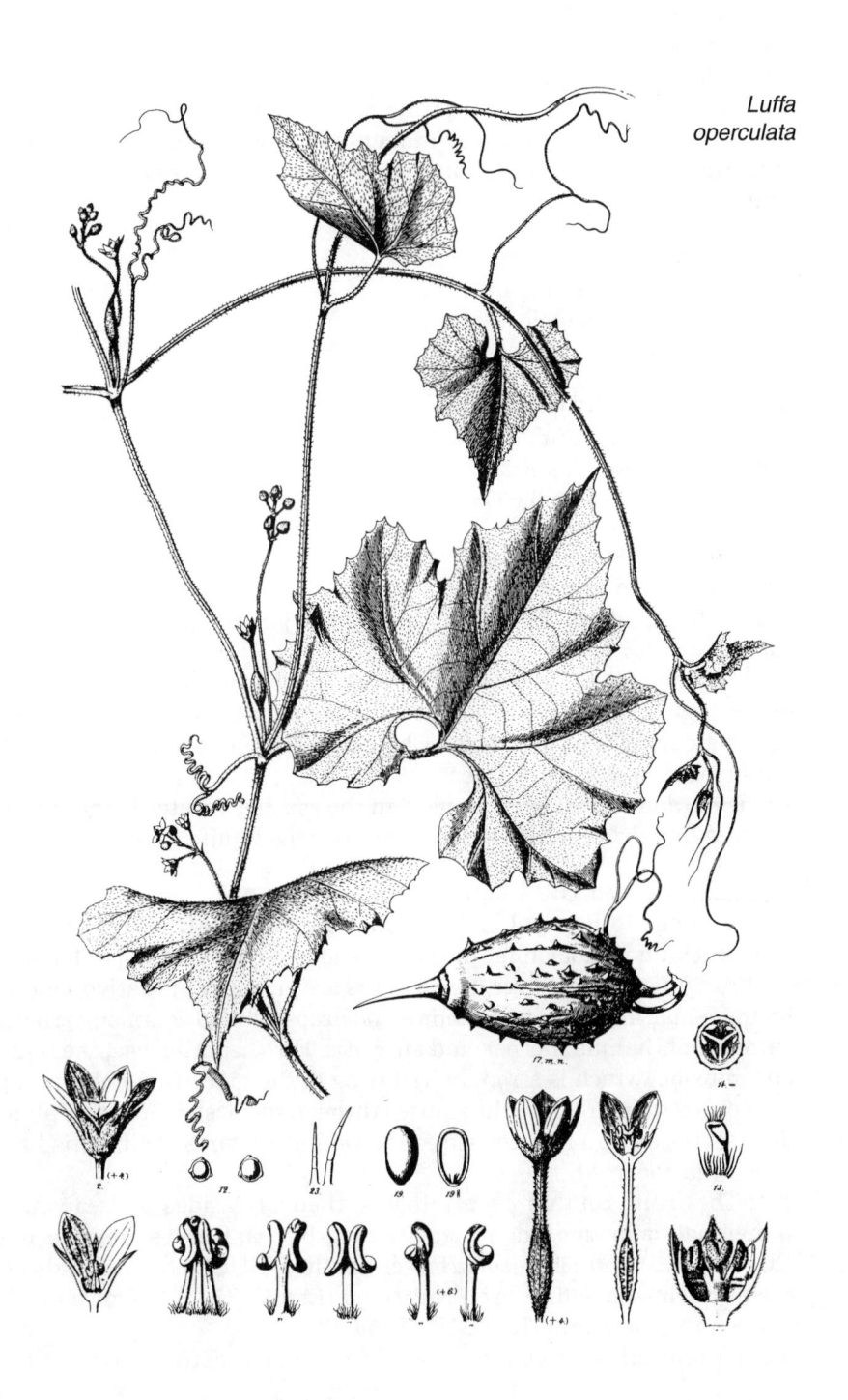

Luffa operculata

CUCURBITACEAE

Fevillea uncipetala Kuhlm.
AREA: Pará, forest.
NAMES: Cipó-jatobá, jatobá, pacapiá.
USES: Seeds are bitter, tonic, stomachic, intensely purgative, toxic in higher doses. Recommended for liver ailments and jaundice. The oil pressed from the seeds is purgative, bitter, used topically for treating erysipelas and tetterworm.

Gurania multiflora Cogn.
AREA: Bahia to Rio de Janeiro.
NAME: Pepino-de-papagaio.
USES: Fruit is purgative.

Gurania paulista Cogn.
AREA: Rio de Janeiro and Minas Gerais.
NAME: Bucha-dos-paulistas.
USE: The same as given for *Gurania multiflora*.

Lagenaria siceraria (Molina) Standl.
AREA: Naturalized and cultivated.
NAMES: Cabaça, cabaça-amargosa, cuia, cuieté, jamaru, porongo, purunga, taquera.
USES: The rind of the mature fruit is given as an abortive, though dangerous in high amounts; pulp is a poultice emollient and purgative. Seeds used for curing nephritis. Leaves heated and applied locally are said to aid in labor; also to cure sores.

The hard mature shells are used in the southern states for gourds, to prepare and drink mate (*Ilex paraguariensis*, Aquifoliaceae).

Luffa operculata (L.) Cogn.
AREA: Amazonia to Rio de Janeiro, Minas Gerais and Mato Grosso.
NAMES: Buchinha, cabacinha, purga-do-joão-paes, purga-dos-paulistas.
USES: Fruit juice is vermifuge. Dried fruits are violently purgative, emetic, hydrago-gue, indicated for jaundice and dropsy, chlorosis, amen-orrhoea, chronic ophthalmia, herpes and sinusitis. For the latter use, the aqueous infusion, which is strongly irritating to the mucous membranes, is introduced (diluted!) into the sinuses through the nostrils, causing abundant secretion as a first consequence. Definitive cures of sinusitis have thus been reported.
CHEM.: The fruits contain cucurbitacins, their glycosides and saponins. Individual compounds identified are cucurbitacin B and elaterin A (Ref: CUCU 8), as well as isocucurbitacin B (Ref: CUCU 9). Glycosides of cucurbitacins have also been identified (Ref: CUCU 10). One saponin aglycon is gypsogenin (Ref: CUCU 11).
PHARM.: A protective effect of aqueous and ethanolic extracts against car-

bon tetrachloride-induced liver injury in rats has been demonstrated (Ref: CUCU 12).

Melothria fluminensis Gardn.
AREA: Pará to Santa Catarina and Mato Grosso.
NAMES: Abóbora-do-mato, cereja-de-purga, guardião, melão-de-morcego, taiuiá-miúdo.
USES: Berries are drastic. Juice of leaves is used as eye-drops to cure albugo.

Melothrianthus smilacifolius (Cogn.) M. Crovetto
AREA: Minas Gerais and Rio de Janeiro.
NAMES: Azougue-dos-pobres, cipó-azougue.
USES: Roots and leaves are depurative, antirheumatic, remedy for syphilis and dermatoses.

The popular designation "azougue-dos-pobres," meaning "mercury of the poor," was assigned to the plant at a time when mercury compounds were in favor among the few then-known drugs against syphilis.

Momordica charantia L.
AREA: Pantropical; ruderal in Brazil.
NAMES: Erva-de-são-caetano, melão-de-são-caetano.
USES: Roots and leaves are antirheumatic, resolvent, antidiarrhoeic. Leaf infusion is used for leukemia and menstrual colics; heated leaves are emollient. Leaves are anthelmintic and antidiabetic. Fruits also are anthelmintic. Leaf juice is purgative and employed to combat scabies. In veterinary medicine, used to treat the gapes of poultry.
CHEM. & PHARM.: The blood sugar lowering properties of the fruit have been confirmed and are attributed to a polypeptide of molecular weight 11,000 (Ref: CUCU 13).

Sicana odorifera Naud.
AREA: Ceará to Minas Gerais.
NAMES: Coroá, cruá, curuá, melão-de-caboclo.
USES: Infusion of fruit rind and seeds is recommended for uterine hemorrhages.

Sicyos polyacanthus Cogn.
AREA: Throughout Brazil.
NAME: Pó-de-mico.
USES: Fruits are drastic; externally applied as a resolvent.

Trianosperma diversifolia Cogn.
AREA: Espírito Santo to São Paulo.
NAME: Abobrinha-do-mato.
USES: Fruit is bitter, antidiabetic.

CUCURBITACEAE

Trianosperma glandulosa Mart.
AREA: Amazonia.
NAMES: Abobrinha-do-mato, cabeça-de-negro, taiuiá.
USES: Root is purgative, used for dropsy, ancylostomiasis, absence of menses, epilepsy and leprosy. Leaves used in poultices for ulcers and scurvy. Roots and berries are depurative. Other species of the same genus, such as *T. trilobata* Cogn. (Rio de Janeiro) display the same properties.

Wilbrandia ebracteata Cogn.
AREA: From Rio de Janeiro southward.
NAME: Taiuiá.
USES: Roots are bitter, purgative, antisyphilitic, used against rheumatism and dropsy. In the drug market, the roots are frequently labelled as *Cayaponia tayuya* (above).

Wilbrandia verticillata (Vell.) Cogn.
AREA: From the northeast southward, to Minas Gerais, Espírito Santo and São Paulo.
NAMES: Abobrinha-do-mato, anapinta, azougue, azougue-do-brasil, azougue-dos-pobres, cabacinha, cabeça-de-negro, cipó-azougue.
USES: Tuberous roots are bitter, antisyphilitic, purgative, depurative, febrifuge, emmenagogue; recommended as antirheumatic, for arthritis, dropsy and erysipelas.

Wilbrandia spp.
CHEM. & PHARM.: Sixteen cucurbitacins were isolated from the roots of *W. ebracteata* (Ref: CUCU 14). C-glycosyl-flavones were shown to be present in roots and fruits (Ref: CUCU 15). Further work was performed on a species of the northeast, either *W. verticillata* or a close relative (Ref: CUCU 16,17). This material was shown to possess considerable anti-inflammatory activity and to contain two *nor*-cucurbitacin glucosides. A purified fraction containing these two compounds showed cytotoxicity and significant antitumor activity against Walker 256 carcinosarcoma (Ref: CUCU 18).

Cucurbitaceae – References

CUCU 1. Lavie, D. & E. Glotter. 1971. The cucurbitacines, a group of tetracyclic triterpenes. In: Herz, W., H. Grisebach & G.W. Kirby, eds.: *Progr. Chem. Org. Nat. Prod. 29*: 307-362.

CUCU 2. Farias, M.R. & E. P. Schenkel. 1987. Caracterização de cucurbitacinas em espécies vegetais conhecidas popularmente como taiuiá. *Ciência e Cultura* (São Paulo) *39*: 970-973.

CUCU 3. Bauer, R., L.H. Barganza, O. Seligmann & H. Wagner. 1985. Cucurbitacins and flavone C-glycosides from *Cayaponia tayuya*. *Phytochemistry 24*: 1587-1591.

CUCU 4. Rios, J.L., R.M.Giner, M.J. Jiménez, G. Wickmann & J.L. Hancke. 1990. A study on the anti-inflammatory activity of *Cayaponia tayuya* root. *Fitoterapia 61*: 275-278.
CUCU 5. Dunhill, M.P. & L. Fowden. 1965. Amino acids of seeds of the Cucurbitaceae. *Phytochemistry 4*: 933-944.
CUCU 6. Fang, S. L.Li, C. Niu & K. Tseng. 1961. Chemical studies of *Cucurbita moschata* Duch. I. The isolation and structural studies of cucurbitine, a new amino acid. *Sci. Sinica* (Peking) *10*: 845-851.
CUCU 7. Tulloch, A.P. & L. Bergter. 1979. Analysis of the conjugated trienoic acid containing oil from *Fevillea trilobata* by ^{13}C nuclear magnetic resonance spectroscopy. *Lipids 14*: 996-1002.
CUCU 8. Kloss, P. 1966. Die Bitterstoffe der *Luffa operculata*. *Arch. Pharm. 299*: 351-355.
CUCU 9. Matos, F.J.A. & O.R. Gottlieb. 1967. Isocucurbitacina B, constituinte citotóxico da *Luffa operculata*. *An. Acad. Brazil. Ci.* 39: 245-247.
CUCU 10. Kloss, P. & H. Schindler. 1966. Dünnschichtchromatographische Methode zur Prüfung von Cucurbitaceen—Tinkturen. *Pharm. Ztg. 111*: 772-775.
CUCU 11. Djerassi, C., A. Bowers, S. Burstein, H. Estrada, J. Grossman, J. Herrman, A.J. Lemin, A. Manjarrez & S.C. Pakrashi. 1956. Terpenoids, XXII. Triterpenes from some Mexican and South American plants. *J. Am. Chem. Soc. 78*: 2312-2315.
CUCU 12. Araujo Silva, E., V. S. Rao & M. C Fonteles. 1987. Protective effect of *Luffa operculata* (L.) Cogn. in experimental liver injury. *Oréades* (Belo Horizonte) *8*: 467-474.
CUCU 13. Khanna, P., S.C. Jain, A. Panagariya & V.P. Dixit. 1981. Hypoglycemic activity of polypeptide-p from a plant source. *J. Nat. Prod. 44*: 648-655.
CUCU 14. Farias, M.R., E. P. Schenkel, R. Mayer & G. Rücker. 1993. Cucurbitacins as constituents of *Wilbrandia ebracteata*. *Planta Medica 59*: 272-275.
CUCU 15. Santos, R.I., M.A. dos Santos & E.P. Schenkel. 1989. C-glycosylflavones from *Wilbrandia ebracteata* Cogn. *Brazilian-Sino Symposium on Chemistry and Pharmacology of Natural Products* (Rio de Janeiro). Summaries of papers, p. 94.
CUCU 16. Almeida, F.R.C., V.S.N. Rao & M.E.O. Matos. 1989. Inhibition of formaldehyde-induced arthritis by a purified fraction prepared from *Wilbrandia* (cf.) *verticillata* which contains novel norcucurbitacin glucosides. *Brazilian J. Med. Biol. Res. 22*: 1397-1399.
CUCU 17. Matos, M.E.O., M.I.L. Machado, A.A. Craveiro, F.J.A. Matos & R. Braz-Filho. 1991. *Nor*-cucurbitacin glucosides from *Wilbrandia* species. *Phytochemistry 30*: 1020-1023.
CUCU 18. Rao, V.S.N., F.R.C. Almeida, A.P. Moraes, J.V. Silva, S.C. Nascimento & M.O. Moraes. 1991. Evaluation of the purified fraction of *Wilbrandia* (cf.) *verticillata* for antitumor activity. *Mem. Inst. Oswaldo Cruz* (Rio de Janeiro) *86*, Suppl. II: 43-45.

CYATHEACEAE

Cyathea armata (Sw.) Domin
AREA: All forest stretches in Brazil.
NAMES: Pau-cardoso, rabo-de-bugio, rabo-de-macaco, samambaia-açu.
USE: Pith and young leaves are bechic.

Cyathea microdonta (Desv.) Domin
AREA: Atlantic forest in Serra do Mar and Serra da Mantiqueira, from Bahia southward.
NAMES: Avenca-grande, rabo-de-bugio, samambaia-açu.
USES: Young leaves are expectorant and styptic for hemoptyses.

CYPERACEAE

Bulbostylis capillaris Clarke
AREA: Throughout Brazil.
NAME: Alecrim-da-praia.
USE: Antirheumatic.

Cyperus corymbosus Rottb.
AREA: Cosmopolitan; widespread in Brazil.
NAMES: Piripirioca, priprioca.
USES: Root decoction used in baths against fever; internally employed as contraceptive.
CHEM.: A sesquiterpene alcohol has been described (Ref: CYPE 1).

Cyperus gracilescens Roem. & Schult.
AREA: Amazonia.
NAMES: Capiscaba-mirim, junça-miúda, junco-miúdo, tiririca.
USES: Bulbs are analeptic, aphrodisiac, recommended for snake bites.

Cyperus ligularis L.
AREA: Tropical America; ruderal.
NAMES: Capim-açu, manibu, flecha-de-urubu.
USES: Root infusion is diuretic. Stem juice is applied to the eyes for treating pterygium.

Cyperus rotundus L.
AREA: Cosmopolitan; ruderal, invasive; one of the worst weeds in Brazil.
NAME: Tiririca.
USES: Bulbs and roots are balsamic, stimulant, diaphoretic, diuretic, anthelmintic.
CHEM.: The essential oil of the rhizomes contains mono- and sesquiterpenoids, with alpha-cyperone, a sesquiterpene ketone, as the major constituent [30-50%] (Ref: CYPE 2,4,6,7). Fatty oil has been analyzed (Ref: CYPE 3), as well as the sugars (Ref: CYPE 5).
PHARM.: The essential oil of the tubers has estrogenic activity. The active substance is a hydrocarbon, cyperene I, at least in part responsible and also antispasmodic on the uterus (Ref: CYPE 8).

Cyperus sesquiflorus (Torrey) Mattf. & Kükent.
AREA: Southern Brazil.
NAMES: Capim-cheiroso, capim-de-cheiro, capim-cidreira, capim-limão, jaçapé.
USES: Leaf and bulb infusion is calmative, stomachic, aromatic sudorific, carminative, antispasmodic, stimulant; also used to lessen dyspnea and flatulence.

Hypolytrum laxum Schrad.
AREA: Amazonia to Maranhão.
NAMES: Capim-navalha-mole, navalha-miúda, tiririca.
USES: Roots are emollient, stomachic, diuretic, emmenagogue.

Kyllinga pungens Link
AREA: Amazonia.
NAME: Capim-de-um-só-botão.
USES: Roots are aromatic, used for colds, flu and fevers.

Mariscus flavus Vahl
AREA: Northeastern Brazil.
NAME: Capim-açu.
USE: Root infusion is diuretic.

Mariscus jacquinii H.B.K.
AREA: Amazonia to Rio de Janeiro.
NAMES: Cálamo-branco, junco.
USES: Tubers are tonic, carminative, indicated for stomach problems.

Remirea maritima Aubl.
AREA: On sandy terrain, along the seashore.
NAMES: Barba-de-boi, cipó-da-praia, carrapicho-de-cavalo, paraturá.
USES: Rhizomes are sudorific, diuretic, antiblennorrhagic.
CHEM.: Several phenolic ketones have been isolated (Ref: CYPE 9,10,11).

Scleria pratensis L.
AREA: Amazonia to Bahia.
NAME: Tiririca.
USES: Tea from leaves and roots is employed against colic and gastralgia.

Cyperaceae – References

CYPE 1. Garbarino, J.A., V. Gambaro & M.C. Chamy. 1985. The structure of corymbolone, an eudesmane sesquiterpenoid keto-alcohol from *Cyperus corymbosus*. *J. Nat. Prod. 48*: 323-325.

CYPE 2. Hedge, B.J. & B.S. Rao. 1935. The essential oil from the rhizomes of *Cyperus rotundus* Linn. *J. Soc. Chem. Ind. 54*: 387-389.

CYPE 3. Asenjo, C.F. 1941. Some of the constituents of the tubers of "Coqui" (*Cyperus rotundus* L.). I. Preliminary examination of the tuber and composition of the fatty oil. *J. Am. Pharm. Assoc. 30*: 216-218.

CYPE 4. Asenjo, C.F. 1942. Some of the constituents of the tubers of "Coqui" (*Cyperus rotundus* L.). II. The volatile oil. *J. Am. Pharm. Assoc. 30*: 628-629.

CYPE 5. Asenjo, C.F. 1942. Some of the constituents of the tubers of "Coqui" (*Cyperus rotundus* L.). III. The sugars. *J. Am. Pharm. Assoc. 31*: 88-89.

CYPE 6. McQuillin, F.J. 1951. The structure of β cyperone. *J. Chem. Soc.*: 716-718.

CYPE 7. Kapadia, V.H., N.G. Naik, M.S. Wadia & S. Dev. 1967. Sesquiterpenoids of *Cyperus rotundus*. *Tetrahedron 47*: 4661-4667.

CYPE 8. Indira, M., M. Sirsi, S. Radomir & K.L. Sukh Dev. 1956. The occurrence of some estrogenic substances in plants. Part. I. Estrogenic activity of *Cyperus rotundus* L. *J. Sci. Ind. Res.* (India) *15C*: 202-204.
CYPE 9. Allan, R.D., R.L. Correll & R.J. Wells. 1969. Two new phenolic ketones from *Remirea maritima*. *Tetrahedron Lett.*: 4673-4674.
CYPE 10. Allan, R.D., R.J. Wells & J.K. MacLeod. 1970. Further phenolic ketones from *Remirea maritima*. *Tetrahedron Lett.*: 3945-3946.
CYPE 11. d'Albuquerque, I.L., O. Gonçalves de Lima, J.F. de Mello, G.M. Maciel & M.A. Moraes e Souza. 1971. Substâncias antimicrobianas de plantas superiores. XXXIV. Observações sobre a ação antimicrobiana de substância identificada como diidroxiparaquinona, isolada de *Remirea maritima* (Cyperaceae), da zona litorânea norte de Olinda. *Rev. Inst. Antibioticos* (Recife) *11*: 15-19.

DENNSTAEDTIACEAE

Pteridium aquilinum (L.) Kuhn

AREA: Ruderal in many places, cosmopolitan.

NAMES: Feto-águia, pluma, pluma-grande, samambaia, samambaia-das-queimadas, samambaia-das-roças, samambaia-das-taperas. English: bracken fern.

USES: Infusion of leaves is bechic and antirheumatic. Decoction of rhizome used for soothing cough in tubercular patients.

CHEM. & PHARM.: Plant is toxic to cattle, horses and laboratory animals (Ref: DENN 1). Fresh leaves contain the cyanogenic glycoside prunasin, the glucoside of mandelonitrile (Ref: DENN 2). A carcinogenic component has been identified (Ref: DENN 3).

Dennstaedtiaceae – References

DENN 1. Tokarnia, C.H., Döbereiner & C.F.C. Canella. 1967. Ocorrência da intoxicação aguda pela "samambaia" (*Pteridium aquilinum* (L.) Kihn) em bovinos no Brasil. *Pesq. Agropec. Bras.* 2: 329-336.
DENN 2. Kofod, H. & R. Eyjolfsson. 1966. The isolation of the cyanogenic glycoside prunasin from *Pteridium aquilinum* (L.) Kuhn. *Tetrahedron Lett.*: 1289-1291.
DENN 3. Matoba, M., E. Saito, K. Saito, K. Koyama, S. Natori, T. Matsushima & M. Takimoto. 1987. Assay of ptaquiloside, the carcinogenic principle of bracken, *Pteridium aquilinum*, by mutagenicity testing in *Salmonella thyphimurium*. *Mutagenesis* 2: 419-423.

DILLENIACEAE

Curatella americana L.

AREA: Amazonia to Minas Gerais and Mato Grosso, cerrado and forest.

NAMES: Cajueiro-branco, caimbé, lixeira, sambaíba.

USES: Bark is astringent, suitable for washing ulcers. Leaves also are used to clean sores.

CHEM.: The bark contains betulinic acid (Ref: DILL 1). Extraction of the

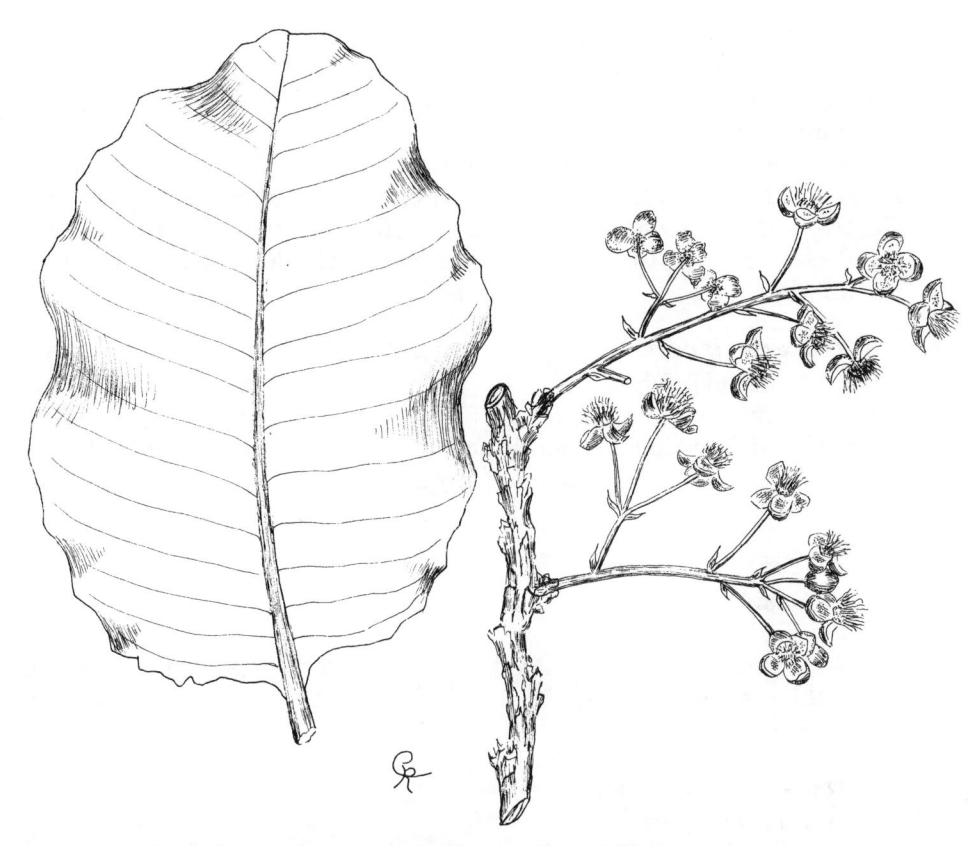

Curatella americana. LEFT: Leaf. RIGHT: Two inflorescences.

leaves yielded the flavonol glycoside avicularin and gallic acid (Ref: DILL 2).

Davilla rugosa Poir.
AREA: Amazonia to Rio Grande do Sul, along littoral.
NAMES: Cambaibinha, capa-homem, cipó-caboclo, cipó-capa-homem, cipó-de-caboclo, cipó-de-carijá, cipó-vermelho, carijó, folha-de-lixa, muiraqueteca, muiratetec, sambaibinha.
USES: Strong stimulant, depurative, aphrodisiac, sometimes suspected to be poisonous. Roots are tonic, astringent and purgative. Branches employed for constipation and jaundice, also diuretic. Leaves recommended for orchitis and epididymitis, lymphangitis, aphthae, hemorrhoids, swelling of the legs, varicose veins and phlebitis. Seeds are emetocathartic.
CHEM.: All *Davilla* species contain rhamnetin and isorhamnetin; almost all contain leucoanthocyanins and 4'-methylkaempferol (Ref: DILL 3).

Doliocarpus rolandri Gmel.
AREA: Throughout Brazil.
NAMES: Cipó-caboclo-venenoso, cipó-d'agua, cipó-vermelho, muiraqueteca, muiracutua, sambaíba.
USES: The abundant sap is diuretic, prescribed for jaundice, cystitis and bladder catarrh. Bark is astringent and febrifuge, reportedly very active against malarial fevers. Leaves are diuretic and laxative. Leaf decoction used to ameliorate oedema of the legs and for treating aphthae.

Tetracera aspera Willd.
AREA: Amazonia, forest.
NAMES: Cipó-vermelho, tigarea.
USES: Wood decoction is sudorific and antisyphilitic. Infusion of the leaves employed to treat chlorosis, scurvy and malarial fevers; in gargles for aphthae.

Tetracera breyniana Schl.
AREA: Bahia and Espírito Santo, forest.
NAME: Cipó-vermelho.
USES: Decoction of branches and leaves used for lymphangitis, swelling of the legs and orchitis. The smoke of the burnt plant is recommended for the same purposes.

Tetracera volubilis L.
AREA: Amazonia, forest.
NAMES: Cipó-de-caboclo, cipó, vermelho.
USES: Leaves and seeds are antipyretic, diaphoretic and antisyphilitic.

Dilleniaceae – References
DILL 1. Matos, F.J.A., M.P. de Souza, & P.A. Rouquayrol. 1968. Triterpenóides de plantas do nordeste brasileiro. *An. Assoc. Bras. Quim.* 27: 161.
DILL 2. El-Azizi, M.M., A.M. Ateya, G.H. Svoboda, P.L. Schiff Jr., D.J. Slatkin & J.S. Knapp. 1980. Chemical constituents of *Curatella americana* (Dilleniaceae). *J. Pharm. Sci.* 69: 360-361.
DILL 3. Kubitzki, K. 1968. Flavonoids and sytematics of the Dilleniaceae. *Ber. Deut. Bot. Ges.* 81: 238-251.

DIOSCOREACEAE

Dioscorea basiclavicaulis Rizz. & Mattos
AREA: Stony caatinga of northeastern Minas Gerais.
NAME: Japecanga.
USES: The fresh mass obtained from rubbing the base of the stem is applied to boils to make them mature.

Dioscorea glandulosa Klotz.
AREA: Bahia to Santa Catarina.
NAMES: Cará-de-folha-colorida, cará-liso, cará-sem-barba, caratinga.
USE: Leaves are emollient.

Dioscorea laxiflora Mart.
AREA: Occurs throughout Brazil.
NAMES: Cará-de-sapo, caratinga-brava, caratinga-do-mato, cascos.
USES: Dry tubers employed against leprosy.
CHEM. This and some other Brazilian *Dioscorea* species were found to contain about 1% diosgenin in their tubers (Ref: DIOS 1).

(X) ***Dioscorea silvestris*** Vell.
AREA: Rio de Janeiro, on rocks and in sunny places.
NAME: Cará-de-pedra.
USES: Recommended against asthma and whooping cough and for nervous diseases.

Dioscoreaceae – Reference

DIOS 1. Guimarães, I.S.S. 1973. Estudo químico de Dioscoreas brasileiras. I. Diosgenina em *Dioscorea laxiflora* var. *cincinata* e *D. trilinguis. An. Acad. Bras. Ci. 45*: 377-380.

DRYOPTERIDACEAE

Rumohra adiantiformis (G. Forst.) Ching
AREA: Ceará to Rio Grande do Sul, forest.
NAME: Calaguala.
USES: Rhizome is depurative and antispasmodic.

EBENACEAE

Diospyros paralea Steud.
AREA: Amazonia, forest.
NAME: Parala.
USE: Decoction of bark is antipyretic.

EPHEDRACEAE

Ephedra americana Willd.
AREA: Amazonia.
NAMES: Morango-do-acre, pingo-pingo.
USE: Fruits and branches are used for stopping hemorrhage.

Ephedra triandra Tul.
AREA: Abundant mainly in the beach sands of Rio Grande do Sul.
NAMES: Cipó-da-areia, orango-do-campo.
USES: Leaves are diaphoretic and antirheumatic. Fruits are mucilaginous, slightly acid and useful for febrile conditions.

EQUISETACEAE

Equisetum giganteum L.
AREA: In swampy areas in the Amazon region, Minas Gerais and Mato Grosso.
NAMES: Cavalinha, cavalinho, cola-de-cavalo, lixa-vegetal.
USES: Stems are astringent, diuretic, styptic, antidysenteric and antigonorrhoeic. Tincture used externally and internally to consolidate bone fractures.

Several closely related species are reputed to have the same medicinal properties. Examples are *E. martii* Milde (Rio de Janeiro and Minas Gerais) and *E. ramosissimum* Desf. (Rio Grande do Sul).

CHEM.: The epidermis of all *Equisetum* species is extremely rich in silica (Ref: EQUI 1), justifying their use as an abrasive and the popular name "lixa-vegetal," i.e., vegetable sandpaper.

Equisetaceae – Reference

EQUI 1. Molisch, H. 1923. *Mikrochemie der Pflanze*. Verlag Gustav Fischer, Jena. 3rd edition. (Pp. 74-81).

ERIOCAULACEAE

Leiothrix flavescens (Bong.) Ruhl.
AREA: Goiás to São Paulo and Rio de Janeiro, campo.
NAME: Sempreviva.
USE: Plant boiled in olive oil is prescribed as a remedy for scabies.

ERYTHROXYLACEAE

Erythroxylum anguifugum Mart.
AREA: Goiás, Minas Gerais and Mato Grosso.
NAME: Fruta-de-pomba.
USES: Root used against snakebite. The smoke of the burning wood is said to drive away snakes (hence the species epithet).

Erythroxylaceae

Erythroxylum campestre St.-Hil.
AREA: Bahia to São Paulo and Mato Grosso, cerrado.
NAMES: Cabelo-de-negro, fruta-de-tucano.
USE: Roots are purgative.

Erythroxylum cataractarum Spruce
AREA: Amazonia, forest.
NAME: Ipadu-mirim.
USES: Uses are the same as those of *Erythroxylum coca* (see below), but considered less active.

Erythroxylum coca Lam.
AREA: Amazonia, forest; mostly cultivated by Indians.

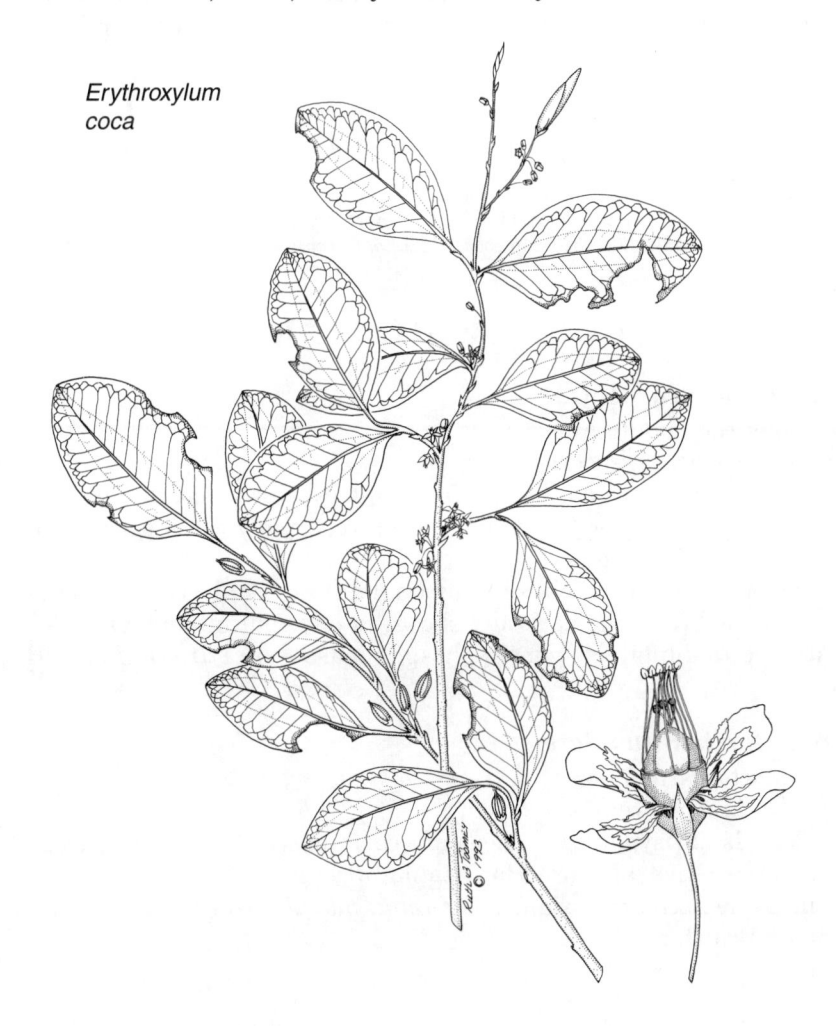

Erythroxylum coca

MEDICINAL PLANTS OF BRAZIL

NAMES: Coca, ipadu.

USES: Coca leaves, though much in evidence because of abuse of cocaine, can hardly be listed as a Brazilian medicinal plant in the sense of the present review. The custom of chewing the leaves, with or without the admixture of ashes from certain plants, as a stimulant to increase endurance and diminish hunger sensation and body fatigue, is mostly extra-Brazilian and, in the Amazon region, restricted to Indian tribes. Actual popular use is that of a tea taken to help digestion, as a remedy for asthma and to promote sweating.

CHEM.: The Amazonian (lowland) coca is considered a distinct variety, *E. coca* Lam. var. *ipadu* Plowman (Ref: ERYT 1). Of 31 species and varieties analyzed, var. *ipadu* showed the lowest cocaine content (Ref: ERYT 2). A complete review on Amazonian coca, comprising the history, distribution, botany, chemistry and other aspects, has been published (Ref: ERYT 3).

Erythroxylaceae – References

ERYT 1. Plowman, T. 1979. The identity of Amazonian and Trujillo coca. *Botanical Museum Leaflets, Harvard University* 27: 45-68.

ERYT 2. Plowman, T. & L. Rivier. 1983. Cocaine and cinnamoylcocaine content of thirty-one species of *Erythroxylum* (Erythroxylaceae). *Ann. Bot.* (London) 51: 641-659.

ERYT 3. Plowman, T. 1981. Amazonian coca. *J. Ethnopharmacol.* 3: 195-225.

EUPHORBIACEAE

Croton cajucara Benth.

AREA: Along the middle Amazon.

NAMES: Casca-sacaca, sacaca.

USES: Bark is aromatic, used in perfumery; leaves used as a tea in liver ailments and to lower blood cholesterol; reportedly carcinogenic, but without scientific evidence.

CHEM.& PHARM.: Essential oil contains linalol (Ref: EUPH 1). Diterpenes were isolated from the bark and shown to have antiinflammatory activity and to inhibit bee-venom phospholipase A_2 *in vitro* (Ref: EUPH 2).

Croton floribundus Spreng.

AREA: Piauí to Paraná, forest.

NAMES: Capixingui, velame-de-cheiro.

USES: Bark is antisyphilitic. Leaves are carminative, antiscorbutic, vulnerary, purgative, also used for healing ulcers.

The same uses are assigned to *Croton moritibensis* Baill. of northeastern Brazil.

Croton hemiargyreus M. Arg.
AREA: Northeast, caatinga.
NAMES: Marmeleiro, marmeleiro-preto.
USES: Roots and bark employed against metrorrhagia and herpes. Bast is indicated for upset stomach.

Croton salutaris Casar.
AREA: São Paulo and Rio de Janeiro, forest.
NAMES: Cambraia, sangue-de-drago.
USES: The red sap from the trunk bark is used for dressing wounds which have stopped bleeding, for protection against bacterial and fungal infections. Leaves are depurative, febrifuge and stomachic.
CHEM.: Stems and leaves contain the dienone alkaloid salutaridine (Ref: EUPH 3,4) which is an important intermediate in the biosynthesis of morphine alkaloids (Ref: EUPH 4).

Croton sincorensis Mart.
AREA: Northeast, caatinga.
NAME: Marmeleiro-branco.
USES: The same as those of *C. hemiargyreus* M. Arg.
CHEM.: The leaves yield 2% of essential oil which contains over 20% of guaiazulene (Ref: EUPH 5).

Croton sonderianus M. Arg.
AREA: Northeast, caatinga; in secondary growth and as an invading weed.
NAMES: Marmeleiro, marmeleiro-preto.
USES: Bark is aromatic, used in an infusion as a stomachic.
CHEM.: All parts are rich in essential oil, resembling pine oil in composition. Main components are á-pinene and ß-caryophyllene (Ref: EUPH 6,7). Its use as an industrial solvent has been suggested. Fixed constituents are diterpenes of different classes from roots and heartwood (Ref: EUPH 8,9,10).

Croton triqueter Lam.
AREA: Pará and Bahia to São Paulo, campo and forest margin.
NAMES: Morrão-de-candeia, velame.
USES: To treat syphilitic lesions.

Croton urucurana Baill.
AREA: Rio de Janeiro to Rio Grando do Sul, forest.
NAMES: Sangue-de-drago, urucurana, velame.
USE: Bark is astringent.

Croton zehntneri Pax & Hoffm.
AREA: Piauí to Bahia, campo and forest margin.

EUPHORBIACEAE

NAMES: Catinga-de-mulata, cravinho, canela-de-cunhã, canela-de-velho, canelinha.
USES: Very aromatic; tea from leaves and shoots is invigorating and calmative, sleep inducing. Also for indigestion.
CHEM.: The species shows considerable chemical variation in the composition of the essential oil of the leaves. Notable constituents are cineol, estragol, anethol, eugenol and methyl-eugenol, compounds which are dominant according to variety (Ref: EUPH 11,12).

Other *Croton* species, generally known as 'velame,' are used for fevers, stomach disorders and as depuratives. Examples are: *C. cascarilla* (L.) Bennet, *C. glabellus* L. and *C. paniculatus* M.Arg.

Dalechampia ficifolia Lam.
AREA: Distributed almost throughout Brazil.
NAMES: Caapuçara, cipó-tripa-de-galinha, tamiarana.
USES: Roots are tonic and apt to ease menstrual flow.

Dalechampia scandens L.
AREA: Amazonia.
NAME: Urtiga.
USES: Tea from roots is used to relieve itches and inflammations.

Euphorbia caecorum Mart.
AREA: Northeastern and central Brazil, campo, cerrado and caatinga.
NAMES: Erva-de-andorinha, erva-de-santa-luzia.
USES: Juice and decoction used against afflictions of the eyes, particularly to treat hardening of the cornea. Erva-de-santa-luzia, the popular name of this and some other species of *Euphorbia* (see below) is an allusion to this use, Santa Luzia being the patron saint for eyecare.

Euphorbia cotinoides Miq.
AREA: Amazonia.
NAMES: Açacu-i, leiteira, maleiteira.
USES: Latex from the leaves is mixed with honey and employed to alleviate syphilitic pains. Roots are purgative.

Euphorbia papillosa St.-Hil., which occurs in southern Brazil, has identical uses there.

Euphorbia hirta L.
AREA: Widespread as a ruderal.
NAMES: Caá-cambuí, caá-cica, erva-andorinha, erva-de-santa-luzia.
USES: Juice and decoction are hydragogue, diuretic, drastic, vulnerary, anti-asthmatic, useful for eye afflictions, mainly corneal ulcers and opacity. All parts are used against snakebite.
CHEM. & PHARM.: Triterpenes (Ref: EUPH 13) and flavonoids (Ref: EUPH

14,15) are reported. Antispasmodic action has been verified (Ref: EUPH 16,17) and shikimic acid identified as one responsible constituent (Ref: EUPH 18). Antidiarrhoeic activity is attributed to the presence of quercitrin (Ref: EUPH 19) and sedative, anxiolytic, analgesic, antipyretic and anti-inflammatory properties have been verified (Ref: EUPH 20,21).

Euphorbia hyssopifolia L.
AREA: Northeast to São Paulo.
NAMES: Burra-leitera, erva-andorinha, erva-de-leite, erva-de-santa-luzia, pau-de-leite.
USES: Latex is caustic, to be used with great care. Prescribed to reduce hardening of the cornea and to remove film from the eyes. Crushed herb for treating amenorrhoea and for speeding up the expulsion of a dead foetus.

Euphorbia phosphorea Mart.
AREA: Bahia and, rarely, Paraíba; caatinga.
NAMES: Cananã, cipó-de-fogo, madacaru-de-leite, pau-de-leite.
USES: Latex is applied locally to remove warts and check malignant ulcers from spreading.

Euphorbia thymifolia L.
AREA: Introduced, but widespread as a ruderal.
NAMES: Acuralzinho, bacuralzinho, erva-de-santa-luzia.
USES: Anthelmintic. Latex employed to remove corneal opacity.
CHEM. & PHARM.: Extracts of *E. thymifolia* and *E. prostrata* are antifungal (Ref: EUPH 22,23) and insecticidal (Ref: EUPH 24). Phorbol esters, triterpenoids and flavonoids have been identified (Ref: EUPH 25,26,27,28).

Euphorbia tirucalli L.
AREA: Introduced from Africa as a garden plant; escaped and naturalized in many places, mainly along the littoral.
NAMES: Árvore-de-coral, árvore-de-são-sebastião, avelós, coroa-de-cristo, forquilha.
USES: Latex is extremely caustic. Used for cleaning phagedenic ulcers. Said to cause blindness when in contact with the eyes.
CHEM.: Latex is rich in triterpenes (Ref: EUPH 29,31,32). Highly irritating — even tumor-promoting — esters of the diterpene phorbol, present in many Euphorbiaceae, also exist in this species (Ref: EUPH 30,33,34).

Hura crepitans L.
AREA: Amazonia, forest; mainly on river banks.
NAMES: Açacu (formerly spelled 'assacu' and encountered thus in the older literature), areeiro, uaçacu.

USES: Latex is caustic, used for treating sloughing ulcers, elephantiasis and leprosy. In small doses antirheumatic and anthelmintic. Bark and leaves are also used against rheumatism and hanseniasis and, though toxic, are considered cathartic, emetic, hydragogue, rubefacient. The seeds are violently purgative, too toxic to have their use recommended.

Jatropha curcas L.
AREA: Throughout Brazil, except the extreme south.
NAMES: Figo-do-inferno, mandobi-guaçu, pião-branco, pinhão, pinhão-de-purga, pinhão-do-inferno, pinhão-do-paraguai, pinhão-manso.
USES: Bark and latex are hemostatic, purgative, used to treat cuts, sinusitis and other inflammations, dropsy and hematoma. Latex used to remove film from eyes. Roots are diuretic and employed against snakebite.
CHEM.: Most studies are concerned with the toxalbumin, curcin, contained in the seeds (Ref: EUPH 35,36,37,39). Flavonoids have also been identified (Ref: EUPH 39).

Jatropha pohliana M. Arg., from northeastern Brazil, has the same indications as *J. curcas*.

Jatropha elliptica (Pohl) M. Arg.
AREA: Pernambuco to São Paulo, campo.
NAMES: Garanhoto, jalapão, medicineiro, raiz-de-cobra, raiz-de-lagarto, raiz-de-laranja, raiz-de-teiú, teiú-iba, teim, tejuíba, tiú.
USES: Roots are purgative; recommended for hydropsy, jaundice, rheumatism, delayed menses, tumors and syphilis. Reputedly active against snakebite.

Jatropha gossypiifolia L.
AREA: Northeast; also ruderal.
NAMES: Erva-purgante, jalapão, mamoninha, pinhão-roxo, raiz-de-teiú.
USES: Seeds are purgative, indicated for rheumatism, intestinal obstruction, hydropsy. Latex is mixed with sulfur to treat erysipelas.
CHEM.: Produces jatrophone, a macrocyclic diterpenoid with tumor inhibiting properties (Ref: EUPH 40). Flavonoids, including a flavonoid C-glycoside, have also been encountered (Ref: EUPH 41).

Jatropha multifida L.
AREA: Bahia to São Paulo; occasionally ruderal.
NAMES: Árvore-de-bálsamo, árvore-de-coral, coral, coral-dos-jardins, flor-de-coral.
USES: Latex is bitter, drastic, rubefacient, applied on ulcers and as dressing for cuts. Leaves are purgative. Seeds are purgative, febrifuge, antisyphilitic when roasted. Oil from seeds is also drastic, useful as a parasiticide.

EUPHORBIACEAE

Jatropha urens L.
AREA: Common in Brazil, caatinga and as a ruderal.
NAMES: Arre-diabo, cansanção, cansanção-de-leite, pinha-queimadeira, ucansanção, urtiga.
USES: Latex applied for eye diseases, including cataract. Roots tonic, diuretic, antileucorrhoeic, for cystitis, chronic metrorrhagia and menstrual disorders. Root decoction said to stimulate both the genital and urinary tracts. Decoction of leaves and twigs is diuretic, anti-algesic, anti-inflammatory. Contused leaves are to be applied on tumors. Seeds are strong purgative.

Joannesia heveoides Ducke
AREA: Amazonia, forest.
NAME: Castanha-de-arara.
USES: Kernels are vomitive and purgative.

Joannesia princeps Vell.
AREA: Pará to São Paulo, forest.
NAMES: Andá-açu, boleira, cotieira, coco-de-purga, fruta-de-arara, purga-de-gentio, purga-dos-paulistas.
USES: Bark used as an antidiarrhoeic and for treating cuts, but toxic. Seed oil is cathartic and hydragogue (e.g., for ascites).

Julocroton humilis Diedr.
AREA: Goiás to São Paulo, campo.
NAME: Velame-do-campo.
USE: Depurative.

Julocroton stipularis M. Arg.
AREA: Goiás and Minas Gerais, cerrado.
NAME: Turubi.
USES: Roots are recommended for skin conditions.

Mabea fistulifera Mart.
AREA: Minas Gerais to São Paulo and Mato Grosso, forest.
NAMES: Canudeiro, canudo-de-pito, mamona-do-mato, raiz-de-teiú.
USES: Bark is bitter, resolvent, tonic, febrifuge. Seed oil is antipyretic. Bruised leaves are applied on old ulcers to clean them and induce regeneration of fresh tissue.

Maprounea brasiliensis L.
AREA: Bahia to São Paulo, cerrado.
NAME: Marmeleiro-do-campo.
USES: Though venomous, the root-bark, in alcoholic infusion, is taken before meals as an appetite stimulant.

EUPHORBIACEAE

Omphalea diandra M. Arg.
AREA: Amazonia, swamp forest along littoral.
NAMES: Caiaté, castanha-comadre-de-azeite, castanha-caetá, castanna-de-azeite, castanha, caiaté, castanha-de-cotia, castanha-de-peixe, comadre-de-azeite.
USES: Oil is purgative, a good substitute for castor oil. Leaves used for treating old ulcers.

Phyllanthus acutifolius Spreng.
AREA: Eastern states of Brazil.
NAMES: Arrebenta-pedras, erva-pombinha, quebra-pedras.
USES: This, as well as the other *Phyllanthus* species known by the same popular designations, has a high reputation for dissolving and eliminating kidney and bladder stones.

Phyllanthus conami Sw.
AREA: Amazonia to São Paulo.
NAMES: Conabi, conambi, conami.
USES: Roots are diuretic and narcotic, useful for urinary afflictions. Bark is bitter, tonic, slightly laxative, depurative, parasiticide.

Phyllanthus diffusus Klotz.
AREA: Throughout Brazil, except the southern states.
NAME: Erva-pombinha.
USES: Root is bitter, astringent, diuretic, recommended against jaundice.

Phyllanthus niruri L.
AREA: Cosmopolitan, common in Brazil both in cultivation and spontaneous.
NAMES: Arranca-pedras, arrebenta-pedras, erva-pombinha, malva-pedra, quebra-pedra.
USES: Root tea used for urinary disorders. Leaves are diuretic, diaphoretic, deobstruent, bitter tonic, highly valued for the elimination of kidney and bladder stones. Also for diabetes, jaundice and malarial fevers. Fruit juice is antidiabetic.
See also uses given for *P. acutifolis* Spreng.
CHEM.: Chemical studies have shown the presence of flavonoids (Ref: EUPH 44,45,46), lignans (Ref: EUPH 44,47) and their glycosides (Ref: EUPH 48,49).
PHARM.: Experiments in rats showed significant increase in diuresis and sodium and creatine excretion. In human subjects, persistent ingestion (3 months) of the tea furthered the elimination of kidney stones (Ref: EUPH 50).

In some cases nomenclatural differences make the evaluation of published results difficult. Thus, *P. amarus* Thonn. & Schum. is often considered a variety of *P. niruri*; and *P. lathyroides* M. Arg. a subspecies. Extracts of *P. niruri* have shown anti-hepatitis B activity, both *in vitro* and *in vivo* (Ref: EUPH 51,52).

Phyllanthus nobilis M. Arg.
AREA: Amazonia.
NAMES: Catuaba, pérola-vegetal.
USES: Tonic, stimulant and aphrodisiac.

Phyllanthus sellowianus M. Arg.
AREA: Rio Grande do Sul, on river banks and, principally, on small river islands.
NAMES: Quebra-pedra, sarandi, sarandi-branco, sarandi-vermelho.
USES: Tea used for eliminating kidney and bladder stones.
CHEM. & PHARM.: Several compounds with analgesic and antispasmodic action have been isolated (Ref: EUPH 53,54). A complete overview of the biological activities of *Phyllanthus* species has been published (Ref: EUPH 55).

Phyllanthus tenellus Roxb.
AREA: Rio de Janeiro.
NAMES: Arrebenta-pedras, erva-pombinha, quebra-pedras.
USES: A tea is employed for dissolving calculi of the urinary tract.
See also uses given for *P. acutifolis* Spreng.
CHEM. & PHARM.: Extracts and isolated steroids show marked analgesic activity (Ref: EUPH 42,43).

Sapium hamatum Pax & Hoffm.
AREA: Amazonia, forest.
NAMES: Árvore-de-leite, curupitá, marupitá.
USES: Toxic latex is applied on warts, malignant tumors and elephantiasis. Infusion of leaves is used to combat syphilitic symptoms, mainly the subcutaneous manifestations.

Sebastiania klotzschiana M. Arg.
AREA: Rio de Janeiro and Minas Gerais.
NAME: Branquilho.
USES: Decoction of the bark is used for treating blennorrhagia and leucorrhoea.

Sebastiania macrocarpa M. Arg.
AREA: Northeastern Brazil.
NAMES: Brandão, purga-de-leite.
USES: The latex, dissolved in water with sugar, is reputedly a remedy for dropsy and syphilis; it is considered to be the most violent of the

purgatives. Bark infusion is said to be efficient against skin eruptions, eczema, troubles of menstruation and leucorrhoea.

Sebastiania potamophila Pax, also from northeastern Brazil, is known for similar properties.

Tragia volubilis L.
AREA: Neotropical; introduced to palaeotropics and now cosmopolitan, frequently encountered in Brazil.
NAMES: Cipó-de-leite, cipó-urtiguinha, tamiarana, urtiguinha-de-cipó.
USES: Root used as an appetite stimulant, diuretic, sudorific and for venereal diseases. Juice mixed with salt is applied for treating skin diseases.

Euphorbiaceae – References

EUPH 1. Campbell, V.A., G.C. Corrêa, J.G.S. Maia, M. Leão da Silva, O.R. Gottlieb, M.C. Marx and M.T. Magalhães. 1971. Oleos essenciais de Amazônia contendo linalol. *Acta Amaz. 1*: 45-47.

EUPH 2. Ichihara, Y., K. Takeya, Y. Hitotsuyanagi, H. Morita, S. Okuyama, M. Suganama, H. Fujiki, M. Motidome & H. Itokawa. 1992. Cajucarinolide and isocajucarinolide: Antiinflammatory diterpenes from *Croton cajucara*. *Planta Medica 58*: 549-551.

EUPH 3. Barnes, R.A. & O.M. Soeiro. 1981. The alkaloids of *Croton salutaris*. *Phytochemistry 20*: 543-544.

EUPH 4. Barton, D.H.R., G.W. Kirby, W. Steglich, G.M. Thomas, A.R. Battersby, T.A. Dobson & R. Ramuz. 1965. Investigations on the biosynthesis of morphine alkaloids. *J. Chem. Soc.*: 2423-2438.

EUPH 5. Mendes, P.H. 1960. Personal communication.

EUPH 6. Craveiro, A.A., E.R. Silveira, F.J.A. Matos & J.W. Alencar. 1978. Essential and fatty oils of *Croton sonderianus*. *Rev. Latinoamer. Quím. 9*: 95-97.

EUPH 7. Craveiro, A.A., A.G. Fernandes, C.H.S. Andrade, F.J.A. Matos, J.W. Alencar & M.I.L. Machado. 1981. OLEOS ESSENCIAIS DE PLANTAS DO NORDESTE. (Federal University of Ceará, Fortaleza). 209 pp.

EUPH 8. Craveiro, A.A., E.R. Silveira, R. Braz Filho & I.P. Mascarenhas. 1981. Sonderianin, a furanoid diterpene from *Croton sonderianus*. *Phytochemistry 20*: 852-854.

EUPH 9. Craveiro, A.A. & E.R. Silveira. 1982. Two cleistanthane diterpenes from *Croton sonderianus*. *Phytochemistry 21*: 2571-2574.

EUPH 10. McChesney, J.D. & E.R. Silveira. 1990. *Ent*-clerodanes of *Croton sonderianus*. *Fitoterapia 61*: 172-175.

EUPH 11. Craveiro, A.A., C.H.S. Andrade, F.J.A. Matos & J.W. Alencar. 1978. Anise-like flavor of *Croton* aff. *zehntneri* Pax et Hoffm. *J. Agr. Food Chem. 26*: 772-773.

EUPH 12. Craveiro, A.A., A.S. Rodrigues, C.H.S. Andrade, F.J.A. Matos, J.W. Alencar & M.I.L. Machado. 1981. Volatile constituents of Brazilian Euphorbiaceae. Genus *Croton*. *J. Nat. Prod. 44*: 602-608.

EUPH 13. Atallan, A.M. & H.J. Nicholas. 1972. Triterpenoids and steroids of *Euphorbia pilulifera* L. *Phytochemistry 11*: 1860.

EUPH 14. Blanc, P. & G. de Saqui-Sannes. 1972. Les flavonoides d'*Euphorbia hirta*. *Plantes Méd. Phytothér. 6*: 106-109.

EUPH 15. Krishna Rao, C.V. & S. Ganapathy. 1983. Investigation of *Euphorbia pilulifera* L. *Fitoterapia 44*: 265-267.

EUPH 16. Hellerman, R.C. & L.W. Hazleton. 1950. The antispasmodic action of *Euphorbia pilulifera*. *J. Am. Pharm. Assoc. (Sci. Ed.) 39*: 142-146.

EUPH 17. Hallet, F.P. & L.M. Parks. 1953. Observations on the antispasmodic principle of *Euphorbia pilulifera*. *J. Am. Pharm. Assoc. 42*: 607-609.

EUPH 18. El Nagger, L., J.L. Beal, L.M. Parks & K.N. Salman. 1978. A note on the isolation and identification of two pharmacologically active constituents of *Euphorbia pilulifera* L. *Lloydia 41*: 73-75.

EUPH 19. Galvez, J., A. Zarzuelo, M.E. Crespo, M.D. Lorente, M.A. Ocete & J. Jiménez. 1993. Antidiarrhoeic activity of *Euphorbia hirta* extract and isolation of an active flavonoid constituent. *Planta Medica 59*: 333-336.

EUPH 20. Lanhers, M.-C., J. Fleurentin, P. Cabalion, A. Rolland, P. Dorfman, R. Mislin & J.-M. Pelt. 1990. Behavioral effects of *Euphorbia hirta* L.: sedative and anxyolytic properties. *J. Ethnopharmacol. 29*: 189-198.

EUPH 21. Lanhers, M.-C., J. Fleurentin, P. Dorfman, F. Mortier & J.-M. Pelt. 1991. Analgesic, antipyretic and antiinflammatory properties of *Euphorbia hirta*. *Planta Medica 57*: 225-231.

EUPH 22. Rao, V.R. & I. Gupta. 1970. In vitro studies on the antifungal activity of some indigenous drugs on *Trichophyton mentagrophytes*. *Indian J. Pharmacol. 2*: 29-30.

EUPH 23. Pal, S. & I. Gupta. 1971. In vitro studies of the antifungal activity of chotidudhi plant (*Euphorbia prostrata* and *E. thymifolia*). *Indian J. Pharmacol. 3*: 27.

EUPH 24. Heal, R.F. & E.F. Rogers. 1950. A survey of plants for insecticidal activity. *Lloydia 13*: 89-162.

EUPH 25. Nagase, M. 1941. On the flavonol glucoside from *Euphorbia thymifolia* L. *J. Agric. Chem. Soc. Japan, Bull. 17*: 50.

EUPH 26. Gupta, D.R. & S.K. Garg. 1966. Chemical examination of *Euphorbia thymifolia* Linn. *Indian J. Appl. Chem. 29*: 39-40.

EUPH 27. Subramanian, S.S., S. Najarajan & N. Sulochana. 1971. Flavonoids of some euphorbiaceous plants. *Phytochemistry 10*: 2548-2549.

EUPH 28. Agarwal, R. & R.K. Baslas. 1981. Chemical examination of the aerial parts of *Euphorbia thymifolia*. *Indian J. Pharm. Sci. 43*: 182-183.

EUPH 29. Haines, D.W. & F.L. Warren. 1949. *Euphorbia* resins. (II). Isolation of taraxasterol and a new triterpene, triucallol, from *Euphorbia tirucalli*. *J. Chem. Soc.*: 2554-2556.

EUPH 30. Khan, A.Q., N.S.H. Kazmi, Z. Ahmed & A. Malik. 1989. Euphorcinol: a new pentacyclic triterpene from *Euphorbia tirucalli*. *Planta Medica 55*: 290-291.

EUPH 31. Khan, A.Q., Z. Ahmed, N. Kazmi & A. Malik. 1987. Further triterpenes from stem bark of *Euphorbia tirucalli*. *Planta Medica 53*: 577.

EUPH 32. Khan, A.Q., T. Rasheed, S.N. Kazmi, Z. Ahmed & A. Malik. 1988. Cycloeuphordenol, a new triterpene from *Euphorbia tirucalli*. *Phytochemistry 27*: 2279-2281.

EUPH 33. Kinghorn, A.D. 1979. Characterization of an irritant 4-deoxy-phorbol diester from *Euphorbia tirucalli*. *J. Nat. Prod. 42*: 112-115.

EUPH 34. Fürstenberger, G. & E. Hecker. 1986. On the active principles of the Euphorbiaceae, XII. Highly unsaturated irritant diterpene esters from *Euphorbia tirucalli* originating from Madagascar. *J. Nat. Prod. 49*: 386-397.

EUPH 35. Mourgue, M., R. Baret, R. Kassab & J. Reynaud. 1961. Étude des proteines de la graine de *Jatropha curcas* L. *Bull. Soc. Chim. Biol. 43*: 505-516.

EUPH 36. Mourgue, M., J. Delphant, R. Baret & R. Kassab. 1961. Étude de la toxalbumine (curcine) des graines de *Jatropha curcas*. *Bull. Soc. Chim. Biol. 43*: 517-531.

EUPH 37. Stirpe, F., A. Pession-Brizi, E. Lorenzoni, P. Strocchi, L. Montanaro & S. Sperti. 1976. Studies on the properties from the seeds of *Croton tiglium* and *Jatropha curcas*. Toxic properties and inhibition of protein synthesis in vitro. *Biochem. J. 156*: 1-6.

EUPH 38. Hufford, D.C. & B.O. Oguntimein. 1978. Nonpolar constituents of *Jatropha curcas*. *Lloydia 41*: 161.

EUPH 39. Sankara, S.S., S. Najarajan & N. Sulochana. 1971. Flavonoids of some euphorbiaceous plants. *Phytochemistry 10*: 1548-1549.

EUPH 40. Kupchan, S.M., C.W. Siegel, M.J. Matz, J.A. Saenz Renauld, R.C. Haltiwanger & R.F. Bryan. 1970. Jatrophone, a novel macrocyclic diterpenoid tumor inhibitor from *Jatropha gossypiifolia*. *J. Am. Chem. Soc. 92*: 4476-4477.

EUPH 41. Subramanian, S.S., S. Nagarajan & N. Sulochana. 1971. Flavonoids of the leaves of *Jatropha gossypiifolia*. *Phytochemistry 10*: 1690.

EUPHORBIACEAE / FABACEAE

EUPH 42. Gorski, F., C.R. Corrêa, V. Cechinel Filho, R.A. Yunes & J.B. Calixto. 1993. Potent antinociceptive activity of the hydroalcoholic extract from *Phyllanthus corcovadensis*. *J. Farm. Pharmacol. 45*: 1046-1049.

EUPH 43. Santos, A.R.S., R. Niero, V. Cechinel Filho, R.A. Yunes, M.G. Pizzolatti, F. Delle Monache & J.B. Caixto. 1995. Antinociceptive properties of steroids isolated from *Phyllanthus corcovadensis* in mice. *Planta Medica 61*: 329-332.

EUPH 44. Stanislas, E., R. Rouffiac & J.J. Foyard. 1967. Constituants de *Phyllanthus niruri* L. (Eurphorbiaceae). *Plantes Méd. Phytothér. 1*: 136-141.

EUPH 45. Nara, T. K., J. Cleye, L.L. de Cerval & E. Stanislas. 1977. Flavonoïdes de *Phyllanthus niruri* L., *P. urinaria* L. et *P. orbiculatus* L. Rich. *Plantes Méd. Phytothér. 11*: 82-86.

EUPH 46. Chauhan, J.S., M. Sultan & S.K. Srivastasa. 1977. Two new glycoflavones from the roots of *Phyllanthus niruri*. *Planta Medica 32*: 217.

EUPH 47. Anjaneyulu, A.S.R., K.J. Rao, L.R. Row & C. Subrahmanyan. 1973. Crystalline constituents of Euphorbiaceae. XII. Isolation and structural elucidation of three new lignans from the leaves of *Phyllanthus niruri* Linn. *Tetrahedron 29*: 1291-1298.

EUPH 48. Pettit, G.R. & D.E. Shaufelberger. 1988. Ioslation and structure of the cytostatic lignan glycoside phllanthostatin A-1. *J. Nat. Prod. 51*: 1104-1112.

EUPH 49. Gupta, D.R. & B. Ahmed. 1984. Nirurin, a new prenylated flavonone glycoside from *Phyllanthus niruri*. *J. Nat. Prod. 47*: 958-963.

EUPH 50. Santos, D.R. 1990. *Chá de "quebra-pedra" (Phyllanthus niruri) na litíase urinária em humanos e ratos*. Thesis, Escola Paulista de Medicina (São Paulo).

EUPH 51. Venkateswaran, P.S., I. Millman & B.S. Blumberg. 1987. Effects of an extract from *Phyllanthus niruri* on hepatitis B and woodchuck hepatitis B viruses. *In vitro* and *in vivo* studies. *Proc. Nat. Acad. Sci.* (Washington) *84*: 274-278.

EUPH 52. Thyagaranjan, S.P., S. Subramanian, T.T. Asundari, P.S. Venkateswaran & B.S. Blumberg. 1988. Effect of *Phyllanthus amarus* on chronic carriers of hepatitis B virus. *Lancet*, Oct. 1: 764-766.

EUPH 53. Calixto, J.B., R.A. Yunes, A.S.O. Neto, R.M. Ribeirodo Valle & G.A. Rae. 1984. Antispasmodic effects of alkaloid extracted from *Phyllanthus sellowianus*: A comparative study with papaverine. *Brazilian J. Med. Biol. Res. 17*: 313-321.

EUPH 54. Tempesta, M.S., D.G. Corley, J.A. Beutler, C.J. Metral, R.A. Yunes, C.A. Giacomozzi & J.B. Calixto. 1988. Phyllanthimide, a new alkaloid from *Phyllanthus sellowianus*. *J. Nat. Prod. 51*: 617-618.

EUPH 55. Unander, D.W., G.L. Webster & B.S. Blumberg. 1990-1995. Usage and bioassays in *Phyllanthus* (Euphorbiaceae): a compilation. *J. Ethnopharmacol.* I.*30*: 233-264 (1990); II.*34*: 97-133 (1991); III.*36*: 103-112 (1991); IV.*45*: 1-118 (1995).

FABACEAE

Abrus precatorius L.

AREA: Tropical cosmopolitan; common in many places; southward to restinga, Rio de Janeiro.

NAME: Jequiriti.

USES: Seeds poisonous, formerly used for sloughing ulcers and conjunctivitis.

CHEM.: Besides a highly toxic albumin, abrin, the seeds contain alkaloids (Ref: FABA 1), steroids (Ref: FABA 2) and isoflavan-quinones (Ref: FABA 3). The roots contain flavonoids (Ref: FABA 4). Both leaves and roots contain sweet-tasting triterpenoids (Ref: FABA 5,6).

PHARM.: Reputed antifertility action of the roots has been confirmed (Ref:

FABACEAE

Acosmium dasycarpum

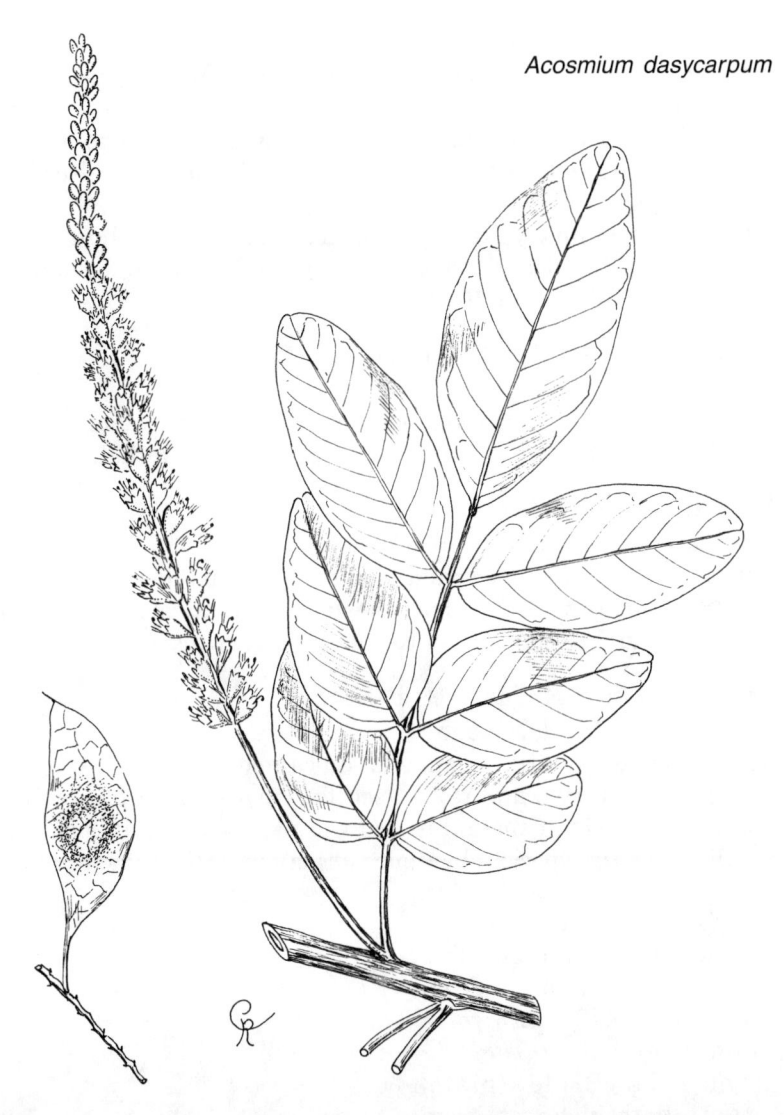

FABA 7). A seed infusion was once used to treat trachoma and corneal opacity; but the practice was abandoned as too dangerous, leading to uncontrollable inflammation and even to loss of eyesight (Ref: FABA 8).

Acosmium dasycarpum (Vog.) Yakovl.
AREA: Central Brazil, cerrado.
NAMES: Chapada, chapadinha.
USES: Bast is somewhat bitter, with effects similar to those of *A. subelegans* (see below), but less active.

FABACEAE

Acosmium subelegans (Mohlenb.) Yakovl.
AREA: Frequent in São Paulo, cerrado; rarer in Minas Gerais and Mato Grosso.
NAMES: Perobinha, perobinha-branca, perobinha-do-campo.
USES: Bast is strongly bitter; sedative and mildly soporific; also prescribed for epilepsy.
CHEM.: Bast contains typical papilionaceous alkaloids of the *Ormosia* type (Ref: FABA 9); also lupeol and a pyrone derivative (11-0-demethyl-yangonin) (Ref: FABA 10).

Andira inermis (Sw.) H.B.K.
AREA: Amazonia, forest.
NAMES: Andirá-uxi, angelim-da-várzea, cumarurana, avineira.
USES: Malodorous bark is purgative, vomitive and anthelmintic.

Andira retusa (Poir.) H.B.K.
AREA: Amazonia to Bahia, forest.
NAMES: Andirá-uxi, cumarurana, morcegueira, uxi-de-morcego, uxirana.
USES: Stinking bark and drupes are vermifuge; their tea is employed to stop colic and stomachache. Kernels are very toxic.

Andira vermifuga Mart. ex Benth.
AREA: Central Brazil, cerrado.
NAMES: Angelim-amargoso, angelim-do-campo.
USES: Powdered bark and wood used for treating skin ulcers. Bark and seeds are used to expel intestinal worms, but are quite poisonous.

Other *Andira* species show similar actions to those mentioned above: *A. humilis* Benth., in cerrado, known as mata-barata; *A. legalis* (Vell.) Tol., the angelim-coco from restinga; *A. fraxinifolia* Benth. and *A. anthelmia* (Vell.) MacBride (plate, right), both in forest, from Bahia to São Paulo. The bark has an extremely disagreeable smell and the seeds have enormous cotyledons, rich in starch but very poisonous.

CHEM.: The anthelmintic principles in all these species is a non-proteinogenic amino acid, N-methyltyrosine (andirine). In addition, the

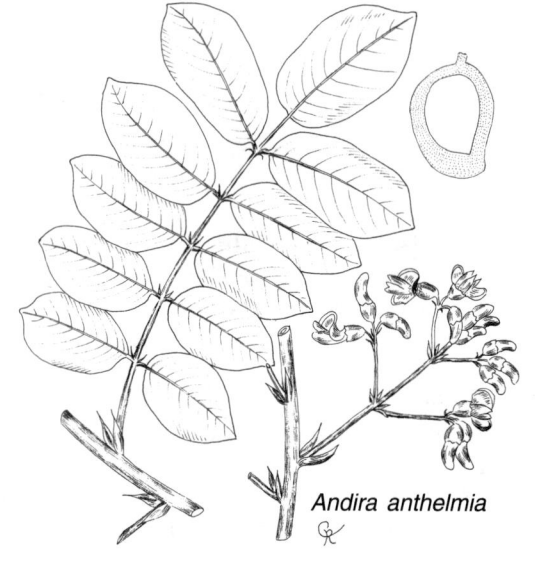

Andira anthelmia

bark of *A. humilis* contains several flavonoids and their glycosides (Ref: FABA 11), the major constituent being the isoflavone biochanin-A (Ref: FABA 12). A pterocarpan, demethylpterocarpin, has been described from *A. inermis* (Ref: FABA 13).

Bowdichia nitida Spruce ex Benth.
AREA: Amazonas and Mato Grosso, forest.
NAMES: Sapupira, sebepira, sucupira.
USES: Bark is depurative, indicated for the treatment of syphilis; decoction for cleaning skin ulcers.
CHEM.: An isoflavone quinone has been isolated (Ref: FABA 14).

Bowdichia virgilioides H.B.K.
AREA: Pará to Mato Grosso, cerrado and dry forest.
NAMES: Cutiuba, paricarana, sucupira, sucupira-açu, sucupira-amarela, sucupira-branca, sucupira-do-campo, sucupira-do-cerrado.
USES: Root tubercles and bark are depurative, antifebrile, antirheumatic, antiluetic, antidiabetic, antidiarrhoeic and used for curing skin conditions. Seed oil is rubbed on skin for articular pain.
CHEM.: Lupeol (Ref: FABA 15) and an alkaloid (Ref: FABA 16) were isolated from bark.

Clitoria guianensis (Aubl.) Benth.
AREA: Amazonia to Mato Grosso and São Paulo, cerrado and campo.
NAME: Espelina-falsa.
USES: Roots and seeds are cathartic, useful against cystitis and urethritis.

Crotalaria verrucosa L.
AREA: Pantropical; Amazonia, ruderal.
NAME: Chocalho-de-cascavel.
USES: Used as a remedy for ringworm and other skin afflictions. Leaf juice reduces salivation.

Dahlstedtia pinnata (Benth.) Malme
AREA: Amazonia to São Paulo, forest.
NAMES: Goraná-timbó, timbó-de-raiz.
USES: To relieve asthma and violent coughs. *D. pentaphylla* (Taub.) Burk. (from Santa Catarina) has similar effects.
CHEM.: A comparative study of flavonoids from the two species has been published (Ref: FABA 17).

Dalbergia gracilis Benth.
AREA: Mato Grosso.
NAMES: Pau-violeta, tripa-de-galinha.
USES: Bark is antidiarrhoeic.

FABACEAE

Dalbergia subcymosa

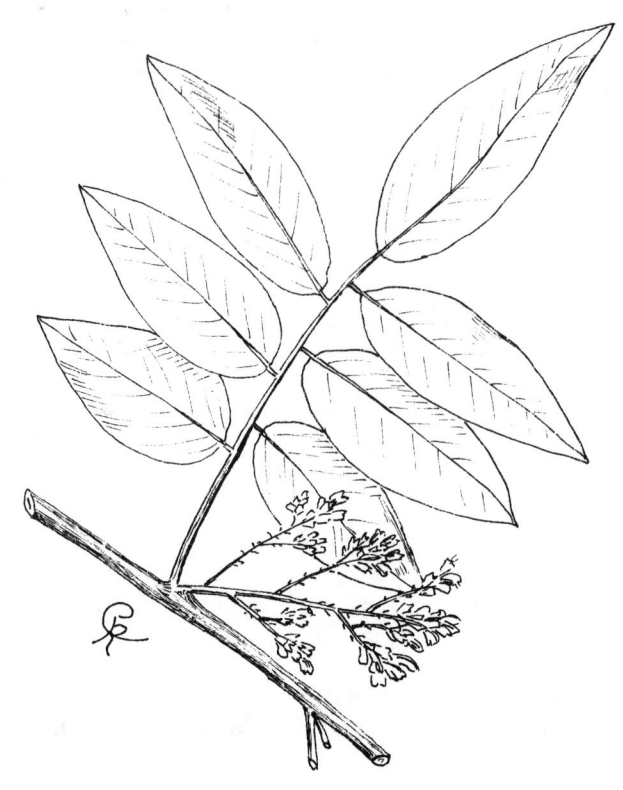

Dalbergia subcymosa Ducke
AREA: Amazonia, forest.
NAME: Verônica.
USES: Bast infusion is anti-inflammatory and bechic. Reported anticancerigenous.

Desmodium axillare (Sw.) DC.
AREA: Throughout Brazil; ruderal.
NAMES: Amendoeirana, amores-o-campo, carrapicho-rasteiro, mandubirana.
USES: Entire plant is used to reduce inflammation and for leucorrhoea.

Desmodium triflorum DC.
AREA: Widespread in Brazil, campo.
NAMES: Amor-do-campo, amorzinho-seco, carrapicho, trevo-do-campo.
USES: Whole plant is laxative, antileucorrhoeic, depurative.

FABACEAE

Dipteryx alata Vog.

AREA: Maranhão to Mato Grosso, cerrado.
NAMES: Baru, coco-feijão, cumarurana, cumbaru, amburana-brava, feijão, cumarurana, cumbaru, amburana-brava, feijão-coco, pau-cumaru.
USES: The drupaceous fruit is good forage, appreciated by cattle. Kernel with analeptic properties, diaphoretic and emmenagogue. It is edible and contains a good quality oil which is considered "medicinal," without further qualification.
CHEM.: Triterpenes have been identified in the bark (Ref: FABA 18).

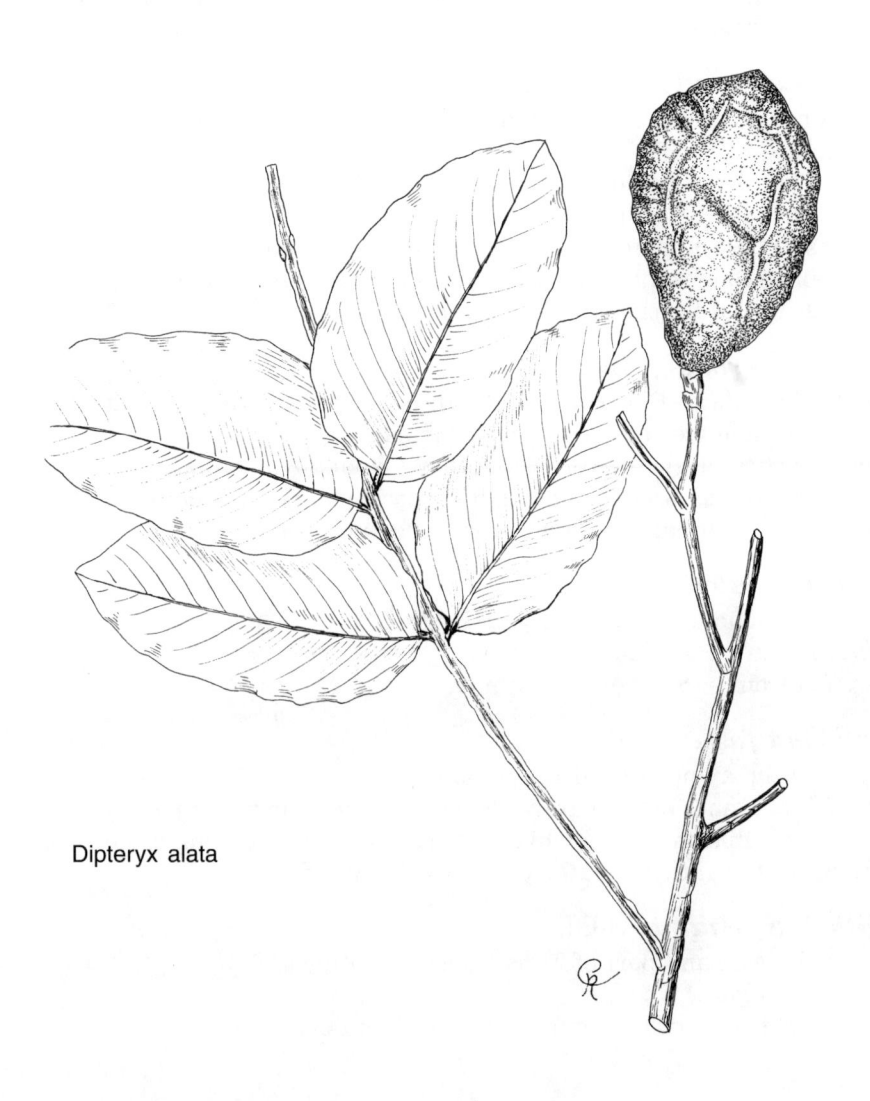

Dipteryx alata

FABACEAE

Dipteryx odorata (Aubl.) Willd.
AREA: Amazonia and Mato Grosso, forest.
NAMES: Cumaru, cumaru-amarelo, cumaru-do-amazonas, cumaru-verdadeiro, fava-tonca (English: tonka bean).
USES: The seeds are fragrant, having the typical smell of coumarin, of which they are the traditional source. Considered antispasmodic, emmenagogue, cardiotonic and antiasthmatic. The oil from the seeds is used to alleviate stomachache and to treat sores in the mouth. Also to fortify the scalp and improve hair growth. Employed in pills against coughs, and in alcohol for rubbing to alleviate pain.
CHEM.: In spite of the seeds being the main commercial article from this tree, chemical studies have been conducted on the bark, which contains triterpenes and isoflavonoids (Ref: FABA 19,20,21,22).

Erythrina corallodendron L.
AREA: Amazonia and Mato Grosso; in forest, and cultivated as an ornamental.
NAMES: Flor-de-coral, mulungu, sananduva, sanandu, suinã.
USES: Bark is calmative, sedative, purgative, diuretic, febrifuge, antiasthmatic. Reputedly good for insomnia; also recommended against whooping cough and liver ailments. Leaves are emollient, used for toothache and for cleaning skin ulcers.

Erythrina crista-galli L.
AREA: Maranhão to Rio Grande do Sul, more frequent in the southern states. In marshes and along river banks.
NAMES: Corticeira, flor-de-coral, mulungu, sananduva, suinã.
USES: Bark extract used as a powerful soporific; bark infusion in gargles against sore throat; also to treat cuts, rheumatism and hepatitis.

Erythrina falcata Benth.
AREA: Maranhão, Bahia and Minas Gerais.
NAMES: Mulungu, sanandu, suinã.
USES: Tea from bark given for asthma.

Erythrina fusca Lour.
AREA: Amazonia and central Brazil, forest.
NAMES: Açacurana, bico-de-arara, feijão-bravo, mulungu, suinã.
USES: Bark infusion used for liver ailments and for inducing sleep. Tea from roots is antirheumatic, purgative in high doses.

Erythrina velutina Willd.
AREA: Northeast and part of Minas Gerais, caatinga.
NAME: Mulungu.
USES: Bark is sudorific, calmative, pectoral and emollient.

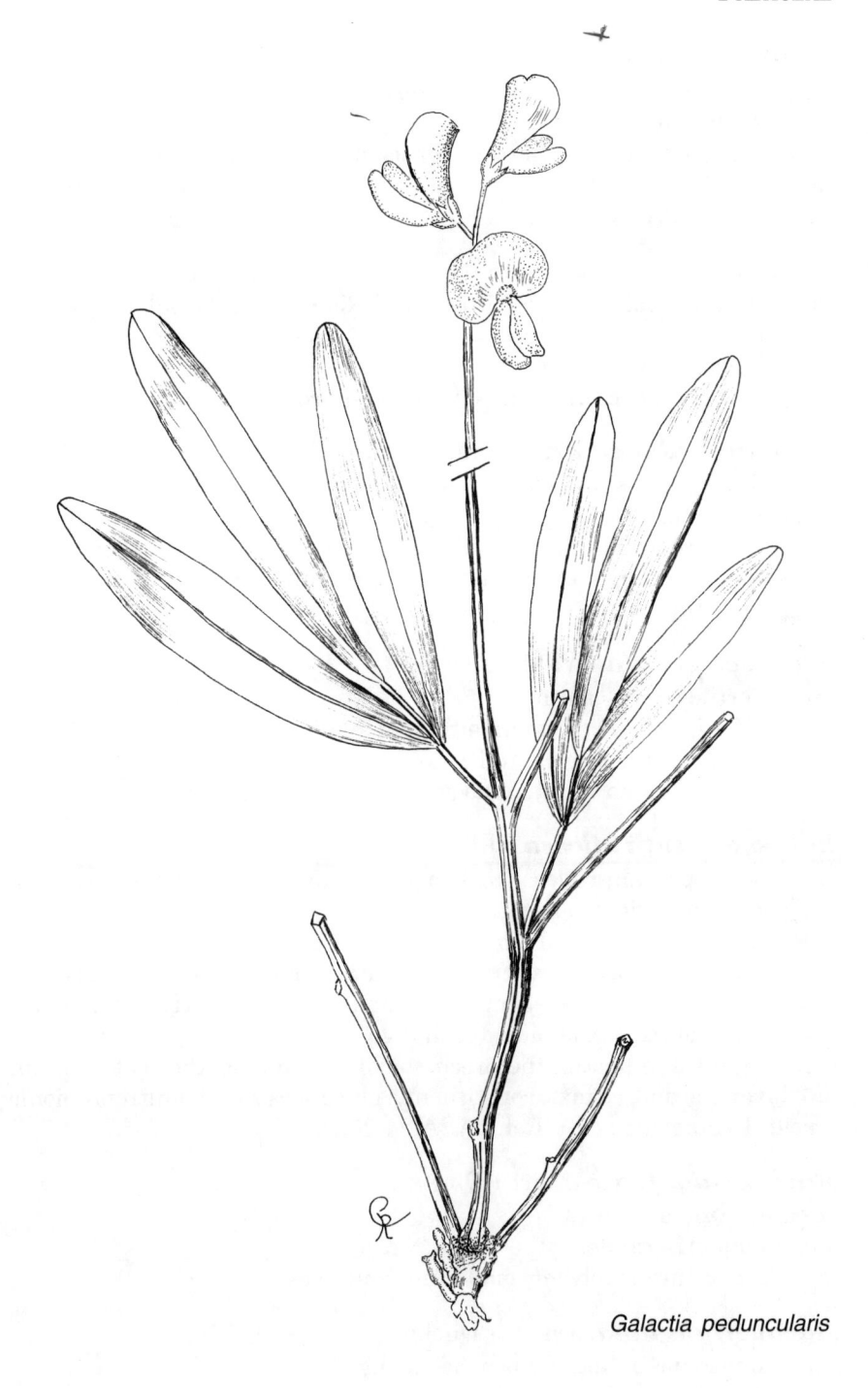

FABACEAE

Galactia peduncularis

FABACEAE

Erythrina verna Vell.
AREA: Minas Gerais and São Paulo, forest and cerradão.
NAME: Mulungu.
USES: Bark is calmative, narcotic, antispasmodic, antitussive.
CHEM.: The bark of all *Erythrina* species is rich in alkaloids. For a review see Ref: FABA 23.

Galactia neesii DC.
AREA: Minas Gerais to Mato Grosso and Rio Grande do Sul, campo and cerrado.
NAME: Feijão-bravo.
USES: Roots in a decoction are said to be aphrodisiac.

Galactia peduncularis (Benth.) Taub.
AREA: Minas Gerais and Goiás, low cerrado.
NAME: Verga-tesa.
USES: A tea from the thick, woody roots is taken as an aphrodisiac. This may be an example of the belief of "signature," due to the suggestive aspect of the roots.

Geoffroea striata (Willd.) Morong
AREA: Northeastern caatinga.
NAMES: Mari, mari-mari, marizeiro, marinheiro, umari.
USES: Tea from the leaves and young shoots is prescribed for delayed menses and as an antidiarrhoeic. Bark is anthelmintic.

Indigofera suffruticosa Mill.
AREA: Cosmopolitan; ruderal in Brazil, mainly in the coastal tracts, escaped from ancient plantations.
NAMES: Anil, anileira, timbó-mirim; English: indigo.
USES: Roots and leaves are antispasmodic, sedative, diuretic, febrifuge, used against jaundice, epilepsy and snakebite. Formerly widely cultivated as source of the blue dye, indigo.
CHEM.: Besides indigotin, the precursor of indigo blue, the roots contain a flavanone and, as toxic constituents, glucose esters of â-nitropropionic acid (hyptagenic acid) (Ref: FABA 24,25,26).

Machaerium ferox (Mart.) Ducke
AREA: Amazonia, forest.
NAME: Juqueri-grande.
USES: Leaves are resolvent, made into poultices.

Machaerium lunatum (L.) Ducke
AREA: Amazonia, on muddy beaches along rivers.
NAME: Aturiá.

FABACEAE

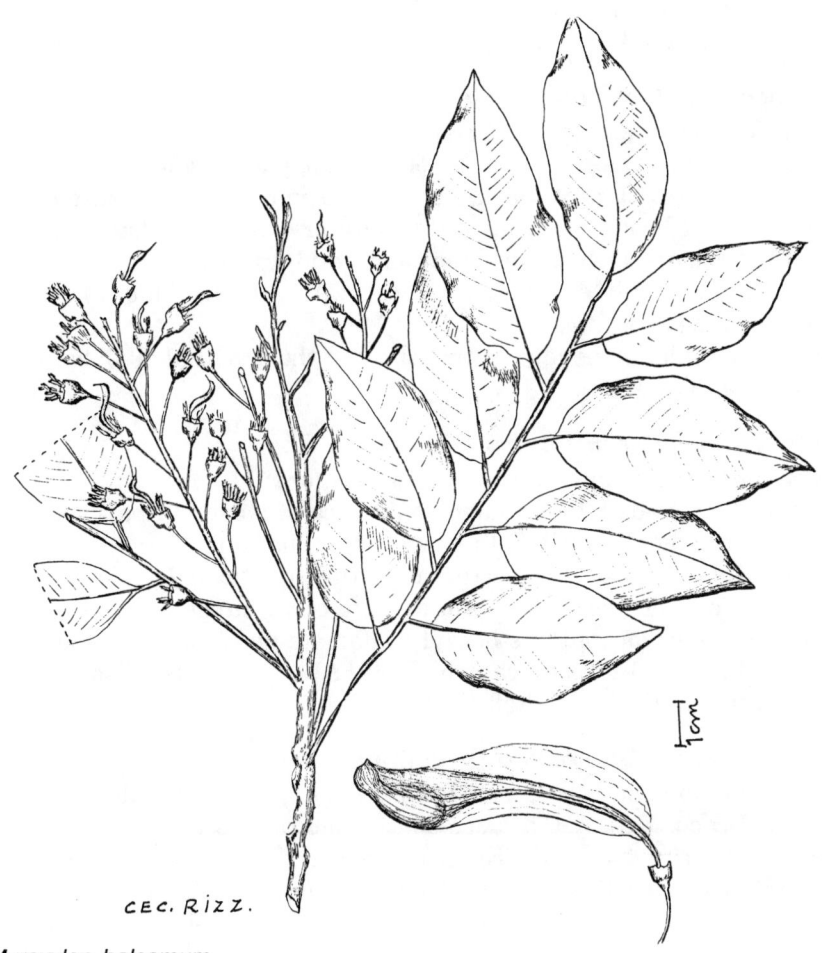

Myroxylon balsamum

USES: Unripe fruits used for abdominal troubles.

Monopteryx uacu Spruce ex Benth.
AREA: Amazonia, forest.
NAME: Uacu.
USES: Kernel is bitter, used to alleviate upset stomach.
CHEM.: The oil of the seeds has been studied (Ref: FABA 27). Isoflavones have been investigated in the genus (Ref: FABA 28).

Mucuna pruriens (L.) DC.
AREA: Throughout Brazil, forest.
NAMES: Fava-café, feijão-café, mucuna, olho-de-burro, pó-de-mico.
USES: Roots are diuretic; seeds are anthelmintic and aphrodisiac, but probably poisonous.

FABACEAE

CHEM. & PHARM.: Alkaloids and their pharmacological action have been described (Ref: FABA 29).

Myrocarpus frondosus Fr. All.
AREA: Southern Bahia to Rio Grande do Sul, forest.
NAMES: Cabriuva, cabriuva-parda, óleo-pardo, pau-bálsamo.
USES: Sap is expectorant. Bark, wood and resin used in a tincture recommended for healing injuries and respiratory ailments; also for cystitis and urethritis. Pods are excitant and antidyspeptic.

The closely related *M. fastigiatus* Fr. All. (Rio de Janeiro) has the same names and uses.
CHEM.: Nerolidol is the major constituent of the essential oil of both species (Ref: FABA 30).

Myroxylon balsamum (L.) Harms
AREA: Amazonia, Bahia and central Brazil, forest.
NAMES: Bálsamo-de-tolu, bálsamo-do-peru, cabriuva, caboriba, caboreíba, óleo-vermelho; English: Tolu balsam, Peru balsam.
USES: Trunk exudate is expectorant, antiasthmatic, balsamic, used for cystitis and blennorrhagia; worked into cough drops.
CHEM.: The balsam contains benzyl cinnamate and benzyl benzoate, besides the sesquiterpene cadinol (Ref: FABA 31,32). Isoflavones were identified in the wood (Ref: FABA 33,34).

Periandra mediterranea (Vell.) Taub.
AREA: Very common throughout Brazil, in campo and cerrado.
NAMES: Alcaçuz-da-terra, alcaçuz-do-cerrado, raiz-doce.
USES: Roots taste like licorice, are resolvent, bechic, expectorant; also used for urinary diseases and abdominal inflammations.
CHEM.: Sweet-tasting triterpenes have been isolated (Ref: FABA 35,36,37).

Psoralea glandulosa L.
AREA: Rio Grande do Sul.
NAME: Congonha.
USES: Leaf infusion is emollient, vulnerary, stimulant, diaphoretic, antiasthmatic and antidiabetic. Also used against enteritis.

Pterodon apparicioi Peders.
AREA: Minas Gerais, gallery forest in Serra do Cipó.
NAME: Sucupira-branca.
USES: Same as those of *Pterodon pubescens*.
CHEM.: Fruits contain isoflavones (Ref: FABA 38,39) and diterpenes (Ref: FABA 40).

FABACEAE

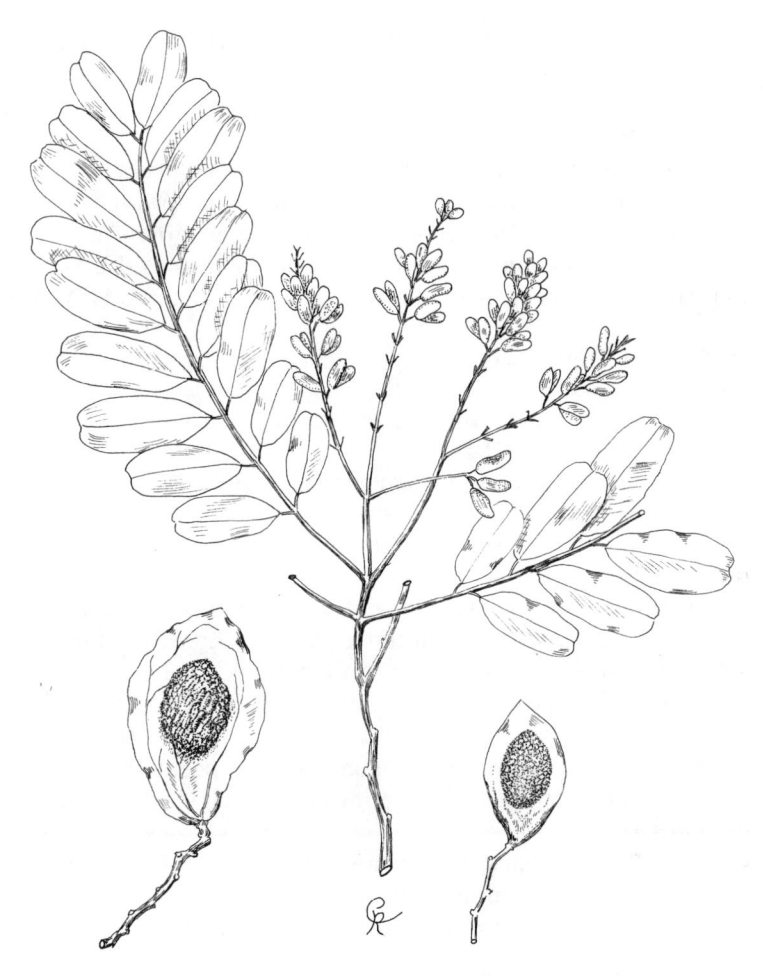

CENTER & LEFT: *Pterodon pubescens.* RIGHT: *Pterodon apparicioi.*

Pterodon pubescens Benth.
AREA: Goiás to Mato Grosso, cerrado.
NAMES: Faveiro, sucupira-branca.
USES: Bark produces a volatile oil which is aromatic, useful for rheumatism. The roots occasionally give rise to a tuberous swelling known as "batata-de-sucupira," which is used against diabetes.
CHEM. & PHARM.: The oil from the fruits inhibits the penetration, into the skin of humans, of schistosome cercariae, the larval stage which causes schistosomiasis (bilharzia). This property can be used for prophylactic

FABACEAE

purposes and was traced to the presence, in the oil, of 14,15-epoxigeranylgeraniol (Ref: FABA 41). Isoflavones have also been described (Ref: FABA 42).

Sophora tomentosa L.
AREA: In sandy beaches along the whole littoral, restinga.
NAMES: Cambuí-da-restinga, comandaíba, feijão-da-praia.
USES: Leaves are diuretic, sudorific, purgative, antipyretic.
CHEM.: Several terpenoids, flavonoids, isoflavonoids and other phenolic compounds have been isolated from the leaves (Ref: FABA 43,44,45).

Sweetia fruticosa Spreng.
AREA: Southern Bahia to São Paulo, forest.
NAMES: Angelim, angelim-pedra, caiçara, canjica, cabo-de-formão, gracuí, sucupira-amarela.
USES: The wood contains a peculiar powder, very much recommended as a fever remedy.

Torresea cearensis Fr. All.
AREA: Maranhão do Minas Gerais and Mato Grosso, forest and caatinga.
NAMES: Amburana, cumaru, cumaru-das-caatingas, cumaru-do-ceará, cumaru-do-nordeste, imburana, imburana-de-cheiro.
USES: Oil extracted from the bark, alone or mixed with the seeds, is used for colds, cough, bronchitis, asthma and lung ailments. Bark is antispasmodic, sedative, emmenagogue. The scented seeds are used as a substitute for those of the genuine cumaru (*Dipteryx odorata*, the tonka bean).
CHEM. & PHARM.: The bark is rich in coumarin (Ref: FABA 46). Extracts tested in laboratory animals and isolated organs showed spasmolytic, anti-inflammatory and bronchodilating effects (Ref: FABA 47).

Vatairea guianensis Aubl.
AREA: Amazonia, forest.
NAMES: Andira-da-várzea, fava-de-empingem, faveira, faveira-amarela.
USES: The seed oil is applied externally to remove freckles and other spots on the skin. The crushed seeds, made into an ointment with oil or vinegar, are used to treat ringworm.

Vataireopsis araroba (Aguiar) Ducke
AREA: Bahia to Minas Gerais and Rio de Janeiro, forest.
NAMES: Angelim-amargoso, angelim-araroba, araroba.
USES: Bark is bitter, purgative. A yellow powder accumulates in cavities in the heartwood, internationally known as "Goa powder" and locally as "pó-da-bahia." It is made up of a mixture of anthraquinones and

FABACEAE

Vataireopsis araroba

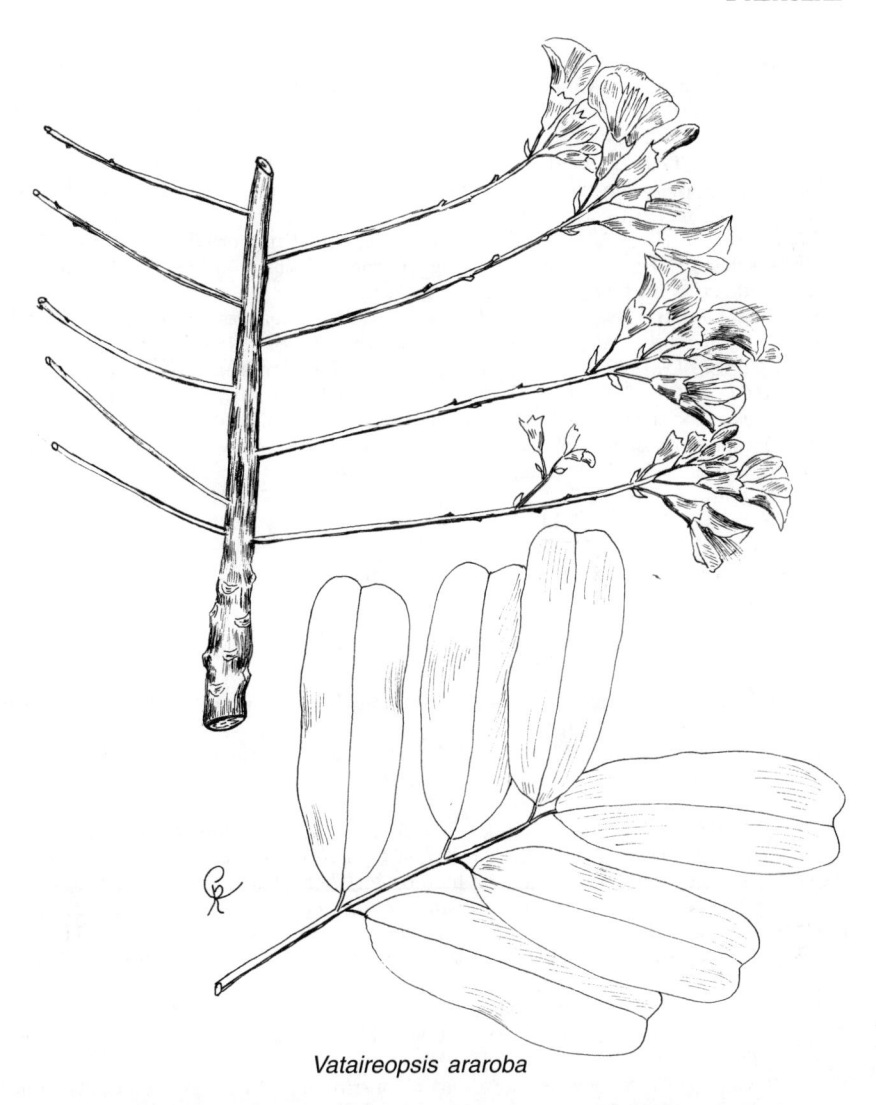

anthranols, called chrysa-robin in pharmacognosy. This is used as a laxative, and topically against skin diseases.

CHEM.: The main constituent of chrysarobin is chrysophanol, an anthraquinone which is also present in the wood of *Vatairea guianensis* (Ref: FABA 48).

Fabaceae – References

FABA 1. Ghosal, S. & S.K. Dutta. 1971. Alkaloids of *Abrus precatorius*. *Phytochemistry 10*: 195-198.

FABA 2. Siddiqui, S., B.S. Siddiqui & Z. Naim. 1978. Studies in the steroidal constituents of the seeds of *Abrus precatorius* Linn. (scarlet variety). *Pak. J. Sci. Ind. Res. 21*: 158-161.

FABACEAE

FABA 3. Lupi, A., F. Delle Monache, G.-B. Marini-Bettòlo, D.L.B. Costa & I.L. d'Albuquerque. 1979. Abruquinones: new natural isoflavanquinones. *Gazz. Chim. Ital. 109*: 9-12.

FABA 4. Bhardwaj, D.K., M.S. Bisht & C.K. Mehta. 1980. Flavonoids from *Abrus precatorius*. *Phytochemistry 19*: 2040-2041.

FABA 5. Chiang, T.-C., H.-M. Chang & C.W. Thomas. 1983. New oleanene-type triterpenes from *Abrus precatorius* and X-ray crystal structure of abrusgenic acid methanol 1:1 solvate. *Planta Medica 49*: 165-169.

FABA 6. Choi, Y.-H., R.A. Hussain, J.M. Pezzuto, A.D. Kinghorn & J.F. Morton. 1989. Abrusosides A-D, four novel sweet-tasting triterpene glycosides from the leaves of *Abrus precatorius*. *J. Nat. Prod. 52*: 1118-1127.

FABA 7. Agarwal, S.S., N. Ghatak & R.B. Arora. 1969. Antiestrogenic activity of alcoholic extract of the roots of *Abrus precatorius* L. *Indian J. Pharm. 31*: 175 -179.

FABA 8. Morton, J.F. 1977. Poisonous and injurious higher plants and fungi. Chapter 71 (pp. 1456-1567) *in*: C.G. Tedeschi, W.G. Eckert & L. G. Tedeschi, eds., FORENSIC MEDICINE, VOL. III, ENVIRONMENTAL HAZARDS. W.B. Saunders Co., Philadelphia.

FABA 9. Paulino Filho, H.F. 1982. Estudo químico da espécie *Acosmium subelegans* (Mohlenb.) Yakovl. Thesis, Federal University of Rio de Janeiro.

FABA 10. Paulino Filho, H.F., J. Muradian & W.B. Mors. 1977. Estudio fitoquímico de la *Acosmium subelegans* (Mohlenb.) Yakovl. Aislamiento y síntesis del 4-metoxi-6-(p-hidroxiestiril)-α-pirona. *Rev. Latinoamer. Quím. 8*: 79-82.

FABA 11. Bautista, A.R.P.L. 1973. Estudo fitoquímico da casca de *Andira humilis* Mart. ex Benth. Thesis, Federal University of Rio de Janeiro.

FABA 12. Bautista, A.R.P.L. & W. B. Mors. 1975. Estudo fitoquímico de *Andira humilis* Mart. ex Benth. I. Biochanin-A, o principal consituinte do órgão subterrâneo. *Bol. Inst. Biol. Bahia 14*: 58-63.

FABA 13. Cocker, W., T. Dahl, C. Dempsey & T.B.H. McMurray. 1962. Extractives from *Andira inermis*. *J. Chem. Soc.*: 4906-4909.

FABA 14. Brown, M.P., R.H. Thomson, B.M. Hausen & M.H. Simatupang. 1974. Über die Inhaltsstoffe von *Bowdichia nitida* Benth.: Erstmalige Isolierung eines Isoflavonchinons. *J. Liebigs Ann. Chem.*: 1295-1300.

FABA 15. Calle, A., J.A. Rivera Umana & E. Moreno. 1983. Isolamiento del lupeol de la cascara de *Bowdichia virgilioides* H.B.K. *Rev. Colomb. Cién. Quím.-Farm. 4*: 93-94.

FABA 16. Torrenegra, R., S. Escarria, P. Bauereiss & H. Achenbach. 1985. Homoormosamine, the major alkaloid of the bark from *Bowdichia virgilioides*. *Planta Medica 50*: 276-277.

FABA 17. Garcez, F.R., S. Scramin, M.C. Nascimento & W.B. Mors. 1988. Prenylated flavonoids as evolutionary indicators in the genus *Dahlstedtia*. *Phytochemistry 27*: 1079-1084.

FABA 18. Kaplan, M.A.C., O.R. Gottlieb, B. Gilbert, I.S. Souza & M.T. Magalhães. 1966. A química das Leguminosas brasileiras. X. Derivados do lupeol em *Dipteryx alata*. *An. Acad. Brasil. Ci. 38*: 419-420.

FABA 19. Nakano, T. & M. Suarez. 1969. Neutral constituents of the bark of *Dipteryx odorata*. *Planta Medica 18*: 79-83.

FABA 20. Hayashi, T. & R.H. Thomson. 1974. Isoflavonoids from *Dipteryx odorata*. *Phytochemistry 13*: 1943-1946.

FABA 21. Nakano, T., J. Alonso, R. Grillet & A. Martín. 1979. Isoflavonoids of the bark of *Dipteryx odorata* Willd. *J. Chem. Soc. Perkin 1*: 2107-2112.

FABA 22. Nakano, T., K. Tori & Y. Yoshimura. 1979. New isoflavones isolated from the bark of *Dipteryx odorata*. *Rev. Latinoam. Quím. 10*: 17-19.

FABA 23. Hargreaves, R.T., R.D. Johnson, D.S. Millington, M.H. Mondal, W. Beavers, L. Becker, C. Young & K.R. Rinehart. 1974. Alkaloids of the American species of *Erythrina*. *Lloydia 37*: 569-580.

FABA 24. Dominguez, X.A., C. Martinez, A. Calero, X.A. Dominguez Jr., M. Hinojosa, A. Zamudio, W.H. Watson & V. Zabel. 1978. Mexican medicinal plants. XXXI. Chemical components from "jiquelite," *Indigofera suffruticosa* Mill. *Planta Medica 34*: 172-175.

FABA 25. Dominguez, X.A., C. Martinez, A. Calero, X.A. Dominguez Jr., M. Hinojosa, A. Zamudio, V. Zabel, W.B. Smith & W.H. Watson. 1978. Louisfieserone, an unusual flavanone derivative from *Indigofera suffruticosa* Mill. *Tetrahedron Lett.*: 429-432.

FABA 26. Garcez, W.S., F.R. Garcez, N.K. Honda & A.J.R. da Silva. 1989. A nitropropanoyl-glucopyranoside from *Indigofera suffruticosa*. *Phytochemistry 28*: 1251-1252.

FABA 27. Pinto, G.P. 1950. O óleo de uacu. Seu estudo químico. *Bol. Téc. Inst. Agron. Norte* (Belém) *21*: 31-62.

FABA 28. Albuquerque, F.B., R. Braz Filho, O.R. Gottlieb, M.T. Magalhães, G.J.S. Maia, A.B. Oliveira, G.G. Oliveira & V.C. Wilberg. 1981. Isoflavone evolution in *Monopteryx*. *Phytochemistry 20*: 235-236.

FABA 29. Ghosal, S. 1971. Alkaloids of *Mucuna pruriens*. Chemistry and Pharmacology. *Planta Medica 24*: 434-436.

FABA 30. Naves, Y.R. 1947. Études sur les matières végétales volatiles. XLIII. Présence de nérolidol dans les huiles essentielles de papilionacées. *Helv. Chim. Acta 30*: 275-277.

FABA 31. Naves, Y.R. 1948. Études sur les matières végétales volatiles. LXI. Présence de nérolidol dans les huiles essentielles de papilionacées. *Helv. Chim. Acta 31*: 408-417.

FABA 32. Naves, Y.R. 1949. Études sur les matières végétales volatiles. XCV. Présence de nérolidol dans les huiles essentielles de papilionacées. *Helv. Chim. Acta 32*: 2181-2185.

FABA 33. Harborne, J.B., O.R. Gottlieb & M.T. Magalhães. 1963. Occurrence of the isoflavone afromosin in cabreúva wood. *J. Org. Chem. 28*: 881-882.

FABA 34. Oliveira, A.B., M.I.L.M. Madruga & O.R. Gottlieb. 1978. Isoflavonoids from *Myroxylon balsamum*. *Phytochemistry 17*: 593-595.

FABA 35. Hashimoto, Y., H. Ishizone & M. Ogura. 1980. Periandrin II and IV, triterpene glycosides from *Periandra dulcis*. *Phytochemistry 19*: 2411-2415.

FABA 36. Hashimoto, Y., Y. Ohta, H. Ishizone, M. Kuriyama & M. Ogura. 1982. Periandrin III, a novel sweet triterpene glycoside from *Periandra dulcis*. *Phytochemistry 21*: 2335-2337.

FABA 37. Hashimoto, Y., H. Ishizone, M. Suganuma, M. Ogura, K. Nakatsu & H. Yoshioka. 1983. Periandrin I, a sweet triterpene glycoside from *Periandra dulcis*. *Phytochemistry 22*: 259-264.

FABA 38. Galina, E. & O.R. Gottlieb. 1974. Isoflavones from *Pterodon aparicioi*. *Phytochemistry 13*: 2593-2595.

FABA 39. Almeida, M.E.L. & O.R. Gottlieb. 1975. Further isoflavones from *Pterodon apparicioi*. *Phytochemistry 14*: 2716.

FABA 40. Fascio, M., W.B. Mors, B. Gilbert, J.R. Mahajan, MB. Monteiro, D. dos Santos Filho & W. Vishnewski. 1976. Diterpenoid furans from *Pterodon* species. *Phytochemistry 15*: 201-203.

FABA 41. Mors, W.B., M.F. Santos Filho, H.J. Monteiro, B. Gilbert & J. Pellegrino. 1967. Chemoprophylactic agent in schistosomiasis: 14,15-epoxigeranylgeraniol. *Science 157*: 950-951.

FABA 42. Braz Filho, R., O.R. Gottlieb & R.M.V. Assumpção. 1971. The isoflavones of *Pterodon pubescens*. *Phytochemistry 10*: 2835-2836.

FABA 43. Delle Monache, F., G. delle Monache, G.-B. Marini-Bettòlo, M.M.F. de Albuquerque, J.F. de Melo & O. Gonçalves de Lima. 1976. Flavonoids of *Sophora tomentosa* (Leguminosae). I. Sophoronol, a new 3-hydroxyflavanone. *Gazz. Chim. Ital. 106*: 935-945.

FABA 44. Komatsu, M., I. Yokoe & Y. Shirataki. 1978. Studies on the constituents of *Sophora* species. XII. Constituents of the aerial parts of *Sophora tomentosa* L. *Chem. Pharm. Bull. 26*: 1274-1278.

FABA 45. Komatsu, M., I. Yokoe & Y. Shirataki. 1978. Studies on the constituents of *Sophora* species. XIII. Constituents of the aerial parts of *Sophora tomentosa* L. (2). *Chem. Pharm. Bull. 26*: 3863-3870.

FABA 46. Liberalli, C.H. & J.F. Lima. 1937. Cumaru do Nordeste. *Rev. Flora Medicinal* (Rio de Janeiro) *3*: 341-379.

FABA 47. Leite, M.G.R., C.L. de Souza, M.A.M. da Silva, L.K.A. Moreira, F.J.A. Matos & G.S.B. Viana. 1993. Estudo farmacológico comparativo de *Mikania glomerata* Spreng. (guaco), *Justicia pectoralis* Jacq. (anador) e *Torresea cearensis* Fr. All. (cumaru). *Rev. Bras. Farm.* 74: 12-15.

FABA 48. Formiga, M.D., O.R. Gottlieb, P.H. Mendes, M. Koketsu, M.E.L. Almeida, M.O.S. Pereira & M.T. Magalhães. 1975. Constituents of Brazilian Leguminosae. *Phytochemistry* 14: 828-829.

FLACOURTIACEAE

Carpotroche brasiliensis (Raddi) Endl.
AREA: Bahia to Minas Gerais and São Paulo.
NAMES: Fruta-de-cotia, fruto-de-babado, fruto-de-macaco, canudo-de-pito, mata-piolho, pau-de-anjo, pau-de-cotia, pau-de-lepra, sapucainha.
USES: Seed oil is insecticidal, parasiticidal, depilatory, useful against dandruff and, principally, used as a remedy for leprosy.
CHEM. & PHARM.: The seed oil ('sapucainha oil') is analogous in properties and chemical composition to the Indian chaulmoogra oil from *Hydnocarpus* and *Oncoba* species, of the same family. Until the 1940s, when the sulfones were discovered as drugs active against leprosy, these two oils were the only acknowledged remedies for the treatment of this disease. The active compounds are glycerides of characteristic fatty acids with a cyclopentenyl ring in the carbon chain: mainly chaulmoogric, hydnocarpic and gorlic acids, all present in sapucainha oil (Ref: FLAC 1,2,3,4,5). Cyanogenetic glycosides were identified in seeds and pericarp (Ref: FLAC 6).

Carpotroche longifolia Benth.
AREA: Amazonia, forest.
NAMES: Cacau-branco, fruta-de-cotia.
USES: Seed oil is insecticidal and parasiticidal. Unripe fruits are reduced to powder and applied in baths to eliminate ticks.

Casearia adstringens Mart.
AREA: Amazonia, forest.
NAME: Quina-do-pará.
USES: For cleaning sloughing ulcers.

Casearia cambessedesii Eichl.
AREA: From Minas Gerais and Rio de Janeiro southward.
NAMES: Guaçatunga, marmeleiro-do-campo, marmeleiro-do-mato.
USES: Leaves are put on wounds and ulcers to hasten healing and cicatrization. Also given against snakebite.

FLACOURTIACEAE

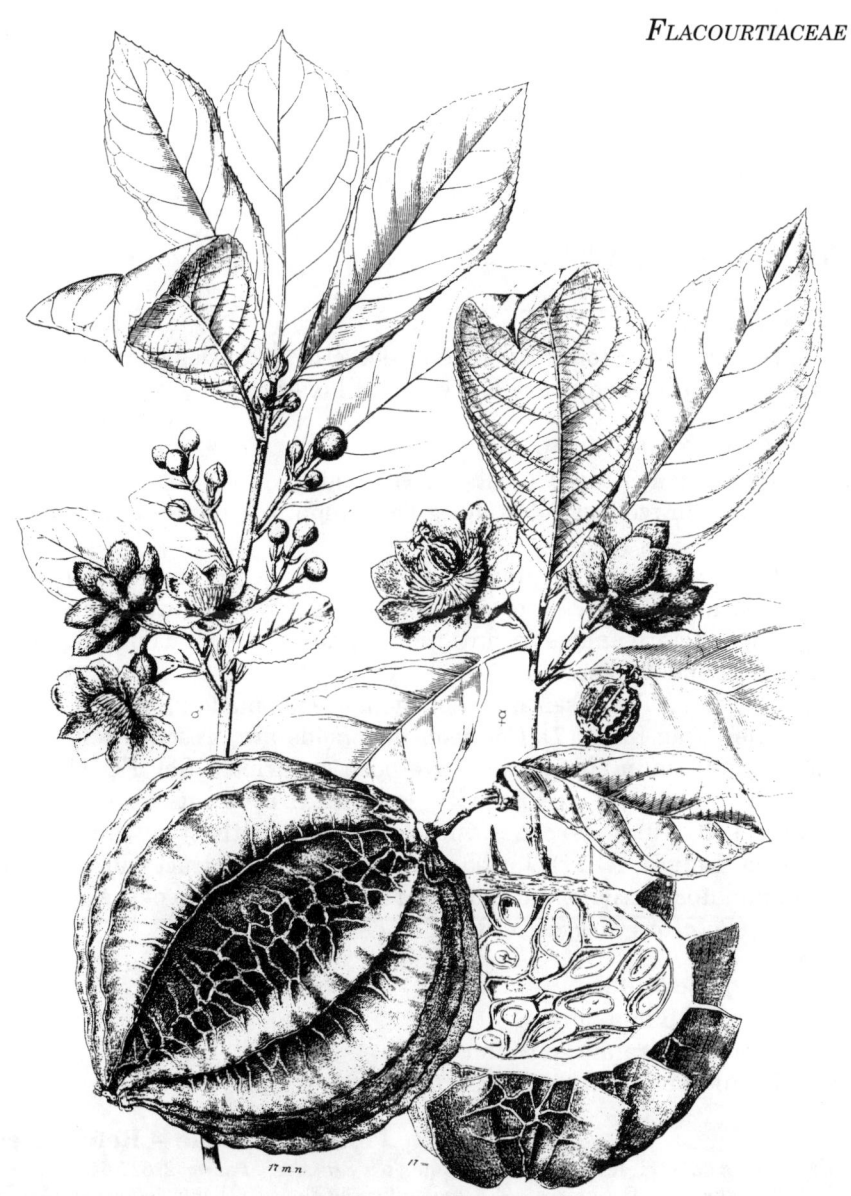

Carpotroche brasiliensis

Casearia guyanensis (Aubl.) Urb.
AREA: Amazonia to Bahia, forest.
NAMES: Café-bravo, café-do-diabo, café-do-mato.
USES: Bark is astringent, used to stop discharges from urethra and vagina.

FLACOURTIACEAE

Casearia inaequilatera Camb.
AREA: From Rio de Janeiro southward, forest.
NAME: Guaçatunga.
USES: To treat skin diseases.

Casearia ovata Willd.
AREA: Amazonia, forest.
NAME: Anavinga.
USES: Bark is bitter, tonic. Infusion or decoction of leaves used to relieve articular pains. Fruits are diuretic and laxative.

Casearia sylvestris Sw.
AREA: Throughout Brazil, forest and cerrado.
NAMES: Café-bravo, erva-de-teiú, guaçatunga, língua-de-teiú, pau-de-lagarto.
USES: Leaves are tonic, depurative, antirheumatic and used against diarrhoea and herpes. Both leaves and bark are employed for wound healing, and are analgesic, anti-inflammatory, as well as used against ill fevers and snakebite.
CHEM. & PHARM.: The essential oil of the leaves is made up principally of terpenes (Ref: FLAC 7). Common flavonoids are present (Ref: FLAC 8). Wound healing properties have been confirmed (Ref: FLAC 9), as well as anti-gastric ulcer activity (Ref: FLAC 10). Acute toxicity is low (Ref: FLAC 10). Diterpenes with anti-tumor activity have been described (Ref: FLAC 11). Tested in mice, the bark extract showed anti-inflammatory activity and protected against the venom of the jararaca snake (*Bothrops jararaca*) (Ref: FLAC 12).

Laetia apetala Jacq.
AREA: Piauí to Bahia, forest.
NAMES: Pau-de-piranha, piranha.
USES: Resin is balsamic, drastic.

Flacourtiaceae – References
FLAC 1. Dias da Silva, R.A. 1926. Sapucainha. *Rev. Bras. Med. Pharm.* 2: 627-643.
FLAC 2. Rothe, O. & D. Surerus. 1931. Indentificação do ácido chaulmoogrico no óleo de *Carpotroche brasiliensis*. *Rev. Soc. Bras. Quím.* 2: 358-365.
FLAC 3. Karyione, T. & Y. Hasegawa. 1934. On the components of sapucainha oil. *J. Pharm. Soc. Japan* 54: 28-29.
FLAC 4. Cole, H.I. & H.T. Cardoso. 1938. Analysis of chaulmoogra oils. I. *Carpotroche brasiliensis* (sapucainha) oil. *J. Am. Chem. Soc.* 60: 614-617.
FLAC 5. Cole, H.I. & H.T. Cardoso. 1938. Analysis of chaulmoogra oils. II. Isolation and properties of gorlic acid, an optically active liquid fatty acid. *J. Am. Chem. Soc.* 60: 612-614.
FLAC 6. Spencer, K.C., D.S. Seigler, L.H. Fikenscher & R. Hegnauer. 1982. Gynocardin and tetraphyllin B from *Carpotroche brasiliensis* (seeds and pericarp). *Planta Medica* 44: 289 (1982).

FLAC 7. Assis Brasil e Silva, G.A. & L. Bauer. 1970. Análise do óleo essencial de *Casearia sylvestris* Sw. *Rev. Bras. Farm. 51*: 327-331.
FLAC 8. Junges, M.J., E.P. Schenkel & C.M.O. Simoes. 1985. Flavonóides de *Casearia sylvestris* Swartz, Flacourtiaceae (erva-de-bugre). *Cad. Farm.* (Porto Alegre) *1*: 95-101.
FLAC 9. Scavone, O., R. Grecchi, S. Panizza & R.A.P. Souza e Silva. 1979. Guaçatonga (*Casearia sylvestris* Swartz): Aspectos botânicos da planta, ensaios fitoquímicos e propriedade cicatrizante da folha. *An. Farm. Quím. S. Paulo 19*: 73-82.
FLAC 10. Basile, A.C., J.A.A. Sertié, S. Panizza, T.T. Oshiro & C.A. Azzolini. 1990. Pharmacological assay of *Casearia sylvestris*. 1. Preventive anti-ulcer activity and toxicity of the leaf crude extract. *J. Ethnopharmacol. 30*: 185-197.
FLAC 11. Itokawa, H., N. Totsuka, K. Takeya, K. Watanabe & E. Obata. 1988. Antitumor principles from *Casearia sylvestris* Sw. (Flacourtiaceae), structure elucidation of new clerodane diterpenes by 2-D NMR spectroscopy. *Chem. Pharm. Bull.* (Japan) *36*: 1585-1588.
FLAC 12. Barbi, N.S., B.M. Ruppelt, N.A. Pereira, M.C. Nascimento & W.B. Mors. 1990. Estudo farmacológico e fitoquímico da casca de *Casearia sylvestris*. *11th Symposium on Medicinal Plants of Brazil and 3rd Natl. Symposium on Pharmacology and Chemistry of Natural Products*, João Pessoa, Brazil, Sept. 1990. Abstracts of Papers, n° 4.02.

GENTIANACEAE

Calolisianthus pendulus (Mart.) Gilg
AREA: Bahia to Paraná.
NAMES: Genciana-brasileira, genciana-do-brasil, raiz-amarga.
USES: Roots are bitter, tonic, antifebrile, antirheumatic, also used for scrofulous afflictions, malarial fever and gastric atony. Serves as a substitute for the European gentian (*Gentiana lutea* L.).

A number of *Lisianthus* species, known by the general name of genciana-da-terra, are employed as substitutes for *C. pendulus*. They occur from Amazonia to São Paulo, mostly in campos. Examples are the following: *L. alpestris* Mart. (Minas Gerais and São Paulo), *L. brevifolius* Gris. (in the same area), *L. campanuloides* Spruce (Amazonia to São Paulo), *L. coerulescens* Aubl. (Amazonia to São Paulo), *L. obtusifolius* Gris. (Rio de Janeiro and Minas Gerais), *L. purpurascens* Aubl. (Amazonia), *L. uliginosus* Gris. (Amazonia to Rio de Janeiro) and *L. viridiflorus* Mart. (Goiás to São Paulo and Mato Grosso). The same holds for *Calolisianthus amplissimus* (Mart.) Gilg (Mato Grosso and São Paulo).

Coutoubea ramosa Aubl.
AREA: Amazonia.
NAME: Diambarana.
USES: Stomachic, anthelmintic.

Coutoubea spicata Aubl.
AREA: Pará to São Paulo.
NAMES: Cutúbeo-brasileira, genciana, genciana-do-brasil, raiz-amargosa.

Gentianaceae

USES: Root used in decoction for a bitter, stomachic, tonic, febrifuge, anthelmintic; also for amenorrhoea.

Curtia tenuifolia (Aubl.) Knobl.
AREA: Amazonia to São Paulo.
NAME: Centáurea-menor.
USES: Bitter, tonic and febrifuge.

Deianira nervosa Cham. & Schl.
AREA: Goiás to São Paulo and Mato Grosso.
NAMES: Centáurea-do-brasil, raiz-amargosa.
USES: Herb is bitter, antidyspeptic, vermifuge and antipyretic. For the latter use it is customary to mix it with orange peels and the fruits of *Xylopia aromatica*.

D. erubescens Cham. & Schl. (Minas Gerais, Mato Grosso, Goiás and São Paulo, campos), known as fel-da-terra, displays the same properties.

Deianira pallescens Cham. & Schl.
AREA: Bahia to São Paulo and Mato Grosso, campo and cerrado.
NAMES: Bico-de-pato, boca-de-sapo.
USES: Roots and flowerheads are bitter, stomachic, tonic and febrifuge. Shoots are used in gargles for sore throat.

Leiphaimos aphylla (Jacq.) Gilg
AREA: Amazonia to Santa Catarina and Mato Grosso; saprophytic herb encountered in rain forest.
NAMES: Batata-cogumelo, genciana-sem-folhas.
USES: Tonic, antidyspeptic, febrifuge and anthelmintic.

Microcolea quadrangularis (Lam.) Gris.
AREA: Rio Grande do Sul.
NAME: Genciana-da-terra.
USES: As a substitute for *Calolisianthus* and *Lisianthus* species.

Schultesia stenophylla Mart.
AREA: Tropical cosmopolitan, distributed throughout Brazil.
NAMES: Fel-da-terra, mata-zombando (meaning "scoffing killer").
USES: Bitter, tonic, febrifuge.
CHEM. & PHARM.: The fresh plant, though said to be toxic to cattle, was found to be innocuous in actual field experiments (Ref: GENT 1). Two iridoid alkaloids of the gentianin type and one new dilactam alkaloid (Ref: GENT 2) have been reported.

Tachia guianensis Aubl.
AREA: Amazonia, forest.

NAMES: Caferana, falso-café, fel-da-terra, jacaré-açu, jacaré-aru, jacuruaru, quássia-do-pará, quina-amargosa, quina-cruzeiro, tinguá-ab, tinguaciba-do-pará, tuparapo, tuparobá, tuparubo.
USES: Root-bark, stem-bark and wood are extremely bitter, antipyretic, vermicidal and antidyspeptic. Used in place of *Cinchona* bark and *Quassia* wood, although the extracts are said to be poisonous.
PHARM.: Crude extracts were shown to be partly active in antimalarial tests performed in *Plasmodium berghei*-infected mice (Ref: GENT 3).

Zygostigma australe (Cham. & Schl.) Gris.
AREA: São Paulo to Rio Grande do Sul, campo.
NAME: Gentiana-da-terra.
USES: As a substitute for *Calolisianthus* and *Lisianthus* species.

Gentianaceae – References

GENT 1. Canella, C.F.C., C.H. Tokarnia & J. Döbereiner. 1966. Experimentos com plantas tidas como tóxicas realizados em bovinos no nordeste do Brasil, com resultados negativos. *Pesquisa Agropecuária Brasileira 1*: 345-352.

GENT 2. Nóbrega, E.M., A.A. Craveiro, J.T. Welch, T. Nicolson & J.A. Zubieta. 1988. New alkaloid from *Schultesia guianensis*. *J. Nat. Prod. 51*: 962-965.

GENT 3. Carvalho, L.H., M.G.L. Brandão, D. Santos-Filho, J.C.C. Lopes & A.U. Krettli. 1991. Antimalarial activity of crude extracts from Brazilian plants studied "in vivo" in *Plasmodium berghei*-infected mice and "in vitro" against *Plasmodium falciparum* in culture. *Braz. J. Med. Biol. Res. 24*: 1113-1123.

GESNERIACEAE

Sinningia allagophylla (Mart.) Wiehl.
AREA: Rio de Janeiro to Rio Grande do Sul, forest and high campos.
NAMES: Batata-do-campo, batatinha-do-campo.
USES: Tuber is employed for a tonic and emollient.

HELICONIACEAE

Heliconia angusta Vell.
AREA: Pará to Alagoas, forest.
NAME: Bananeirinha-do-mato.
USES: Rhizome is anti-gonorrhoeic. Seeds are antidiarrhoeic.

Heliconia bihai L.
AREA: Amazonia to Santa Catarina, forest.
NAMES: Bananeira-brava, bananeirinha-do-mato.
USES: Rhizome is astringent and diuretic.

HELICONIACEAE

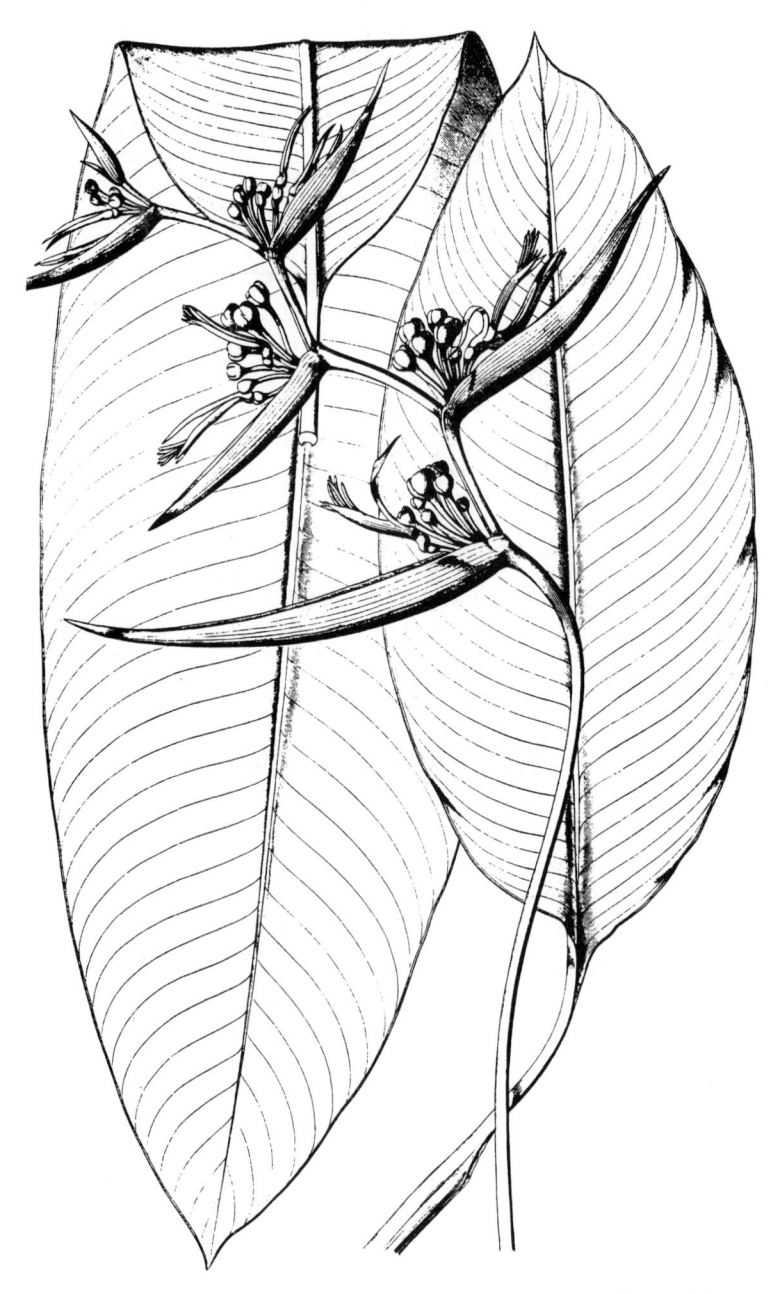

Heliconia angusta

HIPPOCRATEACEAE

Hippocratea volubilis L.
AREA: Amazonia to São Paulo, forest and restinga.
NAME: Cipó-preto.
USE: Used as a bechic.

Peritassa calypsoides (Camb.) A.C. Sm.
AREA: Rio de Janeiro, São Paulo and Rio Grande do Sul, forest and restinga.
NAMES: Bacupari-cipó, cipó-de-copacabana, saputá, tapicuru.
USES: Leaves taken as an antiphlogistic.

Salacia impressifolia (Miers) A.C. Sm.
AREA: Amazonia, forest.
NAMES: Boca-de-velha, saputá, uaimiuru.
USES: Antirheumatic and antiasthmatic.

Tontelea brachypoda Miers
AREA: Minas Gerais and Goiàs to São Paulo and Mato Grosso, forest; once common in Rio de Janeiro city.
NAMES: Abacate-do-mato, castanha-mineira.
USES: Seeds are extremely bitter; used as tea or infusion for a stomachic and antidyspeptic.
CHEM.: Prestimerin, tingenone and other "celastroids" were described in an unidentified *Salacia* species from northeastern Brazil (Ref: HIPP 1). For information on these substances, see *Maytenus* spp. (Celastraceae).

Hippocrateaceae – Reference

HIPP 1. Delle Monache, F., G.-B. Marini-Bettólo, M. Pomponi, J.F. Melo, O. Gonçalves de Lima & R.H. Thomson. 1979. New triterpene quinone methides from Hippocrateaceae. *J. Chem. Soc. Perkin 1*: 3127-3131.

HUMIRIACEAE

Humiria balsamifera (Aubl.) St.-Hil.
AREA: Amazonia to Minas Gerais and Rio de Janeiro, forest and restinga.
NAMES: Umiri, umiri-de-cheiro, umiri-do-pará, umirizeiro.
USES: Bark is aromatic. The sap or resin which exudes from the bark acquires a viscous consistency, being known as "bálsamo-de-umiri." It serves as an anthelmintic, balsamic and expectorant and is also considered a substitute for Peru balsam. A decoction of the bark is used to heal chronic sores.
CHEM.: The bark contains 3% of bergenin, an isocoumarin derivative (Ref: HUMI 1).

HUMIRIACEAE

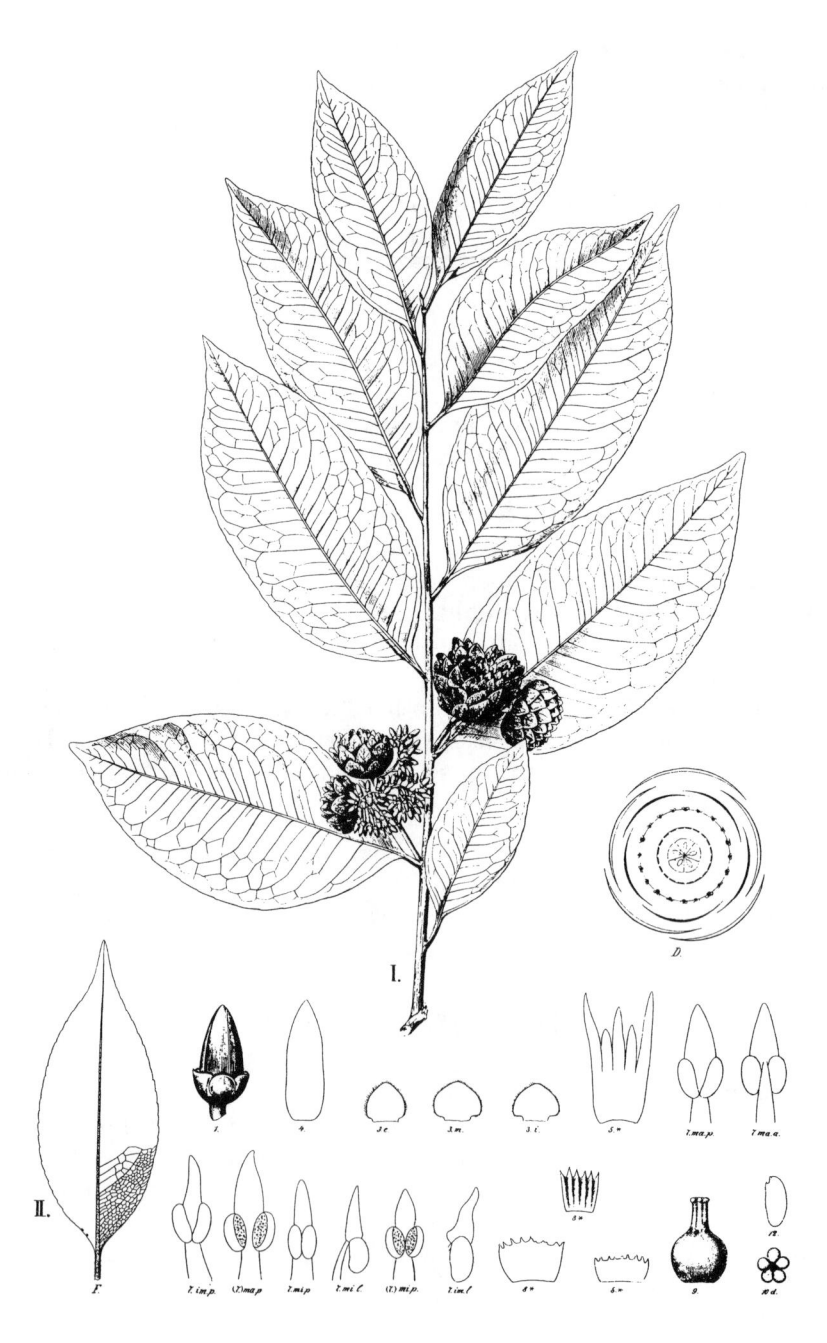

Saccoglottis guianensis

Saccoglottis guianensis Benth.
AREA: Amazonia to Maranhão, forest.
NAMES: Acuá, axuá, uachuá, uaxuá.
USES: Reported as an antirheumatic and for the treatment of gout.

Humiriaceae – Reference

HUMI 1. Dean, B.M. & J. Walker. 1958. A new source of bergenin. *Chem. and Ind.*: 1696-1697.

HYPOXIDACEAE

Hypoxis decumbens L.
AREA: From Bahia to Minas Gerais and São Paulo, ruderal, frequently found invading lawns.
NAME: Falsa-tiririca.
USE: Bulb is prescribed for blennorrhagia.

ICACINACEAE

Citronella congonha (Mart.) Howard
AREA: Minas Gerais to Rio Grande do Sul, forest.
NAMES: Congonha, congonha-de-bugre, congonha-do-sertão, congonha-falsa, erva-de-anta, falso-mate, mate.
USES: Infusion is aromatic, stimulant, diuretic; used as a substitute for mate (*Ilex paraguariensis*, Aquifoliaceae).

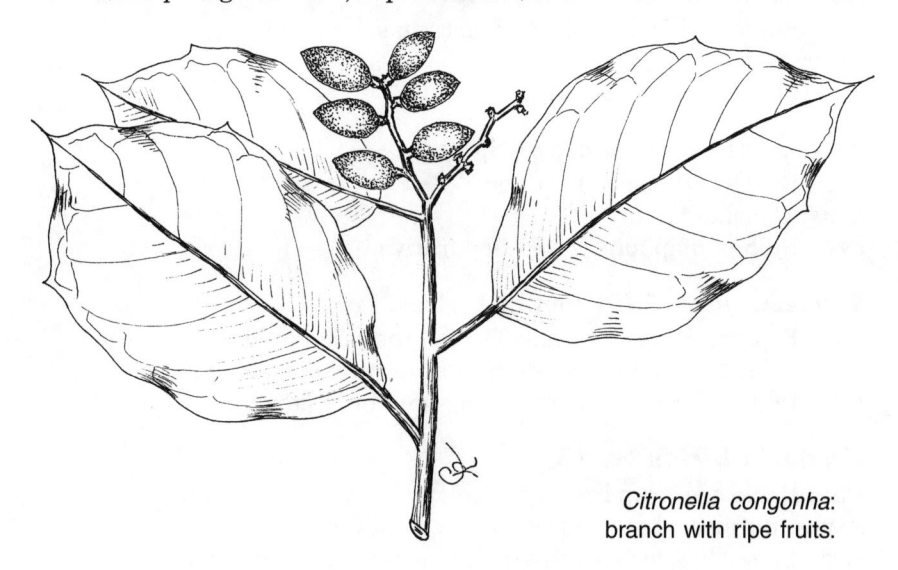

Citronella congonha: branch with ripe fruits.

Citronella mucronata (R. & Pav.) Don
AREA: Goiás to São Paulo and Mato Grosso, forest.
NAMES: Congonha-do-sertão, congonha-verdadeira, erva-de-anta-com-espinho.
USES: Same as for *Citronella congonha*.

IRIDACEAE

Cipura paludosa Aubl.
AREA: Almost throughout Brazil.
NAMES: Alho-da-campina, alho-do-campo, alho-do-mato, cebolinha-do-campo.
USES: Bulb is used for the regulation of delayed menses; also for gonorrhoea.

Cypella herbertii Herb.
AREA: Southern campos.
NAMES: Batatinha-purgative, ruibarbo-do-campo.
USES: Bulb decoction is purgative; in high doses it causes colic.

Eleutherine plicata Herb.
AREA: Dry campos in the state of Pará.
NAMES: Lírio-folha-de-palmeira, marupá-piranga, marupazinho.
USES: Rhizome employed against gastralgia, hysteria and diarrhoea.

Nothoscordum striatum Kunth
AREA: Bahia to Rio Grande do Sul, campo.
NAME: Alho-silvestre.
USE: Bulb used as a vermifuge.

Sisyrinchium vaginatum Spreng.
AREA: Rio Grande do Sul, campo.
NAME: Canchalágua.
USES: Bulb is diaphoretic and depurative.

Trimezia juncifolia Benth. & Hook.
AREA: Espírito Santo to Minas Gerais and São Paulo.
NAMES: Baririçô, batatinha-de-purga, lírio-roxo-do-campo.
USES: Bulb is laxative, indicated mainly for children.

Trimezia lurida Salisb.
AREA: Bahia to Paraná.
NAMES: Barariçô, batatinha-amarela, capim-rei.
USES: Prescribed for constipation, hemorrhoids and dartre.

Iridaceae

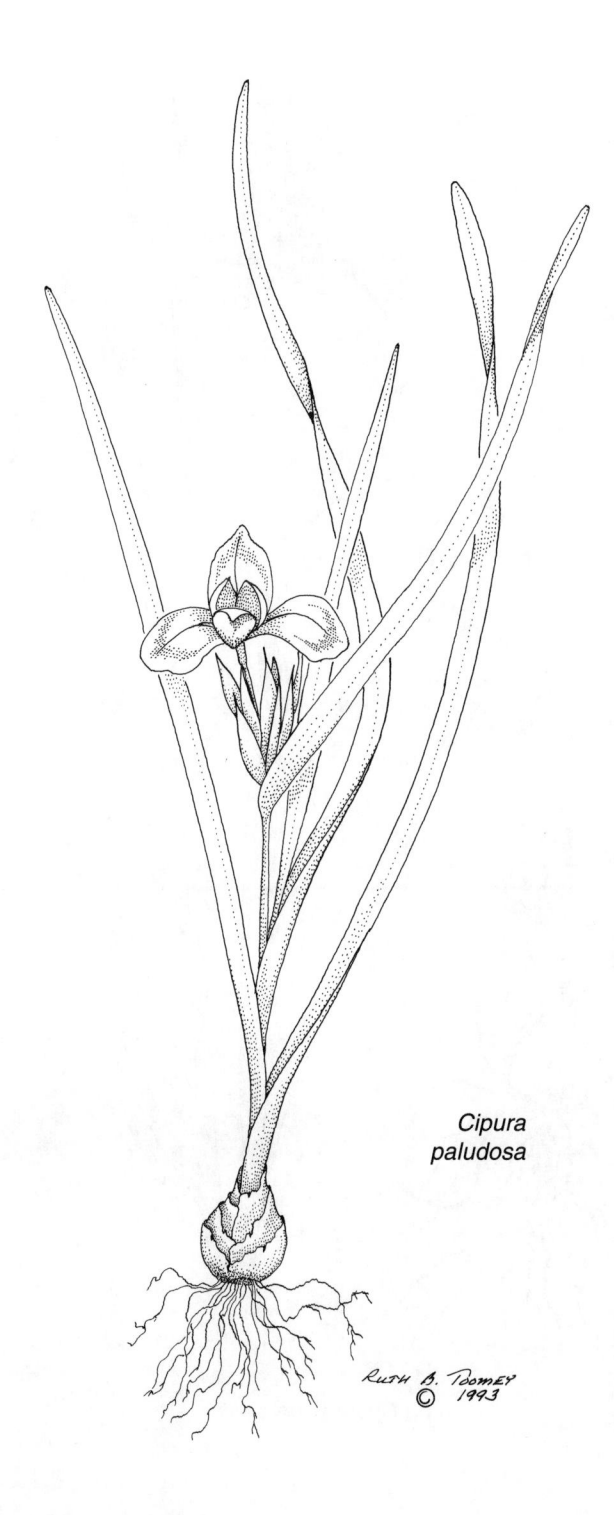

*Cipura
paludosa*

IRIDACEAE

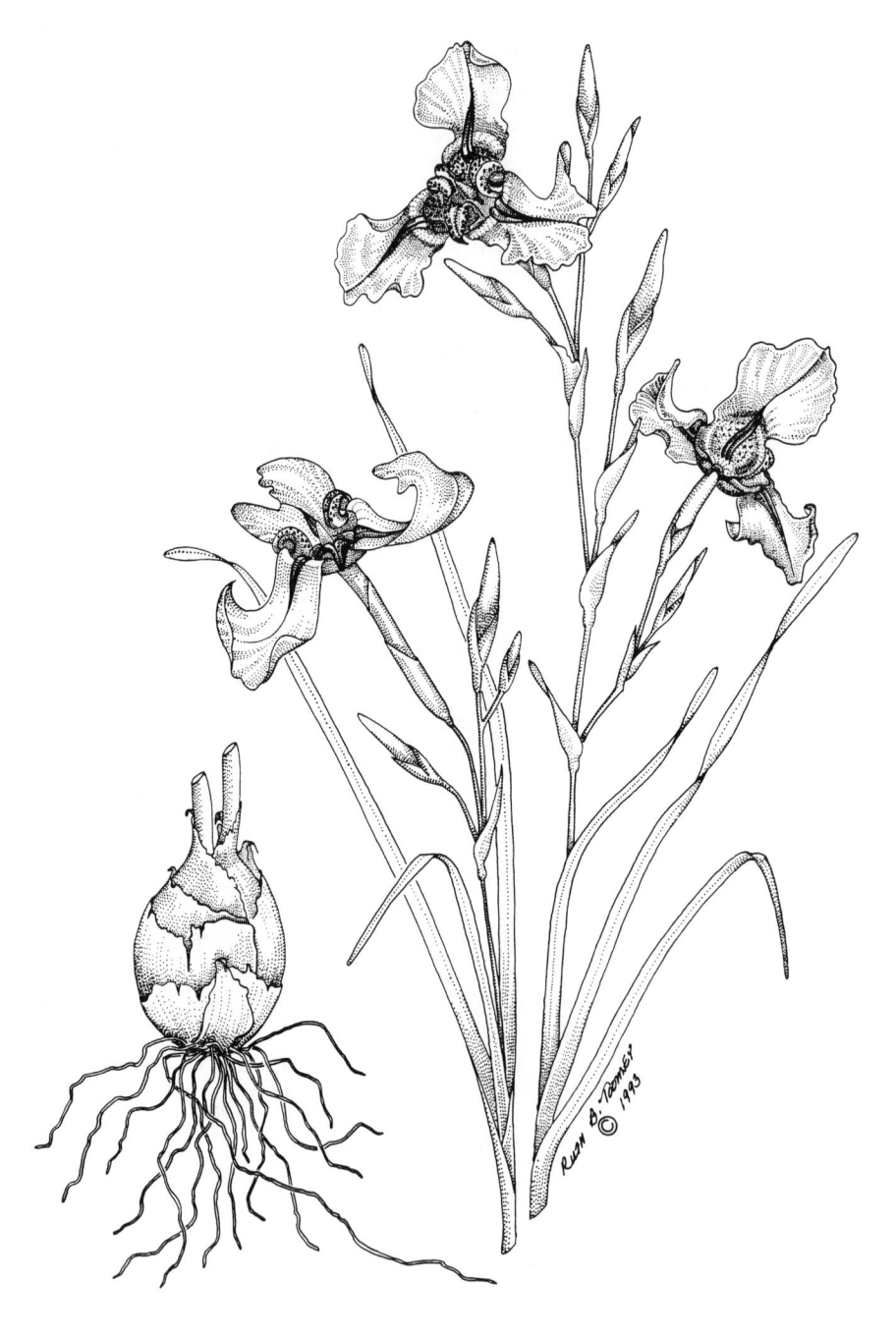

Cypella herbertii

ISOETACEAE

Isoetes martii

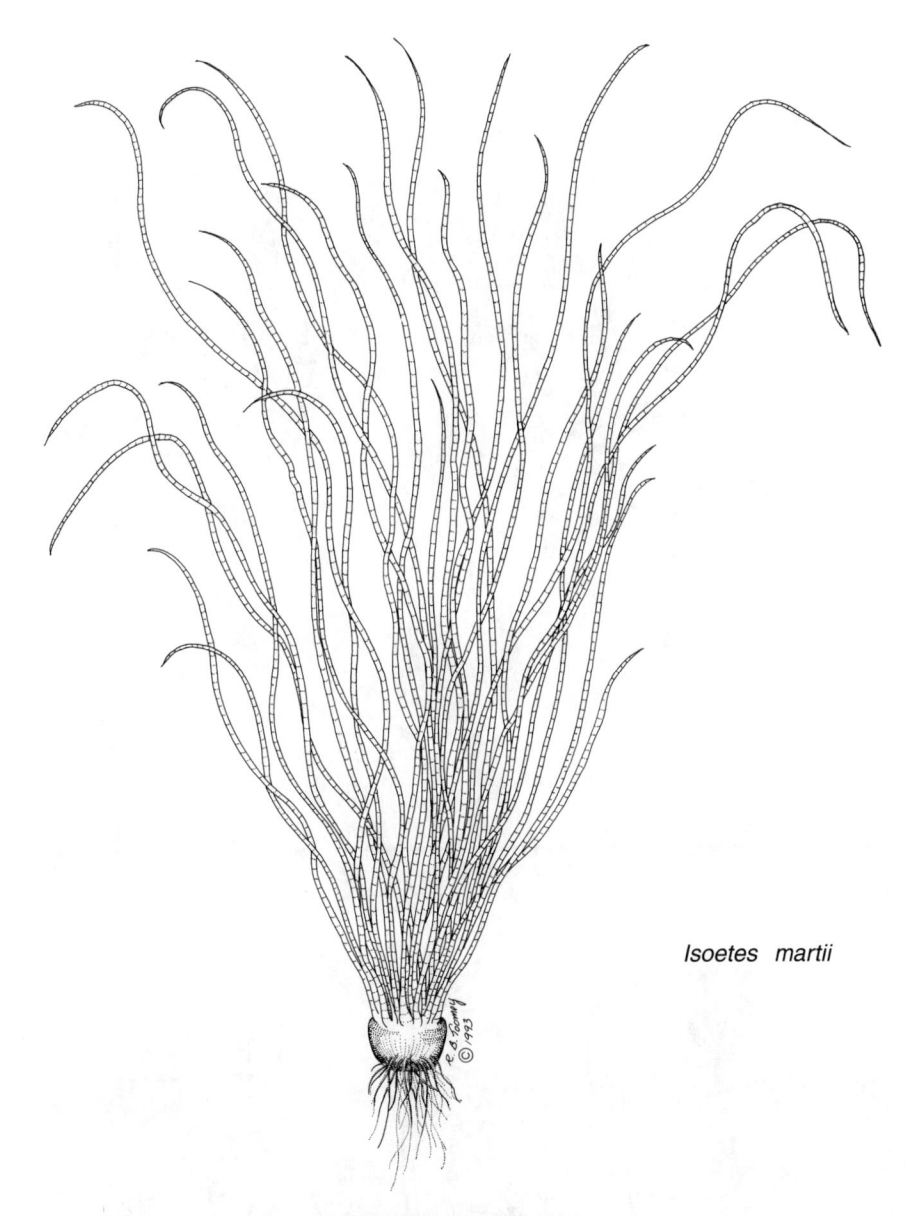

ISOETACEAE

Isoetes martii A. Braun
AREA: Widespread in puddles and ponds in Brazil.
NAME: Batatinha-d'água.
USE: Rhizome used for treating snakebite.

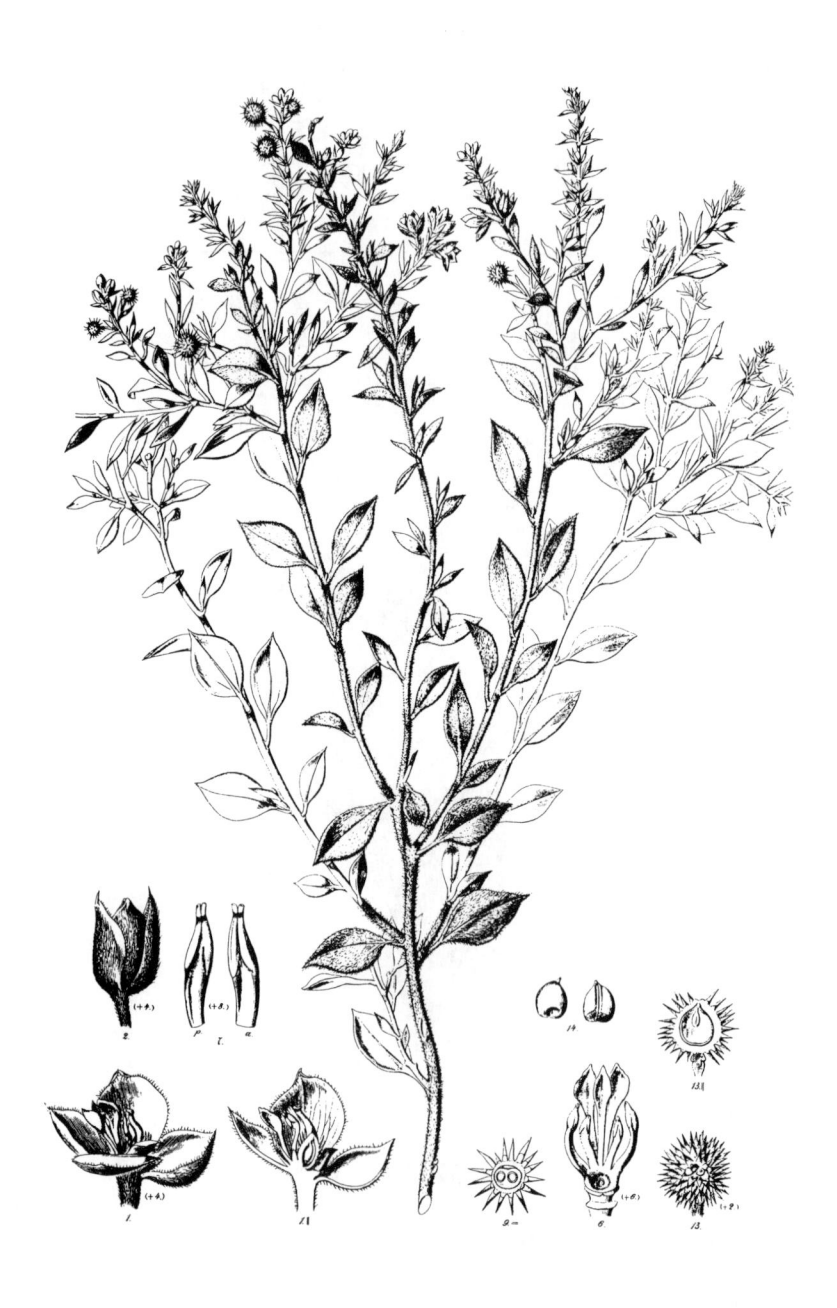

Krameria argentea

KRAMERIACEAE

Krameria argentea Mart.
AREA: Amazonia to Pernam-buco and Goiás.
NAMES: Carrapicho-do-ceará, ratanhia, ratanhia-da-terra, ratanhia-do-ceará.
USES: Root and bark are strongly antidysenteric.
CHEM.: Catechin in root bark (Ref: KRAM 1).

Krameria spartioides Berg
AREA: Northeastern Brazil and Mato Grosso.
NAMES: Ratanhia, ratânia.
USES: Roots are astringent and antidiarrhoeic.

Krameria tomentosa St.-Hil.
AREA: Amazonia to northeast Brazil.
NAMES: Carrapicho-de-cavalo, ratanhia-da-terra.
USES: Powerful astringent used for diarrhoea, hemorrhage, stomatitis, chronic vaginal and urethral catarrhs and in fissures of anus and nipples.

All three mentioned species are considered substitutes for the genuine Peruvian rhatany, *K. triandra* R. & Pav.

Krameriaceae – Reference

KRAM 1. Nierenstein, M. 1931. Rhatany catechin. *J. Chem. Soc.*: 2809.

LAMIACEAE

Coleus barbatus Benth.
AREA: Originally from India, but at present with a large distribution, including in Brazil; grown in gardens as a household remedy.
NAMES: Boldo, falso-boldo, malva-santa.
USES: Tea for stomachache, digestive, hepatic.
CHEM. & PHARM.: *C. barbatus* is often considered a synonym of *C. forskohlii* (Willd.) Briq. The first binomial is maintained here for the species occurring in Brazil, since specimens from Africa were shown to be quite different in chemical composition (Ref: LAMI 1). Compounds isolated from *C. barbatus* are for the most part diterpenes belonging to different structural series (Ref: LAMI 2,3,4,5,6,7,8,9). The labdane diterpene forskolin has raised much interest as a potential drug against hypertension. Its presence in the roots of Brazilian specimens is suspected but has not been confirmed (Ref: LAMI 10). However, hypotensive action in animals has also been shown in at least one of the abietane diterpenoids from Brazilian material (Ref: LAMI 5). An-

other compound of the same class showed antitumor activity (Ref: LAMI 4). A concise review of the subject, including the potentialities of forskolin, has been published (Ref: LAMI 11).

Cunila microcephala Benth.
AREA: Southern campos.
NAME: Poejo.
USES: Infusion for a stimulant, antispasmodic, emmenagogue and antifebrile; also to relieve chronic coughs and as a pulmonary stimulant.

Cunila spicata L.
AREA: São Paulo to Rio Grande do Sul, campo.
NAME: Poejo.
USES: Bechic and sudorific.

Glechon ciliata Benth.
AREA: Minas Gerais to Rio Grande do Sul.
NAME: Mangerona.
USES: Diaphoretic and to combat catarrh.

Glechon spathulata Benth.
AREA: Rio Grande do Sul, campo.
NAME: Mangerona-do-campo.
USES: Stimulant, sudorific and pectoral.

Hyptis atrorubens Poit.
AREA: Pantropical; Amazonia to Bahia, ruderal.
NAME: Hortelã-brava.
USES: Diaphoretic, bechic and antispasmodic.

Hyptis crenata Pohl
AREA: Amazonia to Minas Gerais, campo.
NAMES: Malva-de-marajó, salsa-de-marajó, salva, salva-de-marajó.
USES: Aromatic, stimulant, tonic, sudorific and emmenagogue; also for sore throat, ophthalmia, arthritis and constipation.

Hyptis fasciculata Benth.
AREA: Bahia to Rio Grande do Sul, campo and cerrado.
NAME: Marroio.
USES: Recommended for gout, spasms and respiratory troubles.

Hyptis incana Briq.
AREA: Amazonia.
NAME: Salva-de-marajó.
USES: Used against stomach pains.

LAMIACEAE

Hyptis multiflora Pohl
AREA: Amazonia to São Paulo.
NAME: Betônica-brava.
USES: For gout and dyspepsy; also as tonic.

Hyptis mutabilis (Rich.) Briq.
AREA: Found throughout Brazil.
NAMES: Alafavaca-de-caboclo, alfavacão, mangericão, sambacão, sambacaitá, sambacuité, sambaité.
USES: Tonic, carminative, stomachic. Juice prescribed to remove corneal opacity. Contused leaves reputedly are efficient in curing sores caused by the sting of blowflies, especially on cattle.
CHEM.: Essential oil from the leaves is of varying composition, containing caryophyllene, cineole or alpha-phellandrene as the major component (Ref: LAMI 12,13).

Hyptis plectranthoides Benth.
AREA: Amazonas to Minas Gerais, campo.
NAME: Vassourinha-doce.
USE: Employed as an eyewash.

Hyptis spicigera Lam.
AREA: Bahia, Espírito Santo and Goiás.
NAME: Mentrasto.
USES: Calmative and vulnerary.

Hyptis suaveolens Poit.
AREA: Found almost everywhere in Brazil; in campo, cerrado and as a ruderal.
NAMES: Bamburral, mentrasto-grande.
USES: Bechic, sudorific, antispasmodic and to relieve fits of gout.
CHEM.: The essential oil of the leaves contains cineole as the main constituent (Ref: LAMI 12,13). Non-volatile components include triterpenes (Ref: LAMI 14).

Hyptis umbrosa Salzm.
AREA: Ceará to São Paulo.
NAME: Bamburral.
USES: Stomachic, tonic, carminative, diaphoretic, expectorant and to alleviate headache.

Keithia denudata Benth.
AREA: Minas Gerais, Goiás and São Paulo, campo.
NAME: Poejo-do-campo.
USES: Flower infusion is expectorant and sudorific; also indicated for heart problems. The whole plant is extremely aromatic.

LAMIACEAE

Leonotis nepetaefolia R. Br.
AREA: Neotropical; common in the coastal states of Brazil as a ruderal.
NAMES: Cordão-de-frade, cordão-de-são-francisco, pau-de-praga, rubim.
USES: Antispasmodic, antiasthmatic, tonic, stomachic, antirheumatic, antithermic, antidiarrhoeal, diuretic; recommended for malignant ulcers, incipient elephantiasis and in gynecology against bleeding.
CHEM.: Diterpenes (Ref: LAMI 15,16) and a new coumarin (Ref: LAMI 17) have been isolated.
PHARM.: A study has been done on the effects of stem extracts on smooth and cardiac muscles of laboratory animals (Ref: LAMI 18).

Leonurus sibiricus L.
AREA: Cosmopolitan; ruderal in Brazil.
NAMES: Ana-da-costa, chá-de-frade, cordão-de-são-francisco, erva-de-macaé, erva-do-santo-filho, erva-dos-zangões, erva-macaé, estrela, lavadeira, levantina, marroio, pau-para-tudo, quinino-dos-pobres, rubim, sertão.
USES: Gastralgia, dyspepsia and malarial fever. Flowers employed for treating bronchitis and whooping cough.
CHEM.: Stachydrin has been reported (Ref: LAMI 19).

Leucas martinicensis (Jacq.) R. Br.
AREA: Tropical cosmopolitan; thrives in all Brazilian campos.
NAMES: Catinga-de-mulata, cordão-de-frade, cordão-de-são-francisco, pau-de-praga.
USES: Plant is aromatic, tonic, antispasmodic, useful for neuralgia. Applied locally against tumors. Infusion or decoction of leaves is sudorific and carminative, active in cases of gout and arthritis.

Marsypianthes chamaedrys (Vahl) O. Ktze.
AREA: Ruderal herb, occurring from Amazonia to southern Brazil.
NAMES: Alfavaca-de-cheiro, boia-caá, erva-de-cobra, erva-de-paracari, hortelã-do-brasil, hortelã-do-campo, paracari, paracuru, rabugem-de-cachorro.
USES: Aromatic, carminative, antispasmodic, febrifuge, used in hot baths for articular rheumatism. Tea from roots used for anemia and cephalalgia. Juice of plant taken both internally and externally against snakebite; rubbed on skin against mosquito stings.
PHARM.: Anti-inflammatory and analgesic action confirmed (Ref: LAMI 20).

Mentha crispa L.
AREA: Widespread, though introduced from Europe, particularly in the northeast.
NAMES: Hortelã-de-folha-miúda, hortelã-de-panela, hortelã-rasteira.

USES: The leaves are stomachic and carminative. Dried and reduced to a fine powder, they are prescribed against intestinal protozoa — amoebae and giardia — administered in gelatin capsules or mixed with honey. Cures have been attested in a high percentage of cases, the activity having been confirmed in clinical tests (Ref: LAMI 21).

Ocimum fluminensis Vell.
AREA: Ceará to Rio de Janeiro.
NAMES: Alfavaca, alfavaca-de-cheiro, santa-maria.
USES: Excitant, sudorific, antitussive and against colds; in baths used for rheumatism.

Ocimum micranthum Willd.
AREA: Neotropical; frequent in Brazil.
NAMES: Alfavaca, alfavaca-do-campo, mangericão-grande.
USES: Leaf decoctions are used to treat insect and scorpion stings; diuretic, diaphoretic, carminative, antispasmodic, antiasthmatic. Also used for influenza, common cold, bronchitis, cough and whooping cough.

Other species with the same applications are *O. nudicaule* Benth. and *O. sellowii* Benth., both occurring from São Paulo to Rio Grande do Sul.

Peltodon longipes St.-Hil.
AREA: Southern Brazil, campo and ruderal.
NAMES: Alfavaca-de-cheiro, hortelã-do-campo, santa-maria.
USES: Stimulant and emmenagogue.

Peltodon radicans Pohl
AREA: Common ruderal, throughout Brazil.
NAMES: Hortelã-do-mato, paracari, rabugem-de-cachorro.
USES: Carminative, pectoral, sedative for cough and asthma. For treating dermatoses. Used against scorpion sting and snakebite.
CHEM.: Contains ursolic acid (Ref: LAMI 22).

Lamiaceae – References

LAMI 1. Tandon, J.S., S.B. Katti, P. Rüedi & C.H. Eugster. 1979. Crocetin-dialdehyde from *Coleus forskohlii* Briq., Labiatae. *Helv. Chim. Acta* 62: 2706-2707.

LAMI 2. Wang. A.H.-J., I.C. Paul, R. Zelnik, K. Mizuta & D. Lavie. 1973. Structure and absolute stereochemistry of the diterpenoid barbatusin. *J. Am. Chem. Soc.* 95: 598-600.

LAMI 3. Wang, A.H.-J., I.C. Paul, R. Zelnik, D. Lavie & E.C. Levy. 1974. Structure and stereochemistry of cyclobarbatusin, a diterpenoid containing a four-numbered ring. *J. Am. Chem. Soc.* 96: 580-581.

LAMI 4. Zelnik, R., D. Lavie, E.C. Levy, A.H.-J. Wang & I.C. Paul. 1977. Barbatusin and cyclobarbatusin, two novel diterpenoids from *Coleus barbatus* Benth. *Tetrahedron 33*: 1457-1467.

LAMI 5. Kelecom, A. 1983. Isolation, structure determination, and absolute configuration of Barbatusol, a new bioactive diterpene with a rearranged abietane skeleton from the labiate *Coleus barbatus*. *Phytochemistry* 23: 1677-1679.

LAMI 6. Kelecom, A. 1984. An abietane diterpene from the labiate *Coleus barbatus*. *Phytochemistry 23*: 1677-1679.

LAMI 7. Kelecom, A. & T.C. dos Santos. 1985. Cariocal, a new seco-abietane diterpene from the labiate *Coleus barbatus*. *Tetrahedron Lett. 26*: 3659-3662.

LAMI 8. Kelecom, A., T.C. dos Santos & W.L.B. Medeiros. 1986. On the structure and absolute configuration of (-)-20-deoxocarnosol. *An. Acad. Bras. Ci. 58*: 53-59.

LAMI 9. Kelecom, A. & W.L.B. Medeiros. 1980. Revision of the stereo-chemistry at C-6 of the 6-hydroxycarnosol, a diterpene from the false boldo *Coleus barbatus* Benth. (Labiatae). *An. Acad. Brasil. Ci. 58*: 369-374.

LAMI 10. Castellón, A.F., M.R. Vale, M.I.L. Machado & F.J.A. Matos. 1987. Alguns constiuintes químicos de *Coleus barbatus* Benth. cultivado em Fortaleza (CE). *Ciência e Cultura* (S. Paulo) *39* (Supl.): 535.

LAMI 11. Valdés III, L.J., S.G. Mislankar & A.G. Paul. 1987. *Coleus barbatus* (=*C. forskohlii*) (Lamiaceae) and the potential new drug Forskolin (Coleonol). *Economic Botany 41*: 474-483.

LAMI 12. Craveiro, A.A., A.G. Fernandes, C.H.S. Andrade, F.J.A. Matos, J.W. Alencar & M.I.L. Machado. 1981. *Oleos Essenciais de Plantas do Nordeste*. Federal University of Ceará (Fortaleza), p. 68.

LAMI 13. Luz, A.I.R., M.G.B. Zoghbi, L.S. Ramos, J.G.S. Maia & M.L. da Silva. 1984. Essential oils of some Amazonian Labiatae. 1. Genus *Hyptis*. *J. Nat. Prod. 47*: 745-747.

LAMI 14. Misra, T.N., R.S. Sing, T.N. Ojha & J. Upadhyay. 1981. Chemical constituents of *Hyptis suaveolens*. Part. I. Spectral and biological studies on a triterpene acid. *J. Nat. Prod. 44*: 735-738.

LAMI 15. Baghy, M.O., C.R. Smith & I.A. Watt. 1965. Labdallenic acid. A new allenic acid from *Leonotis nepetaefolia* seed oil. *J. Org. Chem. 30*: 422.

LAMI 16. Machand, P.S. 1973. Methoxynepetofolin, a new labdane diterpene from *Leonotis nepetaefolia*. *Tetrahedron Lett. 21*: 1907.

LAMI 17. Purushothanan, K.K., S. Vasanth, J.D. Connoly & C. Labbe. 1976. 4,6,7-Trimethoxy-5-methoxychromen-2-one: a new coumarin from *Leonotis nepetaefolia*. *J. Chem. Soc. Perkin 1*: 2594.

LAMI 18. Calixto, J.B., R. A. Yunes & G.A. Rae. 1991. Effect of crude extracts from *Leonotis nepetaefolia* (Labiatae) on rat and guinea-pig smooth muscle and rat cardiac muscle. *J. Pharmacol. 43*: 529-534.

LAMI 19. Murakami, S. 1943. Stachydrin in *Leonurus sibiricus*. *Acta Phytochim.* (Japan) *13*: 161-184.

LAMI 20. Pereira, E.F.R. & N.A. Pereira. 1988. Atividade antiinflamatória e analgésica de um extrato etanólico do paracari ou boia-caá (*Marsypianthes hyptoides* Mart., Lamiaceae). *An. Acad. Brasil. Ci. 60*: 263-264.

LAMI 21. Santana, C.F., E.R. Almeida, E.R. dos Santos & I.A. Souza. 1992. Action of *Mentha crispa* hydroalcoholic extracts in patients bearing intestinal protozoa. *Fitoterapia 63*: 409-410.

LAMI 22. Zelnik, R., A.K. Matida & S. Panizza. 1978/79. Chemistry of the Brazilian Labiatae. The occurrence of ursolic acid in *Peltodon radicans* Pohl. *Mem. Inst. Butantan 42*: 357-361.

LAURACEAE

Aiovea brasiliensis Meissn.

AREA: Amazonia to Bahia, forest.

NAME: Amajouva.

USES: The crushed leaves are used to cure ulcers.

Aiovea meissneri Mez

AREA: Ceará to Alagoas, forest.
NAMES: Canela-amarela-de-cheiro, louro-amarelo-de-cheiro.
USES: Bark is depurative, antirheumatic. Infusion of wood is reputedly stomachic.

Aniba canelilla (H.B.K.) Mez

AREA: Amazonia, forest on dry soil.
NAMES: Casca-do-maranhão, casca-preciosa, folha-preciosa, preciosa.
USES: Bark and leaf are excitant, eupeptic, antispasmodic, pectoral, calmative; recommended for dropsy, arthritis, chronic catarrh, syphilis, leucorrhoea, aerophagy and heart ailments.
CHEM.: The strong cinnamon smell of the bark is due to a peculiar nitrocompound, 1-nitro-2-phenylethane (Ref: LAUR 1). Other volatile constituents are eugenol and methyl-eugenol (Ref: LAUR 2).

Aniba permollis (Nees) Mez

AREA: Amazonia, forest.
NAMES: Aiúba, ajuba, aniúba, au-uva.
USES: Bark is aromatic. Wood decoction reputedly is depurative and antirheumatic. Seeds are stomachic and carminative.
CHEM.: Alpha-pyrones have been identified (Ref: LAUR 3).

Aniba puchury-minor (Mart.) Mez

AREA: Amazonia, forest.
NAMES: Puxuri-bravo, puxuri-do-maranhão, puxuri-mirim, puxuri-pequeno.
USES: Bark is aromatic. Seeds are used for dyspepsy, diarrhoea and leucorrhoea.

Aniba rosaeodora Ducke

AREA: Amazonia, forest. Threatened due to over-exploitation for the extraction of "rosewood oil."
NAME: Pau-rosa.
USES: Medicinally, the oil from the wood, soaked up in cotton-wool, is used to relieve pain after tooth extractions. The main industrial use, however, is in perfumery.
CHEM.: Main component of the essential oil steam-distilled from the wood is the sesquiterpene alcohol linalol. Fixed constituents are mainly pyrones, including one pseudo-alkaloid, anibine (Ref: LAUR 4,5); another pseudo-alkaloid is a nitrogen containing diaryl ketone, duckein (Ref: LAUR 6). The chemistry of the essential oils of many *Aniba* species has been investigated (Ref: LAUR 31).

The tree occurring in the state of Pará is often considered a distinct species, *A. duckei* Kosterm.

LAURACEAE

Cassytha filiformis L.
AREA: Cosmopolitan, widespread in Brazil.
NAMES: Cipó-chumbo, erva-chumbo, erva-de-chumbo.
USES: Small branches are made into an agreeable drink for improving the blood and against hemorrhage.
CHEM.: Contains aporphine and oxoaporphine bases (Ref: LAUR 7), apart from dulcitol (Ref: LAUR 8).

Cryptocarya guyanensis Meissn.
AREA: Pará, forest.
NAME: Coaxicó.
USES: Fruits are used as an excitant and carminative.

Cryptocarya mandioccana Meissn.
AREA: Espírito Santo and Rio de Janeiro, forest.
NAME: Cajati.
USES: Bark is bitter and aromatic, prescribed for colics and dysentery.

Cryptocarya minima Mez
AREA: Rio de Janeiro, forest.
NAMES: Canela-abacate, canela-do-brejo, louro-abacate.
USES: Decoction of the leaves is used to clean ulcers. Seeds for a tonic.

Cryptocarya moschata Nees & Mart. ex Nees
AREA: Bahia to Rio Grande do Sul, forest.
NAMES: Noz-moscada-do-brasil (meaning Brazilian nutmeg).
USES: Fruits are carminative and excitant.
CHEM.: The essential oil of the leaves contains linalol as the main constituent (Ref: LAUR 9).

Dicypellium caryophyllatum Nees & Mart.
AREA: Amazonia, forest. Almost extinct due to over-exploitation. This exploitation goes back to colonial times, when the bark was exported to Europe in great quantities for use as a flavoring.
NAMES: Caneleira-cravo, craveiro-do-maranhão, louro-cheiroso, louro-cravo, cravo-do-mato, pau-cravo, cravinho.
USES: Bark reminiscent of cinnamon as to scent, and of cloves as to flavor; tonic, stimulant, also employed as spice.
CHEM.: The essential oil contains eugenol as its main constituent, accompanied by smaller amounts of methyleugenol (Ref: LAUR 10,11).

Licaria camara (Schomb.) Kosterm.
AREA: Amazonia, forest.
NAMES: Cambará-de-cheiro, itaúba-camará.
USES: The grated fruits, made into a tea, are excitant, aromatic, carminative, antispasmodic, and antidiarrhoeic.

Licaria canella (Meissn.) Kosterm.
AREA: Amazonia, forest.
NAME: Canela-caixeta.
USES: Infusion from wood is recommended for rheumatism.
CHEM.: Wood contains neolignans (Ref: LAUR 12,13).

Licaria puchury-major (Mart.) Kosterm.
AREA: Amazonia, forest.
NAMES: Louro-puxuri, pixurim, puxuri, puxurim.
USES: Grated seeds are aromatic, tonic, stimulant, used for dyspepsy, dysentery and leucorrhoea, as well as a calmative to treat insomnia, nervousness and irritability.
CHEM.: Seeds (Ref: LAUR 14,17), leaves (Ref: LAUR 15) and wood (Ref: LAUR 16) contain arylpropanoids, mainly safrol, eugenol and methyleugenol, besides terpene alcohols, such as cineol and terpineol.
PHARM.: An essential oil fraction from the seeds reduced motor activity and anesthetized mice and protected the animals against transcorneal electroshock. A hydrolate from the same material also reduced motor activity but did not anesthetize and did not protect against convulsions induced by electric shock (Ref: LAUR 17).

Mezilaurus crassiramea (Meissn.) Taub. ex Mez
AREA: Goiás, cerrado.
NAME: Canela-de-goiás.
USE: Leaves employed as an antileucorrhoeic.

Nectandra canescens Nees
AREA: Amazonia to Minas Gerais and São Paulo, forest.
NAMES: Caneleira-do-mato, louro-bravo, mucataia.
USES: Wood decoction is considered depurative. Bark is aromatic, excitant.

Nectandra globosa (Aubl.) Mez
AREA: Amazonia to Bahia, forest.
NAMES: Canela-preta, cedro-preto, louro-vermelho.
USES: Bark is aromatic, tonic, carminative and excitant.

Nectandra leucantha Nees
AREA: Alagoas to Santa Catarina, forest.
NAMES: Canela-amarela, canela-da-capoeira, canela-mirim, canela-seca.
USES: Root-bark is tonic. Leaves are antiblennorhagic and antileucorrhoeic. Fruits used against leucorrhoea and flatulence.

Nectandra leucothyrsus Meissn.
AREA: Minas Gerais and Rio de Janeiro to Santa Catarina, forest.

LAURACEAE

NAMES: Anhuiba-do-brejo, canela-branca, canela-da-vargem, canela-de-catarro, louro-anhuiba.
USES: Gum from bark used to treat ulcers.

Nectandra pichurim (H.B.K.) Mez
AREA: Amazonia and central Brazil, forest.
NAMES: Louro-pixurim, noz-moscada-do-pará, puxuri.
USES: Leaves and berries are aromatic, employed to soothe colics and upset stomach.
CHEM.: Isoboldine has been identified (Ref: LAUR 18).

Nectandra puberula Nees
AREA: Alagoas to São Paulo and Mato Grosso.
NAMES: Canela-amarga, canela-parda, louro-amargoso, louro-preto, pau-de-santa-ana, surineia.
USES: Bark used as appetizer, stomachic, antidyspeptic, and antidysenteric.

Nectandra turbacensis Nees
AREA: Amazonia, forest.
NAME: Cigua.
USES: Fruits are aromatic, carminative, and antispasmodic.
CHEM.: Lignans have been identified (Ref: LAUR 19).

Ocotea cujumary Mart.
AREA: Amazonia, campo and forest.
NAMES: Cujumaru, cuiumaru, cuimari, louro-cujumari.
USES: Bark is aromatic, excitant, useful to help digestion. Berries are aromatic, tonic, used to improve appetite, digestion and bowel movements.

Ocotea cymbarum H.B.K.
AREA: Amazonia, forest.
NAMES: Canela-sassafrás-preta, louro-inhamuí, louro-mamori, hamuí, pau-de-gasolina, pau-de-querosene, pau-sassafrás, sassafrás-do-amazonas, sassafrás-do-pará.
USES: The bark has the same uses as that of the preceding species. From holes bored into the bark and trunk oozes a resinous, oily liquid used for treating various skin diseases, such as pityriasis of the scalp.
CHEM.: The fluid released from the bore-holes in the stem is made up mainly of alpha and beta-pinene, thus being, chemically, an authentic oil of turpentine (Ref: LAUR 19,20). Dimers of eugenol in wood (Ref: LAUR 21,22).

Ocotea guianensis Aubl.
AREA: Amazonia, forest.
NAMES: Cujumari-rana, cujumari-da-guiana, cujumari-mirim, louro-branco, louro-das-guianas, louro-tamancão, tamanqueira.
USES: Bark is aromatic, excitant, used to soften abscesses and swollen glands. Leaves are aromatic, mucilaginous, used for the same purpose. Fruits contain an essential oil used for rheumatic pains.
CHEM.: Ferulic acid esters from the wood (Ref: LAUR 23) and sesquiterpene lactones from the bark (Ref: LAUR 24) have been described.

Ocotea opifera Mart.
AREA: Amazonia, forest.
NAMES: Canela-de-cheiro, caneleira-de-cheiro, louro.
USES: Wood oil is resolvent. Oil from fruit applied for rheumatism, arthritis and paralysis.

Ocotea pretiosa (Nees & Mart.) Benth. & Hook.
AREA: Bahia to Rio Grande do Sul, forest.
NAMES: Canela-cheirosa, canela-funcho, canela-sassafrás, canelinha, casca-cheirosa, casca-preciosa, louro-cheiroso, preciosa, sassafrás.
USES: A southern substitute for the northern *Aniba canelilla*. Root-bark and leaves are used to induce sweating. Diuretic and antirheumatic.
CHEM.: This is the "Brazilian sassafras," safrol representing 84% or more of the essential oil distilled from the wood (Ref: LAUR 25,26). A second variety is known, which contains methyleugenol as its major oil component (Ref: LAUR 27). Several propenyl and allylbenzenes have been extracted from the wood (Ref: LAUR 28).

Ocotea pulchella Mart.
AREA: Espírito Santo to Mato Grosso and Rio Grande do Sul, forest.
NAMES: Canela-do-brejo, canela-lageana, canela-preta, caneleira, canelinha.
USES: Bark and leaves are stomachic, emmenagogue and used to strengthen the womb.

Ocotea rodiei (Schomb.) Mez
AREA: Amazonia, forest.
NAMES: Bebiru, bebiri, canela-bebiru, canela-limão, coração-verde.
USES: Bark is aromatic, bitter, astringent, calmative, tonic, febrifuge, also employed to relieve neuralgia, migraine and arthritic pains.

Ocotea spectabilis (Meissn.) Mez
AREA: Maranhão to São Paulo and Mato Grosso, forest.
NAMES: Canela-braúna, canela-mescla, canela-preta, louro-preto.
USES: Root-bark for a bitter tonic.

LAURACEAE

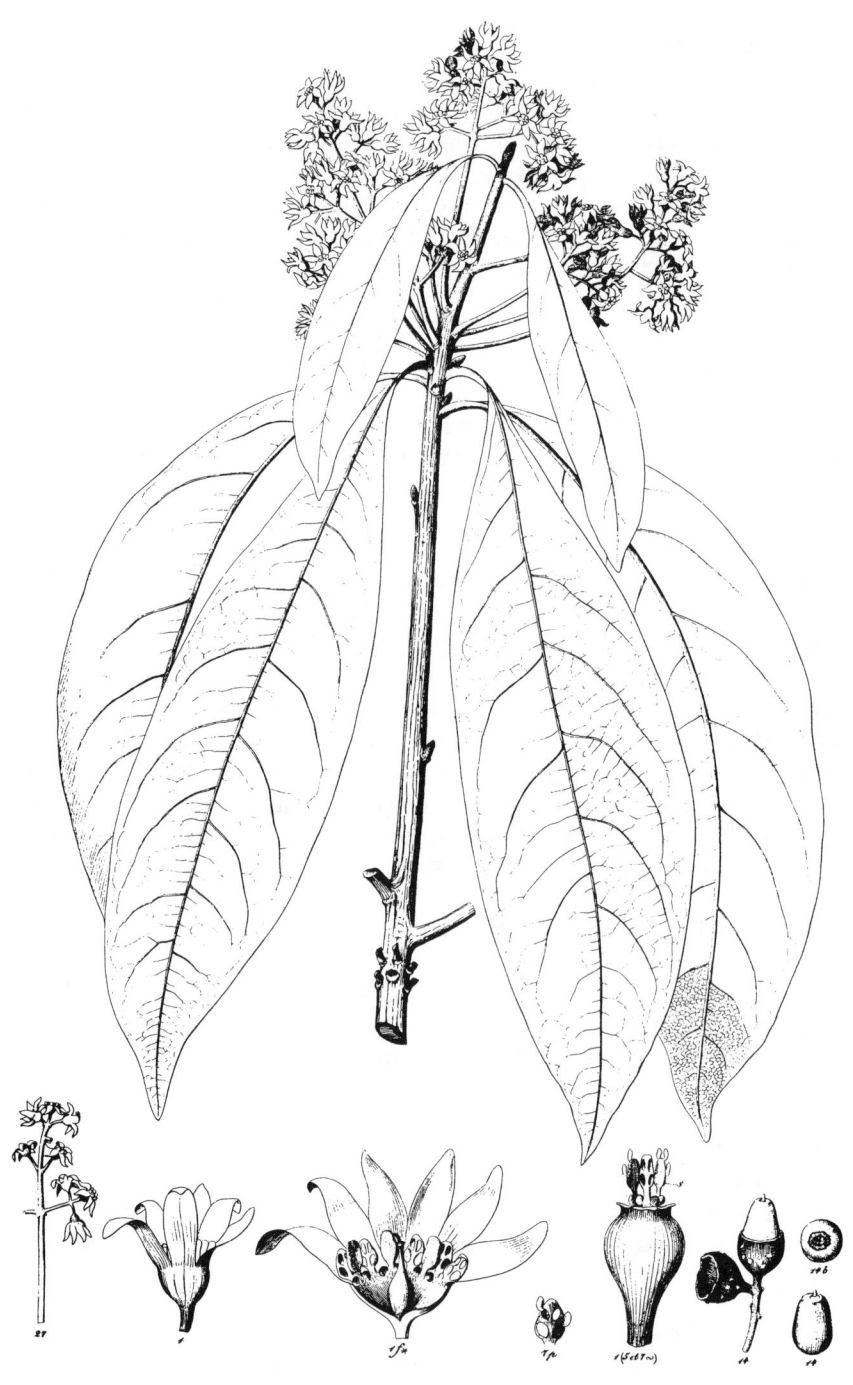

Ocotea pretiosa

Ocotea squarrosa Mart. ex Nees
AREA: Rio de Janeiro, forest.
NAME: Canela-amargosa.
USES: Bark is tonic. Leaves employed for leucorrhoea.

Ocotea teleiandra (Messn.) Mez
AREA: Bahia to Santa Catarina, forest.
NAMES: Canela-iacuá, canela-limão, louro.
USES: Decoction of bark is bitter, used for chest pain. Leaves are diaphoretic.
CHEM.: The essential oil is made predominantly of benzyl benzoate and benzyl salicilate (Ref: LAUR 29). Alkaloids have been identified in extract (Ref: LAUR 30).

Pleurothyrium cuneifolium Nees
AREA: Amazonia, forest.
NAMES: Abacaterana, louro-abacate.
USES: Leaves and young shoots are recommended for liver disorders.

Lauraceae – References

LAUR 1. Gottlieb, O.R. & M.T. Magalhães. 1959. Occurrence of 1-nitro-2-phenylethane in *Ocotea pretiosa* and *Aniba canelilla*. *J. Org. Chem.* 24: 2070-2071.

LAUR 2. Gottlieb, O.R. & M.T. Magalhães. 1960. Essential oil of the bark and wood of *Aniba canelilla*. *Perf. Essent. Oil Record* 51: 69-70.

LAUR 3. Rezende, C.M.A.M., M. V. von Bülow, O.R. Gottlieb, S.L.V. Pinho & A.I. da Rocha. 1971. The 2-pyrones of *Aniba* species. *Phytochemistry* 10: 3167-3172.

LAUR 4. Mors, W.B., O.R. Gottlieb & C. Djerassi. 1957. The chemistry of rosewood. Isolation and structure of anibine and 4-methoxyparacotoin. *J. Am. Chem. Soc.* 79: 4507-4511.

LAUR 5. Mors, W.B., M.T. Magalhães & O.R. Gottlieb. 1962. Naturally occurring aromatic dreivatives of monocyclic alpha-pyrones. In: L. Zechmeister (ed.), PROGRESS IN THE CHEMISTRY OF ORGANIC NATURAL PRODUCTS. Vol. 20, pp. 131-164. Springer-Verlag, Vienna.

LAUR 6. Corrêa, D.B. & O.R. Gottlieb. 1975. Duckein, an alkaloid from *Aniba duckei*. *Phytochemistry* 14: 271-272.

LAUR 7. Cava, M.P., K.V. Rao, V. Kota, E. Douglas & J.A. Weisbach. 1968. Alkaloids of *Cassytha americana* Nees. *J. Org. Chem.* 33: 2443-2446.

LAUR 8. Fuzikawa, F., J. Nakamura & K. Asami. 1940. On the occurrence of dulcitol in *Cassytha filiformis* L. *J. Pharm. Soc. Japan* 60: 209.

LAUR 9. Naves, Y.-R., H. Magalhães Alves, V.H. Arndt, O.R. Gottlieb & M.T. Magalhães. 1963. Études sur les matières végétales volatiles. CLXXXV. Sur les huiles essentielles de deux espèces appartenant au genre *Cryptocarya*. *Helv. Chim. Acta* 46: 1056.

LAUR 10. Alencar, R., R. Alves de Lima, R.G. Campos Corrês, O.R. Gottlieb, M. Leão da Silva, M.C. Marx, J.G.S. Maia, M.T. Magalhães & R.M.V. Assumpção. 1971. Oleos essenciais de plantas brasileiras. *An. Acad. Bras. Ci.* 44 (Supl.): 312-314.

LAUR 11. Craveiro, A.A., A.G. Fernandes, C.H. Souza Andrade, F.J.A. Matos, J.W. Alencar & M.I.L. Machado. 1981. Óleos Essenciais de Lauráceas. *In*: ÓLEOS ESSENCIAIS DE PLANTAS DO NORDESTE. Universidade Federal do Ceará, Fortaleza. p. 76.

LAUR 12. Giesbrecht, A.M., N.C. Franca & O.R. Gottlieb. 1974. The neolignans of *Licaria canella*. *Phytochemistry* 13: 2285-2293.

LAUR 13. Cavalcante, S.H., A.M. Giesbrecht, O.R. Gottlieb, J.C. Mour o & M. Yoshida. 1976. Lanthanide shift reagents in neolignan analysis: Revision of structure of canellin-B. *Phytochemistry* 17: 983-985.

LAUR 14. Gottlieb, O.R. 1956. Estudo do óleo essencial da fava do puxuri. *In*: Estudo de Plantas Odoríferas Brasileiras. *Boletim do Instituto de Química Agrícola* (Rio de Janeiro) nº *43*: 14-17.

LAUR 15. Seabra, A.P., E.C. Guimarães & W.B. Mors. 1967. Estudo do óleo essencial de puxuri por cromatografia gás-líquido. *An. Assoc. Bras. Quím. 26*: 73-78.

LAUR 16. Leão da Silva, M., J.G.S. Maia, C.M.A.M. Rezende & O.R. Gottlieb. 1973. Arylpropanoids from *Licaria puchury-major*. *Phytochemistry 12*: 471-472.

LAUR 17. Carlini, E.A., A.B. de Oliveira & G.G. de Oliveira. 1983. Psychopharmacological effects of the essential oil fraction and of the hydrolate obtained from the seeds of *Licaria puchury-major*. *J. Ethnopharmacol. 8*: 225-236.

LAUR 18. Ferrari, G., O. Fervidi & M. Ferrari. 1971. Occurrence of isoboldine in *Nectandra pichurim*. *Phytochemistry 10*: 465-466.

LAUR 19. Carvalho, M.G., M. Yoshida, O.R. Gottlieb & H.E. Gottlieb. 1987. Lignans from *Nectandra turbacensis*. *Phytochemistry 26*: 265-267.

LAUR 20. Botafogo Gonçalves, N. 1933. Pinen aus der Lauracee *Nectandra elaiophora* Barb. Rodr. *Arch. Pharm. 271*: 461.

LAUR 21. Naves, Y.-R. 1952. Louro inhamuy oil of Amazonas. *Perf. Essent. Oil Record 43*: 38,39,53.

LAUR 22. Diaz, A.P., H.E. Gottlieb & O.R. Gottlieb. 1980. Dehydro-dieugenols from *Ocotea cymbarum*. *Phytochemistry 19*: 681-682.

LAUR 23. Diaz, A.M.P., P.P. Diaz, Z.S. Ferreira, O.R. Gottlieb, R.A. de Lima & S.H. Cavalvante. 1977. The chemistry of Brazilian Lauraceae. XLVII. Ferulic esters from *Endlicheria* and *Ocotea* species. *Acta Amazonica* (Manaus) 7: 292-293.

LAUR 24. Roque, N.F., Z.S. Ferreira, O.R. Gottlieb, R.L. Stephens & E. Wenkert. 1976. The chemistry of Brazilian Lauraceae. Part. I. The structure of ocotealactol, a new eudesmanolide. *Rev. Latinoamer. Quím. 9*: 25-27.

LAUR 25. Machado, R.D. 1945. Algumas cosiderações sobre o óleo de sassafrás. *Bol. Divulgação Instituto Nacional de Oleos* (Rio de Janeiro) nº *3*: 21-30.

LAUR 26. Hickey, M.J. 1948. Investigation of the chemical constituents of Brazilian sassafras oil. *J. Org. Chem. 13*: 443-446.

LAUR 27. Mors, W.B., M.T. Magalhães & O.R. Gottlieb. 1959. Physiological varieties of *Ocotea pretiosa*. *Perf. Essent. Oil Record 50*: 26-27.

LAUR 28. Aiba, O.J., O.R. Gottlieb & M.T. Magalhães. 1976. *In*: "Tabulated phytochemical reports." *Phytochemistry 15*: 2025-2028.

LAUR 29. Naves, Y.-R., O.R. Gottlieb & M.T. Magalhães. 1961. Études sur les matières végétales volatiles. CLXXVII. Sur l'huile essentielle d'*Ocotea teleiandra* (Meissn.) Mez. *Helv. Chim. Acta 44*: 1121-1123.

LAUR 30. Vilegas, J.H.Y. & O.R. Gottlieb. 1992. Benzylisoquinoline alkaloids from *Ocotea teleiandra*. *Rev. Latinoamer. Quím. 23*: 18-19.

LAUR 31. Alpande de Moraes, A., C.M.A.M. Rezende, M.V. von Bülow, J.C. Mourão, O.R. Gottlieb, M.C. Marx, A.I. da Rocha & M.T. Magalhães. 1972. Óleos essenciais de espécies do gênero *Aniba*. *Acta Amazonica 2* (l): 41-44.

LECYTHIDACEAE

Bertholletia excelsa Humb. & Bonpl.
AREA: Amazonia, forest.
NAMES: Castanha-do-pará, castanheira-do-pará (English: Brazil nut).
USES: Tea prepared from fruit used as a cure for gastralgia.

Cariniana legalis (Mart.) O. Ktze.
AREA: Bahia to Rio Grande do Sul and Mato Grosso, forest.

LECYTHIDACEAE

Bertholletia excelsa

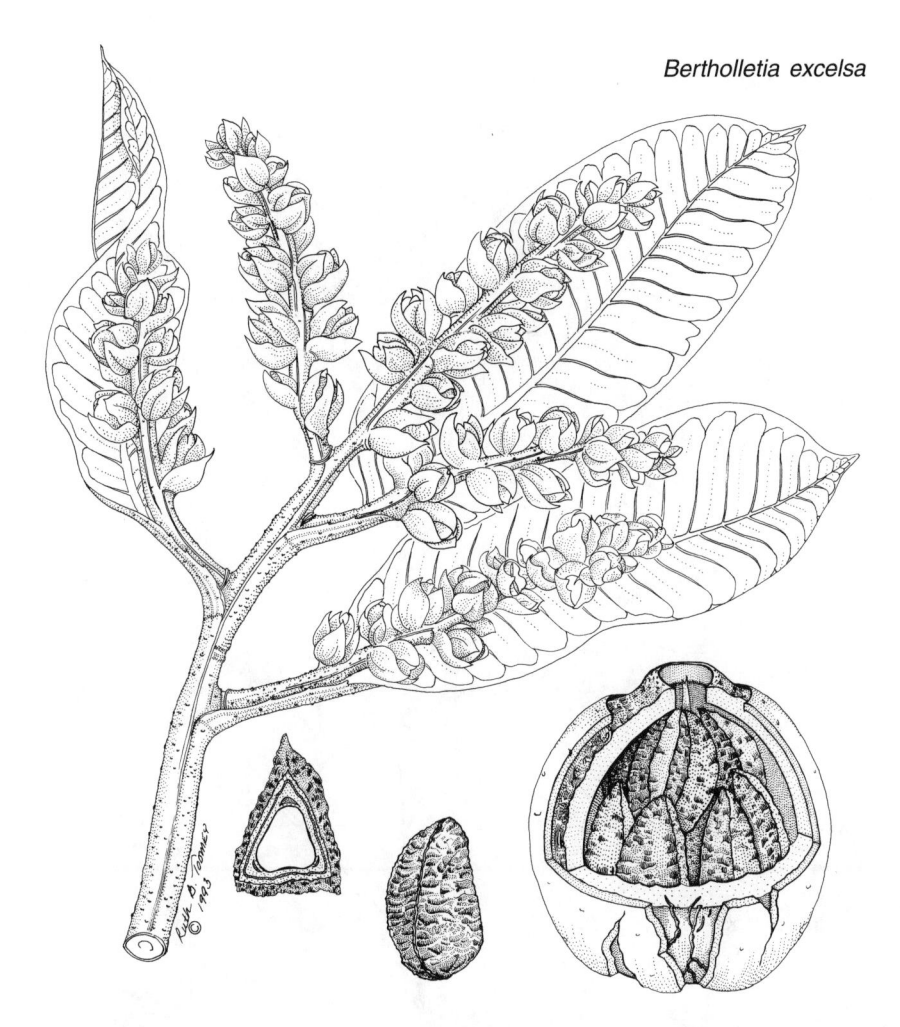

NAMES: Caixão, cengolo-de-porco, estopeira, jequitibá-branco, jequitibá-cedro, jequitibá-rosa.
USES: Bark is astringent, taken for diarrhoea and sore throat.

Gustavia hexapetala (Aubl.) J.E. Smith
AREA: Amazonia, forest.
NAME: Jeniparana.
USES: Root-bark is tonic and laxative, said to be excellent for liver ailments. Leaves externally applied for liver obstruction and to reduce ulcers. Fruits are emetic, thought to be poisonous, sometimes used as a fish poison.

Lecythis amara Aubl.
AREA: Amazonia, forest.

LECYTHIDACEAE

Cariniana legalis

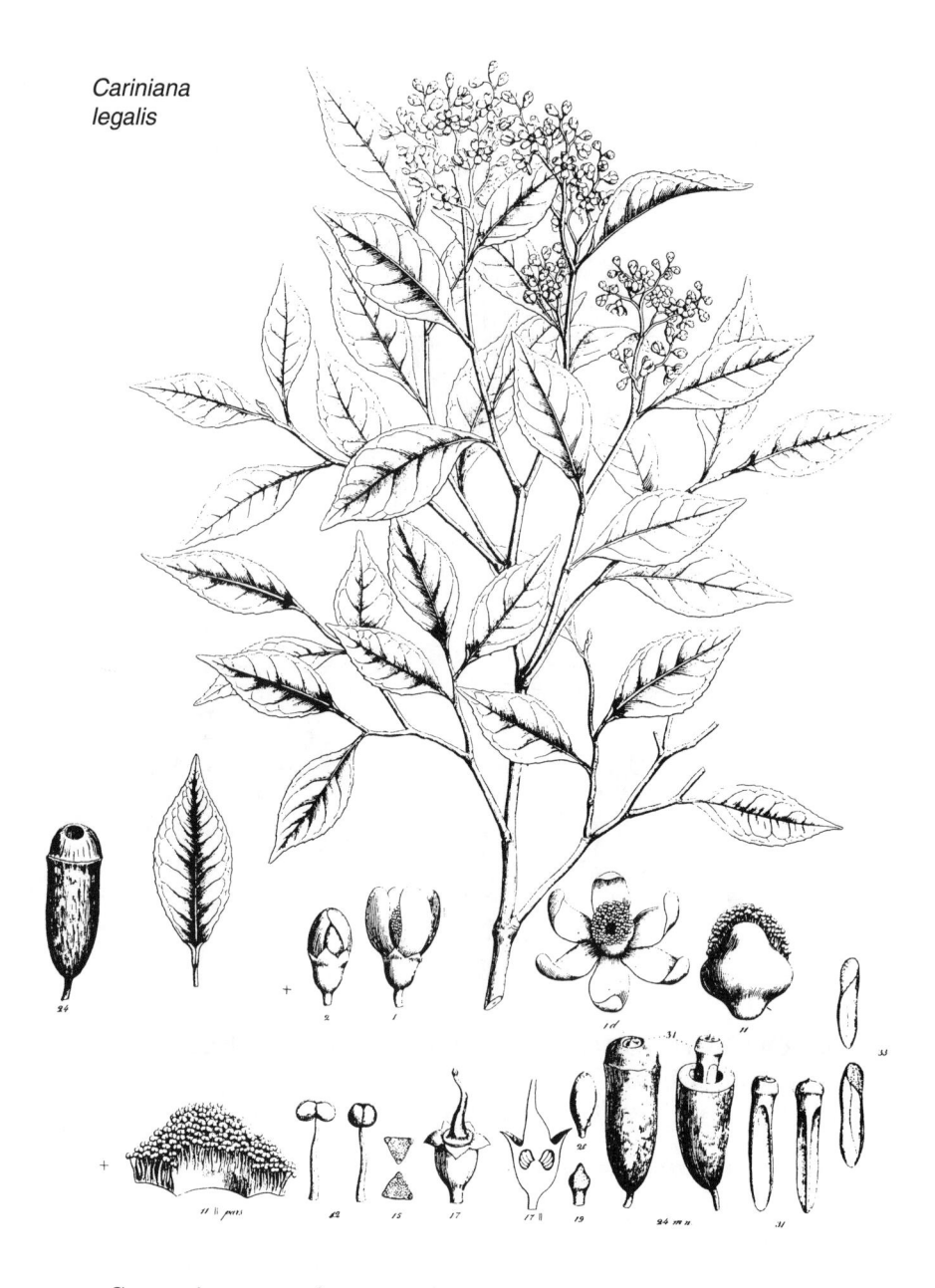

NAMES: Sapucaia, sapucaia-amargosa.
USES: Bark used to check diarrhoea.

Lecythis pisonis Camb.
AREA: Amazonia, forest.

NAME: Castanha-sapucaia.
USES: Tea made from bark is used for coughs; juice from bark to alleviate itch.

LEMNACEAE

Lemna minor L.
AREA: Widely dispersed in ponds.
NAMES: Lentilha-d'água, lentilha-d'água-caparosa, pasta-miúda (English: duckweed).
USES: Whole plants are contused and applied locally to mature tumors.
CHEM.: The composition of the cell wall polysaccharide of this and other Lemnaceae species has been studied, apiose, a branched-chain sugar, being an important constituent (Ref: LEMN 1,2). Flavonoid patterns have been surveyed, revealing a significant presence of C-glycosylflavones (Ref: LEMN 3). Unusual oxygenated fatty acids have been identified (Ref: LEMN 4,5).

Lemnaceae – References

LEMN 1. Duff, R.B. 1965. The occurrence of apiose in *Lemna* (duckweed) and other angiosperms. *Biochem. J. 94*: 768-772.
LEMN 2. van Beusekom, C.F. 1967. Ueber einige Apiose-Vorkommnisse bei den *Helobiae*. *Phytochemistry 6*: 573-576.
LEMN 3. McClure, J.W. & R.E. Alston. 1966. A chemotaxonomic study of Lemnaceae. *Am. J. Bot. 53*: 849-860.
LEMN 4. Previtera, L. & P. Monaco. 1983. Fatty acid composition in *Lemna minor*. Characterization of a novel hydroxy C_{16} acid. *Phytochemistry 22*: 1445-1446.
LEMN 5. Previtera, L. & P. Monaco. 1987. Further oxygenated fatty acids from *Lemna minor*. *J. Nat. Prod. 50*: 807-810.

LILIACEAE

Cordyline dracaenoides Kunth
AREA: Southern Brazil.
NAMES: Coqueiro-de-venus, dracena.
USES: Anti-inflammatory; tea from rhizome used for treatment of rheumatism and arthritis.
CHEM.: Steroids and steroidal saponins in rhizome (Ref: LILI 1).
PHARM.: Antioedematogenic action observed in rhizome extract; root extract is central nervous system (CNS) depressant (Ref: LILI 1).

Herreria salsaparilha Mart.
AREA: Bahia to São Paulo and Mato Grosso, forest.
NAMES: Japecanga, salsa-de-espinho, salsa-do-campo, salsaparrilha.
USES: Roots are depurative, sudorific, diuretic, prescribed to cure dermatoses, syphilis, gout and rheumatism.

LILIACEAE

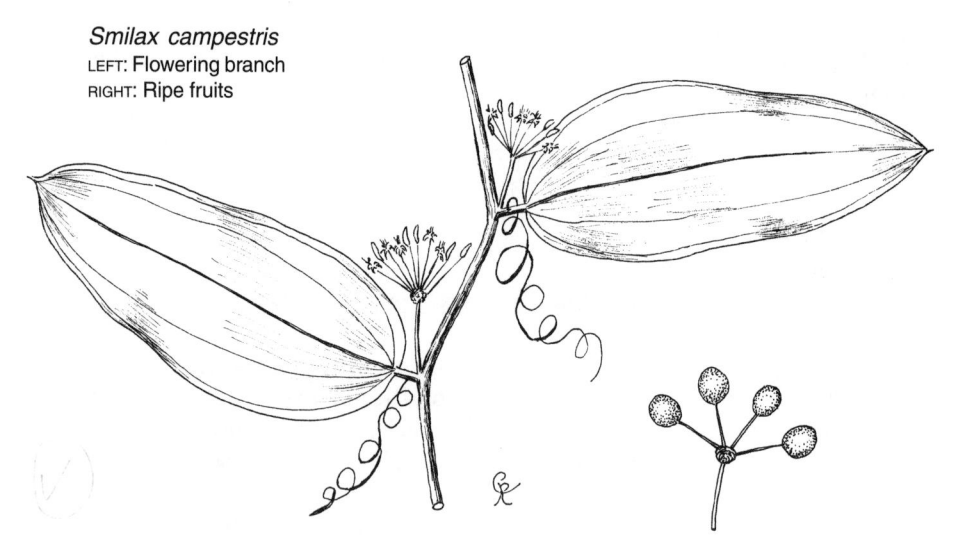

Smilax campestris
LEFT: Flowering branch
RIGHT: Ripe fruits

Smilax campestris Gris.
AREA: Central and southern Brazil, cerrado and campo.
NAME: Japecanga.
USES: Root decoctions are antisyphilitic, anti-goutose and antirheumatic.

Smilax longifolia Rich.
AREA: Amazonia, forest.
NAMES: Cipó-em, japecanga-vermelha, salsa-do-rio-novo, salsaparrilha.
USES: This is one of several *Smilax* species which, under the name "sarsaparilla," were regarded as a remedy for syphilis and rheumatism, scrofula, gout and skin afflictions. It was a Brazilian export article during colonial times and well into the 19th and 20th centuries. Identical in action and uses is *S. brasiliensis* Spreng. (Minas Gerais and São Paulo).
CHEM.: The main characteristic constituents of sarsaparilla roots are glycosides of the steroids smilagenin and sarsasapogenin (Ref: LILI 2).

Smilax oblongifolia Pohl
AREA: Minas Gerais, in open tracts.
NAMES: Cipó-quina, tuia.
USES: Roots are tonic and purgative.

Liliaceae – References
LILI 1. Calixto, J.B., T.C.M. de Lima, G.S. Morato, M. Nicolau, R.N. Takahashi, R.M.R. do Valle, C.C. Schmitt & R.A. Yunes. 1981/1982. Análise química e farmacológica da *Cordyline dracaenoides* (Agavaceae). *Oréades* (Belo Horizonte) *8*: 517-532.
LILI 2. Itoh, T., T. Tamura, T. Tsuhashi & T. Matsumoto. 1977. Steroids of Liliaceae. *Phytochemistry 16*: 140-141.

LOGANIACEAE

Potalia amara Aubl.
AREA: Amazonia and Mato Grosso.
NAMES: Anabi, pau-de-cobra.
USES: Infusion of leaves and twigs is antiluetic; causes vomiting in higher doses. Leaf decoction used for conjunctivitis and other diseases of the eyes. The infusion of wood and bark is highly esteemed as a remedy for snakebite.

Spigelia anthelmia L.
AREA: Amazonia to Goiás.
NAMES: Arapabaca, erva-lombrigueira, lombrigueira.
USES: The whole plant, but especially the root, is cathartic and active in the expulsion of intestinal worms. Care is advised, due to toxicity.
CHEM. & PHARM.: Isoquinoline and one iridoid have been identified as cardiotonically active principles (Ref: LOGA 1).

Spigelia flemingiana Cham. & Schl.
AREA: Amazonia to Bahia.
NAME: Arapabaca.
USES: Diaphoretic and anthelmintic.

Spigelia glabrata Mart.
AREA: Bahia to Rio de Janeiro.
NAMES: Arapabaca, erva-lombrigueira.
USES: Vermifuge, sudorific, febrifuge and excitant.

Strychnos spp.
In spite of being famous for furnishing the raw material for the manufacture of curare, the arrow poison of the Amazonian Indians, *Strychnos* species can hardly be considered "medicinal" in the sense of the present review. Fifty-four species have been recognized in Brazil (Ref: LOGA 2). Only the ones with marginal medicinal utilization are cited below.

Strychnos pseudoquina St.-Hil.
AREA: Minas Gerais to Paraná, cerrado.
NAMES: Falsa-quina, quina-branca, quina-cruzeiro.
USES: Bark is bitter, tonic, febrifuge, prescribed against ailments of the spleen, liver and stomach. Also for malaria.
CHEM.: Alkaloids (Ref: LOGA 3,4) and flavonoids (Ref: LOGA 4) have been described.

Strychnos subcordata Spr. ex Benth.
AREA: Amazonia, forest.

LOGANIACEAE

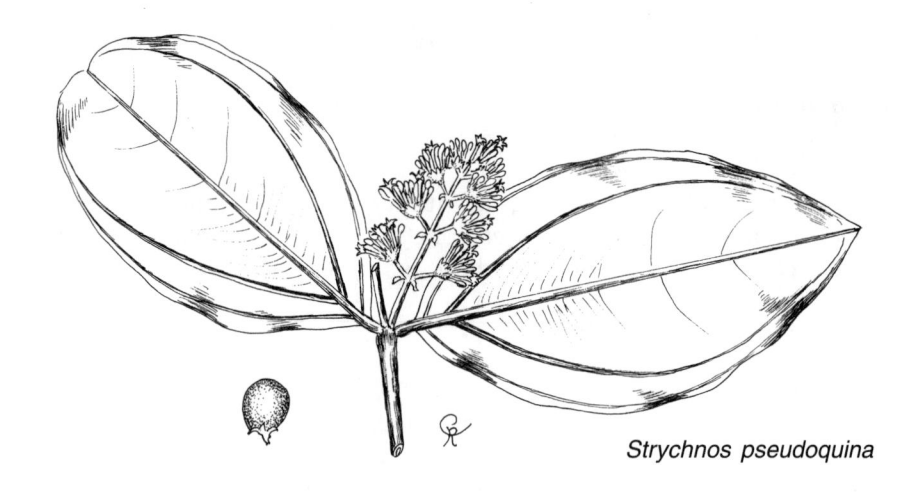

Strychnos pseudoquina

NAMES: Anzol-de-lontra, uirarí-terém.
USES: Root-bark is bitter, stomachic.

Strychnos trinervis (Vell.) Mart.
AREA: Minas Gerais and Rio de Janeiro, forest; also toward the northeast.
NAMES: Capitão-preto, cipó-cruzeiro, quina-cruzeiro, quina-de-cipó, noz-vômica.
USES: Indicated against malarial fever and gastric disturbances; also as a diuretic. Said to be narcotic.
CHEM. & PHARM.: This species and *S. torresiana* Krukoff & Monachino are the only extra-Amazonian species with curare activity (Ref: LOGA 5,6,7). One tertiary (non-curarizing) base, bisnordihydrotoxiferine, was isolated as the major alkaloid from the root-bark. The compound showed

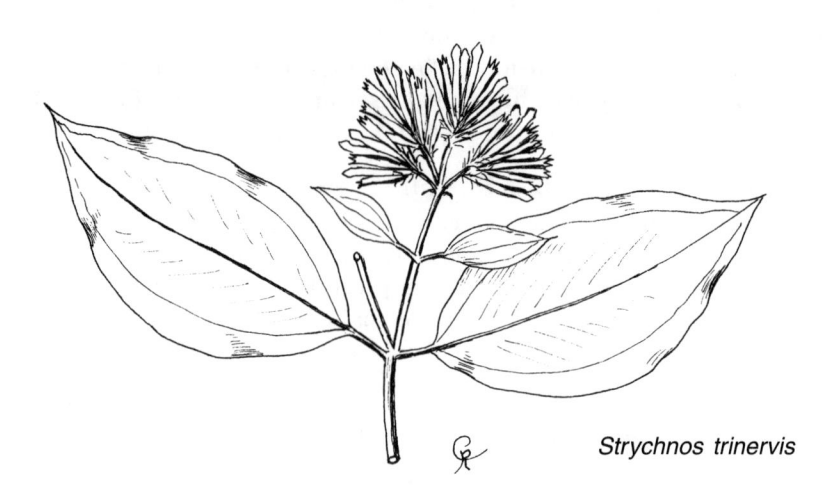

Strychnos trinervis

210   MEDICINAL PLANTS OF BRAZIL

a wide antimicrobial spectrum as well as some cytotoxic activity (Ref: LOGA 8). Other tertiary alkaloids were shown to be strongly spasmolytic (Ref: LOGA 9,10). A review of the alkaloids of American *Strychnos* species has been published (Ref: LOGA 11).

Loganiaceae – References

LOGA 1. Wagner, H., K. Seegert, M.P. Gupta, M. Esposito Avella & P. Solis. 1986. Cardiotone Wirkstoffe aus *Spigelia anthelmia*. *Planta Medica* 52: 376-381.

LOGA 2. Ducke, A. 1955. O genero *Strychnos* no Brasil. *Bol. Téc. Inst. Agron. Norte* (Belém) 30: 5-64.

LOGA 3. Delle Monache, F., A. Poce Tucci & G.B. Marini-Bettòlo. 1969. The occurrence of nor-dihydrotoxiferine in *Strychnos pseudoquina* A. St.-Hil. *Tetrahedron Lett.* 25: 2009-2010.

LOGA 4. Nicolette, M., M.O.F. Goulart, R.A. Lima, A.E. Goulart, F. Delle Monache & G.B. Marini-Bettòlo. 1984. Flavonoids and alkaloids from *Strychnos pseudoquina*. *J. Nat. Prod.* 47: 953-957.

LOGA 5. Couty, L. & J.B. Lacerda. 1880. Sur un nouveau curare, extrait d'une seule plante, le *Strychnos triplinervia*. *J. de Pharm. et Chim.* 1: 34-36.

LOGA 6. Adank, K., D. Bovet, A. Ducke & G.B. Marini-Bettòlo. 1953. Ricerche sugli alcaloidi curarizzanti di varie specie di *Strychnos* del Brasile. Gli alcaloide della *Strychnos trinervis* (Vell.) Mart. *Gazz. Chim. Italiana* 83: 966-982.

LOGA 7. Mello Filho, D.E. 1953. Nova planta curarigênica do Brasil Leste. *Strychnos torresiana* Kruk. & Monac. Thesis, Universidade do Brasil (today Federal University of Rio de Janeiro).

LOGA 8. Melo, M.F.F., C.A.M. Santos, A.A. Chiappeta, J.F. Mello & R. Mukherjee. 1978. Chemistry and pharmacology of a tertiary alkaloid from *Strychnos trinervis* root bark. *J. Ethnopharmacol.* 19: 319-325.

LOGA 9. Medeiros, C.L.C., G. Thomas & R. Mukherjee. 1991. The source of Ca^{2+} for the spasmolytic actions of longicaudatine, a bisindole alkaloid isolated from *Strychnos trinervis* (Vell.) Mart. (Loganiaceae). *Phytotherapy Res.* 5: 24-28.

LOGA 10. Melo Diniz, M.F.F., B.A. da Silva & R. Mukherjee. 1994. Spasmolytic actions of the new indole alkaloid trinervine from *Strychnos trinervis* root. *Phytomedicine* 1: 205-207.

LOGA 11. Marini-Bettòlo, G.B. & N.G. Bisset. 1972. Chemical studies on the alkaloids of American *Strychnos* species, pp. 195-271. In: Krukoff, B.A. 1972. American species of *Strychnos*. *Lloydia* 35: 193-271.

LORANTHACEAE

Phoradendron crassifolium (Pohl) Eichl.

AREA: Throughout Brazil, forest. All members of this family are hemiparasites growing on a large variety of trees.

NAMES: Erva-de-passarinho, erva-de-passarinho-de-folha-grande.

USES: Employed in decoction for treating leg swelling.

Phthirusa adunca (Meyer) Maguire

AREA: Amazonia, forest.

NAME: Erva-de-passarinho.

USES: Leaves in poultice are used to aid consolidation of bone fractures.

Loranthaceae

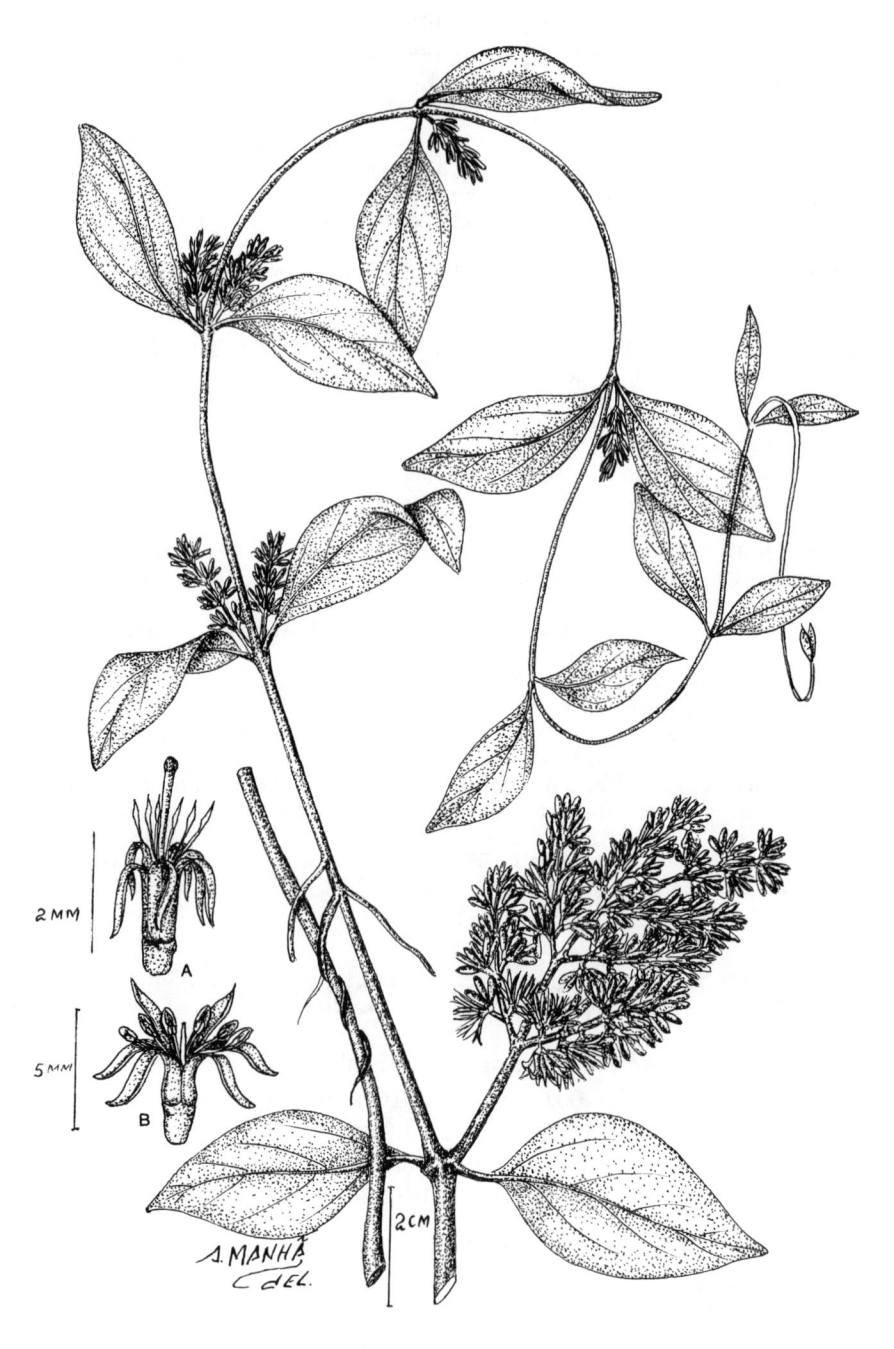

Struthanthus marginatus

Leaves used in baths to treat metritis. Tea is made from leaves for kidney disorders and leucorrhoea; for the latter also used as a vaginal injection. The powdered dry leaves are applied topically to hasten cicatrization of sores.

Struthanthus marginatus (Desf.) Bl.
AREA: Minas Gerais, Rio de Janeiro and São Paulo, in forest and on trees in cities.
NAME: Erva-de-passarinho.
USES: Ointment prepared from the young leaves is used to treat boils caused by cold.

LYTHRACEAE

Cuphea aperta Koehne
AREA: Bahia to Rio de Janeiro, campo.
NAME: Sete-sangrias.
USES: Plant is diuretic.

Cuphea balsamona Cham.
AREA: Throughout Brazil, campo.
NAMES: Balsamona, chagari, erva-de-sangue, sete-sangrias.
USES: Herb is diaphoretic, diuretic, laxative, antisyphilitic, for high blood pressure and arteriosclerosis.
PHARM.: Crude extracts showed hypotensive and anticholinestersic effects in animals and a potentiating activity on smooth muscle contraction (Ref: LYTH 1).

Cuphea ingrata

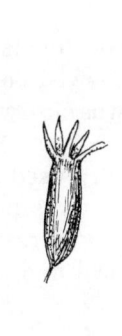

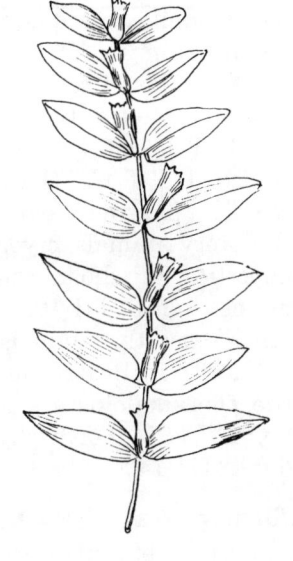

Cuphea carthagenensis (Jacq.) MacBride
AREA: Southern Brazil, campo; cosmopolitan.
NAMES: Sete-sangrias,

sete-sangrias-do-campo.
USES: Diaphoretic and antiluetic.

Cuphea ingrata Cham. & Schl.
AREA: Rio de Janeiro to Rio Grande do Sul, campo and open places near cities.
NAMES: Mata-cana, sete-sangrias.
USES: Diaphoretic, antiluetic, antithermic.

Cuphea melvilla Lindl.
AREA: Everywhere in damp sites.
NAME: Erva-de-bicho.
USES: Very much recommended for piles, as is the related *Cuphea ultriculosa* Hoene.
CHEM.: Oil from the seeds of *Cuphea* species is rich in triglycerides of medium-chain fatty acids ("MCT") (Ref: LYTH 2). Lauric acid (C_{12}), which is one of them, can be obtained in great quantities from other sources (coconut, palm kernel, etc.); but the lower members, like capric acid (C_{10}) and caprylic acid (C_8), which are important in a number of medical, nutritional and dietetic applications, are not easily accessible and their procurement from *Cuphea* species is being considered. Research programs are under way in several countries with the aim of domesticating some of these species (Ref: LYTH 3).

Heimia salicifolia (H.B.K.) Link & Otto
AREA: São Paulo to Rio Grande do Sul, campo.
NAMES: Abre-sol, erva-da-vida, quebra-arado, vassourinha.
USES: Internally as a diaphoretic, diuretic and purgative; externally for wound healing.
CHEM.: Alkaloids of complex chemical structure — macrocyclic lactones — peculiar to the Lythraceae, have been described from this species (Ref: LYTH 4,5,6,7,8). A thorough review of their structure has been published (Ref: LYTH 9).
PHARM.: The pharmacology of some of the alkaloids has been studied. In laboratory animals, cryogenine showed possibly unique tranquilizing properties. Anticholinergic effect was observed in isolated muscle preparations (Ref: LYTH 10,11,12).

In Mexico the plant is reputedly used as an hallucinogenic (Ref: LYTH 13). In Brazil the use as such is unknown. If the assertion is true, the alkaloids are unlikely to be responsible for such an effect (Ref: LYTH 6). For a phytochemical and pharmacological review, see Ref: LYTH 14.

Lafoensia densiflora Pohl
AREA: Cerrado of central Brazil.
NAME: Pacari.

LYTHRACEAE

Lafoensia densiflora

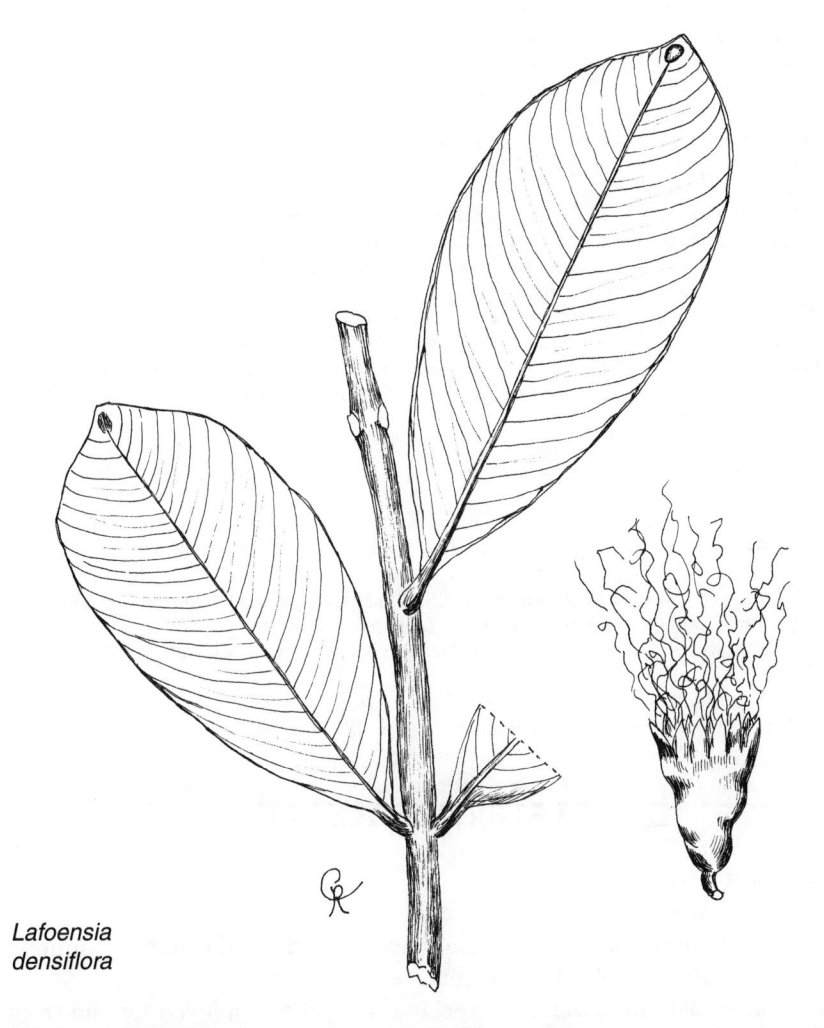

USES: Tea from bark used against snakebite and to cure gastric ulcers; in baths against varicose veins, even if ulcerated.

Lafoensia pacari St.-Hil.
AREA: Minas Gerais to São Paulo and Mato Grosso.
NAMES: Dedaleira-amarela, dedal, magabeira-brava, pacari, pacuri.
USES: Roots are tonic and antifebrile.

Lythraceae – References

LYTH 1. Ericeira, V.R., M.M.R. Martins, C. Souccar & A.J. Lapa. 1984. Atividade farmacológica do extrato etanólico da "sete-sangrias," *Cuphea balsamona* Cham. *VIII Simpósio de Plantas Medicinais do Brasil* (Manaus). Summaries of papers: 35.

LYTH 2. Wolf, R.B., S.A. Graham & R. Kleimann. 1983. Fatty acid composition of *Cuphea* seed oils. *J. Am. Oil Chem. Soc. 60*: 27-28.
LYTH 3. Hirsinger, F. & P.F. Knowles. 1984. Morphological and agronomic description of selected *Cuphea* germplasm. *Econ. Bot. 38*: 439-451.
LYTH 4. Blomster, R.N., A.E. Schwarting & J.M. Bobbit. 1964. Alkaloids of *Heimia salicifolia*. I. A preliminary report. *Lloydia 27*: 15-24.
LYTH 5. Appel, H., A. Rother & A.E. Schwarting. 1965. Alkaloids of *Heimia salicifolia*. II. Isolation of nesodine and lyfoline and their correlation with other Lythraceae alkaloids. *Lloydia 28*: 84-89.
LYTH 6. Douglas, B., J.L. Kirkpatrick, R.F. Raffauf, O. Ribeiro & J.A. Weisbach. 1964. Problems in chemotaxonomy. II. The major alkaloids of the genus *Heimia*. *Lloydia 27*: 25-31.
LYTH 7. El-Olemy, M.M., S.J. Stohs & A.E. Schwarting. 1971. Heimidine, a new alkaloid from *Heimia salicifolia*. *Lloydia 34*: 439-441.
LYTH 8. Dominguez, X.A., J. Marroquín, S. Quintero & B. Vargas. 1975. Two new quinolozidine alkaloids from *Heimia salicifolia*. *Phytochemistry 14*: 1883-1884.
LYTH 9. Ferris, J.P., C.B. Boyce & R.C. Brimer. 1971. Lythraceae alkaloids. VII. The structure and stereochemistry of the biphenyl alkaloids of *Decodon* and *Heimia*. *J. Am. Chem. Soc. 93*: 2942-2953.
LYTH 10. Robichaud, R.C., M.H. Malone & A.E. Schwarting. 1964. Pharmacodynamics of cryogenine, an alkaloid isolated from *Heimia salicifolia* Link & Otto. I. *Arch. Intern. Pharmacodyn. 150*: 220-232.
LYTH 11. Robichaud, R.C., M.H. Malone & O.S. Koserksky. 1965. Pharmacodynamics of cryogenine, an alkaloid isolated from *Heimia salicifolia* Link & Otto. II. *Arch. Intern. Pharmacodyn. 157*: 43-52.
LYTH 12. Kaplan, H.R. & M.H. Malone. 1966. Pharmacologic study of nesodine, cryogenine and other alkaloids of *Heimia salicifolia*. *Lloydia 29*: 348-359.
LYTH 13. Martinez, M. 1959. *Las Plantas Medicinales de México*. 4th edition. Botas, Mexico. (p. 293).
LYTH 14. Malone, M.H. & A. Rother. 1994. *Heimia salicifolia*: a phytochemical and phytopharmacologic review. *J. Ethnopharmacol. 42*: 135-139.

MAGNOLIACEAE

Talauma ovata St.-Hil.

AREA: From Minas Gerais to the south.

NAMES: Araticum-fruta-de-pau, baguaçu, magnólia-da-mata, magnólia-do-brejo, pinha-do-brejo, talaúma.

USES: Bark used for lowering fever; leaf infusion employed for the treatment of diabetes.

CHEM. & PHARM.: Chemical analysis demonstrated the presence of sterols, saponins, alkaloids and tannins. Pharmacological studies failed to demonstrate hypoglycemic effect in normoglycemic, hyper-glycemic or alloxan-diabetic rats. Considerable toxicity was verified, advising against the use of this plant (Ref: MAGN 1).

Magnoliaceae – Reference

MAGN 1. Morato, G.S., J.B. Calixto, L. Cordeiro, T.C.M. de Lima, E.F. Morato, M. Nicolau, G.A. Rae, R.N. Takahashi, R.M.R. Valle & R.A. Yunes. 1989. Chemical and pharmacological studies on *Talauma ovata* St. -Hil. (Magnoliaceae). *J. Ethnopharmacol. 26*: 277-286.

Talauma ovata

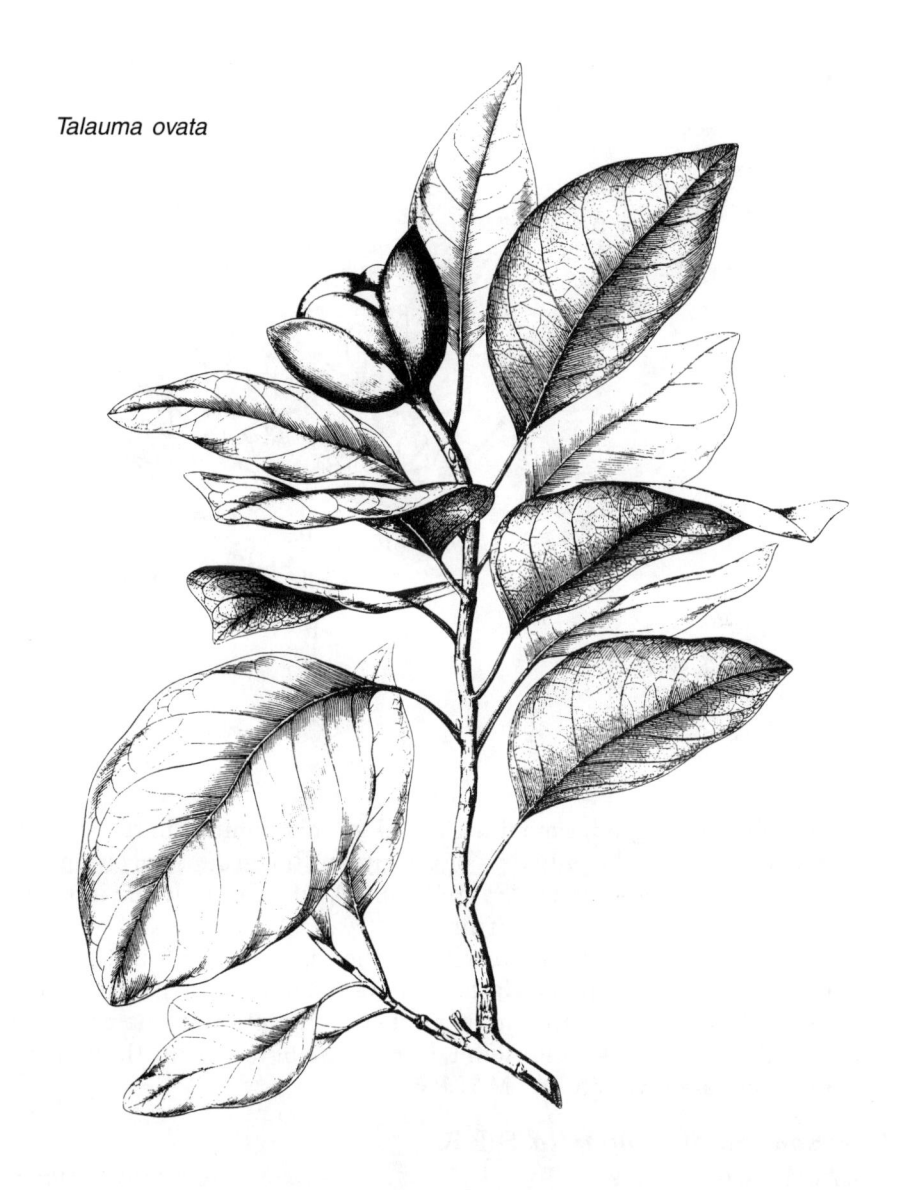

MALPIGHIACEAE

Banisteriopsis caapi (Spr.) Morton
AREA: Amazonia, forest.
NAMES: Caapi, iagê.
USES: The stem-bark is hallucinogenic, used in religious rites by certain Amazonian tribes to reach a state of trance. This use has recently

MALPIGHIACEAE

Banisteriopsis caapi

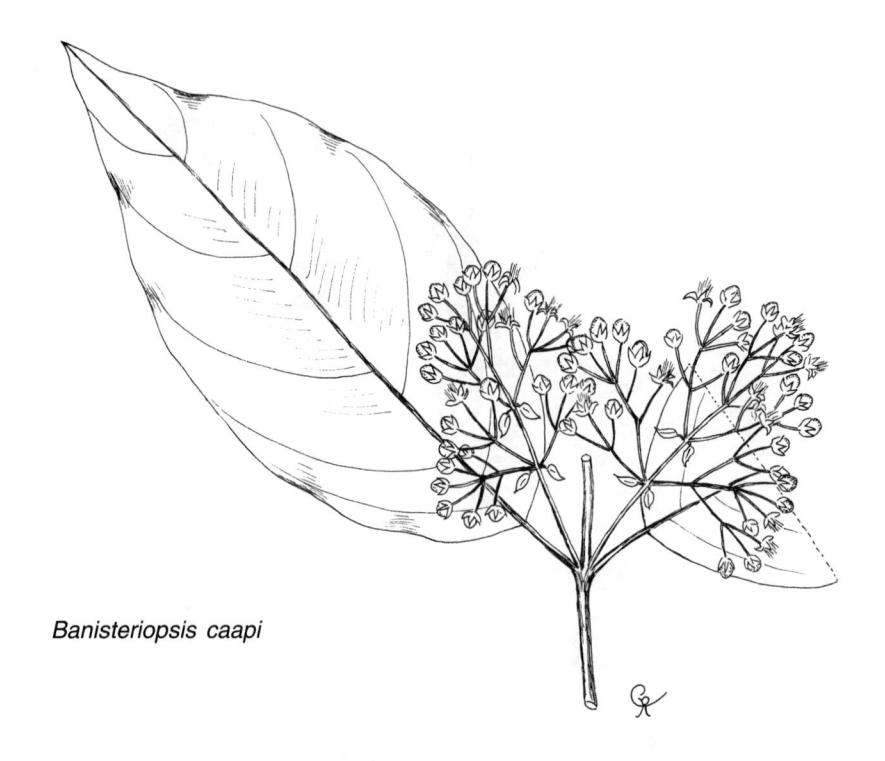

been adopted by groups outside the Indian communities in the state of Acre and even in the outskirts of the city of Rio de Janeiro, organized into pseudoreligious sects ("Santo Daime"), who consume the infusion of the bark as a ceremonial drink.

CHEM.: The ß-carboline base harmine is the major alkaloid in the bark (Ref: MALP 1), accompanied by harmaline and tetrahydro-harmine (Ref: MALP 2), as well as other, minor constituents of the same chemical type (Ref: MALP 3,4). Additional data on use of this plant throughout Amazonia are given in Ref: MALP 5,6,7.

Byrsonima chrysophylla H.B.K.
AREA: Amazonia, forest.
NAMES: Murici, murici-penima, muruchi.
USES: Bark is made into a loch as a cough sedative.

Byrsonima coccolobifolia H.B.K.
AREA: Amazonia to São Paulo, cerrado.
NAMES: Chaparro, matega, mureci.
USES: Bark is indicated as useful in treating tuberculosis.

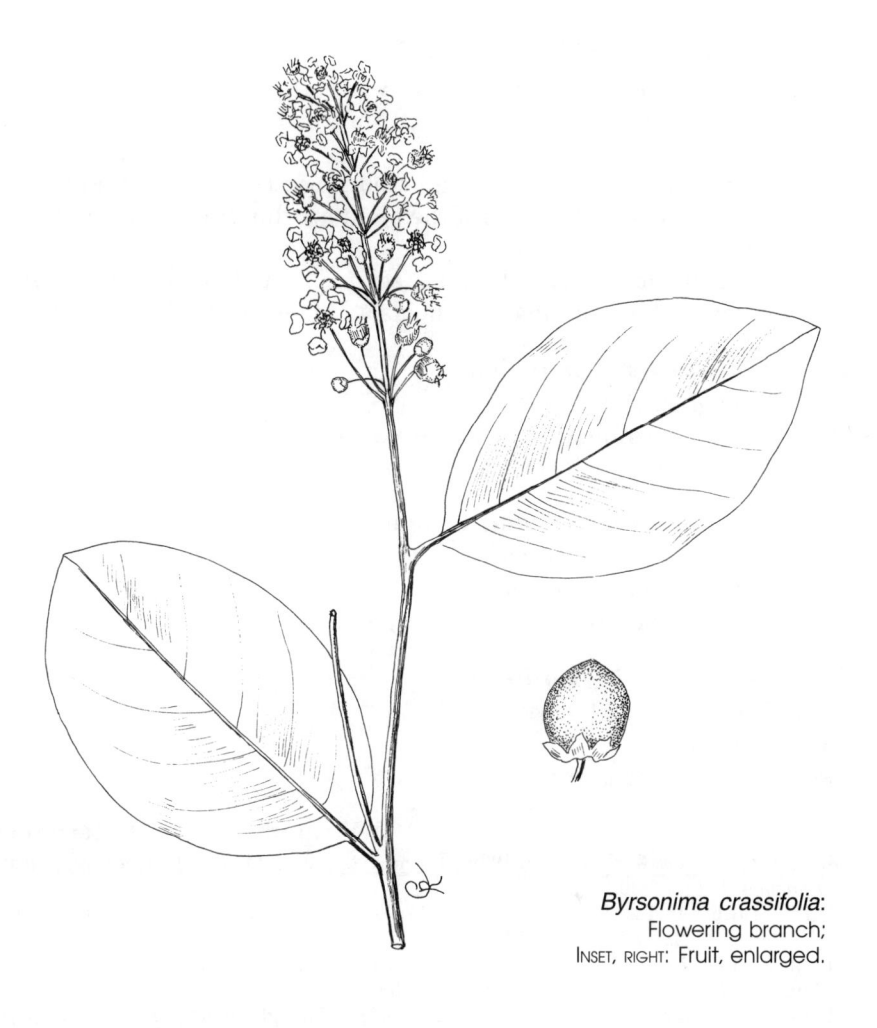

MALPIGHIACEAE

Byrsonima crassifolia:
Flowering branch;
INSET, RIGHT: Fruit, enlarged.

Byrsonima crassifolia H.B.K.
AREA: Amazonia, cerrado.
NAME: Murici-do-campo.
USES: Bark is reportedly active against snakebite and bronchial inflammation.
CHEM.: ß-Amayrin in bark (Ref: MALP 8).

Byrsonima spicata Rich.
AREA: Widespread throughout Brazil.
NAMES: Caá-açu, pau-de-curtume, pessegueiro-de-curtume.
USES: Drupes are astringent, antidysenteric.
CHEM.: ß-Amayrin in bark (Ref: MALP 8).

Malpighiaceae

Byrsonima verbascifolia (L.) Rich.
AREA: Very widespread in Brazil, mainly in cerrado.
NAMES: Douradinha-falsa, murici-açu, murici-da-mata, murici-guaçu, muruchi-rasteiro.
USES: Bark is laxative, astringent and febrifuge. Drupes are mildly laxative and astringent. All parts of the plant are diuretic, emetic and antisyphilitic.
CHEM.: Several triterpenes have been isolated from the bark (Ref: MALP 9). Leaves are rich in tannins, flavonoids and triterpenes (Ref: MALP 10).

Galphimia brasiliensis Juss.
AREA: Throughout Brazil.
NAMES: Guaco, jasmim-amarelo, quaró, resedá-amarelo.
USES: Astringent, emetic, purgative, antifebrile.

Heteropteris aphrodisiaca O. Mach.
AREA: Goiás and Mato Grosso, cerrado.
NAMES: Nú-de-cachorro, nó-de-porco.
USES: Nodose roots are reputedly an aphrodisiac.

Heteropteris syringifolia Gris.
AREA: Southern Brazil, forest.
NAME: Praguá.
USE: Roots are emetocathartic.

Malpighiaceae – References

MALP 1. Chen, A.L. & K.K. Chen. 1939. Harmine, the alkaloid of caapi. *Quart. J. Pharm. Pharmacol.* 12: 30-36.

MALP 2. Hochstein, F.A. & A.M. Paradies. 1957. Alkaloids of *Banisteria caapi* and *Prestonia amazonica*. *J. Am. Chem. Soc.* 79: 5735-5738.

MALP 3. Hashimoto, Y. & K. Kawanishi. 1975. New organic bases from Amazonian *Banisteriopsis caapi*. *Phytochemistry* 14: 1633-1635.

MALP 4. Hashimoto, Y. & K. Kawanishi. 1976. New alkaloids from *Banisteriopsis caapi*. *Phytochemistry* 15: 1550-1560.

MALP 5. Schultes, R.E. & R.F. Raffauf. 1990. THE HEALING FOREST: MEDICINAL AND TOXIC PLANTS OF THE NORTHWEST AMAZONIA. 484 pp. Portland, Oregon: Dioscorides Press.

MALP 6. Schultes, R.E. & R.F. Raffauf. 1992. VINE OF THE SOUL: MEDICINE MEN, THEIR PLANTS AND RITUALS IN THE COLOMBIAN AMAZON. 282 pp. Oracle, Arizona: Synergetic Press.

MALP 7. Schultes, R.E. 1968. Some impacts of Spruce's Amazon explorations on modern phytochemical research. *Rhodora* 70(783): 313-339.

MALP 8. Djerassi, C., A. Bowers, S. Burstein, H. Estrada, J. Grossman, J. Herrán, A.J. Lemin, A. Manjarrez & S.C. Pakrashi. 1956. Terpenoids. XXII. Triterpenes from some Mexican and South American plants. *J. Am. Chem. Soc.* 78: 2312-2315.

MALP 9. Gottlieb, O.R., P.H. Mendes & M.T. Magalhães. 1975. Triterpenoids from *Byrsonima verbascifolia*. *Phytochemistry* 14: 1456.

MALP 10. Dossech, C., C. Moretti, P. Delaveau & A.M. Tessier. 1980. Étude chimique des feuilles de *Byrsonima verbascifolia* Rich. *Plantes Méd. Phytothérap.* 14: 130-142.

MALVACEAE

Hibiscus bifurcatus Cav.
AREA: Throughout Brazil, in meadows.
NAMES: Amandurana, algodoeiro-bravo, algodão-o-brejo, majorana.
USES: Bark is vomitive. Leaves are emollient, anti-inflammatory.

Hibiscus cannabinus L.
AREA: Bahia and Minas Gerais.
NAMES: Cânhamo-brasileiro, papoula-de-são-francisco, umbaru.
USES: Infusion of the roots is said to be aphrodisiac. Leaves are emollient.

Hibiscus sabdariffa L.
AREA: Introduced from Africa, cultivated in gardens; has run wild in many places.
NAMES: Azedinha, caruru-azedo, caruru-da-guiné, quiabo-azedo, quiabo-de-angola, quiabo-róseo, quiabo-roxo, rosela, vinagreira.
USES: Roots are bitter, used as an appetizer. Leaves are emollient, stomachic, febrifuge. Sepals and bracts are acid to the taste, used for seasoning some regional dishes. Also used for lowering fever. Seeds are diuretic, tonic.
CHEM.: Aerial parts contain malic acid (Ref: MALV 1) and hibiscic acid, a lactone of d-allo-hydroxycitric acid (Ref: MALV 2). Flowers contain hibiscitrin, a glucoside of the flavonol hibiscitin (Ref: MALV 3). A sitosterol glycoside has also been described (Ref: MALV 4).

Hibiscus tiliaceus L.
AREA: Tropical cosmopolitan; thrives in Brazil along the coastal region, in restinga and mangrove; moreover, it is much grown as a street tree.
NAME: Algodoeiro-da-praia.
USES: Leaves and flowers are emollient, useful in treating wounds and sores, including chronic ulcers.

Modiolastrum pinnatipartitum (St.-Hil. & Naudin) Krapovickas
AREA: Rio Grande do Sul.
NAME: Mercurial.
USE: Entire plant used as an antisyphilitic.

Sida acuta Burm.
AREA: Widespread, ruderal.
NAMES: Guaxuma, relógio-de-vaqueiro, relógio-vassoura, tupitixá, vassoura-preta, vassourinha.
USES: Plant is tonic, antipyretic, beneficial for hemorrhoids. Roots are bitter, febrifuge, stomachic.

MALVACEAE

CHEM.: Triterpenes (Ref: MALV 5) and alkaloids (Ref: MALV 6,7) have been described.

Sida angustifolia Lam.
AREA: Widespread, ruderal.
NAMES: Relógio, vassourinha-de-relógio.
USES: Recommended for treating bad digestion.

Sida carpinifolia (L. f.) K. Sch.
AREA: Throughout Brazil.
NAMES: Lupiticha, vassoura, vassourinha.
USES: Plant is emollient.
PHARM.: Acetylcholine-like activity has been described (Ref: MALV 8).

Sida macrodon DC.
AREA: Minas Gerais and São Paulo, in open spaces.
NAMES: Carapiá, malva-do-campo.
USES: Tea from the fresh leaves is used, internally and externally, for ulcers in general and specifically for syphilitic manifestations.

Sida micrantha St.-Hil.
AREA: Goiás and Minas Gerais, campo.
NAMES: Guaxima, malvaísco, malva-preta, vassourinha-miuda.
USES: Leaves are pectoral, antiasthmatic and emollient.

Sida rhombea L.
AREA: Cosmopolitan; in Brazil, ruderal and subspontaneous.
NAMES: Guaxima, guaxuma, relógio, tupitixa, vassoura, vassourinha, zanzo.
USES: Roots are diuretic; in decoction for diarrhoea of children, as a substitute for the European "Marsh Mallow" (*Althaea officinalis*). Leaves are mucilaginous, emollient; leaves mixed with salt, and used topically, are said to hasten the maturation of tumors; mixed with sugar, to accelerate wound healing. Ground seeds are taken orally to combat urine retention.

Sida rhombifolia L.
AREA: Widely distributed in Brazil, ruderal, cosmopolitan.
NAMES: Guaxuma, malva-preta, relógio, vassourinha, tupitixa.
USES: Leaves are emollient. Chewed leaves are applied topically to alleviate the pain of insect stings. The mucilage of the leaves suspended in water is said to strengthen hair growth.
CHEM.: Alkaloids have been described (Ref: MALV 7).

Urena lobata L.
AREA: Ruderal and subspontaneous; cosmopolitan.
NAMES: Embira, guaxima-roxa, malvaísco, malva-roxa.
USES: Plant is mucilaginous and emollient. Root infusion is diuretic and used against colics. Decoction of flowers is bechic.

Wissadula periplocifolia Presl.
AREA: Piauí to Minas Gerais, forest.
NAME: Malvaísco.
USES: Leaves are pectoral, and used in gargles against aphthae and laryngitis. Heated on a fire and applied as a poultice, the leaves are considered helpful in treating wounds, cuts, boils and tumors.

Malvaceae – References

MALV 1. Pratt, D.S. 1912. Roselle. *Philippine J. Science* 7: 201-205.
MALV 2. Griebe, C. 1942. Über die Konstitution und den Nachweis von Hibiscussäure [(+)*allo*-Oxycitronensäurelacton)]. *Z. Unters. Lebensmittel* 83: 481-486.
MALV 3. Rao, P.S. & T.R. Seshadri. 1942. Isolation of hibiscitrin from the flowers of *Hibiscus sabdariffa*: constitution of hibiscetin. *Proc. Indian Acad. Sci.* 15A: 148-153.
MALV 4. Osman, A.M., M. El-Garby Younes, & A. Mokhtar. 1975. Sitosterol-ß-D-galactoside from *Hibiscus sabdariffa*. *Phytochemistry* 14: 829-830.
MALV 5. Krishna Rao, R.V., T. Satyanaryana & B.V.K. Rao. 1984. Phytochemical investigation on the roots of *Sida acuta* growing in Waltair. *Fitoterapia* 55: 249-250.
MALV 6. Gunatilaka, A.A.Q., S. Sotheeswaran, S. Balasubramanian, A.I. Chanarasekara & H.T.B. Sriyani. 1980. Studies on medicinal plants of Sri Lanka. III. Pharmacologically important alkaloids of some *Sida* species. *Planta Medica* 39: 66-72.
MALV 7. Prakash, A., R.K. Varma & S. Ghosal. 1981. Alkaloid constituents of *Sida acuta*, *Sida humilis*, *Sida rhombifolia* and *Sida spinosa*. *Planta Medica* 43: 384-388.
MALV 8. Prasad, D.N. & G. Achari. 1966. Acetylcholine-like activity in *Sida carpinifolia*. *Indian J. Pharm.* 28: 241.

MARANTACEAE

Calathea grandiflora Lindl.
AREA: São Paulo and Rio Grande do Sul, forest.
NAMES: Anima-membeca, bananeirinha-do-mato, caeté-açu.
USES: Leaf juice employed in cases of urine retention.

Ischnosiphon arouma Koern.
AREA: Amazonia, forest.
NAMES: Arumá, arumã-membeca.
USES: Rhizome is vulnerary; its starch is indicated for convalescents.

Maranta arundinacea L.
AREA: Widely cultivated from Amazonas to Rio de Janeiro.
NAMES: Agutiguepe, araruta.
USES: In English-speaking countries the plant is known as "West Indian

Arrowroot," valued for Maranta starch from its rhizomes. The starch is of importance in special diets for the newborn, the aged and convalescents. Additionally, the juice of the rhizome is acrid, and employed against the effect of snakebite.

Stromanthe sanguinea Sond.
AREA: Rio de Janeiro, forest.
NAME: Caeté-bravo.
USES: Juice of leaves is recommended for skin eruptions. Rhizome used for treating bladder catarrh.

Thalia geniculata L.
AREA: Amazonia to Minas Gerais, Rio de Janeiro and Mato Grosso, in marshy sites.
NAME: Arumarana.
USES: Rhizome is applied on atonic sores; starch for an analeptic.

MARCGRAVIACEAE

Marcgravia rectiflora Tr. & Planch.
AREA: Minas Gerais, Rio de Janeiro and São Paulo, forest.
NAME: Atepele.
USES: Roots are diuretic and antisyphilitic. Leaves and wood used in baths to cure diseased testes.

MARTYNIACEAE

Craniolaria annua L.
AREA: Mato Grosso.
NAME: Cumba.
USES: Dried roots are used to prepare a bitter, refreshing and laxative beverage. Seeds are depurative.

Craniolaria integrifolia Cham.
AREA: São Paulo and Mato Grosso, campo.
NAME: Cumba.
USES: Reputedly is active against snakebite.

Ibicella lutea (Lindl.) Van Eselt.
AREA: Minas Gerais to Rio Grande do Sul, mata and restinga; also ruderal.
NAMES: Chifre-de-veado, cornos-do-diabo, quingombô-de-espinho.
USES: Seeds are emollient, used to remove opacity of the cornea.

MELASTOMATACEAE

Bellucia grossularioides (L.) Tr.
AREA: Amazonia, forest.
NAMES: Araçá-de-anta, muuba.
USES: Leaves are prescribed for leucorrhoea. Fruits are used to expel intestinal worms.

Clidemia blepharoides DC.
AREA: Bahia, Minas Gerais, Espirito Santo and Rio de Janeiro to Santa Catarina, epiphyte in forest.
NAMES: Anhanga-piri, aninga-pari, aninga-piri.
USES: Leaves used for dressing ulcers.

Leandra lacunosa Cogn.
AREA: Mato Grosso, Distrito Federal to Paraná, forest.
NAME: Aperta-ruão.
USES: Leaves are astringent, used to tighten genitals.

Macairea radula (Bonpl.) DC.
AREA: Bahia; widespread in central Brazilian savannas.
NAME: Capuchinha.
USES: Recommended for scabies and dermatoses in general.

Miconia albicans (Sw.) Tr.
AREA: Amazonia to Paraná, forest edges and cerrado.
NAMES: Canela-de-velha, lacre-branco, olhos de porco.
USES: Leaf infusion is eupeptic.
CHEM. & PHARM.: A benzoquinone derivative (primin) and its corresponding hydroquinone (micoidin) were isolated from wood and roots of an unidentified *Miconia* species from the Brazilian northeast. Primin inhibits the growth of various micro-organisms and showed antitumor activity in mice bearing sarcoma 180, but the antitumor dose borders on the limit of toxicity. On the other hand, micoidin inhibits growth of sarcoma 180 and Yoshida sarcoma at tolerable doses (Ref: MELA 1,2,3,4,5). Both compounds are antifeedants for insects (Ref: MELA 6).

Mouriri apiranga Spruce
AREA: Amazonia, forest.
NAME: Apiranga.
USES: Decoction of bark used for healing wounds.

Mouriri guianensis Aubl.
AREA: Amazonia to Northeast and Mato Grosso.

MELASTOMATACEAE

NAMES: Cruili, cioula, muriri, murta, murta-de-parida.
USES: All of the plant, especially the bark, is very astringent; used in baths after childbirth.

Nepsera aquatica Naud.
AREA: Pará and Maranhão.
NAME: Barba-de-paca.
USE: Leaves prescribed for hematuria.

Tibouchina aspera Aubl.
AREA: Amazonia, forest.
NAME: Margarita.
USES: Leaves and flowers are bechic and sedative.

Tibouchina clavata (Pers.) Wurdack
AREA: Minas Gerais, Rio de Janeiro, São Paulo, Paraná, forest edges, restinga.
NAMES: Orelha-de-gato, orelha-de-onça, pracajá-nambi.
USES: Reputedly effective for throat ailments.
CHEM.: Tannin content has been reported for the stems of several *Tibouchina* species (Ref: MELA 7).

Melastomataceae – References

MELA 1. Gonçalves de Lima, O., I.L. d'Albuquerque, M.M. d'Albuquerque & J.S.B. Coelho. 1959. Substâncias antimicrobianas de plantas superiores. XV. Sobre a ocorrência de antimicrobianos com ação contra *Candida* spp. em cascas do caule e de raizes de "sabiazeira," *Miconia* sp. (Melastomaceae). *Rev. Inst. Antibióticos* (Recife) *2*: 53-61.

MELA 2. Gonçalves de Lima, O., G.B. Marini-Bettòlo, J.S.B. Coelho, I.L. d'Albuquerque, G.M. Maciel, A. Lacerda & D.G. Martins. 1970. Substâncias antimicrobianas de plantas superiores. XXXII. Atividade antimicrobiana e antineoplásica de produto identificado como 2-metoxi-6-n-pentil-p-benzoquinona (primina) isolado de raizes de *Miconia* sp. (Melastomaceae). *Rev. Inst. Antibióticos* (Recife) *10*: 29-34.

MELA 3. Gonçalves de Lima, O., G.B. Marini-Bettòlo, F. Delle Monache, J.S.B. Coelho, I.L. d'Albuquerque, M.S.B. Cavalcanti, D.G. Martins & L. Lins de Oliveira. 1970. Substâncias antimicrobianas de plantas superiores. XXXIII. Primeiras observações sobre a atividade antimicrobiana e antineoplásica de 2-metoxi-6-n-pentil-1, 4-dihidroxibenzeno (miconidina), isolada de extratos de raizes de *Miconia* sp. (Melastomaceae). *Rev. Inst. Antibióticos* (Recife) *10*: 35-39.

MELA 4. Marini-Bettòlo, G.B., F. Delle Monache, O. Gonçalves de Lima & J.S.B. Coelho. 1971. Micoidin, a new hydroquinone from the wood of *Miconia* sp. (Melastomaceae). *Gazz. Chim. Ital. 101*: 41-46.

MELA 5. Pinto, K.V., C.T. Cotias & A.L. Lacerda. 1973. Contibuição ao estudo farmacológico da micoidina. *Rev. Inst. Antibióticos* (Recife) *13*: 47-57.

MELA 6. Barnays, E., A. Lupi, G.B. Marini-Bettòlo & C. Mastrofrancesco. 1984. Antifeedant nature of the quinone primin and its quinol miconidin from *Miconia* spp. *Experientia 40*: 1010-1011.

MELA 7. Moreira, E.A., C. Crecy, T. Nakashima, R. Leonart, T.A. Franke, O.G. Miguel & E.M.O. Sato. 1984. Substâncias tânicas em caules de espécias do gênero *Tibouchina* – Melastomataceae. *Rev. Bras Farm. 65*: 27-33.

MELIACEAE

Cabralea canjerana (Vell.) Mart.
AREA: Bahia to Rio Grande do Sul, forest.
NAMES: Cangerana, pau-de-santo.
USES: Bark of stem and, mainly, of the root is antidyspeptic, febrifuge, emetic, narcotic, abortifacient, antiarthritic; also used for dropsy. Wood extract is employed against dyspepsia and skin afflictions.

Carapa guianensis Aubl.
AREA: Amazonia, forest.
NAME: Andiroba.
USES: The bark is valued for its antidiarrhoeic, anthelmintic, bitter, tonic and antifebrile properties, also used against malarial fevers; externally, against ringworm and exanthema. The seed oil, very bitter, is purgative, antirheumatic, vermicidal, used to cure chronic ulcers, to alleviate insect stings and to kill lice; it is further employed in massages upon the pit of the stomach to relieve gastralgia.
CHEM.: The seeds have yielded two compounds of the limonoid class of tetranortriterpenoids, one of them named andirobin (Ref: MELI 1).

Cedrela fissilis Vell.
AREA: Minas Gerais to Rio Grande do Sul, forest.
NAMES: Cedro, cedro-batata, cedro-branco, cedro-vermelho, cedro-rosa.
USES: Shavings of the wood in a decoction used for cleaning sores and in vapor baths to treat orchitis. Bark is antithermic, emetic, antileucorrhoeic and used for dressing ulcers.
CHEM.: Fruits and seeds contain the limonoid triterpene fissinolide (also called angustinolide) (Ref: MELI 2,3,4).

Cedrela odorata L.
AREA: Amazonia to central Brazil, forest.
NAMES: Cedro, cedro-do-amazonas.
USES: Bark and leaves are indicated in baths for body pains, colds, grippe and fever.
CHEM.: Two limonoids (tetranortriterpenes) have been isolated from wood (Ref: MELI 5,6). Other triterpenoids have been described (Ref: MELI 7).

Guarea spiciflora Juss.
AREA: Rio de Janeiro and São Paulo, forest.
NAMES: Jitó, marinheiro-de-folha-larga, utuapoca.
USES: Bark is used for hydropsy, syphilis and dermatoses.

Guarea trichilioides L.
AREA: Amazonia to São Paulo and Mato Grosso, forest.

MELIACEAE

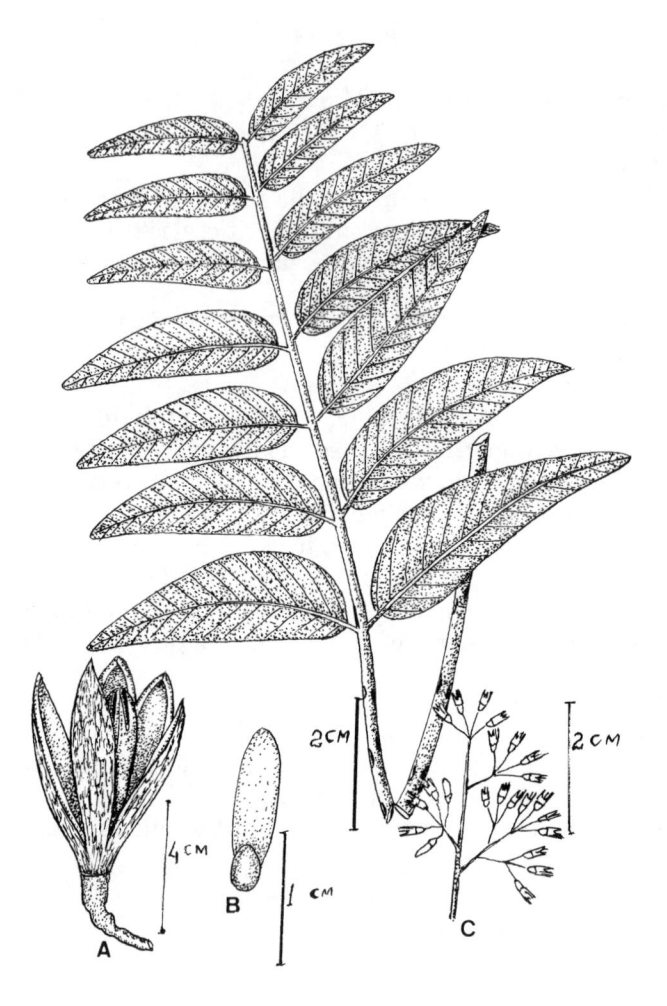

NAMES: Açafroa, bilreiro, cedrão, camboatá, canjerana, carrapeta, gitó, jataíba, marinheiro, macaqueiro.

USES: Bark is bitter, astringent, purgative, anthelmintic, febrifuge, abortifacient. The root-bark, besides having the same properties, is also used for dropsy and gout and, in baths, for arthritic swellings. The seeds, macerated in alcoholic beverages, are also indicated in rheumatic conditions and arthritis. Infusion of the leaves is purgative and emetic.

CHEM. & PHARM.: Ethanolic extract of the seeds had anti-inflammatory action confirmed (Ref: MELI 8). Several limonoids with cell growth inhibitory activity were isolated from the root-bark (Ref: MELI 9). Crude extracts of leaves and fruits showed antiviral activity against pseudorabies virus (Ref: MELI 10).

Guarea tuberculata Vell.
AREA: Ceará to Paraná, forest.
NAMES: Ataúba, camboatá, calcanhar-de-cotia, jitó.
USES: Roots are purgative. Bark is depurative, purgative and antisyphilitic.

Trichilia barraensis DC.
AREA: Amazonia, forest.
NAMES: Tuapoca, tuampoca, utuapoca.
USE: Bark used for an emetocathartic.

Trichilia cathartica Mart.
AREA: Pernambuco to Minas Gerais, forest.
NAMES: Jitó, marinheiro.
USES: Roots and stem-bark are purgative and used for malaria.

Trichilia catigua Juss.
AREA: Goiás to Rio Grande do Sul and Mato Grosso, forest.
NAMES: Caatiguá, catiguá.
USES: Bark is externally applied for rheumatism and dropsy, internally as a purgative and tonic. Also insecticidal.

Trichilia catuaba (Silva) Rizz.
AREA: Southern Bahia, forest.
NAME: Catuaba.
USES: Bark steeped in sugar cane brandy is reputedly an aphrodisiac.

Trichilia hirta L.
AREA: Amazonia, forest.
NAME: Carrapeta.
USE: Root is a strong purgative.

Meliaceae – References

MELI 1. Ollis, W.D., A.D. Ward, M. Meirelles de Oliveira & R. Zelnik. 1970. Andirobin. *Tetrahedron 26*: 1637-1645.

MELI 2. Zelnik, R. & C.M. Rosito. 1966. Fissinolide. *Tetrahedron Lett.*: 6441-6444.

MELI 3. Lavie, D., E.C. Levy, C. Rosito & R. Zelnik. 1970. Studies on tetranortriterpenoids from *Cedrela angustifolia* Sessé and Moc. *Tetrahedron 26*: 219-226.

MELI 4. Taylor, D.A.H. & F.W. Wehrli. 1973. The structure of fissinolide and angustidienolide, limonoids from species of Meliaceae. *J. Chem. Soc.*: 1599-1602.

MELI 5. Bevan, C.W., J.W. Powell & D.A.H. Taylor. 1963. West African timbers, Part VI. Petroleum extracts from species of the genera *Khaya, Guarea, Carapa*, and *Cedrela*. *J. Chem. Soc.*: 980-982.

MELI 6. Adeoye, S.A.& D.A. Bekoe. 1965. The molecular structure of *Cedrela odorata* substance B. *J. Chem. Soc., Chem. Comm.*: 301-302.

MELI 7. Campos, A.M., F.S. Oliveira, M.I.L. Machado, R. Braz Filho & F.J.A. Matos. 1991. Triterpines from *Cedrela odorata*. *Phytochemistry 30*: 1225-1229.

MELI 8. Oga, S., J.A. Sertié, A. Basile & S. Hanada. 1981. Antiinflammatory effect of crude extract from *Guarea guidona*. *Planta Medica 42*: 310-312.

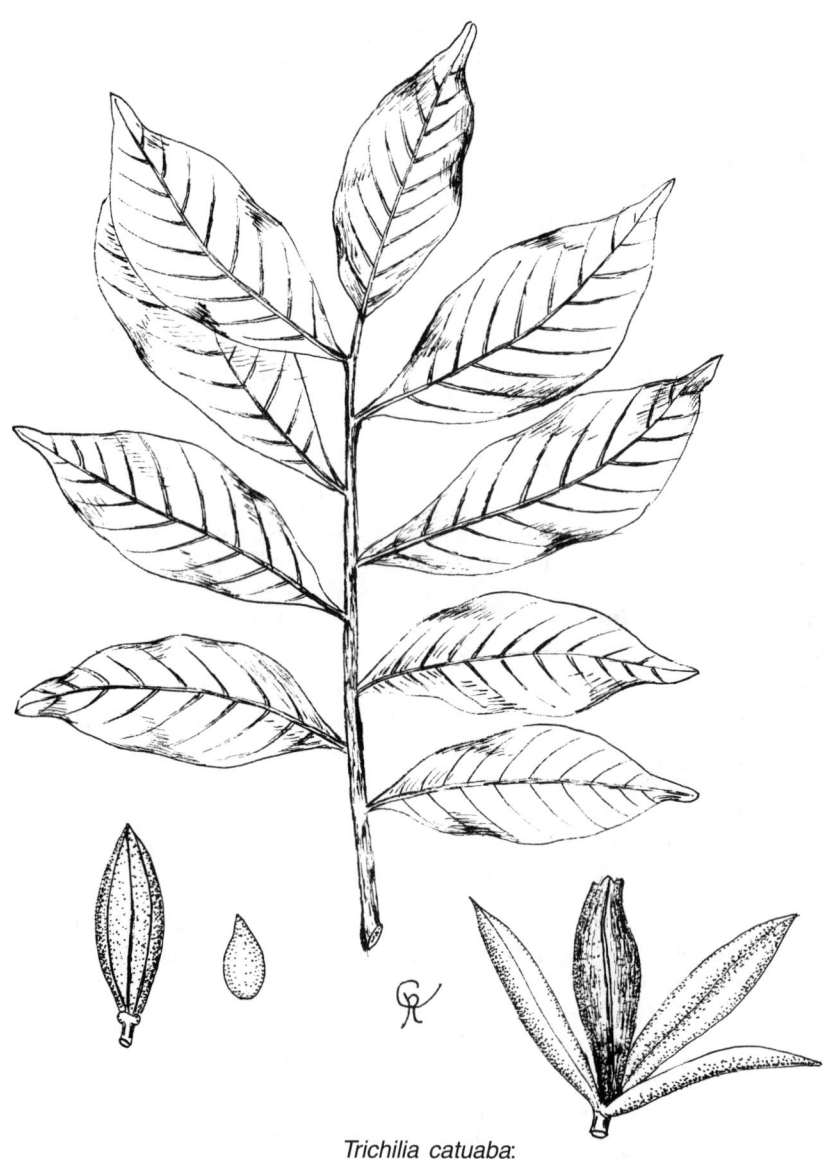

Trichilia catuaba:
A. Vegetative branch; B. Unripe capsule; C. Ripe opened capsule; D. Seed.

MELI 9. Lukacòva, V., J. Polonsky, C. Moretti, G.R. Pettit & J.M. Schmidt. 1982. Isolation and structure of 14,15 -epoxiprieurianin from the South American tree *Guarea guidona*. *J. Nat. Prod.* 45: 288-294.

MELI 10. Simoni, I.C., V. Munford, J.D. Felicio & A.P. Lins. 1996. Antiviral activity of crude extracts of *Guarea guidona*. *Braz. J. Med. Biol. Res.* 29: 647-650.

MENISPERMACEAE

Abuta candicans Rich.
AREA: Amazonia, forest.
NAMES: Abútua, cipó-amargoso.
USES: Roots and branches extemely bitter, reputed to be tonic and excitant, but poisonous in higher doses.

Abuta concolor Poepp. & Endl.
AREA: Amazonia, forest.
NAMES: Abuta, abútua, bútua, caapeba, parreira-brava.
USES: Roots and stem bark are antipyretic, indicated for contusions and ophthalmia; also reputedly effective in expelling calculi from kidneys.

Abuta rufescens Aubl.
AREA: Amazonia to Rio de Janeiro, forest.
NAMES: Abútua, bútua, parreira-brava, pané.
USES: Roots are bitter, tonic, stomachic, antidyspeptic; also emmenagogue, diuretic and for liver disorders, bladder ailments and flatulence. Reputedly effective against snakebite.
CHEM.: Alkaloids of peculiar structure have been isolated from the vine (Ref: MENI 1,2,3).

Abuta selloana Eichl.
AREA: Rio de Janeiro, Minas Gerais and São Paulo, forest.
NAMES: Abútua, bútua, baga-de-caboclo, uva-de-gentio.
USES: Roots are tonic, antithermic and diuretic.

Chondodendron platyphyllum (Mart.) Miers
AREA: Espírito Santo to Paraná, forest.
NAMES: Abútua-da-terra, abútua-grande, abútua-preta, baga-da-praia, jabuticaba-de-cipó, orelha-de-onça, parreira-brava, uva-do-mato.
USES: Root is prescribed to combat anemia, chlorosis, gastric disorders, renal lithiasis, malaria, menstrual colics, dysmenorrhoea and orchitis. Abortifacient in high doses; rather toxic.
CHEM. & PHARM.: *Chondodendron platyphyllum* and *C. tomentosum* (the latter an extra-Brazilian species) are the main curare-yielding Menispermaceae, source of the so-called tubocurares. This not being a medicinal property, it is not mentioned in the above descriptions. For a review of these alkaloids, see Ref: MENI 4. Calabash curares, different in chemical structure, are made from *Strychnos* species (Loganiaceae).

Cissampelos fasciculata Benth.
AREA: Espírito Santo to São Paulo.
NAMES: Abútua, batata-brava, batata-da-uva-do-mato, batata-caapeba, bútua.

MENISPERMACEAE

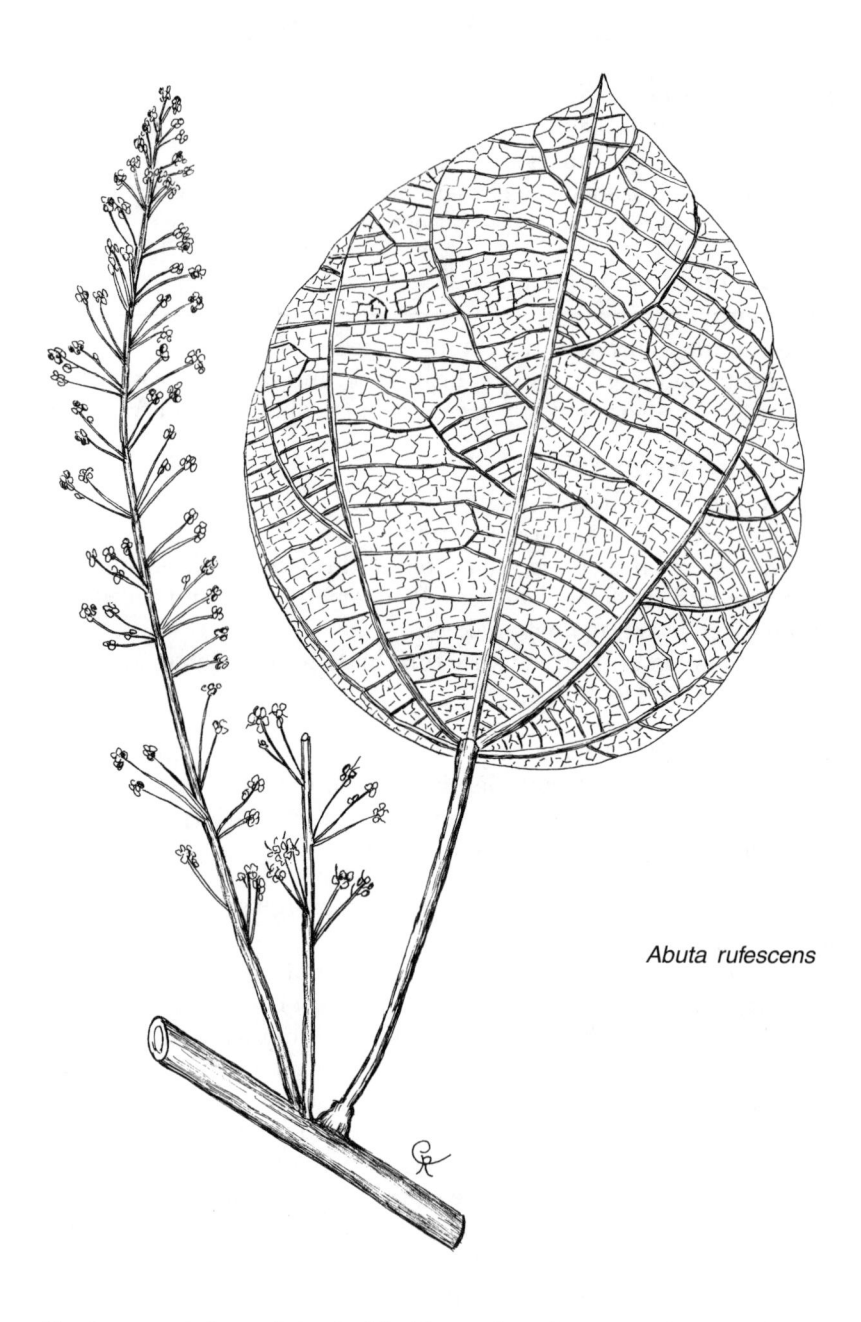

Abuta rufescens

USES: Roots are astringent, tonic, febrifuge, given in cases of metrorrhagia, leucorrhoea and cystitis. Leaves are antidiarrhoeic, antileucorrhoeic and antigonorrhoeic.

Cissampelos fluminensis Eichl.

AREA: Amazonia and Rio de Janeiro, forest.
NAMES: Abútua-do-rio, parreira-brava-do-rio.
USES: Employed against bladder stones.

Cissampelos glaberrima St.-Hil.

AREA: Minas Gerais and Rio de Janeiro to Paraná and Mato Grosso.
NAMES: Abutinha, abútua, butinha, caapeba, catojé, ciparoba, cipó-de-cobra, erva-de-nossa-senhora, parreira-brava-lisa, parreira-caapeba.
USES: Roots are tonic, febrifuge, sudorific, stomachic, lithontriptic, antiasthmatic and used against snakebite. Also used in homeopathy to treat asthma, dyspepsia and urinary problems.
CHEM.: Two alkamides and one alkaloid were isolated from the roots (Ref: MENI 5,6).

Cissampelos ovalifolia DC.

AREA: Throughout Brazil; frequent in the cerrado.
NAMES: Abútua-pequena, orelha-de-onça.
USES: Tuberous roots are bitter, tonic, diaphoretic, diuretic, resolvent, vulnerary; also used against infectious diseases and renal lithiasis.
CHEM. & PHARM.: An isolated alkaloid showed neuromuscular blocking and local anaesthetic activity (Ref: MENI 7).

Cissampelos pareira L.

AREA: In most parts of Brazil, forest.
NAMES: Abútua, cipó-de-cabras, cipó-de-gota, erva-de-nossa-senhora, orelha-de-onça, parreira-brava.
USES: Roots are tonic, diuretic, febrifuge, antidysenteric, antidysmenorrhoeic, emmenagogue, and recommended for cystitis and liver ailments.
CHEM. & PHARM.: Several alkaloids have been isolated, belonging mainly to the bisbenzylisoquinoline type and exhibiting high cytotoxic activity (Ref: MENI 8,9,10,11,12,13,14,15).

Cissampelos sympodialis Eichl.

AREA: Alagoas to Minas Gerais.
NAME: Orelha-de-onça.
USES: Root decoction is bitter, tonic, diuretic, resolvent, indicated for leucorrhoea and amenorrhoea, as well as to improve breathing in crises of asthma and bronchitis.
CHEM. & PHARM.: An alkaloid of the morphinane type has been identified in the leaves (Ref: MENI 16). Bronchodilatory activity has been confirmed in root extracts (Ref: MENI 17).

MENISPERMACEAE

Cocculus filipendula Mart.
AREA: Bahia to Minas Gerais and Rio de Janeiro, forest.
NAME: Abútua-miúda.
USES: Tuberous root is bitter, very poisonous. Indicated for delayed menses and liver and bladder afflictions.

Sciadotenia paraensis (Eichl.) Diels
AREA: Amazonia, forest.
NAME: Abútua.
USES: Roots are made into a beverage offered to women after childbirth. Also for kidney disease and diarrhoea.

Menispermaceae – References

MENI 1. Cava, M.P., K.T. Buck & I. da Rocha. 1972. Azafluoranthene alkaloids. A new structural type. *J. Am. Chem. Soc. 94*: 5931.

MENI 2. Cava, M.P., K.T. Buck, I. Noguchi, M. Srinavasan, M.G. Rao & A.I. da Rocha. 1975. The alkaloids of *Abuta imene* and *Abuta rufescens*. *Tetrahedron 31*: 1667-1669.

MENI 3. Silverton, J.V., C. Kabuto, K.T. Buck & M.P. Cava. 1977. Structure of imerubrine, a novel condensed tropolone-isoquinoline alkaloid. *J. Am. Chem. Soc. 99*: 6708-6712.

MENI 4. Wintersteiner, O. 1959. The chemistry of the *Chondodendron* alkaloids. *In*: Bovet, D., et al., eds. *Curare and Curare-like Agents*. Amsterdam: Elsevier. (Pp. 153-162.)

MENI 5. Rosario, S.L., A.J. Ribeiro da Silva & J.P. Parente. 1996. Alkamides from *Cissampelos glaberrima*. *Planta Medica 62*: 376-377.

MENI 6. Barbosa-Filho, J.M., E.V.L. da Cunha, M.L. Cornélio, C.S. Dias & A.I. Gray. 1997. Cissaglaberrimine, an aporphine alkaloid from *Cissampelos glaberrima*. *Phytochemistry 44*: 959-961.

MENI 7. Gorinsky, C., D.K. Luscombe & P.J. Nicholls. 1972. Neuromuscular blocking and local anaesthetic activity of warifteine hydrochloride, an alkaloid isolated from *Cissampelos ovalifolia* D.C. *J. Pharmacol. 24* (Suppl.): 147.

MENI 8. Srivastava, R.M. & M.P. Khare. 1964. Über wasserlösliche Alkaloide aus der Wurzelrinde von *Cissampelos pareira* L. *Chem. Ber. 97*: 2732-2741.

MENI 9. Kupchan, S.M., A.C. Patel & E. Fujita. 1965. Tumor inhibitors. VI. Cissampareine, new cytotoxic alkaloid from *Cissampelos pareira*. Cytotoxicity of bisbenzylisoquinoline alkaloids. *J. Pharm. Sci. 54*: 580-583.

MENI 10. Kupchan, S.M., S. Kubota, E. Fujita, S. Kobayashi, J.H. Block & S.A. Telang. 1966. Tumor inhibitors. XV. The structure and configuration of cissampareine, a novel bisbenzylisoquinoline alkaloid. *J. Am. Chem. Soc. 88*: 4212-4218.

MENI 11. Haynes, L.J., E.J. Herbert & J.R. Plimmer. 1966. (++)-4"-0-Methylcurine from *Cissampelos pareira* L. *J. Chem. Soc.*: 615-617.

MENI 12. Bhatnagar, A.K. & S.P. Popli. 1967. Chemical examination of the roots of *Cissampelos pareira* L. V. Structure and stereochemistry of hyatidin. *Experientia 23*: 242-243.

MENI 13. Bhatnagar, A.K., S. Bhattacharji, A.C. Roy & S.P. Popli. 1967. Chemical examination of the roots of *Cissampelos pareira*. *J. Org. Chem. 32*: 819-820.

MENI 14. Dwuma-Badu, D., J.S.K. Ayim, C.A. Mingle, A.N. Tackie, D.J. Slatkin, J.E. Knapp & P.L. Schiff, Jr. 1975. Alkaloids of *Cissampelos pareira*. *Phytochemistry 14*: 2520-2521.

MENI 15. Ahmad, R., M.A. Malik & M. Zia-Ul-Haq. 1992. Alkaloids of *Cissampelos pareira*. *Fitoterapia 63*: 282.

MENI 16. Freitas, M.R., J.L. Alencar, E.V.L. Cunha, J.M. Barbosa-Filho & A.I. Gray. 1995. Milonine, a novel 8, 14-dihydromorphinandienone alkaloid from the leaves of *Cissampelos sympodialis* Eichl. *Phytochemistry 40*: 1553-1555.

MENI 17. Thomas, G., C.C. Araújo, M.F. Agra, M.F.F. Diniz, M. Bachelat & B.B. Vargaftig.

1995. Preliminary studies on the hydroalcoholic extract of the root of *Cissampelos sympodialis* Eichl. in guinea-pig tracheal strips and bronchoalveolar leucocytes. *Phytotherapy Res. 9*: 473-477.

MENYANTHACEAE

Nymphoides indica (L.) O. Ktze.

AREA: Observed in most parts of Brazil, in stagnant puddles and lagoons, neotropical.

NAMES: Aguapé-de-flor-miúda, aperana, golfo, muraré, soldanela, soldanela-d'água.

USES: Leaf infusion is bitter, tonic, antidyspeptic, antifebrile and anticatarrhal; also used for removing intestinal parasites.

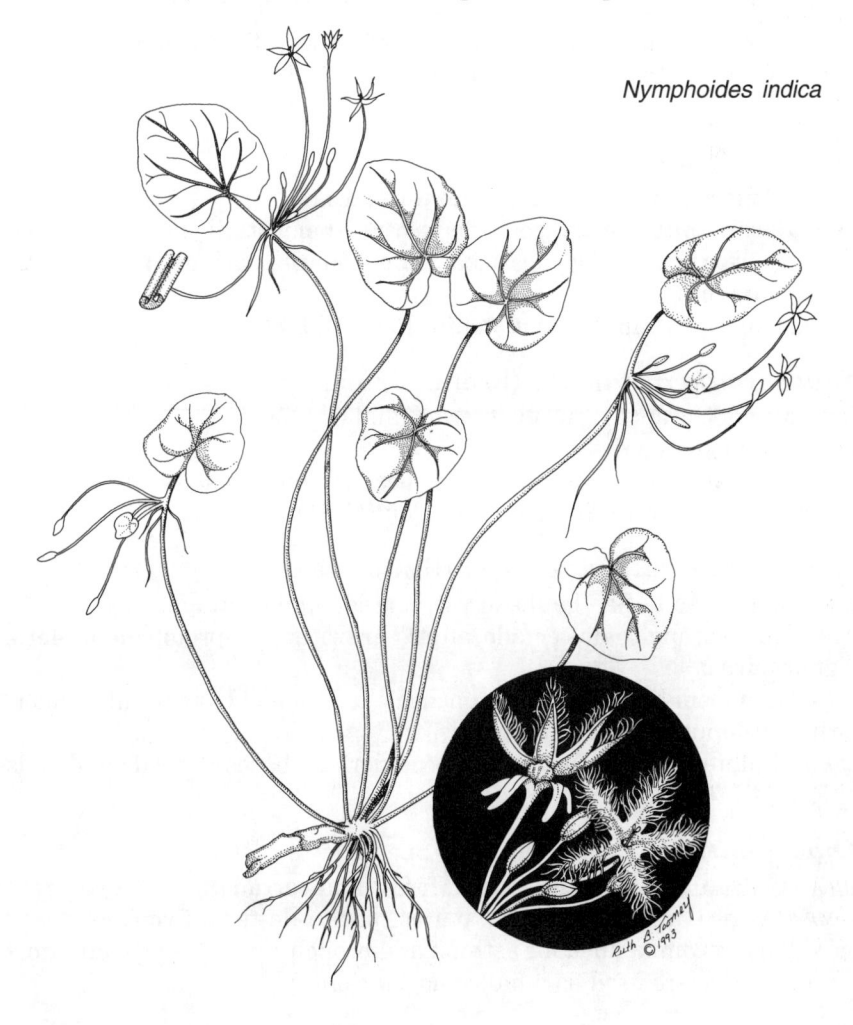

Nymphoides indica

MIMOSACEAE

Acacia paniculata Willd.
AREA: Amazonia to Paraná, forest.
NAMES: Barbadinho, sessenta-feridas, unha-de-gato.
USES: Leaves are antirheumatic, used mainly against arthralgia.

Albizzia lebbeck (L.) Benth.
AREA: Cosmopolitan; much cultivated in streets and public parks.
NAMES: Coração-de-negro, ébano-oriental.
USES: Bark used for diarrhoea, dysentery and piles. Leaves for ophthalmia. Flowers applied locally to mature boils and alleviate skin eruptions. Seeds reduced to a powder are indicated for scrofula.
CHEM.: The seeds contain saponins (Ref: MIMO 1,2,3) and a non-proteinogenic amino acid, albizziin (Ref: MIMO 4). The gum which exudes from the bark has been studied (Ref: MIMO 5).

Anadenanthera colubrina (Vell.) Brenan
AREA: Maranhão to Paraná, forest.
NAMES: Angico, angico-branco, cambuí-branco.
USES: Bark is bitter, astringent, depurative, hemostatic; used to ameliorate leucorrhoea and gonorrhoea. Gum from the bark used for respiratory ailments.
CHEM.: Seeds contain 2.1% bufotenin (Ref: MIMO 6).

Anadenanthera falcata (Benth.) Brenan
AREA: Minas Gerais to Paraná, cerrado and dry forest.
NAMES: Angico, pau-de-boaz.
USES: The gum-resin from the bark is used for pulmonary afflictions.
CHEM.: The seeds contain bufotenin (Ref: MIMO 7).

Anadenanthera macrocarpa (Benth.) Brenan
AREA: Maranhão to São Paulo, forest, cerrado and caatinga.
NAMES: Angico, angico-do-cerrado, angico-bravo, angico-preto, cambuí-fero, guarapiraca.
USES: Gum from bark used for bronchitis. Infusion of bark is anti-hemorrhagic, depurative and pectoral.
CHEM.: Bufotenin and other tryptamine-derived bases in seeds and pods (Ref: MIMO 8).

Anadenanthera peregrina (L.) Speg.
AREA: Amazonia and central Brazil, forest and cerrado.
NAMES: Angico, angico-vermelho, paricá, paricá-da-terra-firme.
USES: Bark recommended for asthma and bronchitis. Seeds ground into a fine powder are used as a hallocinogenic snuff.

MIMOSACEAE

CHEM.: Bufotenin and other indole bases were identified in seeds and bark (Ref: MIMO 9,10,11,12). A ß-carboline base, which is a monoamine oxidase inhibitor, is also present, and may potentiate the hallucinogenic effects of the tryptamines (Ref: MIMO 13,14).

Calliandra tweedii Benth.
AREA: Rio Grande do Sul.
NAMES: Pente-de-macaco, quebra-foice, topete-de-cardeal.
USES: Infusion of the flowers is employed to cure ophthalmia.

Entada paranaguana B. Rodr.
AREA: Amazonia, forest.
NAMES: Jipico, jipoca, jipooca (formerly spelled with G instead of J).
USES: Roots foam abundantly in water when crushed, due to high saponin content. The resulting emulsion is used against dandruff.

Entada polyphylla Benth.
AREA: On the banks of the Amazon river.
NAMES & USES: The same as for *Entada paranaguana* B. Rodr.

Entada polystachya (Jacq.) DC.
AREA: Neotropical; Amazonia, forest.
NAME: Cipó-da-beira-mar.
USES: Roots are prescribed for venereal diseases.

Inga alba (Sw.) Willd.
AREA: Amazonia, forest.
NAME: Ingá-xixi.
USE: Bark is strongly vomitive.

Inga lateriflora Miq.
AREA: Amazonia, forest.
NAME: Ingá-xixi.
USES: Bark is macerated in water to cure sores.

Inga setigera DC.
AREA: Amazonia, forest.
NAME: Ingá-de-flor-amarela.
USES: The flesh of the pods is used against bronchitis. Bark decoction is used to relieve aphthae and laryngitis.

Mimosa acutistipula Benth.
AREA: Ceará to Bahia, caatinga.
NAMES: Jurema, jurema-preta.
USES: Same as given for *M. hostilis* Benth.

Mimosaceae

Mimosa bimucronata (DC.) O. Ktze.
AREA: Pernambuco to Rio Grande do Sul, along coastal tracts.
NAMES: Espinheira, espinheiro-de-cerca, espinho-de-cerca, espinho-roxo, espinho-de-maricá, maricá, unha-de-gato.
USES: Infusion of young shoots is used to relieve asthma, asthmatic bronchitis and recurrent fevers. Leaves are mucilaginous and emollient.

Mimosa caesalpiniaefolia Benth.
AREA: Maranhão to Ceará, forest.
NAME: Sabiá.
USES: Bark is used for a bechic.
CHEM.: Bark contains the triterpene morolic acid (Ref: MIMO 15).

Mimosa hostilis Benth.
AREA: Northeastern Brazil, caatinga.
NAMES: Espinheiro, espinheiro-preto, jurema, jurema-preta.
USES: Some Indian people used the bark to prepare an intoxicating beverage, known as "vinho de jurema" (jurema wine), which produces a pleasant excitement and, subsequently, fantastic, though agreeable, dreams.
CHEM.: The bark contains N,N,-dimethyltryptamine (Ref: MIMO 6).

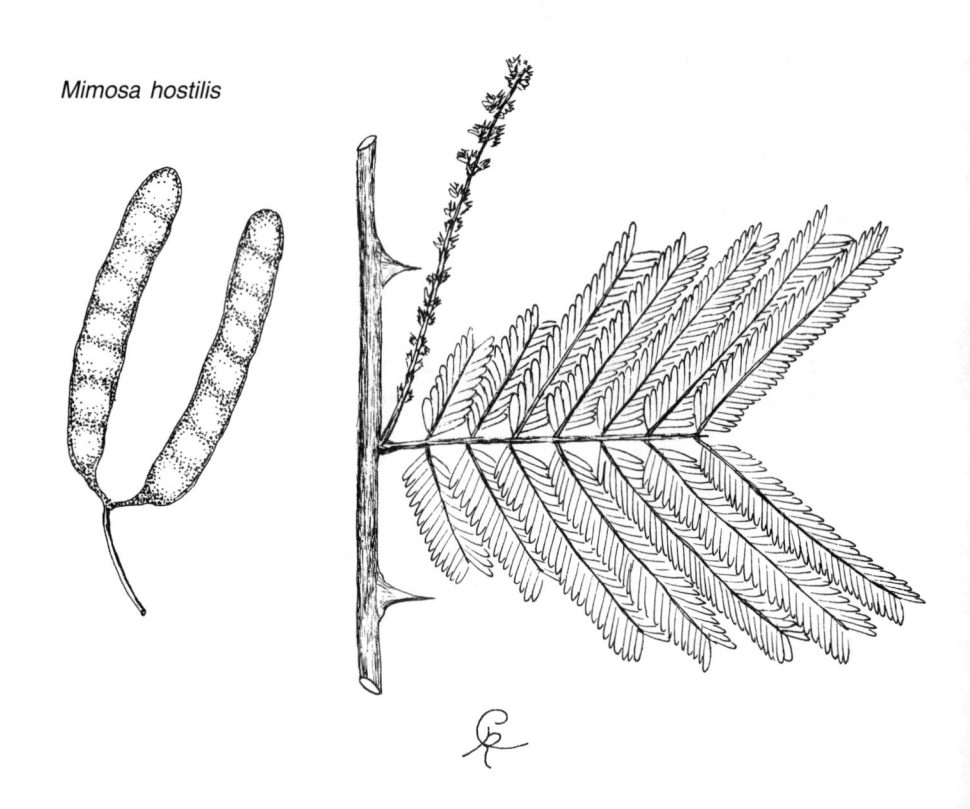

Mimosa hostilis

MIMOSACEAE

Mimosa verrucosa

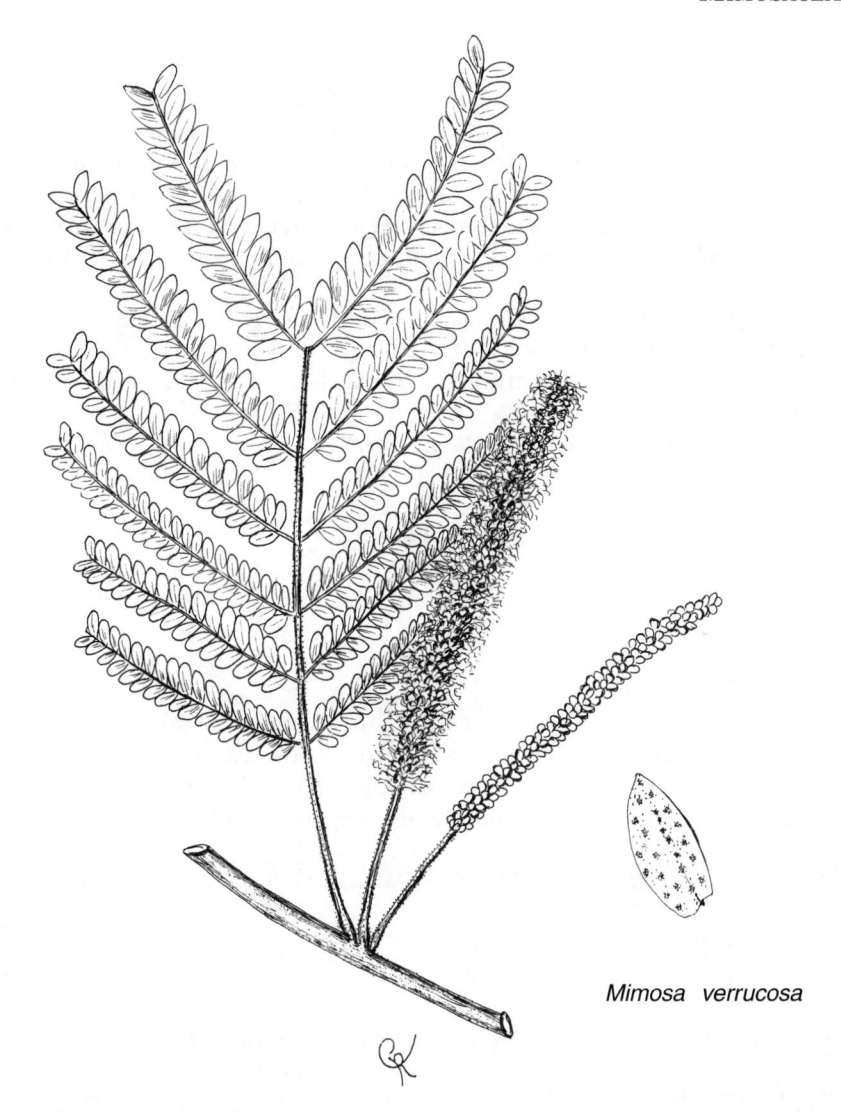

Mimosa invisa Mart.
AREA: Tropical, sparsely distributed in Brazil.
NAME: Malícia-de-mulher.
USES: Diuretic and to expel bladder stones.

Mimosa malacocentra Mart.
AREA: Pernambuco to Rio de Janeiro, caatinga and wasteland.
NAMES: Avoador, calumbi, espinho-de-cerca, jurema, jureminha, rompe-gibão, unha-de-gato.
USES: Baths with a decoction of the leaves are used for rheumatism and boils.

MIMOSACEAE

Mimosa pudica L.
AREA: Amazonia to São Paulo, as a ruderal plant.
NAMES: Dormideira, juquiri, malícia-de-mulher, sensitiva, vergonha.
USES: Roots are irritating, purgative, emetic, employed in baths against swollen joints due to rheumatism. Also for diphtheria. Flowers in baths are used to treat tumors and leucorrhoea or in cataplasms for scrofula. Infusion of leaves is bitter, tonic, purgative and used for gonorrhoea.

Mimosa velloziana Mart.
AREA: Bahia to São Paulo and Mato Grosso, campo.
NAMES: Dorme-maria, dormideira, dormideira-grande, malícia-das-mulheres, sensitiva.
USES: Similar to those given for *M. pudica* L.

Mimosa verrucosa Benth.
AREA: Throughout the northeastern caatinga.
NAME: Jurema.
USES: Bark is sedative, narcotic (see *M. hostilis*), bitter, astringent.

Parapiptadenia rigida (Benth.) Brenan
AREA: São Paulo to Rio Grande do Sul, forest.
NAMES: Angico-branco, angico-cedro, angico-de-curtume, angico-do-banhado, angico-rosa, angico-verdadeiro, angico-dos-montes, guarucaia.
USES: Bark is bitter, reputed against leucorrhoea, diarrhoea and ulcers. Tincture of leaves stops hemorrhage. Gum is expectorant.

Parkia oppositifolia (Spruce) Benth.
AREA: Amazonia, forest.
NAMES: Arara-tucupé, paricá, visgueiro.
USES: Bark is astringent, used against hemorrhage and to cure wounds and ulcers.
CHEM.: The stem bark contains methyl salicylate (Ref: MIMO 16).

Parkia pectinata Benth.
AREA: Amazonia, forest.
NAMES: Paricá, visguero.
USES: Same as given for *Parkia oppositifolia* (Spruce) Benth.

Parkia pendula Benth. ex Walp.
AREA: Amazonia, forest.
NAME: Cordão-de-são-francisco.
USES: Bark used in baths to treat inflammations, itch, vaginal flow and swelling. Dry powdered bark is placed on wounds for cicatrization.

MIMOSACEAE

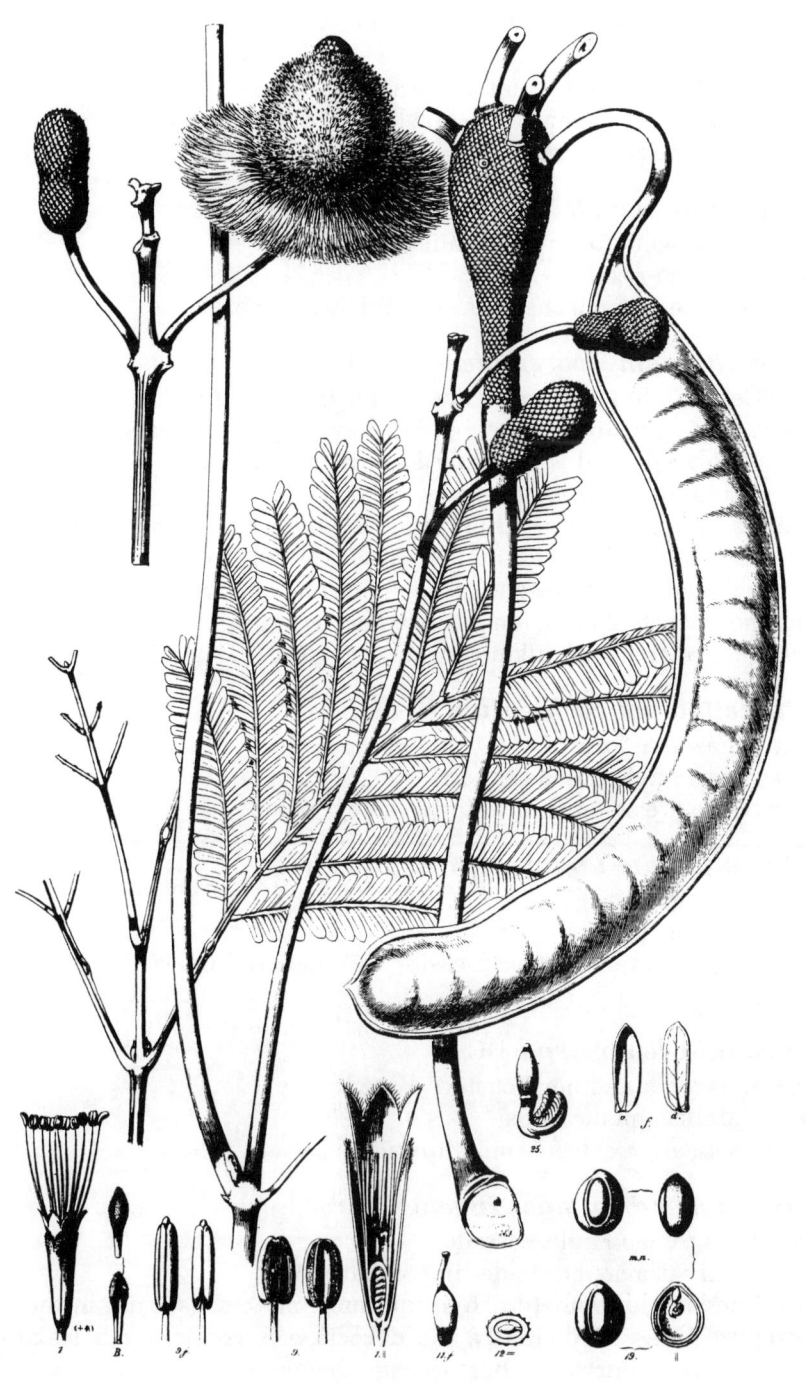

Parkia oppositifolia

MIMOSACEAE

Pentaclethra macroloba (Willd.) O. Ktze.
AREA: Amazonia, forest.
NAMES: Mulateiro, pau-mulato, pracaxi.
USES: Bark is astringent. Seeds and bark are recommended for snakebite and to cicatrize ulcers.

Piptadenia polyptera Benth.
AREA: Rio de Janeiro, on mountains.
NAME: Espinho-roxo.
USES: Gum-resin from the bark is given as a pectoral.

Pithecellobium avaremotemo Mart.
AREA: Ceará to Rio de Janeiro and Minas Gerais, forest.
NAMES: Angico, avaremotemo, bordão-de-velho, guaipipocaíba.
USES: Powdered wood is prescribed to dry chronic ulcers. Bark decoction in vaginal baths for astringency.
CHEM. & PHARM.: Several other *Pithecellobium* species of the Brazilian northeast have been examined, although none of them is of popular medicinal use. The presence of saponins and alkaloids was verified and all the extracts showed inhibitory action on smooth and striated muscle, roughly related with alkaloidal content (Ref: MIMO 17).

Pithecellobium cochleatum (Willd.) Mart.
AREA: Amazonia, forest.
NAME: Lágrima-de-nossa-senhora.
USES: Seeds are steeped in water as an eyewash.

Pithecellobium unguis-cati (L.) Benth.
AREA: Amazonia.
NAME: Avaramo.
USES: Bark is bitter, used for dressing chronic sores; internally used as an antithermic.

Schrankia leptocarpa DC.
AREA: Amazonia and northeastern Brazil.
NAMES: Malícia, malícia-roxa.
USES: Roots are resolvent and diuretic.

Stryphnodendron adstringens (Mart.) Cov.
AREA: Pará to São Paulo, cerrado.
NAMES: Barbatimão, barba-de-timão, ibatimó.
USES: The bark, extremely rich in tannins, finds its main use in the tanning of hides. Medicinally, the decoction is recommended against leucorrhoea, diarrhoea, hemorrhage, hemorrhoids and for cleansing wounds and sores. Also as eye-drops against conjunctivitis. The fluid

Stryphnodendron coriaceum

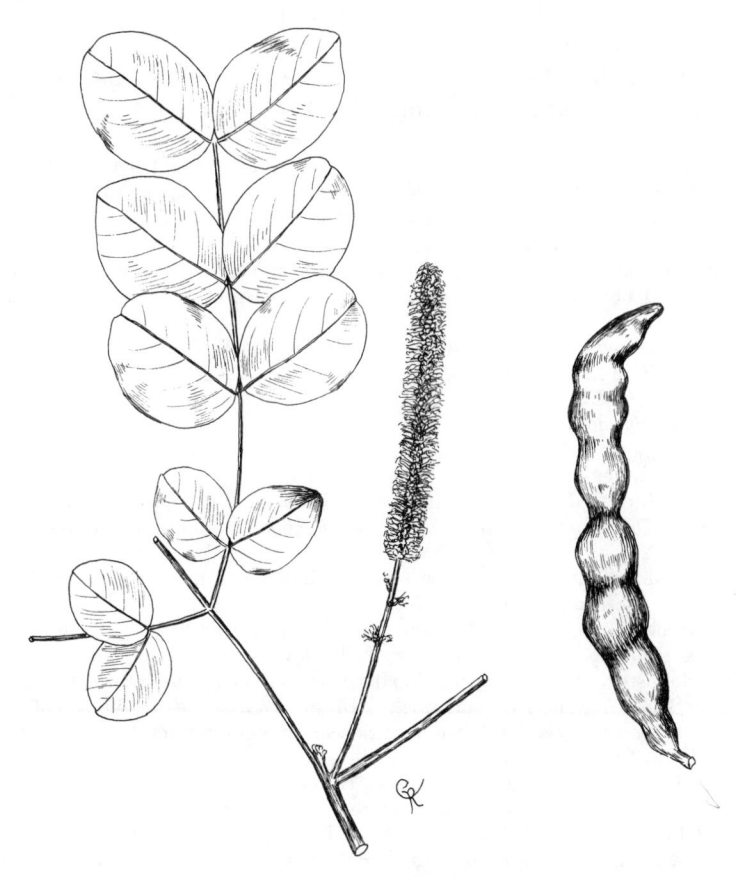

extract, taken by mouth, was shown to be effective as hypoglycemic and for eliminating uric acid (Ref: MIMO 18). In the cancer hospital of the city of Jaú, state of São Paulo, an ointment prepared from the decoction of the bark is being used successfully for preventing burns resulting from radiation treatment.

Stryphnodendron coriaceum Benth.
AREA: Northeastern caatinga.
NAME: Barbatimão.
USES: Plant is toxic. Bark is hemostatic, emetic, depurative; its decoction is used for cleaning ulcers, in vaginal baths and for gonorrhoea.

Mimosaceae

CHEM.: Plant is rich in saponins. Aglycons (sapogenins) belong to the ß-amyrin class of triterpenes (Ref: MIMO 19).

Stryphnodendron polyphyllum Mart.
AREA: Minas Gerais and Rio de Janeiro, forest.
NAMES: Barbatimão.
USES: Bark employed to stop hemorrhage and regulate vaginal flow.
PHARM.: Abortifacient in rats (Ref: MIMO 20).

Mimosaceae – References

MIMO 1. Varshney, I.P., G. Badhwar, A.A. Khan & A. Shrivastawa. 1971. Saponins and sapogenins of *Sesbania grandiflora* seeds, *Albizzia lebbeck* pods and *Psidium guajava* fruits. *Ind. J. Appl. Chem.* 34: 214-216.

MIMO 2. Varshney, I.P., G. Handa, H.C. Srivastava & T.N. Krishnamurthy. 1973. Partial structure of lebbekanin-A, a new saponin from the seeds of *Albizzia lebbeck* Benth. *Ind. J. Chem.* 11: 1094-1096.

MIMO 3. Varshney, I.P., G. Badhwar, H.C. Srivastava & T.N. Krishnamurthy. 1973. Lebbekanin-C, a new saponin from *Albizzia lebbeck* pods. *Planta Medica* 24: 183-189.

MIMO 4. Kraus, G.-J. & H. Reinbothe. 1970. Die Aminosäuren der Gattung *Albizzia* Durazz. *Biochem. u. Physiol. der Pflanzen* 161: 243-250.

MIMO 5. Farooqui, M.I.H. & K.N. Kaul. 1962. Chemical examination of siris (*Albizzia lebbeck* Benth.) gum. *J. Sci. Indus. Res.* 21B (9): 454-455.

MIMO 6. Pachter, L.J., D.E. Zacharias & O. Ribeiro. 1959. Indole alkaloids of *Acer saccharum*, *Dictyoloma incanescens*, *Piptadenia colubrina* and *Mimosa hostilis*. *J. Org. Chem.* 24: 1285.

MIMO 7. Giesbrecht, A.M. 1960. A ocorrência de bufotenina nas sementes de *Piptadenia falcata*. *An. Ass. Bras. Quím.* 19: 117-119.

MIMO 8. Iacobucci, G.A. & E.A. Rúveda. 1964. Bases derived from tryptamine in Argentine *Piptadenia* species. *Phytochemistry* 3: 465-467.

MIMO 9. Holmstedt, B. 1965. Tryptamine derivatives in epená, an intoxicating snuff used by some South American Indian tribes. *Arch. Int. Pharmacodyn.* 156: 285-305.

MIMO 10. Stromberg, V.S. 1954. The isolation of bufotenine from *Piptadenia peregrina* seeds. *J. Am. Chem. Soc.* 76: 170.

MIMO 11. Fish, M.S., N.M. Johnson & E.C. Horning. 1955. *Piptadenia* alkaloids. Indole bases of *P. peregrina* (L.) Benth. and related species. *J. Am. Chem. Soc.* 77: 5892-5895.

MIMO 12. Legler, G. & R. Tschesche. 1963. Die Isolierung von N-Methyltryptamin und 5-Methoxy-N, N-Dimethyltryptamin aus der Rinde von *Piptadenia peregrina*. *Naturwiss.* 50: 94-95; Also: Pereira, N.A. 1957. Obtenção da bufotenina das sementes de *Piptadenia peregrina* Benth. *Rev. Bras. Farm.* 38:139-142.

MIMO 13. Agurell, S., B. Holmstedt, J.E. Lindgren & R.E. Schultes. 1968. Identification of two beta-carboline alkaloids in South American hallucinogenic plants. *Biochem. Pharmacol.* 17: 2487-2488.

MIMO 14. Agurell, S., B. Holmstedt, J.E. Lindgren & R.E. Schultes. 1969. Alkaloids in certain species of *Virola* and other South American plants of ethnopharmacological interest. *Acta Chem. Scand.* 23: 903-916.

MIMO 15. Alencar, J.W., P.A. Roquayrol & F.J.A. Matos. 1970. Ácido morólico em *Mimosa caesalpiniaefolia*. *An. Acad. Bras. Ci.* 42 (Supl.): 93-95.

MIMO 16. Alencar, J.W., R. Alves de Lima, R.G. Campos Corrêa, O.R. Gottlieb, M. Leão da Silva, J. Marx, J.G.S. Maia, M.T. Magalhães & R.M. Viegas Assumpção. 1971. Óleos essenciais de plantas brasileiras. *Acta Amazonica* 1(3): 41-43. Also in *An. Acad. Brasil. Ci.* 44 (Supl.): 312-314 (1972).

MIMO 17. Barros, G.S., M.P. Souza, M.C. Madeiras & F.J.A. Matos. 1973. Some chemical and pharmacological properties of four Brazilian *Pithecellobium* species. *Rev. Bras. Pesq. Med. Biol.* 6: 71-76.

MIMO 18. Malhado Filho, J. 1946. Barbatimão. *Arquivos de Biologia* (São Paulo) *30*: 51.
MIMO 19. Tursch, B., E. Tursch, I.T. Harrison, G.B.T.C. Brazão da Silva, H.J. Monteiro, B. Gilbert, W.B. Mors & C. Djerassi. 1963. Terpenoids. LIII. Demonstration of ring conformational changes in the triterpenes of the beta-amyrin class isolated from *Stryphnodendron coriaceum*. *J. Org. Chem. 28*: 2390-2394.
MIMO 20. Guerra, M.O., F.C. Araujo, V.M. Peters & A.T.L. Andrade. 1980. Aborto em ratas após administração de barbatimão (*Stryphnodendron polyphyllum* M.). *Rev. Bras. Pesq. Med. Biol. 13*: 111-113.

MONIMIACEAE

Mollinedia schottiana (Spr.) Perk.
AREA: Rio de Janeiro and Santa Catarina, forest.
NAME: Erva-santa.
USES: Strong antispasmodic, useful for colics.

Siparuna brasiliensis (Spr.) DC.
AREA: Rio de Janeiro and São Paulo, forest.
NAMES: Cidreira, cidrilha, limão-bravo, limão-do-mato, limãozinho, erva-cidreira-do-mato, negramina.
USES: Leaves are excitant, antispasmodic, aromatic, stomachic, carminative; used for sore throat in gargles, syrups and lozenges. Also to dress contusions.

Siparuna camporum (Tul.) DC.
AREA: Amazonia, campo, especially near the Tocantins river, state of Amazonas.
NAME: Erva-cidreira-dos-campos.
USES: Excitant, aromatic, stomachic, carminative, emmenagogue, pectoral.

Siparuna cujabana (Mart.) DC.
AREA: Minas Gerais and Mato Grosso.
NAME: Limoeiro-bravo.
USES: Leaves used to dress contusions and for making cough drops.
CHEM.: Essential oil has been analyzed (Ref: MONI 1).

Siparuna guianensis Aubl.
AREA: Amazonia, forest.
NAMES: Capitiú, erva-santa, fedorento, negramina.
USES: Leaves and flowers are aromatic, stimulant, febrifuge, carminative, antidyspeptic, diuretic; used in baths against muscle spasms and headache.
CHEM.: Contains the oxoaporphine alkaloids liriodenine and cassamedine (Ref: MONI 2). Essential oil has been analyzed (Ref: MONI 3).

Monimiaceae / Moraceae

Siparuna laurifolia (H.B.K.) DC.
AREA: Amazonia, forest.
NAME: Capitiú-do-amazonas.
USES: Aromatic. Leaves and fruits are prescribed in baths against rheumatism.

Monimiaceae – References

MONI 1. Lima, R.A., R.M. Pinheiro, J.E. Paula, A.A. Craveiro, J.W. Alencar & M.I.L. Machado. 1979. Oleos essendiais de plantas do Distrito Federal. Parte I. O óleo essencial de *Siparuna cujabana* (Mart.) DC. *Rev. Bras. Geog. 41*: 110.

MONI 2. Braz Filho, R., S.J. Gabriel, C.M.R. Gomes, O.R. Gottlieb, M.D.G.A. Bichara & J.G.S. Maia. 1979. Oxoaporphine alkaloids from *Fusea longifolia* and *Siparuna guianensis*. *Phytochemistry 15*: 1187-1188.

MONI 3. Antonio, T.M., G.R. Waller & C.J. Mussinan. 1984. Composition of essential oil from the leaves of *Siparuna guianensis* (Monimiaceae). *Chem. & Ind.* : 514-515.

MORACEAE

Brosimum acutifolium Huber
AREA: Amazonia, forest.
NAMES: Mercúrio-da-terra-firme, mercúrio-vegetal, muira-piranga, mururé.
USES: Latex is depurative, though toxic in large doses. The same properties are attributed to *B. obovata* Ducke (Amazonia).

Brosimum gaudichaudii Tréc.
AREA: Central Brazil; Piauí to São Paulo.
NAMES: Amoreira-do-mato, apê-do-sertão, conduru, mama-cadela.
USES: An extract of the root bark is used topically to treat vitiligo.
CHEM.: The active constituents are the furocoumarins bergapten and psoralen (Ref: MORA 1,2).

Brosimum parinarioides Ducke
AREA: Amazonia, forest.
NAME: Amapá.
USES: Latex is said to strengthen the body.

Brosimum potabile Ducke
AREA: Amazonia, forest.
NAME: Amapá-de-várzea, amapá-doce, leiteira.
USES: Latex is appreciated as a fortifier, tonic.

Brosimum utile (H.B.K.) Pittier
AREA: Amazonia, forest.
NAME: Mururé.
USES: Latex is antipyretic.

CHEM.: All the above-mentioned *Brosimum* species contain furo- and pyranocoumarins (Ref: MORA 3).

Cecropia hololeuca Miq.
AREA: Rio de Janeiro, forest.
NAMES: Embaúba, embaúba-prateada.
USES: Leaves are a strong diuretic; tonic, astringent, emmenagogue, used for leucorrhoea, amenorrhoea, dysmenorrhoea and dysentery. Also for acute respiratory ailments, asthma and whooping cough. Said to possess digitalic properties.

Cecropia leucocoma Miq.
AREA: Amazonia, forest.
NAME: Embaúba-branca.
USES: Tea from roots and leaves is employed for stomach ailments.

Cecropia palmata Willd.
AREA: Amazonia to the Northeast; forest and second growth.
NAMES: Árvore-da-preguiça, embaúba, embaúba-branca, torém.
USES: Trunk pith and sprouts are vulnerary, hemostatic, antileucorrhoeic, antiblennorrhagic, antidiarrhoeic and antidiabetic. Young leaves are stimulant and diuretic.

Clarisia racemosa Ruiz & Pav.
AREA: Amazonas to Minas Gerais and Rio de Janeiro.
NAMES: Guariuba, oiticica, oiticica-cica, oiticica-vermelha.
USES: Bark decoction is applied externally for skin diseases.

Coussapoa asperifolia Tréc.
AREA: Amazonia, forest.
NAME: Caimbé.
USES: Latex is used to dress sloughing ulcers.

Dorstenia asaroides Gardn.
AREA: Amazonia, forest.
NAMES: Apii, caapiá.
USES: Rhizomes and fruits are tonic, stimulant, sudorific, diuretic, antimenorrhoeic, antifebrile, antianemic, antidiarrhoeic, antiophidic; also used against gangrene, for typhoid fever, digestive atony and respiratory problems. An ingredient in compresses to consolidate bone fractures.

Dorstenia brasiliensis Lam.
AREA: Ceará to São Paulo, forest.
NAMES: Caapiá, caapiá-açu, caiapiá, carapiá, conta-de-cobra, contraerva, figueirinha, liga-liga, liga-osso, taropé, tiú.

USES: Rhizome is antiseptic, stimulant, diaphoretic, tonic, purgative, bechic, diuretic, emmenagogue, antimalarial, for chronic diarrhoea, dysentery, orchitis, leucorrhoea, rheumatism, dermatoses, chlorosis. Internally and externally against snakebite; in compresses to solidify fractured bones.

CHEM.: The rhizomes contain the same furocoumarins as in *D. cayapia* and, in addition, psoralen (Ref: MORA 4,5).

Dorstenia cayapia Vell.

AREA: From Piauí to Mato Grosso, Goiás, Minas Gerais and São Paulo.
NAMES: Caapiá, caiapiá, carapiá.
USES: The same as those of the above species.
CHEM.: The rhizomes contain bergapten and a furocoumarin with a monoterpenoid substituent (Ref: MORA 6).

Dorstenia reniformis Pohl

AREA: Amazonia and central Brazil.
NAMES: Apeí.
USES: Roots used in syrup against cough.

Ficus gomelleira Kunth & Bouché

AREA: Espírito Santo to Rio Grande do Sul, forest.
NAMES: Gameleira, gameleira-branca.
USES: Latex is vermifuge, especially active against *Ancylostoma*, purgative; also for hydropsy and inflammation of the liver and spleen. Bark is tonic, depurative, antisyphilitic; externally applied for rheumatic and arthritic ailments. Also for washing ulcers. Used topically in powder form to reduce hernias. Leaves are resolvent; infusion against bladder catarrh.

Ficus insipida Willd.

AREA: Amazonia to Rio de Janeiro, forest.
NAMES: Apuí-açu, caxinguba, coaxinguba, figueira-do-mato, gameleira-branca, gameleira-roxa, lombrigueira.
USES: Latex is anthelmintic, but drastic, even corrosive; recommended for ancylostomiasis and jaundice. Also said to be aphrodisiac and to aid memory.
CHEM.: The leaves contain psoralen and several triterpenes, including a lactone of iso-hopene skeleton (Ref: MORA 7).

Ficus maxima P. Mill.

AREA: Pará to Ceará, forest.
NAMES: Caxinguba, coaxinguba, figueira-brava, figueira-de-lombrigueiro, gameleira-roxa, guaxinduba-preta.
USES: Latex is vermifuge, but its use is dangerous.

MORACEAE

Ficus trigona L. f.
AREA: Pará, forest.
NAME: Apuí.
USES: Infusion of root, bark and leaves has sedative properties.

Maclura brasiliensis Endl.
AREA: Bahia to Rio de Janeiro, forest.
NAMES: Espinheiro-amarelo, espinheiro-branco, espinheiro-bravo, tataíba, tatajuba-do-brejo.
USES: Latex prescribed in cases of suppuration. Fruits used in gargle for throat afflictions.

Maclura tinctoria (L.) D. Don
AREA: Frequent throughout Brazil, forest.
NAMES: Espinho-branco, moreira, oiticicia, tajuba, tatajuba, taúba (English: dyer's mulberry).
USES: Latex used for cicatrization of wounds and to soothe toothache.
CHEM.: The yellow coloring matter of the wood is the flavonol morin, accompanied by the benzophenone maclurin (Ref: MORA 8).

Maquira sclerophylla (Ducke) C. C. Berg
AREA: Amazonia, high forest.
NAMES: Muirá-tinga, rapé-dos-índios.
USES: The powdered seeds and bark are used by Indians in religious ceremonies in the form of a snuff which induces stimulation and euphoria.
CHEM. & PHARM.: Cardiac glycosides have been isolated, confirming the observation of digitalis-like effects (Ref: MORA 9,10).

Naucleopsis amara Ducke
AREA: Amazonia, forest.
NAMES: Bálsamo, quina.
USES: The bitter latex is given to treat malaria. It is probably one of the dart poisons used by the Chocó Indians of western Colombia, containing cardioactive glycosides (Ref: MORA 11).

Sorocea bonplandii (Baill.) Burger
AREA: Rio de Janeiro to Rio Grande do Sul, forest.
NAMES: Árvore-de-chocalho, bainha-de-espada, cincho.
USES: Bark used for ringworm. Latex is anthelmintic. Due to the similarity of the leaves, these are frequently used to adulterate *Maytenus ilicifolia* (Celastraceae).

Moraceae – References

MORA 1. Araujo Lima. O, & O. Ribeiro, 1967. Ocorrência de bergapteno na Morácea *Brosimum gaudichaudii*. *An. Assoc. Bras. Quím.* 26: 67-71.
MORA 2. Vilegas, W., Pozetti, G.L. and J.H.Y. Vilegas. 1993. Coumarins from *Brosimum gaudichaudii*. *J. Nat. Prod.* 56: 416-417.
MORA 3. Gottlieb, O.R., M. Leão da Silva & J.G.S. Maia. 1972. Distribution of coumarins in Amazonian *Brosimum* species. *Phytochemistry* 11: 3479-3480.
MORA 4. Bauer, L. & I.B. Noll. 1986. Furocumarinas em *Dorstenia brasiliensis*. *Caderno de Farmácia* (Porto Alegre) 2: 163-170.
MORA 5. Kuster, R.M., Bernardo, R.R., da Silva, A.J.R., Parente, J.P. & W.B. Mors. 1994. Furocoumarins from the rhizomes of *Dorstenia brasiliensis*. *Phytochemistry* 36: 221-223.
MORA 6. Llabres, G., M. Baiwar, W. Vilegas, G.L. Pozetti & J.H.Y. Vilegas. 1992. A^1 and ^{13}C NMR study of a novel naturally occurring furocoumarin from *Dorstenia cayapia*. *Spectrochimica Acta 48A*: 1347-1353.
MORA 7. Lopes, D., C.T. Villela, M.A.C. Kaplan & J.P.P. Carauta. 1993. Moretenolactone, a â-lactone hopanoid from *Ficus insipida*. *Phytochemistry* 34: 279-280.
MORA 8. Morris, Q.L., T.B. Gage & S.H. Wender. 1951. The isolation and purification of morin. *J. Am. Chem. Soc.* 73: 3340-3341.
MORA 9. Carvalho, J.E. & A.J. Lapa. 1990. Pharmacology of an Indian snuff obtained from Amazonian *Maquira sclerophylla*. *J. Ethnopharmacol.* 30: 43-54.
MORA 10. Carvalho, J.E., L.M.B. Torres & A.J. Lapa. 1991. Cardiac glycosides isolated from the Indian snuff, *Maquira sclerophylla* Ducke. *Mem. Inst. Oswaldo Cruz* (Rio de Janeiro) 86: 235-236.
MORA 11. Shresta, T., B. Kopp & N.G. Bisset. 1992. The Moraceae-based dart poisons of South America. Cardiac glycosides of *Maquira* and *Naucleopsis* species. *J. Ethnopharmacol.* 37: 129-143.

MYRISTICACEAE

Virola macrophylla (Spr. ex Benth.) Warb.
AREA: Amazonia, forest.
NAMES: Cananga, ucuuba (formerly spelled 'ucuhuba').
USES: Decoction of leaves applied externally against rheumatism.

Virola oleifera (Schott) A.C. Smith
AREA: Bahia to Rio Grande do Sul, forest.
NAMES: Bicuíba, bicuíba-vermelha, bocuba.
USES: Bark used for dysentery, hemoptysis, leucorrhoea and blennorrhagia; reduced to a dry powder to apply on the navel of newborns. Seeds are stomachic, antidyspeptic, stimulant, antiasthmatic, antispasmodic and also used against snakebite; oil from seeds used for skin disease, erysipelas, sores, rheumatism and neuralgia.

Virola sebifera Aubl.
AREA: Amazonia and central Brazil, forest and cerrado.
NAMES: Ucuuba, ucuuba-da-terra-firme, ucuuba-vermelha.
USES: Exudate from the bark and a bark infusion are recommended against dyspepsy, intestinal colics, erysipelas, inflammations; externally for

MYRISTICACEAE

Virola surinamensis

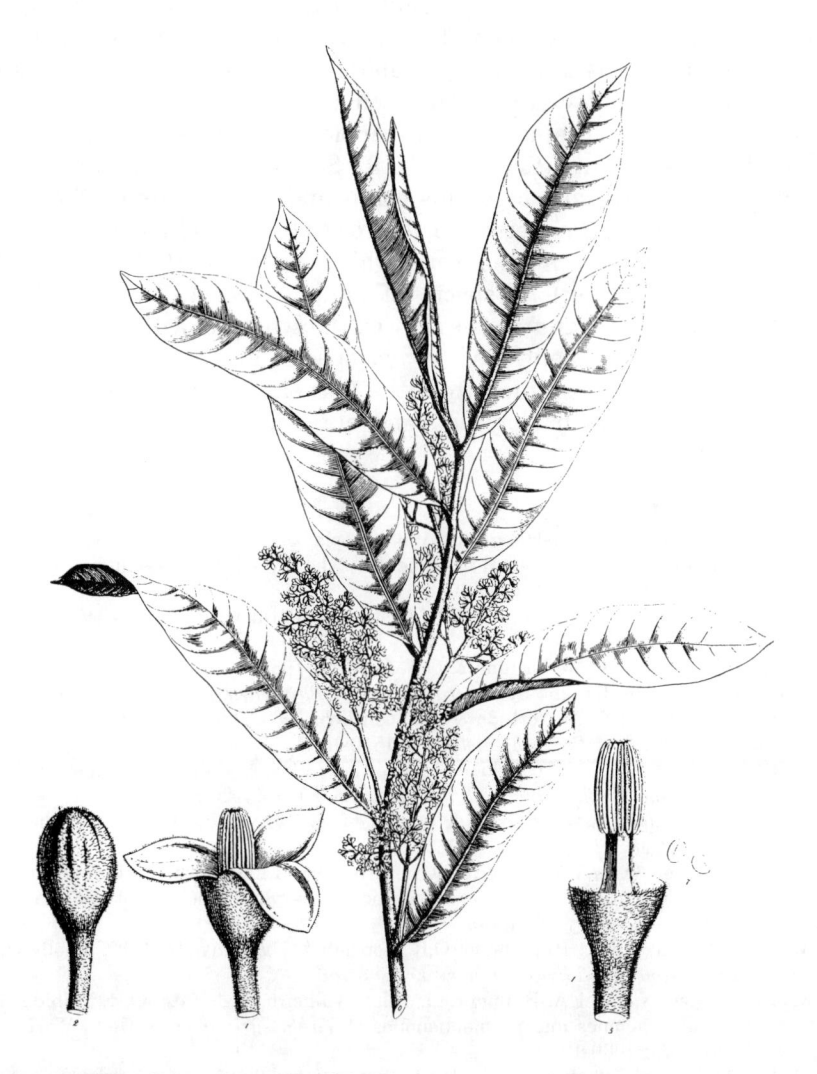

contusions and for cleaning ulcers.

CHEM.: This, like other species from this family, furnishes an exudate from the bark which is worked into preparations with psychotropic properties by several Indian tribes (Ref: MYRI 1). They are, however, not counted among the medicinals. N,N-dimethyltryptamine (Ref: MYRI 2) is a representative of the compounds which are responsible for such action. The leaves and seeds contain lignans and neolignans (Ref: MYRI 3,4,5,6).

MYRISTICACEAE

Virola surinamensis (Rol.) Warb.
AREA: Amazonia to Pernambuco, forest.
NAMES: Árvore-do-sebo, bicuíba, ucuuba, ucuuba-cheirosa, ucuuba-branca.
USES: Bark resin is a resolvent. Bark decoction helps in cases of sloughing ulcers, erysipelas, infections, wounds. Tea from leaves used for stomach troubles. Tallow from seeds used as rubs for aphthae and piles.
CHEM.: The wood contains diarylpropanoids (Ref: MYRI 7) and the leaves contain neolignans (Ref: MYRI 8,9). Several neolignans are counted among the naturally occurring compounds which protect the skin of mammals against penetration of cercaria (the infecting larval stage) of *Schistosoma mansoni*, the worm which causes South American schistosomiasis. Of over forty species of plants tested, the hexane extract of the leaves of *V. surinamensis* showed the strongest activity (Ref: MYRI 8). The last two mentioned *Virola* species are producers of ucuuba ("ucuhuba") fat, obtained from the kernels. The value of this tallow derives from its high trimyristin and laurodimyristin content (Ref: MYRI 10,11,12).

Myristicaceae – References

MYRI 1. Schultes, R.E. & B. Holmstedt. 1968. De plantis toxicariis e mundo novo tropicale commentationes. II. The vegetal ingredients of the myristicaceous snuffs of the Northwest Amazon. *Rhodora 70*: 113-160.
MYRI 2. Corothie, E. & T. Nakano. 1969. Constituents of the bark of *Virola sebifera*. *Planta Medica 17*: 184-188.
MYRI 3. Lopes, L.M.X., M. Yoshida & O.R. Gottlieb. 1982. 1,11-Diarylundecan-1-one and 4-aryltetralone neolignans from *Virola sebifera*. *Phytochemistry 21*: 751-755.
MYRI 4. Lopes, L.M.X., M. Yoshida & O.R. Gottlieb. 1983. Dibenzylbutyrolactone lignans from *Virola sebifera*. *Phytochemistry 22*: 1516-1518.
MYRI 5. Lopes, L.M.X., M. Yoshida & O.R. Gottlieb. 1984. Aryltetralone and arylindanone neolignans from *Virola sebifera*. *Phytochemistry 23*: 2021-2024.
MYRI 6. Lopes, L.M.X., M. Yoshida & O.R. Gottlieb. 1984. Further lignoids from *Virola sebifera*. *Phytochemistry 23*: 2647-2652.
MYRI 7. Gottlieb, O.R., A.A. Loureiro, M.S. Carneiro & A.I. da Rocha. 1973. The chemistry of Brazilian Myristicaceae. II. The distribution of diarylpropanoids in Amazonian *Virola* species. *Phytochemistry 12*: 1830.
MYRI 8. Barata, L.E.S., P.M. Baker, O.R. Gottlieb & E.A. Rúveda. 1987. Neolignans of *Virola surinamensis*. *Phytochemistry 17*: 783-786.
MYRI 9. Lopes, N.P., E.F.A. Blumenthal, A.J. Cavalheiro. M.J. Kato & M. Yoshida. 1996. Neolignans, γ-lactones and propiophenones of *Virola surinamensis* (Rol.) Warb. *Phytochemistry 43*: 1089-1092.
MYRI 10. Michler, W. & A. Sampaio. 1883. Investigações chimicas dos productos naturaes do Brasil. Materia graxa de ucuhuba. *Revista de Engenharia do Rio de Janeiro 5*: 119-121.
MYRI 11. Steger, A. & J. van Loon. 1935. Ucuhubafett. *Rec. Trav. Chim. Pays-Bas 54*: 149-157.
MYRI 12. Culp, T.W., R.D. Harlow, C. Litchfield & R. Reiser. 1965. Analysis of triglycerides by consecutive chromatographic technique. II. Ucuhuba kernel fat. *J. Am. Oil Chem. Soc. 42*: 974-978.

MYRSINACEAE

Cybianthus detergens Mart.
AREA: Ceará to São Paulo.
NAMES: Farinha-seca, jacaré-do-mato.
USES: Decoction of roots and bark used in treating tinea and certain skin ailments, in baths and lotions.

MYRTACEAE

Blepharocalyx salicifolius (H.B.K.) Berg
AREA: Rio Grande do Sul.
NAMES: Guabiroba, guabiroba-do-rio-grande-do-sul.
USES: Leaves are astringent, useful for bladder catarrh, mucous diarrhoea, leucorrhoea, urethritis and rectal prolapse.

Calyptranthes aromatica St.-Hil.
AREA: Rio de Janeiro and Minas Gerais.
NAME: Craveiro-da-terra.
USES: Leaves are excitant, antispasmodic, efficient to expel tapeworms. Bark is carminative, serving as a condiment. Floral buds are used as a substitute for cloves.

Calyptranthes variabilis Berg
AREA: Minas Gerais to Rio Grande do Sul, campo.
NAMES: Craveiro-do-campo, cravo-do-campo.
USES: Plant is aromatic and excitant.

Campomanesia aurea Berg
AREA: Rio Grande do Sul, campo.
NAMES: Araçá-rasteiro, guabiroba, guabiroba-do-campo.
USES: Antidiarrhoeic and used against bladder and urethral catarrh. *C. xanthocarpa* Berg (São Paulo to Rio Grande do Sul) has similar uses.

Eugenia brasiliensis Lam.
AREA: Southern Brazil, sometimes cultivated.
NAMES: Grumixama, grumixaba, ibaporoiti.
USES: Bark and leaves are aromatic, astringent, reputedly useful as diuretic and against rheumatism.

Eugenia dysenterica DC.
AREA: Minas Gerais and Goiás, cerrado.
NAME: Cagaiteira.
USES: Berries are tasty, mildly laxative in higher doses.

MYRTACEAE

Eugenia dysenterica

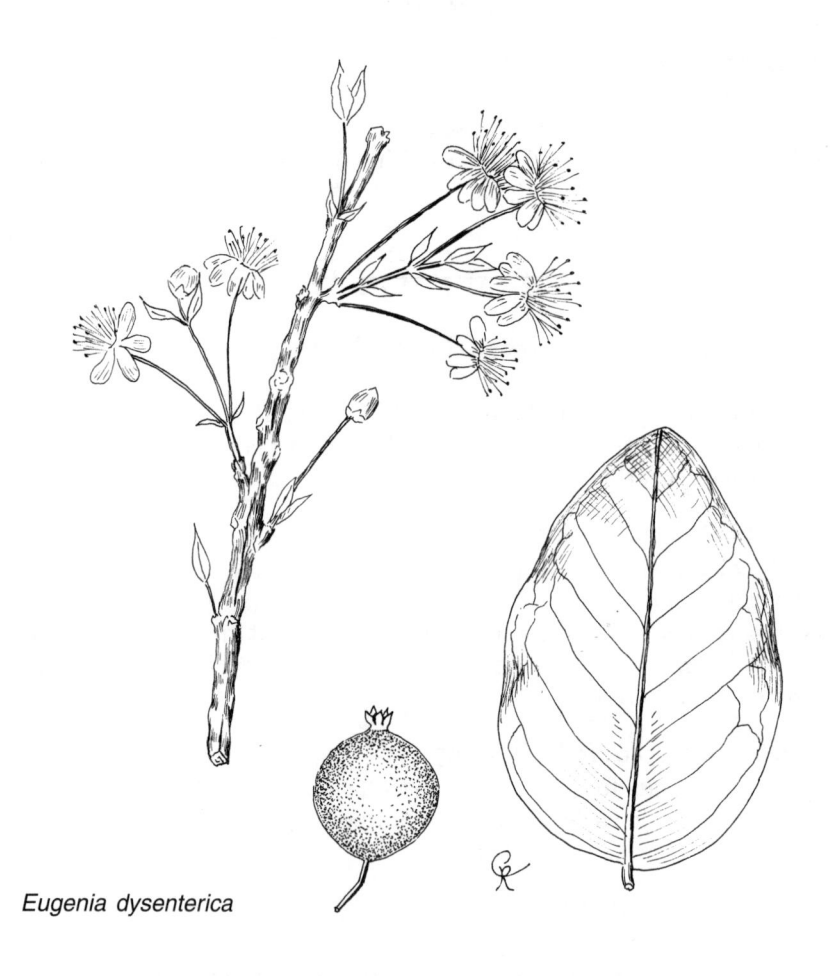

Eugenia sulcata Spring
AREA: Rio de Janeiro.
NAMES: Pitanga, pitangueira-selvagem, pitangui.
USES: Infusion of leaves as a febrifuge and antidiarrhoeic, especially for children.

Eugenia supra-axillaris Spring
AREA: Rio de Janeiro.
NAMES: Fruta-de-tatu, tatu-cáa.
USES: Leaf decoction in clyster as antidiarrhoeic.

Eugenia uniflora L.
AREA: Along coastal sands, restinga.

MYRTACEAE

NAMES: Ibipitanga, jinja, pitanga, pitangueira, pitanga-vermelha, pitangatuba.
USES: Leaves are aromatic, excitant, febrifuge, antirheumatic, good for common cold and flu; used in enema to check diarrhoea.
CHEM.: Several sesquiterpenes have been isolated from the essential oils of fruits and leaves, and their structures determined (Ref: MYRT 1,2,3).
PHARM.: Flavonoids were found to be responsible for the xanthine oxidase inhibitory activity of the plant extract (Ref: MYRT 4), a property also verified in other Myrtaceae (Ref: MYRT 5). Action on lipid metabolism was investigated in monkeys, but the leaf extract showed no cholesterol lowering activity in experimental hypocholesterolemia (Ref: MYRT 6). Antibacterial activity has been verified (Ref: MYRT 7).

Marlierea tomentosa Camb.
AREA: São Paulo to Rio Grande do Sul, prevailing in moist sites.
NAMES: Guaparonga, guaporanga, vapuronga.
USES: Bark is astringent and antidysenteric.

Myrcia amazonica DC.
AREA: Amazonia, forest.
NAME: Pedra-ume-caá.
USES: Baths and a tea from the leaves are used as a cure for leukemia.

Myrcia lanceolata Camb.
AREA: Amazonia.
NAME: Murta-parida.
USES: Tea from leaves used for stomachache and against pains during labor.

Myrcia sphaerocarpa DC.
AREA: Amazonia to Rio de Janeiro, forest.
NAME: Pedra-ume-caá.
USES: Reputedly an efficient antidiabetic.
PHARM.: It was shown in the isolated rat ileum that the leaf extract inhibits the absorption of glucose from a perfused solution. This effect is duplicated by a purified glycopeptide fraction from the same extract (Ref: MYRT 8). However, in clinical trials leaf extracts showed no hypoglycemic effect, neither in normal human subjects nor in type II diabetic patients (Ref: MYRT 9).

Myrcia tingens Berg
AREA: Rio de Janeiro and São Paulo, forest.
NAMES: Cuipuna, paipuna.
USES: Bark is astringent, employed for cleaning chronic ulcers.

MYRTACEAE

Pseudocaryophyllus sericeus Berg
AREA: Minas Gerais to São Paulo, forest.
NAME: Craveiro-da-terra.
USES: The whole plant is aromatic, with a clove-like scent. The flower buds are indicated as a substitute for cloves.

Psidium arboreum Vell.
AREA: Rio de Janeiro to Paraná, forest.
NAMES: Araçá-pelea, araçazeiro-grande, goiabeira-brava, goiabeira-do-mato.
USES: Leaves prescribed for diarrhoea, hemoptyses and suppuration.

Psidium cattleyanum Sabine
AREA: Throughout Brazil; native to littoral, frequently grown as a fruit tree.
NAMES: Araçá, araçá-do-campo, araçá-iba, araçá-de-pedra, araçazeiro.
USES: Roots are diuretic, antidiarrhoeic and recommended as effective to stop hemorrhages.

Psidium cinereum Mart.
AREA: Minas Gerais and São Paulo, forest.
NAME: Araçá-cinzento.
USES: Berries used for hemorrhage.

Psidium guajava L.
AREA: Both native and cultivated; neotropical; much used as a fruit tree.
NAMES: Goiabeira; other vernacular names are without relevance (English: guava).
USES: Most important are the young sprouts, highly regarded as an antidiarrhoeic, especially for children. Prepared in the form of a tea, they are equally recommended against inflammations of the mouth and pharyngitis. Also used, but less important, are the roots, bark and flower buds. Bark is astringent, indicated for leucorrhoea and cholera morbus and for dressing wounds. Unripe fruits are anthelmintic.
CHEM.: Flavonoids (Ref: MYRT 10) and triterpenes (Ref: MYRT 11) were identified in the leaves.
PHARM.: Suppression of locomotor activity in mice, by the leaf extracts, has been investigated (Ref: MYRT 12). Study of the same extracts and their flavonoid constituents on the guinea-pig ileum showed inhibition of contractions, pointing to a possible explanation for the antidiarrhoeic activity (Ref: MYRT 13).

Myrtaceae – References
MYRT 1. Rücker, G., G.A. Assis Brasil e Silva & L. Bauer. 1971. Die Struktur des Isofuranodiens aus *Stenocalyx michelii* (Myrtaceae). *Phytochemistry* 10: 221-224.

MYRT 2. Rücker G., G.A. Assis Brasil e Silva, L. Bauer & M. Schikarski. 1977. Neue Inhaltstoffe aus *Stenocalyx michelii*. *Planta Medica 31*: 322-327.
MYRT 3. Weyerstahl, P., H. Marschall - Weyerstahl, C. Christiansen, B.O. Oguntimein & A.O. Adeoye. 1988. Volatile constituents of *Eugenia uniflora* leaf oil. *Planta Medica 54*: 546-549.
MYRT 4. Schmeda-Hirschmann, G., C. Theoduloz, L. Franco, E. Ferro & A.R. de Arias. 1987. Preliminary pharmacological studies on *Eugenia uniflora* leaves: Xanthine oxidase inhibitory acitivity. *J. Ethnopharmacol. 21*: 183-186.
MYRT 5. Theoduloz C., L. Franco, E. Ferro & G. Schmeda-Hirschmann. 1988. Xanthine oxidase inhibitory activity of Paraguayan Myrtaceae. *J. Ethnopharmacol. 24*: 179-183.
MYRT 6. Ferro, E., A. Schinini, M. Maldonado, J. Rosnar & G. Schmeda-Hirschmann. 1988. *Eugenia uniflora* leaf extract and lipid metabolism in *Cebus spella* monkeys. *J. Ethnopharmacol. 24*: 321-325.
MYRT 7. Fadeyi, M.O. & U.E. Akpan. 1989. Antibacterial activities of the leaf extracts of *Eugenia uniflora* Linn. (synonym *Stenocalyx michelii* Linn.), Myrtaceae. *Phytotherapy Research 3*: 154-155.
MYRT 8. Grüne, U. 1979. Sobre o princípio antidiabético da pedra-hume-caá, *Myrcia multiflora* (Lam.) DC. Thesis, Federal University of Rio de Janeiro.
MYRT 9. Russo, E.M.K., A.A.J. Reichelt, J.R. De-Sá, R.P. Furlanetto, R.C.S. Moisés, T.S. Kasamatsu & A.R. Chacra. 1990. Clinical trial of *Myrcia uniflora* and *Bauhinia forficata* leaf extracts in normal and diabetic patients. *Braz. J. Med. Biol. Res. 23*: 11-20.
MYRT 10. Seshadri, T.R. & K. Vasishta. 1965. Polyphenols of the leaves of *Psidium guajava* – quercetin, guaijaverin, leucocyanidin and amritoside. *Phytochemistry 4*: 989-992.
MYRT 11. Osman, A.M., M.E. Younes & A.E. Sheta. 1974. Triterpenoids of the leaves of *Psidium guajava*. *Phytochemistry 13*: 2015-2016.
MYRT 12. Lutterodt, G.D. & A. Maleque. 1988. Effects on mice locomotor activity of a narcotic-like principle from *Psidium guajava* leaves. *J. Ethnopharmacol. 24*: 219-231.
MYRT 13. Lutterodt, G.D. 1989. Inhibition of gastrointestinal release of acetylcholine by quercetin as a possible mode of action of *Psidium guajava* leaf extracts in the treatment of acute diarrhoeal disease. *J. Ethnopharmacol. 25*: 235-247.

NYCTAGINACEAE

Andradea floribunda Fr. All.
AREA: Rio de Janeiro and Espírito Santo, forest.
NAME: Batão, casca-doce, tapaciriba, tapaciriba-amarela.
USES: Excitant, diaphoretic and antirheumatic in baths.

Boerhavia coccinea Mill.
AREA: Amazonia to Paraná, as a ruderal.
NAME: Batata-de-porco, bredo-de-porco, celidônia, erva-tostão, ipecacuanha-falsa, pega-pinto, selidônia, solidônia, tangará, tangaraca.
USES: Starchy roots are valued for treating jaundice, hepatitis and liver ailments in general. Also recommended as a diuretic and hypotensive. In poultices, against snakebite.
CHEM.: Some ill-defined chemical compounds have been described in thepast. Recent research has shown the presence of sitosterol (Ref: NYCT 1), an alkaloid (Ref: NYCT 2), one phytoecdysone (Ref: NYCT 3), a nucleoside (Ref: NYCT 4) and rotenoids (Ref: NYCT 5).

PHARM.: Early reports stress diuretic action (Ref: NYCT 6). Hepato-protective acitivity has been confirmed, as well as a strong choleretic activity (Ref: NYCT 7); and anticonvulsant properties of the root bark have been described (Ref: NYCT 8). Inhibition of plant viruses by the root extract has been studied (Ref: NYCT 9).

Boerhavia erecta L.
AREA: Minas Gerais and Goiás.
NAME: Erva-tostão-de-minas.
USES: Aerial parts are purgative.

Boerhavia paniculata Rich.
AREA: Amazonia to Rio Grande do Sul, ruderal.
NAMES: Bredo-de-porco, erva-tostão, solidônia, tanrigudinho.
USES: Root is purgative, antianemic and used for liver ailments and jaundice. Leaves also used for jaundice and liver diseases.
CHEM.: A preliminary investigation showed the presence of sitosterol in the root extract (Ref: NYCT 10).

Neea theifera Oersted
AREA: Minas Gerais, São Paulo and Mato Grosso, cerrado.
NAMES: Caparosa, caparosa-do-campo.
USES: Astringent, antidysenteric and used to stop enterorrhagia.

Pisonia aculeata L.
AREA: Cosmopolitan; in Brazil, occurring mainly along the coast, from Rio de Janeiro to São Paulo.
NAMES: Cipó-mole, espora-de-galo, tapaciriba.
USES: Root is purgative. Decoction of both bark and leaves, used externally or internally, relieves rheumatism and venereal diseases.

Pisonia alcalina Fr. All.
AREA: Northeastern caatinga.
NAMES: Mangue-branco, tapaciriba-branca.
USES: Bark from fresh root is emetocathartic; purgative when dried. *P. subcordata* Sw. shows similar action.

Pisonia cordifolia Mart.
AREA: Pernambuco.
NAME: Cumichá.
USES: Bark is prescribed for healing dermal ulcers and scabies.

Torrubia olfersiana (Link, Klotzsch & Otto) Standl.
AREA: Rio de Janeiro, forest.
NAME: Flor-de-pérolas.

USES: Root decoction employed internally as laxative and externally as antirheumatic.

Nyctaginaceae – References

NYCT 1. Misra, A.N. & H.P. Tiwari. 1971. Constituents of roots of *Boerhaavia diffusa*. *Phytochemistry 10*: 3318-3319.

NYCT 2. Basu, N.K., S.B. Leal & S.N. Sharma. 1947. Investigations of Indian medicinal plants. I. *Quart. J. Pharm. Pharmacol. 20*: 38-42.

NYCT 3. Suri, O.P., R. Kant, R.S. Jamwal, K.A. Suri & C.K. Atal. 1982. *Boerhaavia diffusa* L., a new source of phytoecdysones. *Planta Medica 44*: 180-181.

NYCT 4. Ojewole, J.A.O. & S.K. Adesina. 1983. Effect of hypoxanthine-9-L-arabinofuroside, a nucleoside from the roots of *Boerhaavia diffusa* L. (Nyctaginaceae), on isolated coronary artery of the goat. *Fitoterapia 54*: 163-169.

NYCT 5. Messana, I., F. Ferrari & A.E. Goulart Sant'Ana. 1986. Two new 12a-hydroxyrotenoids from *Boerhaavia coccinea*. *Phytochemistry 25*: 2688-2689.

NYCT 6. Aragão, E.M.B. 1909. De la *Boerhavia hirsuta* Willd., "tangaraca," employée comme diuretique. *Progrès Médical 23* (25): 386.

NYCT 7. Chandan, B.K., A.K. Sharma & K.K. Anand. 1991. *Boerhaavia diffusa*: a study of its hepatoprotective activity. *J. Ethnopharmacol. 31*: 299-307.

NYCT 8. Adesina, S.K. 1979. Anticonvulsant properties of the root bark of *Boerhaavia diffusa* L. *Quart. J. Crude Drug Res. 17*: 84-86.

NYCT 9. Verna, H.N. & L.P. Awasthi. 1979. Isolation of the virus inhibitor from the root extract of *Boerhaavia diffusa* inducing systemic resistance in plants. *Can. J. Bot. 57*: 1214-1217.

NYCT 10. Loureiro, H. 1988. Estudo químico de *Boerhaavia diffusa* var. *paniculata* (Rich.) Kuntze. *28° Congr. Bras. Quím.* (Porto Alegre), summaries of papers.

NYMPHAEACEAE

Cabomba piauhyensis Gard.
AREA: Piauí, in stagnant waters.
NAMES: Mururé, redondinho.
USES: Leaves are astringent, indicated for dysentery and piles.

Nymphaea ampla DC.
AREA: Widely distributed, aquatic.
NAMES: Aguapé-da-flor-branca, aguapé-do-grande.
USES: Leaves are vulnerary and emollient. Decoction of the flowers is said to be aphrodisiac; the seed oil has the same reputation.

Nymphaea rudgeana G. Meyer
AREA: Throughout Brazil, aquatic.
NAMES: Aguapé-da-flor-amarela, aguapé-da-meia-noite, apé, mururé, golfo, uapé.
USES: Leaves employed for treating ulcerated wounds and contusions, emollient, in baths for hemorrhoids.

Victoria amazonica (Poepp.) Sower.
AREA: Amazonia, aquatic.

Nymphaea rudgeana

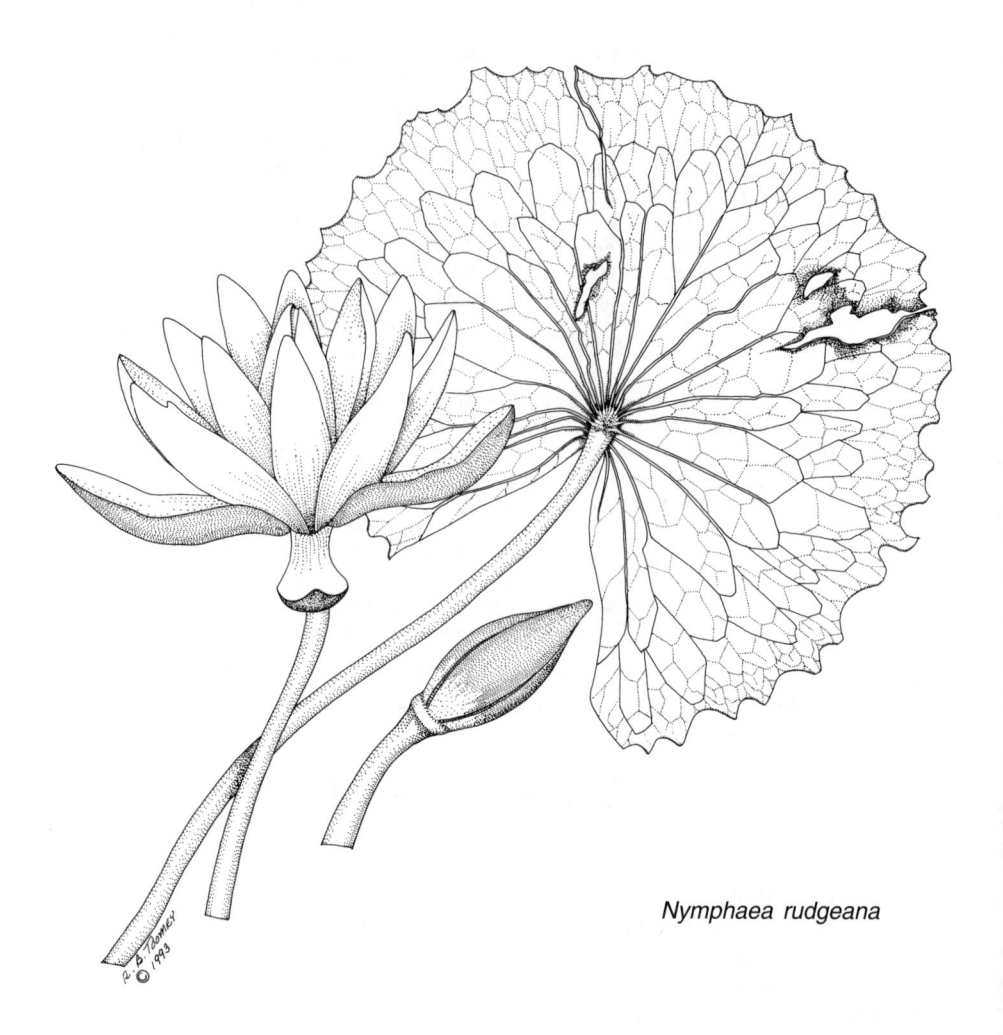

NAMES: Forno-do-jacaré, vitória-régia.
USES: Leaves used for contusions, articular pains, inflammations and hemorrhoids; customarily, they are applied in poultices, mixed with andiroba oil.

OCHNACEAE

Luxemburgia glazioviana Gilg.
AREA: Rio de Janeiro.
NAMES: Congonha-do-campo, congonha-do-mato, mate-do-campo.
USES: Tea from leaves is aromatic and sudorific.

OCHNACEAE

Victoria amazonica, Nymphaeaceae

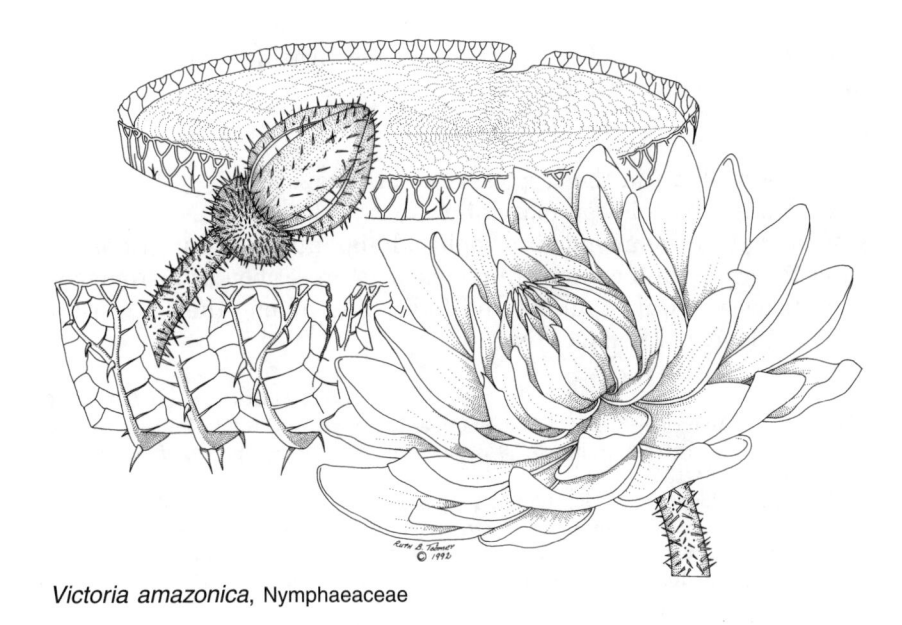

Luxemburgia polyandra St.-Hil.
AREA: Minas Gerais, campo.
NAME: Same as for *L. glazioviana* Gilg.
USES: Same as for *L. glazioviana* Gilg.

Ouratea guianensis Aubl.
AREA: Amazonia, forest.
NAME: Jabotapitá.
USES: Roots and pericarp of fruit are bitter, stomachic and digestive.

Ouratea hexasperma (St.-Hil.) Baill.
AREA: Piauí, Ceará and Minas Gerais, cerrado.
NAME: Sucupira.
USES: For healing wounds.

Ouratea jabotapita Engl.
AREA: Widespread in Brazil; neotropical.
NAMES: Batiputá, jabotapitá.
USES: Bark is tonic and a vermifuge. Oil from seeds useful for treating erysipelas, ulcers and rheumatic conditions.

Ouratea parviflora (DC.) Baill.
AREA: Ceará to São Paulo, cerrado.
NAMES: Batiputá, jabotapitá.
USES: Bark used as in the preceding species; also to regulate menstrual flow.

CHEM.: *Ouratea* species are rich in tannins. Proanthocyanidins and catechins of an unidentified species from the Brazilian Northeast have been studied (Ref: OCHN 1,2,3,4).

Sauvagesia erecta L.
AREA: Cosmopolitan in the tropics; ruderal, campo.
NAMES: Adima, erva-de-são martinho.
USES: Diuretic; recommended for ophthalmia, intestinal infections, cystitis, fever and pulmonary afflictions; also prescribed as a stomachic.
CHEM.: Leaves contain tannins and flavonoids, among them several C-glycosylflavones (Ref: OCHN 5).

Ochnaceae – References
OCHN 1. Delle Monache, F., I.L. d'Albuquerque, F. Ferrari & G.B. Marini-Bettòlo. 1967. Su di una nuova catechina: la 3,5,7,3',5'-pentaossi-4'-metossi(-)epicatechina. *Annali di Chimica 57*: 1364-1367.

OCHN 2. Delle Monache, F., I.L. d'Albuquerque & G.B. Marini-Bettòlo. 1967. Su di una nuova proantocianidina dimera de *Ouratea*. *Annali di Chimica 57*: 1364-1367.

OCHN 3. Delle Monache, F., I.L. d'Albuquerque, F. Ferrari & G.B. Marini-Bettòlo. 1967. A new catechin and dimeric proanthocyanidin from *Ouratea* sp. *Tetrahedron Letters*: 4211-4214.

OCHN 4. Delle Monache, F., F. Ferrari, I.L. d'Albuquerque & G.B. Marini-Bettòlo. 1970. Stereochimica delle proantocianidine da *Ouratea* sp. (Ochnaceae). *Il Farmaco, Ed. Sci. 25*: 96-105.

OCHN 5. Paris, R.R., M.N. Alexis, G. Faugeras & H. Jacquemin. 1978. Plantes de la Guyane Française. V. Sur les polyphénols du *Sauvagesia erecta* L. Ochnacées. *Plantes Médicinales et Phytothérapie 12* (1): 36-41.

OLACACEAE

Ptychopetalum olacoides Benth.
AREA: Amazonia, forest.
NAMES: Marapuama, muirapuama, muiratã.
USES: Stems and roots have the reputation of a powerful aphrodisiac. Also indicated for partial paralyses, dyspepsy, menstrual disturbances and rheumatism.
CHEM.: Fixed constituents identified are fatty acid esters, mainly those of behenic acid, a behenic acid ester of a sterol, and lupeol (Ref: OLAC 1,2,3). The essential oil of the roots has been analyzed. Major components are α-pinene, α-humulene, ß-pinene, ß-caryo-phyllene, camphene and camphor (Ref: OLAC 4).
PHARM.: Blood pressure lowering activity of the extracts has been verified in rabbits, corresponding to nicotinic excitation (Ref: OLAC 5,6).

Ptychopetalum uncinatum Anselm.
AREA: Amazonia, forest.

OLACACEAE

NAMES: Marapuama, muirapuama, muiratã.
USES: The same as for *Ptychopetalum olacoides* Benth.
CHEM.: Similar to *Ptychopetalum olacoides* Benth., except that this species is less rich in lupeol (Ref: OLAC 3).

Ximenia americana L.
AREA: Along the Brazilian coast, restinga.
NAMES: Ameixa, ameixa-de-espinho, ameixa-do-brasil.
USES: Bark is astringent, used externally for dressing wounds; powdered bark serves to hasten cicatrization. Seed oil is purgative.
CHEM.: Seed contains sambunigrin, the glucoside of mandelo-nitrile (Ref: OLAC 7). Seeds and roots produce fats containing acetylenic fatty acids (Ref: OLAC 8,9).

Ximenia coriacea Engl.
AREA: Bahia and Minas Gerais, caatinga and cerrado.
NAMES: Ameixa, ameixa-brava.
USES: The same as for *Ximenia americana* L. Also used to regulate menstrual flow.

Olacaceae – References

OLAC 1. Auterhoff, H. & E. Pankow. 1968. Inhaltsstoffe von Muira-Puama. I. *Arch. Pharm. 301*: 481-489.
OLAC 2. Pankow, E. & H., Auterhoff. 1969. Inhaltsstoffe von Muira-Puama. II. *Arch. Pharm. 302*: 209-212.

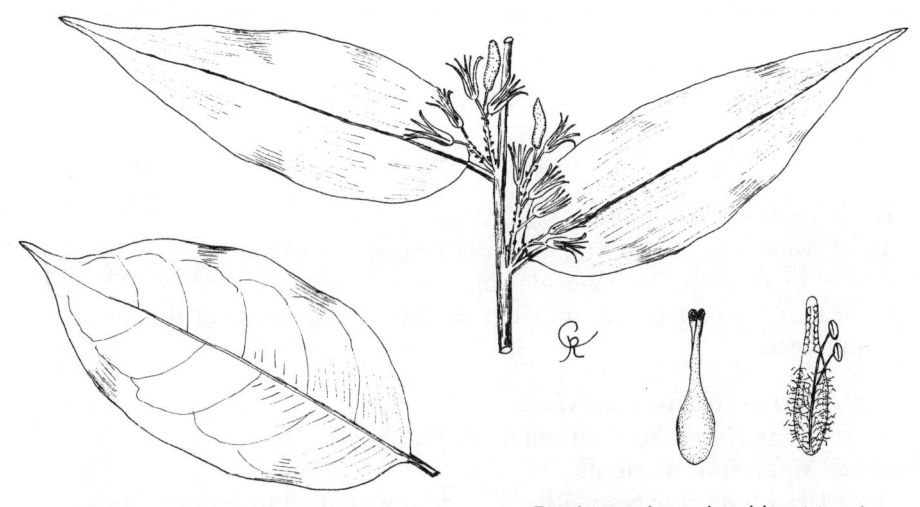

Ptychopetalum olacoides (above),
Ptychopetalum uncinatum (leaf, left)

OLAC 3. Auterhjoff, H. & B. Momberger. 1971. Lipophile Inhaltsstoffe von Muira-Puama. *Arch. Pharm. 304*: 223-228.
OLAC 4. Bucek, E.U., G. Fournier & H. Dadoun. 1987. Volatile constituents of *Ptychopetalum olacoides* root oil. *Planta Medica 53*: 231.
OLAC 5. Olofsson, E. 1927. Action de l'extrait de *Liriosma ovata* sur la tension artérielle, vaisseaux et respiration du lapin. *Compt. Rend. Soc. Biol. 97*: 1639-1640.
OLAC 6. Raymond-Hamet, R. 1932. Action physiologique de l'extrait de Muira-Puama. *Compt. Rend. Soc. Biol. 109*: 1064-1067.
OLAC 7. Finnemore, H., J.M. Cooper & L.J. Harris. 1938. The cyanogenetic constituents of Australian and other plants. VII. *J. Soc. Chem. Ind. 57*: 162-169.
OLAC 8. Hatt, H.H., A.C.K. Triffett & P.C. Wailes. 1959. Acetylenic acids from the fats of Santalaceae and Olacaceae -seed and root oils from *Exocarpus cupressiformis*. *Austral. J. Chem. 12*: 190-195.
OLAC 9. Hatt, H.H., A.C.K. Triffett & P.C. Wailes. 1960. Acetylenic acids from fats of the Olacaceae and Santalaceae. IV. The occurrence of *trans*-ll-*trans* 13-ocatadecadien-9-ynoic acid in plant lipids. *Austral. J. Chem. 13*: 488-497.

ONAGRACEAE

Ludwigia natans (H.B.K.) Ell.
AREA: Pernambuco and Bahia, in still waters.
NAMES: Mururé, saracura.
USES: Indicated for hemoptysis, diarrhoea and for healing wounds.

Ludwigia peruviana (L.) Hara
AREA: Amazonia to São Paulo, in moist places.
NAME: Cruz-de-malta.
USES: Leaves are emollient, employed in cataplasms to mature abscesses and tumors.

Ludwigia repens (L.) Hara
AREA: Tropical cosmopolitan, in rivers and ponds.
NAMES: Cruz-de-malta, mururé.
USES: Reputed to be efficient for treating afflictions of the scalp.

Ludwigia suffruticosa (L.) Gomes
AREA: Tropical cosmopolitan, in humid sites.
NAMES: Cruz-de-malta, mãos-de-sapo.
USES: Plant is astringent; infusion used to soothe pains of the stomach and head.

Oenothera catharinensis Camb.
AREA: Minas Gerais to Rio Grande do Sul, campo.
NAMES: Caparosa, minuana.
USES: Used to improve appetite. Externally applied to dress wounds.

OPILIACEAE

Agonandra brasiliensis Miers
AREA: Piauí to Minas Gerais, cerrado and dry forest.
NAMES: Cerveja-de-pobre, guararema, pau-d'alho-do-campo, pau-marfim, tatu.

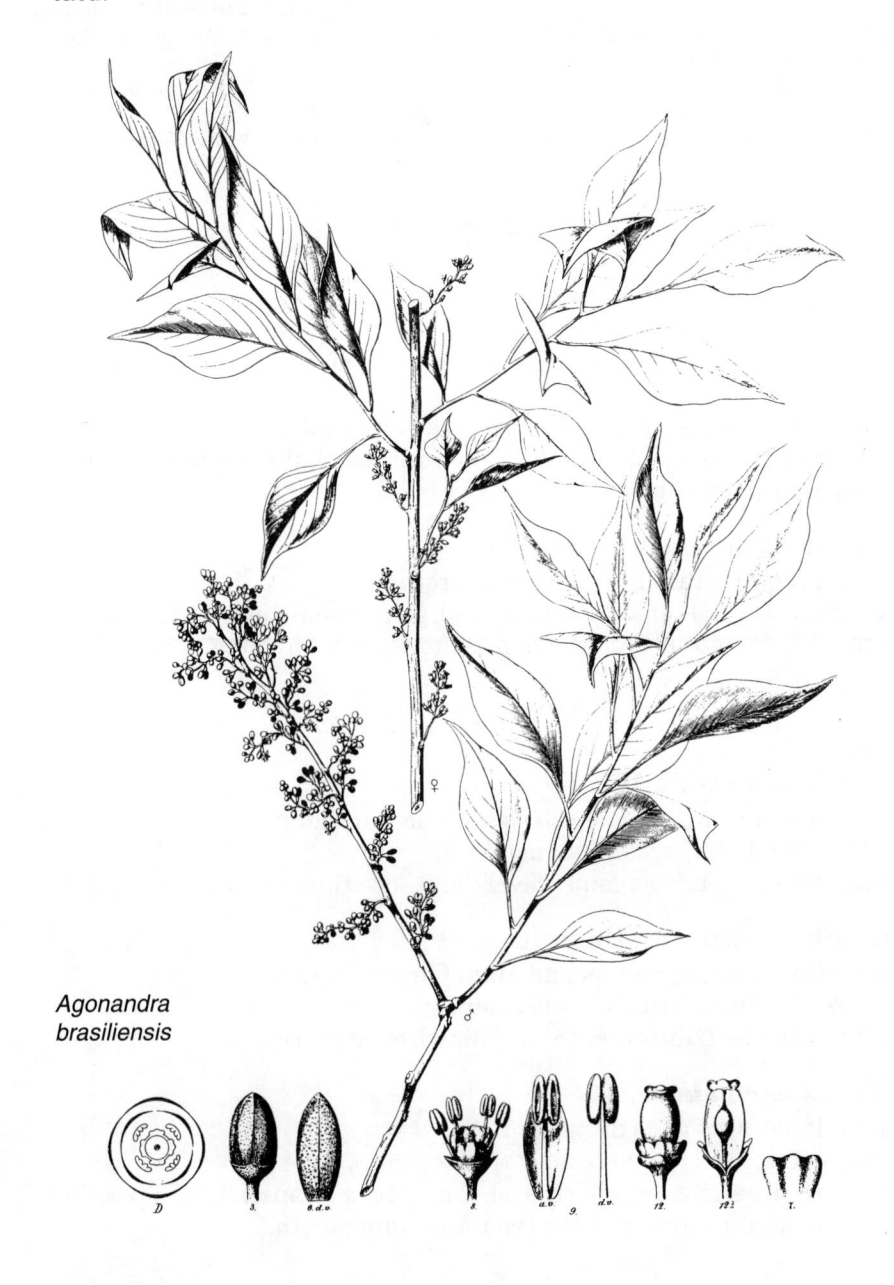

Agonandra brasiliensis

Opiliaceae / Oxalidaceae

USES: Roots are rich in saponin, used to make a frothing drink known as "the poor man's beer." Leaves used in baths, against rheumatism.
CHEM.: Seeds contain a high proportion (over 50%) of a viscous oil, which has been analyzed for its fatty acid composition (Ref: OPIL 1).
PHARM.: Extract of bark is strongly molluscicidal (Ref: OPIL 2,3).

Opiliaceae – References

OPIL 1. Gurgel, L.& T. Amorim. 1929. Óleo de pau-marfim (*Agonandra brasiliensis* Miers). *Mem. Inst. de Chimica* (Rio de Janeiro) *2*: 21-38.
OPIL 2. Silva, M.J.M., M.P. Souza & M. Z. Rouquayrol. 1971. Atividade moluscicida de plantas do Nordeste brasileiro. II. *Rev. Bras. Farm. 52*: 117-123.
OPIL 3. Kloos, H. & F.S. McCullough. 1982. Plant molluscicides. *Planta Medica 46*: 195-209.

ORCHIDACEAE

Cyrtopodium andersoni R. Br.
AREA: Widespread along sandy coast.
NAMES: Bisturi-do-mato, bisturi-vegetal, cola-de-sapateiro, rabo-de-tatu, sumaré, sumaré-da-pedra.
USES: Pseudobulbs are rich in starch-like material which is administered for hemoptyses and to prepare an anticatarrhal syrup; also for healing infected wounds.

Cyrtopodium punctatum Lindl.
AREA: Frequent throughout Brazil, forest.
NAMES: Bisturi-do-mato, bisturi-vegetal, sumaré-da-mata, sumaré-do-pau.
USES: Juice of pseudobulbs is applied to sores to promote cicatrization.

OXALIDACEAE

Oxalis amara St.-Hil.
AREA: Santa Catarina and Rio Grande do Sul, campo.
NAMES: Azedinha, azedinha-amargosa.
USES: Recommended against fevers and sore throat.

Oxalis cordata St.-Hil.
AREA: Goiás, Minas Gerais and Mato Grosso, campo.
NAMES: Azedinha, azedinha-do-campo.
USES: Same as *Oxalis amara* St.-Hil.; also for scurvy.

Oxalis corniculata L.
AREA: Ruderal of wide dispersion.
NAMES: Azedinha, pé-de-pombo, três-corações, trevo.
USES: Antithermic, antidiarrhoeic, for rectal prolapse. Juice prescribed to eliminate warts. Fruits used for cleaning teeth.

Oxalis martiana Zucc.

AREA: Well represented everywhere in Brazil, mainly in back yards and kitchen gardens.
NAME: Caruru-de-sapo.
USES: Decoction of the bulblets mixed with a small amount of rust is prescribed as a medicine for chlorosis, leucorrhoea and amenorrhoea. The formation of iron oxalate may be a rationale for the cure of iron deficiency. Decoction of the leaves is used to treat slight fevers and sore throat.

Many other species of *Oxalis* thrive in Brazilian territory, mostly in campos. Their uses are mostly the same, i.e., as antithermic and against sore throat. The following can be cited, among others: *O. articulata* Sav., *O. bahiensis* Prog., *O. bipartita* St.-Hil., *O. chrysantha* Prog., *O. eriocarpa* DC., *O. triangularis* St.-Hil. and *O. oxyptera* Prog.

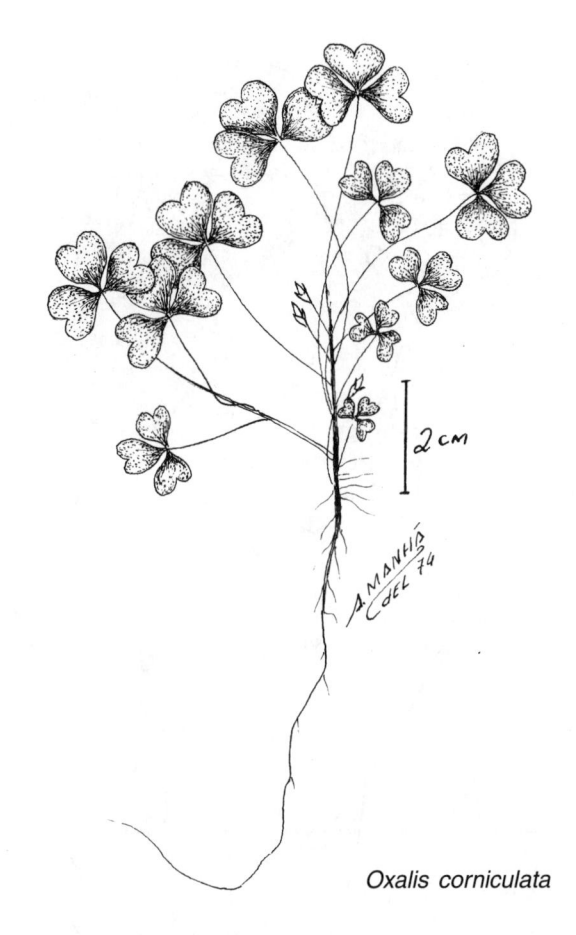

Oxalis corniculata

PASSIFLORACEAE

Passiflora alata Dryand.

AREA: Neotropical, much cultivated in Brazil.
NAMES: Flor-da-paixão, maracujá.
USES: Roots are sedative, narcotic, antihysteric; leaves are mildly soporific.
CHEM.: The dry extract obtained from the leaves contains minute amounts of β-carboline type alkaloids and flavonoids (Ref: PASS 1). C-glycosylflavonoids were identified (Ref: PASS 2).

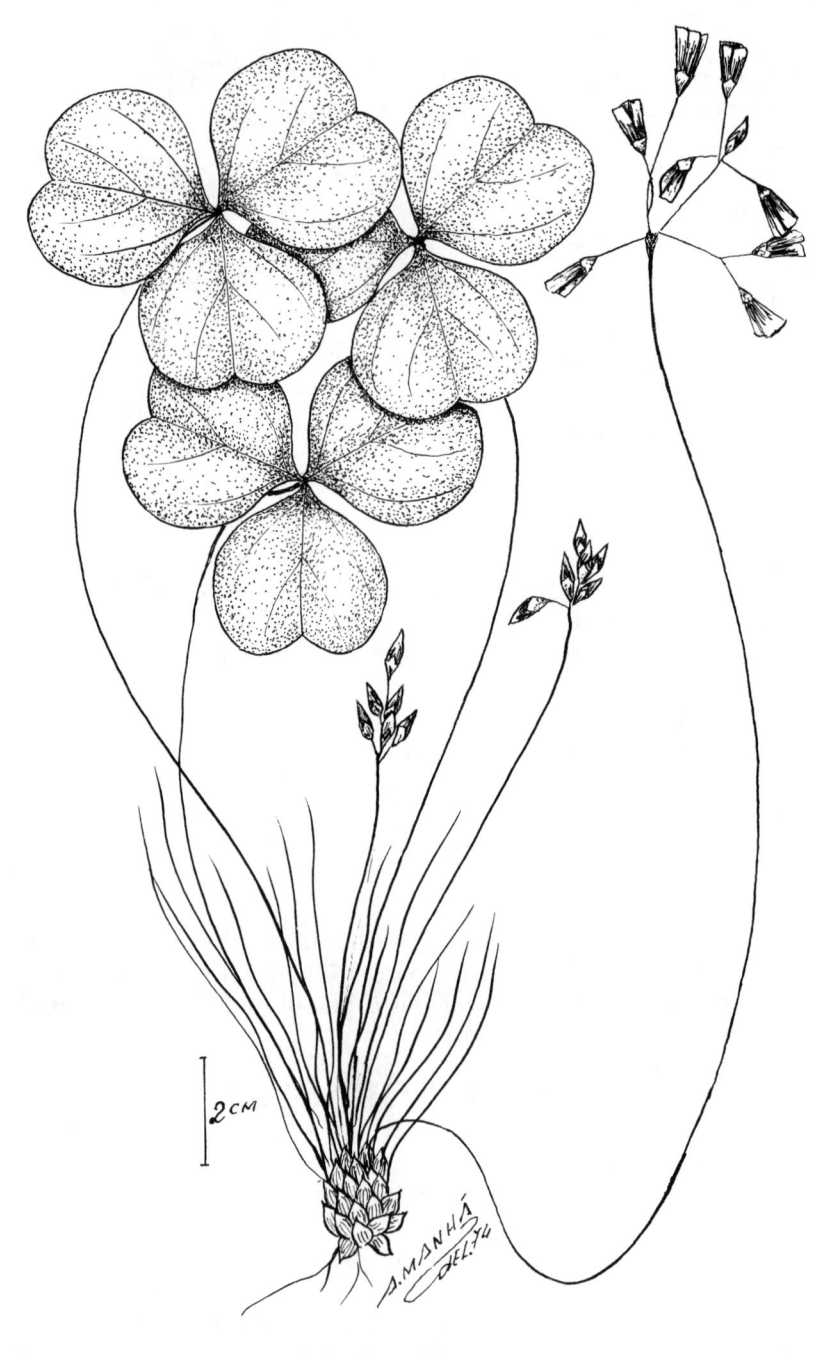

Oxalis martiana

PHARM.: Intraperitoneal injection of the extract reduced the spontaneous motor activity and prolonged the sodium pentobarbital induced sleeping time in mice. Anticonvulsant action was also demonstrated (Ref: PASS 1).

Passiflora amethystina Mikan
AREA: Minas Gerais to Santa Catarina, forest.
NAME: Flor-da-paixão.
USES: Leaves are antifebrile and produce a soothing action on dermal inflammations.

Passiflora caerulea L.
AREA: Ceará to Rio Grande do Sul, forest.
NAMES: Flor-da-paixão, maracujá, maracujá-azul, maracujá-de-cobra.
USES: Same as given for *P. amethystina*; also for bronchitis.

Passiflora coccinea Aubl.
AREA: Amazonia, forest.
NAMES: Maracujá-do-mato, maracujá-poranga.
USES: Tea from leaves is recommended for cardiac troubles.
CHEM.: Contains cyanogenic glycoside (Ref: PASS 3).

Passiflora edulis Sims
AREA: Neotropical, much grown in Brazil.
NAMES: Flor-da-paixão, maracujá, maracujá-comum, maracujá-doce, maracujá-de-ponche, maracujá-mirim, maracujá-peroba, maracujá-roxo.
USES: Tea from leaves is calmative, especially indicated for the respiratory system and for treating insomnia. Roots are sedative, antihysteric and vermifuge.
CHEM.: Leaves contain a triterpene glycoside (Ref: PASS 4) and a cyanogenic glycoside (Ref: PASS 5). The biosynthesis and metabolism of the b-carboline alkaloid harman were investigated in this species (Ref: PASS 6). Investigation of the aroma constituents of the fruits identified over 150 compounds in trace amounts (Ref: PASS 7,14,15).
PHARM.: The calmative properties of the tea from the leaves were experimentally confirmed (Ref: PASS 8). Psychopharmacological effects have been studied (Ref: PASS 9).

Passiflora foetida L.
AREA: Dispersed throughout Brazil.
NAMES: Maracujá-catinga, maracujá-de-estalo, maracujá-fedorento.
USES: Leaves are tonic and antiblennorrhagic.
CHEM.: C-glycosylflavonoids have been described from this species (Ref: PASS 10).

PASSIFLORACEAE

Passiflora gardneri Mast.
AREA: Piauí, caatinga.
NAME: Maracujá-do-piauí.
USES: Leaves are emmenagogue and antispasmodic.

Passiflora laurifolia L.
AREA: Amazonia, frequent in secondary growth.
NAMES: Maracujá, maracujá-comum.
USES: Leaves are bitter, astringent. Roots used as a vermifuge.

Passiflora macrocarpa Mast.
AREA: Occasionally cultivated.
NAMES: Maracujá, maracujá-açu, maracujá-mamão, maracujá-melão.
USES: Leaves are calmative, emmenagogue and antispasmodic. Roots are said to be narcotic, even poisonous.

Passiflora mucronata Lam.
AREA: Bahia to Rio de Janeiro, forest.
NAMES: Flor-da-paixão, sururu.
USES: Seeds are vermicidal.

Passiflora spp.
CHEM. & PHARM.: Compounds identified in *Passiflora* species are mainly β-carboline alkaloids (harman, harmine, harmol, harmalol, harmaline and other bases), flavonoids, coumarins and caffeic acid derivatives. Leaves and roots (but not the ripe fruits) frequently contain hydrocyanic acid liberating glycosides, as has been shown in most of the above mentioned species.

The species which has been most thoroughly investigated is the North American *P. incarnata* L. It appears that the hypotensive and sedative properties which determine the medicinal use cannot be attributed to any of the identified constituents individually (Ref: PASS 11). Either it is the complex of substances which is active in a synergistic way (Ref: PASS 12) or the active compound or compounds have not yet been identified (Ref: PASS 13).

Passifloraceae – References

PASS 1. Oga, S., P.C.D. de Freitas, A.C.S. da Silva & S. Hanada. 1984. Pharmacological trial of crude extract of *Passiflora alata*. *Planta Medica 50*: 303-306.

PASS 2. Ululeben, A., S. Oksuz, T.J. Mabry, G. Dellamonica & J. Chopin. 1982. C-glycosylflavonoids from *Passiflora pittieri, P. alata, P. ambigua* and *Adenia mannii*. *J. Nat. Prod. 45*: 783.

PASS 3. Spencer, K.C. & D.S. Seigler. 1985. Passicoccin: A sulphated cyanogenic glucoside from *Passiflora coccinea*. *Phytochemistry 24*: 2615- 2617.

PASS 4. Bombardelli, E., A. Bonati, B. Gabetta, E.M. Martinelli & G. Mustich. 1975. Passiflorine, a new glycoside from *Passiflora edulis*. *Phytochemistry 14*: 2661-2665.

PASS 5. Spencer, K.C. & D.S. Seigler. 1963. Cyanogenesis of *Passiflora edulis*. *J. Agric. Food Chem. 31*: 794-796.

PASS 6. Slaytor, M. & I. J. McFarlane. 1968. The biosynthesis and metabolism of harman in *Passiflora edulis*. I. *Phytochemistry* 7: 605-611.
PASS 7. Winter, M. & R. Klöti. 1972. Über das Aroma der gelben Passionsfrucht (*Passiflora edulis* f. *flavicarpa*). *Helv. Chim. Acta* 55: 1916-1921.
PASS 8. Matos, F.J.A. (Fortaleza, Ceará): personal communication.
PASS 9. Vale, N.B. & J.R. Leite. 1983. Efeitos psicofarmacológicos de preparações de *Passiflora edulis* (Maracujá). *Ciência e Cultura* (São Paulo) 35: 11-24.
PASS 10. Ululeben, A., G. Topcu, T.J. Mabry, G. Dellamonica & J. Chopin. 1982. C-glycosylflavonoids from *Passiflora foetida* var. *hispida* and *P. foetida* var. *hibiscifolia*. *J. Nat. Prod.* 45: 103.
PASS 11. Fellows, E.J. & C. S. Smith. 1938. The chemistry of *Passiflora incarnata*. *J. Am. Pharm. Assoc.* 27: 565-573.
PASS 12. Lutomski, J. & T. Wrocinski. 1960. Pharmacodynamic properties of *Passiflora incarnata* preparations. The effect of alkaloid and flavonoid components on pharmacodynamic properties of the raw material. *Biul. Inst. Roslin Leczniczych* 6: 176-184. (with German summary).
PASS 13. Speroni, E. & A. Minghetti. 1988. Neuropharmacological activity of extracts from *Passiflora incarnata*. *Planta Medica* 54: 488-491.
PASS 14. Parliment, T.H. 1972. Some volatile constituents of passion fruit. *J. Agr. Chem.* 20: 1043-1045.
PASS 15. Murray, K.E. & J. Shipton. 1972. Volatile constituents of passion fruit, *Passiflora edulis*. *Aust. J. Chem.* 25: 1921-1923.

PHYTOLACCACEAE

Gallesia gorazema (Vell.) Moq.
AREA: Cearà to São Paulo, littoral and forest.
NAMES: Guararema, pau-d'alho.
USES: Exudate from trunk is antispasmodic and antitussive. Contused wood, mixed with leaves and flowers, is used in baths, and considered useful against rheumatism, dartre and hydropsy. Leaves applied in the form of poultices are said to mature prostate tumors. Decoction of bark, branches and leaves is occasionally used as anthelmintic. An extract of the leaves has a reputation as an anticonvulsive and has been used for hysterical fits.

Microtea debilis Sw.
AREA: Amazonia, forest.
NAME: Erva-mijona.
USE: Against urine retention.
CHEM.: Rich in saponins (Ref: PHYT 1).

Petiveria alliacea L.
AREA: Amazonia to Rio de Janeiro and Mato Grosso.
NAMES: Erva-pipi, erva-de-guiné, erva-d'alho, guiné, pipi, tipi.
USES: Herb, of garlic-like, slightly nauseating smell, is considered sudorific, diuretic, antispasmodic, emmenagogue, antirheumatic, stimulant, abortifacient, and odontalgic. Alcoholature (alcoholic tincture) in mas-

sages in cases of convulsions in children. The roots are the more active part, being poisonous in repeated doses.

CHEM.: Organic sulfur compounds have been identified as responsible for the smell and antimicrobial properties (Ref: PHYT 2,3,4).

PHARM.: Phagocytose stimulating activity has been verified (Ref: PHYT 5); also antimitotic action on sea urchin egg development (Ref: PHYT 6).

Seguieria americana L.
AREA: Espírito Santo to Paranà and Minas Gerais.
NAMES: Cipó-de-alho, ibirarema, pau-d'alho, segurelha-brava, ubirarema.
USES: Twigs and leaves are diuretic, antidropsy, antirheumatic; also used against ringworm and for liver afflictions.

Phytolaccaceae – References
PHYT 1. Wong, W. 1976. Some folk medicinal plants from Trinidad. *Econ. Bot. 30*: 103-142.
PHYT 2. von Szczpznski, C., P. Zgorzelak & G.A. Hoyer. 1972. Isolierung, Strukturaufklärung und Synthese einer antimikrobiell wirksamen Substanz aus *Petiveria alliacea* L. *Arzneimittelforsch. 22*: 1975-1976.
PHYT 3. Adesogan, E.K. 1974. Trithiolaniacin, a novel trithiolane from *Petiveria alliacea*. *J. Chem. Soc. Chem. Commun.* 906-907.
PHYT 4. Delaveau, P., P. Lallouette & A.M. Tessier. 1980. Drogues végétales stimulant l'activité phagocitaire du système réticulo-endotelial. *Planta Medica 40*: 49-54.
PHYT 5. Sousa, J.R., A.J. Demmer, J.A. Pinheiro, E. Breitmaier & B.K. Cassels. 1990. Dibenzyltrisulphide and *trans*-N-methyl-4-methoxyproline from *Petiveria alliacea*. *Phytochemistry 29*: 3653-3655.
PHYT 6. Malpezzi, E.L.A., S.C. Davino, L.V. Costa, J.C. Freitas, A.M. Giesbrecht & N.C. Roque. 1994. Antimitotic action of extracts of *Petiveria alliacea* on sea urchin egg development. *Braz. J. Med. Biol. Res. 27*: 749-754.

PIPERACEAE

Ottonia corcovadensis Miq.
AREA: Maranhão to Rio de Janeiro, forest.
NAMES: Chà-bravo, falso-jaborandi, jaborandi, zebradim.
USES: Twigs, leaves and roots are chewed to soothe toothache. Spikes are carminative and stomachic.
CHEM.: Several amides have been isolated; one of them, piperovatine, is responsible for the numbing action the plant has on the tongue and mucous membranes of the mouth (Ref: PIPE 1).

Ottonia jaborandi (Vell.) Kunth
AREA: Rio de Janeiro to Paranà, forest.
NAMES: Jaborandi-da-mata-virgem, jaborandi-do-mato.
USES: Roots are sialagogue, diuretic, diaphoretic, chewed to soothe toothache.
CHEM.: An amide has been isolated and identified (Ref: PIPE 2).

PIPERACEAE

Peperomia elongata Miq.
AREA: Amazonia.
NAMES: Elixir-paregórico, erva-de-soldado.
USES: Herb decoction is used for stomachache; also hemostatic, antidysenteric, antiblennorrhagic and antileucorrhoeic.

Peperomia hederacea Miq.
AREA: Rio de Janeiro and Santa Catarina, forest.
NAME: Caroá-caá.
USES: Herb juice is used for treating rheumatism due to syphilis. Tincture from flowers is tonic and antidyspeptic.

Peperomia pellucida H.B.K.
AREA: Throughout Brazil as a ruderal herb.
NAMES: Alfavaca-de-cobra, comida-de-jaboti, erva-de-jaboti, maria-mole, ximbuí.

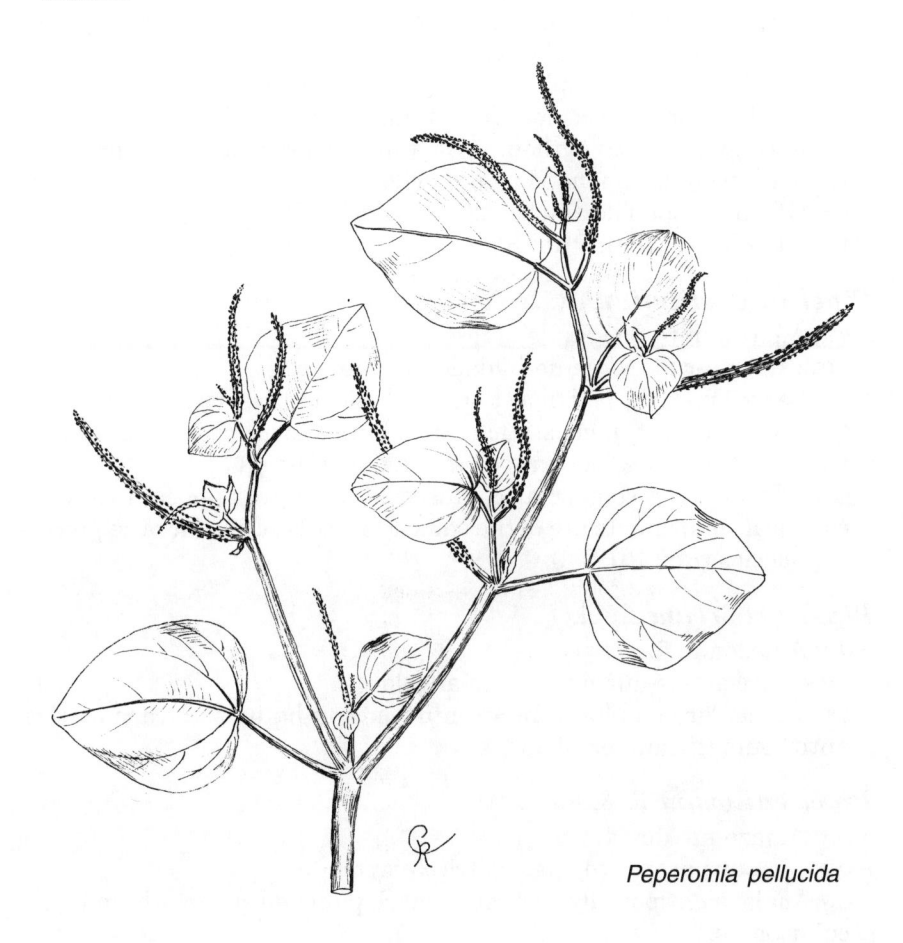

Peperomia pellucida

PIPERACEAE

USES: Entire plant or roots are emollient, antipruriginous, diuretic, antitussive and used for sore throat. Also reputed as an active remedy against coronary arteriosclerosis suitable for preventing heart attack.

Peperomia rotundifolia H.B.K.
AREA: Throughout Brazil, forest.
NAME: Salvavidas.
USES: Tonic and stomachic.

Peperomia transparens Miq.
AREA: Minas Gerais and Rio de Janeiro, forest.
NAMES: Erva-de-vidro, língua-de-sapo.
USES: Pectoral, expectorant and diuretic.

Piper aduncum L.
AREA: Amazonia and Pernambuco to Espírito Santo.
NAMES: Aperta-ruão, erva-de-jaboti, matico-falso, pimenta-longa, jaborandi-do-mato, pimenta-de-macaco.
USES: Roots externally applied for erysipelas, internally as a stimulant and cholagogue. Leaves used in the same way as the roots, and also as an astringent, for strengthening the womb to prevent uterine prolapse. Leaves once recommended against cholera.
CHEM.: Phenylpropanoid and benzoic acid derivatives have been described from the leaves (Ref: PIPE 3).

Piper angustifolium R. & Pav.
AREA: Amazonia to São Paulo, forest.
NAMES: Aperta-ruão, erva-de-soldado, matico.
USES: Leaves used for bad digestion, balsamic and resolvent; their decoction is astringent, hemostatic and recommended for wound healing, treatment of sores, leucorrhoea and menhorrhagia.
CHEM.: From older, somewhat confused literature, it appears that the chemical components are of the same type as described for the preceding species (Ref: PIPE 3).

Piper arboreum Aubl.
AREA: Amazonia, forest.
NAMES: Alecrim-de-angola, pau-de-angola.
USES: Leaves are employed in an infusion and baths as a carminative, antirheumatic and emollient.

Piper callosum R. & Pav.
AREA: Amazonia, forest.
NAMES: Elixir-paregórico, óleo-elétrico, ventre-livre.
USES: Analgesic, especially against stomach pain and rheumatic and muscular pains.

PIPERACEAE

Piper cavalcantei Yunck.
AREA: Amazonia, forest.
NAME: Elixir-paregórico.
USES: Leaf tea used to relieve stomach pain.
CHEM.: Essential oil has been studied (Ref: PIPE 4).

Piper ceanothifolium H.B.K.
AREA: Minas Gerais and Rio de Janeiro, forest.
NAME: Jaborandi-falso.
USES: Roots are stomachic, sialagogue, diuretic; macerated in brandy, taken against snakebite. Tincture of inflorescences aromatic, excitant.

Piper colubrinum Link
AREA: Amazonia to Rio de Janeiro, forest.
NAME: Jaborandi-manso.
USES: Roots are aromatic, similar to ginger; calmative for colics and intestinal gases. Leaf and root infusion used for rheumatic pains.

Piper elongatum Vahl
AREA: Ceará and Bahia, forest.
NAMES: Aperta-ruão-do-ceará, erva-de-soldado, matico, pimenta-de-folha-larga, pimenta-matico.
USES: Leaves are diaphoretic, antihemorrhagic and antileucorrhoeic.

Piper eucalyptifolium (Miq.) Rudge
AREA: Amazonia, forest.
NAMES: Alfavaca-de-cobra, betis, jaborandi.
USES: Roots and leaves used for muscular pains, colics and flatulent dyspepsia.

Piper geniculatum Sw.
AREA: Amazonia to Mato Grosso and Santa Catarina, forest.
NAMES: Fruta-de-morcego, jaborandi-do-rio, jaborandi-falso, nhaborandi, pali, palim.
USES: Roots reputed as a useful alexipharmic against plant poisons, including curare. Also used as a tonic, stomachic, odontalgic, expectorant, sudorific, diuretic and antithermic.

Piper gigantifolium Jacq.
AREA: Ceará, in moist places on mountains.
NAME: Coração.
USES: Spike infusion is carminative and stomachic.

Piper marginatum Jacq.
AREA: Throughout Brazil, in forest.

PIPERACEAE

NAMES: Caapeba-cheirosa, bitre, malvarisco, nhandi, nhandu, pau-d'angola, pimenta-do-mato, pimenta-dos-índios.
USES: Roots are carminative, sialagogue, reputedly effective against snakebite. Leaves are tonic, stomachic, antispasmodic, recommended for liver ailments and in baths after childbirth. Leaves placed in oil, used against swellings. Fruits are aromatic, excitant.
CHEM.: Chemical components, both fixed and volatile, have been studied extensively (Ref: PIPE 5,6,7,8,9). The essential oil contains about 40% anethole. C-glycosylflavones have been described from the leaves. Other components are propiophenones and benzoic acid derivatives.
PHARM.: The essential oil is active against cercariae of schistosomes (Ref: PIPE 10).

Piper mikanianum (Kunth) Steud.
AREA: Minas Gerais and Rio de Janeiro, forest.
NAME: Pariparoba.
USES: Emmenagogue and for metrorrhagia.

Piper mollicomum Kunth
AREA: Bahia to Rio de Janeiro, forest.
NAME: Jaborandi-manso.
USES: Roots are resolvent. Fruiting spikes are excitant and stomachic.

Piper parthenium Mart.
AREA: Rio Grande do Sul.
NAME: Pariparoba-do-rio-grande.
USES: Roots are emmenagogue and antileucorrhoeic. Used to regulate menstrual flow.

Piper reticulatum L.
AREA: Throughout Brazil.
NAME: Jaborandi-falso.
USES: Roots are aromatic, stomachic, sialagogue; leaves are diuretic and excitant.

Piper rohrii C. DC.
AREA: Bahia to Rio de Janeiro, forest.
NAMES: Caapeba, pariparoba.
USES: Used to relieve liver ailments.

Piper tuberculatum Jacq.
AREA: Northeastern Brazil, forest.
NAMES: Pimenta-darta, pimenta-longa.
USES: Roots are pungent, aromatic, antiophidic. Leaves are aromatic and sedative. Spikes are stimulant, carminative.
CHEM.: Leaves contain a cinnamic acid derivative (Ref: PIPE 11) and an

PIPERACEAE

unusual dimeric alkaloid (Ref: PIPE 12).
PHARM.: Plant is molluscicidal (Ref: PIPE 13).

Pothomorphe peltata L.
AREA: Amazonia, forest.
NAMES: Caapeba, caapeba-do-norte, caá-peuá, catajé, malvarisco, pariparoba.
USES: Juice used for burns. Roots, leaves and spikes are diuretic, antigonorrhoeic, vermifuge and vulnerary.

Pothomorphe umbellata (L.) Miq.
AREA: Neotropical; widespread in Brazil, forest.
NAMES: Caapeba, capeba, lençol-de-santa-bárbara, malvaísco, malvavisco, pariparoba.
USES: Diuretic, antipyretic, also against malaria. Prescribed for liver ailments, inflammations, swellings, erysipelas and filariasis. Also to treat contusions and sores. Anti-epileptic. Decoction of the roots is prescribed for liver and spleen diseases; decoction externally used for the same purposes, mixed with almond oil.
CHEM. & PHARM.: Nerolidylcatechol has been isolated and identified (Ref: PIPE 14). Extracts were found to have high antioxidant activity (Ref: PIPE 15).

Antimalarial tests conducted with *Plasmodium berghei* infected mice, both orally and subcutaneously, confirmed anti-malarial activity (Ref: PIPE 16). The same was not true for the related *Pothomorphe peltata*. Assays proved absence of mutagenicity for both these species (Ref: PIPE 17). The two taxa are sometimes regarded as conspecific, cf. Howard, R.A. 1988. *Flora of the Lesser Antilles 4*: 12-14.

Piperaceae – References

PIPE 1. Costa, S.S. & W. B. Mors. 1981. Amides of *Ottonia corcovadensis*. *Phytochemistry* 20: 1305-1307.

PIPE 2. Giesbrecht, A.M., M.A. Alvarenga, O.R. Gottlieb & H.E. Gottlieb. 1981. (2E,4E)-N-isobutyl-9-piperonyl-nona-2, 4-dienoic amide from *Ottonia anisum*. *Planta Medica* 43: 375-377.

PIPE 3. Orjaba, J., C.A.J. Erdelmeier, A.D. Wright, B. Baumgartner, T. Rali, & O. Sticher. 1989. Biologically active phenylpropene and benzoic acid derivatives from *Piper aduncum* leaves. *Planta Medica* 55: 619-620.

PIPE 4. Alencar, R. , R. Alves de Lima, R.G. Campos Corrêa, O.R. Gottlieb, M.C. Marx, M. Leão da Silva, J.G.S. Maia, M.T. Magalhães & R.M.V. Assumpção. 1971. Óleos essenciais de plantas brasileiras. *Acta Amazonica 1(3)*: 41-43.

PIPE 5. Foungbé, S., F. Tillequin, M. Paris, H.Jacquemin & R.R. Paris. 1976. Sur une Pipéracée de Guyane, le *Piper marginatum* Jacq. *Ann. Pharm. Franç. 34*: 339-343.

PIPE 6. Tillequin, F., M. Paris, H. Jacquemin & R.R. Paris. 1978. Flavonoïdes de *Piper marginatum*. Isolement d'un nouvel hétéroside flavonique, le marginatoside. *Planta Medica 33*: 46-52.

PIPE 7. Puentes de Diaz, A.M. & O.R. Gottlieb. 1979. Propiophenones from *Piper marginatum*. *Planta Medica 35*: 190-191.

PIPE 8. Ramos, L.S., M. Leão da Silva, A.I.R. Cruz, M.G.B. Zoghbi & J.G.S. Maia. 1986. Essential oil of *Piper marginatum*. *J. Nat. Prod. 49*: 712-713.

PIPE 9. Maxwell, A. & D. Rampersad. 1988. Prenylated 4-hydroxybenzoic acid derivatives from *Piper marginatum*. *J. Nat. Prod.* **51**: 370-373.
PIPE 10. Frischkorn, C.G.B. & H.E. Frischkorn. 1978. Cercaricidal activity of some essential oils of plants from Brazil. *Naturwiss.* **65**: 480-483.
PIPE 11. Simmonds, N.W. & R. Stevens. 1956. Occurrence of the methylene-dioxy bridge in the phenolic components of plants. *Nature* **178**: 752-753.
PIPE 12. Braz Filho, R., M.P. de Souza & M.E.O. Matos. 1981. Piplartine-dimer A, a new alkaloid from *Piper tuberculatum*. *Phytochemistry* **20**: 345-346.
PIPE 13. Kloos, H. & F.S. McCullough. 1982. Plant molluscicides. *Planta Medica* **46**: 195-209.
PIPE 14. Kyjoa, A., A.M. Giesbrecht, M.K. Akisue, O.R. Gottlieb & H.E. Gottlieb. 1980. 4-Nerolidylcatechol from *Pothomorphe umbellata*. *Planta Medica* **39**: 85-87.
PIPE 15. Barros, S.B.M., D.S. Teixeira, A.E. Aznar, J.A. Moreira Jr., I. Ishi & P.C.D. Freitas. 1996. Antioxidant activity of ethanolic extracts of *Pothomorphe umbellata* (L.) Miq. (pariparoba). *Ciência e Cultura* (São Paulo) **48**:114-116.
PIPE 16. Amorim, C.Z., C.A. Flores, B.E. Gomes, A.D. Marques & R.S.B. Cordeiro. 1988. Screening for antimalarial activity in the genus *Pothomorphe*. *J. Ethnopharmacol.* **24**: 101-106.
PIPE 17. Felzenszwalb, I., J.O. Valsa, A.C. Araujo & R. Alcantara Gomes. 1987. Absence of mutagenicity of *Pothomorphe umbellata* and *Pothomorphe peltata* in the salmonella/mammalian-microsome mutagenicity test. *Braz. J. Med. Biol. Res.* **20**: 403-405.

PLANTAGINACEAE

Plantago brasiliensis Sims
AREA: Rio Grande do Sul, campo.
NAME: Tanchagem.
USES: Used as a gargle to alleviate throat ailments.

Plantago guilleminiana Dcne.
AREA: Southern and eastern campos.
NAME: Tanchagem.
USES: Decoction of leaves in gargle used as a cure for sore throat. Roots are febrifuge and tonic.

Plantago myosurus Lam.
AREA: Rio Grande do Sul, campo.
NAME: Tanchagem-miúda.
USE: Given as gargle for tonsillitis.

PLUMBAGINACEAE

Limonium brasiliense (Boiss.) O. Ktze.
AREA: Santa Catarina and Rio Grande do Sul, in humid sites along the coastal belt.
NAMES: Baicuru, guaicuru.
USES: Plant is strongly astringent, used for acute and chronic diarrhoea as well as enterorrhagia; also for dropsy, enlargement of lymphatic

glands, rheumatism and to normalize menstrual flow.

CHEM.: Roots contains gallotannins, flavonoids and saponins (Ref: PLUM 1,2).

PHARM.: Root extract is bacteriostatic (Ref: PLUM 1,2) and anti-inflammatory (Ref: PLUM 3).

Plumbago scandens L.

AREA: Amazonia to São Paulo and Mato Grosso.

NAMES: Caataia, caapononga, folha-de-louro, erva-do-diabo, jasmim-azul, louco, queimadura.

USES: Roots are used to soothe pains in the ears and teeth, also for swollen joints and as a purgative. Root-juice is used for eliminating warts. Leaves are caustic, efficient against felon. In veterinary medicine the leaves are used to cauterize ulcers in horses.

CHEM.: Roots and leaves produce plumbagin (Ref: PLUM 4,5), a naphthoquinone derivative characteristic of most species of this genus.

PHARM.: Plumbagin was shown to be strongly active against the growth of a variety of fungi (Ref: PLUM 5).

Plumbaginaceae – References

PLUM 1. Rosito, J.F. 1975. *Contribução à análise das raizes de Limonium brasiliense* (Boiss.) Kuntze. Thesis, Federal University of Rio Grande do Sul.

PLUM 2. Moura, T.F.A. de L. 1984. *Sobre o Limonium brasiliense* (Boiss.) Kuntze, *Plumbaginaceae, o baicuru da Farmacopéia Brasileira I* . Thesis, Federal University of Rio Grande do Sul.

PLUM 3. Moura, T.F.A. de L., E.P. Schenkel, E.E.S. Schapoval, C.M.O. Simões & R.I. dos Santos. 1965. Estudos farmacológicos preliminares das raizes de *Limonium brasiliense* (Boiss.) Kuntze, Plumbaginaceae (Baicuru). *Cadernos de Farmácia* (Porto Alegre) *1*: 45-54.

PLUM 4. Harborne, J.B. 1967. Comparative biochemistry of the flavonoids. IV. Correlations between chemistry, pollen morphology and systematics in the family Plumbaginaceae. *Phytochemistry* 6: 1415-1418.

PLUM 5. Gonçalves de Lima, O., I.L. d'Albuquerque, G.M. Maciel & M.C.N. Maciel. 1968. Substâncias antimicrobianas de plantas superiores. XXVII. Isolamento de plumbagina de *Plumbago scandens* L. *Rev. Inst. Antibióticos* (Recife) *8*: 95-97.

POACEAE

Andropogon bicornis L.

AREA: Pará to São Paulo and Mato Grosso.

NAMES: Capim-amargoso, capim-d'agua, capim-de-bezerro, capim-mole, capim-peba, capim-rabo-de-raposa, capim-vassoura, capim-sapê, sapê.

USES: Decoction of roots is diuretic, emollient and diaphoretic.

Andropogon condensatus H.B.K. is very similar to the above, exists over the same range and is used in the same way.

POACEAE

Andropogon minarum Kunth
AREA: Maranhão to São Paulo.
NAME: Capim-açu.
USE: Seeds are diuretic.

Aristida pallens Cav.
AREA: Minas Gerais to Rio Grande do Sul, campo and wasteland.
NAMES: Barba-de-bode, capim-barba-de-bode, capim-de-bode.
USES: Leaves and roots are a mild laxative; used for treatment of enlarged liver.

Avena quadridentata Doell
AREA: Minas Gerais, campo.
NAMES: Aveia-da-terra, aveia-do-campo, aveia-do-mato.
USES: Caryopses used for stopping hemoptysis.

Chloris distichophylla (Nees) Lag.
AREA: Pernambuco to Rio Grande do Sul and Mato Grosso, campo.
NAMES: Capim-batatal, capim-cebola, cocorobó, graminha-de-araraquara, pé-de-galinha.
USES: Leaves are febrifuge; fruits are diuretic.

Chloris polydactyla Sw.
AREA: Pernambuco to Rio Grande do Sul and Mato Grosso, in campos and along roads.
NAMES: Capim-branco, capim-guiamum, pé-de-galinha.
USES: Rhizome employed against uterine disorders.

Cymbopogon schoenanthus (L.) Spreng.
AREA: Cultivated and often naturalized.
NAMES: Capim-cidreira, capim-limão, capim-santo (English: lemon grass).
USES: Leaf tea is tonic, carminative, calmative and weakly soporific. Used for gastric disturbances and against slight fevers.
CHEM.: Essential oil of leaves contains citral (mixture of geranial and neral) as the major constituent (47–70%), followed by myrcene (16–37%) (Ref: POAC 1).
PHARM.: The tea has been tested orally in animals as to central nervous system depressant effect, but the results were negative (Ref: POAC 2). The tea, as used in Brazilian folk medicine, is atoxic and lacks hypnotic or anxiolytic properties (Ref: POAC 3,4). Only following intraperitoneal injection were such effects observed (Ref: POAC 2). More recently it has been reported that the tea induces dipyrone-like analgesia in rodents (Ref: POAC 5). ß-myrcene was shown to be the active substance, being a potent peripheral analgesic drug (Ref: POAC 6). ß-myrcene has low acute toxicity in rats and mice (Ref: POAC 7).

POACEAE

Elionurus bilinguis (Trin.) Hack.
AREA: Minas Gerais, campo.
NAME: Capim-jasmin-da-serra.
USE: Antirheumatic.

Elionurus candidus (Trin.) Hack.
AREA: Minas Gerais to Rio Grande do Sul, campo.
NAMES: Barba-de-bode, capim-amargoso, capim-limão.
USES: Infusion or syrup made from the inflorescences is taken for chronic bronchitis, cystitis and gonorrhoea.

The very closely related *Elionurus latiflorus* Nees occurs in the same area and has the same common names and uses.

Gynerium parviflorum Nees
AREA: Piauí to São Paulo.
NAMES: Cana-brava, cana-do-rio, cana-ubá, flexa, parimá, ubá.
USES: Rhizome is diuretic and excitant; its decoction is used externally to strengthen the hair and promote hair growth.

The closely related *Gynerium sagittatum* (Pers.) Beauv. (Amazonia to Mato Grosso) has similar uses.

Hackelochloa granularis (L.) O. Ktze.
AREA: Piauí to Minas Gerais, ruderal.
NAMES: Capim-mimoso, mimosinho.
USES: Roots are considered good for liver and spleen.

Imperata brasiliensis Trin.
AREA: Alagoas to Rio Grande do Sul, ruderal, weed.
NAMES: Agreste, capim-agreste, capim-massapê, capim-sapê, jucapê, massapê, sapê.
USES: Rhizome is diuretic and resolvent. In pastures it is used to reinvigorate exhausted horses.

Another "sapê" is *Imperata contracta* Hitch., distributed throughout Brazil, with the same uses.

Luziola peruviana Pers.
AREA: Piauí to Rio Grande do Sul.
NAMES: Arroz-das-águas, arroz-do-brejo, arroz-silvestre, capim-arroz.
USES: Caryopses are edible like rice; as a medicine, the caryopses are emollient.

Melinis minutiflora Beauv.
AREA: Throughout Brazil as pasture grass and ruderal.
NAMES: Capim-catinguento, capim-gordo, capim-gordura, capim-melado.
USES: Diuretic and antidysenteric.

POACEAE

Panicum brevifolium L.
AREA: Amazonia to São Paulo and Minas Gerais.
NAMES: Andacá, capim-chuvisco, capim-mimoso, taquari-do-mato, vindecaá.
USE: Roots are diuretic.

Panicum megiston Schult.
AREA: Amazonia to Bahia and Mato Grosso.
NAMES: Capim-açu, capim-da-praia-açu, capim-gigante, capim-lixa, capim-taboquinha.
USE: Roots are diuretic.

Panicum petrosum Trin.
AREA: Alagoas to São Paulo in stony campos.
NAME: Barba-de-bode.
USES: Mild laxative, diuretic; externally applied as emollient for swollen liver.

Panicum trichanthum Nees
AREA: Amazonia to Goiás.
NAMES: Andacaá, capim-andacaá, capim-mimoso, capim-vindecaá.
USES: Rhizome is aromatic, emollient, excitant and diuretic.

Pappophorum mucronulatum Nees
AREA: Piauí to Bahia.
NAME: Capim-amargoso.
USE: Leaves used for flatulence.

Paspalum extenuatum Nees
AREA: Piauí to Bahia.
NAMES: Capim-mão-de-sapo, capim-de-sapo.
USES: To cure skin diseases.

Sacciolepis myuros (Lam.) Chase
AREA: Pará to São Paulo, ruderal.
NAMES: Amonjeaba, capim-amonjeaba.
USES: Emollient, indicated for orchitis.

Setaria scandens Schrad.
AREA: Pará to São Paulo.
NAMES: Capim-mimoso-de-cacho, capim-rabo-de-raposa, capim-rabo-de-rato.
USES: Leaves recommended for treating eczema.

Poaceae – References

POAC 1. Matos, F.J.A., J.W. Alencar, A.A. Craveiro & M.C. Fonteles. 1984. Distinção química e farmacológica de clones de *Cymbopogon citratus* cultivados no Ceará e em São Paulo. *Ciência e Cultura* (São Paulo) *36*: 546.

POAC 2. Carlini, E.A., J.D.P. Contar, A.R. Silva-Filho, N.G. Silveira-Filho, M.L. Frochtengarten & O.F.A. Bueno. 1986. Pharmacology of lemongrass (*Cymbopogon citratus* Stapf). I. Effects of teas prepared from the leaves on laboratory animals. *J. Ethnopharmacol. 17*: 37-64.

POAC 3. Formigoni, M.L.O.S., H.M. Lodder, O. Gianotti Filho, T.M.S. Ferreira & E.A. Carlini. 1986. Pharmacology of lemongrass (*Cymbopogon citratus* Stapf). II. Effects of daily two month administration in male and female rats and in offspring exposed "in utero." *J. Ethnopharmacol. 17*: 65-74.

POAC 4. Leite, J.R., M.L.V. Seabra, E. Maluf, K. Assolant, D. Suchecki, S. Tufik, S. Klepaca, H.M. Calil & E.A. Carlini. 1986. Pharmacology of lemongrass (*Cymbopogon citratus* Stapf). III. Assessment of eventual toxic, hypnotic and anxiolytic effects on humans. *J. Ethnopharmacol. 17*: 75-83.

POAC 5. Lorenzetti, B.B., C.E.P. Souza, S.J. Sarti, D. Santos-Filho & S.H. Ferreira. 1988. Atividade analgésica periférica de *Cymbopogon citratus* ("Capim-cidreira"). *III Reunião Anual da Federação das Sociedades de Biologia Experimental* (Caxambú, Minas Gerais), Summaries of papers: 203.

POAC 6. Lorenzetti, B.B., C.E.P. Souza, S.J. Sarti, D. Santos-Filho & S.H. Ferreira. 1991. Myrcene mimics the peripheral activity of lemongrass tea. *J. Ethnopharmacol. 34*: 43-48.

POAC 7. Paumgarten, F.J.R., I.F. Delgado, E.N. Alves, A.C.M.A. Nogueira, R.C. De-Farias & D. Neubert. 1990. Single dose toxicity study of ß-myrcene, a natural analgesic substance. *Brazilian J. Med. Biol. Res. 23*: 873-877.

POLYGALACEAE

Bredemeyera floribunda Willd.

AREA: Maranhão to São Paulo.

NAMES: Botica-inteira, marfim-de-ramá, pau-caixão, pau-rendoso, raiz-de-joão-da-coasta, cabão-de-bugre.

USES: All parts of the plant are used in aqueous infusion or decoction to treat furunculosis and skin diseases in general, as well as insect stings. Also as an antifebrile and for high blood pressure. Alcoholic infusion used against snakebite.

CHEM.: The roots are extremely rich in triterpenoid saponins, which have been the object of chemical studies (Ref: POLYGA 1,2,3,4,5). Industrialization of the plant as a substitute for *Quillaja* and *Saponaria* saponins has been considered.

PHARM.: The root extract was shown to exert a dramatic regenerating effect on the mucous membrane of the stomach wall containing lesions induced by alcohol (Ref: POLYGA 6).

Polygala angulata DC.

AREA: Pará to São Paulo, campo.

NAMES: Ipecacuanha, poaia, poaia-do-campo.

USES: This is one of several known "false poaias." The roots are emetic and antipyretic and are used in the same way and for the same purposes as the genuine ipecacuanha (*Cephaelis ipecacuanha* Rich., Rubiaceae).

Polygala comata Mart.
AREA: Pará to São Paulo, campo.
NAME: Poaia.
USES: Root is vomitive and bechic.

Polygala klotzschii Chodat
AREA: São Paulo.
NAMES: Laranja-brava, laranjinha, limãozinho.
USES: Leaves are sudorific, pectoral and anticatarrhal.

Polygala paniculata L.
AREA: Coastal sands from Bahia to Rio Grande do Sul and Mato Grosso.
NAME: Barba-de-são-pedro.
USES: Herb is antiblennorrhagic, vomitive, purgative, diuretic; also recommended for snakebite.
CHEM.: Several coumarins have been described (Ref: POLYGA 7).
PHARM.: Hexane and chloroform extracts showed molluscicidal and antifungal activity (Ref: POLYGA 7). The properties of the root saponins have been compared to those of senega root, *Polygala senega* L. (Ref: POLYGA 8).

Polygala spectabilis DC.
AREA: Pará.
NAME: Caá-membeca.
USES: Bechic, expectorant; soothing in baths for hemorrhoids. Tea prescribed as a cure for amoebic dysentery.
CHEM.: The aerial parts yielded three highly oxygenated xanthones, besides stigmasterol (Ref: POLYGA 9).

Polygala timoutou Aubl.
AREA: Throughout Brazil.
NAMES: Timutu.
USES: Roots are emetic, diuretic and emmenagogue.

Polygalaceae – References

POLYGA 1. Tschesche, R. & A.K. Sen Gupta. 1960. Über Triterpene. VI. Sapogenine von *Bredemeyera floribunda*. *Chem. Ber.* 93: 1903-1907.

POLYGA 2. Tschesche, R., E. Henckel & G. Snatzke. 1963. Über Triterpene. X. Die Struktur der Bredemolsäure und die Partialzynthese ihres Methylesters aus Oleanolsäuremethylester. *Tetrahedron Lett.*: 613-617.

POLYGA 3. Tschesche, R. & H. Striegler. 1965. Über Triterpene. XVI. Die Identität der Tenuifolsäure mit Senegenin. *Naturwissenschaft* 52: 303.

POLYGA 4. Daros, M.R., F.J.A. Matos & J.P. Parente. 1996. A new triterpenoid saponin, bredmeyeroside B, from the roots of *Bredemeyera floribunda*. *Planta Medica* 62: 523-527.

POLYGA 5. Pereira, B.M.R., M.R. Daros, J.P. Parente & F.J.A. Matos. 1996. Bredemeyeroside C, a new saponin from *Bredemeyera floribunda*. *Fitoterapia 67*: 323-328.
POLYGA 6. Rao, V.S., G.S.B. Viana, M.G.T. Gadelha & E.R. Silveira. 1990. Experimental evaluation of *Bredemeyera floribunda* in acute gastric lesions induced by ethanol, acetylsalycylic acid and histamine. *Fitoterapia 61*: 9-12.
POLYGA 7. Hamburger, M., M. Gupta & K. Hostettmann. 1985. Coumarins from *Polygala paniculata*. *Planta Medica 51*: 215-217.
POLYGA 8. Siqueira, N.C.S. 1983/84. Contribuição aos estudos farmacológicos de *Polygala paniculata* da flora do Rio Grande do Sul. *Tribuna Farmacêutica* (Curitiba) *51/52*: 32-38.
POLYGA 9. Andrade, C.H.S., R. Braz Filho, O.R. Gottlieb & E.R. Silveira. 1977. The chemistry of Brazilian Polygalaceae. 1. Xanthones from *Polygala spectabilis* L. *Lloydia 40*: 344-346.

POLYGONACEAE

Coccoloba arborescens (Vell.) How.
AREA: Bahia, Rio de Janeiro, Minas Gerais and Santa Catarina, mainly in restinga.
NAMES: Tangaraca-açu.
USES: Juice from fruits used against diarrhoea and leucorrhoea.

Coccoloba laevis Casar.
AREA: Rio Grande do Norte to Rio de Janeiro and Mato Grosso, forest, restinga and cerrado.
NAMES: Baga-da-praia, curatá, guajabara.
USES: Root and stem bark are astringent, indicated against gonorrhoea and leucorrhoea; leaf decoction useful for treating piles.

Coccoloba marginata Benth.
AREA: Amazonia to Goiás and Bahia, forest and cerrado.
NAME: Cabuçu, guajabara, guajuriva.
USES: Roots are antidiarrhoeic, antileucorrhoeic and used in gargles for sore throat.

Coccoloba mollis Casar.
AREA: Amazonia to São Paulo and Mato Grosso, forest, cerrado and campo.
NAME: Cauaçu, pau-de-vassoura.
USES: Decoction of root and stem bark used against gonorrhoea and leucorrhoea. Decoction of leaves employed in sit-baths to alleviate bleeding hemorrhoids.

Muehlenbeckia sagittifolia (Ort.) Meissn.
AREA: Rio Grande do Sul.
NAME: Salsa, salsa-do-rio-grande, salsaparrilha.
USES: Decoction of the plant is depurative, indicated for syphilis.
CHEM.: Aerial parts contain tannins and anthraquinones (Ref: POLYGO 1).

POLYGONACEAE

Polygonum acuminatum H.B.K.
AREA: Distributed throughout South America, from Amazonia to Uruguay.
NAME: Capiçaba, cataia, erva-de-bicho, paia-marioba, pimenta-d'agua.
USES: Herb is recommended against piles, intestinal worms, leucorrhoea, dysentery and arthritic ailments.

Polygonum hydropiperoides Michx.
AREA: Eastern and southern Brazil to Rio Grande do Sul, in marshes.
NAME: Potincoba.

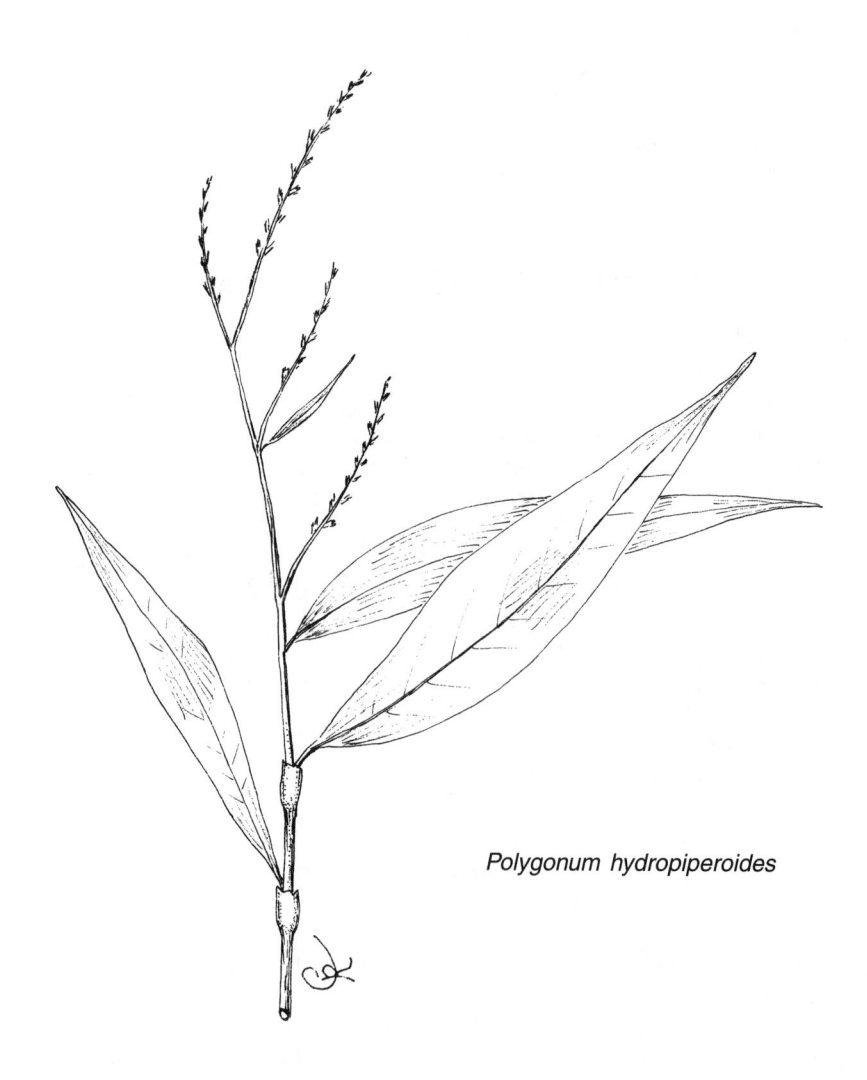

Polygonum hydropiperoides

USES: Juice in cataplasm acts like a sinapism (mustard plaster). Fresh leaves applied locally are antirheumatic. Dried leaves are diuretic.

Polygonum punctatum Elliot
AREA: Much of Brazil in moist places.
NAME: Capitiçova, erva-de-bicho, persicária-do-brasil.
USES: Herb is astringent, stimulant, diuretic, vermicide, antigonorrhoeal, antihemorrhoidal; also applied to skin ulcers, erysipelas, arthritis, bleeding diarrhoea and malignant ulcers.

Polygonum spectabile Mart.
AREA: Pará to Mato Grosso and Rio Grande do Sul, in moist, sandy sites.
NAMES: Capitiçova, erva-de-bicho, persicária-do-brasil.
USES: Recommended for hemorrhoids, worms, gonorrhoea, skin ulcers, erysipelas and rheumatism; also a stimulant and diuretic.

Rumex brasiliensis Link
AREA: Minas Gerais, Rio de Janeiro and São Paulo.
NAMES: Azeda-graúda, labaça.
USES: Juice is resolvent and antisyphilitic. Roots are bitter, tonic, febrifuge, diuretic and used against intestinal catarrh.

Triplaris macrocalyx Casar.
AREA: Rio de Janeiro, coastal woodland, restinga.
NAME: Pau-paraíba.
USE: Used for treating snakebite.

Triplaris noli-tangere Wedd.
AREA: Mato Grosso.
NAME: Formigueira.
USES: Decoction is said to be excitant to the nervous system and to aid in treatment of lymphangitis.

Triplaris weigeltiana (Reichb.) O. Ktze.
AREA: Amazonia and Mato Grosso, forest; also cultivated as an ornamental.
NAMES: Pau-de-novato, tachi, tachi-preto-da-várzea, tachizeiro, tangarana.
USES: Bark used against diarrhoea and piles.

Polygonaceae – Reference
POLYGO 1. Silva, G.A. de A.B. 1974. *Contribuição ao estudo farmacognóstico de Muehlenbeckia sagittifolia Meiss.* Thesis, Federal University of Rio Grande do Sul.

POLYPODIACEAE

Microgramma vaccinifolia (Langsd. & Fisch.) Copel.
AREA: Ruderal, very common on trees in streets.
NAMES: Cipó-peludo, erva-de-lagarto, erva-silveira, erva-silvina, erva-teresa.
USES: Powerful astringent and hemostatic, formerly employed to arrest hemoptyses in tuberculous patients.

Phlebodium aureum (L.) J.E. Smith
AREA: Throughout Brazil, forest.
NAME: Avenca-dourada.
USES: Rhizome used for expelling taenia and to treat respiratory troubles. Leaves are antihemorrhagic.

Phlebodium decumanum (Willd.) J. Smith
AREA: Amazonia, forest.
NAME: Guaririnha.
use: Antitussive syrup is made from the roots.

Polypodium brasiliense Poir.
AREA: Frequent throughout Brazil, forest and restinga.
NAME: Pluma.
USE: Leaf infusion is bechic.

For other medicinally employed ferns closely related to Polypodiaceae, see the families Adiantaceae and Dennstaedtiaceae.

PONTEDERIACEAE

Eichhornia crassipes Solms
AREA: Floating on fresh water irrespective of geography or climate.
NAMES: Aguapé, aguapé-de-flor-roxa, baronesa, mururé, paraci, pavoá; (English: water hyacinth).
USES: Tea of leaves is depurative.

Pontederia cordifolia Mart.
AREA: Alagoas to Rio de Janeiro, aquatic.
NAMES: Aguapé, rainha-dos-lagos.
USES: For treating skin ailments.

PORTULACACEAE

Portulaca grandiflora Hook.
AREA: From Minas Gerais southward; ruderal, cosmopolitan; much cultivated in gardens.

NAMES: Amor-crescido, beldroega-de-flor-grande, flor-de-onze-horas, onze-horas, perexi, cavalheiro-das-onze-horas.
USES: Herb juice is emollient and diuretic; applied topically against dermal afflictions.

Portulaca oleracea L.
AREA: Cosmopolitan; ruderal throughout Brazil.
NAMES: Beldroega, beldroega-pequena, caaponga, ora-pro-nobis (English: purslane).
USES: Leaves are edible; used as a diuretic and vermifuge; also for cystitis, against hemoptyses and renal colics, burns and ulcers. Seeds are emmenagogue, diuretic and anthelmintic.
CHEM.: The plant is exceptionally rich in oxalic acid and potassium salts (nitrate, chloride, sulfate) (Ref: PORT 1). It also contains catecholamine derivatives — (-)-noradrenaline, DOPA and dopamine — in high concentrations (Ref: PORT 2,3).
PHARM.: Besides the hypertensive effect of the aqueous extract due to the presence of catecholamines, a skeletal muscle relaxant property has been demonstrated (Ref: PORT 4,5,6).

Portulaca pilosa L.
AREA: Almost throughout Brazil.
NAME: Amor-crescido.
USES: Herb is diuretic, emmenagogue, used against liver ailments, malaria and ulcers. Contused leaves in compresses are applied topically to treat burns and erysipelas. Used as a tea for "strengthening the blood," for cleaning sores and to check diarrhoea. Also employed as shampoo against hair loss; to strengthen hair growth.

Talinum racemosum (L.) Rohr.
AREA: From Minas Gerais southward, as a ruderal herb.
NAME: Beldroega-grande.
USES: Leaves are mucilaginous, edible; used to soften corns. Seeds are emmenagogue.

Portulacaceae – References

PORT 1. Yasuhe, M. & Y. Honda. 1944. Components of Portulacaceae plants. *J. Pharm. Soc. Japan* 64: 177-178.
PORT 2. Feng, P.C., L.Y. Haynes & K.E. Magnus. 1961. High concentration of (-)-noradrenaline in *Portulaca oleracea*. *Nature* 191: 1108.
PORT 3. Smith, T.A. 1977. Phenylethylamine and related compounds in plants. *Phytochemistry* 1: 9-18.
PORT 4. Okwuasaba, F., C. Ejcke & O. Parry. 1986. Skeletal muscle relaxant properties of the aqueous extract of *Portulaca oleracea*. *J. Ethnopharmacol.* 17: 139-160.
PORT 5. Okwuasaba, F., C. Ejcke & O. Parry. 1987. Effects of extracts of *Portulaca oleracea* on skeletal muscle *in vitro*. *J. Ethnopharmacol.* 21: 55-63.
PORT 6. Parry, O., F. Okwuasaba & C. Ejcke. 1988. Effects of an aqueous extract of *Portu-

laca oleracea leaves on smooth muscle and rat blood pressure. *J. Ethnopharmacol. 22*: 33-44.

PORT 7. Nickell, L.G. 1959. Antimicrobial activity of vascular plants. *Econ. Bot. 13*: 281-283.

PORT 8. Adesina, S.K. 1982. Studies on some plants used as anticonvulsants in Amerindian and African traditional medicine. *Fitoterapia 53*: 147-162.

PRIMULACEAE

Samolus valerandi L.
AREA: Rio Grande do Sul.
NAME: Baicuri-açu, morrião-d'água.
USES: Herb is antiscorbutic and eaten as an appetizer, though somewhat toxic.

RANUNCULACEAE

Anemone decapetala L.
AREA: Southern Brazil.
NAMES: Anêmone, Anêmone-de-dez-folhas.
USES: Herb, though noxious, is indicated for skin diseases.

Clematis campestris St.-Hil.
AREA: Minas Gerais to Rio Grande do Sul, campo.
NAMES: Barba-de-velho, cipó-barba-branca, cipó-do-reino, iride-branca.
USES: Plant is tart, narcotic; poisonous.

Clematis denticulata Vell.
AREA: Rio Grande do Sul, campo.
NAMES: Barba-branca, barba-de-velho.
USES: Leaves are rubefacient and antirheumatic; young shoots said to be useful for rabies and bites of poisonous animals.

Clematis dioica L.
AREA: Most of Brazil.
NAMES: Barba-de-velho, cipó-cruz, cipó-do-reino, cipó-prata, erva-de-gato.
USES: Thought to be narcotic and venomous, at least for cattle. Fresh leaves are rubefacient, even vesicant, recommended for dermal ailments and removal of spots on skin. Dry leaves are inactive. Decocted in sea water they are considered purgative for cases of hydropsy, scrofula and syphilis. Root is drastic.

Ranunculus apiifolius Pers.
AREA: Southern Brazil.
NAMES: Cipó-do-banhado, botão-de-ouro, ranúnculo-aipo.

USES: Dermatoses and persistent cough.

Ranunculus bonariensis Poir.
AREA: Rio Grande do Sul.
NAME: Ranúnculo.
USE: Narcotic.
CHEM. & PHARM.: Ranunculaceae are used as medicinals in many countries, in spite of their pronounced toxicity. Lactones of the anemonin type are characteristic constituents of the genera *Anemone, Clematis* and *Ranunculus*. None of the these Brazilian species has ever been analyzed.

RHABDODENDRACEAE

Rhabdodendron amazonicum (Spr. ex Benth.) Hub.
AREA: Amazonia, forest.
NAMES: Cachaceiro, muirapuama (not to be confused with *Ptychopetalum olacoides* and *P. uncinatum*, Olacaceae).
USES: Leaves used in baths for strengthening the body.

RHAMNACEAE

Ampelozizyphus amazonicus Ducke
AREA: Amazonia, forest and secondary growth.
NAMES: Cerveja-de-índio, saracura-muirá.
USES: A suspension made from the roots, foaming and tasting like beer, is used as a preventive and cure for malaria.
CHEM.: Five triterpenes and triterpenoid saponins were isolated from the roots (Ref: RHAM 1).
PHARM.: Experiments in mice inoculated with *Plasmodium berghei* showed no antimalarial activity, leading to the conclusion that the drug is not a blood schizonticide. A possible effect against sporozoites or tissue schizonts is not excluded (Ref: RHAM 2).

Colletia paradoxa (Spr.) Escalante
AREA: Southern Brazil, campo.
NAMES: Coroa-de-cristo, curro, quina.
USES: Root bark is tonic, febrifuge and cardioactive.
CHEM.: Alkaloids (Ref: RHAM 3) and triterpenoids (Ref: RHAM 4) have been described. The epicuticular wax has been studied (Ref: RHAM 5).

Discaria americana Gill. & Hook.
AREA: Rio Grande do Sul, campo.

RHAMNACEAE

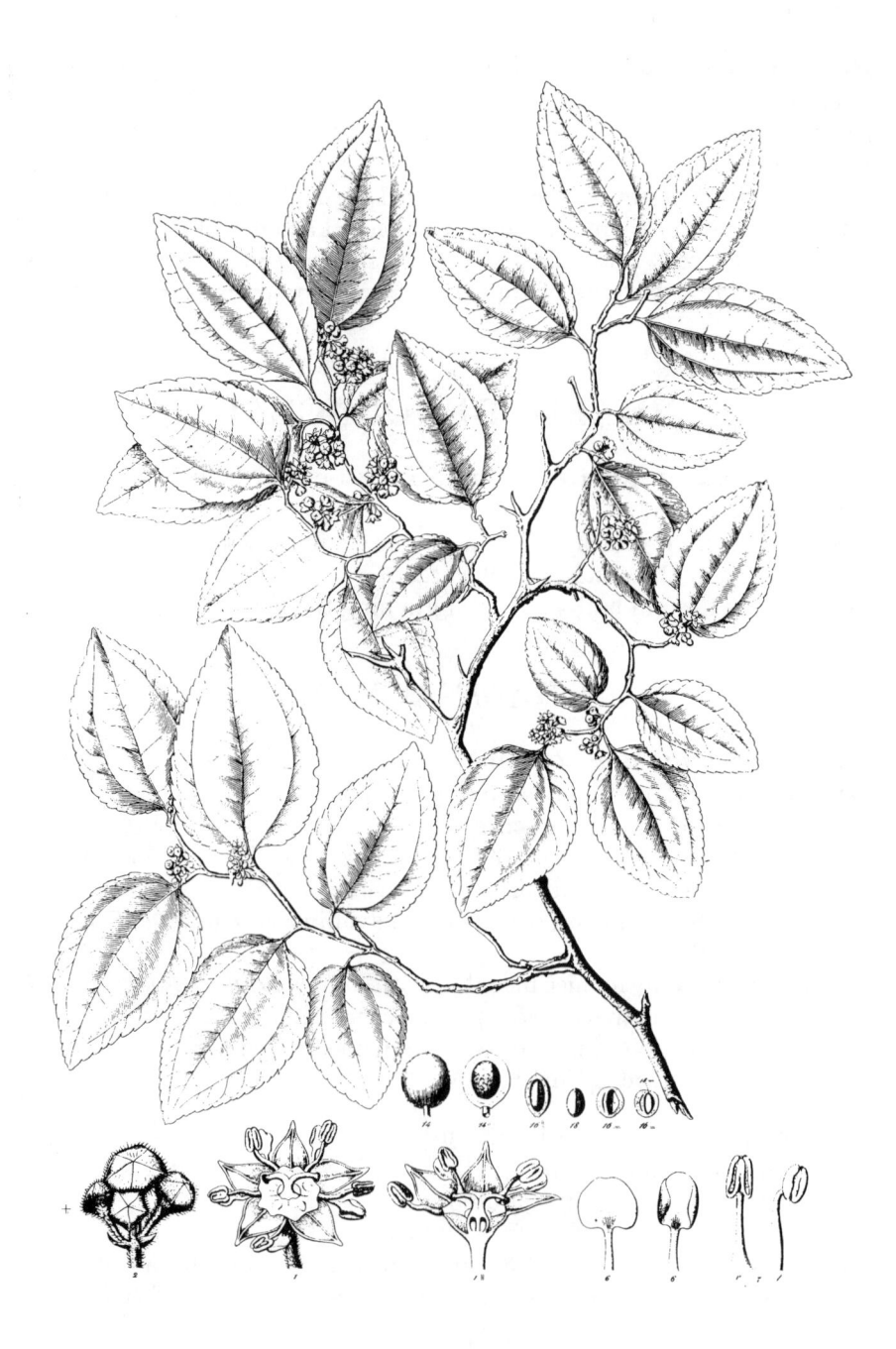

Zizyphus joazeiro

RHAMNACEAE

NAMES: Brusca, quina-do-campo, quina-do-rio-grande.
USES: Roots and bark are tonic and antithermic. This species is sometimes erroneously cited as *D. febrifuga* Mart.

Reisseckia smilacina (Sm.) Steud.
AREA: Rio de Janeiro, common in restinga.
NAME: Cipó-de-lavadeira.
USE: Roots used in remedy for syphilis.

Scutia buxifolia Reiss.
AREA: Paraná to Rio Grande do Sul.
NAMES: Canela-de-espinho, coronilha, espinho-de-touro.
USES: A tincture made from the bark is used for heart and circulatory ailments, and as a substitute for digitalis.
CHEM.: Contains peptide alkaloids, which are typical of this and a few other plant families (Ref: RHAM 6,7,8,9,10).

Zizyphus joazeiro Mart.
AREA: Northeastern caatinga, from Piauí to Minas Gerais.
NAMES: Joazeiro, juá, juazeiro, laranjinha-de-vaqueiro.
USES: Infusion of leaves used for a stomachic. The bast is extremely rich in saponin; its aqueous infusion is widely employed as a hair tonic, to treat skin sores and for brushing teeth; also as a febrifuge.
CHEM.: Triterpenes and saponins have been described (Ref: RHAM 11).
PHARM.: Antifebrile activity has been confirmed in rabbits (Ref: RHAM 12).

Rhamnaceae – References
RHAM 1. Brandão, M.G.L., M.-A. Lacaille-Dubois, M.A. Teixeira & H. Wagner. 1992. Triterpene saponins from the roots of *Ampelozizyphus amazonicus*. *Phytochemistry 31*: 352-354.
RHAM 2. Botelho, M.G.A., H.F. Paulino Filho & A.U. Krettli. 1987. Quimioterapia experimental antimalárica usando a Rhamnaceae *Ampelozizyphus amazonicus* Ducke, vulgarmente denominada "cerveja-de-índio," contra o *Plasmodium berghei*. *Oreades* (Belo Horizonte) *8*: 437-442.
RHAM 3. Theumann, D. & J. Comin. 1966. Plantas argentinas. XXIV. Bases quaternarias de *Colletia paradoxa*. *An. Asoc. Quím. Arg. 54*: 217-219.
RHAM 4. Merkuza, V.M., O.A. Mascaretti, R. Crohare & E.A. Rúveda. 1971. Triterpenoids from *Discaria longispina* and *Colletia paradoxa*. *Phytochemistry 10*: 908-910.
RHAM 5. Moyna, P. 1983. Epicuticular wax of *Colletia paradoxa*. *Phytochemistry 22*: 1283-1285.
RHAM 6. Wasicky, R., M. Wasicky & R. Joachimovits. 1964. Erstuntersuchungen an "Coronilha" — *Scutia buxifolia* Reissek. *Planta Medica 12*: 13-26.
RHAM 7. Tschesche R., R. Welters & H.-W. Fehlhaber. 1967. Scutianin, ein cyclisches Peptid-Alkaloid aus *Scutia buxifolia* Reiss. *Chem. Ber. 100*: 323-334.
RHAM 8. Tschesche, R., E. Ammermann & H.-W. Fehlhaber. 1971. Alkaloide aus Rhamnaceen. X. Scutianin-B, ein weiteres Peptidalkaloid aus *Scutia buxifolia* Reiss. *Tetrahedron Lett.*: 4405-4408.

RHAM 9. Merkuza, V.M., M. González Sierra, O.A. Mascaretti, E.A. Rúveda, C.J. Chang & E. Wenkert. 1974. Peptide alkaloids of *Discaria longispina* and *Scutia buxifolia*. *Phytochemistry 13*: 1279-1282.
RHAM 10. Tschesche, R. & D. Hillebrand. 1976. Scutianin-G, ein weiteres cyclopeptidalkaloid aus *Scutia buxifolia*. *Phytochemistry 16*: 1817-1818.
RHAM 11. Barbosa Filho, J.M., J.A. Trigueiro, U.O. Cheriyan & J. Bhattacharyya. 1985. Constituents of the stem-bark of *Zizyphus joazeiro*. *J. Nat. Prod. 48*: 152-153.
RHAM 12. Nunes, P.H.M., L.C. Marinho, M.L.R.L. Nunes & E.O. Soares. 1987. Antipyretic activity of an aqueous extract of *Zizyphus joazeiro* Mart. (Rhamnaceae). *Braz. J. Med. Biol. Res. 20*: 599-601.

RHIZOPHORACEAE

Rhizophora mangle L.
AREA: Tropical cosmopolitan, in typical formations ("mangroves") on tidal flats, along the seacoast.
NAMES: Mangue, mangue-vermelho (English: red mangrove).
USES: Highly tanniferous bark is prescribed for diarrhoea and hemorrhage.

ROSACEAE

Margyricarpus setosus Ruiz & Pav.
AREA: Rio Grande do Sul.
NAME: Fruta-de-perdiz.
USES: Diuretic, recommended to eliminate gall bladder and urinary calculi; also tonic and emmenagogue.

Prunus subcoriacea (Chod. & Hassl.) Hoehne
AREA: Minas Gerais to Rio Grande do Sul, forest.
NAMES: Pessegueiro-bravo, pessegueiro-do-mato.
USES: Leaf infusion used for treating pulmonary afflictions, asthma.

Rubus brasiliensis Mart.
AREA: Minas Gerais and Rio de Janeiro to Paraná, on mountains.
NAMES: Amora-brava, amora-branca, amora-preta, amora-verde, amoreira-do-brasil, amoreira-do-mato.
USES: Fruits are eaten early in the morning to check bleeding diarrhoea.

RUBIACEAE

Alibertia edulis (Rich.) Rich.
AREA: Amazonia and central Brazil, cerrado.

RUBIACEAE

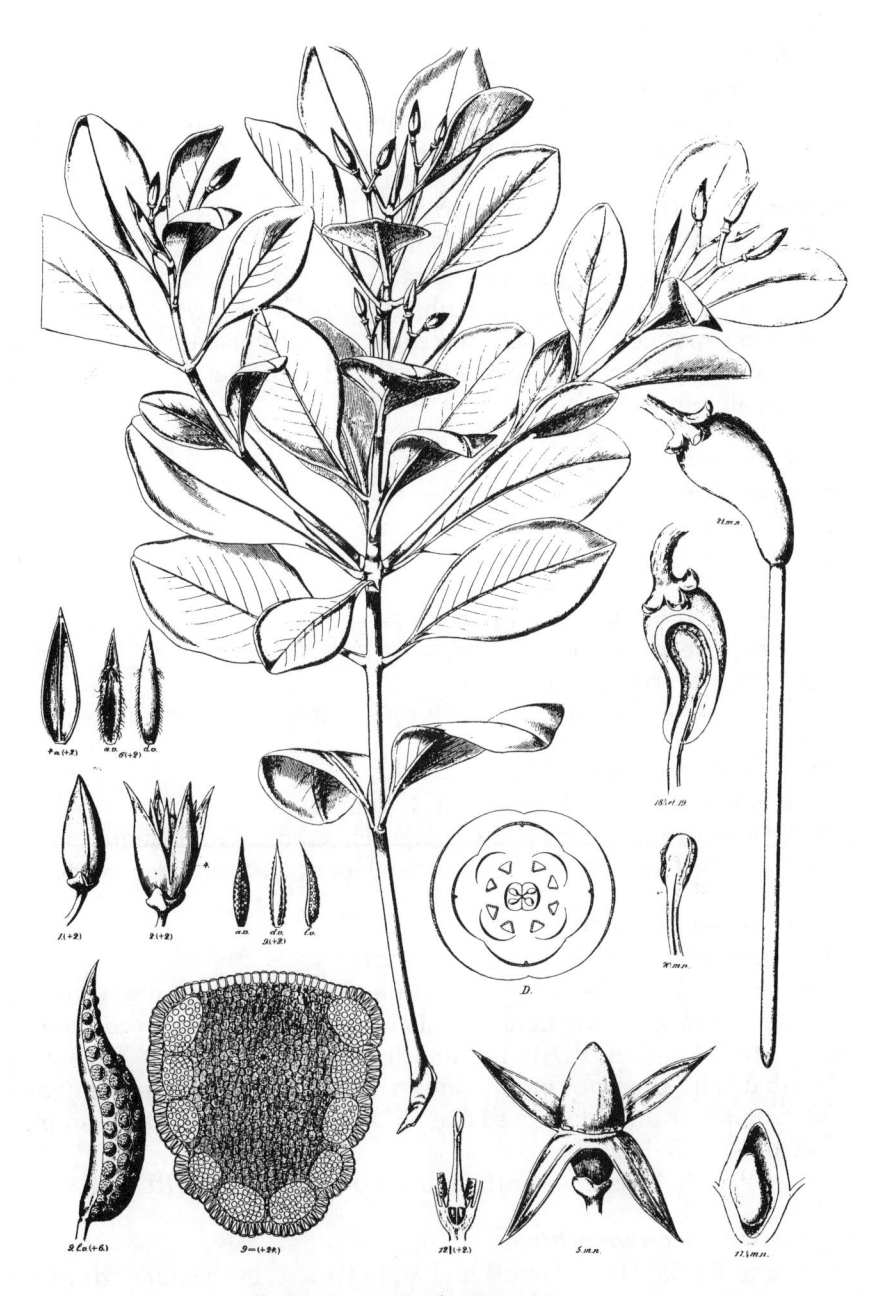

Rhizophora mangle, Rhizophoraceae

NAMES: Marmelada, marmelada-de-cachorro, purui.
USES: Leaves used in baths to reduce hernia.

RUBIACEAE

Bathysa cuspidata Hook.
AREA: Rio de Janeiro and Minas Gerais, forest.
NAME: Quina-do-mato.
USES: Bark used for a bitter tonic, indicated for anemia, malaria, ancylostomiasis and recovery after illness.

Borreria asclepiadea Cham. & Schl.
AREA: Goiás to Rio Grande do Sul, campo.
NAMES: Poaia-do-campo, poaia-rasteira.
USES: As a substitute for ipecacuanha (*Cephaelis ipecacuanha*); also the following species, which bear the same vernacular names: *B. capitata* (Ruiz & Pav.) DC. (Bahia to São Paulo) and *B. latifolia* K. Sch. (Pará to Rio de Janeiro).

Borreria poaya (St.-Hil.) DC.
AREA: Southern Brazil, campos.
NAMES: Poaia-do-arador, poaia-rasteira.
USES: Roots are emetocathartic.

Borreria tenella Cham. & Schl.
AREA: Widespread, campo and cerrado.
NAMES: Poaia-do-cerrado, rubim.
USES: Roots are emetic, purgative, diuretic, antihydropic and antiophidic.

Borreria verbenoides Cham. & Schl.
AREA: São Paulo do Rio Grande do Sul, campo.
NAMES: Guaicuru, poaia-de-haste-comprida, sabugueiro-do-mato.
USES: Root used against diseases of the urinary tract and gonorrhoea.

Borreria verticillata (L.) Meyer
AREA: Frequent throughout Brazil; ruderal.
NAMES: Cordão-de-frade, erva-botão, poaia, poaia-comprida, poaia-rosário.
USES: Roots are vomitive; in an infusion against diarrhoea in children.
CHEM.: Alkaloids (Ref: RUBI 1,2) and iridoids (Ref: RUBI 3) have been isolated. The presence of emetine in the roots was claimed in early work, but was later disproved (Ref: RUBI 1). A revision has been published (Ref: RUBI 4).
PHARM.: The alkaloids have antimicrobial properties (Ref: RUBI 5,6).

Cephaelis ipecacuanha Rich.
AREA: Pará, Bahia, Minas Gerais and Mato Grosso, in the undergrowth of rain forest.
NAMES: Ipeca, ipecacuanha, poaia. (English: ipecac.)
USES: Roots are emetic, expectorant, antidysenteric and diaphoretic.
CHEM. & PHARM.: The roots contain emetine and cephaeline as the main

alkaloids, besides other minor bases. These are used in medicine as expectorants and for treating amebiasis (Ref: RUBI 7,8).

Chiococca alba (L.) Hitch.

AREA: Almost throughout Brazil.

NAMES: Cainca, cainana, casinga, cipó-cruz, cruzeirinha, dambê, poaia, purga-preta, quina-de-raiz-preta, raiz-de-frade, raiz-de-quina, raiz-de-serpentária.

USES: Root-bark is toxic; used nonetheless as a diuretic, purgative, hydragogue, emmenagogue, febrifuge, antiasthmatic and antihydropic. Also prescribed for snakebite, dartre and ailments of the lymphatic system.

CHEM.: Qualitative tests indicated the presence of cardiotonic glycosides, saponins, tannins and flavonoids (Ref: RUBI 9). Alkaloids (Ref: RUBI 10) and a triterpene (Ref: RUBI 11) were isolated.

PHARM.: Anti-inflammatory activity of the extract was verified (Ref: RUBI 9).

Coutarea hexandra (Jacq.) K. Sch.

AREA: Throughout Brazil, in forests.

NAMES: Amora-do-mato, murta-do-mato, quina-brava, quina-de-pernambuco, quina-do-pará, quina-do-piauí.

USES: Bark is bitter, tonic, for treating malaria as a substitute for *Cinchona* bark.

CHEM.: The plant is rich in 4-arylcoumarins (neoflavonoids) and their glycosides (Ref: RUBI 12,13,14,15,16).

PHARM.: One of the constituents has been shown to exert a relaxing effect on the trachea (Ref: RUBI 17). The extract has anti-inflammatory properties (Ref: RUBI 18).

Declieuxia aristolochia M. Arg.

AREA: Minas Gerais and São Paulo, campo.

NAMES: Erva-de-parida, ervinha-de-parida.

USES: Herb is applied in cases of delayed menstrual flow.

Declieuxia cordigera Mart. & Zucc.

AREA: Minas Gerais and São Paulo, campo.

NAMES: Cruzeiro, flor-de-santa-cruz, sete-sangrias.

USES: Roots and leaves used in infusion for malaria.

Diodia polymorpha Cham. & Schl.

AREA: Bahia to Santa Catarina, along the littoral.

NAMES: Poaia-do-campo, vassourinha, vassoura.

USES: Used as a substitute for *Cephaelis ipecacuanha*.

RUBIACEAE

Exostemma australe St.-Hil.
AREA: Eastern and southern Brazil, forest.
NAMES: Cauaçu, quina-de-santa-catarina, quina-do-mato, quina-do-paraná.
USES: Bark is bitter, tonic and antipyretic.

Genipa americana L.
AREA: Neotropical; Amazonia to São Paulo and Mato Grosso, forest.
NAMES: Jenipá, jenipapeirol, jenipapo (old spelling: genipapo).
USES: Roots are purgative and antigonorrhoeic. Bark is cathartic and antidiarrhoeic, used in dressings to cure sores of different origins; also for pharyngitis. Leaf decoction is antidiarrhoeic and antisyphilitic. Pulp of the unripe fruit is used for syphilitic manifestations and to treat navel rupture in newborns. Ripe berries are aromatic and stomachic, used in alcoholic beverages. Berries are diuretic and recommended against anemia, jaundice, dropsy, spleen and liver disorders and asthma. The clear juice of the unripe fruits darkens when exposed to the air, turning first blue, then black, and has been used extensively by the Indians to paint their bodies in war or for ceremonial purposes.
CHEM.: An iridoid, genipin, has been isolated from the Brazilian plant (Ref: RUBI 19,20) (not Mexican, as stated in Ref: RUBI 21). Two compounds of the same class, genipic and genipinic acids (but not genipin) were found in a specimen from Puerto Rico (Ref: RUBI 21). These substances inhibited the growth of a variety of bacteria, one fungus, one alga and one protozoan (Ref: RUBI 21). The same species from Panama yielded geniposidic acid, a glucoside of genipin (Ref: RUBI 22).

Guettarda angelica Mart.
AREA: Piauí to São Paulo, forest.
NAMES: Angélica, angélica-brava, angélica-do-mato, angélica-mansa.
USES: Wood, bark and root-bark are aromatic, tonic, stomachic and febrifuge. Recommended for puerperal fever and delayed menses; said to be abortive.
CHEM.: Triterpenoids have been isolated (Ref: RUBI 23).

Guettarda argentea Lam.
AREA: Amazonia.
NAME: Angélica.
USES: Bark is astringent and tonic.

Guettarda uruguayensis Cham. & Schl.
AREA: Bahia to Rio Grande do Sul.
NAME: Veludinha.
USES: Bark is astringent and tonic.

Ladenbergia hexandra Klotz.
AREA: Minas Gerais, Rio de Janeiro and São Paulo, forest.
NAMES: Quina-de-folha-larga, quina-do-rio-de-janeiro, quina-quina.
USES: Bark is bitter, used as a tonic.

Ladenbergia lambertiana Klotz.
AREA: Amazonia.
NAME: Quina-do-rio-negro.
USES: Bark is bitter, used as a tonic.

Lipostoma campanuliflorum D. Don
AREA: The southern seacoast.
NAME: Poaia-da-areia.
USES: As a substitute for ipecacuanha (*Cephaelis ipecacuanha*). Similar to this is *L. capitata* D. Don (Bahia to São Paulo).

Machaonia brasiliensis Cham. & Schl.
AREA: Parà to Goiàs and Mato Grosso.
NAMES: Coral, poaia-da-praia, poaia-de-cipó, poaia-do-mato, poaia-do-rio.
USES: The same as those given for *Cephaelis ipecacuanha*.

Manettia ignita (Vell.) K. Sch.
AREA: Ceará to Rio Grande do Sul.
NAMES: Coral, poaia-da-praia, poaia-de-cipó, poaia-de-minas, poaia-do-mato, poaia-do-rio, poejo-do-mato.
USES: Root-bark is emetic, antidysenteric; a substitute for ipecacuanha (*Cephaelis ipecacuanha*).

Oldenlandia corymbosa L.
AREA: Amazonia.
NAME: Caá-chira.
USES: Herb is vermicidal, especially the flowering summits; stomachic, antipyretic, for jaundice. Leaves are expectorant.

Rubiaceae – References

RUBI 1. Pousset, J.-L., J. Kerharo, G. Maynart, X. Monseur, A. Cavé & R. Goutarel. 1973. La borrerine: nouvel alcaloïde isolé du *Borreria verticillata*. *Phytochemistry* 12: 2308-2310.

RUBI 2. Pousset, J.-L., A. Cavé, A. Chiaroni & C. Riche. 1977. A novel bis-indole alkaloid. X-Ray crystal structure determination of borreverine and its rearrangement product on deacetylation. *J. Chem. Soc. Chem. Comm.*: 261-262.

RUBI 3. Sainty, D., F. Bailleul, P. Delaveau & H. Jacquemin. 1981. Iridoïdes de *Borreria verticillata*. *Planta Medica* 42: 260-264.

RUBI 4. Saxton, J.E. 1983. Alkaloids of *Aristotelia* species. *Chem. Heterocyclic Comp.* 25: 47-62.

RUBI 5. Maynart, G., J.-L. Pousset, S. Mboup & F. Denis. 1980. Action antibactérienne de la borreverine, alcaloïde isolé de *Borreria verticillata* (Rubiacées). *Compt. Rend. Soc. Biol.* 174: 925-928.

RUBI 6. Baldé, A.M., A. Gergely, L.A. Pieters, M. Claeys, D.A. Vanden Berghe & A. J. Vlietinck. 1989. Antimicrobial alkaloids from *Borreria verticillata*. *Planta Medica* 55: 652.

RUBI 7. Pailer, M. 1951. Brechwurz-Alkaloide. In: L. Zechmeister (ed.), *Progr. Chem. Org. Nat. Prod.* 8: 278-309.

RUBI 8. Wiegrebe, W., W.J. Kramer & M. Shamma. 1984. The emetine alkaloids. *J. Nat. Prod.* 47: 397-408.

RUBI 9. Schapoval, E.E.S., E.P. Schenkel, C.M.G. Chaves, I.L. Schenkel, A. Zanata, L.A. Mentz & B.E. Irgang. 1983. Ensaios químicos e farmacológicos com a *Chiococca alba* (L.) Hitch. Nota prévia. *Anais 2º Simpronat (João Pessoa)*: 289-294.

RUBI 10. El Abbadi, N., B. Weniger, A. Lobstein, J.C. Quirion & R. Anton. 1989. New alkaloids of *Chiococca alba*. *Planta Medica* 55: 603-604.

RUBI 11. Bhattacharyya, J. & E.V.L. Cunha. 1992. A triterpenoid from the root-bark of *Chiococca alba*. *Phytochemistry* 31: 2546-2547.

RUBI 12. Reher, G. & L. Kraus. 1982. Charakterisierung eines neuen 4-Arylcoumarinderivates aus Copalchirinde. *Planta Medica* 45: 145-146.

RUBI 13. Delle Monache, G., B. Botta, A. Serafim-Neto & R. Alves de Lima. 1983. 4-Arylcoumarins from *Coutarea hexandra*. *Phytochemistry* 22: 1657-1658.

RUBI 14. Iinuma, M., T. Tanaka, K. Hamada, M. Mizuno, F. Azai, G. Reher & L. Kraus. 1987. Revised structure of neoflavone in *Coutarea hexandra*. *Phytochemistry* 26: 3096-3097.

RUBI 15. D'Agostino, M., V. De Feo, F. De Simone & C. Pizza. 1989. A 4-arylcoumarin from *Coutarea hexandra*. *Phytochemistry* 28: 1773.

RUBI 16. Delle Monache, G., B. Botta, V. Vinceguerra & E. Gács-Baitz. 1989. A new neoflavonoid from *Coutarea hexandra*. *Heterocycles* 29: 355-357.

RUBI 17. Araujo, C.C., G. Thomas & M.Q. Paulo. 1988. Effects of 5,7,2',5'-tetraacetoxy-4-phenylcoumarin in guinea pig tracheal preparations. *Planta Medica* 54: 494-497.

RUBI 18. Almeida, E.R., C.F. de Santana & J.F. de Mello. 1991. Anti-inflammatory activity of *Coutarea hexandra*. *Fitoterapia* 62: 447-448.

RUBI 19. Djerassi, C., J.D. Gray & F.A. Kingl. 1960. Naturally occurring oxygen heterocycles. IX. Isolation and characterization of genipin. *J. Org. Chem.* 25: 2174-2177.

RUBI 20. Djerassi, C., T. Nakano, A.N. James, L.H. Zalkov, E.J. Eisenbraun & J.N. Schoolery. 1961. The structure of genipin. *J. Org. Chem.* 26: 1192-1206.

RUBI 21. Tallent, W.H. 1964. Two new antibiotic cyclopentanoid monoterpenes of plant origin. *Tetrahedron* 20: 1781-1787.

RUBI 22. Guarnaccia, R., K.M. Madyastha, E. Tegtmeyer & C.J. Coscia. 1972. Geniposidic acid, an iridoid glucoside from *Genipa americana*. *Tetrahedron Lett.* 50: 5125-5127.

RUBI 23. Souza, M.P., M.E.O. Matos, M.I.L. Machado, R. Braz Filho, I. Vencato & Y.P. Mascarenhas. 1984. Triterpenoids from *Guettarda angelica*. *Phytochemistry* 23: 2589-2592.

RUTACEAE

Cusparia febrifuga Humb.

AREA: Northeast and Minas Gerais, forest.

NAMES: Amarelinho-da-serra, amarelo, angustura.

USES: Bark is bitter, tonic, digestive, stimulant and antidysenteric. Leaves are febrifuge. Commercially, the bark used to be an ingredient of the bitter "angostura" liqueurs, but has been replaced with other bitter ingredients (Ref: RUTA 18).

CHEM.: Cusparin (Ref: RUTA 1) and galipin (Ref: RUTA 2) are the major bitter alkaloids of the bark.

RUTACEAE

Cusparia toxicaria Spr. ex Engl.
AREA: Amazonia to Bahia, forest.
NAMES: Angustura-venenosa.
USES: Bark is febrifuge and emmenagogue, but toxic.

Esenbeckia febrifuga Juss.
AREA: Minas Gerais to São Paulo, restinga and forest.
NAMES: Angustura, grumarim, laranja-brava, laranjeira-do-mato, laranjeiro-da-terra, mendanha, quina-laranjeira, quina-do-mato, três-folhas, três-folhas-vermelha.
USES: Bark and leaves are bitter, aromatic, tonic, febrifuge; leaves used in decoction prescribed for healing bubo, constipation, dyspepsia and malaria.
PHARM.: Crude extracts tested in mice showed partly antimalarial activity (Ref: RUTA 3).

Esenbeckia intermedia Mart.
AREA: Rio de Janeiro, São Paulo and Mato Grosso, forest.
NAMES: Angustura, apogitaguará, pitaguará.
USES: Bark is bitter, tonic, febrifuge; recommended as a substitute for quina bark (*Cinchona*).

Galipea dichotoma Sald.
AREA: Rio de Janeiro, forest.
NAME: Arapoca-amarela.
USES: Bark is anthelmintic.

Galipea multiflora Schult.
AREA: Goiás to Santa Catarina, forest.
NAMES: Angustura, chupa-ferro, guaruga, guaximinga.
USES: Bark is astringent, bitter, tonic; both bark and fresh leaf decoction are employed against bubo.

Hortia brasiliensis Vand.
AREA: Bahia to Goiás, cerrado.
NAME: Quina-do-campo.
USES: Bark is bitter, tonic, stomachic and antifebrile.

Metrodorea pubescens St.-Hil. & Tul.
AREA: Minas Gerais, Rio de Janeiro and São Paulo, forest and secondary growth.
NAMES: Caputuna, caputuva, cataguá, laranjeira-do-mato, limoeiro-do-mato.
USES: Bark used for a tonic and antipyretic.

RUTACEAE

Monnieria trifolia Loefl.
AREA: Amazonia to southern Brazil, frequently as a weed.
NAMES: Alfavaca-brava, alfavaca-de-cobra, jaborandi-de-três-folhas, jaborandi-do-pará, maricotinha, pimenta-de-cobra, pimenta-de-lagarta.
USES: Plant is tonic, bitter; leaves are emmenagogue, diuretic, resolvent, pectoral and good for reducing hernia; juice is applied for otalgia and colics. Roots are aromatic, febrifuge, diaphoretic, expectorant and used for ophthalmia. Seeds used for diseases of the eyes and against snakebite. Shoots in baths used in cases of flu, colds and headache.
CHEM.: Alkaloids of the furoquinoline type (Ref: RUTA 4,5,6) and C-glycosylflavones (Ref: RUTA 7) have been isolated.

Pilocarpus pinnatifolius Lem.
AREA: Maranhão to Santa Catarina and Mato Grosso, forest.
NAMES: Jaborandi, jaborandi-do-norte, cataí-guaçu, ibirataí, pimenta-de-cachorro.
USES: Leaves are diaphoretic, diuretic, sialagogue, strongly miotic.
CHEM. & PHARM.: The leaves of this and several other *Pilocarpus* species are the sources of commercial pilocarpine, an alkaloid used in ophthalmology in the treatment of glaucoma. A review on historical and pharmacological aspects has been published (Ref: RUTA 8).

Raputia alba (Nees & Mart.) Engl.
AREA: Rio de Janeiro and Minas Gerais, forest.
NAME: Arapoca-branca.
USES: Bark is bitter, excitant and antithermic.

Raputia aromatica Aubl.
AREA: Amazonia, forest.
NAME: Arapoca-de-cheiro.
USES: Bark is excitant, stomachic and febrifuge.

Raputia magnifica Engl.
AREA: Ceará, to Rio de Janeiro.
NAMES: Arapoca, amarelinho, gema-de-ovo, cocão.
USES: Bark is bitter, stomachic and febrifuge.

Zanthoxylum hyemale St.-Hil.
AREA: Southern states of Brazil, forest.
NAMES: Coentrilho, tembetari, tembetaru.
USES: Bark is bitter, tonic, stimulant. Decoction of bark and roots, as well as juice from the leaves, is recommended for inflammation of the eyes and ears.

Zanthoxylum pterota H.B.K.
AREA: Amazonia, forest.
NAME: Espinheiro.
USES: Bark is sudorific, circulatory and a nerve stimulant; used in poultice against skin problems and afflictions of the scalp. Leaf juice used in rubs to relieve pains and against earache when mixed with castor oil. Powdered bark is used as a condiment.

Zanthoxylum rhoifolium Lam.
AREA: Frequent throughout Brazil, forest, cerrado and restinga.
NAMES: Guaritá, juva, maminha-de-porca, mamica-de-cadela, laranjinha, limãozinho, espinho-de-vintém, juvevê, tamanqueira, tamanqueira-da-terra-firme, tinguaciba, tinguciba, tembetaru.
USES: Roots are bitter, indicated for toothache; bast is bitter, antifebrile, stomachic, antidyspeptic, antispasmodic and antiblennorrhagic.

Zanthoxylum tingoassuiba St.-Hil.
AREA: In the coastal sands, restinga.
NAMES: Laranjinha-do-mato, tembetaru, tinguaciba.
USES: Bark is a stimulant for digestion, antithermic and prescribed against colics.
CHEM.: Several alkaloids of benzophenanthridine skeleton have been isolated from the bark (Ref: RUTA 9,10,11).
PHARM.: One of the alkaloids showed strong hypotensive properties in dogs and antifibrillatory effect in rats (Ref: RUTA 12). Nitidine proved to have white blood cell lowering and antileukemic properties (Ref: RUTA 13,14). The same substance was shown to inhibit reverse transcriptase (Ref: RUTA 15) and to have antiviral activity (Ref: RUTA 16). It has recently been shown to be a potent inhibitor of Human Immunodeficiency Virus type 1 (HIV-1) reverse transcriptase (Ref: RUTA 17).

Rutaceae – References
RUTA 1. Späth, E. & O. Brunner. 1924. Über die Angostura Alkaloide. I. Synthese des Cusparins. *Ber. Deut. Chem. Ges. 57*: 1243-1251.

RUTA 2. Späth, E. & H. Eberstaller. 1924. Über die Angostura Alkaloide. II. Synthese des Galipins. *Ber. Deut. Chem. Ges. 57*: 1687-1690.

RUTA 3. Carvalho, L.H., M.G.L. Brandão, D. Santos-Filho, J.C.C. Lopes & A.U. Krettli. 1991. Antimalarial activity of crude extracts from Brazilian plant studies "in vivo" in *Plasmodium berghei*-infected mice and "in vitro" against *Plasmodium falciparum* in culture. *Braz. J. Med. Biol. Res. 24*: 1113-1123.

RUTA 4. Fouraste, I., J. Gleye & E. Stanislas. 1973. Alcaloïdes des feuilles de *Monnieria trifolia*. *Plantes Méd. Phytothér. 7*: 216-224.

RUTA 5. Moulis, C., J. Gleye, I. Fouraste & E. Stanislas. 1981. Nouvelles furoquinoléines de *Monnieria trifolia*. *Planta Medica 42*: 400-402.

RUTA 6. Bhattacharyya, J., L.M. Serur & U.O. Cheriyan. 1984. Isolation of the alkaloids of *Monnieria trifolia*. *J. Nat. Prod. 47*: 379-381.

RUTA 7. Keite, A., J. Gleye, E. Stanislas & I. Fouraste. 1985. C-Glycosylflavones from *Monnieria trifolia*. *J. Nat. Prod. 48*: 675-676.

RUTA 8. Holmstedt, B., S. H. Wassén & R.E. Schultes. 1979. Jaborandi: An interdisciplinary appraisal. *J. Ethnopharmacol. 1*: 3-21.
RUTA 9. Antonaccio, L.D. 1958. Os alcalóides da *Fagara tingoassuiba. An. Acad. Brasil. Ciênc. 30*: 159-163.
RUTA 10. Riggs, N.V., L. Antonaccio & L. Marion. 1961. A new quaternary aporphine from *Fagara tingoassuiba* Hoehne. *Canad. J. Chem. 39*: 1330-1335.
RUTA 11. Menezes, M.M.M. & N.A. Pereira. 1987. Obtençãode de alcalóides farmacologicamente ativos da tinguaciba (*Fagara tingoasssuiba*) I. Fagara base. *Rev. Bras. Farm. 68*: 71-77.
RUTA 12. Pereira, N.A., H. Moussatché & L.D. Antonaccio. 1961. Sobre algumas propriedades farmacodinâmicas de um alcalóide (tingoassuibina) da *Fagara tingoassuiba. Ciência e Cultura* (São Paulo) *13*: 186-187.
RUTA 13. Paulo, L.G. & N.A. Pereira. 1978. Propriedades leucopenizantes da nitidina obtida da *Fagara tingoassuiba* (Rutácea). *Ciência e Cultura* (São Paulo) *32* (Supl.): 171.
RUTA 14. Wall, M.E., M.C. Wani & H.L. Taylor. 1971. Plant anti-tumor agents. VIII. Isolation and structure of anti-tumor alkaloids from *Fagara macrophylla. Proc. 162nd Natl. Meeting American Chemical Society*: Abstract MEDI 34.
RUTA 15. Kakiuchi, N., M. Hattori, H. Ishii & T. Namba. 1987. Effect of benzo [c] phenanthridine alkaloids on reverse transcriptase and their binding property to nucleic acids. *Planta Medica 48*: 22-27.
RUTA 16. Lagrota, M.H.C., M.D. Wigg, L.O.B. Pereira, N.A. Pereira & J. Ciribelli-Guimarães. 1982. Atividade antiviral de substâncias naturais. I. Nitidina e ajmalina. *Rev. Bras. Farm. 63*: 88-94.
RUTA 17. Tan, G.T., J.M. Pezzuto, A.D. Kinghorn & S.H. Hughes. 1991. Evaluation of natural products as inhibitors of human immunodeficiency virus type 1 (HIV-1) reverse transcriptase. *J. Nat. Prod. 54*: 143-154.
RUTA 18. POTTER'S NEW CYCLOPAEDIA. 1988: pp. 12-13 and J.B. Harbone, H. Baxter & G.P. Moss. DICTIONARY OF PLANT TOXINS, 1997: p. 105. John Wiley.

SALVINIACEAE

Azolla caroliniana Willd.
AREA: Amazonia, aquatic, in rivers.
NAMES: Aguapé, mururé-rendado.
USES: The musk-scented dried leaves are said to be aphrodisiac.

SANTALACEAE

Acanthosyris spinescens (Mart. & Endl.) Gris.
AREA: Southern Brazil.
NAME: Sombra-de-touro.
USES: Decoction of leaves is used to combat high fevers and applied externally to dress ulcers.

Jodina rhombifolia Hook. & Arn.
AREA: Rio Grande do Sul.
NAMES: Cancerosa, cancorosa-de-três-pontas, erva-cancerosa, erva-cancorosa, sombra-de-touro.
USES: Roasted and powdered leaves are applied over infected wounds,

chronic ulcers and certain cancerous growths. Internally taken for gastric troubles and against common cold. Decoction of bark is astringent, used against dysentery.

CHEM.: The seed oil glycerides contain acetylenic fatty acids (Ref: SANT 1).

Santalaceae – Reference

SANT 1. Hopkins, C.Y., M.J. Chisholm & W.J. Cody. 1969. Fatty acid components of some Santalaceae seed oils– References. *Phytochemistry* 8: 161-165.

SAPINDACEAE

Cardiospermum grandiflorum Sw.
AREA: Throughout Brazil.
NAMES: Balãozinho, ensacadinha.
USES: Roots and leaves are prescribed to cure hoarse coughs and whooping cough.
CHEM.: A sulfur-containing cyanogenic glucoside has been described (Ref: SAPI 1).

Cupania racemosa Radlk.
AREA: Bahia to São Paulo, forest.
NAME: Camboatá.
USES: Decoction of the roots and leaves used for whooping cough.

Dodonaea viscosa Jacq.
AREA: Tropical cosmopolitan; throughout Brazil, but mostly in the coastal region.
NAMES: Erva-de-veado, faxina-vermelha, vassoura-do-campo, vassoura-vermelha.
USES: Wood decoction used for lowering fever. Bark is astringent. Leaves and their resinous exudate are aromatic, a bitter astringent, sudorific, purgative and febrifuge; used in cataplasms in the treatment of flatulence, rheumatism, gout and venereal diseases. Sap applied for clearing tumors.
CHEM.: Flavonoids and other polyphenols have been found in the leaves and their viscous exudate (Ref: SAPI 2,3,4). Also diterpenoids (Ref: SAPI 5,6,7). Tannoids from bark (Ref: SAPI 8). Saponin esters with antiexudative, phagocytosis-enhancing and molluscicidal properties have been isolated from the seeds (Ref: SAPI 9).

Magonia pubescens St.-Hil.
AREA: Ceará to Mato Grosso, cerrado.
NAMES: Assapeixe, tinguí, tinguí-açu, tinguí-de-cola, tinguí-do-cerrado, timbó-açu, timbopeba.
USES: Bark decoction is used for cleaning chronic ulcers. In veterinary medicine, a bark infusion is used to heal ulcers in horses.

SAPINDACEAE

Matayba purgans Radlk.
AREA: Amazonia, forest.
NAME: Ituá.
USE: Ground seeds are taken as a purgative.

Paullinia cupana Kunth
AREA: Amazonia, forest, both native and cultivated by Indians. Also cultivated on a large, commercial scale in the states of Amazonas, Pará and Bahia.
NAME: Guaraná.
USES: Seeds are a general stimulant, considered a panacea against a number of ailments, such as neuralgia, migraine, fever and nervousness. Also taken as a tonic, diuretic, slight aphrodisiac, cardioactive, intestinal antiseptic and excitant. Traditionally, the ground seeds are pounded and worked into a dough, sometimes together with manioc flour. The resulting mass is molded into loaves or sticks which, on drying, become very hard. The powder obtained from these by grating is suspended in water, yielding a bitter beverage which, swallowed in the morning, acts as a general stimulant for many hours. On long journeys it helps to suppress the sensation of hunger. For a detailed account on guaraná, its production and uses, see Ref: SAPI 10.
CHEM.: Seeds are rich in catechin tannins (Ref: SAPI 11) and caffeine (up to 5%) (Ref: SAPI 12). Traces of theobromine (Ref: SAPI 13) and theophyllin (Ref: SAPI 14) are also present, as well as allantoin (Ref: SAPI 15). The caffeine is partially bonded to the catechins. The seed husks are also a rich source of caffeine (Ref: SAPI 16).
PHARM.: Guaraná extracts have been found to inhibit platelet aggregation (Ref: SAPI 17).
  The popular Brazilian soft drinks called "guaraná" contain only minimal amounts of seed extract.

Sapindus saponaria L.
AREA: Eastern part of Brazil, forest.
NAMES: Guitó, pau-de-sebo, sabão-de-soldado, sabonete, saboneteira, saboeiro.
USES: Roots and bark are astringent, tonic. Fruits are rich in saponin; used for curing anemia.

Talisia esculenta Radlk.
AREA: Amazonia, forest.
NAMES: Pitomba-grande-da-mata.
USES: Decoction of roots used against bites of poisonous animals, both internally and locally applied. When mixed with urucum (aril of *Bixa orellana*) and açaí (fruit peel of *Euterpe oleracea*), it is reportedly a remedy for jaundice.

SAPINDACEAE

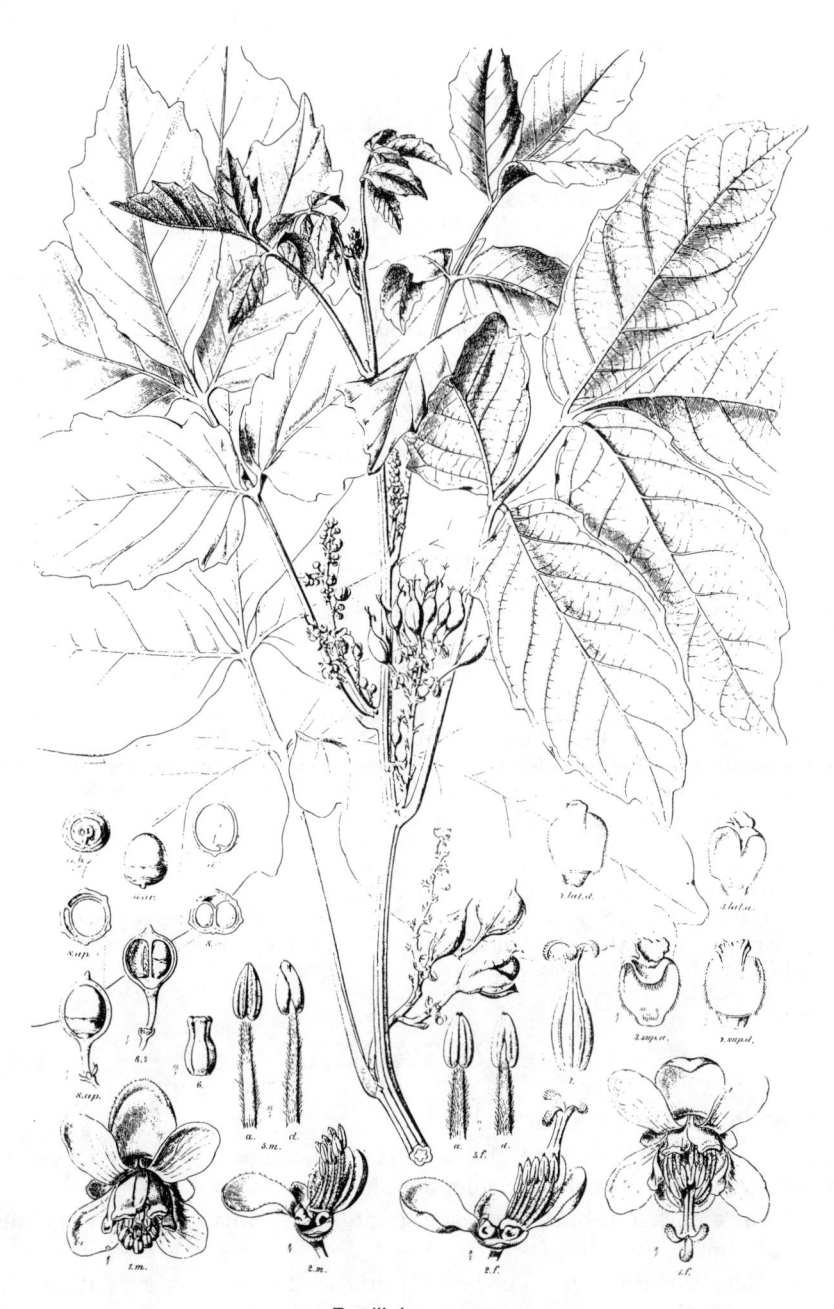

Paullinia cupana

Sapindaceae – References

SAPI 1. Hübel, W. & A. Nahrstedt. 1979. Cardiosperminsulfat, ein schwefelhaltiges cyanogenes Glukosid aus *Cardiospermum grandiflorum*. *Tetrahedron Lett.*: 4395-4397.
SAPI 2. Rao, K.V. 1962. Chemical examination of the leaves of *Dodonaea viscosa*. *J. Indian Chem. Soc. 39*: 561-562.
SAPI 3. Paris, R.R. & A. Nothis. 1970. Plantes de Nouvelle Calédonie. II: Plantes contenand des derivés polyphénoliques. *Plantes Méd. Phytothér. 4*: 63-74.
SAPI 4. Sachdev, K. & D.K. Kulshreshtha. 1983. Flavonoids from *Dodonaea viscosa*. *Phytochemistry 22*: 1253-1256.
SAPI 5. Jefferies, P.R. & T.G. Payne. 1967. Diterpenes of the cascarillin group from *Dodonaea* spp. *Tetrahedron Lett.*: 4777-4782.
SAPI 6. Hsü, H.-Y., Y.P. Chen & H. Kakisawa. 1971. Structure of hautriwaic acid. *Phytochemistry 10*: 2813-2814.
SAPI 7. Sachdev, K. & D.K. Kulshreshtha. 1984. Dodonic acid, a new diterpenoid from *Dodonaea viscosa*. *Planta Medica 50*: 448-449.
SAPI 8. Sastry, K.N.S. & Y. Nayudamma. 1966. Leucocyanidin from *Dodonaea viscosa* bark. *Leather Sci.* (India) *13*: 147.
SAPI 9. Wagner, H., C. Ludwig, L. Grotjahn & M.S.Y. Kahn. 1987. Biologically active saponins from *Dodonaea viscosa*. *Phytochemistry 26*: 697-701.
SAPI 10. Henman, A.R. 1982. Guaraná (*Paullinia cupana* var. *sorbilis*): Ecological and social perspectives on an economic plant of the central Amazon basin. *J. Ethnopharmacol. 6*: 311-338.
SAPI 11. Freudenberg, K., O. Böhme & L. Purrmann. 1922. Raumisomere Catechine. *Ber. Deut. Chem. Ges. 55*: 1734-1747.
SAPI 12. Bertrand, G. & P. de Berredo Carneiro. 1931. Contribution à l'étude chimique de la pâte de guarana. *Bull. Soc. Chim.* (France) *49*: 1093-1096.
SAPI 13. Bertrand, G. & P. de Berredo Carneiro. 1932. Sur l'existence et sur la répartition de la caféine et de la théobromine dans les organes due guarana (*Paullinia cupana* H.B.K.). *Bull. Soc. Chim.* (France) *51*: 284-288.
SAPI 14. Maravalhas, N. 1965. Teofilina e teobromina, metilpurinas constantes nas plantas produtoras de cafeína. In: *Estudos sobre o guaraná e outras plantas produtoras de cafeína*. Instituto Nacional de Pesquisas da Amazônia (Manaus) *10*: 17-25.
SAPI 15. Alves, M.H.L., W.B. Mors & S.S. Costa. 1986. Alantoína, um componente do extrato etanólico das sementes de *Paullinia cupana* H.B.K. (Guaraná). *9th Symposium on Medicinal Plants of Brazil*, Rio de Janeiro, Summary of papers, p. 96.
SAPI 16. Maravalhas, N. 1965. Casca de guaraná — matéria-prima para cafeína — método industrial de extração. In: *Estudos sobre o guaraná e outras plantas produtoras de cafeína*. Instituto Nacional de Pequisas da Amazônia (Manaus) *10*: 5-11.
SAPI 17. Bydlowski, S.P., R.L. Yunker & M.T.R. Subbian. 1988. A novel property of an aqueous guaraná extract (*Paullinia cupana*): inhibition of platelet aggregation *in vitro* and *in vivo*. *Brazilian J. Med. Biol. Res. 21*: 535-538.

SAPOTACEAE

Bumelia sartorum Mart.

AREA: Piauí to northeastern Minas Gerais, caatinga.
NAMES: Quixaba, quixabeira, rompe-gibão.
USES: Bark and root-bark are astringent, tonic, anti-inflammatory and antidiabetic.
CHEM.: Bassic acid has been isolated from the ethanolic extract; it may be the anti-inflammatory component (Ref: SAPO 1).

PHARM.: The ethanolic extract of the root-bark elicited a hypoglycemic effect in normal and alloxan-induced diabetic rats. In addition, the extract altered glucose tolerance, enhanced glucose uptake in skeletal muscle and significantly inhibited glycogenolysis in the liver in the same laboratory animals with alloxan-induced diabetes (Ref: SAPO 1). At the University Hospital of the Federal University of Paraíba, an antidiabetic remedy has been produced in tablet form and administered on an experimental scale.

Dipholis nigra Gr.
AREA: Southern Brazil.
NAME: Miri.
USES: Bark is bitter, febrifuge.

Lucuma caimito Roem. & Schult.
AREA: Neotropical; much cultivated for its edible fruit.
NAME: Abiu.
USES: Bark is antidysenteric and febrifuge. Latex used to remove albugo.

Lucuma rivicoa Gaertn.
AREA: Amazonia to Ceará and Mato Grosso; neotropical.
NAMES: Cutiti, cutitiribá, oiti-tereba, tutiriba, mititoroba.
USES: Bark is antidysenteric. Flesh of the berries is antidiarrhoeic and used to combat pulmonary catarrh. Seeds are emmenagogue and antidysenteric, highly praised for curing otitis. The same property is ascribed to the bark.

Manilkara bidentata (A. DC.) Chev.
AREA: Amazonia, forest.
NAMES: Balata, balata-verdadeira.
USE: Leaves used for treating paralysis of limbs.

Manilkara zapota (L.) Van Royen
AREA: Cultivated in many parts of Brazil as a fruit tree.
NAMES: Sapoti, sapotizeiro.
USES: Pulverized roots indicated for thrush in babies. Bark is febrifuge and antidiarrhoeic. Crushed seeds in water are employed to expel urinary and gall bladder calculi.

Pouteria laurifolia Radlk.
AREA: Rio de Janeiro, Minas Gerais and São Paulo, forest.
NAMES: Guapeba, guapebeira, tapinhoã-amarelo.
USE: Bark is prescribed for dysentery.

Pouteria obtusifolia Baehni
AREA: Maranhão, forest.
USE: Bark is considered aphrodisiac.

Pouteria salicifolia Hook. & Arn.
AREA: Southern states of Brazil, forest.
NAMES: Mata-olho, sarandi.
USES: Bark is astringent, employed for hemorrhage and dysentery.

Pradosia lactescens (Vell.) Radlk.
AREA: Alagoas to São Paulo, forest.
NAMES: Buranhém, pau-de-remo, pau-doce.
USES: Bark extract is astringent; used as hemostatic and against leucorrhoea, diarrhoea, gonorrhoea, metrorrhagia and hemoptyses, also for asthma, scrofula and dyspepsy.

Sapotaceae – Reference

SAPO 1. Almeida, R.N., J.M. Barbosa Filho & S.R. Naik. 1985. Chemistry and pharmacology of an ethanol extract of *Bumelia sartorum*. *J. Ethnopharmacol.* 14: 173-185.

SCHIZAEACEAE

Anemia phyllitidis (L.) Sw.
AREA: Almost throughout Brazil, forest.
NAME: Avenca-de-espiga.
USE: Expectorant.

SCROPHULARIACEAE

Angelonia integerrima Spreng.
AREA: Rio de Janeiro to Rio Grande do Sul, campo.
NAMES: Angelônia, violeta-de-petrópolis, violeta-do-campo.
USES: Herb is aromatic, stomachic, antispasmodic.

Buchnera aquatica Aubl.
AREA: Throughout Brazil, in marshy places.
NAME: Bacopá.
USES: Herb is rubefacient; indicated for burns, rheumatism, injuries and anthlete's foot. Also in gargles in cases of angina and stomatitis.

Buchnera virgata H.B.K.
AREA: Pernambuco to Rio Grande do Sul, campo,
NAMES: Canguçu, canguçu-preto.

SCROPHULARIACEAE

USES: Infusion from the roots is said to induce a prolonged lethargic sleep.

Capraria biflora

Capraria biflora L.

AREA: Pará to Espirito Santo and Minas Gerais.

NAMES: Balsaminha, chá-da-américa, chá-cravo, chá-da-terra, chá-de-boi, chá-de-marajó, chá-preto.

USES: The whole plant, prepared as a tea, is prescribed against stomach pains and bad digestion; also as a nervous stimulant, febrifuge, diuretic, excitant and digestive.

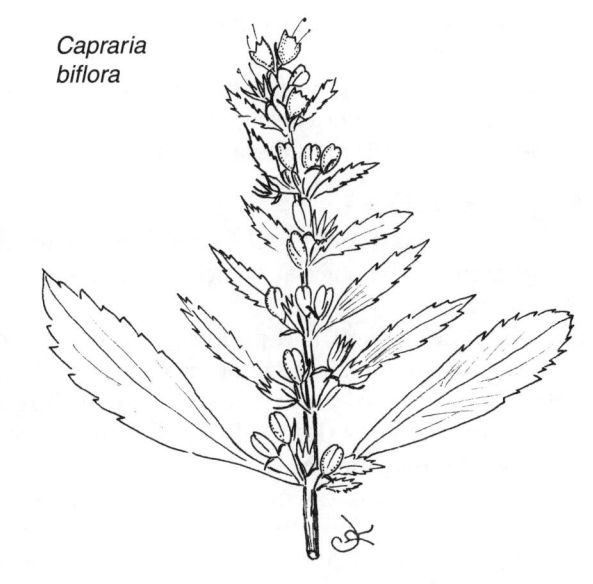

CHEM.: A diterpenoid compound named biflorin, with antimicrobial properties, has been isolated and had its structure determined (Ref: SCRO 1,2,3). Two iridoid glucosides were isolated from the same species collected in Mexico (Ref: SCRO 4).

Conobea aquatica Aubl.

AREA: Throughout Brazil, in moist and swampy sites.
NAME: Pataquera.
USES: Aromatic and excitant.

Conobea scoparioides Benth.

AREA: Amazonia, in puddles and swamps.
NAMES: Pataquera, pataquira, vassourinha-do-campo.
USES: The entire herb is used to alleviate cough.
CHEM.: The essential oil distilled from the leaves contains up to 65% thymol (Ref: SCRO 5).

Lindernia crustacea F. Muell.

AREA: Amazonia, Bahia and Mato Grosso, in still waters.
NAMES: Douradinha-do-campo, douradinha-do-pará, matacana, matucan, orelha-de-onça.
USES: Herb is emetocathartic, diuretic, emmenagogue.

Lindernia diffusa Wettst.

AREA: Amazonia to Mato Grosso and São Paulo, in humid terrain.

SCROPHULARIACEAE

NAMES: Aruaaca, caá-ataia, douradinha, orelha-de-rato, papaterra, purga-de-joão-paes.
USES: Herb is bitter, febrifuge, diuretic, strongly purgative, emetic and emmenagogue. Indicated against ancylostomiasis and against helmintic infestations with manifestation of geophagy.

Scoparia dulcis L.
AREA: In most parts of Brazil, ruderal, as a weed.
NAMES: Tapixava, tupeiçava, tupiçaba, tupixaba, vassourinha, vassourinha-de-botão.
USES: Roots emollient and pectoral, especially for bronchitis. Juice from leaves reputedly is active for erysipelas and ulcers. Leaf tea given for diseases of the urinary tract and as a febrifuge.
CHEM.: Triterpenoids (Ref: SCRO 6,7), one diterpene acid (Ref: SCRO 8) and a cytotoxic flavone (Ref: SCRO 9) have been isolated.
PHARM.: An extract of the plant, under the name of "amellin," was claimed to be a powerful antidiabetic (Ref: SCRO 10). However, this was not confirmed by clinical tests (Ref: SCRO 11). On the other hand, a cardiotonic effect has been demonstrated (Ref: SCRO 12), as well as anti-inflammatory and analgesic properties (Ref: SCRO 13), a triterpene being responsible for the latter (Ref: SCRO 14).

Tetralacrium veroniciforme Turcz.
AREA: Piauí to Bahia.
NAME: Paracari.
USES: Roots are aromatic, bitter and bechic.

Scrophulariaceae – References
SCRO 1. Gonçalves de Lima, O., I.L. d'Albuquerque & P. Loureiro. 1953. Novas observações sobre a biflorina, antibiótico isolado da *Capraria biflora* L. (Scrophulariaceae). *An. Soc. Biol. Pernambuco 11*: 3-9.
SCRO 2. Gonçalves de Lima, O., W. Keller-Schierlein & V. Prelog. 1958. Über das Biflorin. *Helv. Chim. Acta 41*: 1386-1390.
SCRO 3. Comin, J., O. Gonçalves de Lima, H.N. Grant, L.M. Jackman, W. Keller-Schierlein & V. Prelog. 1963. Über die Konstitution des Biflorins, eines o-Chinons der Diterpen-Reihe. *Helv. Chim. Acta 46*: 409-415.
SCRO 4. Heinrich, M. & H. Rimpler. 1989. Harpagide and 8-O-benzoyl-harpagide from the Mixe medicinal plant *Capraria biflora*. *Planta Medica 55*: 626.
SCRO 5. Moraes, A.A., J. Corrêa Mourão, O.R. Gottlieb, J.G.S. Maia & M.T. Magalhães. 1972. Óleos essenciais da Amazônia contendo timol. *An. Acad. Brasil. Ciênc. 44* (Supl.): 315-316.
SCRO 6. Chen, C.-M. & M.-T. Chen. 1976. 6-Methoxybenzoxazolinone and triterpenoids from roots of *Scoparia dulcis*. *Phytochemistry 15*: 1997-1999.
SCRO 7. Mahato, S.B., M.C. Das & N.P. Sahu. 1981. Triterpenoids of *Scoparia dulcis*. *Phytochemistry 20*: 171-173.
SCRO 8. Hayashi, T., M. Kishi, M. Kawasaki, M. Arisawa & N. Morita. 1988. The crystal structure of scopadulcic acid A from Paraguayan crude drug "Typychá Kuratu" (*Scoparia dulcis*). *J. Nat. Prod. 51*: 360-363.

SCRO 9. Hayashi, T., J. Ushida, K. Hayashi, S. Niwayama & M. Morita. 1988. A cytotoxic flavone from *Scoparia dulcis* L. *Chem. Pharm. Bull. 36*: 4849-4851.
SCRO 10. Nath, M.C. & S. R. Banerjee. 1943. The new antidiabetic principle (amellin) occurring in nature. II. Effect on glycosuria and hyperglycemia in cases of human diabetes. *Ann. Biochem. Exptl. Med.* (India) *3*: 55-62.
SCRO 11. Whittaker, H. 1948. Amellin for diabetes. *Brit. Med. J. 1*: 546-547.
SCRO 12. Pereira, N.A. 1949. Contribução ao estudo da tapixava (*Scoparia dulcis* L.). *Rev. Flora Med.* (Rio de Janeiro) *16*: 363-381.
SCRO 13. Freire, S.M.F. J.A.S. Emim, L.M.B. Torres, A.J. Lapa & C. Souccar. 1993. Analgesic and antiinflammatory properties of *Scoparia dulcis* L. *Phytotherapy Research 7*: 408-414.
SCRO 14. Freire, S.M.F., L.M.B. Torres, N.F. Roque, C. Souccar & A.J. Lapa. 1991. Analgesic activity of a triterpene isolated from *Scoparia dulcis* (vassourinha). *Mem. Inst. Oswaldo Cruz 86* (Suppl. II): 149-151.

SELAGINELLACEAE

Selaginella convoluta Spring
AREA: Northeastern caatinga, in lightly shaded places.
NAMES: Jericó, pé-de-papagaio, ressurreição.
USES: Claimed to be strongly diuretic and aphrodisiac.
CHEM.: Contains considerable quantities of trehalose (Ref: SELA 1).

Selaginella erythropus Spring
AREA: Amazonia to Minas Gerais, in shady places of the forest.
NAME: Palminha-das-pedras.
USE: Diuretic.

Selaginella stellata Spring
AREA: Amazonia, forest.
NAME: Samambaia.
USES: Tea is prescribed against stings of spiders and snake bites; also for colds.

Selaginellaceae – Reference
SELA 1. Matos, F.J.A., personal communication.

SIMAROUBACEAE

Marupa francoana Miers
AREA: Pará to Minas Gerais, forest.
NAMES: Marupá, pau-pombo.
USES: Tonic, bitter.

Picramnia bahiensis Turcz.
AREA: Bahia and Sergipe, forest.

SIMAROUBACEAE

NAME: Camboatã-da-baía.
USES: Tonic, bitter.

Picramnia camboita Engl.
AREA: Rio de Janeiro, forest.
NAMES: Camboatã, camboita.
USES: Wood decoction is bitter, tonic, antipyretic.

Picramnia ciliata Mart.
AREA: Rio de Janeiro and São Paulo.
NAMES: Pau-pereira-falso, tariri.
USES: Bitter, tonic, antipyretic.

Picrolemma pseudocoffea Ducke
AREA: Amazonia, forest.
NAME: Caferana.
USE: Tea from roots and leaves is used for gastralgia, malaria and as a general febrifuge.
CHEM. & PHARM.: Three "quassinoids" were isolated; one of them, sergeolide, showed strong activity against chloroquine resistant strains of *Plasmodium falciparum* (Ref: SIMA 1). Another constituent, 15-deacetylsergeolide, has strong antineoplastic properties, among others against one kind of leukemia (Ref: SIMA 2).

Quassia amara L.
AREA: Amazonia and Maranhão, forest.
NAMES: Marubá, marupá, quassia, quina.
USES: Wood is extremely bitter, used in cases of flatulence, diarrhoea, anemia, dyspepsia, fever and gall bladder ailments. Leaves are used in teas and baths for combatting malaria. The tea is also used to rinse the mouth after tooth extraction.
CHEM. & PHARM.: Water extracts of all parts of the plant are used as insecticides in gardens. Quassinoids are present, but here no antimalarial activity could be detected. Alkaloids have been described (Ref: SIMA 3).

Simaba ferruginea St.-Hil.
AREA: Pernambuco to Minas Gerais, cerrado.
NAME: Calunga.
USES: Roots and bark are bitter, tonic, used for dyspepsia, hydropsy, fevers; externally applied for reducing prolapse of the rectum and for cicatrizing wounds.

Simaba glandulifera Gardn.
AREA: Rio de Janeiro, forest.

NAMES: Calunga, paraíba-mirim.
USES: Bark is bitter and antithermic.

Simaba salubris Engl.
AREA: São Paulo.
NAMES: Calumba, calunga.
USES: Bark is bitter and antithermic.

Simarouba amara Aubl.
AREA: Amazonia, forest.
NAMES: Marupá, maruparaíba, paraíba, simaruba.
USES: Bark is extremely bitter, employed for dyspepsia, anemia and fevers. Decoction of roots and bark used for bleeding diarrhoea.
CHEM. & PHARM.: The fruits contain four active quassinoids. Extracts were found active against *Plasmodium falciparum in vitro* and against *P. berghei* in mice (Ref: SIMA 4).

Simarouba versicolor St.-Hil.
AREA: Throughout most of Brazil, cerrado and forest.
NAMES: Marupaís, mata-barata, paraíba, pé-de-perdiz, pau-paraíba.
USES: Bark is bitter, tonic, vermifuge, antianemic and antisyphilitic; poisonous in higher doses.
CHEM. & PHARM.: All parts of all of the above-mentioned species of Simaroubaceae are extremely bitter, due to the presence of chemical compounds known as quassinoids. These substances determine the uses of the plants which are all similar: as tonics and stimulants in bitter beverages and as remedies against fever. They are also strongly insecticidal and vermifuge and are used as such. The chemistry is well covered in two review articles (Ref: SIMA 5,6).

Simaroubaceae – References

SIMA 1. Fandeur T., C. Moretti & J. Polonsky. 1985. *In vitro* and *in vivo* assessment of the antimalarial activity of a new quassinoid, sergeolide. *Planta Medica* 51: 20-23.

SIMA 2. Polonsky J., J. Batnagar & C. Moretti. 1984. 15-Deacetylsergeolide, a potent antileukemic from *Picrolemma pseudocoffea*. *J. Nat. Prod.* 47: 994-996.

SIMA 3. Barbetti, P., G. Grandolini, G. Fardella & I. Chiappini. 1987. Indole alkaloids from *Quassia amara*. *Planta Medica* 53: 289-290.

SIMA 4. O'Neill, M.J., D.H. Bray, P. Boardman, C.W. Wright, J.D. Philipson, D.C. Warhurst, M.P. Gupta, M. Carreya & P. Solis. 1988. Plants as sources of antimalarial drugs. Part 6. Activities of *Simarouba amara* fruits. *J. Ethnopharmacol.* 22: 183-190.

SIMA 5. Polonsky, J. 1973. Quassinoid bitter principles. In: Herz, W., H. Grisebach & G.W. Kirby, eds., PROGRESS IN THE CHEMISTRY OF ORGANIC NATURAL PRODUCTS, vol. 30: 101-150. Springer-Verlag, Vienna and New York.

SIMA 6. Polonsky, J. 1985. Quassinoid bitter principles. II. In: Herz, W., H. Grisebach, G.W. Kirby & C. Tamm, eds., PROGRESS IN THE CHEMISTRY OF ORGANIC NATURAL PRODUCTS, vol. 47: 221-264. Springer-Verlag, Vienna and New York.

SOLANACEAE

Acnistus arborescens (L.) Schl.
AREA: Minas Gerais to São Paulo and Rio de Janeiro.
NAMES: Esporão-de-galo-falso, fruta-de-sabiá, mariana, marianeira.
USES: Roots and leaves are narcotic, used for piles. Leaves are diuretic. Fruits poisonous.
CHEM.: Leaves and stems contain a steroid of the withanolide class (Ref: SOLA 1).

Bassovia lucida Dunal
AREA: Bahia to São Paulo.
NAMES: Coerana, marianeira.
USES: Used to soothe pains in vesical lithiasis.

Brunfelsia uniflora (Pohl) D. Don
AREA: Pará to São Paulo, forest and caatinga, very popular in gardens.
NAMES: Manacá, manacá-cheiroso.
USES: Roots are purgative, emetic, abortifacient, antirheumatic and antiblennorrhagic. In high doses the drug causes delirium, mental confusion, tremor and sleep. The closely related *B. grandiflora* D. Don is occasionally used in the same way.

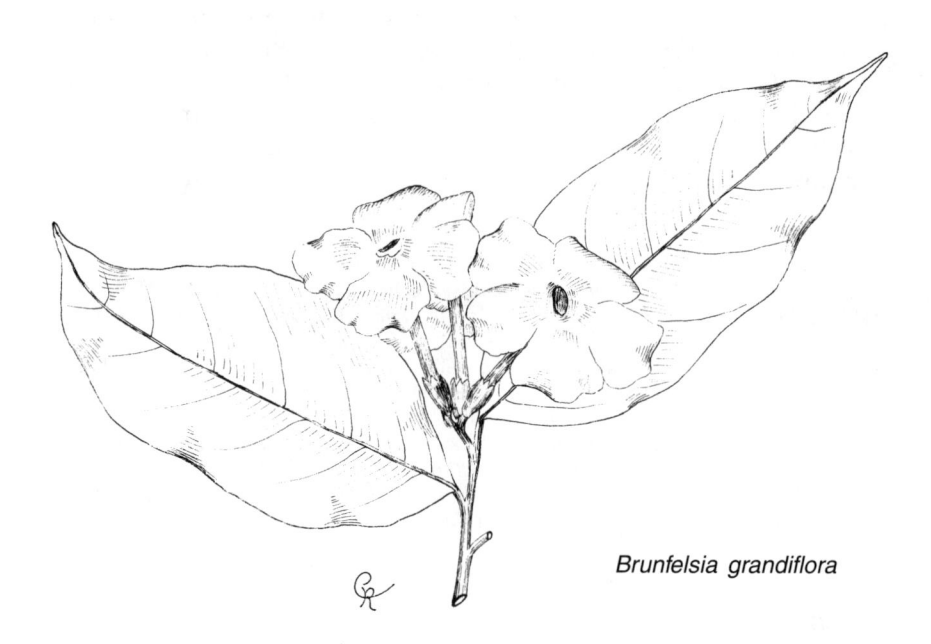

Brunfelsia grandiflora

CHEM.: All parts of *Brunfelsia* species contain the coumarin scopoletin (Ref: SOLA 2,3). A review describes the ethnomedical uses of the genus (Ref: SOLA 4).

Cestrum amictum Schl.
AREA: Southern Brazil.
NAME: Coerana.
USES: Leaves are bitter, febrifuge, applied for hemorrhoids.

Cestrum bracteatum Link & Otto
AREA: Minas Gerais, Rio de Janeiro and São Paulo.
NAME: Coerana.
USES: Fresh leaves are used to clean wounds and ulcers. Bruised leaves mixed with unripe fruits serve for treatment of liver obstruction and bladder catarrh.

Cestrum calycinum Willd.
AREA: Goiàs to Rio Grande do Sul.
NAME: Coerana.
USES: Though poisonous, the plant is employed as an antidysenteric, emollient, sedative and antispasmodic; externally used to treat rheumatism and dermatoses.

Cestrum parqui L'Herit.
AREA: Southern Brazil.
NAME: Coerana.
USES: Indicated for skin afflictions, dyspepsy, catarrh of the bladder, malaria, jaundice, chorea, epilepsy, diarrhoea, rheumatism, liver congestion and, as an ointment, to combat piles.
CHEM.: All parts of the plant contain saponins. Some of the aglycons have been identified as steroidal sapogenins (Ref: SOLA 5,6).

Cestrum pseudoquina Mart.
AREA: Amazonia to Rio Grande do Sul.
NAMES: Quina-da-terra, quina-do-mato, quina-do-pará.
USES: The root-bark is tonic and antipyretic, used in place of the genuine quina (*Cinchona*).

Datura arborea L.
AREA: Subspontaneous in Brazil; frequently cultivated.
NAMES: Açucena-do-brejo, saia-branca, trombeteira, trombeta-branca, zabumba-branca.
USES: The same as those of the thorn-apple, *Datura stramonium* L. Poisoning has been reported (Ref: SOLA 7).

SOLANACEAE

Datura insignis B. Rodr.
AREA: Amazonia, forest; cultivated by the Indians.
NAMES: Maricaua, toé.
USES: Leaves in a decoction are hallucinogenic; taken in religious rites to promote trance states.
CHEM.: The leaves contain up to 0.3% of the alkaloid scopolamine (Ref: SOLA 8).

Datura stramonium L.
AREA: Common in most parts of Brazil, frequently as a ruderal herb.
NAMES: Estramônio, figueira-do-inferno, mata-zombando, trombeta, zabumba (English: thorn-apple).
USES: Seed oil used in rubs as a calmative for local pain. Smoking cigarettes made from the dried leaves is prescribed for asthma. The plant is known to be stupefacient.
CHEM.: The main alkaloid in the plant is hyosciamine, the levo-form of atropine. It is a natural anticholinergic with sedative properties.

Datura suaveolens Humb. & Bonpl.
AREA: Widely distributed in Brazil as subspontaneous and sometimes grown in gardens.
NAMES: Copo-de-leite, saia-branca, trombeta-cheirosa, zabumba-branca.
USES: Leaves are sedative; in higher dose they are narcotic, hallucinogenic, toxic.
CHEM.: Scopolamine is the predominating alkaloid (Ref: SOLA 9,10).
PHARM.: Moderated antiviral activity has been reported (Ref: SOLA 11).

Nicandra physaloides (L.) Gaertn.
AREA: Rio de Janeiro, Minas Gerais and São Paulo.
NAME: Quintilho.
USE: Sedative in small doses.

Physalis angulata L.
AREA: Pará to Rio de Janeiro.
NAMES: Balãozinho, bucho-de-rã, camapu, juá-de-capote, matafome.
USES: Sap is calmative, depurative, active against rheumatic ailments. Berries are resolvent, diuretic. A tea made from the roots also containing urucum (*Bixa orellana*, Bixaceae) and açaí (*Euterpe oleracea*, Arecaceae) is recommended to cure jaundice.
CHEM.: The berries contain acetylcholine (Ref: SOLA 12).

Physalis pubescens L.
AREA: Amazonia to São Paulo and Mato Grosso.
NAMES: Bate-testa, camapu, erva-moura-do-peru, juá-poca.

SOLANACEAE

USES: Narcotic, stimulant, useful in cases of cystitis, otitis, jaundice and herpes. Unripe fruits are laxative and diuretic.

Salpichroa origanifolia (Lam.) Thell.
AREA: Rio Grande do Sul, cultivated.
NAMES: Congonha, grão-de-galo, ovo-de-galo.
USES: Leaves, though venomous, are considered antirheumatic.

Solanum aculeatissimum Jacq.
AREA: Widespread as a ruderal herb.
NAMES: Arrebenta-boi, arrebenta-cavalo, babá, bobó, juá.
USES: Entire plant is prescribed in baths against dermal afflictions, oedema of the legs and intestinal tuberculosis. Said to be toxic.

Solanum agrarium Sendt.
AREA: Piauí, campo.
NAMES: Babá, babão, melancia-da-praia.
USES: Useful for gonorrhoea and orchitis.

Solanum albidum Dun.
AREA: Ceará to Rio Grande do Sul.
NAME: Jurubeba-branca.
USES: Fruits are digestive and, in higher doses, cathartic. *S. ambrosiacum* Vell. (Ceará to Mato Grosso and Rio de Janeiro) is considered a substitute for this species.

Solanum caavurana Vell.
AREA: Piauí to Rio de Janeiro.
NAME: Caavurana.
USE: Prescribed for treating leprosy.

Solanum cernuum Vell.
AREA: Espírito Santo to Rio de Janeiro.
NAMES: Bolsa-de-pastor, braço-de-preguiça, caapuera-branca, panacéia, velame-do-mato.
USES: Roots are hemostatic. Leaves used in infusion as a sudorific, diuretic, depurative, for healing gonorrhoea, dermal diseases and skin ulcers. Roasted leaves produce a tasteful tea which is calmative for persons with heart trouble.

Solanum ciliatum Lam.
AREA: Southern Brazil.
NAMES: Arrebenta-cavalo, juá, juá-vermelho, mata-cavalo.
USES: Leaves are narcotic, lethal for animals.
CHEM.: Unripe or maturing fruits contain 2% or more of solasodine (Ref: SOLA 13).

SOLANACEAE

Solanum grandiflorum Ruiz & Pav.
AREA: Amazonia to São Paulo.
NAMES: Fruta-de-lobo, fumo-bravo, jurubeba-grande, lobeira.
USES: Root infusion is used for hepatitis and jaundice. Syrup from fruits for treating asthma.
CHEM.: Solasodine has been identified (Ref: SOLA 14).

Solanum insidiosum Mart.
AREA: Rio de Janeiro to Rio Grande do Sul; common as ruderal.
NAMES: Juá-bravo, jurubeba-de-espinho.
USES: Root and berries are bitter, prescribed for chronic hepatitis, jaundice and malaria. Leaves applied externally for the dressing of ulcers.

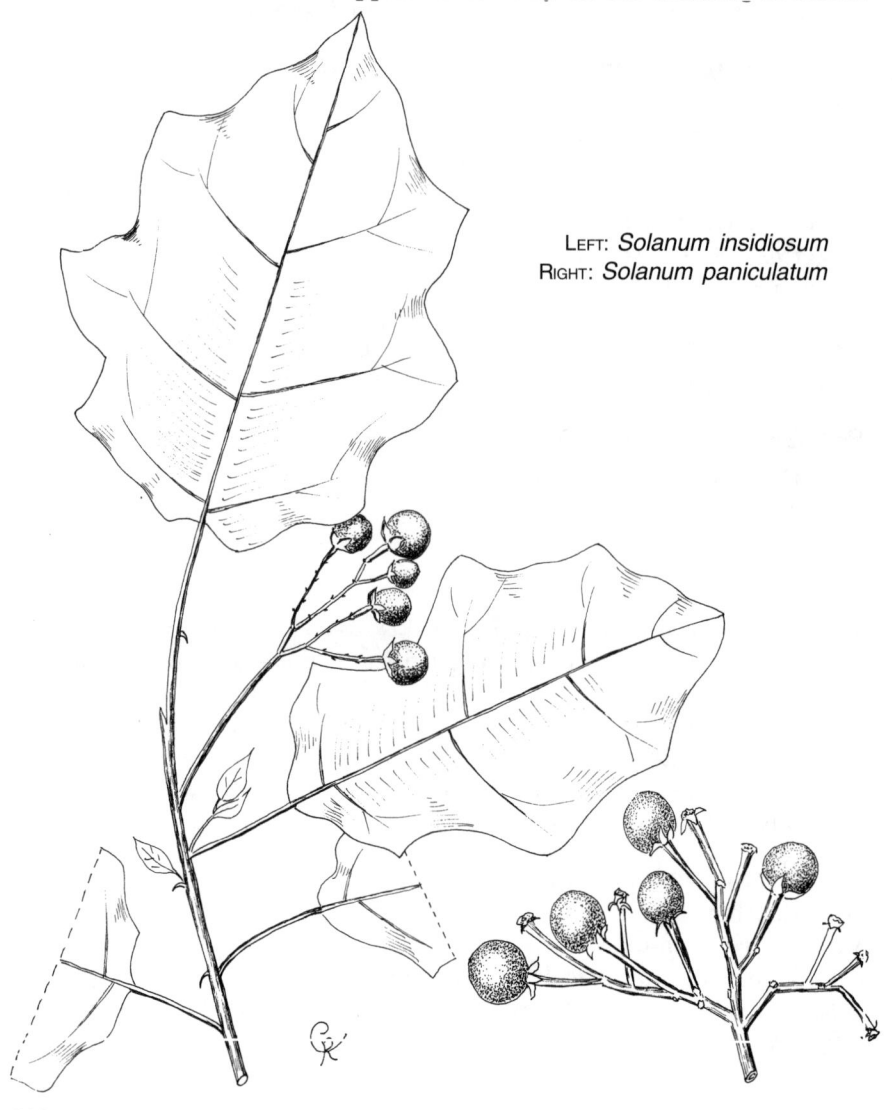

LEFT: *Solanum insidiosum*
RIGHT: *Solanum paniculatum*

Solanum juciri Mart.
AREA: Rio de Janeiro to Santa Catarina.
NAMES: Caruru-de-espinho, jiquirioba, juá, juciri, juqueri.
USES: Fruits are used to relieve liver congestion.
The same uses are made of *S. juripeba* Rich. (Amazonia).

Solanum lycocarpum St.-Hil.
AREA: Central Brazil, mainly in cerrado.
NAMES: Fruta-de-lobo, lobeira.
USES: Juice squeezed from berries is applied externally to cure warts.
CHEM.: Solamargine and solasonine have been identified in the plant (Ref: SOLA 15).

Solanum mammosum L.
AREA: Pará, Ceará and Mato Grosso, cultivated by the Indians; neotropical.
NAMES: Juá-bravo, jurubeba-do-pará, peito-de-moça, peito-de-vaca.
USES: Leaves are bitter, diuretic, aphrodisiac and indicated for psoriasis.
CHEM.: The plant contains solasodine (Ref: SOLA 16).

Solanum martii Sendt.
AREA: Espírito Santo and Minas Gerais.
NAMES: Braço-de-mono, panacéia.
USES: Leaves are diuretic, recommended for cystitis.

Solanum mauritianum Scop.
AREA: Throughout Brazil.
NAMES: Caavitinga, capoeira-branca, convetinga, cuvitinga, fruta-de-guará, fruta-de-lobo, fumo-bravo.
USES: Leaves are diuretic and calmative.

Solanum nigrum L.
AREA: Cosmopolitan; ruderal in most of Brazil.
NAMES: Caraxixi, erva-moura, maria-preta, suê.
USES: Plant is antialgetic, sedative, slightly narcotic, reputedly active against gastralgia, bladder spasms, arthralgia; also is anaphrodisiac, expectorant, emollient, diuretic, depurative and for ulcers. Used externally for psoriasis, eczema and pruritus.

Solanum paniculatum L.
AREA: Amazonia to São Paulo.
NAMES: Jubeba, juripeba, jurubeba, jurubeba-verdadeira, jurubebinha, juuna, juvena.
USES: Roots and berries are bitter, prescribed for chronic hepatitis, jaundice and malaria. Externally, leaves are applied for dressing ulcers.

CHEM.: Solanum-type alkaloids identified by chromatography (Ref: SOLA 17).

PHARM.: Extract of roots showed high toxicity in mice and fish and depressor effect on cardiorespiratory activity in cats (Ref: SOLA 18,19).

Solanum pseudoquina St.-Hil.
AREA: Paraná and São Paulo.
NAME: Quina-de-são-paulo.
USES: Bark is antipyretic.
CHEM. & PHARM.: Solanum-type alkaloids have been isolated, one of them with convulsive action (Ref: SOLA 20,21).

Solanum variabile Mart.
AREA: Rio de Janeiro to Rio Grande do Sul.
NAME: Jupicanga.
USES: Roots and leaves are tonic, diuretic, recommended for treating liver ailments and jaundice.

Solanum verbascifolium L.
AREA: Cosmopolitan; sparsely dispersed in Brazil.
NAMES: Cuvitinga, funcho-brabo, fruta-de-lobo.
USES: Heated leaves applied to the forehead are a remedy for migraine. Also an emollient when placed on ulcers and boils.

CHEMISTRY OF SOLANUM ALKALOIDS: The alkaloids of *Solanum* species are of steroidal nature, present as aglycons (sapogenins) of saponins. When available in large enough quantities, they serve as raw materials for producing steroid hormones through chemical transformation. For reviews, see Ref: SOLA 22,23.

Solanaceae – References

SOLA 1. Barata, L., W.B. Mors, I. Kirson & D. Lavie. 1970. A new withanolide from *Acnistus arborescens* (L.) Schlecht. (Solanaceae) from the state of Guanabara, Brazil. *An. Acad. Brasil. Ci. 42*: 401-407.

SOLA 2. Mors, W.B. & O. Ribeiro. 1957. Occurrence of scopoletin in the genus *Brunfelsia*. *J. Org. Chem. 22*: 978-979.

SOLA 3. Campos, S.M. 1964. Scopoletin in *Brunfelsia* seeds. *An. Acad. Brasil. Ci. 36*: 511-513.

SOLA 4. Plowman, T.C. 1977. *Brunfelsia* in ethnomedicine. *Bot. Mus. Leaflets Harvard Univ. 25*: 289-320.

SOLA 5. Cabham, P.A.S. & F.L. Warren. 1951. Saponins. II. Isolation of gitogenin and digitogenin from *Cestrum parqui*. *J. South African Chem. Inst. 3*: 63-65.

SOLA 6. Bianchi, E., F. Girardi, F. Diaz, R. Sandoval & M. Gonzalez. 1963. Components of the leaves and fruits of *Cestrum parqui*. *Ann. Chim. 53*: 1761-1778.

SOLA 7. Miguel, R. 1959. Poisoning by *Datura arborea*. *Rev. Farm. Bahia 3*: 73-75.

SOLA 8. Rizzini, C.T. & M.L. Bastos. 1956. *Datura insignis* Barb. Rodr.: seus alcalóides. *An. Acad. Brasil. Ci. 28*: 473-483.

SOLA 9. Evans, W.C., & J.F. Lampard. 1972. Alkaloids of *Datura suaveolens*. *Phytochemistry* 11: 3293-3298.
SOLA 10. Akisue, M.K., G. Akisue, F. Oliveira, R. Wasicky & M.L. Saito. 1977. Contribuição ao estudo farmacognóstico de *Datura suaveolens* Humboldt et Bonpland ex Willdenow. *An. Farm. Quím.* (São Paulo) 17: 75-99.
SOLA 11. Van den Berghe, D.A., M. Ieven, F. Mertens, A.J. Vleitinck & E. Lammens. 1978. Screening of higher plants for biological activities. II. Antiviral activity. *Lloydia* 41: 463-471.
SOLA 12. Mello, A.C. & P. Afiatpour. 1985. Presence of acetylcholine in the fruit of *Physalis angulata* (Solanaceae). *Ciência e Cultura*. (São Paulo) 37: 799-805.
SOLA 13. Sigueira, N.C.S., C.B. Alice, L.A. Mentz, G.A. Assis Brasil e Silva & I.C. Halbig. 1988. Determinação de solasodina em algumas espécies do gênero *Solanum* nativas do Rio Grande do Sul. *Rev. Bras. Farm.* 69: 25-28.
SOLA 14. Rippenberger, H. & K. Schreiber. 1981. THE ALKALOIDS: CHEMISTRY AND PHYSIOLOGY. Academic Press, New York.
SOLA 15. Motidome, M., M.E. Leeking & O.R. Gottlieb. 1970. A química das Solanáceas brasileiras. I. A. presença de solamargina e de solasodina no juá e na lobeira. *An. Acad. Brasil. Ci.* 42 (Supl.): 375-376.
SOLA 16. Telek, L., H. Delpin & E. Cabanillas. 1977. *Solanum mammosum* as a source of solasodine in the lowland tropics. *Econ. Bot.* 31: 120-128.
SOLA 17. Siqueira, N.S. & A. Macan. 1976. Cromatografia dos alcalóides do *Solanum paniculatum* L. *Tribuna Farmacêutica* (Curitiba) 44: 101-104.
SOLA 18. Barros, G.S.G., J.E.V. Vieira, M.P. Souza & F.J.A. Matos. 1967 Pharmacological screening of some Brazilian northeastern plants. *Rev. Bras. Farm.* 48: 195-204.
SOLA 19. Barros, G.S.G., F.J.A. Matos, J.E.V. Vieira, M.P. Sousa & M.C. Medeiros. 1969. Pharmacological screening of some Brazilian plants. *J. Pharm. Pharmacol.* 22: 116-122.
SOLA 20. Usubillaga, A., G. Castellano, J. Hidalgo, C. Guevara, P. Martinod & A. Paredes. 1977. Solaquidine, a new steroidal alkaloid from *Solanum pseudoquina*. *Phytochemistry* 16: 1861-1862.
SOLA 21. Oliveira, R.A.G., J. Battacharyya, R. Leonart, L.A.E. Carvalho, M.Q. Paulo & G. Trolin. 1988. Convulsive action of (25S)-iso-solafloridine isolated from *Solanum pseudoquina* bark. *J. Ethnopharmacol.* 24: 155-165.
SOLA 22. Schreiber, K. 1968. Steroid alkaloids. The *Solanum* group. *In*: R.H.F. Manske (ed.), THE ALKALOIDS 10: 1-192. Academic Press, New York.
SOLA 23. Patel, A.V. 1987. A review of naturally-occurring steroidal sapogenins. *Fitoterapia* 58: 61-107.

STERCULIACEAE

Guazuma ulmifolia Lam. var. *tomentella* Schum.
AREA: Amazonia and Mato Grosso, forest.
NAMES: Camacã, pau-de-mutamba.
USES: Bark is prescribed against elephantiasis and certain dermatoses.

Guazuma ulmifolia Lam. var. *ulmifolia*
AREA: Amazonia to Rio Grande do Sul, forest.
NAMES: Embira, embiru, mutamba.
USES: Bark is employed to improve hair growth and to combat parasites of the scalp. Its decoction is reputedly depurative, antisyphilitic, pectoral, antiblennorrhagic and indicated for skin afflictions.

STERCULIACEAE

Helicteres ovata

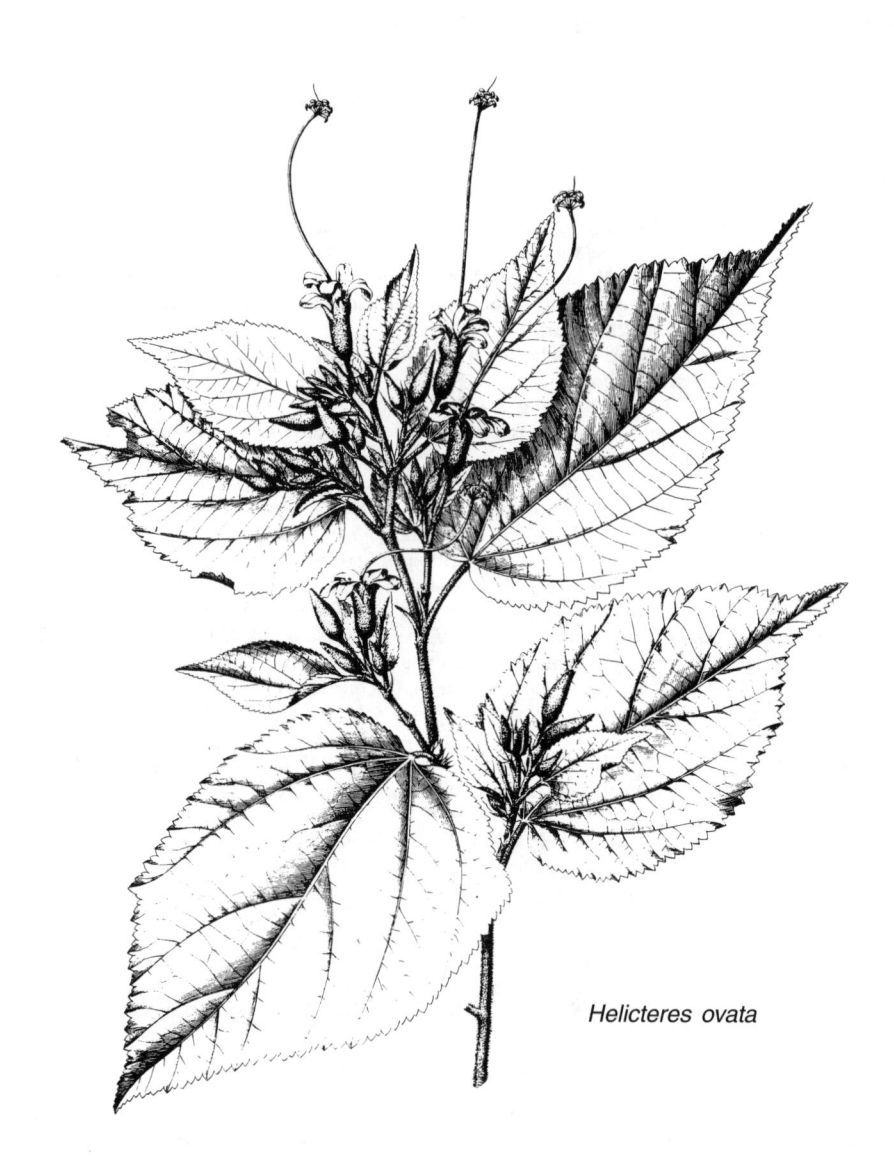

Helicteres ovata Lam.
AREA: Goiás to São Paulo, cerrado and campo.
NAMES: Guaxima, embira-brava, embira-do-mato, rosca, sacarrolha.
USES: Roots are depurative. Flowers are bechic and emollient.

Sterculia apetala (Jacq.) Karst. var. ***elata*** (Ducke) E. Taylor
AREA: Amazonia; neotropical.

NAME: Chichá.
USES: Pectoral, to eliminate catarrh.

Sterculia chicha St.-Hil.
AREA: Southern Brazil.
NAME: Chichá.
USES: The bruised leaves in poultices are resolvent.

Waltheria communis St.-Hil.
AREA: Bahia to Rio Grande do Sul, campo and cerrado.
NAMES: Douradinha, douradinha-do-campo.
USES: Stimulant, emetic, sudorific, diuretic, indicated for dysentery, bronchial catarrh, lung afflictions, cystitis and blennorrhagia.

Waltheria indica L.
AREA: Cosmopolitan; frequent in Brazil.
NAMES: Malva-branca, malva-veludo.
USES: Plant is bechic and antisyphilitic.

Waltheria viscosissima St.-Hil.
AREA: Pará to Mato Grosso, campo.
NAME: Malva-branca.
USES: Bronchial and pulmonary afflictions, also used as an emollient for clearing torpid ulcers.

STYRACACEAE

Styrax ferrugineum Nees & Mart.
AREA: Bahia to São Paulo, cerrado.
NAMES: Benjoeiro, limoeiro-do-campo, pindaíba, pindaibuna.
USES: From the trunk oozes a balsamic resin which may be used as a substitute for storax or benzoin (*Styrax benzoin* Dryander and *S. officinale* L.) from Asia.

Styrax glabratum Schott
AREA: Rio de Janeiro and São Paulo, forest.
NAME: Almíscar.
USES: Resinous exudation from the trunk is balsamic and may be used instead of the Asiatic benzoin.

Styrax pohlii DC., from Minas Gerais to Paraná, known as benjoeiro or árvore do bálsamo, does not differ from the preceding two species as to properties and uses.

SYMPLOCACEAE

Symplocos parviflora Benth.
AREA: Amazonia to Rio Grande do Sul, forest.
NAMES: Pau-de-cangalha, sete-sangrias.
USES: Bark infusion is used to lessen fever.

Symplocos platyphylla (Pohl) Benth.
AREA: Minas Gerais to Rio Grande do Sul, forest.
NAME: Sete-sangrias.
USES: Root-bark is febrifuge, bitter, tonic and astringent.

Symplocos pubescens Klotzsch
AREA: Minas Gerais and São Paulo, forest.
NAMES: Cinzeiro-do-mato, pau-de-cinza, saboeiro, sete-sangrias.
USES: Same as for *S. platyphylla* (Pohl) Benth.

THEACEAE

Laplacea fruticosa (Schr.) Kobuski
AREA: Almost everywhere in forest and restinga.
NAME: Santa-rita.
USE: Bark is astringent, antidiarrhoeic.

Ternstroemia brasiliensis Camb.
AREA: Bahia to Rio Grande do Sul, forest.
USES: Bark is astringent and antidiarrhoeic, like *Laplacea fruticosa*.
CHEM. & PHARM.: A triterpene with antitumor activity has been isolated from the roots. Its complete structure, however, was not elucidated (Ref: THEA 1).

Theaceae – Reference
THEA 1. Maciel, M.C.N., I.E. d'Albuquerque, M.S.B. Cavalcanti, G.M. Maciel, M.C.M. Araújo & A.L. Lacerda. 1979. Estudos preliminares de substância antineoplásica de raizes de *Ternstroemia brasiliensis* Camb. (Theaceae). *Rev. Inst. Antib.* (Recife) *19*: 17-22.

TILIACEAE

Luehea divaricata Mart. & Zucc.
AREA: Bahia to Rio Grande do Sul, forest.
NAME: Açoita-cavalo.
USES: Bark and leaves used for laryngitis and bronchitis.

Luehea rufescens St.-Hil.
AREA: Minas Gerais and Goiás, cerrado and dry forest.
NAMES: Açoita-cavalo, ivitinga.
USES: Leaves are astringent; recommended for diarrhoea, leucorrhoea, blennorrhagia, hemorrhage and arthritis. Roots are depurative.

Muntingia calabura L.
AREA: Amazonia, forest.
NAMES: Calabura, curumi, pau-de-seda.
USES: Flowers are antispasmodic.

Triumfetta rhomboidea Jacq.
AREA: Cosmopolitan, widely dispersed in Brazil.
NAMES: Amor-do-campo, barba-de-boi, carrapicho-da-calçada.
USES: Roots and leaves are mucilaginous and astringent, injected into the urethra in treatment of gonorrhoea.

Triumfetta semitriloba Jacq.
AREA: Cosmopolitan, common in Brazil as a ruderal and weed.
NAMES: Carrapichinho, carrapicho-de-linho, carrapicho-de-calçada, guaxuma, juta-nacional.
USES: Roots and leaves are astringent and diuretic, used for treating blennorrhagia and genital discharges in general.

TROPAEOLACEAE

Tropaeolum pentaphyllum Lam.
AREA: Rio Grande do Sul.
NAMES: Capuchinha, carrapicho, chagas, chagas-miúdas, sapatinho-de-iaiá, sapatinho-do-diabo.
USES: Edible tubers are considered antiscorbutic and depurative.

TURNERACEAE

Turnera diffusa Willd.
AREA: Tropical cosmopolitan, from Amazonia to São Paulo.
NAME: Damiana.
USES: Aromatic and astringent, this plant has the fame of a veritable panacea. Considered tonic and stimulant, it is purported to be effective in cases of alcoholic abuse and in the treatment of dyspepsia and nervous disorders. It is recommended as a stimulant of the appetite and digestion, as well as a diuretic and laxative, and is also prescribed as antisyphilitic, antidiabetic, antimalarial and antileucorrhoeic. It is equally

applied for afflictions of the kidneys and gall bladder, medullary ailments, stomach ulcer and paralysis. Above all, it is reputed as a powerful aphrodisiac.

CHEM.: Plant contains the cyanogenic glycoside tetraphyllin B (Ref: TURN 1). A flavonoid has also been described (Ref: TURN 2).

Turnera guianensis Aubl.
AREA: Amazonia and Ceará.
NAME: Damiana.
USES: Leaves are emollient, especially for maturing boils.

Turnera opifera Mart.
AREA: Minas Gerais and São Paulo, campo.
NAMES: Chanana, damiana.
USES: In general, the same as those of *T. diffusa* Willd., but used principally as a tonic for the genito-urinary organs and for gastric troubles.

Turnera rupestris Aubl.
AREA: Amazonia and Maranhã.
NAME: Chá-da-terra.
USES: Recommended for nervous diseases, stomach weakness and painful menses.

Turnera ulmifolia L.
AREA: Cosmopolitan, widespread in Brazil as a ruderal.
NAMES: Albina, chanana, saca-estrepe.
USES: Herb is astringent, expectorant, tonic, dyspeptic, antidiabetic and antileucorrhoeic. Contused leaves are used to aid the removal of thorns from skin, the same are also applied in a cataplasm for maturing external tumors.
CHEM.: Plant contains the cyanogenic glycoside deidaclin (Ref: TURN 3).

Turneraceae – References

TURN 1. Spencer, K.C. & D.S. Seigler. 1981. Tetraphyllin B from *Turnera diffusa*. *Planta Medica* 43: 175-178.

TURN 2. Dominguez, X.A. & M. Minojosa. 1976. Isolation of 5-hydroxy-7,3,4'-trimethoxyflavone from *Turnera diffusa*. *Planta Medica* 30: 68-71.

TURN 3. Spencer, K.C. & D.S. Seigler. 1980. Deidaclin from *Turnera ulmifolia*. *Phytochemistry* 19: 1863-1864.

TYPHACEAE

Typha domingensis Pers.
AREA: The plant grows in most still waters, puddles and marshes.
NAMES: Espadana, landim, partasana, tabua (English: cattail).
USES: Rhizome is astringent and diuretic.

TYPHACEAE

Typha domingensis

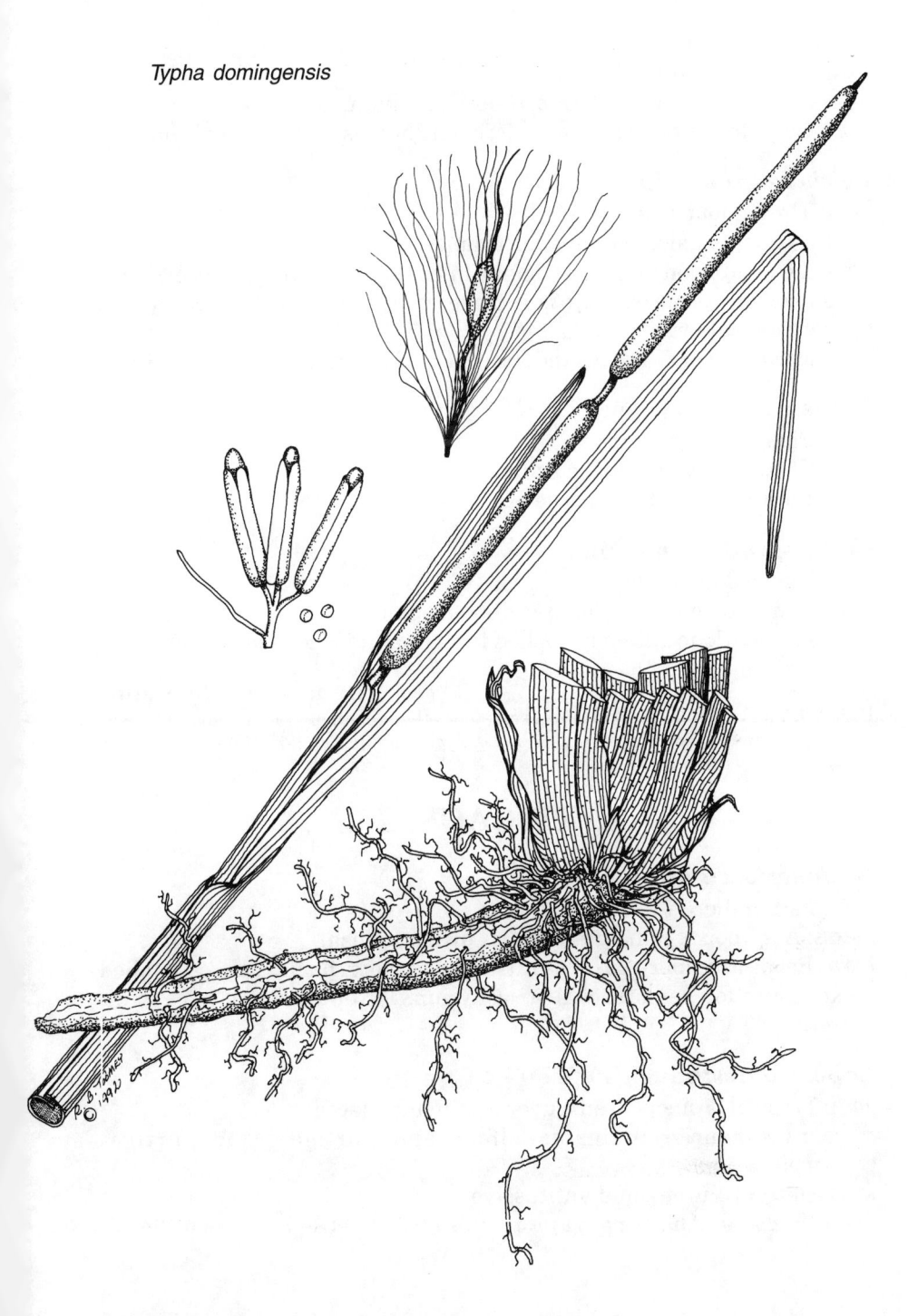

MEDICINAL PLANTS OF BRAZIL

ULMACEAE

Celtis brasiliensis Planch.
AREA: Bahia to São Paulo, forest.
NAMES: Coatindiba, corindiba, corindiúba, crindiúva.
USES: Bark decoction is antithermic; externally used to treat ophthalmia.

Celtis iguanaea Sarg.
AREA: Throughout Brazil, forest.
NAMES: Grão-de-galo, joá-miúdo, irurapia.
USES: Leaf infusion used in vaginal injection for treating leucorrhoea. The boiled, contused fruit is considered a specific for dysentery and intestinal catarrh.
CHEM. & PHARM.: Leaf contains the sugar alcohol quebrachitol (Ref: ULMA 1).

Celtis morifolia Planch.
AREA: Piauí to Rio de Janeiro.
NAMES: Coatindiba, corubá, curubá.
USES: Bark employed against fever.

Celtis spinosissima Miq.
AREA: Rio de Janeiro, forest.
NAMES: Grão-de-galo-miúdo, grãozinho-de-galo.
USES: Root-bark decoction is applied in vaginal injections for leucorrhoea.

Ulmaceae – Reference

ULMA 1. Plouvier, V. 1958. Sur la recherche des ethers methyliques des isnositols dans quelques groupes botaniques. *Compt. Rend. Acad. Sci.* (Paris) *247*: 2423-2426.

URTICACEAE

Boehmeria caudata Sw.
AREA: Pernambuco to Paraná, forest.
NAMES: Assa-peixe, folha-de-santana, urtiga-mansa.
USES: Roots are aperient, depurative, antihemorrhagic. Leaves applied externally for hemorrhoids, as collyrium for ophthalmia; juice is diuretic.

Laportea aestuans (L.) Chew
AREA: Tropical cosmopolitan, ruderal in many places.
NAMES: Cansanção, urtiga-de-folha-grande, urtiga-grande, urtiga-vermelha.
USES: Herb is diuretic and antitussive.
CHEM. & PHARM.: The stinging properties of this nettle have been the ob-

ject of a detailed study (Ref: URTI 1). One leaf placed in an aquarium with snails significantly augments oviposition (Ref: URTI 2).

Parietaria boehmerioides Mart.
AREA: Minas Gerais and Rio de Janeiro.
NAME: Parietária.
USES: Diuretic and antipyretic.

Pilea microphylla (L.) Liebm.
AREA: Cosmopolitan; in Brazil ruderal and as a garden plant.
NAMES: Brilhantina, erva-gorda, folha-gorda, urtiga.
USES: Herb is diuretic and antithermic, recommended in cases of urine retention. Externally, the poultice hastens the maturation of boils.

Urera aurantiaca Wedd.
AREA: São Paulo and Mato Grosso.
NAMES: Cansanção-verdadeiro, puru, urtiga-branca.
USES: Leaves are diuretic.

Urera baccifera Gaud.
AREA: Amazonia to São Paulo, forest.
NAMES: Cansanção, urtiga-brava, urtiga-fogo, urtiga-grande, urtiga-vermelha, urtigão.
USES: A violently stinging nettle. Contused leaves, though very pungent, are used as a resolvent and hemostatic. Their infusion or decoction is prescribed as aperient, diuretic and antileucorrhoeic. Root decoction used for amenorrhoea.

Urera caracasana Jacq.
AREA: Amazonia to São Paulo, forest.
NAMES: Cansanção, caracasana, urtiga-brava.
USES: Leaf juice is taken against hemorrhage and metrorrhagia. Decoction of the leaves prescribed for lung diseases. Bark infusion is antisyphilitic. Roots are diuretic.

Urera subpeltata Miq.
AREA: Pará to Paraná, forest.
NAMES: Cansanção, urtiga-grande, urtigão, uafé.
USES: Bark used for pulmonary diseases.

Urticaceae – References

URTI 1. MacFarlane, W.V. 1903. The stinging properties of *Laportea. Econ. Bot. 17*: 303-311.
URTI 2. Magalães Neto, B., personal communication.

Urera subpeltata, Urticaceae

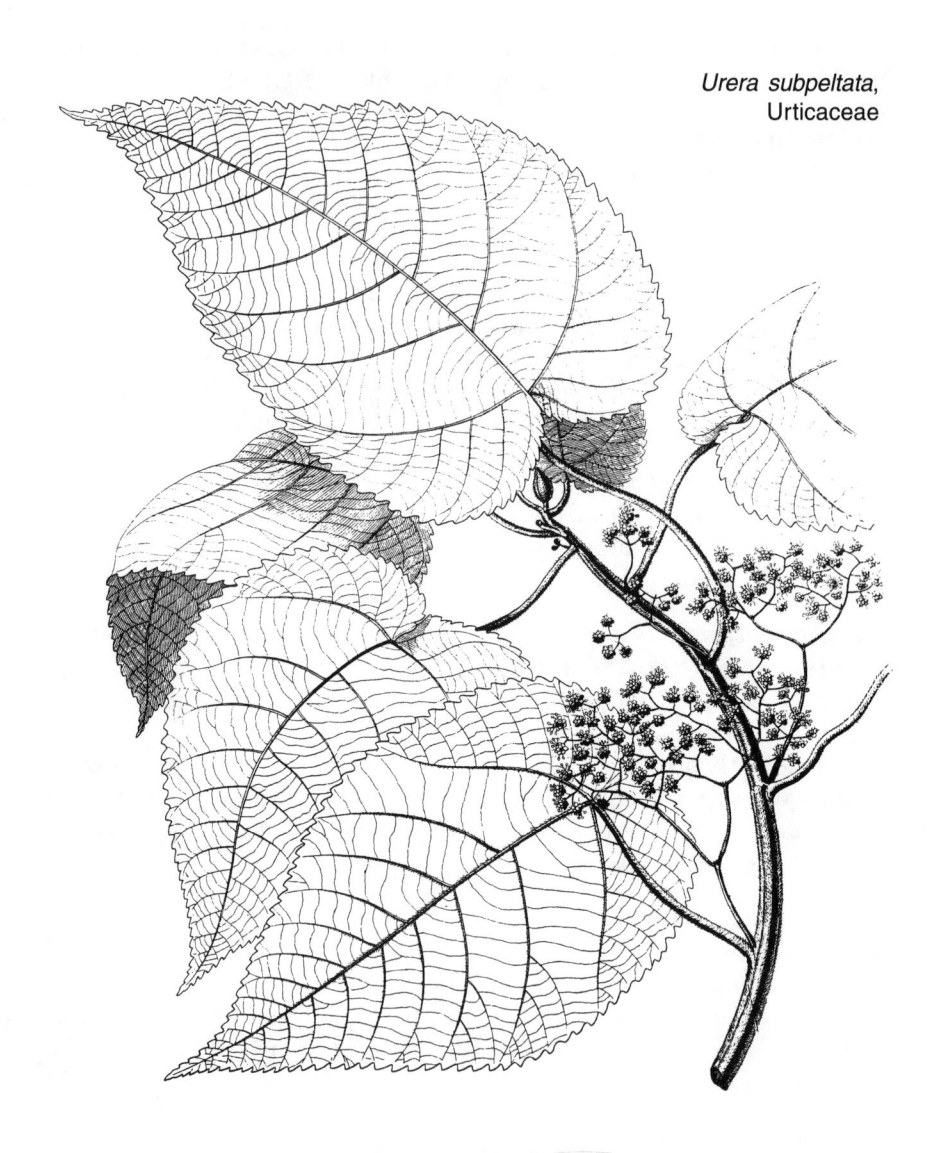

VERBENACEAE

Aloysia triphylla (L'Her.) Britt.
AREA: Neotropical; Rio Grande do Sul, but also much cultivated elsewhere, in gardens.
NAMES: Cidrão, cidrilha, cidró, erva-cidreira, salva-limão.
USES: Leaves and flowers are scented, antispasmodic, digestive, calmatives for nerves and heart, emmenagogue; also taken as a tea to induce sleep.

VERBENACEAE

Amasonia arborea H.B.K.
AREA: Amazonia, forest.
NAMES: Japim-caá.
USES: Infusion of entire plant is used in baths or as enema to check diarrhoea. The juice of the flowers is used as ear drops for earache; also for breast sores. Leaf tea for jaundice and urological disorders.

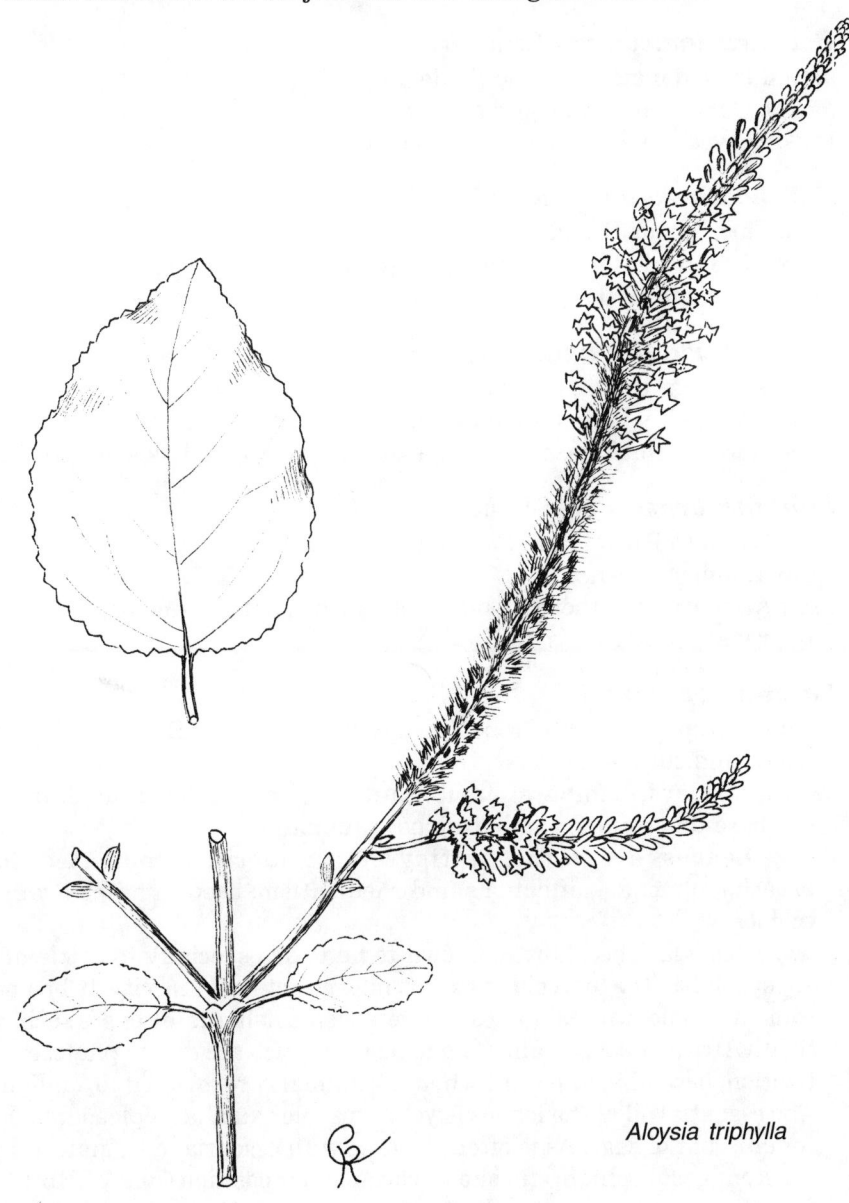

Aloysia triphylla

VERBENACEAE

Avicennia germinans (L.) L.
AREA: In mangroves along the entire coast.
NAMES: Cerebuna, mangue-branco, mangue-amarelo, mangue-manso, pere-siriúba, sereíba-tinga, siriúba.
USES: Bark is hemostatic and antidiarrhoeic; also used to relieve toothache.

Bouchea laetevirens Schauer
AREA: Rio de Janeiro and São Paulo.
NAMES: Gervão-bastardo, gervão-falso.
USES: Leaves are antiemetic and digestive.

Bouchea pseudogervao (St.-Hil.) Cham.
AREA: Throughout Brazil.
NAMES: Gervão-de-folha-grande, gervão-de-folha-larga, gervão-falso.
USES: The same as the preceding species of *Bouchea*.

Glandularia peruviana (L.) Small
AREA: Southern Brazil, campo.
NAMES: Melindre, verbena-melindre.
USES: Herb is febrifuge, stimulant; externally employed as a cicatrizant.

Lantana brasiliensis Link
AREA: Bahia to Paraná and Mato Grosso, campo.
NAME: Cambará-branco.
USES: Aromatic, antithermic, bitter, stomachic, antispasmodic; also used to prepare pectoral syrups.

Lantana camara L.
AREA: Neotropical; mainly from Ceará to Rio Grande do Sul, both spontaneous and cultivated.
NAMES: Camará, cambará, cambará-de-cheiro, cambará-de-chumbo, cambará-de-espinho, cambará-juba, chumbinho.
USES: Leaves are tonic, antipyretic, sudorific, indicated for bronchopulmonary afflictions and rheumatism; used in baths against scabies.
CHEM. & PHARM.: The plant is known to be toxic especially to cattle and sheep. Cattle try to avoid it except in cases of food scarcity. It has become a problem in countries where sheep raising is intense, such as South Africa and Australia. The toxic properties are due to photosensitization, becoming apparent when the animals are exposed to sunlight. The essential oil of the leaves is yellow in color and has a pleasant odor reminiscent of sage. As is often the case with essential oils, material of different geographic origin shows variable composition (Ref: VERB 1,2). The compounds responsible for photosensitization and consequent

VERBENACEAE

Amasonia arborea H.B.K.
AREA: Amazonia, forest.
NAMES: Japim-caá.
USES: Infusion of entire plant is used in baths or as enema to check diarrhoea. The juice of the flowers is used as ear drops for earache; also for breast sores. Leaf tea for jaundice and urological disorders.

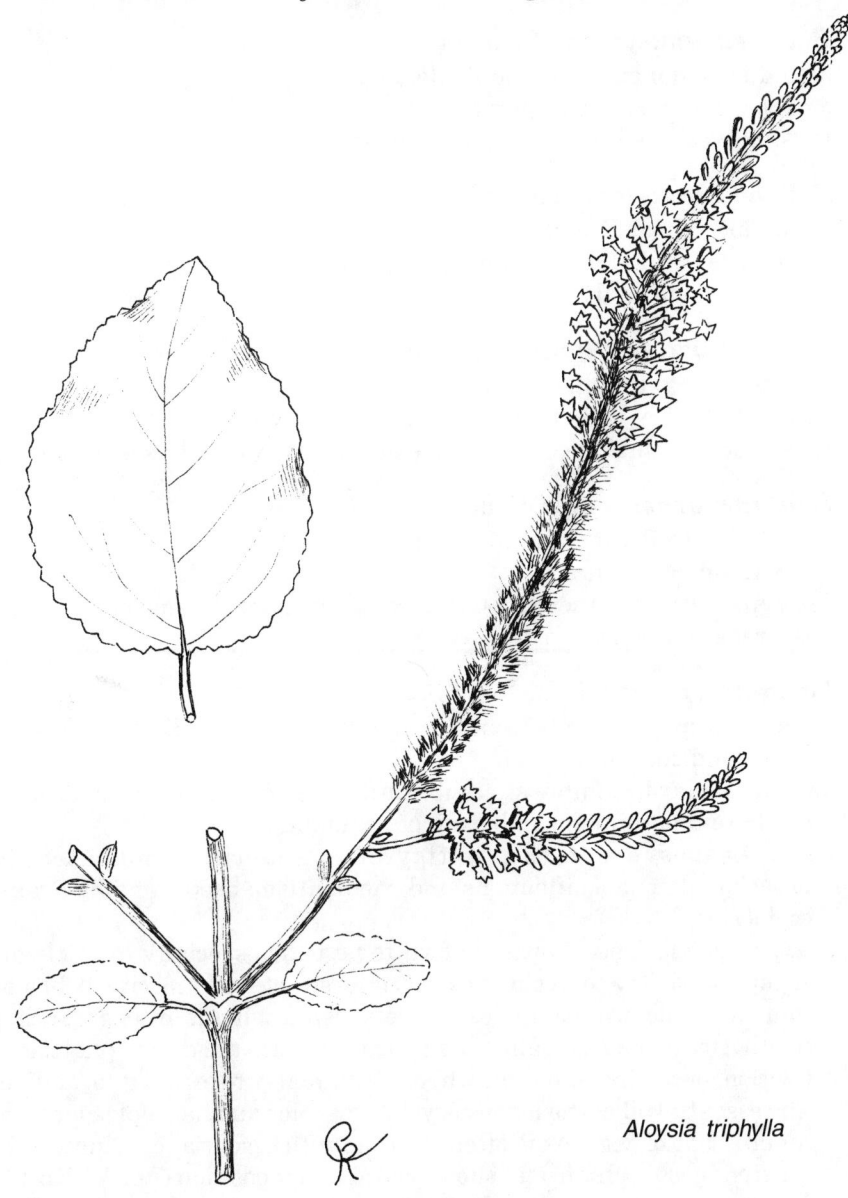

Aloysia triphylla

VERBENACEAE

Avicennia germinans (L.) L.
AREA: In mangroves along the entire coast.
NAMES: Cerebuna, mangue-branco, mangue-amarelo, mangue-manso, pere-siriúba, sereíba-tinga, siriúba.
USES: Bark is hemostatic and antidiarrhoeic; also used to relieve toothache.

Bouchea laetevirens Schauer
AREA: Rio de Janeiro and São Paulo.
NAMES: Gervão-bastardo, gervão-falso.
USES: Leaves are antiemetic and digestive.

Bouchea pseudogervao (St.-Hil.) Cham.
AREA: Throughout Brazil.
NAMES: Gervão-de-folha-grande, gervão-de-folha-larga, gervão-falso.
USES: The same as the preceding species of *Bouchea*.

Glandularia peruviana (L.) Small
AREA: Southern Brazil, campo.
NAMES: Melindre, verbena-melindre.
USES: Herb is febrifuge, stimulant; externally employed as a cicatrizant.

Lantana brasiliensis Link
AREA: Bahia to Paraná and Mato Grosso, campo.
NAME: Cambará-branco.
USES: Aromatic, antithermic, bitter, stomachic, antispasmodic; also used to prepare pectoral syrups.

Lantana camara L.
AREA: Neotropical; mainly from Ceará to Rio Grande do Sul, both spontaneous and cultivated.
NAMES: Camará, cambará, cambará-de-cheiro, cambará-de-chumbo, cambará-de-espinho, cambará-juba, chumbinho.
USES: Leaves are tonic, antipyretic, sudorific, indicated for bronchopulmonary afflictions and rheumatism; used in baths against scabies.
CHEM. & PHARM.: The plant is known to be toxic especially to cattle and sheep. Cattle try to avoid it except in cases of food scarcity. It has become a problem in countries where sheep raising is intense, such as South Africa and Australia. The toxic properties are due to photosensitization, becoming apparent when the animals are exposed to sunlight. The essential oil of the leaves is yellow in color and has a pleasant odor reminiscent of sage. As is often the case with essential oils, material of different geographic origin shows variable composition (Ref: VERB 1,2). The compounds responsible for photosensitization and consequent

icterus where shown to be triterpenoids (Ref: VERB 3,4), which have had their chemical structure investigated (Ref: VERB 5,6,7,8). The pathology of the intoxication has been studied (Ref: VERB 9,10). More recently, verbascoside, a glucoside of caffeic acid, was isolated from the plant and was shown to be a specific inhibitor of protein kinase C, an enzyme important in cell proliferation and differentiation. *In vitro* growth of tumor cells was checked by this compound (Ref: VERB 11).

Lantana lilacina Desf.
AREA: São Paulo to Rio Grande do Sul, campo.
NAME: Cambará-rosa.
USES: Leaves and flowers are aromatic, used in an infusion and syrup for cold and bronchitis.

Lantana macrophylla Schauer
AREA: Bahia.
NAME: Cambará-de-folha-grande.
USES: Plant is bechic and emmenagogue.

Lantana microphylla Cham.
AREA: Ceará to Paraná, campo.
NAMES: Alecrim-bravo, alecrim-do-campo.
USES: Leaves are aromatic, febrifuge, antirheumatic. Flowers recommended for catarrhal afflictions. Fruits are tonic and stimulant.

Several other *Lantana* species have similar properties and uses, as, for instance, *L. mixta* L. (Rio de Janeiro and São Paulo) and *L. pseudothea* (St.-Hil.) Schauer (Minas Gerais and São Paulo).

Lippia alba (Mill.) N.E. Brown
AREA: Neotropical; frequent in Brazilian coastal region.
NAMES: Alecrim-do-campo, chá-do-tabuleiro, cidrilha, erva-cidreira, salsa-branca, salsa-limão, salva-branca, salva-limão.
USES: Leaf tea is sudorific, antispasmodic, stomachic and emmenagogue.
CHEM.: The essential oil has been variously analyzed (Ref: VERB 12,13). Again, the composition varies considerably depending on the geographical origin and other factors.

Lippia gratissima (Gill. & Hook.) Troncoso
AREA: Minas Gerais to Rio Grande do Sul, stony campo.
NAME: Cidrão.
USES: Leaves and flowering summits used for common cold and flu; also as a stomachic and against bladder pains.

Stachytarpheta cayennensis (Rich.) Vahl
AREA: Neotropical; from Amazonia to Rio Grande do Sul.

Verbenaceae

NAMES: Gervão-das-taperas, gervão-roxo, rinchão, verbena-falsa.
USES: Sudorific, stimulant, febrifuge, diuretic, tonic, used to soothe chest pains and stomachache; also for cleaning ulcers.

Stachytarpheta dichotoma Vahl
AREA: Pará and Bahia to São Paulo.
NAMES: Gervão, rinchão, verbena-falsa.
USES: Leaves are aromatic, laxative (mainly for children), used for piles.

Stachytarpheta elatior Schrad.
AREA: Bahia to Minas Gerais, in marshy places.
NAMES: Erva-santa, gervão-do-alagadiço.
USES: Hot infusion is used to mitigate the symptoms of malaria.

Stachytarpheta jamaicensis (L.) Vahl
AREA: Neotropical; Brazil: Amazonia.
NAMES: Gervão-verdadeiro.
USES: Leaf infusion is stimulant, digestive, tonic, febrifuge, diaphoretic, anthelmintic, emetic, cathartic, emmenagogue, antihydropic, antisyphilitic; also used to treat yellow fever and chronic hepatitis.
CHEM.: Choline and three flavonic glucuronides have been described from the leaves (Ref: VERB 14).

Verbena bonariensis L.
AREA: Rio de Janeiro to Rio Grande do Sul, campo.
NAME: Cambará-de-capoeira.
USE: Antiasthmatic.

Verbena erinoides Lam.
AREA: Southern Brazil, campo.
NAME: Gervão-cheiroso.
USES: Antiasthmatic, diaphoretic, tonic, stimulant for digestion, febrifuge.

Vitex agnus-castus L.
AREA: Cosmopolitan; Brazil: Amazonia.
NAMES: Alecrim-de-angola, alecrim-do-norte, pau-de-angola.
USES: Leaf tea is prescribed for rheumatism, diarrhoea, gastralgia, amenorrhoea and bronchitis. Leaves crushed in fat are applied topically for influenza and colds.

Vitex gardneriana Schauer
AREA: Piauí to Rio de Janeiro, forest.
NAMES: Gerimato, gerimataia.
USES: Appetizer, excitant, calmative; in baths it is antirheumatic and antihydropic.

Vitex montevidensis Cham.

AREA: Bahia to Rio Grande do Sul and Mato Grosso, forest.
NAMES: Azeitona-brava, azeitona-do-mato, sombra-de-touro, tarumã, tarumã-romã.
USES: Fruits are mucilaginous, pectoral and used to treat venereal diseases.

Verbenaceae – References

VERB 1. Ahmed, Z.F., A.M. El-Moghazy Shoaib, G.M. Wassel & S.M. El-Sayyad. 1971. Phytochemical study of *Lantana camara*. I. *Planta Medica* 21: 282-288.

VERB 2. Craveiro, A.A., C.H.S. Andrade, F.J.A. Matos, J.W. Alencar & M.I.L. Machado. 1980. Óleos essenciais de novas espécies de verbenáceas do nordeste. *Ciência e Cultura* (São Paulo) 32 (Supl.): 469.

VERB 3. Louw, P.G.J. 1943. Lantanin, the active principle of *Lantana camara* L. I. Isolation and preliminary results on the determination of its constitution. *Onderstepoort J. Vet. Sci. and Animal Ind.* (South Africa) 18: 197-202.

VERB 4. Louw, P.G.J. 1948. Lantadene A, the active principle of *Lantana camara*. II. Isolation of lantadene B, and the oxygen functions of lantadene A and lantadene B. *Ondestepoort J. Vet. Sci. and Animal Ind.* (South Africa) 23: 233-238.

VERB 5. Barton, D.H.R., P. de Mayo, E.W. Warnhoff, O. Jeger & J.W. Perold. 1954. Triterpenoids. Part XIX. The constitution of lantadene B. *J. Chem. Soc.*: 3689-3692.

VERB 6. Barton, D.H.R., P. de Mayo & J.C. Orr. 1956. Triterpenoids. Part XXIII. The nature of lantadene A. *J. Chem. Soc.*: 4160-4162.

VERB 7. Barua, A.K., P. Chakrabarti, S.P. Dutta, D.K. Mukherjee & B.C. Das. 1971. Triterpenoids. XXXVII. The structure and stereochemistry of lantanolic acid — a new triterpenoid from *Lantana camara*. *Tetrahedron* 27: 1141-1147.

VERB 8. Barua, A.K., P. Chakrabarti, M.K. Chowdhury, A. Basak & K. Basu. 1976. The structure and stereochemistry of lantanilic acid, the â, â-dimethylacryloyl ester of lantaninilic acid isolated from *Lantana camara*. *Phytochemistry* 15: 987-989.

VERB 9. Seawright, A.A. 1963. Studies on experimental intoxication of sheep with *Lantana camara*. *Austr. Vet. J.* 9: 340-344.

VERB 10. Seawright, A.A. & J.G. Allen. 1972. Pathology of the liver and kidneys in *Lantana* poisoning of cattle. *Austr. Vet. J.* 48: 323-333.

VERB 11. Herbert, J.M., J.P. Maffrand, K. Taoubi, J.M. Angereaux, I. Fouraste & J. Gleye. 1991. Verbascoside isolated from *Lantana camara*, an inhibitor of protein kinase C. *J. Nat. Prod.* 54: 1595-1600.

VERB 12. Craveiro, A.A., J.W. Alencar, F.J.A. Matos, C.H.S. Andrade & M.I.L. Machado. 1981. Essential oils from Brazilian Verbenaceae, genus *Lippia*. *J. Nat. Prod.* 44: 598-601.

VERB 13. Ramos, L.S., J.G.S. Maia, M. Leão da Silva, A.I.R. Luz & M.G.B. Zoghbi. 1982. Óleos essenciais, oleaginosas e látices da Amazônia. 12. Estudo da composição química de algumas espécies da família Verbenaceae. *Ciência e Cultura* (São Paulo) 34 (Supl.): 511.

VERB 14. Duret, S., H. Jacquemin, & R.R. Paris. 1976. Plantes malagaches. XIX. Sur la composition chimique de *Stachytarpheta jamaicensis* (L.) Vahl, Verbenacées. *Plantes Méd. Phytothér.* 10: 96-104.

VIOLACEAE

Alsodeia flavescens (Aubl.) Spreng.

AREA: Amazonia.

VIOLACEAE

Anchietea pyrifolia

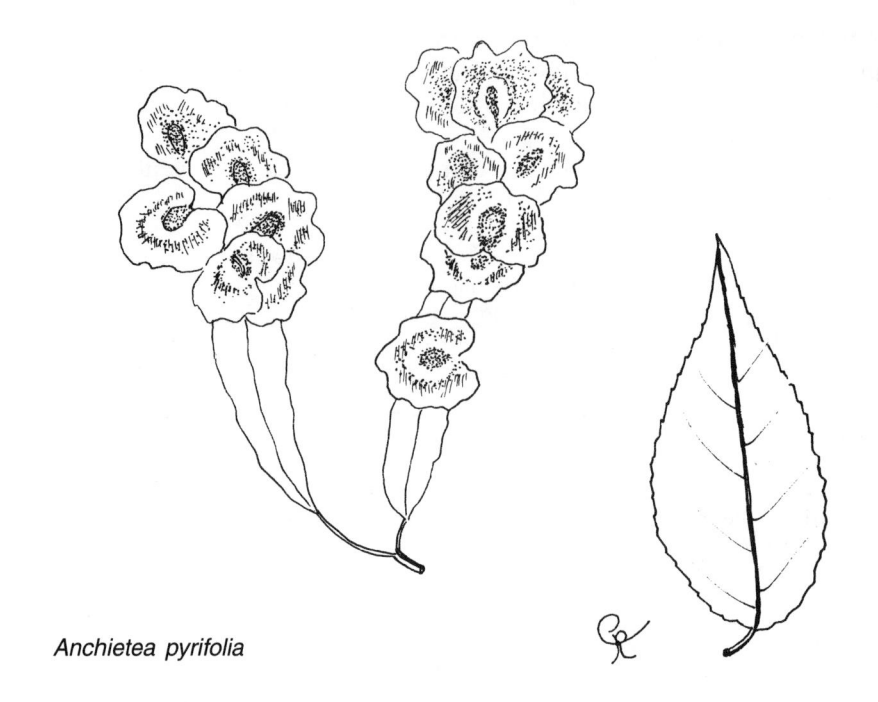

NAME: Jacamim-renepeá.
USES: Bark is febrifuge. Leaves are bitter, astringent.

Anchietea pyrifolia (Mart.) G. Don
AREA: Goiás to Rio Grande do Sul, forest.
NAMES: Cipó-suma, paraguaia, piraguaia, piriguara, purunara.
USES: Depurative, especially for dermal diseases and, among these, more indicated for syphilitic lesions. Its decoction acts as a mild purgative and sialagogue. Also prescribed for infantile whooping cough.
CHEM. & PHARM.: The reserve material in the roots was identified as inulin (Ref: VIOL 1). Triterpenoids have been isolated from the whole plant (Ref: VIOL 2).

Corynostylis hybanthus (L.) Mart. & Zucc.
AREA: Amazonia.
NAMES: Ipecacuanha, piraguaia.
USE: Roots are emetic.

Hybanthus atropurpureus Taub.
AREA: Goiás to São Paulo, campo.
NAMES: Apanha-saia, ganha-saia, purga-de-veado, purga-de-vento.
USES: Roots are purgative and depurative, but their use is said to be dangerous.

Hybanthus ipecacuanha (L.) Baill.
AREA: Neotropical; Maranhão to São Paulo, in the coastal belt and campo.
NAMES: Ipecacuanha-branca, poaia-branca, poaia-da-praia, purga-de-campo.
USES: Roots are emetocathartic, employed in the same manner as the genuine ipecacuanha (Rubiaceae), although devoid of emetine and also otherwise chemically unrelated.
CHEM.: Like a number of other members of the Violaceae, the roots contain methyl salicylate (Ref: VIOL 3). Their reserve material has also been described as inulin (Ref: VIOL 4).

Ionidium poaya St.-Hil.
AREA: Goiás and Minas Gerais, campo.
NAMES: Poaia, purga-do-campo.
USES: This species, like the preceding one, belongs to the so-called "false poaias," which, although unrelated, are used for the same purposes as the genuine ipecacuanha, *Cephaelis ipecacuanha* Rich. (Rubiaceae).

Violaceae – References

VIOL 1. Kraus, G. 1879. Inulin bei Violaceae. *Sitzungsber. Naturforsch. Ges. Halle 1879*: 6-8.
VIOL 2. Matida, A.K., M.M. Nakada, A.S.S. Andreoni & R. Zelnik. 1992. Triterpenoids from *Anchietea salutaris. Fitoterapia 63*: 271.
VIOL 3. Desmoulières, A. 1904. Occurrence naturelle de l'acide salycilique en certaines plantes des Violacées. *J. Pharm. Chim. 19*: 121-125.
VIOL 4. Beauvisage, M. 1889. L'inuline das les *Ionidium*. Étude anatomique du faux ipecacuanha blanc du Brésil, *Ionidium ipecacuanha* Vent. *Bull. Soc. Bot. Lyon* [2] *6*: 12-23.

VITACEAE

Cissus palmata Poir.
AREA: Rio Grande do Sul, forest.
NAME: Salsa-moura.
USES: Roots are depurative and antirheumatic.

Cissus salutaris H.B.K.
AREA: Bahia to São Paulo, forest.
NAME: Uva-do-campo.
USE: Roots are recommended for dropsy.

Cissus sicyoides L.
AREA: Neotropical; throughout Brazil, sometimes cultivated as an ornamental.
NAMES: Anil-trepador, cipó-pucá, cipó-puci, cortina-de-pobre, pucá.
USES: Tea from leaves is drunk for heart problems, tachycardia, hydropsy,

VITACEAE / WINTERACEAE

high blood pressure and anemia. In the Amazon the sap is used for epilepsy.

PHARM.: Preliminary experiments have indicated positive results against convulsions induced in laboratory animals by metrazol and electric shock (Ref: VITA 1,2).

Vitaceae – References

VITA 1. Elisabetsky, E. & H. Santana. 1984. Avaliação psicofarmacológica de um anticonvulsivante caseiro. *Ciência e Cultura* (São Paulo) *36* (7): 990-991.

VITA 2. Elisabetsky, E., M.P. Carrera, K.M.C. Teixeira, A.H. Müller & B.A.S. Moura. 1988. Estudo pré-clínico da ação anticonvulsivante do *Cissus sicyoides*. *X Simpósio de Plantas Medicinais do Brasil*, São Paulo. Summary of papers: 6/08.

VOCHYSIACEAE

Callisthene major Mart.
AREA: Central Brazil; dry forest and cerrado.
NAMES: Carvoeira, itapicuru, itapiúva, jacará-mirim, pau-terra-do-mato, tiriba.
USES: Bark used in baths, for the treatment of chronic lymphangitis.

Vochysia thyrsoidea Pohl
AREA: Ceará to São Paulo; cerrado and campo.
NAMES: Goma-arábica, gomeira, pau-de-vinho, vinheiro-do-campo.
USES: Bark employed for treating afflictions of the respiratory tract.
CHEM.: Bark contains ellagic acid derivatives (Ref: VOCH 1).

Vochysiaceae – Reference

VOCH 1. Corrêa, D.B., E. Birchal, J.E. Vale Aquilar & O.R. Gottlieb. 1975. Ellagic acids from Vochysiaceae. *Phytochemistry 14*: 1138-1139.

WINTERACEAE

Drimys winteri Forst.
AREA: Neotropical, observed thoughout Brazil, forest.
NAMES: Canela-amarga, capororoca-picante, casca-d'anta, cataia, paratudo, pau-para-tudo.
USES: Bark is stomachic, antiscorburic, antispasmodic (for intestinal colic), sudorific, antidiarrhoeic, tonic, antidyspeptic, for chronic catarrh; also used for invigorating a person during convalescence.
CHEM. & PHARM.: Sesquiterpenoids of *Drimys winteri* have been extensively investigated. Comprehensive overviews of the early studies have been published (Ref: WINT 1,2). For more recent findings see Ref: WINT 3,4.

Drimys winteri

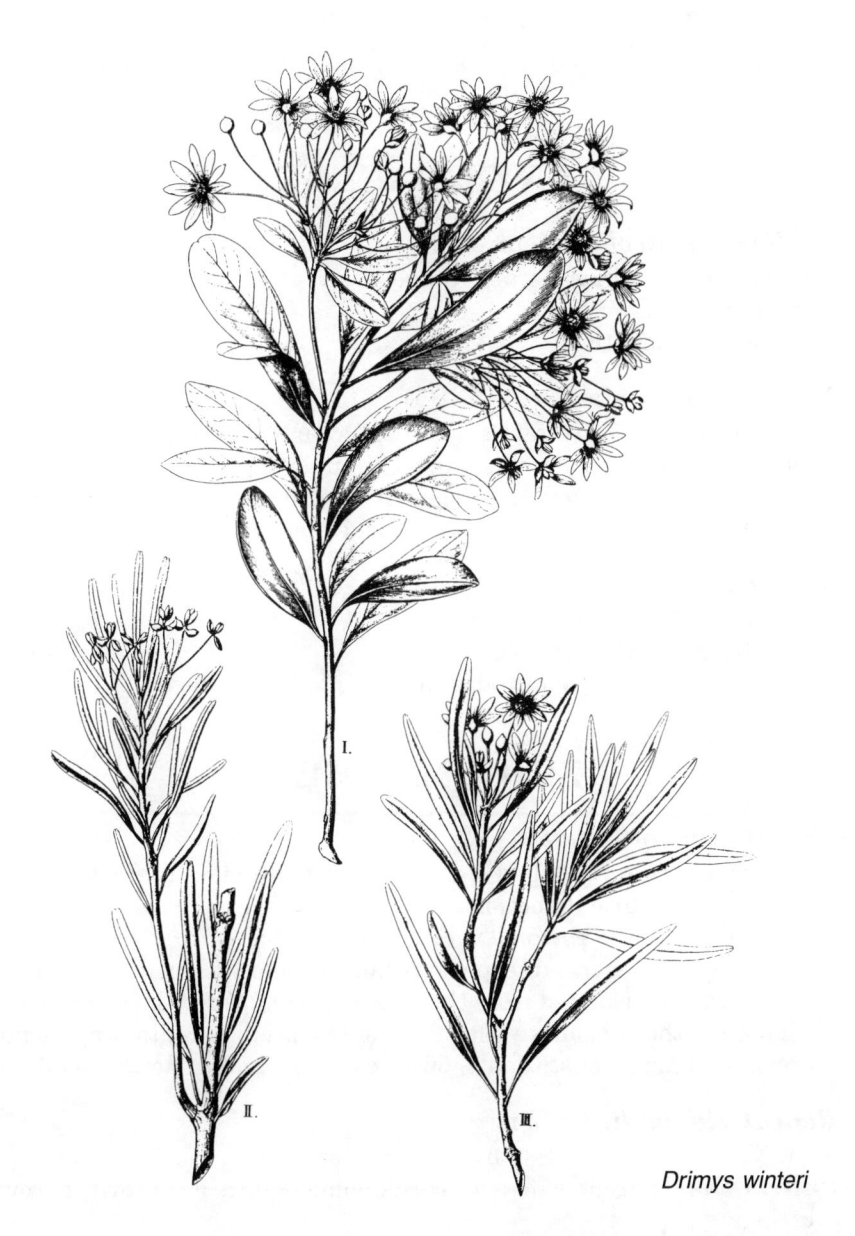

Winteraceae – References

WINT 1. Appel, H.H., C.J.W. Brooks & K.H. Overton. 1959. Constitution and stereochemistry of drimenol, a novel bicyclic sesquiterpenoid. *J. Chem. Soc.* 3322-3332.

WINT 2. Appel, H.H., J.D. Connolly, K.H. Overton & R.P.M. Bond. 1960. Sesquiterpenoids. Part II. The constitution and stereochemistry of drimenin, isodrimenin and confertifolin. *J. Chem. Soc.*: 4685-4692.

WINT 3. Aasen, A.J., T. Nishida, C.R. Enzell & H.H. Appel. 1977. The structure of (11ξ, 12ξ)-11, 12-di (7-drimen-11-oxy) -11,12-epoxy-7-drimene. *Acta Chem. Scand., B 31*: 51-55.
WINT 4. Cortés, M. & M.L. Oyarzún. 1981. Tadeonal and isotadeonal from *Drimys winteri*. *Fitoterapia 52*: 33-35.

XYRIDACEAE

Abolboda poarchon Seub.
AREA: Goiás and Minas Gerais; campo.
NAME: Capim-rei.
USE: Roots are laxative.

Xyris laxifolia Mart.
AREA: Amazonia to Rio Grande do Sul, in swampy terrain.
NAMES: Botão-de-ouro, erva-de-empigem, jupicaí.
USES: Roots are emetocathartic. The contused aerial parts serve for dressings in hanseniasis, dartre, eczema and ringworm.

Xyris pallida Mart.
AREA: Amazonia to Ceará.
NAMES: Botão-de-ouro, maiaca.
USES: Used for the same purposes as *Xyris laxifolia* Mart.

ZINGIBERACEAE

Hedychium coronarium Koenig
AREA: Cosmopolitan; widely dispersed in Brazil in marshy tracts.
NAMES: Açucena, lírio-do-brejo.
USE: Starch from the rhizome is considered bechic.
CHEM. & PHARM.: Several diterpenes, some of them with cytotoxic properties, have been isolated from the rhizomes (Ref: ZING 1,2). Steam distillation of the rhizomes yields 0.1% of essential oil containing monoterpenes as main constituents, 60% being eucalyptol (Ref: ZING 3).

Renealmia exaltata L. f.
AREA: Neotropical; in forests in eastern Brazil.
NAMES: Cana-do-brejo, café-açu, cardamomo-do-brasil, pacová, pacová-catinga.
USES: Seeds are aromatic, anthelmintic. Rhizome is tonic, stomachic, carminative; infusion for cleaning ulcers.

Renealmia occidentalis Sweet
AREA: Amazonia to São Paulo and Mato Grosso, forest.

NAMES: Cana-branca, cana-do-mato, cardamomo-da-terra, cuité-açu, capitiú, paco-seroca, pacová.

USES: Rhizome is carminative, stomachic, tonic, antisyphilitic and used to cure old ulcers. Seeds are aromatic, sour, indicated to allay flatulence accompanied by colic; also given as an abortifacient.

Renealmia sylvestris Horan. (Amazonia to Rio de Janeiro) displays the same properties. These *Renealmia* species are frequently used as substitutes for the genuine cardamom (*Elettaria cardamomum* (L.) Maton, from Asia), an herb of the same family.

The Zingiberaceae formerly included the family Costaceae, which is treated herein under the latter name.

Zingiberaceae – References

ZING 1. Itokawa, H., H. Morita, I. Katon, K. Takeya, A.J. Cavalheiro, R.C.B. de Oliveira, M. Ishige & M. Motidome. 1988. Cytotoxic diterpenes from the rhizomes of *Hedychium coronarium*. *Planta Medica* 54: 311-315.

ZING 2. Itokawa, H., H. Morita, K. Takeya & M. Motidome. 1988. Diterpenes from rhizomes of *Hedychium coronarium*. *Chem. Pharm. Bull.* (Japan) 36: 2682-2684.

ZING 3. Gottlieb, O.R. & M.T. Magalhães. 1960. Eucaliptol no óleo essencial do rizoma do lírio do brejo. *In*: "Estudo de Plantas Odoriferas Brasileiras. III. Canela sassafrás, cascapreciosa, lírio do brejo." *Bol. Inst. Química Agrícola* (Rio de Janeiro) 60: 17-22.

NOTES & SYNONYMS

ADIANTACEAE. *Adiantopsis chlorophylla* (Sw.) Fée includes *Cheilanthes chlorophylla* Sw.
The fern family Adiantaceae was formerly included in Polypodiaceae.
AMARANTHACEAE. *Pfaffia jubata* Mart. includes *Gomphrena jubata* Moq.
AMARYLLIDACEAE. *Hippeastrum puniceum* (Lam.) Kuntze includes *Hippeastrum equestre* (L.) Herbert.
Hymenocallis tubiflora Salisb. includes *Pancratium guianensis* Ker-Gawl.
ANACARDIACEAE. *Spondias mombin* L. includes *Spondias lutea* L.
Myracroduon urundeuva Fr. All. includes *Astronium urundeuva* (Fr. All.) Engl.
ANNONACEAE. *Annona glabra* L. includes *Annona palustris* L.
APIACEAE. *Apium sellowianum* Wolf includes *Apium australe* Thouars.
Hydrocotyle bonariensis Lam. is sometimes included in *Hydrocotyle umbellata* L.
APOCYNACEAE. *Himatanthus drastica* (Mart.) Woods. includes *Plumeria drastica* Mart.
Himatanthus fallax (M. Arg.) Woods. includes *Plumeria fallax* M. Arg.
Himatanthus lancifolia (M. Arg.) Woods. includes *Plumeria lancifolia* M. Arg.
Himatanthus phagedaenica (Mart.) Woods. includes *Plumeria phagedaenica* Mart.
Himatanthus sucuuba (Spr. ex M. Arg.) Woods. includes *Plumeria sucuuba* Spr. ex M. Arg.
Mandevilla velutina (Mart. ex Stadelm.) Woods. var. *velutina*, a Brazilian plant (cf. *Ann. Missouri Bot. Gard.* 20: 732. 1933), is not to be confused with the Mexican and Central American "loroco" *Fernaldia pandurata* (A. DC.) Woods. (cf. *Econ. Bot.* 44(3): 301-310. 1990), a synonym of which is *Mandevilla velutina* K. Schum. (cf. *Ann. Missouri Bot. Gard.* 20: 777. 1933).
ARACEAE. Information from D.H. Nicolson: *Anthurium affine* Schott includes *Anthurium crassinervium* (Jacq.) Schott, which is an error for *Anthurium crassinervium* (Jacq.) G. Don (in Sweet, HORT. BRIT. ed. 3, 633. 1839). That name, as well as other "bird's nest anthuriums," apparently is misapplied. This problem has been approached by S. Mayo (*Kew Bull.* 36: 714-715. 1982), indicating that *Anthurium affine* Schott (of eastern Brazil) is probably the correct name for this plant.
Caladium bicolor (Aiton) Vent. var. *poecile* (Schott) Engler includes *Caladium poecile* Schott.
Caladium sororium Schott is doubtfully distinct from *Caladium bicolor* (Aiton) Vent.
Dieffenbachia seguine (Jacq.) Schott includes *Dieffenbachia picta* Schott.
Monstera adansonii Schott includes *Monstera pertusa* (L.) DeVries (1839), non (Roxb.) Schott (1830).
Montrichardia linifera is probably an ecological variant of *Montrichardia arborescens* (L.) Schott.
Philodendron hederaceum (Jacq.) Schott var. *hederaceum* includes *Philodendron cordatum* hort., non Vellozo, according to Croat, *Ann. Missouri Bot. Gard.* 84: 311-704 (1997).
Philodendron pedatum (Hook.) Kunth includes *Philodendron laciniatum* (Vell.) Engler.
Xanthosoma striatipes (Kunth & Bouché) Madison includes *Caladium striatipes* (Kunth & Bouché) Schott.

NOTES & SYNONYMS

ARECACEAE. In addition to comments from L.R. Noblick, the following reference was used by the authors as a guide to botanical nomenclature: Pio Corrêa, M. 1987. BRAZILIAN PALMS. Translated and edited by Pinheiro, C.U.B. and M.J. Balick. *Contrib. New York Bot. Gard.* 17: 1-50 + 38 figs.

Attalea spectabilis Mart. is an uncertain species which may be an *Orbignya* but whose holotype may have been destroyed. It is possibly identical to *Orbignya spectabilis* (Mart.) Burret, which is known from Pará.

Copernicia prunifera (Mill.) Moore includes *Copernicia cerifera* Mart.

Elaeis oleifera (H.B.K.) Cortez includes *Elaeis melanococca* Gaertn. and *Corozo oleifera* (H.B.K.) Bailey.

Orbignya phalerata Mart. is intended, in this volume, to include *Orbignya martiana* B. Rodr. As noted by Anderson, Overal & Henderson (1988; Ref: AREC 2), "*O. phalerata* is the principal species of the babassu complex and ranges from eastern Bolivia through northern and central Brazil to the Guianas... Frequently cited names such as *O. martiana* Barb. Rodr., *O. speciosa* (Mart.) Barb. Rodr., and *O. barbosiana* Burret have recently been reduced to synonymy under *O. phalerata* (Anderson & Balick, 1988)." Prior to conclusions based on fieldwork, as noted by Anderson & Balick (1988; Ref: AREC 1), *Orbignya martiana* was the earliest, validly published name definitely referable to babassu." Another dimension of complexity in babassu nomenclature is demonstrated by the acceptance of *Attalea speciosa* Mart. ex Spreng. as the correct name, in Henderson, A. 1995. THE PALMS OF THE AMAZON. 362 pp. New York and Oxford: Oxford University Press (p. 153), which is also maintained in Henderson, A., Galeano, G. and R. Bernal. 1995. FIELD GUIDE TO THE PALMS OF THE AMERICAS. 352 pp. Princeton, New Jersey: Princeton University Press (p. 163). It should be noted that *Orbignya phalerata* Mart. is not the same plant as *Scheelea phalerata* (Mart. ex Spreng.) Burret (Synonym: *Attalea phalerata* Mart. ex Spreng.), the most common attaleoid palm of the Pantanal region of Mato Grosso do Sul, Brazil. *Scheelea phalerata* (Mart. ex Spreng.) Burret should not be confused with *Scheelea princeps* (Mart.) Karst., which is a Bolivian species.

ASCLEPIADACEAE. *Marsdenia amylacea* (Barb. Rodr.) Malme includes *Elcomarhiza amylacea* Barb. Rodr.

ASTERACEAE. *Acmella oleracea* (L.) R.K. Jansen includes *Spilanthes oleracea* L.

Acmella repens (Walt.) L.C. Rich. includes *Spilanthes americana* (Mutis) Hieron. This plant is frequently cited in Brazil as *Spilanthes acmella*. However, this "*S. acmella* auct." is quite distinct from *S. acmella* (L.) Murr., which is not found in Brazil.

Ayapana triplinerve (Vahl) King & Robinson includes *Eupatorium triplinerve* Vahl and *Eupatorium ayapana* Vent.

Baccharidastrum triplinerve (Less.) Cabr. includes *Conyza triplinervia* Less.

Baccharis trimera (Less.) DC. includes *Baccharis genistelloides* Pers.

Chromolaena hirsuta (Hook. & Arn.) King & Robinson includes *Eupatorium bartisiifolium* DC. and *Eupatorium subhastatum* Hook. & Arn.

Chromolaena laevigata (Lam.) King & Robinson includes *Eupatorium laevigatum* Lam.

Cyrtocymura scorpioides (Lam.) Robinson includes *Vernonia scorpioides* Lam.

Eclipta prostrata (L.) L. includes *Eclipta alba* (L.) Hassk. and *Eclipta erecta* Lam.

Egletes viscosa (L.) Less. includes *Cotula viscosa* L.

Elephantopus mollis H.B.K. includes *Elephantopus scaber* L.

Gochnatia polymorpha (Less.) Cabr. includes *Moquinia polymorpha* DC.

Isostigma megapotamicum (Spr.) Sherff includes *Isostigma peucedanifolium* Less.

Mikania parviflora (Aubl.) Karst. includes *Mikania amara* Willd.

Noticastrum diffusum (Pers.) Cabr. includes *Aster montevidensis* (Spr.) Gris.

Pluchea suaveolens (Vell.) O. Ktze. includes *Epaltes brasiliensis* DC., *Pluchea quitoc* DC., and *Pluchea sagittalis* (Lam.) Cabr.

Raulinoreitzia tremula (Hook. & Arn.) King & Robinson includes *Eupatorium tremulum* Hook. & Arn.

Solidago chilensis Meyen includes *Solidago microglossa* DC.

Sphagneticola trilobata (L.) Pruski includes *Wedelia trilobata* (L.) Hitch. and *Wedelia paludosa* DC.

Stomatanthes oblongifolius (Spr.) Robinson includes *Eupatorium oblongifolium* (Spr.) Bak.

Unxia camphorata L.f. includes *Melampodium camphoratum* (L.f.) Benth. & Hook.

Vernonanthura brasiliana (L.) Robinson includes *Vernonia brasiliana* (L.) Druce.

BALANOPHORACEAE. *Helosis cayennensis* (Swartz) Spreng. includes *Helosis guyanensis* Rich., according to Hansen, B. 1980. *Flora Neotropica*, Monograph No. 23, Balanophoraceae, pp. 35-41.

BIGNONIACEAE. *Adenocalymma alliacea* (Lam.) Miers includes *Bignonia alliacea* Lam. and *Pseudocalymma alliacea* (Lam.) Sandw.

Sparattosperma leucanthum (Vell.) K. Sch. includes *Sparattosperma vernicosum* Bur. & K. Sch.

Tabebuia ipe (Mart.) Standl. includes *Tabebuia avellanedae* Lour.

CAESALPINIACEAE. *Senna latifolia* (Meyer) Ir. & Barn. includes *Cassia sclerocarpa* Vog.

CAMPANULACEAE. *Centropogon cornutus* (L.) Druce includes *Centropogon surinamensis* (L.) Presl.

Hippobroma longiflora (L.) G. Don includes *Lobelia longiflora* L., *Isotoma longiflora* (L.) Presl, and *Laurentia longiflora* (L.) Endl.

CARICACEAE. *Jacaratia spinosa* (Aubl.) A. DC. includes *Jacaratia dodecaphylla* (Vell.) A. DC.

CLADONIACEAE. *Cladonia miniata* Mey. includes *Cladonia sanguinea* Mart.

CLUSIACEAE. *Hypericum brasiliense* Choisy includes *Hypericum laxiusculum* St.-Hil.

COMMELINACEAE. *Tradescantia spathacea* Sw. includes *Rhoeo spathacea* (Sw.) Stearn and *Rhoeo discolor* (L'Her.) Hance.

CONVOLVULACEAE. *Calonyction aculeatum* (L.) House includes *Ipomoea bona-nox* L.

COSTACEAE. *Costus cuspidatus* (Nees & Mart.) Maas includes *Costus igneus* N.E. Brown.

CRASSULACEAE. *Kalanchoe brasiliensis* Cambess. includes *Kalanchoe crenata* (Andrews) Haworth (non R. Hamet) and *Kalanchoe integra* (Medic.) Kuntze var. *verea* (Jacq.) Cuf. Wickens, G.E. 1987. Crassulaceae, in R.M. Polhill, ed., FLORA OF TROPICAL EAST AFRICA. maintains *K. crenata* as the valid designation for *K. brasiliensis* (pp. 42-45). The name *Kalanchoe crenata* (Baker) R. Hamet is a synonym of *K. laxiflora* Baker.

Kalanchoe pinnata (Lam.) Pers. includes *Bryophyllum pinnatum* (Lam.) Oken and *Bryophyllum calycinum* Salisb.

CUCURBITACEAE. *Cayaponia espelina* (Manso) Cogn. includes *Perianthopodus espelina* Manso.

Cayaponia martiana (Cogn.) Cogn. includes *Trianosperma ficifolia* Cogn. and *Trianosperma martiana* Cogn.

Lagenaria siceraria (Molina) Standl. includes *Lagenaria vulgaris* Serr.

Melothrianthus smilacifolius (Cogn.) M. Crovetto includes *Apodanthera smilacifolia* Cogn.

CYATHEACEAE. *Cyathea armata* (Sw.) Domin includes *Alsophila armata* (Sw.) Presl.

Cyathea microdonta (Desv.) Domin includes *Alsophila microdonta* Desv.

CYPERACEAE. *Cyperus sesquiflorus* (Torrey) Mattf. & Kükent. is sometimes synonymized with *Kyllinga odorata* Vahl.

NOTES & SYNONYMS

DENNSTAEDTIACEAE. The fern family Dennstaedtiaceae was formerly included in Polypodiaceae.

DRYOPTERIDACEAE. *Rumohra adiantiformis* (G. Forst.) Ching includes *Aspidium capense* Willd.

EUPHORBIACEAE. *Croton triqueter* Lam. includes *Julocroton triqueter* (Lam.) M. Arg.

Euphorbia hirta L. includes *Euphorbia pilulifera* L., *fide* Howard, R.A. 1989. FLORA OF THE LESSER ANTILLES 5: 25, wherein *E. hirta* is treated as *Chamaesyce hirta* (L.) Millsp.; the placement in *Chamaesyce* is accepted by Webster, G.L. 1991. Euphorbiaceae, in Nicolson, D.H., Flora of Dominica, Part 2: Dicotyledoneae. *Smithsonian Contributions to Botany* 77: 82, but conversely is accepted as *Euphorbia hirta* by Correll, D.C. and H.B. Correll. 1982. FLORA OF THE BAHAMA ARCHIPELAGO, pp. 809-910.

Julocroton Mart. is currently considered a synonym of *Croton* L.; appropriate transfers of the two *Julocroton* species treated herein await publication by specialists.

Phyllanthus tenellus Roxb. includes *Phyllanthus corcovadensis* M. Arg.

FABACEAE. *Acosmium dasycarpum* (Vog.) Yakovl. includes *Sweetia dasycarpa* Vog.

Erythrina fusca Lour. includes *Erythrina glauca* Willd.

Erythrina verna Vell. includes *Erythrina mulungu* Mart.

Periandra mediterranea (Vell.) Taub. is frequently cited as *Periandra dulcis* Mart.

GENTIANACEAE. *Curtia tenuifolia* (Aubl.) Knobl. includes *Schnebleria tenuifolia* (Aubl.) G. Don.

Schultesia stenophylla Mart. includes *Schultesia guianensis* Malme.

Zygostigma australe (Cham. & Schl.) Gris. includes *Zygostigma uniflorum* Gris.

GESNERIACEAE. *Sinningia allagophylla* (Mart.) Wiehl. includes *Gesneria allagophylla* Mart.

HELICONIACEAE. *Heliconia angusta* Vell. includes *Heliconia brasiliensis* Hook.

HIPPOCRATEACEAE. *Peritassa calypsoides* (Camb.) A.C. Sm. includes *Salacia calypsoides* Camb. and *Salacia silvestris* Steud.

Salacia impressifolia (Miers) A.C. Sm. includes *Salacia grandiflora* Peyr.

Tontelea brachypoda Miers includes *Salacia brachypoda* (Miers) Peyr.

HUMIRIACEAE. *Humiria balsamifera* (Aubl.) St. Hil. possibly includes *Humiria floribunda* (Spr.) Mart. Information given for *H. balsamifera* also applies to *H. floribunda*.

ICACINACEAE. *Citronella congonha* (Mart.) Howard includes *Villaresia congonha* (Mart.) Miers.

Citronella mucronata (R. & Pav.) Don includes *Villaresia mucronata* R. & Pav.

LAMIACEAE. *Coleus barbatus* Benth. is often included in *Coleus forskohlii* (Willd.) Briq.

Keithia denudata Benth. is sometimes synonymized with *Rhabdocaulon denudatus* (Benth.) Epling.

Marsypianthes chamaedrys (Vahl) O. Ktze. includes *Marsypianthes hyptoides* Mart.

LAURACEAE. *Aiovea brasiliensis* Meissn. includes *Aydendron tenellum* Meissn.

Cassytha filiformis L. includes *Cassytha americana* Nees.

Cryptocarya minima Mez includes *Aydendron floribundum* Meissn.

Licaria camara includes *Acrodiclidium camara* Schomb.

Ocotea cymbarum H.B.K. includes the synonyms *Nectandra barcellensis* Meissn. and *Nectandra elaiophora* B. Rodr.

LECYTHIDACEAE. *Gustavia hexapetala* (Aubl.) J.E. Smith includes *Gustavia brasiliana* DC.

Lecythis amara Aubl. includes *Chytroma amara* Aubl.

Lecythis pisonis Camb. includes *Lecythis usitata* Miers.

LILIACEAE. *Smilax longifolia* Rich. includes *Smilax papyracea* Duham. The genus *Smilax* is sometimes placed in a separate family: Smilacaceae.

Notes & Synonyms

LOGANIACEAE. *Strychnos subcordata* Spr. ex Benth. includes *Strychnos ericetina* Barb. Rodr.

Strychnos trinervis (Vell.) Mart. includes *Strychnos triplinervia* Mart.

MALVACEAE. *Modiolastrum pinnatipartitum* (St. Hil. & Naudin) Krapovickas probably includes *Modiolastrum jaeggianum* Schumann.

Hibiscus tiliaceus L., according to Fryxell, P.A., *Syst. Bot. Monogr.* 25: 217-218 (1988), is the plant cultivated as a street tree in the neotropics, whereas *Hibiscus pernambucensis* Arruda is a distinct native species, not the cultivated entity.

Plants attributed to *Sida rhombea* L. are probably conspecific with *Sida rhombifolia* L., which is also in the text.

MARTYNIACEAE. *Ibicella lutea* (Lindl.) Van Eselt. includes *Martynia lutea* Lindl., *Martynia montevidensis* Cham. and *Proboscidea lutea* (Lindl.) Stapf.

MELASTOMATACEAE. *Macairea radula* (Bonpl.) DC. includes *Macairea sericea* Cogn.

Tibouchina clavata (Pers.) Wurdack includes *Tibouchina holosericea* (Sw.) Baill.

MELIACEAE. *Cabralea canjerana* (Vell.) Mart. includes *Cabralea glaberrima* Juss., *Cabralea laevis* DC. and *Cabralea multijuga* DC.

Cedrela fissilis Vell. includes *Cedrela angustifolia* Sessé & Moc.

Guarea trichilioides L. includes *Guarea guidona* (L.) Sleum.

MENISPERMACEAE. *Abuta rufescens* Aubl. includes *Abuta splendida* Kr. & Mold.

MENYANTHACEAE. *Nymphoides indica* (L.) O. Ktze. includes *Nymphoides humboldtianum* (Kunth) O. Ktze.

MIMOSACEAE. Most *Anadenanthera* species were formerly included in the genus *Piptadenia*.

Anadenanthera colubrina (Vell.) Brenan includes *Piptadenia colubrina* Benth.

Mimosa bimucronata (DC.) O. Ktze. includes *Mimosa sepiaria* Benth.

Parapiptadenia rigida (Benth.) Brenan includes *Piptadenia rigida* Benth.

Stryphnodendron adstringens (Mart.) Cov. includes *Stryphnodendron barbatimam* (Vell.) Mart.

MONIMIACEAE. *Mollinedia schottiana* (Spr.) Perk. includes *Mollinedia brasiliensis* Schott.

Siparuna brasiliensis (Spr.) DC. includes *Citriosma apiosyce* Tul.

MORACEAE. *Ficus gomelleira* Kunth & Bouché includes *Ficus doliaria* Mart.

Ficus insipida Willd. includes *Ficus anthelmintica* Mart., *Ficus helminthagoga* Dugand and *Ficus vermifuga* Miq.

Ficus trigona L.f. includes *Ficus fagifolia* Miq.

Maclura sclerophylla (Ducke) C.C. Berg includes *Olmedioperebea sclerophylla* Ducke.

Maclura tinctoria (L.) D. Don includes *Chlorophora tinctoria* (L.) Gaud.

Sorocea bonplandii (Baill.) Burger includes *Sorocea ilicifolia* Miq.

MYRTACEAE. *Eugenia uniflora* L. is sometimes cited as *Stenocalyx michelii* Berg.

Myrcia sphaerocarpa DC. includes *Myrcia multiflora* (Lam.) DC.

Psidium cattleyanum Sabine includes *Psidium littorale* Raddi and *Psidium variabile* Berg. Both *P. cattleyanum* and *P. littorale* were published in 1820, and thus it is difficult to decide which name has priority. Different researchers prefer one or the other, and sometimes an author uses both names on different occasions.

Psidium cinereum Mart. includes *Psidium incanescens* Mart., the latter from Minas Gerais to Rio Grande do Sul.

NYCTAGINACEAE. *Boerhavia coccinea* Mill. includes *Boerhavia repens* L., *Boerhavia diffusa* L. and *Boerhavia hirsuta* Willd.

Boerhavia paniculata Rich. is sometimes included in *Boerhavia coccinea* Mill.

NOTES & SYNONYMS

Torrubia olfersiana (Link, Klotzsch & Otto) Standl. includes *Guapira olfersiana* (Link, Klotzsch & Otto) Lundell. The plant also has been accorded the rank of synonym of the eastern Brazilian *Guapira opposita* (Vell.) Reitz, FLORA ILUSTRADA CATARINENSE (Fasciculo Nictaginaceas) *32* (1970) var. *opposita.*

NYMPHAEACEAE. *Victoria amazonica* (Poepp.) Sower. includes *Victoria regia* Lindl.

OLACACEAE. *Ptychopetalum olacoides* Benth. includes citations of *Liriosma ovata* Miers in the early literature of the family.

ONAGRACEAE. The genus *Ludwigia* L. was previously designated as *Jussiaea* L.

PASSIFLORACEAE. *Passiflora macrocarpa* Mast. includes *Passiflora quadrangularis* L.

PIPERACEAE. *Ottonia jaborandi* (Vell.) Kunth includes *Ottonia anisum* Spreng.

Pothomorphe peltata (L.) Miq. includes *Piper peltatum* L. and *Lepianthes peltata* (L.) Raf.

PLUMBAGINACEAE. *Limonium brasiliense* (Boiss.) O. Ktze. includes *Statice brasiliensis* Boiss.

POACEAE. *Cymbopogon schoenanthus* (L.) Spreng. includes *Cymbopogon citratus* Stapf and *Andropogon schoenanthus* L.

POLYGONACEAE. *Polygonum punctatum* Elliot includes *Polygonum acre* L.

Triplaris weigeltiana (Reichb.) O. Ktze. includes *Triplaris surinamensis* Cham.

POLYPODIACEAE. *Microgramma vaccinifolia* (Langsd. & Fisch.) Copel. includes *Polypodium vaccinifolium* Langsd. & Fisch.

Phlebodium aureum (L.) J.E. Smith includes *Polypodium aureum* L.

Phlebodium decumanum (Willd.) J. Smith includes *Polypodium decumanum* Willd.

RHAMNACEAE. *Reisseckia smilacina* (Sm.) Steud. includes *Reisseckia cordifolia* Steud.

RUBIACEAE. *Chiococca alba* (L.) Hitch. includes *Chiococca brachiata* Ruiz & Pavon.

Manettia ignita (Vell.) K. Sch. includes *Manettia cordifolia* Mart.

RUTACEAE. *Zanthoxylum* L. includes the genus *Fagara* Duham.

SAPINDACEAE. *Magonia pubescens* St.-Hil. includes *Magonia glabrata* St.-Hil.

SAPOTACEAE. *Manilkara zapota* (L.) Van Royen includes *Pouteria sapota* (Jacq.) Moore & Stearn and *Achras zapota* L.

SCHIZAEACEAE. *Anemia phyllitidis* (L.) Sw. includes *Anemia fraxinifolia* Raddi.

SOLANACEAE. *Acnistus arborescens* (L.) Schl. includes *Acnistus cauliflorus* Schott and *Dunalia arborescens* (L.) Sleumer.

Solanum nigrum L. includes *Solanum americanum* Mill.

STERCULIACEAE. *Guazuma ulmifolia* Lam. var. *tomentella* Schum. includes *Guazuma tomentosa* H.B.K.

Sterculia apetala (Jacq.) Karst. var. *elata* (Ducke) E. Taylor includes *Sterculia elata* Ducke.

URTICACEAE. *Laportea aestuans* (L.) Chew includes *Fleurya aestuans* (L.) Miq.

VERBENACEAE. *Aloysia triphylla* (L'Her.) Britt. includes *Aloysia virgata* (Ruiz & Pavon) Juss., *Aloysia citriodora* (Cav.) Ort. and *Lippia citriodora* H.B.K.

Lippia alba (Mill.) N.E. Brown includes *Lippia geminata* Kunth.

VIOLACEAE. *Anchietea pyrifolia* (Mart.) G. Don includes *Anchietea salutaris* St.-Hil.

Hybanthus ipecacuanha (L.) Baill. includes *Ionidium ipecacuanha* (L.) Vent.

ZINGIBERACEAE. *Hedychium coronarium* Koenig includes *Hedychium flavescens* Carey.

Glossary

ABORTIFACIENT – a drug or material that causes the expulsion of the fetus.
ABORTIVE – effecting an abortion.
ABRASIVE – causing abrasion; a substance used for abrading, grinding or polishing.
ABSCESS – localized collection of pus or liquid derived from blood in any part of the body.
ADENITIS – inflammation of a gland.
AEROPHAGY (aerophagia) – spasmodic swallowing of air, followed by eructations.
ALBUGO – a white opacity of the cornea of the eye.
ALBUMINURIA – the excretion of abnormal amounts of albumin in the urine.
ALEXIPHARMIC – an antidote, warding off the ill effects of a poison.
ALOPECIA – baldness, loss of hair.
AMEBIASIS (amoebiasis) – the state of being infected with amoebae, especially with *Entamoeba histolytica*.
AMENORRHOEA – the absence of menstrual bleeding.
AMYGDALITIS – inflammation of the tonsils.
ANALEPTIC – a drug which acts as a stimulant of the central nervous system.
ANALGESIC (antialgesic) – an agent causing the loss of sensitivity to pain.
ANAPHRODISIAC – a substance or drug which suppresses the sexual urge.
ANASARCA – generalized massive edema.
ANCYLOSTOMIASIS – disease caused by infection with *Ancylostoma* or *Necator* hookworms.
ANEMIA – an abnormal decrease in red blood cells.
ANGINA – various conditions characterized by painful or cramping spasms.
ANTHELMINTIC – a drug which kills or causes destruction and expulsion of intestinal worms. The same as Vermifuge.
ANTHRAX – an often fatal, infectious disease spread from animals to humans, caused by *Bacillus anthracis*.
ANTIANEMIC – a drug which increases the count of red blood cells or their hemoglobin content.
ANTIASTHMATIC – affording relief of asthma; an agent that relieves the spasms of asthma.
ANTIBLENNORRHAGIC – curing or relieving gonorrhoea; see BLENNORRHAGIA.
ANTICANCERIGENOUS – see CARCINOSTATIC.
ANTICHOLESTERASIC – a substance which inhibits the action of cholinesterase.
ANTIDIABETIC – hypoglycemic; a material which lowers the concentration of sugar in the blood.
ANTIDIARRHOEIC – a drug or substance that acts against diarrhoea.

GLOSSARY

ANTIDYSENTERIC – preventing, alleviating or curing dysentery.
ANTIDYSPEPTIC – acting against dyspepsia or indigestion.
ANTIEMETIC – having the effect of suppressing vomiting.
ANTIFUNGAL – destructive to fungi, or suppressing their reproduction or growth; effective against fungus infections.
ANTIGOUTOSE – drug that acts to alleviate the gout.
ANTIHEPATOTOXIC – drug that acts to alleviate toxicity to liver cells.
ANTIHYDROPIC – an agent that prevents or relieves dropsical conditions.
ANTIHYSTERIC – preventing or relieving hysteria.
ANTI-INFLAMMATORY – counteracting or suppressing inflammation. The same as Antiphlogistic.
ANTILUETIC – *see* ANTISYPHILITIC.
ANTIMALARIAL – an agent that is therapeutically effective against malaria.
ANTIODONTALGIC – a substance used against toothache.
ANTIOPHIDIC – active against snake venom.
ANTIPHLOGISTIC – *see* ANTI-INFLAMMATORY.
ANTIPOISON – a remedy for counteracting a poison. The same as Alexipharmic.
ANTIPYRETIC – an agent that prevents or reduces fever.
ANTIRABIES – a drug or substance which prevents or cures rabies.
ANTISCORBUTIC – any substance that prevents or cures scurvy.
ANTISEPTIC – a substance that inhibits the growth and development of microorganisms without necessarily destroying them.
ANTISPASMODIC – spasmolytic; a drug or agent that prevents or relieves spasms or the involuntary and irregular contractions of the body muscles.
ANTISYPHILITIC – a drug which is effective against or a remedy for syphilis. The same as Antiluetic.
ANTITHERMIC – antipyretic; a substance that reduces fever; also antifebrile, febrifuge.
ANTITUSSIVE – a drug that reduces or prevents cough.
ANURIA – the absence of urine production.
APERIENT – a mild laxative.
APHRODISIAC – an agent or substance that causes the stimulation of sexual passion and libido.
APHTHA (plural: APHTHAE) – an ulcer of the mucous membrane, usually oral.
AROMATIC – a medicinal substance with a spicy fragrance and stimulant qualities.
ARTERIOSCLEROSIS – hardening of the walls of the arteries.
ARTHRALGIA – neuralgia or pain in the joints.
ARTHRITIS – inflammation of joints.
ASCITES – effusion of serous fluid into the abdominal cavity, often a complication of cirrhosis of the liver.
ASTHMA – a chronic respiratory disease, often derived from allergies, and accompanied by labored breathing, chest constriction and coughing.
ASTRINGENT – a substance that contracts the body tissues to check the discharge of secretion or arrest capillary bleeding. The same as Styptic.

Glossary

Athlete's Foot – a fungal infection of the foot, causing itching, blisters, and cracking of the skin.
Balsamic – soothing, of the nature of a balsam.
Bechic – a tonic or other remedy that controls coughing.
Beriberi – a thiamine deficiency disease of the peripheral nervous system, characterized by partial paralysis of the extremities, emaciation and anemia.
Biliary – pertaining to bile, a yellowish liquid secreted by the liver and stored in the gall bladder.
Bitter – a medicinal agent that has a bitter taste, used as an appetizer.
Blennorrhagia – gonorrhoea; an inordinate secretion and discharge of mucus, through the urethra.
Bronchitis – an illness caused by inflammation of the bronchial mucous membrane.
Bronchopulmonary – relating to the bronchi and lungs.
Bubo – an inflamed swelling of a lymphatic gland, especially in the armpit or groin.
Calmative – sedative.
Cancer – an abnormal mass of tissue cells having potentially unlimited growth.
Carcinoma – a malignant tumor derived from epithelial tissue; the most frequent form of cancer.
Carcinostatic – anticancerigenous; tending to check the growth of cancerous tissue.
Cardioactive – having an effect upon the heart; said especially of drugs; see Cardiotonic.
Cardiotonic – having a tonic or stimulating effect on the heart.
Caries – the decay or death of a bone, in which it becomes softened, discolored, and porous; most commonly applied to tooth decay.
Carminative – a drug or substance which prevents formation of, or promotes expulsion of, flatus.
Cataract – an opacity of the lens of the eye, causing partial or total blindness.
Catarrh – inflammation of mucous membranes, especially of the nose and throat.
Cathartic – an agent which causes bowel movement.
Cephalalgia – headache.
Chlorosis – an anemic disorder, generally occurring in female puberty, characterized by greenish-yellow color of the skin due to hemoglobin deficiency of the red blood cells.
Cholagogue – a drug which stimulates the flow of bile.
Cholera – an acute, specific, infectious disease caused by *Vibrio* bacteria resulting in profuse, effortless diarrhoea, vomiting, collapse, muscular cramps, and suppression of urine.
Choleretic – stimulating the production of bile by the liver.
Chorea – a nervous disorder, especially of children, marked by uncontrollable and irregular movements of the muscles of the arms, legs and face.
Colic – acute paroxysmal stomach pain, caused by spasm, obstruction or distention of the intestines.
Conjunctivitis – inflammation of the conjunctive membrane of the eye.

CONSTIPATION – condition of bowels in which defecation is irregular and difficult.
CONTUSION – bruise; an injury in which the skin is not broken, but blood vessels beneath are disrupted, causing a hematoma under the skin.
CONVULSION – violent irregular motion of limbs or body due to involuntary contraction of muscles.
CYSTITIS – inflammation of the urinary bladder.
DARTRE – herpes, or any skin disease resembling it.
DEOBSTRUENT – that which causes the removal of an obstruction.
DEPILATORY – having the ability to remove hair.
DEPURATIVE – a drug or agent that induces the excretion and removal of waste material from the blood; blood purifier.
DERMATITIS – see DERMATOSIS.
DERMATOSIS – inflammation of the skin causing discomforts such as eczema; same as dermatitis.
DIAPHORETIC – a drug causing an increase in perspiration as a result of the stimulation of the sweat glands.
DIARRHOEA (diarrhea) – a common symptom of gastrointestinal disease resulting in increased frequency of stool discharge.
DIGESTIVE – pertaining to digestion; digestant.
DIURETIC – a drug that has the ability to increase the volume of urine secreted by the kidneys.
DRASTIC – an agent which causes violent bowel movements; same as purgative.
DROPSY (hydropsy) – a leakage of the watery part of the blood into any of the tissues or cavities of the body. *See* ASCITES, HYDRAGOGUE.
DYSENTERY – a disease caused by bacteria or protozoa, causing inflammation of the mucous membrane and glands of the large intestine, accompanied by painful diarrhoea and blood evacuations.
DYSMENORRHOEA – painful menstruation.
DYSPEPSIA – indigestion.
DYSPNEA – shortness of breath.
ECZEMA – acute or chronic, non-contagious inflammation of the skin, accompanied by itching.
EDEMA – an excessive accumulation of fluid in tissue spaces.
EMETIC – a drug or agent which induces vomiting.
EMETOCATHARTIC – an agent that is both emetic and cathartic.
EMMENAGOGUE – a drug that stimulates the menstrual flow.
EMOLLIENT – a substance applied externally to soften the surface tissues, or internally to soothe inflamed or irritated surfaces.
ENEMA – a liquid preparation injected into the rectum resulting in quick complete emptying of the large bowel.
ENTERITIS – inflammation of the intestine.
ENTEROCOLITIS – inflammation involving both the small intestine and the colon.
ENTERORRHAGIA – gastric bleeding.
EPIDIDYMITIS – inflammation of the epididymis, a portion of the spermatic duct system of the testis.

Glossary

Epilepsy – a nervous disorder involving temporary loss of consciousness with or without convulsions and muscular spasms.

Erysipelas – an acute inflammation of the skin and subcutaneous tissues, characterized by serious toxic symptoms, high fever and prostration.

Eupepsia – good digestion.

Eupeptic – pertaining to, characterized by, or promoting eupepsia.

Exanthema – a skin eruption.

Excitant – see Analeptic.

Expectorant – a drug that promotes the ejection of mucous or other secretions from the upper respiratory tract by coughing.

Febrifuge – antithermic.

Felon – a painful inflammation at the fingertip, near the nail root; same as Whitlow.

Filariasis – infestation of tissue with filariae (parasitic nematode worms) resulting in lymphatic obstruction causing elephantiasis (enlargement of legs and scrotum).

Flatulence – the presence of an excessive amount of gas in the stomach and intestines.

Flatus – excessive intestinal gas.

Furunculosis – a condition marked by the presence of furuncles (boils, or deep staphylococcal folliculitis).

Galactagogue – a drug that induces or increases the secretion of milk.

Gastralgia – stomachache.

Gastric Ulcers – ulcers in the stomach.

Geophagy – the practice of eating soil or earth.

Gingivitis – inflammation of the gums.

Glaucoma – a condition of the eye characterized by increased intraocular pressure.

Gout – paroxysmal disease with painful inflammation of smaller joints due to deposits of calcium urate and excessive uric acid in the blood.

Grippe – influenza.

Haemoptysis (hemoptysis) – spitting of blood from the bronchi, larynx, lungs or trachea.

Hair Tonic – substance that stimulates hair growth.

Hanseniasis – chronic contagious disease due to infection with mycobacteria. The same as Leprosy.

Helminthicide – see Anthelmintic.

Hematoma – a localized swelling filled with blood.

Hematuria – the discharge of blood in the urine.

Hemorrhoid – an enlarged and often dilated blood vessel of the anal canal or the lower portion of the alimentary tract; piles.

Hemostatic – a drug or substance that arrests hemorrhage.

Hepatitis – inflammation of the liver.

Herpes – an acute inflammation of the skin characterized by the appearance of groups of vesicles.

Hydragogue – a cathartic that induces a watery purge of the gastrointestinal tract.

GLOSSARY

HYDROCOELE – a pathological accumulation of fluids in a cavity, especially in the scrotum.

HYDROPHOBIA – rabies.

HYDROPSY – *see* DROPSY.

HYPERCHOLESTEROLEMIA – a greater than normal amount of cholesterol in the blood.

HYPERTENSION – high blood pressure.

HYPOCHOLESTEREMIC (hypocholesterolemic) – causing lowering of cholesterol in blood and vessels.

HYPOCHOLESTEROLEMIA – a less than normal amount of cholesterol in the blood. The presence of cholesterol in the blood, a normal condition, is termed 'cholesterolemia.'

HYPOGLYCEMIC – abnormally low level of blood sugar; an agent causing lowering of blood sugar.

HYPOTENSIVE – an agent causing lowering of blood pressure.

HYSTERIA – a psychoneurosis characterized by lack of control over acts and emotions.

INFLAMMATION – the condition into which tissues enter as a reaction to injury.

INFLUENZA – an acute, infectious viral disease characterized by inflammation of the respiratory tract, fever, muscular pain and irritation of the intestinal tract; the same as grippe.

INSOMNIA – sleeplessness.

JAUNDICE – yellowness of the skin, mucous membranes and secretions due to bile pigments in the blood.

KIDNEY AILMENTS – diseases of the kidneys.

KIDNEY STONE – calculus occurring in the kidney.

LARYNGITIS – inflammation of the membrane lining of the larynx.

LAXATIVE – a drug having the action of loosening the bowels, stimulating defecation.

LEISHMANIASIS – skin diseases derived from infection by *Leishmania* flagellates.

LEPROSY – *see* HANSENIASIS.

LEUCORRHOEA – a whitish, viscid discharge from the vagina and uterine cavity.

LITHIASIS – the pathological formation of calculi (stones) in the body, as in gall bladder or kidney.

LITHONTRIPTIC – related to the breaking up of kidney stones.

LYMPHANGITIS – inflammation of lymphatic vessels.

LYMPHOADENITIS – inflammation of lymph nodes.

MALARIA – disease caused by protozoa of the genus *Plasmodium* and transmitted by the *Anopheles* mosquito, characterized by intermittent spells of fever.

MASTICATORY – *see* SIALAGOGUE.

MENORRHAGIA – abnormally heavy menstrual flow.

MENSTRUAL DISORDERS – dysmenorrhoea; spasmodic or continuous pain during the menstrual period.

METRORRHAGIA – uterine bleeding, usually of normal amount, occurring at irregular intervals.

MIOTIC – a medication causing constriction of the pupil of the eye.

MOLLUSCICIDAL – destructive to snails and other molluscs.

Glossary

Mucilaginous – gummy, gelatinous substance used to soothe mucous membranes.
Narcotic – drug or substance that relieves pain and induces drowsiness, sleep, stupor or insensibility.
Neuralgia – sudden severe pain radiating along the course of a nerve, without the occurrence of demonstrable structural changes.
Odontalgic – pertaining to or marked by toothache.
Ophthalmia – inflammation of the conjunctiva of the eye or the eyeball.
Orchitis – inflammation of the testes.
Palpitation – a rapid pulsation or throbbing of the heart.
Panacea – a universal remedy.
Pectoral – pertaining to the chest.
Pharyngitis – inflammation of the pharynx.
Phlebitis – inflammation of a vein.
Pian – the same as yaws.
Piles – see Hemorrhoid.
Pityriasis – skin diseases characterized by epidermal shedding of flaky scales.
Prurigo – a chronic, inflammatory skin disease characterized by eruption and severe itching.
Pruritis – severe itching, usually of undamaged skin.
Psoriasis – a chronic, noncontagious skin disease characterized by inflammation and white, scaly patches.
Pterygium – a winglike structure in the eye growing in the interpalpebral fissure, extending from the conjunctiva and covering a part of the cornea, causing vision disturbance; also, a forward growth of the cuticle over the nail.
Puerperal Fever – an infection occurring in a woman during childbirth; childbed fever.
Purgative – see Drastic.
Rachitism – rickets.
Renal Lithiasis – the presence of kidney stones.
Resolutive – see Resolvent.
Resolvent – an agent promoting the resolution (subsidence) of a lesion, such as an inflammatory exudate.
Restorative – a medication or treatment that promotes a restoration of strength and vigor.
Revulsant – a substance causing an irritant reaction for purposes of counterirritant therapy.
Rheumatism – a general term indicating diseases of muscle tendons, joints, bone or nerves, resulting in discomfort, pain and sometimes disability.
Rickets – infantile scurvy.
Ringworm – common contagious disease produced by fungi that affects the skin, hair or nails.
Rubefacient – a substance that causes redness of the skin. The same as ruberary.
Scabies – a contagious parasitic disease of the skin caused by the mite *Sarcoptes scabi*.
Sciatica – neuralgic pain in the hip or thigh areas.

Glossary

SCROFULA – tuberculosis of the lymphatic glands, especially of the neck, in which the glands become enlarged.

SCURVY – a nutritional disorder caused by deficiency of Vitamin C, characterized by extreme weakness, spongy gums, and a tendency to develop hemorrhages under the skin, from the mucous membranes and under the periosteum.

SIALAGOGUE – a drug or substance chewed to increase salivation; masticatory.

SOPORIFIC – a drug that causes deep sleep.

SORE – a popular term for almost any lesion of the skin or mucous membrane.

SPLENITIS – inflammation of the spleen; a condition that is usually produced by pyemia (septicemia caused by abscess-producing bacteria).

STIMULANT – a drug or agent that causes increased functional activity.

STOMACHIC – a drug or substance which stimulates the functional activity of the stomach.

STOMATITIS – inflammation of the mucous tissue of the mouth.

STYPTIC – see ASTRINGENT.

SUDORIFIC – a drug or agent producing sweating.

TACHYCARDIA – excessively rapid heartbeat.

TAENIFUGE – anthelmintic that acts against tapeworm.

TETANUS – an acute, infectious disease (often entering the body through wounds) caused by the bacillus *Clostridium tetani*, characterized by rigidity and spasmodic contraction of the voluntary muscles.

TETTERWORM – ringworm.

THRUSH – an oral infection caused by the fungus *Candida albicans*, characterized by white eruptions in the mouth.

TINEA – any of several fungus diseases, such as athlete's foot and ringworm.

TONIC – a drug that invigorates or improves the normal tone of an organ or of the patient generally.

TRACHOMA – a viral disease of the conjunctiva and cornea, producing photophobia, pain and lacrimation (weeping of tears), and characterized by redness, inflammation, and follicular and papillary hypertrophy of the conjunctiva.

ULCER – an external or internal, open sore secreting pus, other than a wound.

URETHRITIS – inflammation of the urethra.

UROGENITAL – pertaining to both the urinary and genital functions.

VASOCONSTRICTOR – a drug causing constriction of the blood vessels.

VERMIFUGE (vermicide) – see ANTHELMINTIC.

VESICANT (vesicatory) – a drug or agent that produces blisters on the skin.

VITILIGO – a skin disease characterized by whitish nonpigmented areas surrounded by hyperpigmented borders.

VOMITIVE – an agent that causes vomiting; see EMETIC.

VULNERARY – a remedy used for treating wounds.

WART – a common skin tumor often cused by a virus infection.

WHITLOW – any inflammation around the nail of a finger or toe.

YAWS – an infectious skin disease caused by the spirochaete *Treponema pertenue*, characterized by multiple red pimples.

ILLUSTRATION CREDITS

Original illustrations by Cecilia Rizzini, Ruth B. Toomey and Anna V. Di Carlo.

Illustrations were also:
Reproduced with permission from: Mors, W.B. & C.T. Rizzini. 1966. USEFUL PLANTS OF BRAZIL. San Francisco, London, Amsterdam: Holden-Day Inc. Illustrations by Cecilia Rizzini.

Reproduced with permission from: *Leandra,* published by the Department of Botany, Institute of Biology, Federal University of Rio de Janeiro. Illustrations by Atídio Manhã.

Reproduced from: Little, E.L. & F.H. Wadsworth. 1964. COMMON TREES OF PUERTO RICO AND THE VIRGIN ISLANDS. Agriculture Handbook No. 249. Washington, D.C.: USDA Forest Service.

Reproduced from: Martius, K.F.P. von, Eichler, A.W. & I. Urban. 1840-1906. FLORA BRASILIENSIS. Leipzig.

Page xxii: Brazilian Indian. Original Amerindian illustration by Anna V. Di Carlo based on: Debret, J.B. 1834-1839. Voyage Pittoresque et Historique au Brésil. As represented in: Cronau, R. 1892. AMERIKA: DIE GESCHICHTE SEINER ENTDECKUNG (Vol. 2, p. 233). Leipzig: Abel & Müller).

Page xxiv: Mauá Indian. Original Amerindian illustration by Anna V. Di Carlo based on: Ferreira, Alexandre Rodrigues. VIAGEM FILOSÓFICA PELAS CAPITANIAS DO GRÃO PARÁ, RIO NEGRO, MATO GROSSO E CUIABÁ, 1783-1792. Iconografia, Vol. I: Geologia e Antropologia (Plate 109). Rio de Janeiro: Conselho Federal de Cultura (1971).

Page xxv: *Top*: Mura Indian inhaling narcotic paricá powder. Original Amerindian illustration by Anna V. Di Carlo based on: Ferreira, A.R., *op. cit.,* Plate 121 (1971). *Bottom*: Mura Indian, state of Amazonas. Original Amerindian illustration by Anna V. Di Carlo based on: Spix, J.B. von & K.F.P. von Martius. 1823-1831. VIAGEM PELO BRASIL. Vol. 4. Rio de Janeiro: Imprensa Nacional (1938).

Page xxvi: Jurupixuna Indian. Original Amerindian illustration by Anna V. Di Carlo based on: Ferreira, A.R., *op. cit.,* Plate 104 (1971).

Page xxvii: Coeruna Indian. Original Amerindian illustration by Anna V. Di Carlo based on: Spix, J.B. von & K.F.P. von Martius, *op. cit.* (1823-1831). As represented in: Zerries, O., 1980. UNTER INDIANERN BRASILIENS: SAMMLUNG SPIX UND MARTIUS 1817-1820 (p. 65, Taf. 17). Innsbruck: Pinguin-Verlag; and in Helbig, J., *op. cit.,* Taf. 15 (1994).

Page xxviii: Juri Indian. Original Amerindian illustration by Anna V. Di Carlo based on: Spix, J.B. von & K.F.P. von Martius. 1823-1831. REISE IN BRASILIEN. ATLAS. Munich. As represented in: Striker, I.A. 1977. EARLY VISIONS OF IMPERIAL BRAZIL (Page S-6). Washington, D.C.: Organization of American States; Zerries,

ILLUSTRATION CREDITS

O., *op. cit.,* p. 20, Taf. 4 (1980); and in Helbig, J. 1994. BRASILIANISCHE REISE 1817-1820: CARL FRIEDRICH PHILIPP VON MARTIUS ZUM 200. Geburtstag (Taf. 47). München: Hirmer Verlag.

Page xxix: Mayoruna Indian. Original Amerindian illustration by Anna V. Di Carlo based on: Spix, J.B. von & K.F.P. von Martius, *op. cit.* (1823-1831). As represented in: Zerries, O., *op. cit.,* p. 123, Taf. 59 (1980); Marcoy, P. 1875. TRAVELS IN SOUTH AMERICA. Vol. 2. New York: Scribner, Armstrong & Co.; and in Helbig, J., *op. cit.,* Taf. 11 & p. 265 (1994).

Page xxx: Mauhé Indian. Original Amerindian illustration by Anna V. Di Carlo based on: Spix, J.B. von and K.F.P. von Martius, *op. cit.* (1823-1831). As represented in: Zerries, O., *op. cit.,* p. 179, Taf. 67 (1980); and in Helbig, J., *op. cit.,* Taf. 14 (1994).

Page xxxi: Botocudos Indian. Original Amerindian illustration by Anna V. Di Carlo based on: Cronau, R., *op. cit.,* Vol. 2, p. 221 (1892).

Page xxxiii: Mongoyo Indian. Original Amerindian illustration by Anna V. Di Carlo based on: Debret, J.B., *op. cit.* (1834-1839). As represented in: Cronau, R., *op. cit.,* p. 217 (1892).

Page xxxiv: Indian of the Rio Xingu. Original Amerindian illustration by Anna V. Di Carlo based on: Ribeiro, B.G. 1957. BASES PARA UMA CLASSIFICAÇÃO DOS ADORNOS PLUMARIOS DOS INDIOS DO BRASIL. Arquivos do Museu Nacional (Rio de Janeiro) 43: 59-119 (p. 108, Plate 4).

Page xxxvii: Karajá Indian. Original Amerindian illustration by Anna V. Di Carlo based on: Ribeiro, B.G., *op. cit.,* p. 112, Plate 8 (1957).

Page xxxviii: Bororo Indian. Original Amerindian illustration by Anna V. Di Carlo based on: Ribeiro, B.G., *op. cit.,* p. 113, Plate 9 (1957).

Page 8: *Anacardium occidentale* (Anacardiaceae): Little, E.L. & F.H. Wadsworth. COMMON TREES OF PUERTO RICO AND THE VIRGIN ISLANDS.

Page 17: *Xylopia aromatica* (Annonaceae): Mors, W.B. & C.T. Rizzini. USEFUL PLANTS OF BRAZIL. p.72, fig.9-1.

Page 22: *Dipladenia fragrans* (Apocynaceae): Martius, K.F.P. von, Eichler, A.W. & I. Urban. FLORA BRASILIENSIS.

Page 25: *Top – Hancornia speciosa:* Mors, W.B. & C.T. Rizzini. USEFUL PLANTS OF BRAZIL p. 5, fig.1-2. *Bottom – Parahancornia amapa* (Apocynaceae). Original illustrations by Cecilia Rizzini.

Page 32: *Ilex paraguariensis* (Aquifoliaceae): *Leandra 3*: 15, fig.2 (1972). Original illustration by Atídio Manhã.

Page 34: *Caladium bicolor* (Araceae). Original illustration by Ruth B. Toomey.

Page 38: *Philodendron pedatum* (Araceae). Original illustration by Ruth B. Toomey.

Page 41: *Copernicia prunifera* (Arecaceae). Original illustration by Ruth B. Toomey.

Page 42: *Euterpe oleracea* (Arecaceae). Original illustration by Ruth B. Toomey.

Page 44: *Mauritia flexuosa* (Arecaceae). Original illustration by Ruth B. Toomey.

Page 47: *Aristolochia cymbifera* (Aristolochiaceae). Original illustration by Ruth B. Toomey.

Page 49: *Aristolochia trilobata* (Aristolochiaceae). Original illustration by Ruth B. Toomey.

Page 55: *Baccharis trimera* (Asteraceae): Martius, K.F.P. von, Eichler, A.W. & I.

ILLUSTRATION CREDITS

Urban. FLORA BRASILIENSIS.
Page 63: *Mikania glomerata* (Asteraceae): Martius, K.F.P. von, Eichler, A.W. & I. Urban. FLORA BRASILIENSIS.
Page 66: *Senecio brasiliensis* (Asteraceae): Martius, K.F.P. von, Eichler, A.W. & I. Urban. FLORA BRASILIENSIS.
Page 74: *Helosis cayennensis* (Balanophoraceae). Original illustration by Ruth B. Toomey.
Page 75: *Begonia paulensis* (Begoniaceae): Martius, K.F.P. von, Eichler, A.W. & I. Urban. FLORA BRASILIENSIS.
Page 77: *Berberis laurina* (Berberidaceae): Martius, K.F.P. von, Eichler, A.W. & I. Urban. FLORA BRASILIENSIS.
Page 79: *Anemopaegma arvense* (Bignoniaceae). Original illustration by Cecilia Rizzini.
Page 92: *Tillandsia aeranthos* (Bromeliaceae). Original illustration by Ruth B. Toomey.
Page 94: *Protium brasiliense* (Burseraceae): Martius, K.F.P. von, Eichler, A.W. & I. Urban. FLORA BRASILIENSIS.
Page 96: *Brasilopuntia brasiliensis* (Cactaceae). Original illustration by Ruth B. Toomey.
Page 98: *Bauhinia forficata* (Caesalpiniaceae). Original illustration by Cecilia Rizzini.
Page 101: *Caesalpinia echinata* (Caesalpiniaceae): Martius, K.F.P. von, Eichler, A.W. & I. Urban. FLORA BRASILIENSIS.
Page 103: *Hymenaea courbaril* (Caesalpiniaceae): Mors, W.B. & C.T. Rizzini. USEFUL PLANTS OF BRAZIL, p.43, fig.5-1.
Page 107: *Senna rugosa* (Caesalpiniaceae). Original illustration by Cecilia Rizzini.
Page 117: *Maytenus ilicifolia* (Celastraceae): *Leandra 3*: 27, fig.1 (1972). Original illustration by Atídio Manhã.
Page 127: *Tradescantia spathacea* (Commelinaceae). Original illustration by Ruth B. Toomey.
Page 137: *Luffa operculata* (Cucurbitaceae): Martius, K.F.P. von, Eichler, A.W. & I. Urban. FLORA BRASILIENSIS.
Page 145: *Curatella americana* (Dilleniaceae). Original illustration by Cecilia Rizzini.
Page 149: *Erythroxylium coca* (Erythroxylaceae). Original illustration by Ruth B. Toomey.
Page 161: *Acosmium dasycarpum* (Fabaceae). Original illustration by Cecilia Rizzini.
Page 162: *Andira anthelmia* (Fabaceae). Original illustration by Cecilia Rizzini.
Page 164: *Dalbergia subcymosa* (Fabaceae). Original illustration by Cecilia Rizzini.
Page 165: *Dipteryx alata* (Fabaceae). Original illustration by Cecilia Rizzini.
Page 167: *Galactia peduncularis* (Fabaceae). Original illustration by Cecilia Rizzini.
Page 169: *Myroxylon balsamum* (Fabaceae): Mors, W.B. & C.T. Rizzini. USEFUL PLANTS OF BRAZIL, p.45, fig.5-2
Page 171: *Right – Pterodon apparicioi* (Fabaceae). *Left and center – Pterodon pubescens* (Fabaceae). Original illustrations by Cecilia Rizzini.
Page 173: *Vataireopsis araroba* (Fabaceae). Original illustration by Cecilia Rizzini.
Page 177: *Carpotroche brasiliensis* (Flacourtiaceae): Martius, K.F.P. von, Eichler,

ILLUSTRATION CREDITS

A.W. & I. Urban. FLORA BRASILIENSIS.XIII, 1, Tab 88.
Page 182: *Heliconia angusta* (Heliconiaceae): Martius, K.F.P. von, Eichler, A.W. & I. Urban. FLORA BRASILIENSIS.
Page 184: *Saccoglottis guianensis* (Humiriaceae): Martius, K.F.P. von, Eichler, A.W. & I. Urban. FLORA BRASILIENSIS.
Page 185: *Citronella congonha* (Icacinaceae). Original illustration by Cecilia Rizzini.
Page 187: *Cipura paludosa* (Iridaceae). Original illustration by Ruth B. Toomey.
Page 188: *Cypella herbertii* (Iridaceae). Original illustration by Ruth B. Toomey.
Page 189: *Isoetes martii* (Isoetaceae). Original illustration by Ruth B. Toomey.
Page 190: *Krameria argentea* (Krameriaceae): Martius, K.F.P. von, Eichler, A.W. & I. Urban. FLORA BRASILIENSIS.
Page 202: *Ocotea pretiosa* (Lauraceae): Martius, K.F.P. von, Eichler, A.W. & I. Urban. FLORA BRASILIENSIS.
Page 205: *Bertholletia excelsa* (Lecythidaceae). Original illustration by Ruth B. Toomey.
Page 206: *Cariniana legalis* (Lecythidaceae): Martius, K.F.P. von, Eichler, A.W. & I. Urban. FLORA BRASILIENSIS.
Page 208: *Smilax campestris* (Liliaceae). Original illustration by Cecilia Rizzini.
Page 210: Top – *Strychnos pseudoquina* (Loganiaceae); bottom – *Strychnos trinervis* (Loganiaceae). Original illustrations by Cecilia Rizzini.
Page 212: *Struthanthus marginatus* (Loranthaceae): *Leandra* 2: 84, fig.4 (1972). Original illustration by Atídio Manhã.
Page 213: *Cuphea ingrata* (Lythraceae). Original illustration by Cecilia Rizzini.
Page 215: *Lafoensia densiflora* (Lythraceae). Original illustration by Cecilia Rizzini.
Page 217: *Talauma ovata* (Magnoliaceae): Martius, K.F.P. von, Eichler, A.W. & I. Urban. FLORA BRASILIENSIS. XIII, 1, Tab 28.
Page 218: *Banisteriopsis caapi* (Malpighiaceae). Original illustration by Cecilia Rizzini.
Page 219: *Byrsonima crassifolia* (Malpighiaceae). Original illustration by Cecilia Rizzini.
Page 228: *Cedrela fissilis* (Meliaceae): *Leandra* 3: 42, fig.4 (1972). Original illustration by Atídio Manhã.
Page 230: *Trichilia catuaba* (Meliaceae). Original illustration by Cecilia Rizzini.
Page 232: *Abuta rufescens* (Menispermaceae). Original illustration by Cecilia Rizzini.
Page 235: *Nymphoides indica* (Menyanthaceae). Original illustration by Ruth B. Toomey.
Page 238: *Mimosa hostilis* (Mimosaceae). Original illustration by Cecilia Rizzini.
Page 239: *Mimosa verrucosa* (Mimosaceae). Original illustration by Cecilia Rizzini.
Page 241: *Parkia oppositifolia* (Mimosaceae): Martius, K.F.P. von, Eichler, A.W. & I. Urban. FLORA BRASILIENSIS.
Page 243: *Stryphnodendron coriaceum* (Mimosaceae). Original illustration by Cecilia Rizzini.
Page 251: *Virola surinamensis* (Myristicaceae): Martius, K.F.P. von, Eichler, A.W. & I. Urban. FLORA BRASILIENSIS.
Page 254: *Eugenia dysenterica* (Myrtaceae). Original illustration by Cecilia

ILLUSTRATION CREDITS

Rizzini.

Page 260: *Nymphaea rudgeana* (Nymphaeaceae). Original illustration by Ruth B. Toomey.

Page 261 *Victoria amazonica* (Nymphaeaceae). Original illustration by Ruth B. Toomey.

Page 263: *Above – Ptychopetalum olacoides* (Olacaceae). *Leaf left – Ptychopetalum uncinatum* (Olacaceae). Original illustrations by Cecilia Rizzini.

Page 265: *Agonandra brasiliensis* (Opiliaceae): Martius, K.F.P. von, Eichler, A.W. & I. Urban. FLORA BRASILIENSIS.

Page 267: *Oxalis corniculata* (Oxalidaceae): *Leandra 4-5*: 84, fig.1 (1974). Original illustration by Atídio Manhã.

Page 268: *Oxalis martiana* (Oxalidaceae): *Leandra 4-5*: 85, fig.2 (1974). Original illustration by Atídio Manhã.

Page 273: *Peperomia pellucida* (Piperaceae). Original illustration by Cecilia Rizzini.

Page 286: *Polygonum hydropiperoides* (Polygonaceae). Original illustration by Cecilia Rizzini.

Page 292: *Zizyphus joazeiro* (Rhamnaceae): Martius, K.F.P. von, Eichler, A.W. & I. Urban. FLORA BRASILIENSIS.

Page 295: *Rhizophora mangle* (Rhizophoraceae): Martius, K.F.P. von, Eichler, A.W. & I. Urban. FLORA BRASILIENSIS.

Page 307: *Paullinia cupana* (Sapindaceae): Martius, K.F.P. von, Eichler, A.W. & I. Urban. FLORA BRASILIENSIS.

Page 311: *Capraria biflora* (Scrophulariaceae). Original illustration by Cecilia Rizzini.

Page 316: *Brunfelsia grandiflora* (Solanaceae). Original illustration by Cecilia Rizzini.

Page 320: *Left – Solanum insidiosum* & *right – Solanum paniculatum* (Solanaceae). Original illustrations by Cecilia Rizzini.

Page 324: *Helicteres ovata* (Sterculiaceae): Martius, K.F.P. von, Eichler, A.W. & I. Urban. FLORA BRASILIENSIS.

Page 329: *Typha domingensis* (Typhaceae). Original illustration by Ruth B. Toomey.

Page 332: *Urera subpeltata* (Urticaceae): Martius, K.F.P. von, Eichler, A.W. & I. Urban. FLORA BRASILIENSIS.

Page 333: *Aloysia triphylla* (Verbenaceae). Original illustration by Cecilia Rizzini.
Page 338: *Anchietea pyrifolia* (Violaceae). Original illustration by Cecilia Rizzini.
Page 341: *Drimys winteri* (Winteraceae): Martius, K.F.P. von, Eichler, A.W. & I. Urban. FLORA BRASILIENSIS.

Editor's Acknowledgements

Many colleagues generously extended their botanical expertise and other forms of assistance during the preparation of this volume. For comments on the taxonomy and nomenclature of various plant families, thanks are accorded to members of the Department of Botany, National Museum of Natural History, Smithsonian Institution, Washington, D.C.: Pedro Acevedo (Sapindaceae), Laurence Dorr (Malvaceae, Sterculiaceae), Christian Feuillet (Aristolochiaceae), W. John Kress (Costaceae, Heliconiaceae), David Lellinger (Ferns and Fern Allies), Dan Nicolson (Araceae), John Pruski (Asteraceae), Harold Robinson (Asteraceae), Laurence Skog (Gesneriaceae), Dieter Wasshausen (Acanthaceae), and John Wurdack (Melastomataceae). Other specialists who read portions of the manuscript include: Lynn Gillespie (Euphorbiaceae), Scott Mori (Lecythidaceae), Larry Noblick (Arecaceae), and Paulo Windisch (Ferns).

In addition, I am grateful to a number of Smithsonian staff who supplied information, materials or otherwise helped to facilitate this endeavor, including: Robert Faden (*Tradescantia spathacea*), Pamela Keef, Shirley Maina (Floristics Program), Robert Read, Ruth Schallert, Christian Tuccinardi, and Diane Wilson.

The contributions of two talented artists from the Smithsonian Behind the Scenes Volunteer Program, who prepared the Amerindian illustrations accompanying the Foreword (Anna DiCarlo), and drawings of plants for the text (Ruth B. Toomey), are gratefully acknowledged.

Finally, I wish to record my deep appreciation to the Irvine family of Reference Publications, Inc., for the support they have given during the preparation of this book. Keith Irvine created the opportunity for a Brazilian component in the series and maintained his deep involvement over many years; Aline Irvine (Algonac, Michigan) continues his mission; and Ms. Lilou Irvine (New Windsor, New York) generously channeled her considerable skills in computer technology towards production of this volume.

Dr. Robert A. DeFilipps
Washington, DC

Medicinal Index*

A

Abdominal Troubles
Machaerium lunatum (L.) Ducke, Fabaceae 168
Mikania officinalis Mart., Asteraceae 62
Abortifacient (Abortive)
Ananas comosus (L.) Merrill, Bromeliaceae 90
Aristolochia esperanzae
  O. Kuntze, Aristolochiaceae 48
Aristolochia trilobata L., Aristolochiaceae 48
Bromelia antiacantha Bertol., Bromeliaceae 91
Bromelia pinguin L., Bromeliaceae 91
Brunfelsia uniflora (Pohl) D. Don, also
  B. grandiflora D. Don, Solanaceae 316
Cabralea canjerana (Vell.) Mart., Meliaceae 227
Chenopodium ambrosioides L., Chenopodiaceae ... 118
Chondodendron platyphyllum
  (Mart.) Miers, Menispermaceae 231
Eryngium foetidum L., Apiaceae 19
Guarea trichilioides L., Meliaceae 227
Guettarda angelica Mart., Rubiaceae 298
Lagenaria siceraria
  (Molina) Standl., Cucurbitaceae 138
Petiveria alliacea L., Phytolaccaceae 271
Pluchea suaveolens (Vell.) O. Ktze., Asteraceae 64
Renealmia occidentalis Sweet, also
  Renealmia sylvestris Horan., Zingiberaceae 342
Senna occidentalis (L.) Link, Caesalpiniaceae 105
Senna quinqueangulata
  (Rich.) Ir. & Barn., Caesalpiniaceae 106
Tanacetum vulgare L., Asteraceae 67
–in rats
Stryphnodendron polyphyllum Mart.,
  Mimosaceae (PHARM.) 244
Abscesses
Anisolobus cururu (Mart.) M. Arg., Apocynaceae 21
Annona reticulata L., Annonaceae 13
Annona spinescens Mart., Annonaceae 13
Cochlospermum regium (Mart. & Schl.)
  Pilg., Cochlospermaceae 125
Hylocereus undatus (Haw.) Br. & Rose, Cactaceae .. 95
Ipomoea pes-caprae (L.) R. Br., Convolvulaceae .. 130
Ludwigia peruviana (L.) Hara, Onagraceae 264
Ocotea guianensis Aubl., Lauraceae 201
Acid
Ephedra triandra Tul., Ephedraceae 148
Acrid
Maranta arundinacea L., Marantaceae 223
Adenitis. *See* **Glandular Conditions**
Aerophagy
Aniba canelilla (H.B.K.) Mez, Lauraceae 197

Aged, special diet for
Maranta arundinacea L., Marantaceae 223
AIDS. *See* **HIV-1**
Albugo. *See* **Corneal Opacity**
Albuminuria
Mikania hirsutissima DC., Asteraceae 62
Mikania setigera
  Schultz-Bip. ex Baker, Asteraceae 62
Alcoholism
Turnera diffusa Willd., Turneraceae 327
Turnera opifera Mart., Turneraceae 328
Alexipharmic. *See* **Poison Antidote**
Amebiasis (Amoebicide)
Bauhinia guianensis Aubl., Caesalpiniaceae 99
Borreria asclepiadea Cham. & Schl.,
  substitute for *Cephaelis ipecacuanha* Rich.,
  Rubiaceae (PHARM.) 296
Calea pinnatifida (R. Br.) Less., Asteraceae 57
Carica papaya L., Caricaceae (CHEM. & PHARM.) 113
Cephaelis ipecacuanha Rich., Rubiaceae (PHARM.) 296
Couma macrocarpa B. Rodr., Apocynaceae 23
Diodia polymorpha Cham. & Schl., substitute
  for *Cephaelis ipecacuanha* Rich.,
  Rubiaceae (PHARM.) 297
Hybanthus ipecacuanha (L.) Baill., Violaceae, same
  use as *Cephaelis ipecacuanha* Rich., Rubiaceae .. 339
Ionidium poaya St.-Hil., Violaceae, same use
  as *Cephaelis ipecacuanha* Rich., Rubiaceae 339
Licania macrophylla Benth., Chrysobalanceae 120
Lipostoma campanuliflorum D. Don, also
  substitute for *Cephaelis ipecacuanha* Rich.,
  Rubiaceae (PHARM.) 299
Machaonia brasiliensis Cham. & Schl., Rubiaceae 299
Manettia ignita (Vell.) K. Sch., substitute
  for *Cephaelis ipecacuanha* Rich.,
  Rubiaceae (PHARM.) 299
Mentha crispa L., Lamiaceae 194
Amenorrhoea
Ageratum conyzoides L., Asteraceae 53
Aristolochia esperanzae
  O. Kuntze, Aristolochiaceae 48
Arrabidaea chica (H.B.K.) Bur., Bignoniaceae 78
Cayaponia tayuya (Mart.) Cogn., Cucurbitaceae 135
Cecropia hololeuca Miq., Moraceae 247
Cissampelos sympodialis Eichl., Menispermaceae . 233
Coutoubea spicata Aubl., Gentianaceae 179
Dracontium asperum K. Koch, Araceae 35
Euphorbia hyssopifolia L., Euphorbiaceae 153
Luffa operculata (L.) Cogn., Cucurbitaceae 138
Operculina alata (Ham.) Urb., Convolvulaceae ... 131
Operculina macrocarpa Urb., Convolvulaceae 131
Oxalis martiana Zucc., Oxalidaceae 267

---

* This index includes a number of listings relating to Antidotes, Poisons, and Toxic substances. The authors, editor and publisher have provided these listings as a report of use and a general guide to the text, not as a recommendation for casual use. Toxicity or antidotal qualities are often related to the part of the plant used, its preparation and application or consumption. Such details are not provided herein.

Swartzia chrysantha B. Rodr., Caesalpiniaceae 107
Urera baccifera Gaud., Urticaceae 331
Vitex agnus-castus L., Verbenaceae 336

Amoebicide. *See* **Amebiasis**

Amygdalitis. *See* **Tonsillitis**

Anal Fissures
Krameria tomentosa St.-Hil., Krameriaceae 191

Analeptic. *See* **Excitant**

Analgesic
Casearia sylvestris Sw., Flacourtiaceae 178
Euphorbia hirta
  L., Euphorbiaceae (CHEM. & PHARM.) 152
Jatropha urens L., Euphorbiaceae 155
Mikania glomerata Spreng., Asteraceae 61
Philodendron hederaceum (Jacq.) Schott
  var. *hederaceum*, Araceae 36
Phyllanthus tenellus
  Roxb., Euphorbiaceae (CHEM. & PHARM.) 157
Piper callosum R. & Pav., Piperaceae 274
Scoparia dulcis L., Scrophulariaceae (PHARM.) 312

Anaphrodisiac
Solanum nigrum L., Solanaceae 321

Anasarca. *See also* **Edema**
Monstera obliqua Miquel, Araceae 36
Tradescantia diuretica Mart., Commelinaceae 128

Ancylostomiasis. *See also* **Anthelmintic**
Bathysa cuspidata Hook., Rubiaceae 296
Bromelia antiacantha Bertol., Bromeliaceae 91
Ficus gomelleira Kunth & Bouché, Moraceae 248
Ficus insipida Willd., Moraceae 248
Lindernia diffusa Wettst., Scrophulariaceae 311
Trianosperma glandulosa Mart., Cucurbitaceae 140
Trianosperma trilobata Cogn., Cucurbitaceae 140

Anemia. *See also* **Chlorosis**
Acanthospermum australe
  (Loefl.) O. Ktze., Asteraceae 51
Arrabidaea chica (H.B.K.) Bur., Bignoniaceae 78
Baccharis articulata (Lam.) Pers., Asteraceae 54
Bathysa cuspidata Hook., Rubiaceae 296
Boerhavia paniculata Rich., Nyctaginaceae 258
Chondodendron platyphyllum
  (Mart.) Miers, Menispermaceae 231
Cissus sicyoides L., Vitaceae 339
Clibadium surinamense L., Asteraceae 58
Dorstenia asaroides Gardn., Moraceae 247
Genipa americana L., Rubiaceae 298
Hymenaea courbaril L., Caesalpiniaceae 103
Marsypianthes chamaedrys
  (Vahl) O. Ktze., Lamiaceae 194
Orbignya phalerata Mart., Arecaceae 43
Quassia amara L., Simaroubaceae 314
Sapindus saponaria L., Sapindaceae 306
Simarouba amara Aubl., Simaroubaceae 315
Simarouba versicolor St.-Hil., Simaroubaceae 315

Angina
Buchnera aquatica Aubl., Scrophulariaceae 310
Chenopodium ambrosioides L., Chenopodiaceae ... 118
Dieffenbachia seguine (Jacq.) Schott, Araceae 35

Animal Bites.
See also Antidotes, Bites, Poison, Stings
Clematis denticulata Vell., Ranunculaceae 290

Anthelmintic (Vermifuge). *See also*
Ancylostomiasis, Filariasis,
Parasiticide, Schistosomiasis, Taenifuge
Allamanda cathartica L., Apocynaceae 20
Ambrosia artemisiifolia L., Asteraceae 53
Anacardium occidentale L., Anacardiaceae 7
Ananas comosus (L.) Merrill, Bromeliaceae 90
Andira inermis (Sw.) H.B.K., Fabaceae 162
Andira retusa (Poir.) H.B.K., Fabaceae 162
Andira vermifuga Mart. ex Benth., Fabaceae 162
Annona glabra L., Annonaceae 13
Aristolochia triangularis Cham., Aristolochiaceae ... 48
Baccharis trimera (Less.) DC., Asteraceae 54
Bellucia grossularioides
  (L.) Tr., Melastomataceae 225
Bidens pilosa L., Asteraceae 57
Bocagea alba St.-Hil., Annonaceae 14
Bocagea viridis St.-Hil., Annonaceae 14
Bromelia antiacantha Bertol., Bromeliaceae 91
Bromelia pinguin L., Bromeliaceae 91
Butia yatay (Mart.) Becc., Arecaceae 39
Caesalpinia bonduc (L.) Roxb., Caesalpiniaceae 99
Caladium bicolor (Aiton) Vent., Araceae 34
Calyptranthes aromatica St.-Hil., Myrtaceae 253
Caraipa grandifolia Mart., Clusiaceae 121
Carapa guianensis Aubl., Meliaceae 227
Carica papaya L., Caricaceae 113
Chenopodium ambrosioides L., Chenopodiaceae ... 118
Chenopodium hircinum Schrad., Chenopodiaceae . 119
Cocos nucifera L., Arecaceae 40
Couma utilis (Mart.) M. Arg., Apocynaceae 23
Coutoubea ramosa Aubl., Gentianaceae 179
Coutoubea spicata Aubl., Gentianaceae 179
Cucurbita pepo L., Cucurbitaceae 136
Cyperus rotundus L., Cyperaceae 142
Deianira nervosa Cham. & Schl., also
  D. erubescens Cham. & Schl., Gentianaceae 180
Duguetia riparia Hub., Annonaceae 14
Euphorbia thymifolia L., Euphorbiaceae 153
Ficus gomelleira Kunth & Bouché, Moraceae 248
Ficus insipida Willd., Moraceae 248
Ficus maxima P. Mill., Moraceae 248
Flaveria bidentis (L.) Ktze., Asteraceae 60
Galipea dichotoma Sald., Rutaceae 301
Gallesia gorazema (Vell.) Moq., Phytolaccaceae ... 271
Geoffroea striata (Willd.) Morong, Fabaceae 168
Guarea trichilioides L., Meliaceae 227
Himatanthus lancifolia
  (M. Arg.) Woods., Apocynaceae 26
Himatanthus phagedaenica
  (Mart.) Woods., Apocynaceae 26
Himatanthus sucuuba (Spr.) Woods., Apocynaceae . 26
Humiria balsamifera
  (Aubl.) St.-Hil., Humiriaceae 183
Hura crepitans L., Euphorbiaceae 153
Hylocereus undatus (Haw.) Br. & Rose, Cactaceae .. 95
Hymenaea courbaril L., Caesalpiniaceae 103
Jacaratia spinosa (Aubl.) A. DC., Caricaceae 113
Leiphaimos aphylla (Jacq.) Gilg, Gentianaceae 180
Lindernia diffusa Wettst., Scrophulariaceae 311
Luffa operculata (L.) Cogn., Cucurbitaceae 138
Mammea americana L., Clusiaceae 123

MEDICINAL INDEX: ANTHELMINTIC – APHRODISIAC

Momordica charantia L., Cucurbitaceae 139
Mucuna pruriens (L.) DC., Fabaceae 169
Nothoscordum striatum Kunth, Iridaceae 186
Oldenlandia corymbosa L., Rubiaceae 299
Ouratea jabotapita Engl., Ochnaceae 261
Ouratea parviflora (DC.) Baill., Ochnaceae 261
Passiflora edulis Sims, Passifloraceae 269
Passiflora laurifolia L., Passifloraceae 270
Passiflora mucronata Lam., Passifloraceae 270
Philodendron bipinnatifidum Schott, Araceae 36
Philodendron selloum Koch, Araceae 37
Philodendron speciosum Schott, Araceae 37
Pluchea suaveolens (Vell.) O. Ktze., Asteraceae 64
Polygonum acuminatum H.B.K., Polygonaceae 286
Polygonum punctatum Elliot, Polygonaceae 287
Polygonum spectabile Mart., Polygonaceae 287
Portulaca oleracea L., Portulacaceae 289
Pothomorphe peltata L., Piperaceae 277
Psidium guajava L., Myrtaceae 256
Renealmia exaltata L. f., Zingiberaceae 342
Senna occidentalis (L.) Link, Caesalpiniaceae 105
Senna quinqueangulata
  (Rich.) Ir. & Barn., Caesalpiniaceae 106
Simarouba versicolor St.-Hil., Simaroubaceae 315
Sorocea bonplandii (Baill.) Burger, Moraceae 249
Spigelia anthelmia L., Loganiaceae 209
Spigelia glabrata Mart., Loganiaceae 209
Spigelia flemingiana Cham. & Schl., Loganiaceae . 209
Stachytarpheta jamaicensis (L.) Vahl, Verbenaceae 336
Tachia guianensis Aubl., Gentianaceae 180
Tagetes minuta L., Asteraceae 67
Tanacetum vulgare L., Asteraceae 67
Anthrax
  Heliotropium elongatum Willd., Boraginaceae 88
  Ilex paraguariensis St.-Hil., Aquifoliaceae 31
Antialgesic. *See* **Analgesic**
Antialgetic
  Solanum nigrum L., Solanaceae 321
Anticancer. *See also* **Cancer**
  Dalbergia subcymosa Ducke, Fabaceae 164
  Maytenus spp., Celastraceae (CHEM. & PHARM.) 116
  Tabebuia spp., Bignoniaceae 83
Antidiarrhoeic. *See* **Diarrhoea**
Antidote. *See* **Poison Antidote.** *See also*
  Cassava Poison Antidote, Curare Antidote, Dart Antidote, Fish Poison Antidote, Plant Poison Antidote, Snakebite Antidote, Toxic
Antiemetic
  Bouchea laetevirens Schauer, Verbenaceae 334
  Bouchea pseudogervao
    (St.-Hil.) Cham., Verbenaceae 334
Antifungal
  Euphorbia thymifolia
    L., Euphorbiaceae (CHEM. & PHARM.) 153
Antihydropic. *See* **Dropsy**
Antiluetic. *See* **Syphilis**
Antimicrobial
  Maytenus spp., Celastraceae (CHEM. & PHARM.) 116
Antiodontalgic. *See* **Toothache**
Antiophidic
  Borreria tenella Cham. & Schl., Rubiaceae 296

Dorstenia asaroides Gardn., Moraceae 247
Eclipta prostrata (L.) L., Asteraceae 59
Hypericum brasiliense Choisy, Clusiaceae 122
Mandevilla velutina (Mart. ex Stadelm.) Woods.
  var. *velutina*, Apocynaceae 27
Pfaffia jubata Mart., Amaranthaceae 5
Piper tuberculatum Jacq., Piperaceae 276
Antiphlogistic. *See* **Inflammations**
Antipoison. *See* **Poison Antidote**
Antipruriginous
  Peperomia pellucida H.B.K., Piperaceae 273
Antipyretic. *See* **Febrifuge**
Antirheumatic. *See* **Rheumatism, also Joint Pain**
Antiscorbutic
  Bidens graveolens Mart., Asteraceae 56
  Bidens pilosa L., Asteraceae 57
  Cereus peruvianus (L.) Mill., Cactaceae 94
  Croton floribundus Spreng., Euphorbiaceae 150
  Drimys winteri Forst., Winteraceae 340
  Melocactus melocactoides (Hoffm.) DC., Cactaceae . 97
  Rollinia orthopetala DC., Annonaceae 15
  Samolus valerandi L., Primulaceae 290
  Tropaeolum pentaphyllum Lam., Tropaeolaceae ... 327
Antiseptic
  Aristolochia trilobata L., Aristolochiaceae 48
  Copaifera officinalis (Jacq.) L., Caesalpiniaceae 102
  Dorstenia brasiliensis Lam., Moraceae 247
  Paullinia cupana Kunth, Sapindaceae 306
Antispasmodic. *See* **Spasmodic**
Antisyphilitic (Antiluetic). *See* **Syphilis**
Antithermic. *See* **Febrifuge**
Antitussive. *See* **Coughs**
Antiulcerogenic Effect
  Maytenus spp., Celastraceae (CHEM. & PHARM.) 116
Anuria
  Cybistax antisyphilitica
    (Mart.) Mart., Bignoniaceae 80
Anxiolytic
  Euphorbia hirta
    L., Euphorbiaceae (CHEM. & PHARM.) 152
Aperient
  Boehmeria caudata Sw., Urticaceae 330
  Hydrocotyle bonariensis Lam., Apiaceae 19
  Hydrocotyle leucocephala
    Cham. & Schlecht., Apiaceae 20
  Urera baccifera Gaud., Urticaceae 331
Aphrodisiac
  Acanthospermum hispidum DC., Asteraceae 52
  Anacardium occidentale L., Anacardiaceae 7
  Anemopaegma arvense (Vell.) Stapf, Bignoniaceae . 78
  Anemopaegma spp.: *A. album* Mart., *A. glaucum*
    Mart. & *A. scabriusculum* Mart., Bignoniaceae 78
  Anthurium oxycarpum Poepp., Araceae 33
  Astrocaryum murumuru Mart., Arecaceae 39
  Azolla caroliniana Willd., Salviniaceae 304
  Bixa orellana L., Bixaceae 85
  Cyperus gracilescens
    Roem. & Schult., Cyperaceae 142
  Davilla rugosa Poir., Dilleniaceae 145
  Ficus insipida Willd., Moraceae 248

Swartzia chrysantha B. Rodr., Caesalpiniaceae 107
Urera baccifera Gaud., Urticaceae 331
Vitex agnus-castus L., Verbenaceae 336

Amoebicide. *See* **Amebiasis**

Amygdalitis. *See* **Tonsillitis**

Anal Fissures
Krameria tomentosa St.-Hil., Krameriaceae 191

Analeptic. *See* **Excitant**

Analgesic
Casearia sylvestris Sw., Flacourtiaceae 178
Euphorbia hirta
  L., Euphorbiaceae (CHEM. & PHARM.) 152
Jatropha urens L., Euphorbiaceae 155
Mikania glomerata Spreng., Asteraceae 61
Philodendron hederaceum (Jacq.) Schott
  var. *hederaceum*, Araceae 36
Phyllanthus tenellus
  Roxb., Euphorbiaceae (CHEM. & PHARM.) 157
Piper callosum R. & Pav., Piperaceae 274
Scoparia dulcis L., Scrophulariaceae (PHARM.) 312

Anaphrodisiac
Solanum nigrum L., Solanaceae 321

Anasarca. *See also* **Edema**
Monstera obliqua Miquel, Araceae 36
Tradescantia diuretica Mart., Commelinaceae 128

Ancylostomiasis. *See also* **Anthelmintic**
Bathysa cuspidata Hook., Rubiaceae 296
Bromelia antiacantha Bertol., Bromeliaceae 91
Ficus gomelleira Kunth & Bouché, Moraceae 248
Ficus insipida Willd., Moraceae 248
Lindernia diffusa Wettst., Scrophulariaceae 311
Trianosperma glandulosa Mart., Cucurbitaceae 140
Trianosperma trilobata Cogn., Cucurbitaceae 140

Anemia. *See also* **Chlorosis**
Acanthospermum australe
  (Loefl.) O. Ktze., Asteraceae 51
Arrabidaea chica (H.B.K.) Bur., Bignoniaceae 78
Baccharis articulata (Lam.) Pers., Asteraceae 54
Bathysa cuspidata Hook., Rubiaceae 296
Boerhavia paniculata Rich., Nyctaginaceae 258
Chondodendron platyphyllum
  (Mart.) Miers, Menispermaceae 231
Cissus sicyoides L., Vitaceae 339
Clibadium surinamense L., Asteraceae 58
Dorstenia asaroides Gardn., Moraceae 247
Genipa americana L., Rubiaceae 298
Hymenaea courbaril L., Caesalpiniaceae 103
Marsypianthes chamaedrys
  (Vahl) O. Ktze., Lamiaceae 194
Orbignya phalerata Mart., Arecaceae 43
Quassia amara L., Simaroubaceae 314
Sapindus saponaria L., Sapindaceae 306
Simarouba amara Aubl., Simaroubaceae 315
Simarouba versicolor St.-Hil., Simaroubaceae 315

Angina
Buchnera aquatica Aubl., Scrophulariaceae 310
Chenopodium ambrosioides L., Chenopodiaceae ... 118
Dieffenbachia seguine (Jacq.) Schott, Araceae 35

Animal Bites.
See also **Antidotes, Bites, Poison, Stings**
Clematis denticulata Vell., Ranunculaceae 290

Anthelmintic (Vermifuge). *See also*
Ancylostomiasis, Filariasis,
Parasiticide, Schistosomiasis, Taenifuge
Allamanda cathartica L., Apocynaceae 20
Ambrosia artemisiifolia L., Asteraceae 53
Anacardium occidentale L., Anacardiaceae 7
Ananas comosus (L.) Merrill, Bromeliaceae 90
Andira inermis (Sw.) H.B.K., Fabaceae 162
Andira retusa (Poir.) H.B.K., Fabaceae 162
Andira vermifuga Mart. ex Benth., Fabaceae 162
Annona glabra L., Annonaceae 13
Aristolochia triangularis Cham., Aristolochiaceae ... 48
Baccharis trimera (Less.) DC., Asteraceae 54
Bellucia grossularioides
  (L.) Tr., Melastomataceae 225
Bidens pilosa L., Asteraceae 57
Bocagea alba St.-Hil., Annonaceae 14
Bocagea viridis St.-Hil., Annonaceae 14
Bromelia antiacantha Bertol., Bromeliaceae 91
Bromelia pinguin L., Bromeliaceae 91
Butia yatay (Mart.) Becc., Arecaceae 39
Caesalpinia bonduc (L.) Roxb., Caesalpiniaceae 99
Caladium bicolor (Aiton) Vent., Araceae 34
Calyptranthes aromatica St.-Hil., Myrtaceae 253
Caraipa grandifolia Mart., Clusiaceae 121
Carapa guianensis Aubl., Meliaceae 227
Carica papaya L., Caricaceae 113
Chenopodium ambrosioides L., Chenopodiaceae ... 118
Chenopodium hircinum Schrad., Chenopodiaceae . 119
Cocos nucifera L., Arecaceae 40
Couma utilis (Mart.) M. Arg., Apocynaceae 23
Coutoubea ramosa Aubl., Gentianaceae 179
Coutoubea spicata Aubl., Gentianaceae 179
Cucurbita pepo L., Cucurbitaceae 136
Cyperus rotundus L., Cyperaceae 142
Deianira nervosa Cham. & Schl., also
  D. erubescens Cham. & Schl., Gentianaceae 180
Duguetia riparia Hub., Annonaceae 14
Euphorbia thymifolia L., Euphorbiaceae 153
Ficus gomelleira Kunth & Bouché, Moraceae 248
Ficus insipida Willd., Moraceae 248
Ficus maxima P. Mill., Moraceae 248
Flaveria bidentis (L.) Ktze., Asteraceae 60
Galipea dichotoma Sald., Rutaceae 301
Gallesia gorazema (Vell.) Moq., Phytolaccaceae ... 271
Geoffroea striata (Willd.) Morong, Fabaceae 168
Guarea trichilioides L., Meliaceae 227
Himatanthus lancifolia
  (M. Arg.) Woods., Apocynaceae 26
Himatanthus phagedaenica
  (Mart.) Woods., Apocynaceaae 26
Himatanthus sucuuba (Spr.) Woods., Apocynaceae . 26
Humiria balsamifera
  (Aubl.) St.-Hil., Humiriaceae 183
Hura crepitans L., Euphorbiaceae 153
Hylocereus undatus (Haw.) Br. & Rose, Cactaceae .. 95
Hymenaea courbaril L., Caesalpiniaceae 103
Jacaratia spinosa (Aubl.) A. DC., Caricaceae 113
Leiphaimos graphita (Jacq.) Gilg, Gentianaceae 180
Lindernia diffusa Wettst., Scrophulariaceae 311
Luffa operculata (L.) Cogn., Cucurbitaceae 138
Mammea americana L., Clusiaceae 123

Momordica charantia L., Cucurbitaceae 139
Mucuna pruriens (L.) DC., Fabaceae 169
Nothoscordum striatum Kunth, Iridaceae 186
Oldenlandia corymbosa L., Rubiaceae 299
Ouratea jabotapita Engl., Ochnaceae 261
Ouratea parviflora (DC.) Baill., Ochnaceae 261
Passiflora edulis Sims, Passifloraceae 269
Passiflora laurifolia L., Passifloraceae 270
Passiflora mucronata Lam., Passifloraceae 270
Philodendron bipinnatifidum Schott, Araceae 36
Philodendron sellowm Koch, Araceae 37
Philodendron speciosum Schott, Araceae 37
Pluchea suaveolens (Vell.) O. Ktze., Asteraceae 64
Polygonum acuminatum H.B.K., Polygonaceae 286
Polygonum punctatum Elliot, Polygonaceae 287
Polygonum spectabile Mart., Polygonaceae 287
Portulaca oleracea L., Portulacaceae 289
Pothomorphe peltata L., Piperaceae 277
Psidium guajava L., Myrtaceae 256
Renealmia exaltata L. f., Zingiberaceae 342
Senna occidentalis (L.) Link, Caesalpiniaceae 105
Senna quinqueangulata
  (Rich.) Ir. & Barn., Caesalpiniaceae 106
Simarouba versicolor St.-Hil., Simaroubaceae 315
Sorocea bonplandii (Baill.) Burger, Moraceae 249
Spigelia anthelmia L., Loganiaceae 209
Spigelia glabrata Mart., Loganiaceae 209
Spigelia flemingiana Cham. & Schl., Loganiaceae . 209
Stachytarpheta jamaicensis (L.) Vahl, Verbenaceae 336
Tachia guianensis Aubl., Gentianaceae 180
Tagetes minuta L., Asteraceae 67
Tanacetum vulgare L., Asteraceae 67

Anthrax
  Heliotropium elongatum Willd., Boraginaceae 88
  Ilex paraguariensis St.-Hil., Aquifoliaceae 31

Antialgesic. *See* **Analgesic**

Antialgetic
  Solanum nigrum L., Solanaceae 321

Anticancer. *See also* **Cancer**
  Dalbergia subcymosa Ducke, Fabaceae 164
  Maytenus spp., Celastraceae (CHEM. & PHARM.) 116
  Tabebuia spp., Bignoniaceae 83

Antidiarrhoeic. *See* **Diarrhoea**

Antidote. *See* **Poison Antidote.** *See also* **Cassava Poison Antidote, Curare Antidote, Dart Antidote, Fish Poison Antidote, Plant Poison Antidote, Snakebite Antidote, Toxic**

Antiemetic
  Bouchea laetevirens Schauer, Verbenaceae 334
  Bouchea pseudogervao
    (St.-Hil.) Cham., Verbenaceae 334

Antifungal
  Euphorbia thymifolia
    L., Euphorbiaceae (CHEM. & PHARM.) 153

Antihydropic. *See* **Dropsy**

Antiluetic. *See* **Syphilis**

Antimicrobial
  Maytenus spp., Celastraceae (CHEM. & PHARM.) 116

Antiodontalgic. *See* **Toothache**

Antiophidic
  Borreria tenella Cham. & Schl., Rubiaceae 296

Dorstenia asaroides Gardn., Moraceae 247
Eclipta prostrata (L.) L., Asteraceae 59
Hypericum brasiliense Choisy, Clusiaceae 122
Mandevilla velutina (Mart. ex Stadelm.) Woods.
  var. *velutina*, Apocynaceae 27
Pfaffia jubata Mart., Amaranthaceae 5
Piper tuberculatum Jacq., Piperaceae 276

Antiphlogistic. *See* **Inflammations**
Antipoison. *See* **Poison Antidote**
Antipruriginous
  Peperomia pellucida H.B.K., Piperaceae 273
Antipyretic. *See* **Febrifuge**
Antirheumatic. *See* **Rheumatism, also Joint Pain**
Antiscorbutic
  Bidens graveolens Mart., Asteraceae 56
  Bidens pilosa L., Asteraceae 57
  Cereus peruvianus (L.) Mill., Cactaceae 94
  Croton floribundus Spreng., Euphorbiaceae 150
  Drimys winteri Forst., Winteraceae 340
  Melocactus melocactoides (Hoffm.) DC., Cactaceae . 97
  Rollinia orthopetala DC., Annonaceae 15
  Samolus valerandi L., Primulaceae 290
  Tropaeolum pentaphyllum Lam., Tropaeolaceae 327
Antiseptic
  Aristolochia trilobata L., Aristolochiaceae 48
  Copaifera officinalis (Jacq.) L., Caesalpiniaceae 102
  Dorstenia brasiliensis Lam., Moraceae 247
  Paullinia cupana Kunth, Sapindaceae 306
Antispasmodic. *See* **Spasmodic**
Antisyphilitic (Antiluetic). *See* **Syphilis**
Antithermic. *See* **Febrifuge**
Antitussive. *See* **Coughs**
Antiulcerogenic Effect
  Maytenus spp., Celastraceae (CHEM. & PHARM.) 116
Anuria
  Cybistax antisyphilitica
    (Mart.) Mart., Bignoniaceae 80
Anxiolytic
  Euphorbia hirta
    L., Euphorbiaceae (CHEM. & PHARM.) 152
Aperient
  Boehmeria caudata Sw., Urticaceae 330
  Hydrocotyle bonariensis Lam., Apiaceae 19
  Hydrocotyle leucocephala
    Cham. & Schlecht., Apiaceae 20
  Urera baccifera Gaud., Urticaceae 331
Aphrodisiac
  Acanthospermum hispidum DC., Asteraceae 52
  Anacardium occidentale L., Anacardiaceae 7
  Anemopaegma arvense (Vell.) Stapf, Bignoniaceae . 78
  Anemopaegma spp.: *A. album* Mart., *A. glaucum*
    Mart. & *A. scabriusculum* Mart., Bignoniaceae 78
  Anthurium oxycarpum Poepp., Araceae 33
  Astrocaryum murumuru Mart., Arecaceae 39
  Azolla caroliniana Willd., Salviniaceae 304
  Bixa orellana L., Bixaceae 85
  Cyperus gracilescens
    Roem. & Schult., Cyperaceae 142
  Davilla rugosa Poir., Dilleniaceae 145
  Ficus insipida Willd., Moraceae 248

APHRODISIAC – AROMATIC: MEDICINAL INDEX

Galactia neesii DC., Fabaceae 168
Galactia peduncularis (Benth.) Taub., Fabaceae ... 168
Hedyosmum brasiliense Mart., Chloranthaceae 119
Heteropteris aphrodisiaca
   O. Mach., Malpighiaceae 220
Hibiscus cannabinus L., Malvaceae 221
Lophophytum mirabile
   Schott & Endl., Balanophoraceae 73
Mucuna pruriens (L.) DC., Fabaceae 169
Nymphaea ampla DC., Nymphaeaceae 259
Paullinia cupana Kunth, Sapindaceae 306
Pfaffia paniculata (Mart.) Kuntze, Amaranthaceae 5
Phyllanthus nobilis M. Arg., Euphorbiaceae 157
Pouteria obtusifolia Baehni, Sapotaceae 310
Ptychopetalum olacoides Benth., Olacaceae 262
Ptychopetalum uncinatum Anselm., Olacaceae 262
Scybalium fungiforme
   Schott & Endl., Balanophoraceae 74
Secondatia floribunda DC., Apocynaceae 28
Selaginella convoluta Spring, Selaginellaceae 313
Solanum mammosum L., Solanaceae 321
Trichilia catuaba (Silva) Rizz., Meliaceae 229
Turnera diffusa Willd., Turneraceae 327
Turnera opifera Mart., Turneraceae 328
Tynanthus cognatus (Cham.) Miers, Bignoniaceae .. 84
Xylopia aromatica (Lam.) Mart., Annonaceae 15
Xylopia frutescens Aubl., Annonaceae 16

Aphthae. *See also* Ulcers
Anacardium occidentale L., Anacardiaceae 7
Annona marcgravii Mart., Annonaceae 13
Ayapana triplinerve
   (Vahl) King & Robinson, Asteraceae 53
Begonia hirtella Link, Begoniaceae 76
Bromelia arenaria Ule, Bromeliaceae 91
Bromelia pinguin L., Bromeliaceae 91
Cladonia miniata Mey., Cladoniaceae 120
Davilla rugosa Poir., Dilleniaceae 145
Doliocarpus rolandri Gmel., Dilleniaceae 146
Eryngium pristis Cham. & Schlecht., Apiaceae 19
Hypericum connatum Lam., Clusiaceae 122
Inga setigera DC., Mimosaceae 237
Rollinia sylvatica (St.-Hil.) Mart., Annonaceae 15
Tetracera aspera Willd., Dilleniaceae 146
Virola surinamensis (Rol.) Warb., Myristicaceae ... 252
Wissadula periplocifolia Presl., Malvaceae 223

Appetite Improver
Ilex paraguariensis St.-Hil., Aquifoliaceae 31
Maprounea brasiliensis L., Euphorbiaceae 155
Ocotea cujumary Mart., Lauraceae 200
Odontadenia speciosa Benth., Apocynaceae 27
Oenothera catharinensis Camb., Onagraceae 264
Senna occidentalis (L.) Link, Caesalpiniaceae 105
Senna quinqueangulata
   (Rich.) Ir. & Barn., Caesalpiniaceae 105
Tragia volubilis L., Euphorbiaceae 158
Turnera diffusa Willd., Turneraceae 327
Turnera opifera Mart., Turneraceae 328

Appetizer
Acmella oleracea (L.) R.K. Jansen, Asteraceae 52
Acmella repens (Walt.) L.C. Rich., Asteraceae 52
Capparis cynophallophora L., Capparaceae 111
Cleome speciosa H.B.K., Capparaceae 112
Hibiscus sabdariffa L., Malvaceae 221

Nectandra puberula Nees, Lauraceae 200
Samolus valerandi L., Primulaceae 290
Senna obtusifolia
   (L.) Ir. & Barn., Caesalpiniaceae 105
Vitex gardneriana Schauer, Verbenaceae 336

Arnica Substitute
Chionolaena latifolia (Benth.) Baker, Asteraceae 57
Heterothalamus alienus (Spr.) O. Ktze., Asteraceae 60
Solidago chilensis Meyen, Asteraceae 65

Aromatic
Achyrocline satureioides (Lam.) DC., Asteraceae 52
Ageratum conyzoides L., Asteraceae 53
Ambrosia artemisiifolia L., Asteraceae 53
Angelonia integerrima Spreng., Scrophulariaceae .. 310
Aniba permollis (Nees) Mez, Lauraceae 197
Aniba puchury-minor (Mart.) Mez, Lauraceae 197
Annona muricata L., Annonaceae 13
Astrocaryum murumuru Mart., Arecaceae 39
Calophyllum brasiliense Camb., Clusiaceae 120
Calyptranthes variabilis Berg, Myrtaceae 253
Cinnamodendron axillare
   (Nees & Mart.) Endl., Canellaceae 110
Citronella congonha (Mart.) Howard, Icacinaceae . 185
Citronella mucronata
   (R. & Pav.) Don, Icacinaceae 186
Cleome polygama L., Capparaceae 112
Conobea aquatica Aubl., Scrophulariaceae 311
Croton cajucara Benth., Euphorbiaceae 150
Croton sonderianus M. Arg., Euphorbiaceae 151
Croton zehntneri Pax & Hoffm., Euphorbiaceae ... 151
Cryptocarya mandioccana Meissn., Lauraceae 198
Cyperus sesquiflorus
   (Torrey) Mattf. & Kükent., Cyperaceae 142
Dodonaea viscosa Jacq., Sapindaceae 305
Esenbeckia febrifuga Juss., Rutaceae 301
Eugenia brasiliensis Lam., Myrtaceae 253
Eugenia uniflora L., Myrtaceae 254
Galinsoga parviflora Cav., Asteraceae 60
Genipa americana L., Rubiaceae 298
Gomphrena officinalis Mart., Amaranthaceae 4
Guatteria nigrescens Mart., Annonaceae 14
Guatteria scandens Ducke, Annonaceae 15
Guettarda angelica Mart., Rubiaceae 298
Hedyosmum brasiliense Mart., Chloranthaceae 119
Heterothalamus alienus (Spr.) O. Ktze., Asteraceae 60
Humiria balsamifera (Aubl.) St.-Hil., Humiriaceae 183
Hypericum brasiliense Choisy, Clusiaceae 122
Hypericum teretiusculum St.-Hil., Clusiaceae 122
Hyptis crenata Pohl, Lamiaceae 192
Keithia denudata Benth., Lamiaceae 193
Kyllinga pungens Link, Cyperaceae 143
Lantana brasiliensis Link, Verbenaceae 334
Lantana lilacina Desf., Verbenaceae 335
Lantana microphylla Cham., also *L. mixta* L.,
   L. pseudothea (St.-Hil.) Schauer, Verbenaceae 335
Leucas martinicensis (Jacq.) R. Br., Lamiaceae ... 194
Licaria camara (Schomb.) Kosterm., Lauraceae ... 198
Licaria puchury-major (Mart.)
   Kosterm., Lauraceae 199
Luxemburgia glazioviana Gilg, Ochnaceae 260
Luxemburgia polyandra St.-Hil., Ochnaceae 261
Marsypianthes chamaedrys
   (Vahl) O. Ktze., Lamiaceae 194

Melampodium divaricatum (Rich.) DC., Asteraceae 61
Mikania officinalis Mart., Asteraceae 62
Monnieria trifolia Loefl., Rutaceae 302
Nectandra canescens Nees, Lauraceae 199
Nectandra globosa (Aubl.) Mez, Lauraceae 199
Nectandra pichurim (H.B.K.) Mez, Lauraceae 200
Nectandra turbacensis Nees, Lauraceae 200
Ocotea cujumary Mart., Lauraceae 200
Ocotea cymbarum H.B.K., Lauraceae 200
Ocotea guianensis Aubl., Lauraceae 201
Ocotea rodiei (Schomb.) Mez, Lauraceae 201
Panicum trichanthum Nees, Poaceae 282
Piper ceanothifolium H.B.K., Piperaceae 275
Piper colubrinum Link, Piperaceae 275
Piper marginatum Jacq., Piperaceae 275
Piper reticulatum L., Piperaceae 276
Piper tuberculatum Jacq., Piperaceae 276
Pluchea suaveolens (Vell.) O. Ktze., Asteraceae 64
Pseudocaryophyllus sericeus Berg, Myrtaceae 256
Pterodon appariciol Peders., Fabaceae 170
Pterodon pubescens Benth., Fabaceae 171
Renealmia exaltata L. f., Zingiberaceae 342
Renealmia occidentalis Sweet, also
 Renealmia sylvestris Horan., Zingiberaceae 342
Siparuna brasiliensis (Spr.) DC., Monimiaceae 245
Siparuna camporum (Tul.) DC., Monimiaceae 245
Siparuna guianensis Aubl., Monimiaceae 245
Siparuna laurifolia (H.B.K.) DC., Monimiaceae 246
Stachytarpheta dichotoma Vahl, Verbenaceae 336
Tagetes minuta L., Asteraceae 67
Tanacetum vulgare L., Asteraceae 67
Tetralacrium veroniciforme
 Turcz., Scrophulariaceae 312
Tournefortia volubilis L., Boraginaceae 90
Turnera diffusa Willd., Turneraceae 327
Turnera opifera Mart., Turneraceae 328
Vernonanthura brasiliana
 (L.) H. Robinson, Asteraceae 67
Xylopia aromatica (Lam.) Mart., Annonaceae 15
Xylopia frutescens Aubl., Annonaceae 16
Xylopia sericea St.-Hil., Annonaceae 16

Arteriosclerosis.
See also Circulatory Problems
Costus spiralis (Jacq.) Roscoe, Costaceae 132
Cuphea balsamona Cham., Lythraceae 213
Echinodorus grandiflorus
 (Cham. & Schl.) Mich., Alismataceae 2
Echinodorus pubescens Mart., Alismataceae 2
Peperomia pellucida H.B.K., Piperaceae 273

Arthralgia
Acacia paniculata Willd., Mimosaceae 236
Aristolochia cymbifera
 Mart. & Zucc., Aristolochiaceae 46
Solanum nigrum L., Solanaceae 321

Arthritis. See also Gout, Joint Pain
Aniba canelilla (H.B.K.) Mez, Lauraceae 197
Buddleja brasiliensis Jacq. ex Spr., Buddlejaceae 93
Buddleja stachioides Cham., Buddlejaceae 93
Cabralea canjerana (Vell.) Mart., Meliaceae 227
Copernicia prunifera (Mill.) H. Moore, Arecaceae .. 40
Cordyline dracaenoides Kunth, Liliaceae 207
Echinodorus macrophyllus
 (Kunth) Mich., Alismataceae 2

Ficus gomelleira Kunth & Bouché, Moraceae 248
Guarea trichilioides L., Meliaceae 227
Himatanthus sucuuba (Spr.) Woods., Apocynaceae . 26
Hyptis crenata Pohl, Lamiaceae 192
Leucas martinicensis (Jacq.) R. Br., Lamiaceae 194
Luehea rufescens St.-Hil., Tiliaceae 327
Monstera adansonii Schott, Araceae 36
Ocotea opifera Mart., Lauraceae 201
Ocotea rodiei (Schomb.) Mez, Lauraceae 201
Philodendron pedatum (Hook.) Kunth, Araceae 37
Polygonum acuminatum H.B.K., Polygonaceae 286
Polygonum punctatum Elliot, Polygonaceae 287
Wilbrandia verticillata
 (Vell.) Cogn., Cucurbitaceae 140

Articular Pain. See Joint Pain

Ascites. See also Hydragogue
Cayaponia cabocla (Vell.) Mart., Cucurbitaceae ... 135
Cayaponia pilosa Cogn., Cucurbitaceae 135
Dichorisandra affinis Mart., Commelinaceae 128
Dichorisandra leucophthalmos
 Hook., Commelinaceae 128
Joannesia princeps Vell., Euphorbiaceae 155

Asthma
Anadenanthera peregrina (L.) Speg., Mimosaceae 236
Aristolochia cordigera Willd., Aristolochiaceae 46
Aristolochia cymbifera
 Mart. & Zucc., Aristolochiaceae 46
Bromelia antiacantha Bertol., Bromeliaceae 91
Buddleja brasiliensis Jacq. ex Spr., Buddlejaceae 93
Caesalpinia ferrea Mart. ex Tul., Caesalpiniaceae . 100
Cayaponia espelina
 (Manso) Cogn., Cucurbitaceae 135
Cecropia hololeuca Miq., Moraceae 247
Chiococca alba (L.) Hitch., Rubiaceae 297
Cissampelos glaberrima St.-Hil., Menispermaceae 233
Cissampelos sympodialis Eichl., Menispermaceae . 223
Cleome spinosa Jacq., Capparaceae 112
Dahlstedtia pentaphylla (Taub.) Burk, Fabaceae ... 163
Dahlstedtia pinnata (Benth.) Malme, Fabaceae 163
Datura arborea L., Solanaceae 317
Datura stramonium L., Solanaceae 318
Dioscorea silvestris Vell., Dioscoreaceae 147
Dipteryx odorata (Aubl.) Willd., Fabaceae 166
Dracontium asperum K. Koch, Araceae 35
Dracontium polyphyllum L., Araceae 36
Eclipta prostrata (L.) L., Asteraceae 59
Erythrina corallodendron L., Fabaceae 166
Erythrina falcata Benth., Fabaceae 166
Erythroxylum cataractarum
 Spruce, Erythroxylaceae 149
Erythroxylum coca Lam., Erythroxylaceae 149
Euphorbia hirta L., Euphorbiaceae 152
Genipa americana L., Rubiaceae 298
Heliotropium elongatum Willd., Boraginaceae 88
Himatanthus lancifolia
 (M. Arg.) Woods., Apocynaceae 26
Hippeastrum vittatum
 (L'Hérit.) Herb., Amaryllidaceae 6
Hippobroma longiflora (L.) G. Don [including
 Lobelia longiflora L.], Campanulaceae 109
Leonotis nepetaefolia R. Br., Lamiaceae 194
Mimosa bimucronata (DC.) O. Ktze., Mimosaceae 238
Myroxylon balsamum (L.) Harms, Fabaceae 170

ASTHMA – ASTRINGENT: MEDICINAL INDEX

Ocimum micranthum Willd., Lamiaceae 195
Parahancornia amapa (Hub.) Ducke, Apocynaceae 27
Peltodon radicans Pohl, Lamiaceae 195
Pradosia lactescens (Vell.) Radlk., Sapotaceae 310
Prunus subcoriacea (Chod. & Hassl.)
  Hoehne, Rosaceae 294
Psoralea glandulosa L., Fabaceae 170
Salacia impressifolia
  (Miers) A.C. Sm., Hippocrateaceae 183
Sida micrantha St.-Hil., Malvaceae 222
Solanum grandiflorum Ruiz & Pav., Solanaceae ... 320
Torresea cearensis Fr. All., Fabaceae 172
Verbena bonariensis L., Verbenaceae 336
Verbena erinoides Lam., Verbenaceae 336
Virola oleifera (Schott) A.C. Smith, Myristicaceae . 250

Astringent

Alsodeia flavescens (Aubl.) Spreng., Violaceae 337
Anacardium occidentale L., Anacardiaceae 7
Anadenanthera colubrina
  (Vell.) Brenan, Mimosaceae 236
Annona muricata L., Annonaceae 13
Annona reticulata L., Annonaceae 13
Annona squamosa L., Annonaceae 13
Aspidosperma polyneuron M. Arg., Apocynaceae 21
Astronium fraxinifolium Schott, Anacardiaceae 9
Ayapana triplinerve
  (Vahl) King & Robinson, Asteraceae 53
Bauhinia langsdorffiana Bong., Caesalpiniaceae 99
Berberis laurina Thunb., Berberidaceae 76
Blepharocalyx salicifolius
  (H.B.K.) Berg, Myrtaceae 253
Bumelia sartorum Mart., Sapotaceae 308
Byrsonima spicata Rich., Malpighiaceae 219
Byrsonima verbascifolia (L.) Rich., Malpighiaceae 220
Cabomba piauhyensis Gard., Nymphaeaceae 259
Calea pinnatifida (R. Br.) Less., Asteraceae 57
Calophyllum brasiliense Camb., Clusiaceae 120
Cariniana legalis (Mart.) O. Ktze., Lecythidaceae .. 204
Casearia guyanensis (Aubl.) Urb., Flacourtiaceae . 177
Cecropia hololeuca Miq., Moraceae 247
Chrysobalanus icaco L., Chrysobalanaceae 119
Cissampelos fasciculata Benth., Menispermaceae . 231
Clusia rosea Jacq., Clusiaceae 122
Coccoloba laevis Casar., Polygonaceae 285
Conocarpus erecta L., Combretaceae 126
Croton urucurana Baill., Euphorbiaceae 151
Curatella americana L., Dilleniaceae 144
Cuscuta racemosa Mart., Convolvulaceae 130
Cyathea microdonta (Desv.) Domin, Cyatheaceae . 141
Davilla rugosa Poir., Dilleniaceae 145
Dodonaea viscosa Jacq., Sapindaceae 305
Doliocarpus rolandri Gmel., Dilleniaceae 146
Echinodorus macrophyllus
  (Kunth) Mich., Alismataceae 2
Equisetum giganteum L., Equisetaceae 148
Eugenia brasiliensis Lam., Myrtaceae 253
Galipea multiflora Schult., Rutaceae 301
Galphimia brasiliensis Juss., Malpighiaceae 220
Guarea trichilioides L., Meliaceae 227
Guettarda argentea Lam., Rubiaceae 298
Guettarda uruguayensis
  Cham. & Schl., Rubiaceae 298
Heliconia bihai L., Heliconiaceae 181

Helosis cayennensis
  (Swartz) Spreng., Balanophoraceae 73
Hymenaea courbaril L., Caesalpiniaceae 103
Hypericum brasiliense Choisy, Clusiaceae 122
Ilex acrodonta Reiss., Aquifoliaceae 31
Jacaranda caroba (Vell.) DC., Bignoniaceae 80
Jodina rhombifolia Hook. & Arn., Santalaceae 304
Krameria spartioides Berg, Krameriaceae 191
Krameria tomentosa St.-Hil., Krameriaceae 191
Laplacea fruticosa (Schr.) Kobuski, Theaceae 326
Leandra lacunosa Cogn., Melastomataceae 225
Limonium brasiliense
  (Boiss.) O. Ktze., Plumbaginaceae 278
Lithraea molleoides (Vell.) Engl., Anacardiaceae 9
Ludwigia suffruticosa (L.) Gomes, Onagraceae 264
Luehea rufescens St.-Hil., Tiliaceae 327
Marlierea tomentosa Camb., Myrtaceae 255
Microgramma vaccinifolia
  (Langsd. & Fisch.) Copel., Polypodiaceae 288
Mimosa verrucosa Benth., Mimosaceae 240
Mouriri guianensis Aubl., Melastomataceae 225
Myrcia tingens Berg, Myrtaceae 255
Neea theifera Oersted, Nyctaginaceae 258
Ocotea rodiei (Schomb.) Mez, Lauraceae 201
Parkia oppositifolia (Spruce) Benth., Mimosaceae 240
Parkia pectinata Benth., Mimosaceae 240
Passiflora laurifolia L., Passifloraceae 270
Pentaclethra macroloba
  (Willd.) O. Ktze., Mimosaceae 242
Philodendron imbe Schott, Araceae 36
Philodendron ochrostemon Schott, Araceae 37
Phyllanthus diffusus Klotz., Euphorbiaceae 156
Piper aduncum L., Piperaceae 274
Piper angustifolium R. & Pav., Piperaceae 274
Pithecellobium avaremotemo Mart., Mimosaceae .. 242
Polygonum punctatum Elliot, Polygonaceae 287
Pouteria salicifolia Hook. & Arn., Sapotaceae 310
Pradosia lactescens (Vell.) Radlk., Sapotaceae 310
Protium icicariba (DC.) March., Burseraceae 94
Psidium guajava L., Myrtaceae 256
Raulinoreitzia tremula (Hook. & Arn.)
  King & Robinson, Asteraceae 64
Rollinia exalbida (Vell.) Mart., Annonaceae 15
Rollinia salicifolia Schl., Annonaceae 15
Sapindus saponaria L., Sapindaceae 306
Schinus molle L., Anacardiaceae 9
Senna multijuga Rich. var. *verrucosa*
  (Vog.) Ir. & Barn., Caesalpiniaceae 105
Sparattosperma leucanthum
  (Vell.) K. Sch., Bignoniaceae 82
Spondias macrocarpa Engl., Anacardiaceae 10
Spondias mombin L., Anacardiaceae 10
Symplocos platyphylla
  (Pohl) Benth., Symplocaceae 326
Symplocos pubescens Klotzsch, Symplocaceae 326
Tabebuia ipe (Mart.) Standl., Bignoniaceae 83
Tabebuia umbellata (Sond.) Sandw., Bignoniaceae .. 83
Ternstroemia brasiliensis Camb., Theaceae 326
Triumfetta rhomboidea Jacq., Tiliaceae 327
Triumfetta semitriloba Jacq., Tiliaceae 327
Turnera diffusa Willd., Turneraceae 327
Turnera opifera Mart., Turneraceae 328
Turnera ulmifolia L., Turneraceae 328

MEDICINAL INDEX: ASTRINGENT – BITTER

Typha domingensis Pers., Typhaceae 328
Vouacapoua americana Aubl., Caesalpiniaceae 108
Ximenia americana L., Olacaceae 263
Ximenia coriacea Engl., Olacaceae 263

Athlete's Foot
Buchnera aquatica Aubl., Scrophulariaceae 310
Hedyosmum brasiliense Mart., Chloranthaceae 119
Kalanchoe brasiliensis Camb., Crassulaceae 133

Atony, Gastric
Calolisianthus pendulus
   (Mart.) Gilg, Gentianaceae 179

B

Bacterial Infections
Croton salutaris Casar., Euphorbiaceae 151

Bactericide
Conocarpus erecta L., Combretaceae 126
Mikania glomerata Spreng., Asteraceae 61

Bacteriostatic
Limonium brasiliense (Boiss.) O. Ktze.,
   Plumbaginaceae (CHEM & PHARM.) 278

Baldness
Adiantum trapeziforme L., Adiantaceae 1
Anthurium affine Schott, Araceae 33
Scheelea phalerata
   (Mart. ex Spreng.) Burret, Arecaceae 45

Balsamic
Clusia rosea Jacq., Clusiaceae 122
Copaifera officinalis (Jacq.) L., Caesalpiniaceae 102
Cyperus rotundus L., Cyperaceae 142
Humiria balsamifera
   (Aubl.) St.-Hil., Humiriaceae 183
Hymenaea courbaril L., Caesalpiniaceae 103
Laetia apetala Jacq., Flacourtiaceae 178
Myracroduon urundeuva
   Fr. All., Anacardiaceae 9
Myroxylon balsamum (L.) Harms, Fabaceae 170
Piper angustifolium R. & Pav., Piperaceae 274
Styrax ferrugineum Nees & Mart., Styracaceae 325
Styrax glabratum Schott, Styracaceae 325
Styrax pohlii DC., Styracaceae 325

Bechic. *See* Coughs

Benzoin Substitute
Styrax ferrugineum Nees & Mart., Styracaceae 325
Styrax glabratum Schott, also
   Styrax pohlii DC., Styracaceae 325

Beriberi
Cocos nucifera L., Arecaceae 40

Bilharzia. *See* Schistosomiasis

Biliar Calculi
Sparattosperma leucanthum
   (Vell.) K. Sch., Bignoniaceae 82

Biliary Obstructions
Silybum marianum Gaertn., Asteraceae 65
Symphonia globulifera L. f., Clusiaceae 123

Bites. *See also* Poison, Stings, Snakebite
Clematis denticulata Vell., Ranunculaceae 290
Talisia esculenta Radlk., Sapindaceae 306

Bitter
Abuta candicans Rich., Menispermaceae 231
Abuta rufescens Aubl., Menispermaceae 231
Acanthospermum australe
   (Loefl.) O. Ktze., Asteraceae ....
Acanthospermum hispidum DC., Asteraceae 52
Achyrocline satureioides (Lam.) DC., Asteraceae 52
Acosmium dasycarpum (Vog.) Yakovl., Fabaceae .. 162
Acosmium subelegans
   (Mohlenb.) Yakovl., Fabaceae 162
Ageratum conyzoides L., Asteraceae 53
Allagoptera campestris (Mart.) Kuntze, Arecaceae .. 39
Alsodeia flavescens (Aubl.) Spreng., Violaceae 337
Anadenanthera colubrina
   (Vell.) Brenan, Mimosaceae 236
Anisosperma passiflora Manso, Cucurbitaceae 135
Aristolochia trilobata L., Aristolochiaceae 48
Aspidosperma discolor Benth., Apocynaceae 21
Aspidosperma polyneuron M. Arg., Apocynaceae ... 21
Baccharis articulata (Lam.) Pers., Asteraceae 54
Bathysa cuspidata Hook., Rubiaceae 296
Bidens pilosa L., Asteraceae 57
Buddleja brasiliensis Jacq. ex Spr., Buddlejaceae 93
Calea pinnatifida (R. Br.) Less., Asteraceae 57
Calolisianthus pendulus
   (Mart.) Gilg, Gentianaceae 179
Calophyllum brasiliense Camb., Clusiaceae 120
Carapa guianensis Aubl., Meliaceae 227
Casearia ovata Willd., Flacourtiaceae 178
Cayaponia pilosa Cogn., Cucurbitaceae 135
Cayaponia tayuya (Mart.) Cogn., Cucurbitaceae ... 135
Cestrum amictum Schl., Solanaceae 317
Cissampelos ovalifolia DC., Menispermaceae 233
Cissampelos sympodialis Eichl., Menispermaceae . 233
Clibadium surinamense L., Asteraceae 58
Clusia rosea Jacq., Clusiaceae 122
Cocculus filipendula Mart., Menispermaceae 234
Coutarea hexandra (Jacq.) K. Sch., Rubiaceae 297
Coutoubea spicata Aubl., Gentianaceae 179
Craniolaria annua L., Martyniaceae 224
Crataeva tapia L., Capparaceae 112
Cryptocarya mandioccana Meissn., Lauraceae 198
Curtia tenuifolia (Aubl.) Knobl., Gentianaceae 180
Cusparia febrifuga Humb., Rutaceae 300
Deianira erubescens Cham. & Schl., Gentianaceae 180
Deianira nervosa Cham. & Schl., Gentianaceae 180
Deianira pallescens Cham. & Schl., Gentianaceae . 180
Dipholis nigra Gr., Sapotaceae 309
Dodonaea viscosa Jacq., Sapindaceae 305
Egletes viscosa (L.) Less., Asteraceae 59
Eryngium pristis Cham. & Schlecht., Apiaceae 19
Esenbeckia febrifuga Juss., Rutaceae 301
Esenbeckia intermedia Mart., Rutaceae 301
Evolvulus alsinoides L., Convolvulaceae 130
Exostemma australe St.-Hil., Rubiaceae 298
Fevillea uncipetala Kuhlm., Cucurbitaceae 138
Galipea multiflora Schult., Rutaceae 301
Geissospermum laeve (Vell.) Baill., Apocynaceae ... 23
Guarea trichilioides L., Meliaceae 227
Hibiscus sabdariffa L., Malvaceae 221
Hortia brasiliensis Vand., Rutaceae 301
Jacaranda caroba (Vell.) DC., Bignoniaceae 80

BITTER – BLADDER STONES: MEDICINAL INDEX

Jatropha multifida L., Euphorbiaceae 154
Ladenbergia hexandra Klotz., Rubiaceae 299
Ladenbergia lambertiana Klotz., Rubiaceae 299
Lantana brasiliensis Link, Verbenaceae 334
Lindernia diffusa Wettst., Scrophulariaceae 311
Mabea fistulifera Mart., Euphorbiaceae 155
Marupa francoana Miers, Simaroubaceae 313
Melampodium divaricatum (Rich.) DC., Asteraceae 61
Mikania officinalis Mart., Asteraceae 62
Mimosa pudica L., Mimosaceae 240
Mimosa velloziana Mart., Mimosaceae 240
Mimosa verrucosa Benth., Mimosaceae 240
Monnieria trifolia Loefl., Rutaceae 302
Monopteryx uacu Spruce ex Benth., Fabaceae 169
Naucleopsis amara Ducke, Moraceae 249
Nymphoides indica (L.) O. Ktze., Menyanthaceae 235
Ocotea rodiei (Schomb.) Mez, Lauraceae 201
Ocotea spectabilis (Meissn.) Mez, Lauraceae 201
Ocotea teleiandra (Messn.) Mez, Lauraceae 203
Ouratea guianensis Aubl., Ochnaceae 261
Parapiptadenia rigida
   (Benth.) Brenan, Mimosaceae 240
Passiflora laurifolia L., Passifloraceae 270
Phyllanthus conami Sw., Euphorbiaceae 156
Phyllanthus diffusus Klotz., Euphorbiaceae 156
Phyllanthus niruri L., Euphorbiaceae 156
Picramnia bahiensis Turcz., Simaroubaceae 313
Picramnia camboita Engl., Simaroubaceae 314
Picramnia ciliata Mart., Simaroubaceae 314
Pithecellobium unguis-cati
   (L.) Benth., Mimosaceae 242
Quassia amara L., Simaroubaceae 314
Raputia alba (Nees & Mart.) Engl., Rutaceae 302
Raputia magnifica Engl., Rutaceae 302
Rumex brasiliensis Link, Polygonaceae 287
Schultesia stenophylla Mart., Gentianaceae 180
Senna obtusifolia (L.) Ir. & Barn., Caesalpiniaceae 105
Senna occidentalis (L.) Link, Caesalpiniaceae 105
Senna quinqueangulata
   (Rich.) Ir. & Barn., Caesalpiniaceae 106
Sida acuta Burm., Malvaceae 221
Simaba ferruginea St.-Hil., Simaroubaceae 314
Simaba glandulifera Gardn., Simaroubaceae 314
Simaba salubris Engl., Simaroubaceae 315
Simarouba amara Aubl., Simaroubaceae 315
Simarouba versicolor St.-Hil., Simaroubaceae 315
Solanum insidiosum Mart., Solanaceae 320
Solanum mammosum L., Solanaceae 321
Solanum paniculatum L., Solanaceae 321
Solidago chilensis Meyen, Asteraceae 65
Sparattosperma leucanthum
   (Vell.) K. Sch., Bignoniaceae 82
Strychnos pseudoquina St.-Hil., Loganiaceae 209
Strychnos subcordata Spr. ex Benth., Loganiaceae 209
Syagrus comosa Mart., Arecaceae 45
Syagrus oleracea (Mart.) Becc., Arecaceae 45
Symplocos platyphylla
   (Pohl) Benth., Symplocaceae 326
Symplocos pubescens Klotzsch, Symplocaceae 326
Tabebuia impetiginosa
   (Mart.) Standl., Bignoniaceae 83
Tachia guianensis Aubl., Gentianaceae 180
Tanacetum vulgare L., Asteraceae 67

Tetralacrium veroniciforme
   Turcz., Scrophulariaceae 312
Thevetia ahouai (L.) DC., Apocynaceae 28
Tontelea brachypoda Miers, Hippocrateaceae 183
Trianosperma diversifolia Cogn., Cucurbitaceae 139
Vataireopsis araroba (Aguiar) Ducke, Fabaceae 172
Wilbrandia ebracteata Cogn., Cucurbitaceae 140
Wilbrandia verticillata
   (Vell.) Cogn., Cucurbitaceae 140
Zanthoxylum hyemale St.-Hil., Rutaceae 302
Zanthoxylum rhoifolium Lam., Rutaceae 303

Bladder Disease. *See also*
Cystitis; includes Bladder Catarrh
Abuta rufescens Aubl., Menispermaceae 231
Ageratum conyzoides L., Asteraceae 53
Alternanthera achyrantha R. Br., Amaranthaceae 3
Amaranthus spinosus L., Amaranthaceae 3
Amaranthus viridis L., Amaranthaceae 3
Blepharocalyx salicifolius
   (H.B.K.) Berg, Myrtaceae 253
Bomarea spectabilis Schrenk, Amaryllidaceae 6
Campomanesia aurea Berg,
   C. xanthocarpa Berg, Myrtaceae 253
Canna glauca L., Cannaceae 110
Cestrum bracteatum Link & Otto, Solanaceae 317
Cestrum parqui L'Herit., Solanaceae 317
Chamissoa macrocarpa H.B.K., Amaranthaceae 4
Chrysobalanus icaco L., Chrysobalanaceae 119
Cocculus filipendula Mart., Menispermaceae 234
Costus cuspidatus
   (Nees & Mart.) Maas, Costaceae 132
Doliocarpus rolandri Gmel., Dilleniaceae 146
Ficus gomelleira Kunth & Bouché, Moraceae 248
Heliotropium elongatum Willd., Boraginaceae 88
Jacaranda subrhombea DC., Bignoniaceae 81
Lippia gratissima
   (Gill. & Hook.) Troncoso, Verbenaceae 335
Quassia amara L., Simaroubaceae 314
Stromanthe sanguinea Sond., Marantaceae 224
Turnera diffusa Willd., Turneraceae 327
Turnera opifera Mart., Turneraceae 328
Xanthium orientale L., X. spinosum L.
   & X. strumarium L., Asteraceae 67
Xylopia frutescens Aubl., Annonaceae 16

Bladder Spasms
Solanum nigrum L., Solanaceae 321

Bladder Stones (Gallstones).
See also **Biliary Obstructions**
Cissampelos fluminensis Eichl., Menispermaceae .. 233
Costus spicatus (Jacq.) Sw., Costaceae 132
Manilkara zapota (L.) Van Royen, Sapotaceae 309
Margyricarpus setosus Ruiz & Pav., Rosaceae 294
Mimosa invisa Mart., Mimosaceae 239
Phyllanthus acutifolius Spreng., Euphorbiaceae ... 156
Phyllanthus niruri L., Euphorbiaceae 156
Phyllanthus sellowianus M. Arg., Euphorbiaceae .. 157
Phyllanthus tenellus Roxb. [includes
   P. corcovadensis M. Arg.], Euphorbiaceae 157
Pterocaulon virgatum DC., Asteraceae 64
Quassia amara L., Simaroubaceae 314
Sparattosperma leucanthum
   (Vell.) K. Sch., Bignoniaceae 82

MEDICINAL INDEX: BLEEDING – BRONCHOPULMONARY PROBLEMS

Bleeding. *See* **Hemorrhage, Menstruation, Metrorrhagia**
Blennorrhagia. *See also* **Gonorrhoea**
Acanthospermum australe
  (Loefl.) O. Ktze., Asteraceae 51
Amaranthus spinosus L., Amaranthaceae 3
Brunfelsia uniflora (Pohl) D. Don, also
  B. grandiflora D. Don, Solanaceae 316
Canna glauca L., Cannaceae 110
Cecropia palmata Willd., Moraceae 247
Chrysobalanus icaco L., Chrysobalanaceae 119
Cocos nucifera L., Arecaceae 40
Copaifera officinalis (Jacq.) L., Caesalpiniaceae ... 102
Cuscuta racemosa Mart., Convolvulaceae 130
Guazuma ulmifolia Lam.,
  var. *ulmifolia*, Sterculiaceae 323
Hymenaea courbaril L., Caesalpiniaceae 103
Hypoxis decumbens L., Hypoxidaceae 185
Jacaranda subrhombea DC., Bignoniaceae 81
Lithraea molleoides (Vell.) Engl., Anacardiaceae 9
Luehea rufescens St.-Hil., Tiliaceae 327
Myroxylon balsamum (L.) Harms, Fabaceae 170
Nectandra leucantha Nees, Lauraceae 199
Passiflora foetida L., Passifloraceae 269
Peperomia elongata Miq., Piperaceae 273
Polygala paniculata L., Polygalaceae 284
Protium schomburgkianum Engl., Burseraceae 94
Remirea maritima Aubl., Cyperaceae 143
Schinus molle L., Anacardiaceae 9
Sebastiania klotzschiana M. Arg., Euphorbiaceae .. 157
Tillandsia aeranthos
  (Loisel.) L.B. Smith, Bromeliaceae 91
Triumfetta semitriloba Jacq., Tiliaceae 327
Waltheria communis St.-Hil., Sterculiaceae 325
Virola oleifera (Schott) A.C. Smith, Myristicaceae . 250
Zanthoxylum rhoifolium Lam., Rutaceae 303

Blood Pressure.
  See **Hypertension, Hypotension**

Blood Strengthener. *See also* **Depurative**
Cassytha filiformis L., Lauraceae 198
Euterpe oleracea Mart., Arecaceae 42
Polycarpaea corymbosa
  (L.) Lam., Caryophyllaceae 115
Portulaca pilosa L., Portulacaceae 289

Blood Sugar Level, Controls.
  See also **Hypoglycemia**
Chrysobalanus icaco
  L., Chrysobalanaceae (PHARM.) 119

Boils. *See also* **Furunculosis**
Albizzia lebbeck (L.) Benth., Mimosaceae 236
Caryocar coriaceum Wittm., Caryocaraceae 114
Cayaponia tayuya (Mart.) Cogn., Cucurbitaceae 135
Dioscorea basiclavicaulis
  Rizz. & Mattos, Dioscoreaceae 146
Griffinia hyacinthina Ker-Gawl., Amaryllidaceae 6
Heliotropium indicum L., Boraginaceae 89
Hymenocallis tubiflora Salisb. [includes *Pancratium guianensis* Ker-Gawl.], Amaryllidaceae 7
Mimosa malacocentra Mart., Mimosaceae 239
Pilea microphylla (L.) Liebm., Urticaceae 331
Solanum verbascifolium L., Solanaceae 322

Struthanthus marginatus
  (Desf.) Bl., Loranthaceae 213
Turnera guianensis Aubl., Turneraceae 313
Wissadula periplocifolia Presl., Malvaceae 223
Xanthosoma violaceum Schott, Araceae 37

Bone Disease
Symphonia globulifera L. f., Clusiaceae 123

Bone Fractures. *See* **Fractures**

Bowel Movements, Improve
Ocotea cujumary Mart., Lauraceae 200

Breast Sores
Amasonia arborea H.B.K., Verbenaceae 333

Bronchitis
Acanthospermum hispidum DC., Asteraceae 52
Anadenanthera macrocarpa
  (Benth.) Brenan, Mimosaceae 236
Anadenanthera peregrina (L.) Speg., Mimosaceae 236
Ananas comosus (L.) Merrill, Bromeliaceae 90
Aristolochia cordigera Willd., Aristolochiaceae 46
Aspidosperma excelsum Benth., Apocynaceae 21
Bauhinia radiata Vell., Caesalpiniaceae 99
Bixa orellana L., Bixaceae 85
Bromelia antiacantha Bertol., Bromeliaceae 91
Buddleja brasiliensis Jacq. ex Spr., Buddlejaceae ... 93
Byrsonima crassifolia H.B.K., Malpighiaceae 219
Caryocar brasiliense Camb., Caryocaraceae 114
Cayaponia espelina
  (Manso) Cogn., Cucurbitaceae 135
Cissampelos sympodialis Eichl., Menispermaceae . 233
Cleome spinosa Jacq., Capparaceae 112
Copaifera officinalis (Jacq.) L., Caesalpiniaceae 102
Cordia grandiflora DC., Boraginaceae 87
Cordia multispicata Cham., Boraginaceae 88
Elionurus candidus (Trin.) Hack., also
  Elionurus latiflorus Nees, Poaceae 281
Gochnatia polymorpha (Less.) Cabr., Asteraceae 60
Hymenaea courbaril L., Caesalpiniaceae 103
Hymenocallis tubiflora Salisb. [includes *Pancratium guianensis* Ker-Gawl.], Amaryllidaceae 7
Inga setigera DC., Mimosaceae 237
Lantana lilacina Desf., Verbenaceae 335
Leonurus sibiricus L., Lamiaceae 194
Luehea divaricata Mart. & Zucc., Tiliaceae 326
Mimosa bimucronata (DC.) O. Ktze., Mimosaceae 238
Ocimum micranthum Willd., Lamiaceae 195
Parahancornia amapa (Hub.) Ducke, Apocynaceae 27
Passiflora caerulea L., Passifloraceae 269
Scoparia dulcis L., Scrophulariaceae 312
Tagetes erecta L., Asteraceae 67
Torresea cearensis Fr. All., Fabaceae 172
Vitex agnus-castus L., Verbenaceae 336
Waltheria communis St.-Hil., Sterculiaceae 325
Waltheria viscosissima St.-Hil., Sterculiaceae 325

Bronchodilator
Cissampelos sympodialis Eichl.,
  Menispermaceae (CHEM. & PHARM.) 233
Mikania glomerata Spreng., Asteraceae 61
Torresea cearensis Fr. All., Fabaceae 172

Bronchopulmonary Problems.
  See also **Asthma, Catarrh, Tuberculosis**
Caryocar coriaceum Wittm., Caryocaraceae 114
Cladonia pyxidata (L.) Ach., Cladoniaceae 120

BRONCHOPULMONARY PROBLEMS – CARMINATIVE: MEDICINAL INDEX

Lantana camara L., Verbenaceae 334
Stomatanthes oblongifolius
   (Spr.) H. Robinson, Asteraceae 65
Bruises. *See* **Contusions**
Buboes
Esenbeckia febrifuga Juss., Rutaceae 301
Galipea multiflora Schult., Rutaceae 301
Kalanchoe brasiliensis Camb., Crassulaceae 133
Lithraea molleoides (Vell.) Engl., Anacardiaceae 9
Schinus molle L., Anacardiaceae 9
Burns
Apium sellowianum Wolf, Apiaceae 18
Berberis laurina Thunb., Berberidaceae 76
Buchnera aquatica Aubl., Scrophulariaceae 310
Cereus peruvianus (L.) Mill., Cactaceae 94
Kalanchoe brasiliensis Camb., Crassulaceae 133
Portulaca oleracea L., Portulacaceae 289
Portulaca pilosa L., Portulacaceae 289
Pothomorphe peltata L., Piperaceae 277
Senna occidentalis (L.) Link, Caesalpiniaceae 105
Senna quinqueangulata
   (Rich.) Ir. & Barn., Caesalpiniaceae 106
Stryphnodendron adstringens
   (Mart.) Cov., Mimosaceae 242

C

Calculi. *See* **Bladder Stones, Gallstones**
Calmative
Aloysia triphylla (L'Her.) Britt., Verbenaceae 332
Aniba canelilla (H.B.K.) Mez, Lauraceae 197
Annona muricata L., Annonaceae 13
Carica papaya L., Caricaceae 113
Combretum leprosum Mart., Combretaceae 126
Costus spiralis (Jacq.) Roscoe, Costaceae 132
Croton zehntneri Pax & Hoffm., Euphorbiaceae 151
Cymbopogon schoenanthus (L.) Spreng., Poaceae 280
Cyperus sesquiflorus
   (Torrey) Mattf. & Kükent., Cyperaceae 142
Datura arborea L., Solanaceae 317
Datura stramonium L., Solanaceae 318
Erythrina corallodendron L., Fabaceae 166
Erythrina velutina Willd., Fabaceae 166
Erythrina verna Vell., Fabaceae 168
Hyptis spicigera Lam., Lamiaceae 193
Licaria puchury-major
   (Mart.) Kosterm., Lauraceae 199
Ocotea rodiei (Schomb.) Mez, Lauraceae 201
Passiflora edulis Sims, Passifloraceae 269
Passiflora macrocarpa Mast., Passifloraceae 270
Philodendron pedatum (Hook.) Kunth, Araceae 37
Physalis angulata L., Solanaceae 318
Piper colubrinum Link, Piperaceae 275
Pluchea laxiflora Hook. & Arn., Asteraceae 64
Solanum cernuum Vell., Solanaceae 319
Solanum mauritianum Scop., Solanaceae 321
Vitex gardneriana Schauer, Verbenaceae 336
Cancer. *See* **also Carcinoma**
Aspidosperma nigricans Handro, Apocynaceae 21
Copaifera officinalis (Jacq.) L., Caesalpiniaceae 102
Dalbergia subcymosa Ducke, Fabaceae 164
Himatanthus sucuuba (Spr.) Woods., Apocynaceae . 26

Jodina rhombifolia Hook. & Arn., Santalaceae 304
Tabebuia impetiginosa
   (Mart.) Standl., Bignoniaceae 83
Carcinoma. *See also* **Cancer**
Aristolochia spp., Aristolochiaceae 49
Croton cajucara Benth., Euphorbiaceae 150
Orbignya phalerata Mart., Arecaceae 43
Cardio [*See also* Heart Problems]
–active
Colletia paradoxa (Spr.) Escalante, Rhamnaceae ... 291
Dipteryx odorata (Aubl.) Willd., Fabaceae 166
Hylocereus undatus (Haw.) Br. & Rose, Cactaceae .. 95
Paullinia cupana Kunth, Sapindaceae 306
Peschiera laeta (Mart.) Miers, Apocynaceae 27
Spondias macrocarpa Engl., Anacardiaceae 10
Spondias mombin L., Anacardiaceae 10
–tonic
Dipteryx odorata (Aubl.) Willd., Fabaceae 166
Scoparia dulcis L., Scrophulariaceae (PHARM.) 312
Caries
Xylopia frutescens Aubl., Annonaceae 16
Carminative (Flatulence)
Abuta rufescens Aubl., Menispermaceae 231
Ageratum conyzoides L., Asteraceae 53
Aniba permollis (Nees) Mez, Lauraceae 197
Annona squamosa L., Annonaceae 13
Aristolochia cymbifera
   Mart. & Zucc., Aristolochiaceae 46
Aspidosperma excelsum Benth., Apocynaceae 21
Calyptranthes aromatica St.-Hil., Myrtaceae 253
Chenopodium ambrosioides L., Chenopodiaceae ... 118
Croton floribundus Spreng., Euphorbiaceae 150
Cryptocarya guyanensis Meissn., Lauraceae 198
Cryptocarya moschata
   Nees & Mart. ex Nees, Lauraceae 198
Cymbopogon schoenanthus (L.) Spreng., Poaceae 280
Cyperus sesquiflorus
   (Torrey) Mattf. & Kükent., Cyperaceae 142
Dodonaea viscosa Jacq., Sapindaceae 305
Gomphrena mollis Mart., Amaranthaceae 4
Hyptis mutabilis (Rich.) Briq., Lamiaceae 193
Hyptis umbrosa Salzm., Lamiaceae 193
Leucas martinicensis (Jacq.) R. Br., Lamiaceae 194
Licaria camara (Schomb.) Kosterm., Lauraceae 198
Mariscus jacquinii H.B.K., Cyperaceae 143
Marsypianthes chamaedrys
   (Vahl) O. Ktze., Lamiaceae 194
Mentha crispa L., Lamiaceae 194
Nectandra globosa (Aubl.) Mez, Lauraceae 199
Nectandra leucantha Nees, Lauraceae 199
Nectandra turbacensis Nees, Lauraceae 200
Ocimum micranthum Willd., Lamiaceae 195
Ottonia corcovadensis Miq., Piperaceae 272
Pappophorum mucronulatum Nees, Poaceae 282
Peltodon radicans Pohl, Lamiaceae 195
Piper arboreum Aubl., Piperaceae 274
Piper colubrinum Link, Piperaceae 275
Piper eucalyptifolium (Miq.) Rudge, Piperaceae 275
Piper gigantifolium Jacq., Piperaceae 275
Piper marginatum Jacq., Piperaceae 275
Piper tuberculatum Jacq., Piperaceae 276
Pluchea laxiflora Hook. & Arn., Asteraceae 64

Pluchea suaveolens (Vell.) O. Ktze., Asteraceae 64
Quassia amara L., Simaroubaceae 314
Renealmia exaltata L. f., Zingiberaceae 342
Renealmia occidentalis Sweet, also
  Renealmia sylvestris Horan., Zingiberaceae 342
Siparuna brasiliensis (Spr.) DC., Monimiaceae 245
Siparuna camporum (Tul.) DC., Monimiaceae 245
Siparuna guianensis Aubl., Monimiaceae 245
Syagrus oleracea (Mart.) Becc., Arecaceae 45
Xylopia aromatica (Lam.) Mart., Annonaceae 15
Xylopia frutescens Aubl., Annonaceae 16
Xylopia sericea St.-Hil., Annonaceae 16

Carnauba Wax. *See* **Cataplasms**

Cassava Poison Antidote
Bixa orellana L., Bixaceae 85
Fevillea trilobata L., Cucurbitaceae 136
Tabebuia leucoxylon (L.) DC., Bignoniaceae 83

Castor Oil Substitute
Omphalea diandra M. Arg., Euphorbiaceae 156

Cataplasms
Copernicia prunifera (Mill.) H. Moore, Arecaceae .. 40
Mimosa pudica L., Mimosaceae 240
Mimosa velloziana Mart., Mimosaceae 240

Cataract. *See also* **Eye Problems**
Jatropha urens L., Euphorbiaceae 155

Catarrh (Bladder, Intestinal, Bronchial, Pulmonary, Urethral, Vaginal)
Ageratum conyzoides L., Asteraceae 53
Anacardium occidentale L., Anacardiaceae 7
Aniba canelilla (H.B.K.) Mez, Lauraceae 197
Aristolochia birostris Duch., Aristolochiaceae 46
Baccharis dentata (Vell.) G.M. Barroso, Asteraceae 54
Bixa orellana L., Bixaceae 85
Blepharocalyx salicifolius
  (H.B.K.) Berg, Myrtaceae 253
Buddleja stachioides Cham., Buddlejaceae 93
Caesalpinia ferrea Mart. ex Tul., Caesalpiniaceae .. 100
Caesalpinia pyramidalis Tul., Caesalpiniaceae 100
Campomanesia aurea Berg, &
  C. xanthocarpa Berg, Myrtaceae 253
Canna glauca L., Cannaceae 110
Cayaponia espelina
  (Manso) Cogn., Cucurbitaceae 135
Celtis iguanaea Sarg., Ulmaceae 330
Cestrum bracteatum Link & Otto, Solanaceae 317
Cestrum parqui L'Herit., Solanaceae 317
Chrysobalanus icaco L., Chrysobalanaceae 119
Copaifera officinalis (Jacq.) L., Caesalpiniaceae ... 102
Cuscuta racemosa Mart., Convolvulaceae 130
Cyrtopodium andersoni R. Br., Orchidaceae 266
Doliocarpus rolandri Gmel., Dilleniaceae 146
Drimys winteri Forst., Winteraceae 340
Ficus gomelleira Kunth & Bouché, Moraceae 248
Glechon ciliata Benth., Lamiaceae 192
Krameria tomentosa St.-Hil., Krameriaceae 191
Lantana microphylla Cham., also *L. mixta* L., &
  *L. pseudothea (*St.-Hil.) Schauer, Verbenaceae 335
Lucuma rivicoa Gaertn., Sapotaceae 309
Nymphoides indica (L.) O. Ktze., Menyanthaceae . 235
Polygala klotzschii Chodat, Polygalaceae 284
Rumex brasiliensis Link, Polygonaceae 287
Sterculia apetala (Jacq.) Karst.

  var. *elata* (Ducke) E. Taylor, Sterculiaceae 324
Stromanthe sanguinea Sond., Marantaceae 224
Waltheria communis St.-Hil., Sterculiaceae 325
Xylopia frutescens Aubl., Annonaceae 16

Cathartic.
See also **Hydragogue, Purgative**
Clitoria guianensis (Aubl.) Benth., Fabaceae 163
Genipa americana L., Rubiaceae 298
Hippeastrum vittatum
  (L'Hérit.) Herb., Amaryllidaceae 6
Hura crepitans L., Euphorbiaceae 153
Jacaranda copaia (Aubl.) D. Don, Bignoniaceae 80
Joannesia princeps Vell., Euphorbiaceae 155
Senna spp.: *S. alexandrina* Miller
  & *S. italica* Miller, Caesalpiniaceae 107
Solanum albidum Dun., Solanaceae 319
Spigelia anthelmia L., Loganiaceae 209
Stachytarpheta jamaicensis
  (L.) Vahl, Verbenaceae 336
Thevetia ahouai (L.) DC., Apocynaceae 28
Vismia guianensis (Aubl.) Choisy, Clusiaceae 124

Caustic
Dracontium polyphyllum L., Araceae 36
Euphorbia hyssopifolia L., Euphorbiaceae 153
Euphorbia tirucalli L., Euphorbiaceae 153
Himatanthus alba (L.) Woods., Apocynaceae 24
Hura crepitans L., Euphorbiaceae 153
Philodendron speciosum Schott, Araceae 37
Plumbago scandens L., Plumbaginaceae 279
Urospatha caudata
  (Poepp. & Endl.) Schott, Araceae 37

Central Nervous System (CNS) Depressant.
See also **Nervous Disorders**
Cordyline dracaenoides Kunth, Liliaceae (PHARM.) 207

Cephalalgia. *See* **Headache**

Cerebral Palsy
Operculina alata (Ham.) Urb., Convolvulaceae 131
Operculina macrocarpa Urb., Convolvulaceae 131

Chest Problems. *See* **Pectoral**

Chiggers (Chigoes)
Attalea oleifera Barb. Rodr., Arecaceae 39
Protium icicariba (DC.) March., Burseraceae 94

Chigoes. *See* **Chiggers**

Childbirth. *See also* **Foetus Expulsion, Labor, Placenta Expulsion, Pregnancy, Puerperal Fever**
Bidens pilosa L., Asteraceae 57
Chenopodium ambrosioides L., Chenopodiaceae ... 118
Crescentia cujete L., Bignoniaceae 80
Lagenaria siceraria
  (Molina) Standl., Cucurbitaceae 138
Mouriri guianensis Aubl., Melastomataceae 225
Myracroduon urundeuva
  Fr. All., Anacardiaceae 9
Myrcia lanceolata Camb., Myrtaceae 255
Piper marginatum Jacq., Piperaceae 275
Sciadotenia paraensis
  (Eichl.) Diels, Menispermaceae 234

Chlorosis
Aristolochia cymbifera Mart. & Zucc.,
  Aristolochiaceae 46

Chondodendron platyphyllum
  (Mart.) Miers, Menispermaceae 231
Clibadium surinamense L., Asteraceae 58
Crescentia cujete L., Bignoniaceae 80
Dorstenia brasiliensis Lam., Moraceae 247
Dorstenia cayapia Vell., Moraceae 248
Dracontium asperum K. Koch, Araceae 35
Himatanthus lancifolia
  (M. Arg.) Woods., Apocynaceae 26
Luffa operculata (L.) Cogn., Cucurbitaceae 138
Oxalis martiana Zucc., Oxalidaceae 267
Tetracera aspera Willd., Dilleniaceae 146
Cholagogue
Piper aduncum L., Piperaceae 274
Cholera
Baccharis articulata (Lam.) Pers., Asteraceae 54
Mikania parviflora (Aubl.) Karst., Asteraceae 62
Piper aduncum L., Piperaceae 274
Psidium guajava L., Myrtaceae 256
Cholesterol, to lower blood.
See Hypocholesteremic
Chorea
Cestrum parqui L'Herit., Solanaceae 317
Cicatrizant
Ayapana triplinerve
  (Vahl) King & Robinson, Asteraceae 53
Casearia cambessedesii Eichl., Flacourtiaceae 176
Copaifera cearensis Huber
  ex Ducke, Caesalpiniaceae 102
Cyrtopodium punctatum Lindl., Orchidaceae 266
Glandularia peruviana (L.) Small, Verbenaceae ... 334
Kalanchoe brasiliensis Camb., Crassulaceae 133
Maclura tinctoria (L.) D. Don, Moraceae 249
Parkia pendula Benth. ex Walp., Mimosaceae 240
Pentaclethra macroloba
  (Willd.) O. Ktze., Mimosaceae 242
Phthirusa adunca
  (Meyer) Maguire, Loranthaceae 211
Simaba ferruginea St.-Hil., Simaroubaceae 314
Ximenia americana L., Olacaceae 263
Ximenia coriacea Engl., Olacaceae 263
Circulatory Problems. See also
Arteriosclerosis, Heart Problems,
Hypertension, Phlebitis, Varicose Veins,
Vasoconstrictor
Scutia buxifolia Reiss., Rhamnaceae 293
Circulatory Stimulant
Zanthoxylum pterota H.B.K., Rutaceae 303
Clove Substitute
Calyptranthes aromatica St.-Hil., Myrtaceae 253
Pseudocaryophyllus sericeus Berg, Myrtaceae 255
Coffee Substitute
Senna uniflora
  (P. Miller) Ir. & Barn., Caesalpiniaceae 106
Colds
Adenocalymma alliacea (Lam.)
  Miers, Bignoniaceae 78
Ageratum conyzoides L., Asteraceae 53
Aristolochia cordigera Willd., Aristolochiaceae 46
Caryocar brasiliense Camb., Caryocaraceae 114

Cedrela odorata L., Meliaceae 227
Elephantopus mollis H.B.K., Asteraceae 59
Eugenia uniflora L., Myrtaceae 254
Heliotropium elongatum Willd., Boraginaceae 88
Jodina rhombifolia Hook. & Arn., Santalaceae 304
Kyllinga pungens Link, Cyperaceae 143
Lantana lilacina Desf., Verbenaceae 335
Lippia gratissima
  (Gill. & Hook.) Troncoso, Verbenaceae 335
Monnieria trifolia Loefl., Rutaceae 302
Ocimum fluminensis Vell., Lamiaceae 195
Ocimum micranthum Willd., Lamiaceae 195
Selaginella stellata Spring, Selaginellaceae 313
Senna leiophylla
  (Vog.) Ir. & Barn., Caesalpiniaceae 105
Tagetes erecta L., Asteraceae 67
Torresea cearensis Fr. All., Fabaceae 172
Vitex agnus-castus L., Verbenaceae 336
Colic includes: *intestinal, liver, menstrual, renal, uterine*
Ageratum conyzoides L., Asteraceae 53
Anacardium occidentale L., Anacardiaceae 7
Andira retusa (Poir.) H.B.K., Fabaceae 162
Anisosperma passiflora Manso, Cucurbitaceae 135
Chondodendron platyphyllum
  (Mart.) Miers, Menispermaceae 231
Copaifera officinalis (Jacq.) L., Caesalpiniaceae 102
Cryptocarya mandioccana Meissn., Lauraceae 198
Cuscuta racemosa Mart., Convolvulaceae 130
Cypella herbertii Herb., Iridaceae 186
Drimys winteri Forst., Winteraceae 340
Guatteria ouregon (Aubl.) Dun., Annonaceae 14
Mikania cordifolia (L. f.) Willd., Asteraceae 61
Mollinedia schottiana (Spr.) Perk., Monimiaceae .. 245
Momordica charantia L., Cucurbitaceae 139
Monnieria trifolia Loefl., Rutaceae 302
Nectandra pichurim (H.B.K.) Mez, Lauraceae 200
Orbignya phalerata Mart., Arecaceae 43
Piper colubrinum Link, Piperaceae 275
Piper eucalyptifolium (Miq.) Rudge, Piperaceae 275
Portulaca oleracea L., Portulacaceae 289
Renealmia occidentalis Sweet, also
  Renealmia sylvestris Horan., Zingiberaceae 342
Scleria pratensis L., Cyperaceae 143
Tagetes minuta L., Asteraceae 67
Urena lobata L., Malvaceae 223
Virola oleifera (Schott) A.C. Smith, Myristicaceae . 250
Virola sebifera Aubl., Myristicaceae 250
Xylopia frutescens Aubl., Annonaceae 16
Zanthoxylum tingoassuiba St.-Hil., Rutaceae 303
Condiment
Acmella repens (Walt.) L.C. Rich., Asteraceae 52
Calyptranthes aromatica St.-Hil., Myrtaceae 253
Eryngium foetidum L., Apiaceae 19
Xylopia aromatica (Lam.) Mart., Annonaceae 15
Zanthoxylum pterota H.B.K., Rutaceae 303
Conjunctivitis. See also Eye Problems
Abrus precatorius L., Fabaceae 160
Ceiba pentandra (L.) Gaertn., Bombacaceae 86
Ipomoea pentaphylla Jacq., Convolvulaceae 130
Potalia amara Aubl., Loganiaceae 209
Stryphnodendron adstringens
  (Mart.) Cov., Mimosaceae 242

MEDICINAL INDEX: CONSTIPATION – COUGHS

Constipation
Davilla rugosa Poir., Dilleniaceae 145
Esenbeckia febrifuga Juss., Rutaceae 301
Hyptis crenata Pohl, Lamiaceae 192
Operculina alata (Ham.) Urb., Convolvulaceae 131
Operculina macrocarpa Urb., Convolvulaceae 131
Spondias macrocarpa Engl., Anacardiaceae 10
Spondias mombin L., Anacardiaceae 10
Trimezia lurida Salisb., Iridaceae 186

Contraceptive
Cyperus corymbosus Rottb., Cyperaceae 142

Contusions (Bruises)
Abuta concolor Poepp. & Endl., Menispermaceae . 231
Buddleja brasiliensis Jacq. ex Spr., Buddlejaceae 93
Buddleja cambara Arech., Buddlejaceae 93
Calea pinnatifida (R. Br.) Less., Asteraceae 57
Cochlospermum orinocense
  (H.B.K.) Steud., Cochlospermaceae 125
Cochlospermum regium
  (Mart. & Schl.) Pilg., Cochlospermaceae 125
Nymphaea rudgeana G. Meyer, Nymphaeaceae 259
Pothomorphe umbellata (L.) Miq., Piperaceae 277
Siparuna brasiliensis (Spr.) DC., Monimiaceae 245
Siparuna cujabana (Mart.) DC., Monimiaceae 245
Solidago chilensis Meyen, Asteraceae 65
Victoria amazonica
  (Poepp.) Sower., Nymphaeaceae 259
Virola sebifera Aubl., Myristicaceae 250

Convalescents, for
Ischnosiphon arouma Koern., Marantaceae 223
Maranta arundinacea L., Marantaceae 223

Convulsions
Aristolochia cymbifera
  Mart. & Zucc., Aristolochiaceae 46
Gallesia gorazema (Vell.) Moq., Phytolaccaceae ... 271
Petiveria alliacea L., Phytolaccaceae 271

Corneal Opacity (Albugo).
See also Eye Problems
Abrus precatorius L., Fabaceae (PHARM.) 160
Euphorbia caecorum Mart., Euphorbiaceae 152
Euphorbia hirta L., Euphorbiaceae 152
Euphorbia hyssopifolia L., Euphorbiaceae 153
Euphorbia thymifolia L., Euphorbiaceae 153
Hyptis mutabilis (Rich.) Briq., Lamiaceae 193
Ibicella lutea (Lindl.) Van Eselt., Martyniaceae 224
Jatropha urens L., Euphorbiaceae 155
Lucuma caimito Roem. & Schult., Sapotaceae 309
Melothria fluminensis Gardn., Cucurbitaceae 139

Corneal Ulcers. See also Eye Problems
Euphorbia hirta L., Euphorbiaceae 152

Corns
Anacardium occidentale L., Anacardiaceae 7
Astronium fraxinifolium Schott, Anacardiaceae 9
Carica papaya L., Caricaceae 113
Kalanchoe brasiliensis Camb., Crassulaceae 133
Talinum racemosum (L.) Rohr., Portulacaceae 289

Corrosive
Ficus insipida Willd., Moraceae 248

Coughs (Antitussive, Bechic).
See also Whooping Cough
Acanthospermum hispidum DC., Asteraceae 52

Adiantum cuneatum Langsd. & Fisch., Adiantaceae ... 1
Alternanthera brasiliana
  (L.) O. Ktze., Amaranthaceae 3
Ambelania tenuifolia Aubl., Apocynaceae 20
Annona muricata L., Annonaceae 13
Ayapana triplinerve
  (Vahl) King & Robinson, Asteraceae 53
Bauhinia radiata Vell., Caesalpiniaceae 99
Buddleja brasiliensis Jacq. ex Spr., Buddlejaceae 93
Byrsonima chrysophylla H.B.K., Malpighiaceae 218
Caesalpinia bracteosa Tul., Caesalpiniaceae 100
Caesalpinia ferrea Mart. ex Tul., Caesalpiniaceae . 100
Cardiospermum grandiflorum Sw., Sapindaceae ... 305
Cereus peruvianus (L.) Mill., Cactaceae 94
Chaptalia nutans (L.) Polak., Asteraceae 57
Chenopodium ambrosioides L., Chenopodiaceae ... 118
Conobea scoparioides Benth., Scrophulariaceae 311
Cordia ecalyculata Vell., Boraginaceae 87
Cordia magnoliifolia Cham., Boraginaceae 87
Cordia multispicata Cham., Boraginaceae 88
Costus spicatus (Jacq.) Sw., Costaceae 132
Cunila microcephala Benth., Lamiaceae 192
Cunila spicata L., Lamiaceae 192
Cyathea armata (Sw.) Domin, Cyatheaceae 141
Cydista aequinoctialis Miers, Bignoniaceae 80
Dahlstedtia pentaphylla (Taub.) Burk, Fabaceae ... 163
Dahlstedtia pinnata (Benth.) Malme, Fabaceae 163
Dalbergia subcymosa Ducke, Fabaceae 164
Dipteryx odorata (Aubl.) Willd., Fabaceae 166
Dorstenia brasiliensis Lam., Moraceae 247
Dorstenia reniformis Pohl, Moraceae 248
Elephantopus mollis H.B.K., Asteraceae 59
Erythrina verna Vell., Fabaceae 168
Gallesia gorazema (Vell.) Moq., Phytolaccaceae ... 271
Hedychium coronarium Koenig, Zingiberaceae 342
Helicteres ovata Lam., Sterculiaceae 324
Hippocratea volubilis L., Hippocrateaceae 183
Hymenaea courbaril L., Caesalpiniaceae 103
Hyptis atrorubens Poit., Lamiaceae 192
Hyptis suaveolens Poit., Lamiaceae 193
Jacaranda brasiliana (Lam.) Pers., Bignoniaceae ... 80
Kalanchoe pinnata (Lam.) Pers., Crassulaceae 133
Lantana macrophylla Schauer, Verbenaceae 335
Laportea aestuans (L.) Chew, Urticaceae 330
Lecythis pisonis Camb., Lecythidaceae 206
Lithraea molleoides (Vell.) Engl., Anacardiaceae 9
Mikania glomerata Spreng., Asteraceae 61
Mikania parviflora (Aubl.) Karst., Asteraceae 62
Mimosa caesalpiniaefolia Benth., Mimosaceae 238
Myroxylon balsamum (L.) Harms, Fabaceae 170
Ocimum fluminensis Vell., Lamiaceae 195
Ocimum micranthum Willd., Lamiaceae 195
Peltodon radicans Pohl, Lamiaceae 195
Peperomia pellucida H.B.K., Piperaceae 273
Pereskia bleo H.B.K., Cactaceae 97
Periandra mediterranea (Vell.) Taub., Fabaceae ... 170
Phlebodium decumanum
  (Willd.) J. Smith, Polypodiaceae 288
Polygala comata Mart., Polygalaceae 284
Polygala spectabilis DC., Polygalaceae 284
Polypodium brasiliense Poir., Polypodiaceae 288
Pteridium aquilinum (L.) Kuhn, Dennstaedtiaceae . 144
Ranunculus apiifolius Pers., Ranunculaceae 290

Rollinia sylvatica (St.-Hil.) Mart., Annonaceae 15
Schinus molle L., Anacardiaceae 9
Silybum marianum Gaertn., Asteraceae 65
Siparuna cujabana (Mart.) DC., Monimiaceae 245
Sphagneticola trilobata (L.) Pruski, Asteraceae 65
Tagetes erecta L., Asteraceae 67
Tetralacrium veroniciforme
  Turcz., Scrophulariaceae 312
Tibouchina aspera Aubl., Melastomataceae 226
Torresea cearensis Fr. All., Fabaceae 172
Urena lobata L., Malvaceae 223
Waltheria indica L., Sterculiaceae 325

Curare Additive
Dieffenbachia seguine (Jacq.) Schott, Araceae 35

Curare Antidote
Leopoldinia major Wallace, Arecaceae 43
Piper geniculatum Sw., Piperaceae 275

Cuts
Apium sellowianum Wolf, Apiaceae 18
Calea pinnatifida (R. Br.) Less., Asteraceae 57
Caryocar coriaceum Wittm., Caryocaraceae 114
Erythrina crista-galli L., Fabaceae 166
Jatropha curcas L., Euphorbiaceae 154
Jatropha multifida L., Euphorbiaceae 154
Joannesia princeps Vell., Euphorbiaceae 155
Wissadula periplocifolia Presl., Malvaceae 223

Cystitis. *See also* **Bladder Disease**
Aristolochia triangularis Cham., Aristolochiaceae ... 48
Bauhinia forficata Link, Caesalpiniaceae 99
Canna edulis Ker-Gawl., Cannaceae 110
Cissampelos fasciculata Benth., Menispermaceae . 231
Cissampelos pareira L., Menispermaceae 233
Clitoria guianensis (Aubl.) Benth., Fabaceae 163
Copaifera cearensis
  Huber ex Ducke, Caesalpiniaceae 102
Doliocarpus rolandri Gmel., Dilleniaceae 146
Elionurus candidus (Trin.) Hack., also
  E. latiflorus Nees, Poaceae 281
Hymenaea courbaril L., Caesalpiniaceae 103
Jatropha urens L., Euphorbiaceae 155
Myrocarpus frondosus Fr. All., Fabaceae 170
Myroxylon balsamum (L.) Harms, Fabaceae 170
Physalis pubescens L., Solanaceae 318
Portulaca oleracea L., Portulacaceae 289
Sauvagesia erecta L., Ochnaceae 262
Solanum martii Sendt., Solanaceae 321
Spondias macrocarpa Engl., Anacardiaceae 10
Spondias mombin L., Anacardiaceae 10
Waltheria communis St.-Hil., Sterculiaceae 325

D

Dandruff
Aristolochia cymbifera
  Mart. & Zucc., Aristolochiaceae 46
Aristolochia trilobata L., Aristolochiaceae 48
Carpotroche brasiliensis
  (Raddi) Endl., Flacourtiaceae 176
Commelina pohliana Seub., Commelinaceae 127
Elaeis oleifera (H.B.K.) Cortez, Arecaceae 40
Entada paranaguana B. Rodr., Mimosaceae 237

Entada polyphylla Benth., Mimosaceae 237
Monstera adansonii Schott, Araceae 36

Dartre (Skin Disease)
Chiococca alba (L.) Hitch., Rubiaceae 297
Commelina pohliana Seub., Commelinaceae 127
Desmoncus orthacanthos Mart., Arecaceae 40
Dichorisandra affinis Mart., Commelinaceae 128
Dichorisandra leucophthalmos
  Hook., Commelinaceae 128
Dichorisandra spp., Commelinaceae 128
Gallesia gorazema (Vell.) Moq., Phytolaccaceae ... 271
Trimezia lurida Salisb., Iridaceae 186
Xyris laxifolia Mart., Xyridaceae 342
Xyris pallida Mart., Xyridaceae 342

Debility from Chronic Diseases
Anacardium occidentale L., Anacardiaceae 7

Deficiency, Iron
Oxalis martiana Zucc., Oxalidaceae 267

Delirium Inducer
Brunfelsia uniflora (Pohl) D. Don,
  also *B. grandiflora* D. Don, Solanaceae 316

Dentifrice
Oxalis corniculata L., Oxalidaceae 266
Zizyphus joazeiro Mart., Rhamnaceae (PHARM.) 293

Deobstruent
Phyllanthus niruri L., Euphorbiaceae 156

Depilatory (Hair Remover)
Calotropis procera (Ait.) Ait. f., Asclepiadaceae 50
Carpotroche brasiliensis
  (Raddi) Endl., Flacourtiaceae 176

Depurative
Adiantum concinnum Humb. & Bonp., Adiantaceae .. 1
Aiovea meissneri Mez, Lauraceae 197
Alternanthera achyrantha R. Br., Amaranthaceae 3
Anacardium occidentale L., Anacardiaceae 7
Anadenanthera colubrina
  (Vell.) Brenan, Mimosaceae 236
Anadenanthera macrocarpa
  (Benth.) Brenan, Mimosaceae 236
Anchietea pyrifolia (Mart.) G. Don, Violaceae 338
Aniba permollis (Nees) Mez, Lauraceae 197
Boehmeria caudata Sw., Urticaceae 330
Bowdichia nitida Spruce ex Benth., Fabaceae 163
Bowdichia virgilioides H.B.K., Fabaceae 163
Brosimum acutifolium Huber,
  also *B. obovata* Ducke, Moraceae 246
Caraipa minor Huber, Clusiaceae 121
Casearia sylvestris Sw., Flacourtiaceae 178
Cayaponia martiana
  (Cogn.) Cogn., Cucurbitaceae 135
Cayaponia tayuya (Mart.) Cogn., Cucurbitaceae 135
Cissus palmata Poir., Vitaceae 339
Copernicia prunifera (Mill.) H. Moore, Arecaceae .. 40
Cordia coffeoides Warm., Boraginaceae 87
Costus spicatus (Jacq.) Sw., Costaceae 132
Craniolaria annua L., Martyniaceae 224
Cremastus sceptrum Bur. & K. Sch., Bignoniaceae .. 79
Croton salutaris Casar., Euphorbiaceae 151
Croton spp., those known as 'velame' including:
  C. cascarilla (L.) Bennet, *C. glabellus* L. &
  C. paniculatus M. Arg., Euphorbiaceae 152
Cuscuta racemosa Mart., Convolvulaceae 130

MEDICINAL INDEX: DEPURATIVE – DIARRHOEA

Cybistax antisyphilitica
  (Mart.) Mart., Bignoniaceae 80
Davilla rugosa Poir., Dilleniaceae 145
Desmodium triflorum DC., Fabaceae 164
Desmoncus polyacanthos Mart., Arecaceae 40
Echinodorus grandiflorus
  (Cham. & Schl.) Mich., Alismataceae 2
Echinodorus pubescens Mart., Alismataceae 2
Eichhornia crassipes Solms, Pontederiaceae 288
Ficus gomelleira Kunth & Bouché, Moraceae 248
Guarea tuberculata Vell., Meliaceae 229
Guazuma ulmifolia Lam.
  var. *ulmifolia*, Sterculiaceae 323
Helicteres ovata Lam., Sterculiaceae 324
Herreria salsaparilha Mart., Liliaceae 207
Hybanthus atropurpureus Taub., Violaceae 338
Jacaranda micrantha Cham., Bignoniaceae 81
Jacaranda spp., including *J. clausseniana* Casar.,
  J. decurrens Cham., *J. elegans* Mart.,
  J. heterophylla Bur. & Pet., *J. oxyphylla* Cham.,
  J. paucifoliata Mart., *J. puberula* Cham.,
  J. rufa Manso, *J. semiserrata* Cham.
  & *J. tomentosa* R.Br., Bignoniaceae 81
Julocroton humilis Diedr., Euphorbiaceae 155
Luehea rufescens St.-Hil., Tiliaceae 327
Macrosiphonia longiflora
  (Desf.) M. Arg., Apocynaceae 26
Macrosiphonia velame
  (St.-Hil.) M. Arg., Apocynaceae 26
Maytenus ilicifolia Mart., Celastraceae 115
Melothrianthus smilacifolius
  (Cogn.) M. Crovetto,Cucurbitaceae 139
Muehlenbeckia sagittifolia
  (Ort.) Meissn., Polygonaceae 285
Nectandra canescens Nees, Lauraceae 199
Phyllanthus conami Sw., Euphorbiaceae 156
Physalis angulata L., Solanaceae 318
Protium icicariba (DC.) March., Burseraceae 94
Rumohra adiantiformis
  (G. Forst.) Ching, Dryopteridaceae 147
Schinus lentiscifolius March., Anacardiaceae 9
Schinus terebinthifolius Raddi, Anacardiaceae 10
Sisyrinchium vaginatum Spreng., Iridaceae 186
Solanum cernuum Vell., Solanaceae 319
Solanum nigrum L., Solanaceae 321
Sparattosperma leucanthum
  (Vell.) K. Sch., Bignoniaceae 82
Stryphnodendron coriaceum Benth., Mimosaceae . 243
Trianosperma glandulosa Mart., Cucurbitaceae 140
Trianosperma trilobata Cogn., Cucurbitaceae 140
Tropaeolum pentaphyllum Lam., Tropaeolaceae 327
Wilbrandia verticillata
  (Vell.) Cogn., Cucurbitaceae 140

Dermatoses. *See* Skin Disease
Diabetes
Anacardium occidentale L., Anacardiaceae 7
Annona muricata L., Annonaceae 13
Baccharis trimera (Less.) DC., Asteraceae 54
Bauhinia candicans Benth., Caesalpiniaceae 99
Bauhinia forficata Link, Caesalpiniaceae 99
Bidens pilosa L., Asteraceae 57
Bowdichia virgilioides H.B.K., Fabaceae 163
Bumelia sartorum Mart., Sapotaceae 308

Caesalpinia ferrea Mart. ex Tul., Caesalpiniaceae . 100
Calophyllum brasiliense Camb., Clusiaceae 120
Cecropia palmata Willd., Moraceae 247
Chrysobalanus icaco L., Chrysobalanaceae 119
Conocarpus erecta L., Combretaceae 126
Momordica charantia L., Cucurbitaceae 139
Myrcia sphaerocarpa DC., Myrtaceae 255
Pfaffia paniculata (Mart.) Kuntze, Amaranthaceae 5
Phyllanthus niruri L., Euphorbiaceae 156
Psoralea glandulosa L., Fabaceae 170
Pterodon apparicioi Peders., Fabaceae 170
Pterodon pubescens Benth., Fabaceae 171
Talauma ovata St.-Hil., Magnoliaceae 216
Trianosperma diversifolia Cogn., Cucurbitaceae 139
Turnera diffusa Willd., Turneraceae 327
Turnera opifera Mart., Turneraceae 328
Turnera ulmifolia L., Turneraceae 328

Diaphoretic. *See* Sudorific
Diarrhoea
Acanthospermum hispidum DC., Asteraceae 52
Acanthospermum australe
  (Loefl.) O. Ktze., Asteraceae 52
Ageratum conyzoides L., Asteraceae 53
Albizzia lebbeck (L.) Benth., Mimosaceae 236
Amasonia arborea H.B.K., Verbenaceae 333
Aniba puchury-minor (Mart.) Mez, Lauraceae 197
Annona muricata L., Annonaceae 13
Annona reticulata L., Annonaceae 13
Aristolochia cymbifera
  Mart. & Zucc., Aristolochiaceae 46
Aristolochia trilobata L., Aristolochiaceae 48
Arrabidaea chica (H.B.K.) Bur., Bignoniaceae 78
Avicennia germinans (L.) L., Verbenaceae 334
Baccharis articulata (Lam.) Pers., Asteraceae 54
Baccharis notosergila Gris., Asteraceae 54
Begonia hirtella Link, Begoniaceae 76
Blepharocalyx salicifolius
  (H.B.K.) Berg, Myrtaceae 253
Borreria verticillata (L.) Meyer, Rubiaceae 296
Bowdichia virgilioides H.B.K., Fabaceae 163
Caesalpinia ferrea Mart. ex Tul., Caesalpiniaceae . 100
Caesalpinia pyramidalis Tul., Caesalpiniaceae 100
Campomanesia aurea Berg, also
  C. xanthocarpa Berg, Myrtaceae 253
Carapa guianensis Aubl., Meliaceae 227
Cariniana legalis (Mart.) O. Ktze., Lecythidaceae . 204
Casearia sylvestris Sw., Flacourtiaceae 178
Cecropia palmata Willd., Moraceae 247
Cestrum parqui L'Herit., Solanaceae 317
Chrysobalanus icaco L., Chrysobalanaceae 119
Cissampelos fasciculata Benth., Menispermaceae . 231
Coccoloba arborescens
  (Vell.) How., Polygonaceae 285
Coccoloba marginata Benth., Polygonaceae 285
Cocos nucifera L., Arecaceae 40
Connarus suberosus Planch., Connaraceae 129
Copaifera officinalis (Jacq.) L., Caesalpiniaceae ... 102
Cuscuta racemosa Mart., Convolvulaceae 130
Dalbergia gracilis Benth., Fabaceae 163
Dorstenia asaroides Gardn., Moraceae 247
Dorstenia brasiliensis Lam., Moraceae 247
Dorstenia cayapia Vell., Moraceae 248
Drimys winteri Forst., Winteraceae 340

Egletes viscosa (L.) Less., Asteraceae 59
Eleutherine plicata Herb., Iridaceae 186
Eugenia sulcata Spring, Myrtaceae 254
Eugenia supra-axillaris Spring, Myrtaceae 254
Eugenia uniflora L., Myrtaceae 254
Euphorbia hirta L.,
   Euphorbiaceae (CHEM. & PHARM.) 152
Euterpe oleracea Mart., Arecaceae 42
Genipa americana L., Rubiaceae 298
Geoffroea striata (Willd.) Morong, Fabaceae 168
Gomphrena leucocephala Mart., Amaranthaceae 4
Heliconia angusta Vell., Heliconiaceae 181
Helosis cayennensis
   (Swartz) Spreng., Balanophoraceae 73
Joannesia princeps Vell., Euphorbiaceae 155
Krameria spartioides Berg, Krameriaceae 191
Krameria tomentosa St.-Hil., Krameriaceae 191
Laplacea fruticosa (Schr.) Kobuski, Theaceae 326
Lecythis amara Aubl., Lecythidaceae 205
Leonotis nepetaefolia R. Br., Lamiaceae 194
Licaria camara (Schomb.) Kosterm., Lauraceae 198
Limonium brasiliense
   (Boiss.) O. Ktze., Plumbaginaceae 278
Lucilia nitens Less., Asteraceae 61
Ludwigia natans (H.B.K.) Ell., Onagraceae 264
Luehea rufescens St.-Hil., Tiliaceae 327
Lucuma rivicoa Gaertn., Sapotaceae 309
Macfadyena unguis-cati (L.) Gentry, Bignoniaceae . 81
Manilkara zapota (L.) Van Royen, Sapotaceae 309
Mikania hirsutissima DC., Asteraceae 62
Momordica charantia L., Cucurbitaceae 139
Operculina alata (Ham.) Urb., Convolvulaceae 131
Operculina macrocarpa Urb., Convolvulaceae 131
Oxalis corniculata L., Oxalidaceae 266
Parapiptadenia rigida
   (Benth.) Brenan, Mimosaceae 240
Pfaffia glomerata (Spreng.) Peders., Amaranthaceae .. 4
Polygonum punctatum Elliot, Polygonaceae 287
Portulaca pilosa L., Portulacaceae 289
Pradosia lactescens (Vell.) Radlk., Sapotaceae 310
Psidium arboreum Vell., Myrtaceae 256
Psidium cattleyanum Sabine, Myrtaceae 256
Psidium guajava L., Myrtaceae 256
Pyrostegia ignea (Vell.) Pres., Bignoniaceae 82
Quassia amara L., Simaroubaceae 314
Rhizophora mangle L., Rhizophoraceae 294
Rollinia exalbida (Vell.) Mart., Annonaceae 15
Rubus brasiliensis Mart., Rosaceae 294
Sciadotenia paraensis
   (Eichl.) Diels, Menispermaceae 234
Sida rhombea L., Malvaceae 222
Simarouba amara Aubl., Simaroubaceae 315
Spondias macrocarpa Engl., Anacardiaceae 10
Spondias mombin L., Anacardiaceae 10
Stryphnodendron adstringens
   (Mart.) Cov., Mimosaceae 242
Syagrus comosa Mart., Arecaceae 45
Terminalia tanibouca Smith, Combretaceae 126
Ternstroemia brasiliensis Camb., Theaceae 326
Tovomita brasiliensis (Mart.) Walp., Clusiaceae 123
Triplaris weigeltiana
   (Reichb.) O. Ktze., Polygonaceae 287
Vitex agnus-castus L., Verbenaceae 336

Digestive. *See also* **Dyspepsia,**
Eupeptic, Pharyngitis
Aloysia triphylla (L'Her.) Britt., Verbenaceae 332
Alternanthera achyrantha R. Br., Amaranthaceae 3
Ananas comosus (L.) Merrill, Bromeliaceae 90
Baccharis articulata (Lam.) Pers., Asteraceae 54
Baccharis spp., Asteraceae 56
Bixa orellana L., Bixaceae 85
Bouchea laetevirens Schauer, Verbenaceae 334
Bouchea pseudogervao
   (St.-Hil.) Cham., Verbenaceae 334
Caesalpinia microphylla Mart., Caesalpiniaceae ... 100
Capraria biflora L., Scrophulariaceae 311
Coleus barbatus Benth., Lamiaceae 191
Croton zehntneri Pax & Hoffm., Euphorbiaceae 151
Cusparia febrifuga Humb., Rutaceae 300
Dorstenia asaroides Gardn., Moraceae 247
Erythroxylum cataractarum
   Spruce, Erythroxylaceae 149
Erythroxylum coca Lam., Erythroxylaceae 149
Grindelia scorzonerifolia
   Hook. & Arn., Asteraceae 60
Mammea americana L., Clusiaceae 123
Ocotea cujumary Mart., Lauraceae 200
Ocotea cymbarum H.B.K., Lauraceae 200
Ouratea guianensis Aubl., Ochnaceae 261
Piper angustifolium R. & Pav., Piperaceae 274
Sida angustifolia Lam., Malvaceae 222
Solanum albidum Dun., Solanaceae 319
Stachytarpheta jamaicensis
   (L.) Vahl, Verbenaceae 336
Turnera diffusa Willd., Turneraceae 327
Turnera opifera Mart., Turneraceae 328
Verbena erinoides Lam., Verbenaceae 336
Zanthoxylum tingoassuiba St.-Hil., Rutaceae 303

Digestive Tract, prevent diseases of
Operculina alata (Ham.) Urb., Convolvulaceae 131
Operculina macrocarpa Urb., Convolvulaceae 131

Digestive Tract, stimulant
Noticastrum diffusum (Pers.) Cabr., Asteraceae 62

Digitalis Substitute
Cecropia hololeuca Miq., Moraceae 247
Scutia buxifolia Reiss., Rhamnaceae 293

Diphtheria
Mimosa pudica L., Mimosaceae 240
Mimosa velloziana Mart., Mimosaceae 240

Disinfectant
Cordia umbraculifera DC., Boraginaceae 88

Diuretic
Abuta rufescens Aubl., Menispermaceae 231
Abuta selloana Eichl., Menispermaceae 231
Achyranthes ficoidea Lam., Amaranthaceae 3
Acnistus arborescens (L.) Schl., Solanaceae 316
Alternanthera achyrantha R. Br., Amaranthaceae 3
Amaranthus spinosus L., Amaranthaceae 3
Amaranthus viridis L., Amaranthaceae 3
Anacardium occidentale L., Anacardiaceae 7
Andropogon bicornis L., Poaceae 279
Andropogon condensatus H.B.K., Poaceae 279
Andropogon minarum Kunth, Poaceae 280
Apium sellowianum Wolf, Apiaceae 18
Aristolochia triangularis Cham., Aristolochiaceae ... 48

MEDICINAL INDEX: DIURETIC

Aristolochia trilobata L., Aristolochiaceae 48
Baccharis articulata (Lam.) Pers., Asteraceae 54
Begonia hirtella Link, Begoniaceae 76
Bidens cynapiifolia H.B.K., Asteraceae 56
Bixa orellana L., Bixaceae 85
Boehmeria caudata Sw., Urticaceae 330
Boerhavia coccinea Mill., Nyctaginaceae 257
Bomarea salsilloides Roem., Amaryllidaceae 6
Bomarea spectabilis Schrenk, Amaryllidaceae 6
Borreria tenella Cham. & Schl., Rubiaceae 296
Bromelia antiacantha Bertol., Bromeliaceae 91
Bromelia pinguin L., Bromeliaceae 91
Byrsonima verbascifolia (L.) Rich., Malpighiaceae . 220
Canna edulis Ker-Gawl., Cannaceae 110
Canna gigantea Desf., Cannaceae 110
Canna glauca L., Cannaceae 110
Canna lutea Roscoe, Cannaceae 111
Canna warszewiczii Dietr., Cannaceae 111
Capparis cynophallophora L., Capparaceae 111
Capraria biflora L., Scrophulariaceae 311
Caryocar brasiliense Camb., Caryocaraceae 114
Casearia ovata Willd., Flacourtiaceae 178
Cayaponia espelina
 (Manso) Cogn., Cucurbitaceae 135
Cecropia hololeuca Miq., Moraceae 247
Cecropia palmata Willd., Moraceae 247
Chamissoa altissima H.B.K., Amaranthaceae 4
Chamissoa macrocarpa H.B.K., Amaranthaceae 4
Chiococca alba (L.) Hitch., Rubiaceae 297
Chloris distichophylla (Nees) Lag., Poaceae 280
Cissampelos ovalifolia DC., Menispermaceae 233
Cissampelos pareira L., Menispermaceae 233
Cissampelos sympodialis Eichl., Menispermaceae . 233
Citronella congonha (Mart.) Howard, Icacinaceae . 185
Citronella mucronata
 (R. & Pav.) Don, Icacinaceae 186
Cleome speciosa H.B.K., Capparaceae 112
Commelina nudiflora L., Commelinaceae 126
Commelina platyphylla
 Klotz. ex Seub., Commelinaceae 126
Commelina vestita Seub., Commelinaceae 128
Commelina virginica L., Commelinaceae 128
Copernicia prunifera (Mill.) H. Moore, Arecaceae .. 40
Cordia ecalyculata Vell., Boraginaceae 87
Costus spicatus (Jacq.) Sw., Costaceae 132
Crescentia cujete L., Bignoniaceae 80
Crinum scabrum Sims, Amaryllidaceae 6
Cuphea aperta Koehne, Lythraceae 213
Cuphea balsamona Cham., Lythraceae 213
Cuscuta racemosa Mart., Convolvulaceae 130
Cyperus ligularis L., Cyperaceae 142
Cyperus rotundus L., Cyperaceae 142
Davilla rugosa Poir., Dilleniaceae 145
Dichorisandra affinis Mart., Commelinaceae 128
Dichorisandra leucophthalmos
 Hook., Commelinaceae 128
Doliocarpus rolandri Gmel., Dilleniaceae 146
Dorstenia asaroides Gardn., Moraceae 247
Dorstenia brasiliensis Lam., Moraceae 247
Echinodorus grandiflorus
 (Cham. & Schl.) Mich., Alismataceae 2
Echinodorus pubescens Mart., Alismataceae 2
Elephantopus mollis H.B.K., Asteraceae 59

Equisetum giganteum L., Equisetaceae 148
Eryngium elegans Cham. & Schlecht., Apiaceae 19
Eryngium pandanifolium
 Cham. & Schlecht., Apiaceae 19
Eryngium paniculatum
 Cav. & Domb. ex Delar., Apiaceae 19
Eryngium pristis Cham. & Schlecht., Apiaceae 19
Erythrina corallodendron L., Fabaceae 166
Eugenia brasiliensis Lam., Myrtaceae 253
Euphorbia hirta L., Euphorbiaceae 152
Genipa americana L., Rubiaceae 298
Griffinia hyacinthina Ker-Gawl., Amaryllidaceae 6
Gynerium parviflorum Nees, also
 G. sagittatum (Pers.) Beauv., Poaceae 281
Heimia salicifolia
 (H.B.K.) Link & Otto, Lythraceae 214
Heliconia bihai L., Heliconiaceae 183
Heliotropium elongatum Willd., Boraginaceae 88
Heliotropium indicum L., Boraginaceae 89
Heliotropium lanceolatum Loefgr., Boraginaceae 89
Herreria salsaparilha Mart., Liliaceae 207
Hibiscus sabdariffa L., Malvaceae 221
Hydrocotyle bonariensis Lam., Apiaceae 19
Hydrocotyle leucocephala
 Cham. & Schlecht., Apiaceae 20
Hylocereus undatus (Haw.) Br. & Rose, Cactaceae .. 95
Hymenocallis tubiflora Salisb. [includes
 Pancratium guianensis Ker-Gawl.], Amaryllidaceae 7
Hypolytrum laxum Schrad., Cyperaceae 143
Ilex paraguariensis St.-Hil., Aquifoliaceae 31
Imperata brasiliensis Trin., also
 Imperata contracta Hitch., Poaceae 281
Indigofera suffruticosa Mill., Fabaceae 168
Ipomoea acetosifolia
 (Vahl) Roem. & Schult., Convolvulaceae 130
Ipomoea pes-caprae (L.) R. Br., Convolvulaceae .. 130
Iresine polymorpha Mart., Amaranthaceae 4
Jacaranda caroba (Vell.) DC., Bignoniaceae 80
Jatropha curcas L., Euphorbiaceae 154
Jatropha urens L., Euphorbiaceae 155
Laportea aestuans (L.) Chew, Urticaceae 330
Leonotis nepetaefolia R. Br., Lamiaceae 194
Lindernia crustacea F. Muell., Scrophulariaceae ... 311
Lindernia diffusa Wettst., Scrophulariaceae 311
Lithraea molleoides (Vell.) Engl., Anacardiaceae 9
Macfadyena unguis-cati (L.) Gentry, Bignoniaceae .. 81
Marcgravia rectiflora
 Tr. & Planch., Marcgraviaceae 224
Margyricarpus setosus Ruiz & Pav., Rosaceae 294
Mariscus flavus Vahl, Cyperaceae 143
Maytenus obtusifolia Mart., Celastraceae 116
Melampodium divaricatum (Rich.) DC., Asteraceae 61
Melinis minutiflora Beauv., Poaceae 281
Mikania setigera Schultz-Bip. ex Baker, Asteraceae 62
Mimosa invisa Mart., Mimosaceae 239
Monnieria trifolia Loefl., Rutaceae 302
Montrichardia linifera (Arruda) Schott, Araceae ... 36
Mucuna pruriens (L.) DC., Fabaceae 169
Notocactus ottonis (Lem.) Berg., Cactaceae 97
Ocimum micranthum Willd., Lamiaceae 195
Ocotea pretiosa
 (Nees & Mart.) Benth. & Hook., Lauraceae 201
Ottonia jaborandi (Vell.) Kunth, Piperaceae 272

DIURETIC –DROPSY: MEDICINAL INDEX

Panicum brevifolium L., Poaceae 282
Panicum megiston Schult., Poaceae 282
Panicum petrosum Trin., Poaceae 282
Panicum trichanthum Nees, Poaceae 282
Parahancornia amapa (Hub.) Ducke, Apocynaceae 27
Parietaria boehmerioides Mart., Urticaceae 331
Paullinia cupana Kunth, Sapindaceae 306
Peperomia pellucida H.B.K., Piperaceae 273
Peperomia transparens Miq., Piperaceae 274
Petiveria alliacea L., Phytolaccaceae 271
Philodendron imbe Schott, Araceae 36
Philodendron ochrostemon Schott, Araceae 37
Phyllanthus conami Sw., Euphorbiaceae 156
Phyllanthus diffusus Klotz., Euphorbiaceae 156
Phyllanthus niruri L., Euphorbiaceae 156
Physalis angulata L., Solanaceae 318
Physalis pubescens L., Solanaceae 318
Pilea microphylla (L.) Liebm., Urticaceae 331
Pilocarpus pinnatifolius Lem., Rutaceae 302
Piper ceanothifolium H.B.K., Piperaceae 275
Piper geniculatum Sw., Piperaceae 275
Piper reticulatum L., Piperaceae 276
Polygala paniculata L., Polygalaceae 284
Polygala timoutou Aubl., Polygalaceae 284
Polygonum hydropiperoides
  Michx., Polygonaceae 286
Polygonum punctatum Elliot, Polygonaceae 287
Polygonum spectabile Mart., Polygonaceae 287
Portulaca grandiflora Hook., Portulacaceae 288
Portulaca oleracea L., Portulacaceae 289
Portulaca pilosa L., Portulacaceae 289
Pothomorphe peltata L., Piperaceae 277
Pothomorphe umbellata (L.) Miq., Piperaceae 277
Psidium cattleyanum Sabine, Myrtaceae 256
Pterocaulon virgatum DC., Asteraceae 64
Remirea maritima Aubl., Cyperaceae 143
Rhipsalis macrocarpa Miq., Cactaceae 97
Rumex brasiliensis Link, Polygonaceae 287
Sauvagesia erecta L., Ochnaceae 262
Schinus molle L., Anacardiaceae 9
Schrankia leptocarpa DC., Mimosaceae 242
Seguieria americana L., Phytolaccaceae 272
Selaginella convoluta Spring, Selaginellaceae 313
Selaginella erythropus Spring, Selaginellaceae 313
Senna affinis (Benth.) Ir. & Barn., Caesalpiniaceae 104
Senna alata (L.) Roxb., Caesalpiniaceae 104
Senna occidentalis (L.) Link, Caesalpiniaceae 105
Senna quinqueangulata
  (Rich.) Ir. & Barn., Caesalpiniaceae 106
Senna uniflora
  (P. Miller) Ir. & Barn., Caesalpiniaceae 106
Sida rhombea L., Malvaceae 222
Siparuna guianensis Aubl., Monimiaceae 245
Solanum cernuum Vell., Solanaceae 319
Solanum mammosum L., Solanaceae 321
Solanum martii Sendt., Solanaceae 321
Solanum mauritianum Scop., Solanaceae 321
Solanum nigrum L., Solanaceae 321
Solanum variabile Mart., Solanaceae 322
Sophora tomentosa L., Fabaceae 172
Sparattosperma leucanthum
  (Vell.) K. Sch., Bignoniaceae 82
Stachytarpheta cayennensis
  (Rich.) Vahl, Verbenaceae 335

Strychnos trinervis (Vell.) Mart., Loganiaceae 210
Syagrus comosa Mart., Arecaceae 45
Syagrus oleracea (Mart.) Becc., Arecaceae 45
Tagetes minuta L., Asteraceae 67
Tillandsia aeranthos
  (Loisel.) L.B. Smith, Bromeliaceae 91
Tournefortia paniculata Cham., Boraginaceae 89
Tradescantia diuretica Mart., Commelinaceae 128
Tradescantia effusa Mart., Commelinaceae 129
Tradescantia spathacea Sw., Commelinaceae 129
Tragia volubilis L., Euphorbiaceae 158
Triumfetta semitriloba Jacq., Tiliaceae 327
Turnera diffusa Willd., Turneraceae 327
Turnera opifera Mart., Turneraceae 328
Typha domingensis Pers., Typhaceae 328
Urena lobata L., Malvaceae 223
Urera aurantiaca Wedd., Urticaceae 331
Urera baccifera Gaud., Urticaceae 331
Urera caracasana Jacq., Urticaceae 331
Waltheria communis St.-Hil., Sterculiaceae 325

Drastic. *See* **Purgative, Emetic**

Dropsy (Antihydropic, Hydropsy)
Amaranthus spinosus L., Amaranthaceae 3
Amaranthus viridis L., Amaranthaceae 3
Aniba canelilla (H.B.K.) Mez, Lauraceae 197
Aristolochia cymbifera
  Mart. & Zucc., Aristolochiaceae 46
Aristolochia triangularis Cham., Aristolochiaceae ... 48
Borreria tenella Cham. & Schl., Rubiaceae 296
Bromelia antiacantha Bertol., Bromeliaceae 91
Cabralea canjerana (Vell.) Mart., Meliaceae 227
Cayaponia pilosa Cogn., Cucurbitaceae 135
Chiococca alba (L.) Hitch., Rubiaceae 297
Cissus salutaris H.B.K., Vitaceae 339
Cissus sicyoides L., Vitaceae 339
Clematis dioica L., Ranunculaceae 290
Commelina nudiflora L., Commelinaceae 126
Commelina vestita Seub., Commelinaceae 128
Crescentia cujete L., Bignoniaceae 80
Crinum scabrum Sims, Amaryllidaceae 6
Cybistax antisyphilitica
  (Mart.) Mart., Bignoniaceae 80
Dichorisandra affinis Mart., Commelinaceae 128
Dichorisandra leucophthalmos
  Hook., Commelinaceae 128
Dieffenbachia seguine (Jacq.) Schott, Araceae 35
Eryngium foetidum L., Apiaceae 19
Ficus gomelleira Kunth & Bouché, Moraceae 248
Gallesia gorazema (Vell.) Moq., Phytolaccaceae ... 271
Genipa americana L., Rubiaceae 298
Guarea spiciflora Juss., Meliaceae 227
Guarea trichilioides L., Meliaceae 227
Hymenocallis tubiflora Salisb. [including *Pancratium guianensis* Ker-Gawl.], Amaryllidaceae 7
Ipomoea acetosifolia
  (Vahl) Roem. & Schult., Convolvulaceae 130
Jatropha curcas L., Euphorbiaceae 154
Jatropha elliptica (Pohl) M. Arg., Euphorbiaceae .. 154
Jatropha gossypiifolia L., Euphorbiaceae 154
Limonium brasiliense
  (Boiss.) O. Ktze., Plumbaginaceae 278
Luffa operculata (L.) Cogn., Cucurbitaceae 138
Monstera adansonii Schott, Araceae 36

Operculina alata (Ham.) Urb., Convolvulaceae 131
Operculina macrocarpa Urb., Convolvulaceae 131
Philodendron imbe Schott, Araceae 36
Philodendron ochrostemon Schott, Araceae 37
Sebastiania macrocarpa M. Arg., Euphorbiaceae .. 157
Seguieria americana L., Phytolaccaceae 272
Senna affinis (Benth.) Ir. & Barn., Caesalpiniaceae 104
Senna occidentalis (L.) Link, Caesalpiniaceae 105
Senna quinqueangulata
  (Rich.) Ir. & Barn., Caesalpiniaceae 106
Simaba ferruginea St.-Hil., Simaroubaceae 314
Stachytarpheta jamaicensis
  (L.) Vahl, Verbenaceae 336
Tournefortia laevigata Lam., Boraginaceae 89
Tradescantia diuretica Mart., Commelinaceae 128
Tradescantia effusa Mart., Commelinaceae 129
Trianosperma glandulosa Mart., Cucurbitaceae 140
Trianosperma trilobata Cogn., Cucurbitaceae 140
Trichilia catigua Juss., Meliaceae 229
Vitex gardneriana Schauer, Verbenaceae 336
Wilbrandia ebracteata Cogn., Cucurbitaceae 140
Wilbrandia verticillata
  (Vell.) Cogn., Cucurbitaceae 140

Dysentery
Achyrocline satureioides (Lam.) DC., Asteraceae 52
Albizzia lebbeck (L.) Benth., Mimosaceae 236
Annona coriacea Mart., Annonaceae 12
Annona reticulata L., Annonaceae 13
Ayapana triplinerve
  (Vahl) King & Robinson, Asteraceae 53
Bauhinia guianensis Aubl., Caesalpiniaceae 99
Begonia luxurians Scheidw., Begoniaceae 76
Bidens pilosa L., Asteraceae 57
Borreria asclepiadea Cham. & Schl., substitute for
  Cephaelis ipecacuanha Rich., Rubiaceae 296
Byrsonima spicata Rich., Malpighiaceae 219
Cabomba piauhyensis Gard., Nymphaeaceae 259
Caryocar glabrum (Aubl.) Pers., Caryocaraceae 114
Cayaponia espelina
  (Manso) Cogn., Cucurbitaceae 135
Cecropia hololeuca Miq., Moraceae 247
Celtis iguanaea Sarg., Ulmaceae 330
Cephaelis ipecacuanha Rich., Rubiaceae 296
  see also *Polygala angulata* DC., Polygalaceae ... 284
Cestrum calycinum Willd., Solanaceae 317
Cissampelos pareira L., Menispermaceae 233
Cocos nucifera L., Arecaceae 40
Commelina robusta Kunth, Commelinaceae 128
Copaifera officinalis (Jacq.) L., Caesalpiniaceae 102
Cryptocarya mandioccana Meissn., Lauraceae 198
Cusparia febrifuga Humb., Rutaceae 300
Cydista aequinoctialis Miers, Bignoniaceae 80
Diodia polymorpha Cham. & Schl., substitute for
  Cephaelis ipecacuanha Rich., Rubiaceae 297
Dorstenia brasiliensis Lam., Moraceae 247
Equisetum giganteum L., Equisetaceae 148
Hybanthus ipecacuanha (L.) Baill., Violaceae, same
  use as *Cephaelis ipecacuanha* Rich., Rubiaceae .. 339
Ionidium poaya St.-Hil., Violaceae, same use
  as *Cephaelis ipecacuanha* Rich., Rubiaceae 339
Jodina rhombifolia Hook. & Arn., Santalaceae 304
Krameria argentea Mart., Krameriaceae 191

Licaria puchury-major
  (Mart.) Kosterm., Lauraceae 199
Lipostoma campanuliflorum D. Don, also substitute
  for *Cephaelis ipecacuanha* Rich., Rubiaceae 299
Lithraea molleoides (Vell.) Engl., Anacardiaceae 9
Lucuma caimito Roem. & Schult., Sapotaceae 309
Lucuma rivicoa Gaertn., Sapotaceae 309
Machaonia brasiliensis Cham. & Schl., Rubiaceae 299
Manettia ignita (Vell.) K. Sch., Rubiaceae 299
Marlierea tomentosa Camb., Myrtaceae 255
Melinis minutiflora Beauv., Poaceae 281
Nectandra puberula Nees, Lauraceae 200
Neea theifera Oersted, Nyctaginaceae 258
Peperomia elongata Miq., Piperaceae 273
Polygala spectabilis DC., Polygalaceae 284
Polygonum acuminatum H.B.K., Polygonaceae 286
Pouteria laurifolia Radlk., Sapotaceae 309
Pouteria salicifolia Hook. & Arn., Sapotaceae 310
Rollinia sylvatica (St.-Hil.) Mart., Annonaceae 15
Schinus molle L., Anacardiaceae 9
Virola oleifera (Schott) A.C. Smith, Myristicaceae ....
Waltheria communis St.-Hil., Sterculiaceae 325
Xanthium orientale L., *X. spinosum* L.
  & *X. strumarium* L., Asteraceae 67

Dysmenorrhoea
Cecropia hololeuca Miq., Moraceae 247
Chondodendron platyphyllum
  (Mart.) Miers, Menispermaceae 231
Cissampelos pareira L., Menispermaceae 233
Gomphrena macrocephala St.-Hil., Amaranthaceae .. 4

Dyspepsia (Indigestion).
See also Digestive, Eupeptic
Abuta rufescens Aubl., Menispermaceae 231
Achyrocline satureioides (Lam.) DC., Asteraceae 52
Anacardium occidentale L., Anacardiaceae 7
Ananas comosus (L.) Merrill, Bromeliaceae 90
Aniba puchury-minor (Mart.) Mez, Lauraceae 197
Anisolobus cururu (Mart.) M. Arg., Apocynaceae ... 21
Anisosperma passiflora Manso, Cucurbitaceae 135
Annona squamosa L., Annonaceae 13
Aristolochia cymbifera
  Mart. & Zucc., Aristolochiaceae 46
Baccharis articulata (Lam.) Pers., Asteraceae 54
Baccharis dracunculifolia DC., Asteraceae 54
Cabralea canjerana (Vell.) Mart., Meliaceae 227
Cestrum parqui L'Herit., Solanaceae 317
Cissampelos glaberrima St.-Hil., Menispermaceae 233
Croton zehntneri Pax & Hoffm., Euphorbiaceae 151
Deianira nervosa Cham. & Schl., Gentianaceae 180
Drimys winteri Forst., Winteraceae 340
Esenbeckia febrifuga Juss., Rutaceae 301
Gomphrena leucocephala Mart., Amaranthaceae 4
Guatteria ouregon (Aubl.) Dun., Annonaceae 14
Hyptis multiflora Pohl, Lamiaceae 193
Leiphaimos aphylla (Jacq.) Gilg, Gentianaceae 180
Leonurus sibiricus L., Lamiaceae 194
Licaria puchury-major
  (Mart.) Kosterm., Lauraceae 199
Mikania officinalis Mart., Asteraceae 62
Myrocarpus frondosus Fr. All., Fabaceae 170
Nectandra puberula Nees, Lauraceae 200
Nymphoides indica (L.) O. Ktze., Menyanthaceae . 235

Odontadenia speciosa Benth., Apocynaceae 27
Peperomia hederacea Miq., Piperaceae 273
Piper eucalyptifolium (Miq.) Rudge, Piperaceae 275
Pradosia lactescens (Vell.) Radlk., Sapotaceae 310
Ptychopetalum olacoides Benth., Olacaceae 262
Ptychopetalum uncinatum Anselm., Olacaceae 262
Quassia amara L., Simaroubaceae 314
Simaba ferruginea St.-Hil., Simaroubaceae 314
Simarouba amara Aubl., Simaroubaceae 315
Siparuna guianensis Aubl., Monimiaceae 245
Syagrus pseudococos (Raddi) Glassman, Arecaceae 45
Tachia guianenesis Aubl., Gentianaceae 180
Tagetes minuta L., Asteraceae 67
Tontelea brachypoda Miers, Hippocrateaceae 183
Turnera diffusa Willd., Turneraceae 327
Turnera opifera Mart., Turneraceae 328
Turnera ulmifolia L., Turneraceae 328
Virola oleifera (Schott) A.C. Smith, Myristicaceae . 250
Virola sebifera Aubl., Myristicaceae 250
Zanthoxylum rhoifolium Lam., Rutaceae 303

Dyspnea

Cyperus sesquiflorus
 (Torrey) Mattf. & Kükent., Cyperaceae 142

E

Earache. See also Otalgia, Otitis

Amasonia arborea H.B.K., Verbenaceae 333
Canna glauca L., Cannaceae 110
Zanthoxylum hyemale St.-Hil., Rutaceae 302
Zanthoxylum pterota H.B.K., Rutaceae 303

Eczema

Aristolochia cymbifera
 Mart. & Zucc., Aristolochiaceae 46
Berberis laurina Thunb., Berberidaceae 76
Cayaponia tayuya (Mart.) Cogn., Cucurbitaceae 135
Desmoncus orthacanthos Mart., Arecaceae 40
Jacaranda subrhombea DC., Bignoniaceae 81
Monstera adansonii Schott, Araceae 36
Sebastiania macrocarpa M. Arg., Euphorbiaceae .. 157
Setaria scandens Schrad., Poaceae 282
Solanum nigrum L., Solanaceae 321
Xyris laxifolia Mart., Xyridaceae 342
Xyris pallida Mart., Xyridaceae 342

Edema. See also Anasarca

Dieffenbachia seguine (Jacq.) Schott, Araceae 35
Doliocarpus rolandri Gmel., Dilleniaceae 146
Mikania officinalis Mart., Asteraceae 62
Solanum aculeatissimum Jacq., Solanaceae 319

Elemi

Protium icicariba (DC.) March., Burseraceae 94

Elephantiasis

Guazuma ulmifolia Lam.
 var. *tomentella* Schum., Sterculiaceae 323
Hura crepitans L., Euphorbiaceae 153
Leonotis nepetaefolia R. Br., Lamiaceae 194
Sapium hamatum Pax & Hoffm., Euphorbiaceae ... 157

Emetic (Vomitive)

Allamanda cathartica L., Apocynaceae 20
Allamanda doniana M. Arg., Apocynaceae 20
Andira inermis (Sw.) H.B.K., Fabaceae 162

Anisolobus cururu (Mart.) M. Arg., Apocynaceae 21
Annona muricata L., Annonaceae 13
Araujia sericifera Brot., Asclepiadaceae 50
Bixa orellana L., Bixaceae 85
Borreria asclepiadea Cham. & Schl. substitute
 for *Cephaelis ipecacuanha* Rich., Rubiaceae 296
Borreria tenella Cham. & Schl., Rubiaceae 296
Borreria verticillata (L.) Meyer, Rubiaceae 296
Brunfelsia uniflora (Pohl) D. Don,
 also *B. grandiflora* D. Don, Solanaceae 316
Byrsonima verbascifolia (L.) Rich., Malpighiaceae 220
Cabralea canjerana (Vell.) Mart., Meliaceae 227
Caesalpinia bonduc (L.) Roxb., Caesalpiniaceae 99
Caladium bicolor (Aiton) Vent., Araceae 34
Cayaponia martiana
 (Cogn.) Cogn., Cucurbitaceae 135
Cedrela fissilis Vell., Meliaceae 227
Cephaelis ipecacuanha Rich., Rubiaceae 296
Cocos nucifera L., Arecaceae 40
Copaifera officinalis (Jacq.) L., Caesalpiniaceae 102
Corynostylis hybanthus
 (L.) Mart. & Zucc., Violaceae 338
Diodia polymorpha Cham. & Schl., substitute for
 Cephaelis ipecacuanha Rich., Rubiaceae 297
Fevillea trilobata L., Cucurbitaceae 136
Galphimia brasiliensis Juss., Malpighiaceae 220
Guarea trichilioides L., Meliaceae 227
Gustavia hexapetala (Aubl.)
 J.E. Smith, Lecythidaceae 205
Hibiscus bifurcatus Cav., Malvaceae 221
Hippeastrum puniceum (Lam.) Kuntze
 [includes *Hippeastrum equestre*
 (L.) Hebert], Amaryllidaceae 6
Hippeastrum vittatum
 (L'Hérit.) Herb., Amaryllidaceae 6
Hura crepitans L., Euphorbiaceae 153
Hybanthus ipecacuanha (L.) Baill., Violaceae, same
 use as *Cephaelis ipecacuanha* Rich., Rubiaceae .. 339
Hydrocotyle bonariensis Lam., Apiaceae 19
Hydrocotyle leucocephala
 Cham. & Schlecht., Apiaceae 20
Hymenocallis tubiflora Salisb. [includes *Pancratium
 guianensis* Ker-Gawl.], Amaryllidaceae 7
Inga alba (Sw.) Willd., Mimosaceae 237
Ionidium poaya St.-Hil., Violaceae, same use
 as *Cephaelis ipecacuanha* Rich., Rubiaceae 339
Jacaranda copaia (Aubl.) D. Don, Bignoniaceae 80
Joannesia heveoides Ducke, Euphorbiaceae 155
Lindernia diffusa Wettst., Scrophulariaceae 311
Lipostoma campanuliflorum D. Don, Rubiaceae ... 299
Luffa operculata (L.) Cogn., Cucurbitaceae 138
Machaonia brasiliensis Cham. & Schl., Rubiaceae 299
Manettia ignita (Vell.) K. Sch., Rubiaceae 299
Mimosa pudica L., Mimosaceae 240
Mimosa velloziana Mart., Mimosaceae 240
Ochroma pyramidale (Cav.) Urb., Bombacaceae 86
Polygala angulata DC., Polygalaceae 283
Polygala comata Mart., Polygalaceae 284
Polygala paniculata L., Polygalaceae 284
Polygala timoutou Aubl., Polygalaceae 284
Potalia amara Aubl., Loganiaceae 209
Rauwolfia ligustrina
 Willd. ex Roem. & Schult., Apocynaceae 28

MEDICINAL INDEX: EMETIC – EMOLLIENT

Ruellia geminiflora H.B.K., Acanthaceae 1
Ruellia tuberosa L., Acanthaceae 1
Spondias macrocarpa Engl., Anacardiaceae 10
Spondias mombin L., Anacardiaceae 10
Stachytarpheta jamaicensis (L.) Vahl, Verbenaceae 336
Stryphnodendron coriaceum Benth., Mimosaceae . 243
Thevetia ahouai (L.) DC., Apocynaceae 28
Waltheria communis St.-Hil., Sterculiaceae 325

Emetocathartic

Allamanda blanchetii M. Arg., Apocynaceae 20
Borreria poaya (St.-Hil.) DC., Rubiaceae 296
Cayaponia tayuya (Mart.) Cogn., Cucurbitaceae 135
Davilla rugosa Poir., Dilleniaceae 145
Heteropteris syringifolia Gris., Malpighiaceae 220
Hybanthus ipecacuanha (L.) Baill., Violaceae 339
Lindernia crustacea F. Muell., Scrophulariaceae ... 311
Parahancornia amapa (Hub.) Ducke, Apocynaceae 27
Pisonia alcalina Fr. All., also
  P. subcordata Sw., Nyctaginaceae 258
Rauwolfia blanchetii DC., Apocynaceae 28
Trichilia barraensis DC., Meliaceae 229
Xyris laxifolia Mart., Xyridaceae 342
Xyris pallida Mart., Xyridaceae 342

Emmenagogue

Abuta rufescens Aubl., Menispermaceae 231
Adiantum concinnum Humb. & Bonp., Adiantaceae .. 1
Aloysia triphylla (L'Her.) Britt., Verbenaceae 332
Aristolochia cordigera Willd., Aristolochiaceae 46
Aristolochia triangularis Cham., Aristolochiaceae ... 48
Bixa orellana L., Bixaceae 85
Carica papaya L., Caricaceae 113
Cayaponia pilosa Cogn., Cucurbitaceae 135
Cecropia hololeuca Miq., Moraceae 247
Chenopodium ambrosioides L., Chenopodiaceae ... 118
Chiococca alba (L.) Hitch., Rubiaceae 297
Cissampelos pareira L., Menispermaceae 233
Conyza blakei (Cabr.) Cabr., Asteraceae 58
Costus spicatus (Jacq.) Sw., Costaceae 132
Cunila microcephala Benth., Lamiaceae 192
Cusparia toxicaria Spr. ex Engl., Rutaceae 301
Dipteryx alata Vog., Fabaceae 165
Dipteryx odorata (Aubl.) Willd., Fabaceae 166
Dorstenia brasiliensis Lam., Moraceae 247
Egletes viscosa (L.) Less., Asteraceae 59
Elephantopus mollis H.B.K., Asteraceae 59
Eryngium foetidum L., Apiaceae 19
Fevillea trilobata L., Cucurbitaceae 136
Grindelia buphthalmoides DC., Asteraceae 60
Grindelia scorzonerifolia Hook. & Arn., Asteraceae 60
Heliotropium lanceolatum Loefgr., Boraginaceae 89
Himatanthus lancifolia
  (M. Arg.) Woods., Apocynaceae 26
Hypericum teretiusculum St.-Hil., Clusiaceae 122
Hypolytrum laxum Schrad., Cyperaceae 143
Hyptis crenata Pohl, Lamiaceae 192
Ipomoea acetosifolia
  (Vahl) Roem. & Schult., Convolvulaceae 130
Lantana macrophylla Schauer, Verbenaceae 335
Lindernia crustacea F. Muell., Scrophulariaceae ... 311
Lindernia diffusa Wettst., Scrophulariaceae 311
Lippia alba (Mill.) N.E. Brown, Verbenaceae 335
Lithraea molleoides (Vell.) Engl., Anacardiaceae 9
Lucuma rivicoa Gaertn., Sapotaceae 309

Margyricarpus setosus Ruiz & Pav., Rosaceae 294
Monnieria trifolia Loefl., Rutaceae 302
Ocotea pulchella Mart., Lauraceae 201
Passiflora gardneri Mast., Passifloraceae 270
Passiflora macrocarpa Mast., Passifloraceae 270
Peltodon longipes St.-Hil., Lamiaceae 195
Petiveria alliacea L., Phytolaccaceae 271
Piper mikanianum (Kunth) Steud., Piperaceae 276
Piper parthenium Mart., Piperaceae 276
Polygala timoutou Aubl., Polygalaceae 284
Porophyllum ruderale (Jacq.) Cass., Asteraceae 64
Portulaca oleracea L., Portulacaceae 289
Portulaca pilosa L., Portulacaceae 289
Schinus molle L., Anacardiaceae 9
Senna alata (L.) Roxb., Caesalpiniaceae 104
Senna occidentalis (L.) Link, Caesalpiniaceae 105
Senna quinqueangulata
  (Rich.) Ir. & Barn., Caesalpiniaceae 106
Senna uniflora
  (P. Miller) Ir. & Barn., Caesalpiniaceae 106
Siparuna camporum (Tul.) DC., Monimiaceae 245
Stachytarpheta jamaicensis (L.) Vahl, Verbenaceae 336
Talinum racemosum (L.) Rohr., Portulacaceae 289
Tanacetum vulgare L., Asteraceae 67
Torresea cearensis Fr. All., Fabaceae 172
Wilbrandia verticillata
  (Vell.) Cogn., Cucurbitaceae 140

Emollient

Adiantum trapeziforme L., Adiantaceae 1
Amaranthus spinosus L., Amaranthaceae 3
Amaranthus viridis L., Amaranthaceae 3
Andropogon bicornis L., Poaceae 279
Andropogon condensatus H.B.K., Poaceae 279
Blanchetia heterotricha DC., Asteraceae 57
Brasilopuntia brasiliensis (Willd.) Berg., Cactaceae 95
Buddleja brasiliensis Jacq. ex Spr., Buddlejaceae 93
Canna warszewiczii Dietr., Cannaceae 111
Cestrum calycinum Willd., Solanaceae 317
Commelina platyphylla
  Klotz. ex Seub., Commelinaceae 126
Commelina vestita Seub., Commelinaceae 128
Commelina virginica L., Commelinaceae 128
Conocliniopsis prasiifolia
  (DC.) King & Robinson, Asteraceae 58
Copaifera cearensis
  Huber ex Ducke, Caesalpiniaceae 102
Cordia insignis Cham., Boraginaceae 87
Crescentia cujete L., Bignoniaceae 80
Cuscuta racemosa Mart., Convolvulaceae 130
Dichorisandra affinis Mart., Commelinaceae 128
Dichorisandra leucophthalmos
  Hook., Commelinaceae 128
Dioscorea glandulosa Klotz., Dioscoreaceae 147
Elaeis guineensis Jacq., Arecaceae 40
Elephantopus mollis H.B.K., Asteraceae 59
Erythrina corallodendron L., Fabaceae 166
Erythrina velutina Willd., Fabaceae 166
Helicteres ovata Lam., Sterculiaceae 324
Hibiscus bifurcatus Cav., Malvaceae 221
Hibiscus cannabinus L., Malvaceae 221
Hibiscus sabdariffa L., Malvaceae 221
Hibiscus tiliaceus L., Malvaceae 221
Himatanthus sucuuba (Spr.) Woods., Apocynaceae . 26

EMOLLIENT – EUPEPTIC: MEDICINAL INDEX

Hylocereus undatus (Haw.) Br. & Rose, Cactaceae .. 95
Hypolytrum laxum Schrad., Cyperaceae 143
Ibicella lutea (Lindl.) Van Eselt., Martyniaceae 224
Ipomoea acetosifolia
   (Vahl) Roem. & Schult., Convolvulaceae 130
Ipomoea pes-caprae (L.) R. Br., Convolvulaceae .. 130
Iresine polymorpha Mart., Amaranthaceae 4
Kalanchoe pinnata (Lam.) Pers., Crassulaceae 133
Kielmeyera coriacea Mart., Clusiaceae 122
Kielmeyera petiolaris Mart., Clusiaceae 122
Kielmeyera rosea Mart., Clusiaceae 122
Kielmeyera speciosa St.-Hil., Clusiaceae 123
Lagenaria siceraria
   (Molina) Standl., Cucurbitaceae 138
Ludwigia peruviana (L.) Hara, Onagraceae 264
Luziola peruviana Pers., Poaceae 281
Mauritia flexuosa L. f., Arecaceae 43
Mimosa bimucronata (DC.) O. Ktze., Mimosaceae 238
Momordica charantia L., Cucurbitaceae 139
Monstera adansonii Schott, Araceae 36
Nymphaea ampla DC., Nymphaeaceae 259
Nymphaea rudgeana G. Meyer, Nymphaeaceae 259
Oenocarpus distichus Mart., Arecaceae 43
Panicum petrosum Trin., Poaceae 282
Panicum trichanthum Nees, Poaceae 282
Parthenium hysterophorus L., Asteraceae 64
Patagonula americana L., Boraginaceae 89
Peperomia pellucida H.B.K., Piperaceae 273
Pereskia aculeata Mill., Cactaceae 97
Pereskia bleo H.B.K., Cactaceae 97
Piper arboreum Aubl., Piperaceae 274
Portulaca grandiflora Hook., Portulacaceae 288
Psoralea glandulosa L., Fabaceae 170
Scoparia dulcis L., Scrophulariaceae 312
Sesuvium portulacastrum L., Aizoaceae 1
Sida carpinifolia (L. f.) K. Sch., Malvaceae 222
Sida micrantha St.-Hil., Malvaceae 222
Sida rhombea L., Malvaceae 222
Sida rhombifolia L., Malvaceae 222
Sinningia allagophylla
   (Mart.) Wiehl., Gesneriaceae 181
Solanum nigrum L., Solanaceae 321
Solanum verbascifolium L., Solanaceae 322
Tradescantia effusa Mart., Commelinaceae 129
Tradescantia spathacea Sw., Commelinaceae 129
Turnera guianensis Aubl., Turneraceae 328
Urena lobata L., Malvaceae 223
Waltheria viscosissima St.-Hil., Sterculiaceae 325
Xanthium orientale L., *X. spinosum* L.
   & *X. strumarium* L., Asteraceae 67

Endurance, to increase
Erythroxylum cataractarum
   Spruce, Erythroxylaceae 149
Erythroxylum coca Lam., Erythroxylaceae 149

Enema
Chamissoa macrocarpa H.B.K., Amaranthaceae 4
Pfaffia glomerata (Spreng.) Peders., Amaranthaceae .. 5

Enteritis
Cochlospermum regium
   (Mart. & Schl.) Pilg., Cochlospermaceae 125
Crescentia cujete L., Bignoniaceae 80
Psoralea glandulosa L., Fabaceae 170

Enterocolitis
Arrabidaea chica (H.B.K.) Bur., Bignoniaceae 78
Rollinia orthopetala DC., Annonaceae 15

Enterorrhagia
Limonium brasiliense
   (Boiss.) O. Ktze., Plumbaginaceae 278
Neea theifera Oersted, Nyctaginaceae 258

Epididymitis
Davilla rugosa Poir., Dilleniaceae 145

Epilepsy
Acosmium dasycarpum (Vog.) Yakovl., Fabaceae .. 162
Acosmium subelegans
   (Mohlenb.) Yakovl., Fabaceae 162
Cayaponia espelina
   (Manso) Cogn., Cucurbitaceae 135
Cayaponia tayuya (Mart.) Cogn., Cucurbitaceae 135
Cestrum parqui L'Herit., Solanaceae 317
Cissus sicyoides L., Vitaceae 339
Indigofera suffruticosa Mill., Fabaceae 168
Lophophytum mirabile
   Schott & Endl., Balanophoraceae 73
Parkinsonia aculeata L., Caesalpiniaceae 104
Pothomorphe umbellata (L.) Miq., Piperaceae 277
Trianosperma glandulosa Mart., Cucurbitaceae 140
Trianosperma trilobata Cogn., Cucurbitaceae 140

Eruptive Diseases
Fevillea trilobata L., Cucurbitaceae 137

Erysipelas
Acanthospermum australe
   (Loefl.) O. Ktze., Asteraceae 51
Attalea oleifera Barb. Rodr., Arecaceae 39
Clibadium rotundifolium DC., Asteraceae 58
Clibadium surinamense L., Asteraceae 58
Crescentia cujete L., Bignoniaceae 80
Cyrtocymura scorpioides
   (Lam.) H. Robinson, Asteraceae 58
Elaeis guineensis Jacq., Arecaceae 40
Fevillea trilobata L., Cucurbitaceae 136
Fevillea uncipetala Kuhlm., Cucurbitaceae 138
Jatropha gossypiifolia L., Euphorbiaceae 154
Kalanchoe brasiliensis Camb., Crassulaceae 133
Monstera adansonii Schott, Araceae 36
Ouratea jabotapita Engl., Ochnaceae 261
Ouratea parviflora (DC.) Baill., Ochnaceae 261
Philodendron imbe Schott, Araceae 36
Philodendron ochrostemon Schott, Araceae 37
Piper aduncum L., Piperaceae 274
Polygonum punctatum Elliot, Polygonaceae 287
Polygonum spectabile Mart., Polygonaceae 287
Portulaca pilosa L., Portulacaceae 289
Pothomorphe umbellata (L.) Miq., Piperaceae 277
Scoparia dulcis L., Scrophulariaceae 312
Spondias macrocarpa Engl., Anacardiaceae 10
Spondias mombin L., Anacardiaceae 10
Virola sebifera Aubl., Myristicaceae 250
Virola oleifera (Schott) A.C. Smith, Myristicaceae . 250
Virola surinamensis (Rol.) Warb., Myristicaceae ... 252
Wilbrandia verticillata
   (Vell.) Cogn., Cucurbitaceae 140

Eupeptic. *See also* Digestive, Dyspepsia
Aniba canelilla (H.B.K.) Mez, Lauraceae 197
Baccharis dracunculifolia DC., Asteraceae 54

Baccharis spp., Asteraceae 56
Carica papaya L., Caricaceae 113
Miconia albicans (Sw.) Tr., Melastomataceae 225
Xylopia aromatica (Lam.) Mart., Annonaceae 15
Xylopia frutescens Aubl., Annonaceae 16

Euphoria
Maquira sclerophylla
 (Ducke) C. C. Berg, Moraceae 249

Exanthema
Carapa guianensis Aubl., Meliaceae 227

Excitant (Analeptic, Nerve Stimulant)
Abuta candicans Rich., Menispermaceae 231
Anacardium occidentale L., Anacardiaceae 7
Andradea floribunda Fr. All., Nyctaginaceae 257
Aniba canelilla (H.B.K.) Mez, Lauraceae 197
Aristolochia cordigera Willd., Aristolochiaceae 46
Aristolochia trilobata L., Aristolochiaceae 48
Calyptranthes aromatica St.-Hil., Myrtaceae 253
Calyptranthes variabilis Berg, Myrtaceae 253
Campsiandra comosa Benth. var.
 laurifolia (Benth.) Cowan, Caesalpiniaceaae 100
Canna indica L., Cannaceae 111
Capraria biflora L., Scrophulariaceae 311
Cinnamodendron axillare
 (Nees & Mart.) Endl., Canellaceae 110
Cleome polygama L., Capparaceae 112
Cleome speciosa H.B.K., Capparaceae 112
Cleome spinosa Jacq., Capparaceae 112
Conobea aquatica Aubl., Scrophulariaceae 311
Conocliniopsis prasiifolia
 (DC.) King & Robinson, Asteraceae 58
Cryptocarya guyanensis Meissn., Lauraceae 198
Cryptocarya moschata
 Nees & Mart. ex Nees, Lauraceae 198
Cyperus gracilescens
 Roem. & Schult., Cyperaceae 142
Dipteryx alata Vog., Fabaceae 165
Eugenia uniflora L., Myrtaceae 254
Galinsoga parviflora Cav., Asteraceae 60
Gomphrena officinalis Mart., Amaranthaceae 4
Grindelia buphthalmoides DC., Asteraceae 60
Grindelia scorzonerifolia
 Hook. & Arn., Asteraceae 60
Guatteria nigrescens Mart., Annonaceae 14
Guatteria ouregon (Aubl.) Dun., Annonaceae 14
Gynerium parviflorum Nees, also
 G. sagittatum (Pers.) Beauv., Poaceae 281
Hedyosmum brasiliense Mart., Chloranthaceae 119
Heterothalamus alienus (Spr.) O. Ktze., Asteraceae   60
Hippeastrum psittacinum Herb., Amaryllidaceae 6
Hippeastrum puniceum (Lam.) Kuntze [includes
 H. equestre (L.) Hebert], Amaryllidaceae 6
Hymenocallis tubiflora Salisb. [includes *Pancratium
 guianensis* Ker-Gawl.], Amaryllidaceae 7
Hypericum brasiliense Choisy, Clusiaceae 122
Licaria camara (Schomb.) Kosterm., Lauraceae 198
Myrocarpus frondosus Fr. All., Fabaceae 170
Nectandra canescens Nees, Lauraceae 199
Nectandra globosa (Aubl.) Mez, Lauraceae 199
Noticastrum diffusum (Pers.) Cabr., Asteraceae 62
Ocimum fluminensis Vell., Lamiaceae 195
Ocotea cujumary Mart., Lauraceae 200

Ocotea cymbarum H.B.K., Lauraceae 200
Ocotea guianensis Aubl., Lauraceae 201
Panicum trichanthum Nees, Poaceae 282
Paullinia cupana Kunth, Sapindaceae 306
Piper ceanothifolium H.B.K., Piperaceae 275
Piper marginatum Jacq., Piperaceae 275
Piper mollicomum Kunth, Piperaceae 276
Piper reticulatum L., Piperaceae 276
Raputia alba (Nees & Mart.) Engl., Rutaceae 302
Raputia aromatica Aubl., Rutaceae 302
Rollinia orthopetala DC., Annonaceae 15
Siparuna brasiliensis (Spr.) DC., Monimiaceae 245
Siparuna camporum (Tul.) DC., Monimiaceae 245
Spigelia glabrata Mart., Loganiaceae 209
Tagetes minuta L., Asteraceae 67
Thalia geniculata L., Marantaceae 224
Triplaris noli-tangere Wedd., Polygonaceae 287
Virola oleifera (Schott) A.C. Smith, Myristicaceae . 250
Vitex gardneriana Schauer, Verbenaceae 336
Zanthoxylum pterota H.B.K., Rutaceae 303
Zanthoxylum tingoassuiba St.-Hil., Rutaceae 303

Exhaustion (Fatigue)
Erythroxylum cataractarum
 Spruce, Erythroxylaceae 149
Erythroxylum coca Lam., Erythroxylaceae 149
Ilex paraguariensis St.-Hil., Aquifoliaceae 31
Imperata brasiliensis Trin., also
 Imperata contracta Hitch., Poaceae 281
Orbignya phalerata Mart., Arecaceae 43

Expectorant
Adiantopsis chlorophylla (Sw.) Fée, Adiantaceae 1
Anacardium occidentale L., Anacardiaceae 7
Anemia phyllitidis (L.) Sw., Schizaeaceae 310
Borreria asclepiadea Cham. & Schl., substitute for
 Cephaelis ipecacuanha Rich., Rubiaceae 296
Cephaelis ipecacuanha Rich., Rubiaceae 296
 see also *Polygala angulata* DC., Polygalaceae 284
Crescentia cujete L., Bignoniaceae 80
Cyathea microdonta (Desv.) Domin, Cyatheaceae . 141
Diodia polymorpha Cham. & Schl., substitute for
 Cephaelis ipecacuanha Rich., Rubiaceae 297
Humiria balsamifera (Aubl.) St.-Hil., Humiriaceae .. 183
Hybanthus ipecacuanha (L.) Baill., Violaceae, same
 use as *Cephaelis ipecacuanha* Rich., Rubiaceae .. 339
Hymenocallis tubiflora Salisb. [includes *Pancratium
 guianensis* Ker-Gawl.], Amaryllidaceae 7
Hyptis umbrosa Salzm., Lamiaceae 193
Ionidium poaya St.-Hil., Violaceae, same use as
 Cephaelis ipecacuanha Rich., Rubiaceae 339
Keithia denudata Benth., Lamiaceae 193
Lipostoma campaniflorum D. Don, also substitute
 for *Cephaelis ipecacuanha* Rich., Rubiaceae 299
Machaonia brasiliensis Cham. & Schl., Rubiaceae 299
Manettia ignita (Vell.) K. Sch., substitute
 for *Cephaelis ipecacuanha* Rich., Rubiaceae 299
Mikania glomerata Spreng., Asteraceae 61
Monnieria trifolia Loefl., Rutaceae 302
Myrocarpus frondosus Fr. All., Fabaceae 170
Myroxylon balsamum (L.) Harms, Fabaceae 170
Oldenlandia corymbosa L., Rubiaceae 299
Parapiptadenia rigida
 (Benth.) Brenan, Mimosaceae 240
Peperomia transparens Miq., Piperaceae 274

Pereskia aculeata Mill., Cactaceae 97
Periandra mediterranea (Vell.) Taub., Fabaceae ... 170
Piper geniculatum Sw., Piperaceae 275
Polygala spectabilis DC., Polygalaceae 284
Solanum nigrum L., Solanaceae 321
Turnera ulmifolia L., Turneraceae 328
**Expulsion. *See* Foetus Expulsion,
Placenta Expulsion, Childbirth
Eye Inflammation. *See also* Eye Problems**
Bixa orellana L., Bixaceae 85
Cocos nucifera L., Arecaceae 40
Trixis antimenorrhoea (Schrank) Mart., Asteraceae . 67
Vallesia cymbifolia Ortega, Apocynaceae 29
Zanthoxylum hyemale St.-Hil., Rutaceae 302
**Eye Problems. *See also* Cataract,
Conjunctivitis, Corneal Opacity,
Corneal Ulcers, Eye Inflammation,
Eyes (Remove Film), Glaucoma,
Ophthalmia, Pterygium Remover, Trachoma**
Chromolaena hirsuta
   (Hook. & Arn.) King & Robinson, Asteraceae 58
Cocos nucifera L., Arecaceae 40
Euphorbia caecorum Mart., Euphorbiaceae 152
Euphorbia hirta L., Euphorbiaceae 152
Euphorbia tirucalli L., Euphorbiaceae 153
Jatropha urens L., Euphorbiaceae 155
Monnieria trifolia Loefl., Rutaceae 302
Potalia amara Aubl., Loganiaceae 209
Schinus terebinthifolius Raddi, Anacardiaceae 10
Trixis antimenorrhoea (Schrank) Mart., Asteraceae . 67
Vallesia cymbifolia Ortega, Apocynaceae 29
Zanthoxylum hyemale St.-Hil., Rutaceae 302
Eye Pupil Contraction (Miotic)
Pilocarpus pinnatifolius Lem., Rutaceae 302
Eyes (Remove Film)
Euphorbia hyssopifolia L., Euphorbiaceae 153
Jatropha curcas L., Euphorbiaceae 154
Eyewash
Begonia paulensis DC., Begoniaceae 76
Bixa orellana L., Bixaceae 85
Buddleja cambara Arech., Buddlejaceae 93
Commelina sulcata Willd., Commelinaceae 128
Hyptis plectranthoides Benth., Lamiaceae 193
Martinella obovata
   (H.B.K.) Bur. & K. Sch., Bignoniaceae 82
Pithecellobium cochleatum
   (Willd.) Mart., Mimosaceae 242

F

**Fatigue. *See* Exhaustion
Febrifuge (Antipyretic, Antithermic, Fever).
See also Puerperal Fever, Typhoid Fever,
Yellow Fever**
Abuta concolor Poepp. & Endl., Menispermaceae . 231
Abuta selloana Eichl., Menispermaceae 231
Acanthospermum hispidum DC., Asteraceae 52
Acanthosyris spinescens
   (Mart. & Endl.) Gris., Santalaceae 304
Adenocalymma alliacea
   (Lam.) Miers, Bignoniaceae 78

Ageratum conyzoides L., Asteraceae 53
Allagoptera campestris (Mart.) Kuntze, Arecaceae .. 39
Alsodeia flavescens (Aubl.) Spreng., Violaceae 337
Ambrosia artemisiifolia L., Asteraceae 53
Annona reticulata L., Annonaceae 13
Aristolochia cymbifera
   Mart. & Zucc., Aristolochiaceae 46
Aristolochia trilobata L., Aristolochiaceae 48
Aspidosperma desmanthum M. Arg., Apocynaceae . 21
Aspidosperma nitidum Benth., Apocynaceae 21
Aspidosperma polyneuron M. Arg., Apocynaceae 21
Attalea spectabilis Mart., Arecaceae 39
Baccharis articulata (Lam.) Pers., Asteraceae 54
Baccharis dracunculifolia DC., Asteraceae 54
Baccharis spp., Asteraceae 56
Baccharis trimera (Less.) DC., Asteraceae 54
Begonia hirtella Link, Begoniaceae 76
Begonia luxurians Scheidw., Begoniaceae 76
Begonia paulensis DC., Begoniaceae 76
Blanchetia heterotricha DC., Asteraceae 57
Bowdichia virgilioides H.B.K., Fabaceae 163
Brasilopuntia brasiliensis (Willd.) Berg., Cactaceae 95
Bredemeyera floribunda Willd., Polygalaceae 283
Brosimum utile (H.B.K.) Pittier, Moraceae 246
Byrsonima verbascifolia (L.) Rich., Malpighiaceae 220
Cabralea canjerana (Vell.) Mart., Meliaceae 227
Caesalpinia ferrea Mart. ex Tul., Caesalpiniaceae . 100
Calolisianthus pendulus
   (Mart.) Gilg, Gentianaceae 179
Capraria biflora L., Scrophulariaceae 311
Carapa guianensis Aubl., Meliaceae 227
Carica papaya L., Caricaceae 113
Caryocar brasiliense Camb., Caryocaraceae 114
Casearia sylvestris Sw., Flacourtiaceae 178
Cayaponia cabocla (Vell.) Mart., Cucurbitaceae ... 135
Cedrela fissilis Vell., Meliaceae 227
Cedrela odorata L., Meliaceae 227
Celtis brasiliensis Planch., Ulmaceae 330
Celtis morifolia Planch.,Ulmaceae 330
Cestrum amictum Schl., Solanaceae 317
Cestrum pseudoquina Mart., Solanaceae 317
Chiococca alba (L.) Hitch., Rubiaceae 297
Chloris distichophylla (Nees) Lag., Poaceae 280
Cinnamodendron axillare
   (Nees & Mart.) Endl., Canellaceae 110
Cissampelos fasciculata Benth., Menispermaceae . 231
Cissampelos glaberrima St.-Hil., Menispermaceae 233
Cissampelos pareira L., Menispermaceae 233
Clusia panapanari Choisy, Clusiaceae 122
Cocos nucifera L., Arecaceae 40
Colletia paradoxa (Spr.) Escalante, Rhamnaceae ... 291
Conocarpus erecta L., Combretaceae 126
Copaifera multijuga Hayne, Caesalpiniaceae 102
Costus cuspidatus
   (Nees & Mart.) Maas, Costaceae 132
Costus spicatus (Jacq.) Sw., Costaceae 132
Coutoubea spicata Aubl., Gentianaceae 179
Crataeva tapia L., Capparaceae 112
Crescentia cujete L., Bignoniaceae 80
Croton salutaris Casar., Euphorbiaceae 151
Croton spp., those known as 'velame' including:
   C. cascarilla (L.) Bennet, C. glabellus L. &
   C. paniculatus M. Arg., Euphorbiaceae 152

MEDICINAL INDEX: FEBRIFUGE

Cunila microcephala Benth., Lamiaceae 192
Cuphea ingrata Cham. & Schl., Lythraceae 214
Curtia tenuifolia (Aubl.) Knobl., Gentianaceae 180
Cusparia febrifuga Humb., Rutaceae 300
Cusparia toxicaria Spr. ex Engl., Rutaceae 301
Cymbopogon schoenanthus (L.) Spreng., Poaceae 280
Cyperus corymbosus Rottb., Cyperaceae 142
Deianira nervosa Cham. & Schl. (including
   D. erubescens Cham.& Schl.), Gentianaceae 180
Deianira pallescens Cham. & Schl., Gentianaceae . 180
Diospyros paralea Steud., Ebenaceae 147
Dipholis nigra Gr., Sapotaceae 309
Discaria americana Gill. & Hook., Rhamnaceae ... 291
Dodonaea viscosa Jacq., Sapindaceae 305
Doliocarpus rolandri Gmel., Dilleniaceae 146
Dorstenia asaroides Gardn., Moraceae 247
Elephantopus micropappus Less., Asteraceae 59
Elephantopus mollis H.B.K., Asteraceae 59
Ephedra triandra Tul., Ephedraceae 148
Erythrina corallodendron L., Fabaceae 166
Esenbeckia febrifuga Juss., Rutaceae 301
Esenbeckia intermedia Mart., Rutaceae 301
Eugenia sulcata Spring, Myrtaceae 254
Eugenia uniflora L., Myrtaceae 254
Euphorbia hirta L., Euphorbiaceae
   (CHEM. & PHARM.) 152
Euterpe oleracea Mart., Arecaceae 42
Evolvulus alsinoides L., Convolvulaceae 130
Exostemma australe St.-Hil., Rubiaceae 298
Fevillea trilobata L., Cucurbitaceae 136
Galphimia brasiliensis Juss., Malpighiaceae 220
Geissospermum laeve (Vell.) Baill., Apocynaceae 23
Geissospermum sericeum
   Benth. & Hook., Apocynaceae 24
Glandularia peruviana (L.) Small, Verbenaceae ... 334
Gomphrena leucocephala Mart., Amaranthaceae 4
Gomphrena officinalis Mart., Amaranthaceae 4
Guarea trichilioides L., Meliaceae 227
Guettarda angelica Mart., Rubiaceae 298
Hedyosmum brasiliense Mart., Chloranthaceae 119
Heliotropium lanceolatum Loefgr., Boraginaceae 89
Heterothalamus alienus (Spr.) O. Ktze., Asteraceae   60
Heterothalamus psiadioides Less., Asteraceae 60
Hibiscus sabdariffa L., Malvaceae 221
Himatanthus drastica (Mart.) Woods., Apocynaceae 24
Himatanthus sucuuba (Spr.) Woods., Apocynaceae . 26
Hortia brasiliensis Vand., Rutaceae 301
Hylocereus undatus (Haw.) Br. & Rose, Cactaceae .. 95
Indigofera suffruticosa Mill., Fabaceae 168
Jacaranda cuspidifolia Mart., Bignoniaceae 81
Jatropha multifida L., Euphorbiaceae 154
Kyllinga pungens Link, Cyperaceae 143
Lafoensia pacari St.-Hil., Lythraceae 215
Lantana brasiliensis Link, Verbenaceae 334
Lantana camara L., Verbenaceae 334
Lantana microphylla Cham., also L. mixta L.,
   L. pseudothea (St.-Hil.) Schauer, Verbenaceae ... 335
Leiphaimos aphylla (Jacq.) Gilg, Gentianaceae 180
Leonotis nepetaefolia R. Br., Lamiaceae 194
Lindernia diffusa Wettst., Scrophulariaceae 311
Lucuma caimito Roem. & Schult., Sapotaceae 309
Mabea fistulifera Mart., Euphorbiaceae 155
Macfadyena unguis-cati (L.) Gentry, Bignoniaceae . 81

Manilkara zapota (L.) Van Royen, Sapotaceae 309
Marsypianthes chamaedrys
   (Vahl) O. Ktze., Lamiaceae 194
Maytenus boaria Mol., Celastraceae 115
Maytenus communis Reiss., Celastraceae 115
Maytenus ilicifolia Mart., Celastraceae 115
Metrodorea pubescens St.-Hil. & Tul., Rutaceae ... 301
Mikania glomerata Spreng., Asteraceae 61
Mikania officinalis Mart., Asteraceae 62
Mikania parviflora (Aubl.) Karst., Asteraceae 62
Mimosa bimucronata (DC.) O. Ktze., Mimosaceae 238
Monnieria trifolia Loefl., Rutaceae 302
Nymphoides indica (L.) O. Ktze., Menyanthaceae . 235
Ocotea rodiei (Schomb.) Mez, Lauraceae 201
Oldenlandia corymbosa L., Rubiaceae 299
Oxalis amara St.-Hil., Oxalidaceae 266
Oxalis cordata St.-Hil., Oxalidaceae 266
Oxalis corniculata L., Oxalidaceae 266
Oxalis martiana Zucc., Oxalidaceae 267
Oxalis spp., Oxalidaceae 267
Parietaria boehmerioides Mart., Urticaceae 331
Parkinsonia aculeata L., Caesalpiniaceae 104
Passiflora amethystina Mikan, Passifloraceae 269
Passiflora caerulea L., Passifloraceae 269
Paullinia cupana Kunth, Sapindaceae 306
Pfaffia jubata Mart., Amaranthaceae 5
Phyllanthus niruri L., Euphorbiaceae 156
Picramnia camboita Engl., Simaroubaceae 314
Picramnia ciliata Mart., Simaroubaceae 314
Picrolemma pseudocoffea Ducke, Simaroubaceae . 314
Piper geniculatum Sw., Piperaceae 275
Pithecellobium unguis-cati
   (L.) Benth., Mimosaceae 242
Plantago guilleminiana Dcne., Plantaginaceae 278
Polygala angulata DC., Polygalaceae 283
Pothomorphe umbellata (L.) Miq., Piperaceae 277
Quassia amara L., Simaroubaceae 314
Raputia alba (Nees & Mart.) Engl., Rutaceae 302
Raputia aromatica Aubl., Rutaceae 302
Raputia magnifica Engl., Rutaceae 302
Rollinia sylvatica (St.-Hil.) Mart., Annonaceae 15
Ruellia tuberosa L., Acanthaceae 1
Rumex brasiliensis Link, Polygonaceae 287
Sauvagesia erecta L., Ochnaceae 262
Schinus terebinthifolius Raddi, Anacardiaceae 10
Schultesia stenophylla Mart., Gentianaceae 180
Scoparia dulcis L., Scrophulariaceae 312
Senna alata (L.) Roxb., Caesalpiniaceae 104
Senna hirsuta (L.) Ir. & Barn.
   var. puberula Ir. & Barn., Caesalpiniaceae 105
Senna obtusifolia (L.) Ir. & Barn., Caesalpiniaceae 105
Senna occidentalis (L.) Link, Caesalpiniaceae 105
Senna quinqueangulata
   (Rich.) Ir. & Barn., Caesalpiniaceae 106
Senna uniflora
   (P. Miller) Ir. & Barn., Caesalpiniaceae 106
Sida acuta Burm., Malvaceae 221
Silybum marianum Gaertn., Asteraceae 65
Simaba ferruginea St.-Hil., Simaroubaceae 314
Simaba glandulifera Gardn., Simaroubaceae 314
Simaba salubris Engl., Simaroubaceae 315
Simarouba amara Aubl., Simaroubaceae 315
Siparuna guianensis Aubl., Monimiaceae 245

Solanum pseudoquina St.-Hil., Solanaceae 322
Sophora tomentosa L., Fabaceae 172
Spigelia glabrata Mart., Loganiaceae 209
Stachytarpheta cayennensis
    (Rich.)Vahl, Verbenaceae 335
Stachytarpheta jamaicensis (L.) Vahl, Verbenaceae 336
Strychnos pseudoquina St.-Hil., Loganiaceae 209
Sweetia fruticosa Spreng., Fabaceae 172
Symplocos parviflora Benth., Symplocaceae 326
Symplocos platyphylla
    (Pohl) Benth., Symplocaceae 326
Symplocos pubescens Klotzsch, Symplocaceae 326
Tabebuia leucoxylon (L.) DC., Bignoniaceae 83
Tabernaemontana citrifolia L., Apocynaceae 28
Tachia guianenesis Aubl., Gentianaceae 180
Talauma ovata St.-Hil., Magnoliaceae 216
Tetracera volubilis L., Dilleniaceae 146
Thevetia ahouai (L.) DC., Apocynaceae 28
Verbena erinoides Lam., Verbenaceae 336
Vismia guianensis (Aubl.) Choisy, Clusiaceae 124
Vismia japurensis Reich., Clusiaceae 124
Vismia latifolia (Aubl.) Choisy, Clusiaceae 124
Wilbrandia verticillata
    (Vell.) Cogn., Cucurbitaceae 140
Xanthium orientale L.,
    X. spinosum L. & *X. strumarium* L., Asteraceae 67
Zanthoxylum rhoifolium Lam., Rutaceae 303
Zanthoxylum tingoassuiba St.-Hil., Rutaceae 303
Zizyphus joazeiro Mart., Rhamnaceae (PHARM.) 293

Felon. *See* **Whitlow**

Fertility
Himatanthus lancifolia
    (M. Arg.) Woods., Apocynaceae 26

Fever. *See also* **Febrifuge, Malaria,
Puerperal Fever, Typhoid Fever, Yellow
Fever**
Calolisianthus pendulus
    (Mart.) Gilg, Gentianaceae 179
Campsiandra comosa Benth.
    var. *laurifolia* (Benth.) Cowan, Caesalpiniaceae ... 100
Doliocarpus rolandri Gmel., Dilleniaceae 146
Phyllanthus niruri L., Euphorbiaceae 156
Tetracera aspera Willd., Dilleniaceae 146

Filariasis. *See also* **Anthelmintic**
Elaeis guineensis Jacq., Arecaceae 40
Pothomorphe umbellata (L.) Miq., Piperaceae 277

Fish Poison
Clibadium surinamense L., Asteraceae 58
Gustavia hexapetala
    (Aubl.) J.E. Smith, Lecythidaceae 196
Ichthyothere terminalis
    (Spr.) S.F. Blake, Asteraceae 61

Fissures. *See* **Anal Fissures, Nipple Fissures**

Flatulence. *See* **Carminative**

Foetus Expulsion.
See also **Childbirth, Placenta Expulsion**
Chenopodium ambrosioides L., Chenopodiaceae .. 118
Euphorbia hyssopifolia L., Euphorbiaceae 153

Fortifier. *See also* **Strengthener**
Annona ambotay Aubl., Annonaceae 11
Brosimum parinarioides Ducke, Moraceae 246
Brosimum potabile Ducke, Moraceae 246

Dorstenia cayapia Vell., Moraceae 248
Hymenaea courbaril L., Caesalpiniaceae 103
Polycarpaea corymbosa
    (L.) Lam., Caryophyllaceae 115

Fractures
Clusia rosea Jacq., Clusiaceae 122
Dorstenia asaroides Gardn., Moraceae 247
Dorstenia brasiliensis Lam., Moraceae 247
Equisetum giganteum L., Equisetaceae 148
Himatanthus sucuuba (Spr.) Woods., Apocynaceae . 26
Phthirusa adunca (Meyer) Maguire,
    Loranthaceae 211

Freckles
Hydrocotyle bonariensis Lam., Apiaceae 19
Hydrocotyle leucocephala Cham.
    & Schlecht., Apiaceae 20
Vatairea guianensis Aubl., Fabaceae 172

Fungal Infections
Croton salutaris Casar., Euphorbiaceae 151

Furunculosis
Bredemeyera floribunda Willd., Polygalaceae 283

G

Galactagogue
Amaranthus blitum L., Amaranthaceae 3
Araujia sericifera Brot., Asclepiadaceae 50

Gall Bladder Disease. *See also*
Biliary Obstructions, Bladder Stones
Quassia amara L., Simaroubaceae 314
Turnera diffusa Willd., Turneraceae 327
Turnera opifera Mart., Turneraceae 328

Gangrene
Dorstenia asaroides Gardn., Moraceae 247
Protium heptaphyllum (Aubl.) March., Burseraceae 93

Gapes (Bird Disease)
Momordica charantia L., Cucurbitaceae 139

Gargles
Canna glauca L., Cannaceae 110

Gastralgia. *See* **Stomachache**

Gastric Disorders
Turnera opifera Mart., Turneraceae 328

Gastrointestinal Problems
Anisosperma passiflora Manso, Cucurbitaceae 135
Cocos nucifera L., Arecaceae 40
Cymbopogon schoenanthus (L.) Spreng., Poaceae 280
Operculina alata (Ham.) Urb., Convolvulaceae 131
Operculina macrocarpa Urb., Convolvulaceae 131
Swartzia chrysantha B. Rodr., Caesalpiniaceae 107
Turnera opifera Mart., Turneraceae 328

Genital Discharges
Triumfetta semitriloba Jacq., Tiliaceae 327

Genital Pruritus
Dieffenbachia seguine (Jacq.) Schott, Araceae 35

Genital Tract, stimulate
Jatropha urens L., Euphorbiaceae 155

Genitals, to tighten
Leandra lacunosa Cogn., Melastomataceae 225

Genitourinary Problems.
See also **Urogenital Problems, Urethritis**
Turnera opifera Mart., Turneraceae 328

Gentian Substitute
Calolisianthus pendulus
   (Mart.) Gilg, Gentianaceae 179
Geophagy
Lindernia diffusa Wettst., Scrophulariaceae 311
Gingivitis
Ayapana triplinerve
   (Vahl) King & Robinson, Asteraceae 53
Ginseng Substitute
Pfaffia paniculata (Mart.) Kuntze, Amaranthaceae 5
Glandular Conditions (Adenitis).
See also Filariasis
Ocotea guianensis Aubl., Lauraceae 201
Schinus molle L., Anacardiaceae 9
Symphonia globulifera L. f., Clusiaceae 123
Glaucoma. See also Eye Problems
Kalanchoe pinnata (Lam.) Pers., Crassulaceae 133
Gonorrhoea. See also Blennorrhagia
Ageratum conyzoides L., Asteraceae 53
Amaranthus viridis L., Amaranthaceae 3
Anadenanthera colubrina
   (Vell.) Brenan, Mimosaceae 236
Arrabidaea agnus-castus
   (Cham.) DC., Bignoniaceae 78
Borreria verbenoides Cham. & Schl., Rubiaceae ... 296
Canna edulis Ker-Gawl., Cannaceae 110
Canna warszewiczii Dietr., Cannaceae 111
Chaptalia nutans (L.) Polak., Asteraceae 57
Cipura paludosa Aubl., Iridaceae 186
Cissampelos fasciculata Benth., Menispermaceae . 231
Cleome spinosa Jacq., Capparaceae 112
Coccoloba laevis Casar., Polygonaceae 285
Coccoloba mollis Casar., Polygonaceae 285
Commelina nudiflora L., Commelinaceae 126
Copaifera cearensis
   Huber ex Ducke, Caesalpiniaceae 102
Costus spicatus (Jacq.) Sw., Costaceae 132
Elionurus candidus (Trin.) Hack., also
   E. latiflorus Nees, Poaceae 281
Equisetum giganteum L., Equisetaceae 148
Genipa americana L., Rubiaceae 298
Heliconia angusta Vell., Heliconiaceae 181
Lithraea molleoides (Vell.) Engl., Anacardiaceae 9
Mimosa pudica L., Mimosaceae 240
Mimosa velloziana Mart., Mimosaceae 240
Polygonum punctatum Elliot, Polygonaceae 287
Polygonum spectabile Mart., Polygonaceae 287
Pothomorphe peltata L., Piperaceae 277
Pradosia lactescens (Vell.) Radlk., Sapotaceae 310
Protium icicariba (DC.) March., Burseraceae 94
Schinus molle L., Anacardiaceae 9
Solanum agrarium Sendt., Solanaceae 319
Solanum cernuum Vell., Solanaceae 319
Spondias macrocarpa Engl., Anacardiaceae 10
Spondias mombin L., Anacardiaceae 10
Stryphnodendron coriaceum Benth., Mimosaceae . 243
Tabebuia ipe (Mart.) Standl., Bignoniaceae 83
Triumfetta rhomboidea Jacq., Tiliaceae 327
Gout
Aristolochia cymbifera
   Mart. & Zucc., Aristolochiaceae 46

Dieffenbachia seguine (Jacq.) Schott, Araceae 35
Dodonaea viscosa Jacq., Sapindaceae 305
Dracontium asperum K. Koch, Araceae 35
Guarea trichilioides L., Meliaceae 227
Herreria salsaparilha Mart., Liliaceae 207
Hyptis fasciculata Benth., Lamiaceae 192
Hyptis multiflora Pohl, Lamiaceae 193
Hyptis suaveolens Poit., Lamiaceae 193
Jacaranda subrhombea DC., Bignoniaceae 81
Leucas martinicensis (Jacq.) R. Br., Lamiaceae 194
Mikania parviflora (Aubl.) Karst., Asteraceae 62
Monstera obliqua Miquel, Araceae 36
Raphia taedigera (Mart.) Mart., Arecaceae 45
Saccoglottis guianensis Benth., Humiriaceae 185
Smilax campestris Gris., Liliaceae 208
Smilax longifolia Rich. (includes *S. brasiliensis*
   Spreng.), Liliaceae 208
Grippe. See Influenza
Gum Strengthener
Cocos nucifera L., Arecaceae 40

H

Hair Remover. See Depilatory
Hair Restorer (Hair Growth Stimulant)
Eclipta prostrata (L.) L., Asteraceae 59
Guazuma ulmifolia Lam.
   var. *ulmifolia*, Sterculiaceae 323
Gynerium parviflorum Nees, Poaceae 323
Portulaca pilosa L., Portulacaceae 289
Hair Strengthener (Hair Invigorator)
Dipteryx odorata (Aubl.) Willd., Fabaceae 166
Elaeis oleifera (H.B.K.) Cortez, Arecaceae 40
Gynerium parviflorum Nees, also
   Gynerium sagittatum (Pers.) Beauv., Poaceae 281
Sida rhombifolia L., Malvaceae 222
Syagrus oleracea (Mart.) Becc., Arecaceae 45
Hair Tonic
Zizyphus joazeiro Mart., Rhamnaceae 293
Hallucinogen
Anadenanthera peregrina (L.) Speg., Mimosaceae 236
Banisteriopsis caapi (Spr.) Morton, Malpighiaceae 217
Datura insignis B. Rodr., Solanaceae 318
Datura suaveolens Humb. & Bonpl., Solanaceae ... 318
Mimosa acutistipula Benth., Mimosaceae 236
Mimosa hostilis Benth., Mimosaceae 238
Tanaecium nocturnum (B. Rodr.) Bur.
   & K. Sch., Bignoniaceae 84
Hanseniasis. See Leprosy
Headache (Cephalalgia). See also Migraine
Chaptalia nutans (L.) Polak., Asteraceae 57
Crescentia cujete L., Bignoniaceae 80
Hyptis umbrosa Salzm., Lamiaceae 193
Kalanchoe brasiliensis Camb., Crassulaceae 133
Ludwigia suffruticosa (L.) Gomes, Onagraceae 264
Marsypianthes chamaedrys
   (Vahl) O. Ktze., Lamiaceae 194
Monnieria trifolia Loefl., Rutaceae 302
Siparuna guianensis Aubl., Monimiaceae 245
Healing, hasten
Casearia cambessedesii Eichl., Flacourtiaceae 176

Heart Problems.
See also **Arteriosclerosis; Cardio: –active, –tonic; Palpitation; Tachycardia**

Aniba canelilla (H.B.K.) Mez, Lauraceae 197
Aristolochia cymbifera
  Mart. & Zucc., Aristolochiaceae 46
Carica papaya L., Caricaceae (CHEM. & PHARM.) 113
Cissus sicyoides L., Vitaceae 339
Haynaldia exaltata
  (Pohl) Kanitz, Campanulaceae 109
Hylocereus undatus (Haw.) Br. & Rose, Cactaceae .. 95
Keithia denudata Benth., Lamiaceae 193
Passiflora coccinea Aubl., Passifloraceae 269
Peperomia pellucida H.B.K., Piperaceae 273
Scutia buxifolia Reiss., Rhamnaceae 293
Solanum cernuum Vell., Solanaceae 319

Helminthicide. *See also* Anthelmintic
Allamanda cathartica L., Apocynaceae 20

Helmintic infestations
Lindernia diffusa Wettst., Scrophulariaceae 311

Hematoma
Jatropha curcas L., Euphorbiaceae 154

Hematuria
Nepsera aquatica Naud., Melastomataceae 226

Hemoptysis
Astronium fraxinifolium Schott, Anacardiaceae 9
Avena quadridentata Doell, Poaceae 280
Buddleja brasiliensis Jacq. ex Spr., Buddlejaceae 93
Cuscuta racemosa Mart., Convolvulaceae 130
Cyathea microdonta (Desv.) Domin, Cyatheaceae . 141
Cyrtopodium andersoni R. Br., Orchidaceae 266
Helosis cayennensis (Swartz)
  Spreng., Balanophoraceae 73
Ludwigia natans (H.B.K.) Ell., Onagraceae 264
Microgramma vaccinifolia
  (Langsd. & Fisch.) Copel., Polypodiaceae 288
Myracroduon urundeuva
  Fr. All., Anacardiaceae 9
Phlebodium aureum
  (L.) J.E. Smith, Polypodiaceae 288
Portulaca oleracea L., Portulacaceae 289
Pradosia lactescens (Vell.) Radlk., Sapotaceae 310
Psidium arboreum Vell., Myrtaceae 256
Schinus terebinthifolius Raddi, Anacardiaceae 10
Virola oleifera (Schott) A.C. Smith, Myristicaceae . 250

Hemorrhage (Bleeding). *See also* Hemostatic
Anadenanthera macrocarpa
  (Benth.) Brenan, Mimosaceae 236
Begonia luxurians Scheidw., Begoniaceae 76
Boehmeria caudata Sw., Urticaceae 330
Cassytha filiformis L., Lauraceae 198
Cayaponia espelina
  (Manso) Cogn., Cucurbitaceae 135
Cocos nucifera L., Arecaceae 40
Ephedra americana Willd., Ephedraceae 147
Euterpe edulis Mart., Arecaceae 40
Haemadyction gaudichaudii DC., Apocynaceae 24
Helosis cayennensis
  (Swartz) Spreng., Balanophoraceae 73
Krameria tomentosa St.-Hil., Krameriaceae 191
Lithraea molleoides (Vell.) Engl., Anacardiaceae 9
Luehea rufescens St.-Hil., Tiliaceae 327

Parapiptadenia rigida
  (Benth.) Brenan, Mimosaceae 240
Parkia oppositifolia (Spruce) Benth., Mimosaceae 240
Parkia pectinata Benth., Mimosaceae 240
Phlebodium aureum
  (L.) J.E. Smith, Polypodiaceae 288
Piper elongatum Vahl, Piperaceae 273
Portulaca oleracea L., Portulacaceae 289
Pouteria salicifolia Hook. & Arn., Sapotaceae 310
Psidium cattleyanum Sabine, Myrtaceae 256
Psidium cinereum Mart., Myrtaceae 256
Rhizophora mangle L., Rhizophoraceae 294
Schinus molle L., Anacardiaceae 9
Sicana odorifera Naud., Cucurbitaceae 139
Stryphnodendron adstringens
  (Mart.) Cov., Mimosaceae 242
Stryphnodendron polyphyllum
  Mart., Mimosaceae 244
Trixis antimenorrhoea (Schrank) Mart., Asteraceae . 67
Urera caracasana Jacq., Urticaceae 331

Hemorrhoids (Piles)
Acnistus arborescens (L.) Schl., Solanaceae 316
Albizzia lebbeck (L.) Benth., Mimosaceae 236
Boehmeria caudata Sw., Urticaceae 330
Buddleja brasiliensis Jacq. ex Spr., Buddlejaceae 93
Buddleja stachioides Cham., Buddlejaceae 93
Cabomba piauhyensis Gard., Nymphaeaceae 259
Canna lanuginosa Roscoe, Cannaceae 111
Cestrum amictum Schl., Solanaceae 317
Cestrum parqui L'Herit., Solanaceae 317
Coccoloba laevis Casar., Polygonaceae 285
Coccoloba mollis Casar., Polygonaceae 285
Cocos nucifera L., Arecaceae 40
Commelina nudiflora L., Commelinaceae 126
Cuphea melvillea Lindl., Lythraceae 214
Cuphea ultriculosa Hoene, Lythraceae 214
Davilla rugosa Poir., Dilleniaceae 145
Dichorisandra affinis Mart., Commelinaceae 128
Dichorisandra leucophthalmos
  Hook., Commelinaceae 128
Dichorisandra spp., Commelinaceae 128
Macrosiphonia longiflora
  (Desf.) M. Arg., Apocynaceae 26
Nymphaea rudgeana G. Meyer, Nymphaeaceae 259
Peschiera affinis (M. Arg.) Miers, Apocynaceae 27
Peschiera laeta (Mart.) Miers, Apocynaceae 27
Pfaffia glomerata (Spreng.) Peders., Amaranthaceae .. 4
Polygala spectabilis DC., Polygalaceae 284
Polygonum acuminatum H.B.K., Polygonaceae 286
Polygonum punctatum Elliot, Polygonaceae 287
Polygonum spectabile Mart., Polygonaceae 287
Senna alata (L.) Roxb., Caesalpiniaceae 104
Sida acuta Burm., Malvaceae 221
Spondias macrocarpa Engl., Anacardiaceae 10
Spondias mombin L., Anacardiaceae 10
Stachytarpheta dichotoma Vahl, Verbenaceae 336
Stryphnodendron adstringens
  (Mart.) Cov., Mimosaceae 242
Tillandsia usneoides L., Bromeliaceae 91
Tradescantia diuretica Mart., Commelinaceae 128
Trimezia lurida Salisb., Iridaceae 186
Triplaris weigeltiana
  (Reichb.) O. Ktze., Polygonaceae 287

Victoria amazonica
   (Poepp.) Sower., Nymphaeaceae 259
Virola surinamensis (Rol.) Warb., Myristicaceae 252
Xylopia sericea St.-Hil., Annonaceae 16

Hemostatic. *See also* **Hemorrhage**
Anadenanthera colubrina
   (Vell.) Brenan, Mimosaceae 236
Avicennia germinans (L.) L., Verbenaceae 334
Cecropia palmata Willd., Moraceae 247
Combretum leprosum Mart., Combretaceae 126
Elaeis oleifera (H.B.K.) Cortez, Arecaceae 40
Jatropha curcas L., Euphorbiaceae 154
Micrograma vaccinifolia
   (Langsd. & Fisch.) Copel., Polypodiaceae 288
Myracrodruon urundeuva
   Fr. All., Anacardiaceae 9
Peperomia elongata Miq., Piperaceae 273
Piper angustifolium R. & Pav., Piperaceae 274
Pradosia lactescens (Vell.) Radlk., Sapotaceae 310
Protium heptaphyllum (Aubl.) March., Burseraceae 93
Protium icicariba (DC.) March., Burseraceae 94
Solanum cernuum Vell., Solanaceae 319
Stryphnodendron coriaceum Benth., Mimosaceae . 243
Urera baccifera Gaud., Urticaceae 331

Hepatitis
Anisolobus cururu (Mart.) M. Arg., Apocynaceae 21
Bidens pilosa L., Asteraceae 57
Boerhavia coccinea Mill., Nyctaginaceae 257
Coleus barbatus Benth., Lamiaceae 191
Erythrina crista-galli L., Fabaceae 166
Mikania lindleyana DC., Asteraceae 62
Senna occidentalis (L.) Link, Caesalpiniaceae 105
Senna quinqueangulata
   (Rich.) Ir. & Barn., Caesalpiniaceae 106
Solanum grandiflorum Ruiz & Pav., Solanaceae ... 320
Solanum insidiosum Mart., Solanaceae 320
Solanum paniculatum L., Solanaceae 321
Stachytarpheta jamaicensis (L.) Vahl, Verbenaceae 336

Hernia
Alibertia edulis (Rich.) Rich., Rubiaceae 294
Chorisia crispiflora H.B.K., Bombacaceae 86
Echinodorus grandiflorus
   (Cham. & Schl.) Mich., Alismataceae 2
Echinodorus pubescens Mart., Alismataceae 2
Ficus gomelleira Kunth & Bouché, Moraceae 248
Himatanthus alba (L.) Woods., Apocynaceae 24
Himatanthus drastica (Mart.) Woods., Apocynaceae 24
Monnieria trifolia Loefl., Rutaceae 302
Plumeria alba L., Apocynaceae 28
Tillandsia usneoides L., Bromeliaceae 91

Herpes
Caraipa grandifolia Mart., Clusiaceae 121
Caraipa minor Huber, Clusiaceae 121
Casearia sylvestris Sw., Flacourtiaceae 178
Croton hemiargyreus M. Arg., Euphorbiaceae 151
Croton sincorensis Mart., Euphorbiaceae 151
Elephantopus mollis H.B.K., Asteraceae 59
Himatanthus lancifolia
   (M. Arg.) Woods., Apocynaceae 26
Himatanthus phagedaenica
   (Mart.) Woods., Apocynaceaae 26
Luffa operculata (L.) Cogn., Cucurbitaceae 138
Physalis pubescens L., Solanaceae 318

Zschokkea arborescens M. Arg., Apocynaceae 29

HIV-1 (AIDS)
Alexa sp., Fabaceae xxxviii
Zanthoxylum tingoassuiba St.-Hil., Rutaceae 303

Hunger Suppressant
Erythroxylum cataractarum
   Spruce, Erythroxylaceae 149
Erythroxylum coca Lam., Erythroxylaceae 149
Paullinia cupana Kunth, Sapindaceae 306

Hydragogue
Capparis cynophallophora L., Capparaceae 111
Chiococca alba (L.) Hitch., Rubiaceae 297
Euphorbia hirta L., Euphorbiaceae 152
Hura crepitans L., Euphorbiaceae 153
Jacaratia spinosa (Aubl.) A. DC., Caricaceae 113
Joannesia princeps Vell., Euphorbiaceae 155
Luffa operculata (L.) Cogn., Cucurbitaceae 138

Hydrocele
Crescentia cujete L., Bignoniaceae 80

Hydrocyanic Acid Antidote
Bixa orellana L., Bixaceae 85

Hydrophobia. *See* **Rabies**

Hydropsy. *See* **Dropsy**

Hyperacidity
Maytenus ilicifolia Mart., Celastraceae 115

Hypertension
Bredemeyera floribunda Willd., Polygalaceae 283
Carica papaya L., Caricaceae (CHEM. & PHARM.) 113
Cissus sicyoides L., Vitaceae 339
Coleus barbatus
   Benth., Lamiaceae (CHEM. & PHARM.) 191
Cuphea balsamona Cham., Lythraceae 213
Geissospermum laeve (Vell.) Baill., Apocynaceae 23

Hypnotic
Chamaecrista fasciculata
   (Michx.) Greene, Caesalpiniaceae 102

Hypocholesteremic
Bauhinia candicans Benth., Caesalpiniaceae 99
Croton cajucara Benth., Euphorbiaceae 150

Hypoglycemic. *See also* **Blood Sugar Levels, Controls**
Chrysobalanus icaco
   L., Chrysobalanaceae (PHARM.) 119
Stryphnodendron adstringens
   (Mart.) Cov., Mimosaceae 242

Hypotensive
Boerhavia coccinea Mill., Nyctaginaceae 257
Copaifera officinalis (Jacq.) L., Caesalpiniaceae 102

Hysteria
Aristolochia triangularis Cham., Aristolochiaceae ... 48
Aristolochia trilobata L., Aristolochiaceae 48
Eleutherine plicata Herb., Iridaceae 186
Gallesia gorazema (Vell.) Moq., Phytolaccaceae ... 271
Himatanthus lancifolia
   (M. Arg.) Woods., Apocynaceae 26
Mikania cordifolia (L. f.) Willd., Asteraceae 61
Passiflora alata Dryand., Passifloraceae 267
Passiflora edulis Sims, Passifloraceae 269
Schinopsis brasiliensis Engl., Anacardiaceae 9
Stomatanthes oblongifolius
   (Spr.) H. Robinson, Asteraceae 65
Syagrus oleracea (Mart.) Becc., Arecaceae 45

I

Impotence. *See also* **Sexual Impotence**
Anacardium occidentale L., Anacardiaceae 7
Eryngium foetidum L., Apiaceae 19
Indigestion. *See* **Dyspepsia**
Infections. *See also* **Fungal Infections**
Allagoptera campestris (Mart.) Kuntze, Arecaceae .. 39
Cissampelos ovalifolia DC., Menispermaceae 233
Cyrtopodium andersoni R. Br., Orchidaceae 266
Rollinia orthopetala DC., Annonaceae 15
Virola surinamensis (Rol.) Warb., Myristicaceae 252
Inflammations (Antiphlogistic). *See also*
Bronchitis, Catarrh, Dysentery, Enteritis,
Erysipelas, Gout, Hepatitis, Herpes,
Lymphoadenitis, Otitis, Pharyngitis,
Phlebitis, Prurigo, Psoriasis, Stomatitis,
Urethritis, Whitlow
Anacardium occidentale L., Anacardiaceae 7
Ananas comosus (L.) Merrill, Bromeliaceae 90
Annona marcgravii Mart., Annonaceae 13
Bixa orellana L., Bixaceae 85
Bumelia sartorum Mart., Sapotaceae 308
Casearia sylvestris Sw., Flacourtiaceae 178
Chiococca alba (L.) Hitch., Rubiaceae (PHARM.) 297
Cocos nucifera L., Arecaceae 40
Copaifera officinalis (Jacq.) L., Caesalpiniaceae 102
Cordia verbenacea DC., Boraginaceae 88
Cordyline dracaenoides Kunth, Liliaceae 207
Coutarea hexandra
  (Jacq.) K. Sch., Rubiaceae (PHARM.) 297
Cuscuta racemosa Mart., Convolvulaceae 130
Dalbergia subcymosa Ducke, Fabaceae 164
Dalechampia scandens L., Euphorbiaceae 152
Desmodium axillare (Sw.) DC., Fabaceae 164
Dieffenbachia seguine (Jacq.) Schott, Araceae 35
Echites peltata Vell., Apocynaceae 23
Euphorbia hirta
  L., Euphorbiaceae (CHEM. & PHARM.) 152
Heterothalamus psiadioides Less., Asteraceae 60
Hibiscus bifurcatus Cav., Malvaceae 221
Jacaratia spinosa (Aubl.) A. DC., Caricaceae 113
Jatropha curcas L., Euphorbiaceae 154
Jatropha urens L., Euphorbiaceae 155
Kalanchoe pinnata (Lam.) Pers., Crassulaceae 133
Limonium brasiliense
  (Boiss.) O. Ktze., Plumbaginaceae (PHARM.) 278
Lithraea molleoides (Vell.) Engl., Anacardiaceae 9
Macfadyena unguis-cati (L.) Gentry, Bignoniaceae . 81
Mandevilla velutina (Mart. ex Stadelm.) Woods.
  var. *velutina*, Apocynaceae 27
Mikania glomerata Spreng., Asteraceae 61
Mikania lindleyana DC., Asteraceae 62
Orbignya phalerata Mart., Arecaceae 43
Parkia pendula Benth. ex Walp., Mimosaceae 240
Periandra mediterranea (Vell.) Taub., Fabaceae ... 170
Peritassa calypsoides (Camb.)
  A.C. Sm., Hippocrateaceae 183
Philodendron hederaceum (Jacq.) Schott var.
  hederaceum, Araceae 36
Philodendron pedatum (Hook.) Kunth, Araceae 37

Pothomorphe umbellata (L.) Miq., Piperaceae 277
Protium heptaphyllum (Aubl.) March., Burseraceae 93
Psidium guajava L., Myrtaceae 256
Schinus molle L., Anacardiaceae 9
Scoparia dulcis L., Scrophulariaceae (PHARM.) 312
Tabebuia ipe (Mart.) Standl., Bignoniaceae 83
Torresea cearensis Fr. All., Fabaceae 172
Trixis antimenorrhoea (Schrank) Mart., Asteraceae . 67
Vallesia cymbifolia Ortega, Apocynaceae 29
Vernonanthura brasiliana
  (L.) H. Robinson, Asteraceae 67
Victoria amazonica
  (Poepp.) Sower., Nymphaeaceae 259
Virola sebifera Aubl., Myristicaceae 250
Wilbrandia verticillata (Vell.) Cogn.,
  Cucurbitaceae (CHEM. & PHARM.) 140
Zanthoxylum hyemale St.-Hil., Rutaceae 302
Influenza (Grippe)
Cedrela odorata L., Meliaceae 227
Cordia multispicata Cham., Boraginaceae 88
Eugenia uniflora L., Myrtaceae 254
Kyllinga pungens Link, Cyperaceae 143
Lippia gratissima
  (Gill. & Hook.) Troncoso, Verbenaceae 335
Monnieria trifolia Loefl., Rutaceae 302
Ocimum micranthum Willd., Lamiaceae 195
Sphagneticola trilobata (L.) Pruski, Asteraceae 65
Vitex agnus-castus L., Verbenaceae 336
Injuries
Buchnera aquatica Aubl., Scrophulariaceae 310
Canna gigantea Desf., Cannaceae 110
Myrocarpus frondosus Fr. All., Fabaceae 170
Insect Repellent. *See also* **Chiggers, Stings**
Annona squamosa L., Annonaceae 13
Baccharis ramosissima Gardn., Asteraceae 54
Elaeis oleifera (H.B.K.) Cortez, Arecaceae 40
Tanacetum vulgare L., Asteraceae 67
Insecticide
Annona squamosa L., Annonaceae 13
Baccharis ramosissima Gardn., Asteraceae 54
Carpotroche brasiliensis
  (Raddi) Endl., Flacourtiaceae 176
Carpotroche longifolia Benth., Flacourtiaceae 176
Euphorbia thymifolia
  L., Euphorbiaceae (CHEM. & PHARM.) 153
Tanaecium nocturnum
  (B. Rodr.) Bur. & K. Sch., Bignoniaceae 84
Trichilia catigua Juss., Meliaceae 229
Insomnia
Aloysia triphylla (L'Her.) Britt., Verbenaceae 332
Annona squamosa L., Annonaceae 13
Croton zehntneri Pax & Hoffm., Euphorbiaceae 151
Erythrina corallodendron L., Fabaceae 166
Erythrina fusca Lour., Fabaceae 166
Licaria puchury-major
  (Mart.) Kosterm., Lauraceae 199
Passiflora edulis Sims, Passifloraceae 269
Intestinal Gases, calmative for
Piper colubrinum Link, Piperaceae 275
Intestinal Parasites
Nymphoides indica (L.) O. Ktze., Menyanthaceae . 235
Philodendron bipinnatifidum Schott, Araceae 36

MEDICINAL INDEX: INTESTINAL PROBLEMS – KIDNEY STONES

Intestinal Problems. *See also* **Colic, Dysentery, Enteritis, Enterocolitis, Enterorrhagia, Pharyngitis**
Jatropha gossypiifolia L., Euphorbiaceae 154
Mentha crispa L., Lamiaceae 194
Mikania cordifolia (L. f.) Willd., Asteraceae 61
Rollinia orthopetala DC., Annonaceae 15
Sauvagesia erecta L., Ochnaceae 262
Swartzia chrysantha B. Rodr., Caesalpiniaceae 107

Intoxicant
Mimosa acutistipula Benth., Mimosaceae 237
Mimosa hostilis Benth., Mimosaceae 238

Invigorant
Croton zehntneri Pax & Hoffm., Euphorbiaceae 151
Drimys winteri Forst., Winteraceae 340
Imperata brasiliensis Trin., also
   I. contracta Hitch., Poaceae 281

Ipecac (Ipecacuanha) Substitute
Borreria asclepiadea Cham. & Schl.,
   also *B. capitata* DC. &
   B. latifolia K. Sch., Rubiaceae 296
Diodia polymorpha Cham. & Schl., Rubiaceae 297
Hybanthus ipecacuanha (L.) Baill., Violaceae 339
Ionidium poaya St.-Hil., Violaceae 339
Lipostoma campanuliflorum D. Don, also
   L. capitata D. Don, Rubiaceae 299
Machaonia brasiliensis Cham. & Schl., Rubiaceae 299
Manettia ignita (Vell.) K. Sch., Rubiaceae 299
Polygala angulata DC., Polygalaceae 283
Ruellia tuberosa L., Acanthaceae 1

Irritability
Licaria puchury-major
   (Mart.) Kosterm., Lauraceae 199

Irritant
Mimosa pudica L., Mimosaceae 240
Mimosa velloziana Mart., Mimosaceae 240

Itch. *See also* **Prurigo, Pruritus**
Dalechampia scandens L., Euphorbiaceae 152
Elephantopus mollis H.B.K., Asteraceae 59
Jacaranda copaia (Aubl.) D. Don, Bignoniaceae 80
Lecythis pisonis Camb., Lecythidaceae 206
Parkia pendula Benth. ex Walp., Mimosaceae 240

J

Jaundice
Amasonia arborea H.B.K., Verbenaceae 333
Anisosperma passiflora Manso, Cucurbitaceae 135
Astrocaryum aculeatissimum
   (Schott) Burret, Arecaceae 39
Bidens pilosa L., Asteraceae 57
Boerhavia coccinea Mill., Nyctaginaceae 257
Boerhavia paniculata Rich., Nyctaginaceae 258
Bromelia antiacantha Bertol., Bromeliaceae 91
Cestrum parqui L'Herit., Solanaceae 317
Chaptalia nutans (L.) Polak., Asteraceae 57
Cocos nucifera L., Arecaceae 40
Davilla rugosa Poir., Dilleniaceae 145
Doliocarpus rolandri Gmel., Dilleniaceae 146
Euterpe oleracea Mart., Arecaceae 42
Fevillea trilobata L., Cucurbitaceae 136

Fevillea uncipetala Kuhlm.,Cucurbitaceae 138
Ficus insipida Willd., Moraceae 248
Genipa americana L., Rubiaceae 298
Indigofera suffruticosa Mill., Fabaceae 168
Jatropha elliptica (Pohl) M. Arg., Euphorbiaceae .. 154
Lophophytum mirabile
   Schott & Endl., Balanophoraceae 73
Luffa operculata (L.) Cogn., Cucurbitaceae 138
Oldenlandia corymbosa L., Rubiaceae 299
Phyllanthus diffusus Klotz., Euphorbiaceae 156
Phyllanthus niruri L., Euphorbiaceae 156
Physalis angulata L., Solanaceae 318
Physalis pubescens L., Solanaceae 318
Solanum grandiflorum Ruiz & Pav., Solanaceae ... 320
Solanum insidiosum Mart., Solanaceae 320
Solanum paniculatum L., Solanaceae 321
Solanum variabile Mart., Solanaceae 322
Talisia esculenta Radlk., Sapindaceae 306

Joint Pain. *See also* **Arthralgia, Arthritis, Gout, Rheumatism**
Bowdichia virgilioides H.B.K., Fabaceae 163
Casearia ovata Willd., Flacourtiaceae 178
Himatanthus alba (L.) Woods., Apocynaceae 24
Mimosa pudica L., Mimosaceae 240
Mimosa velloziana Mart., Mimosaceae 240
Plumbago scandens L., Plumbaginaceae 279
Plumeria alba L., Apocynaceae 28
Victoria amazonica
   (Poepp.) Sower., Nymphaeaceae 259

K

Kidney Disease
Costus spicatus (Jacq.) Sw., Costaceae 132
Dichorisandra affinis Mart., Commelinaceae 128
Dichorisandra leucophthalmos
   Hook., Commelinaceae 128
Hydrocotyle bonariensis Lam., Apiaceae 19
Hydrocotyle leucocephala
   Cham. & Schlecht., Apiaceae 20
Lagenaria siceraria
   (Molina) Standl., Cucurbitaceae 138
Mikania hirsutissima DC., Asteraceae 62
Mikania setigera Schultz-Bip. ex Baker, Asteraceae 62
Myracroduon urundeuva
   Fr. All., Anacardiaceae 9
Phthirusa adunca
   (Meyer) Maguire, Loranthaceae 211
Sciadotenia paraensis
   (Eichl.) Diels, Menispermaceae 234
Senna hirsuta (L.) Ir. & Barn.
   var. *puberula* Ir. & Barn., Caesalpiniaceae 105
Turnera diffusa Willd., Turneraceae 327
Turnera opifera Mart., Turneraceae 328
Unxia camphorata L. f., Asteraceae 67

Kidney Stones. *See also* **Lithontriptic**
Abuta concolor Poepp. & Endl., Menispermaceae . 231
Bromelia antiacantha Bertol., Bromeliaceae 91
Chamissoa macrocarpa H.B.K., Amaranthaceae 4
Chondodendron platyphyllum
   (Mart.) Miers, Menispermaceae 231
Cissampelos ovalifolia DC., Menispermaceae 233

KIDNEY STONES – LEUCORRHOEA: MEDICINAL INDEX

Elephantopus mollis H.B.K., Asteraceae 59
Manilkara zapota (L.) Van Royen, Sapotaceae 309
Margyricarpus setosus Ruiz & Pav., Rosaceae 294
Phyllanthus acutifolius Spreng., Euphorbiaceae 156
Phyllanthus niruri L., Euphorbiaceae 156
Phyllanthus sellowianus M. Arg., Euphorbiaceae .. 157
Phyllanthus tenellus Roxb., Euphorbiaceae 157
Pterocaulon virgatum DC., Asteraceae 64
Sparattosperma leucanthum
   (Vell.) K. Sch., Bignoniaceae 82

L

Labor
Annona ambotay Aubl., Annonaceae 12
Crescentia cujete L., Bignoniaceae 80
Lagenaria siceraria
   (Molina) Standl., Cucurbitaceae 138

Lactation
Amaranthus viridis L., Amaranthaceae 3
Bidens pilosa L., Asteraceae 57

Laryngitis
Inga setigera DC., Mimosaceae 237
Luehea divaricata Mart. & Zucc., Tiliaceae 326
Spondias macrocarpa Engl., Anacardiaceae 10
Spondias mombin L., Anacardiaceae 10
Wissadula periplocifolia Presl., Malvaceae 223

Laxative. *See also* Aperient
Abolboda poarchon Seub., Xyridaceae 342
Amaranthus spinosus L., Amaranthaceae 3
Annona crassifolia Mart., Annonaceae 12
Annona squamosa L., Annonaceae 13
Aristida pallens Cav., Poaceae 280
Astrocaryum aculeatissimum
   (Schott) Burret, Arecaceae 39
Byrsonima verbascifolia (L.) Rich., Malpighiaceae 220
Casearia ovata Willd., Flacourtiaceae 178
Cassia ferruginea
   (Schrad.) Schrad. ex DC., Caesalpiniaceae 100
Cassia grandis L., Caesalpiniaceae 101
Chamaecrista cathartica
   (Mart.) Ir. & Barn., Caesalpiniaceae 101
Cordia monosperma
   (Jacq.) Roem. & Schult., Boraginaceae 87
Craniolaria annua L., Martyniaceae 224
Cuphea balsamona Cham., Lythraceae 213
Desmodium triflorum DC., Fabaceae 164
Doliocarpus rolandri Gmel., Dilleniaceae 146
Echinodorus macrophyllus
   (Kunth) Mich., Alismataceae 2
Eugenia dysenterica DC., Myrtaceae 253
Gustavia hexapetala
   (Aubl.) J.E. Smith, Lecythidaceae 205
Hippeastrum psittacinum Herb., Amaryllidaceae 6
Hymenaea courbaril L., Caesalpiniaceae 103
Ipomoea acetosifolia
   (Vahl) Roem. & Schult., Convolvulaceae 130
Marsdenia amylacea
   (Barb.-Rodr.) Malme, Asclepiadaceae 51
Operculina alata (Ham.) Urb., Convolvulaceae 131
Operculina macrocarpa Urb., Convolvulaceae 131
Panicum petrosum Trin., Poaceae 282

Phyllanthus conami Sw., Euphorbiaceae 156
Physalis pubescens L., Solanaceae 318
Senna affinis (Benth.) Ir. & Barn., Caesalpiniaceae 104
Senna corymbosa
   (Lam.) Ir. & Barn., Caesalpiniaceae 104
Senna uniflora
   (P. Miller) Ir. & Barn., Caesalpiniaceae 106
Stachytarpheta dichotoma
   Vahl, Verbenaceae 336
Tagetes erecta L., Asteraceae 67
Torrubia olfersiana
   (Link, Klotzsch & Otto) Standl., Nyctaginaceae ... 258
Trimezia juncifolia Benth. & Hook., Iridaceae 186
Turnera diffusa Willd., Turneraceae 327
Turnera opifera Mart., Turneraceae 328
Vataireopsis araroba (Aguiar) Ducke, Fabaceae 172

Leishmaniasis
Marsdenia amylacea
   (Barb.-Rodr.) Malme, Asclepiadaceae 51
Tabebuia serratifolia (Vahl) Nichol., Bignoniaceae .. 83

Leprosy
Anacardium occidentale L., Anacardiaceae 7
Baccharis notosergila Gris., Asteraceae 54
Baccharis trimera (Less.) DC., Asteraceae 54
Carpotroche brasiliensis
   (Raddi) Endl., Flacourtiaceae 176
Commelina nudiflora L., Commelinaceae 126
Dioscorea laxiflora Mart., Dioscoreaceae 147
Hura crepitans L., Euphorbiaceae 153
Schinus terebinthifolius Raddi, Anacardiaceae 10
Solanum caavurana Vell., Solanaceae 319
Trianosperma glandulosa Mart., Cucurbitaceae 140
Trianosperma trilobata Cogn., Cucurbitaceae 140
Xyris laxifolia Mart., Xyridaceae 342
Xyris pallida Mart., Xyridaceae 342

Lethargy
Buchnera virgata H.B.K., Scrophulariaceae 310
Capparis lineata Pers., Capparaceae 111

Leucorrhoea
Ambrosia artemisiifolia L., Asteraceae 53
Anadenanthera colubrina
   (Vell.) Brenan, Mimosaceae 236
Aniba canelilla (H.B.K.) Mez, Lauraceae 197
Aniba puchury-minor (Mart.) Mez, Lauraceae 197
Bellucia grossularioides (L.) Tr., Melastomataceae 225
Bidens pilosa L., Asteraceae 57
Blepharocalyx salicifolius
   (H.B.K.) Berg, Myrtaceae 253
Capparis lineata Pers., Capparaceae 111
Cecropia hololeuca Miq., Moraceae 247
Cecropia palmata Willd., Moraceae 247
Cedrela fissilis Vell., Meliaceae 227
Celtis iguanaea Sarg., Ulmaceae 330
Celtis spinosissima Miq., Ulmaceae 330
Chrysobalanus icaco L., Chrysobalanaceae 119
Cissampelos fasciculata Benth., Menispermaceae . 231
Cissampelos sympodialis Eichl., Menispermaceae . 233
Cleome spinosa Jacq., Capparaceae 112
Coccoloba arborescens
   (Vell.) How., Polygonaceae 285
Coccoloba laevis Casar., Polygonaceae 285
Coccoloba marginata Benth., Polygonaceae 285

Coccoloba mollis Casar., Polygonaceae 285
Copaifera officinalis (Jacq.) L., Caesalpiniaceae 102
Costus spicatus (Jacq.) Sw., Costaceae 132
Desmodium axillare (Sw.) DC., Fabaceae 164
Desmodium triflorum DC., Fabaceae 164
Dorstenia brasiliensis Lam., Moraceae 247
Dorstenia cayapia Vell., Moraceae 248
Jatropha urens L., Euphorbiaceae 155
Licaria puchury-major
   (Mart.) Kosterm., Lauraceae 199
Lithraea molleoides (Vell.) Engl., Anacardiaceae 9
Luehea rufescens St.-Hil., Tiliaceae 327
Melampodium divaricatum (Rich.) DC., Asteraceae 61
Mezilaurus crassiramea
   (Meissn.) Taub. ex Mez, Lauraceae 199
Mimosa pudica L., Mimosaceae 240
Mimosa velloziana Mart., Mimosaceae 240
Nectandra leucantha Nees, Lauraceae 199
Ocotea squarrosa Mart. ex Nees, Lauraceae 203
Oxalis martiana Zucc., Oxalidaceae 267
Parapiptadenia rigida
   (Benth.) Brenan, Mimosaceae 240
Peperomia elongata Miq., Piperaceae 273
Philoxerus portulacoides St.-Hil., Amaranthaceae 5
Phthirusa adunca (Meyer) Maguire, Loranthaceae 211
Piper angustifolium R. & Pav., Piperaceae 274
Piper elongatum Vahl, Piperaceae 275
Piper parthenium Mart., Piperaceae 276
Polygonum acuminatum H.B.K., Polygonaceae 286
Pradosia lactescens (Vell.) Radlk., Sapotaceae 310
Psidium guajava L., Myrtaceae 256
Schinus molle L., Anacardiaceae 9
Sebastiania klotzschiana M. Arg., Euphorbiaceae .. 157
Sebastiania macrocarpa M. Arg., Euphorbiaceae .. 157
Spondias macrocarpa Engl., Anacardiaceae 10
Spondias mombin L., Anacardiaceae 10
Stryphnodendron adstringens
   (Mart.) Cov., Mimosaceae 242
Tabebuia barbata (May) Sandw., Bignoniaceae 82
Turnera diffusa Willd., Turneraceae 327
Turnera opifera Mart., Turneraceae 328
Turnera ulmifolia L., Turneraceae 328
Unxia camphorata L. f., Asteraceae 67
Urera baccifera Gaud., Urticaceae 331
Virola oleifera (Schott) A.C. Smith, Myristicaceae . 250
Xylopia frutescens Aubl., Annonaceae 16

Leukemia
Momordica charantia L., Cucurbitaceae 139
Myrcia amazonica DC., Myrtaceae 255

Lice
Carapa guianensis Aubl., Meliaceae 227
Duguetia furfuracea
   (St.-Hil.) Benth. & Hook., Annonaceae 14

Liniments (Ointments)
Attalea spectabilis Mart., Arecaceae 39

Lithiasis. *See also* Bladder Stones, Kidney Stones
Acmella oleracea (L.) R.K. Jansen, Asteraceae 52
Acmella repens (Walt.) L.C. Rich., Asteraceae 52
Bassovia lucida Dunal, Solanaceae 316
Chondodendron platyphyllum
   (Mart.) Miers, Menispermaceae 231

Cissampelos ovalifolia
   DC., Menispermaceae 233
Costus spicatus (Jacq.) Sw., Costaceae 132

Lithontriptic
Cissampelos glaberrima St.-Hil., Menispermaceae 233

Liver Disease. *See also* Ascites, Cholagogue, Hepatitis, Jaundice
Abuta rufescens Aubl., Menispermaceae 231
Acanthospermum hispidum DC., Asteraceae 52
Alternanthera achyrantha R. Br., Amaranthaceae 3
Anisosperma passiflora Manso, Cucurbitaceae 135
Aristida pallens Cav., Poaceae 280
Baccharis notosergila Gris., Asteraceae 54
Baccharis trimera (Less.) DC., Asteraceae 54
Boerhavia coccinea Mill., Nyctaginaceae 257
Boerhavia paniculata Rich., Nyctaginaceae 258
Caraipa grandifolia Mart., Clusiaceae 121
Cestrum bracteatum Link & Otto, Solanaceae 317
Cestrum parqui L'Herit., Solanaceae 317
Chamaecrista mimosoides
   (L.) Ir. & Barn., Caesalpiniaceae 102
Cissampelos pareira L., Menispermaceae 233
Cocculus filipendula Mart., Menispermaceae 234
Croton cajucara Benth., Euphorbiaceae 150
Cuscuta racemosa Mart., Convolvulaceae 130
Echinodorus grandiflorus
   (Cham. & Schl.) Mich., Alismataceae 2
Echinodorus macrophyllus
   (Kunth) Mich., Alismataceae 2
Echinodorus pubescens Mart., Alismataceae 2
Erythrina corallodendron L., Fabaceae 166
Erythrina fusca Lour., Fabaceae 166
Fevillea trilobata L., Cucurbitaceae 136
Fevillea uncipetala Kuhlm., Cucurbitaceae 138
Ficus gomelleira Kunth & Bouché, Moraceae 248
Genipa americana L., Rubiaceae 298
Gustavia hexapetala
   (Aubl.) J.E. Smith, Lecythidaceae 205
Hackelochloa granularis (L.) O. Ktze., Poaceae ... 281
Hancornia speciosa Gomes, Apocynaceae 24
Heliotropium elongatum Willd., Boraginaceae 88
Hydrocotyle bonariensis Lam., Apiaceae 19
Hydrocotyle leucocephala
   Cham. & Schlecht., Apiaceae 20
Panicum petrosum Trin., Poaceae 282
Piper marginatum Jacq., Piperaceae 275
Piper rohrii C. DC., Piperaceae 276
Pleurothyrium cuneifolium Nees, Lauraceae 203
Portulaca pilosa L., Portulacaceae 289
Pothomorphe umbellata (L.) Miq., Piperaceae 277
Seguieria americana L., Phytolaccaceae 272
Senna affinis (Benth.) Ir. & Barn., Caesalpiniaceae 104
Senna alata (L.) Roxb., Caesalpiniaceae 104
Senna occidentalis (L.) Link, Caesalpiniaceae 105
Senna quinqueangulata
   (Rich.) Ir. & Barn., Caesalpiniaceae 106
Solanum juciri Mart., also
   S. juripeba Rich., Solanaceae 321
Solanum variabile Mart., Solanaceae 322
Strychnos pseudoquina St.-Hil., Loganiaceae 209
Tillandsia usneoides L., Bromeliaceae 91
Xanthium orientale L., *X. spinosum* L.
   & *X. strumarium* L., Asteraceae 67

LIVER DISEASE – MENSTRUATION: MEDICINAL INDEX

Zschokkea arborescens M. Arg., Apocynaceae 29
Lumbar Aches
Xylopia frutescens Aubl., Annonaceae 16
Lung Disease. See also Pneumonia
Buddleja brasiliensis Jacq. ex Spr., Buddlejaceae 93
Cereus jamacaru DC., Cactaceae 95
Torresea cearensis Fr. All., Fabaceae 172
Urera caracasana Jacq., Urticaceae 331
Waltheria communis St.-Hil., Sterculiaceae 325
Lymph Gland Problems.
See also Buboes, Lymphangitis,
Lymphoadenitis, Scrofula
Chiococca alba (L.) Hitch., Rubiaceae 297
Himatanthus lancifolia
  (M. Arg.) Woods., Apocynaceae 26
Limonium brasiliense
  (Boiss.) O. Ktze., Plumbaginaceae 278
Lymphangitis. See also Lymphoadenitis
Callisthene major Mart., Vochysiaceae 340
Davilla rugosa Poir., Dilleniaceae 145
Kalanchoe brasiliensis Camb., Crassulaceae 133
Tetracera breyniana Schl., Dilleniaceae 146
Triplaris noli-tangere Wedd., Polygonaceae 287
Lymphoadenitis
Monstera adansonii Schott, Araceae 36

M

Malaria. See also Quinine Substitute
Ampelozizyphus amazonicus Ducke, Rhamnaceae . 291
Annona foetida Mart., Annonaceae 12
Aristolochia cordigera Willd., Aristolochiaceae 46
Aristolochia esperanzae
  O. Kuntze, Aristolochiaceae 48
Aristolochia triangularis Cham., Aristolochiaceae ... 48
Aspidosperma discolor Benth., Apocynaceae 21
Aspidosperma nitidum Benth., Apocynaceae 21
Bathysa cuspidata Hook., Rubiaceae 296
Berberis laurina Thunb., Berberidaceae 76
Berberis spinulosa St.-Hil., Berberidaceae 76
Calolisianthus pendulus
  (Mart.) Gilg, Gentianaceae 179
Campsiandra comosa Benth. var.
  laurifolia (Benth.) Cowan, Caesalpiniaceae 100
Carapa guianensis Aubl., Meliaceae 227
Cestrum parqui L'Herit., Solanaceae 317
Chamissoa macrocarpa H.B.K., Amaranthaceae 4
Chondodendron platyphyllum
  (Mart.) Miers, Menispermaceae 231
Coutarea hexandra (Jacq.) K. Sch., Rubiaceae 297
Declieuxia cordigera Mart. & Zucc., Rubiaceae ... 297
Doliocarpus rolandri Gmel., Dilleniaceae 146
Dorstenia brasiliensis Lam., Moraceae 247
Esenbeckia febrifuga Juss., Rutaceae 301
Geissospermum laeve (Vell.) Baill., Apocynaceae ... 23
Leonurus sibiricus L., Lamiaceae 194
Macfadyena unguis-cati (L.) Gentry, Bignoniaceae . 81
Maytenus boaria Mol., Celastraceae 115
Mikania parviflora (Aubl.) Karst., Asteraceae 62
Naucleopsis amara Ducke, Moraceae 249
Parkinsonia aculeata L., Caesalpiniaceae 104
Phyllanthus niruri L., Euphorbiaceae 156

Picrolemma pseudocoffea Ducke, Simaroubaceae . 314
Portulaca pilosa L., Portulacaceae 289
Pothomorphe umbellata (L.) Miq., Piperaceae 277
Quassia amara L., Simaroubaceae 314
Senna occidentalis (L.) Link, Caesalpiniaceae 105
Senna quinqueangulata
  (Rich.) Ir. & Barn., Caesalpiniaceae 106
Solanum insidiosum Mart., Solanaceae 320
Solanum paniculatum L., Solanaceae 321
Stachytarpheta elatior Schrad., Verbenaceae 336
Strychnos pseudoquina St.-Hil., Loganiaceae 209
Strychnos trinervis (Vell.) Mart., Loganiaceae 210
Tetracera aspera Willd., Dilleniaceae 146
Trichilia cathartica Mart., Meliaceae 229
Turnera diffusa Willd., Turneraceae 327
Turnera opifera Mart., Turneraceae 328
Malarial Fever. See Malaria
Malignant
–fevers
Cayaponia cabocla (Vell.) Mart., Cucurbitaceae ... 135
–ulcers
Euphorbia phosphorea Mart., Euphorbiaceae 153
Marsh Mallow Substitute
Sida rhombea L., Malvaceae 222
Mate Adulterant
Ilex brevicuspis Reiss., Aquifoliaceae 31
Ilex paraguariensis St. Hil., Aquifoliaceae 31
Mate Substitute
Citronella congonha (Mart.) Howard, Icacinaceae . 185
Citronella mucronata
  (R. & Pav.) Don, Icacinaceae 186
Maytenus Adulterant
Sorocea bonplandii (Baill.) Burger, Moraceae 249
Measles
Bixa orellana L., Bixaceae 85
Medullary Conditions
Turnera diffusa Willd., Turneraceae 327
Turnera opifera Mart., Turneraceae 328
Memory Aid
Ficus insipida Willd., Moraceae 248
Menorrhagia. See also Menstruation
Dorstenia asaroides Gardn., Moraceae 247
Piper angustifolium R. & Pav., Piperaceae 274
Menstruation.
See also Amenorrhea, Dysmenorrhea,
Emmenagogue, Menorrhagia
Achyranthes indica L., Amaranthaceae 3
Ambrosia artemisiifolia L., Asteraceae 53
Chondodendron platyphyllum
  (Mart.) Miers, Menispermaceae 231
Cipura paludosa Aubl., Iridaceae 186
Cocculus filipendula Mart., Menispermaceae 234
Dalechampia ficifolia Lam., Euphorbiaceae 152
Declieuxia aristolochia M. Arg., Rubiaceae 297
Geoffroea striata (Willd.) Morong, Fabaceae 168
Guettarda angelica Mart., Rubiaceae 298
Jatropha elliptica (Pohl) M. Arg., Euphorbiaceae .. 154
Jatropha urens L., Euphorbiaceae 155
Leonotis nepetaefolia R. Br., Lamiaceae 194
Limonium brasiliense
  (Boiss.) O. Ktze., Plumbaginaceae 278

MEDICINAL INDEX: MENSTRUATION – NERVOUS DISORDERS

Mikania cordifolia (L. f.) Willd., Asteraceae 61
Momordica charantia L., Cucurbitaceae 139
Orbignya phalerata Mart., Arecaceae 43
Ouratea parviflora (DC.) Baill., Ochnaceae 261
Piper parthenium Mart., Piperaceae 276
Ptychopetalum olacoides Benth., Olacaceae 262
Ptychopetalum uncinatum Anselm., Olacaceae 262
Sebastiania macrocarpa M. Arg., Euphorbiaceae .. 157
Tagetes minuta L., Asteraceae 67
Trianosperma glandulosa Mart., Cucurbitaceae 140
Trianosperma trilobata Cogn., Cucurbitaceae 140
Turnera rupestris Aubl., Turneraceae 328
Ximenia coriacea Engl., Olacaceae 263

Mental Imbalance Inducer
Brunfelsia uniflora (Pohl) D. Don, also
 B. grandiflora D. Don, Solanaceae 316

Metritis. *See* Uterine Disorders

Metrorrhagia
Cissampelos fasciculata Benth., Menispermaceae . 231
Croton hemiargyreus M. Arg., Euphorbiaceae 151
Croton sincorensis Mart., Euphorbiaceae 151
Jatropha urens L., Euphorbiaceae 155
Myracroduon urundeuva
 Fr. All., Anacardiaceae 9
Piper mikanianum (Kunth) Steud., Piperaceae 276
Pradosia lactescens (Vell.) Radlk., Sapotaceae 310
Urera caracasana Jacq., Urticaceae 331

Migraine
Annona squamosa L., Annonaceae 13
Aristolochia cymbifera
 Mart. & Zucc., Aristolochiaceae 46
Hedyosmum brasiliense Mart., Chloranthaceae 119
Ocotea rodiei (Schomb.) Mez, Lauraceae 201
Paullinia cupana Kunth, Sapindaceae 306
Solanum verbascifolium L., Solanaceae 322

Miotic. *See* Eye Pupil Contraction

Molluscicide
Piper tuberculatum Jacq., Piperaceae 276

Mouth Problems.
See also Stomatitis, Thrush
Acmella oleracea (L.) R.K. Jansen, Asteraceae 52
Acmella repens (Walt.) L.C. Rich., Asteraceae 52
Berberis laurina Thunb., Berberidaceae 76
Dipteryx odorata (Aubl.) Willd., Fabaceae 166
Eryngium pristis Cham. & Schlecht., Apiaceae 19
Psidium guajava L., Myrtaceae 255
Tabebuia umbellata (Sond.) Sandw., Bignoniaceae .. 83

Mouthwash
Quassia amara L., Simaroubaceae 314

Mucilaginous Substance
Acanthospermum australe
 (Loefl.) O. Ktze., Asteraceae 51
Acanthospermum hispidum DC., Asteraceae 52
Amaranthus viridis L., Amaranthaceae 3
Bauhinia langsdorffiana Bong., Caesalpiniaceae 99
Bidens pilosa L., Asteraceae 57
Bromelia arenaria Ule, Bromeliaceae 91
Cordia grandiflora DC., Boraginaceae 87
Ephedra triandra Tul., Ephedraceae 148
Heliotropium curassavicum L., Boraginaceae 88
Mimosa bimucronata (DC.) O. Ktze., Mimosaceae 238

Ocotea guianensis Aubl., Lauraceae 201
Sida rhombea L., Malvaceae 222
Syagrus comosa Mart., Arecaceae 45
Tabebuia ipe (Mart.) Standl., Bignoniaceae 83
Talinum racemosum (L.) Rohr., Portulacaceae 289
Tournefortia elegans Cham., Boraginaceae 89
Triumfetta rhomboidea Jacq., Tiliaceae 327
Urena lobata L., Malvaceae 223
Vitex montevidensis Cham., Verbenaceae 337

Mucous Diarrhoea. *See* Diarrhoea

Mucous Membrane Problems.
See also Catarrh
Acmella oleracea (L.) R.K. Jansen, Asteraceae 52
Acmella repens (Walt.) L.C. Rich., Asteraceae 52
Bromelia arenaria Ule, Bromeliaceae 91

Muscle Pain
Piper callosum R. & Pav., Piperaceae 274
Piper eucalyptifolium (Miq.) Rudge, Piperaceae 275

N

Narcotic.
See also Delerium Inducer, Euphoria, Hallucinogen, Hypnotic, Mental Imbalance Inducer, Soporific, Stupefacient, Trance Inducer, Tremor Inducer
Acnistus arborescens (L.) Schl., Solanaceae 316
Annona reticulata L., Annonaceae 13
Cabralea canjerana (Vell.) Mart., Meliaceae 227
Clematis campestris St.-Hil., Ranunculaceae 290
Clematis dioica L., Ranunculaceae 290
Clibadium leiocarpum Mart., Asteraceae 58
Datura suaveolens Humb. & Bonpl., Solanaceae ... 318
Erythrina verna Vell., Fabaceae 168
Mimosa verrucosa Benth., Mimosaceae 240
Passiflora alata Dryand., Passifloraceae 267
Passiflora macrocarpa Mast., Passifloraceae 270
Phyllanthus conami Sw., Euphorbiaceae 156
Physalis pubescens L., Solanaceae 318
Ranunculus bonariensis Poir., Ranunculaceae 291
Solanum ciliatum Lam., Solanaceae 319
Solanum nigrum L., Solanaceae 321
Strychnos trinervis (Vell.) Mart., Loganiaceae 210

Nausea
Copaifera officinalis (Jacq.) L., Caesalpiniaceae 102

Nephritis. *See* Kidney Disease

Nerve Calmative
Costus spiralis (Jacq.) Roscoe, Costaceae 132

Nerve Sedative. *See also* Sedative
Porophyllum ruderale (Jacq.) Cass., Asteraceae 64

Nerve Stimulant. *See* Excitant

Nervous Disorders. *See also*
Berbiberi, Chorea, Epilepsy, Neuralgia
Dioscorea silvestris Vell., Dioscoreaceae 147
Turnera diffusa Willd., Turneraceae 327
Turnera opifera Mart., Turneraceae 328
Turnera rupestris Aubl., Turneraceae 328
Zanthoxylum pterota H.B.K., Rutaceae 303

NERVOUSNESS – PANACEA: MEDICINAL INDEX

Nervousness
Licaria puchury-major
  (Mart.) Kosterm., Lauraceae 199
Paullinia cupana Kunth, Sapindaceae 306
Neuralgia. See also Sciatica
Aristolochia esperanzae
  O. Kuntze, Aristolochiaceae 48
Leucas martinicensis (Jacq.) R. Br., Lamiaceae 194
Mikania hirsutissima DC., Asteraceae 62
Ocotea rodiei (Schomb.) Mez, Lauraceae 201
Paullinia cupana Kunth, Sapindaceae 306
Philodendron pedatum (Hook.) Kunth, Araceae 37
Schinus terebinthifolius Raddi, Anacardiaceae 10
Virola oleifera (Schott) A.C. Smith, Myristicaceae . 250
Newborn (Infants)
Copaifera officinalis (Jacq.) L., Caesalpiniaceae 102
Maranta arundinacea L., Marantaceae 223
Virola oleifera (Schott) A.C. Smith, Myristicaceae . 250
–navel ruptures in
Genipa americana L., Rubiaceae 298
Nipple Fissures
Clusia grandiflora Splitg., Clusiaceae 121
Clusia insignis Mart., Clusiaceae 121
Krameria tomentosa St.-Hil., Krameriaceae 191
Senna hirsuta (L.) Ir. & Barn.
  var. *puberula* Ir. & Barn., Caesalpiniaceae 105
Nutrition: *newborns, the aged & convalescents*
Maranta arundinacea L., Marantaceae 223

O

Obesity
Orbignya phalerata Mart., Arecaceae 43
Obstructions, removal of internal
Ipomoea acetosifolia
  (Vahl) Roem. & Schult., Convolvulaceae 130
Odontalgic. See Toothache
Ophthalmia. See also Eye Problems
Abuta concolor Poepp. & Endl., Menispermaceae . 231
Albizzia lebbeck (L.) Benth., Mimosaceae 236
Begonia paulensis DC., Begoniaceae 76
Boehmeria caudata Sw., Urticaceae 330
Buddleja cambara Arech., Buddlejaceae 93
Calliandra tweedii Benth., Mimosaceae 237
Celtis brasiliensis Planch., Ulmaceae 330
Chromolaena hirsuta
  (Hook. & Arn.) King & Robinson, Asteraceae 58
Commelina robusta Kunth, Commelinaceae 128
Hyptis crenata Pohl, Lamiaceae 192
Lithraea molleoides (Vell.) Engl., Anacardiaceae 9
Luffa operculata (L.) Cogn., Cucurbitaceae 138
Monnieria trifolia Loefl., Rutaceae 302
Sauvagesia erecta L., Ochnaceae 262
Scheelea phalerata
  (Mart. ex Spreng.) Burret, Arecaceae 45
Schinus molle L., Anacardiaceae 9
Spondias macrocarpa Engl., Anacardiaceae 10
Spondias mombin L., Anacardiaceae 10
Syagrus schizophylla
  (Mart.) Glassman, Arecaceae 46

Vernonanthura brasiliana
  (L.) H. Robinson, Asteraceae 67
Oral Disorders. See Mouth Problems
Orchitis. See also Testicular Problems
Aristolochia cymbifera
  Mart. & Zucc., Aristolochiaceae 46
Aristolochia triangularis Cham., Aristolochiaceae ... 48
Aristolochia trilobata L., Aristolochiaceae 48
Cedrela fissilis Vell., Meliaceae 227
Chondodendron platyphyllum
  (Mart.) Miers, Menispermaceae 231
Cleome spinosa Jacq., Capparaceae 112
Davilla rugosa Poir., Dilleniaceae 145
Dorstenia brasiliensis Lam., Moraceae 247
Dorstenia cayapia Vell., Moraceae 248
Echites macrocalyx M. Arg., Apocynaceae 23
Echites peltata Vell., Apocynaceae 23
Lithraea molleoides (Vell.) Engl., Anacardiaceae 9
Monstera adansonii Schott, Araceae 36
Philodendron bipinnatifidum Schott, Araceae 36
Philodendron imbe Schott, Araceae 37
Philodendron ochrostemon Schott, Araceae 37
Sacciolepis myuros (Lam.) Chase, Poaceae 282
Schinus molle L., Anacardiaceae 9
Solanum agrarium Sendt., Solanaceae 319
Tetracera breyniana Schl., Dilleniaceae 146
Otalgia (Ear Pain). See also Earache
Monnieria trifolia Loefl., Rutaceae 302
Otitis (Ear Inflammation). See also Earache
Capparis urens B. Rodr., Capparaceae 111
Cleome spinosa Jacq., Capparaceae 112
Lucuma rivicoa Gaertn., Sapotaceae 302
Monstera adansonii Schott, Araceae 36
Physalis pubescens L., Solanaceae 318
Zanthoxylum hyemale St.-Hil., Rutaceae 302
Ovarian Disease
Hedyosmum brasiliense Mart., Chloranthaceae 119

P

Pain. See also Analgesic, Muscle Pain
Dipteryx odorata (Aubl.) Willd., Fabaceae 166
Philodendron pedatum (Hook.) Kunth, Araceae 37
Zanthoxylum pterota H.B.K., Rutaceae 303
–articular
Victoria amazonica
  (Poepp.) Sower., Nymphaeaceae 259
–body
Cedrela odorata L., Meliaceae 227
Xylopia frutescens Aubl., Annonaceae 16
–ear & tooth. See also Toothache, Earache
Plumbago scandens L., Plumbaginaceae 279
–vesical lithiasis
Bassovia lucida Dunal, Solanaceae 316
Palpitation. See also Heart Problems
Aristolochia cymbifera
  Mart. & Zucc., Aristolochiaceae 46
Panacea
Gomphrena macrocephala St.-Hil., Amaranthaceae .. 4
Gomphrena officinalis Mart., Amaranthaceae 4
Paullinia cupana Kunth, Sapindaceae 306

MEDICINAL INDEX: PANACEA – POISON ANTIDOTE

Turnera diffusa Willd., Turneraceae 327
Turnera opifera Mart., Turneraceae 328
Paralysis
Cleome gigantea L., Capparaceae 112
Manilkara bidentata (A. DC.) Chev., Sapotaceae .. 309
Mikania hirsutissima DC., Asteraceae 62
Ocotea opifera Mart., Lauraceae 201
Ptychopetalum olacoides Benth., Olacaceae 262
Ptychopetalum uncinatum Anselm., Olacaceae 262
Raphia taedigera (Mart.) Mart., Arecaceae 45
Turnera diffusa Willd., Turneraceae 327
Turnera opifera Mart., Turneraceae 328
Parasites
–intestinal
Nymphoides indica (L.) O. Ktze., Menyanthaceae . 235
Tagetes minuta L., Asteraceae 67
–skin
Senna septentrionalis
 (Viv.) Ir. & Barn., Caesalpiniaceae 106
Parasiticide. See also Anthelmintic
Bidens pilosa L., Asteraceae 57
Carpotroche brasiliensis
 (Raddi) Endl., Flacourtiaceae 176
Carpotroche longifolia Benth., Flacourtiaceae 176
Guazuma ulmifolia Lam.
 var. ulmifolia, Sterculiaceae 323
Jatropha multifida L., Euphorbiaceae 154
Mammea americana L., Clusiaceae 123
Nymphoides indica (L.) O. Ktze., Menyanthaceae . 235
Phyllanthus conami Sw., Euphorbiaceae 156
Senna septentrionalis
 (Viv.) Ir. & Barn., Caesalpiniaceae 106
Tagetes minuta L., Asteraceae 67
Pectoral (Chest Problems)
Acanthospermum hispidum DC., Asteraceae 52
Adiantum concinnum Humb. & Bonp., Adiantaceae .. 1
Adiantum trapeziforme L., Adiantaceae 1
Anadenanthera macrocarpa
 (Benth.) Brenan, Mimosaceae 236
Anemopaegma arvense (Vell.) Stapf, Bignoniaceae . 78
Aniba canelilla (H.B.K.) Mez, Lauraceae 197
Annona muricata L., Annonaceae 13
Astronium fraxinifolium Schott, Anacardiaceae 9
Buddleja cambara Arech., Buddlejaceae 93
Carica papaya L., Caricaceae 113
Clusia rosea Jacq., Clusiaceae 122
Cocos nucifera L., Arecaceae 40
Eclipta prostrata (L.) L., Asteraceae 59
Erythrina velutina Willd., Fabaceae 166
Glechon spathulata Benth., Lamiaceae 192
Guazuma ulmifolia Lam.,
 var. ulmifolia, Sterculiaceae 323
Heliotropium curassavicum L., Boraginaceae 88
Heliotropium elongatum Willd., Boraginaceae 88
Heliotropium indicum L., Boraginaceae 89
Himatanthus alba (L.) Woods., Apocynaceae 24
Hippeastrum vittatum
 (L'Hérit.) Herb., Amaryllidaceae 6
Hymenaea courbaril L., Caesalpiniaceae 103
Lantana brasiliensis Link, Verbenaceae 334
Monnieria trifolia Loefl., Rutaceae 302
Ocotea teleiandra (Messn.) Mez, Lauraceae 203

Peltodon radicans Pohl, Lamiaceae 195
Peperomia transparens Miq., Piperaceae 274
Piptadenia polyptera Benth., Mimosaceae 242
Pluchea suaveolens (Vell.) O. Ktze., Asteraceae 64
Plumeria alba L., Apocynaceae 28
Polygala klotzschii Chodat, Polygalaceae 284
Scoparia dulcis L., Scrophulariaceae 312
Sida micrantha St.-Hil., Malvaceae 222
Siparuna camporum (Tul.) DC., Monimiaceae 245
Stachytarpheta cayennensis
 (Rich.) Vahl, Verbenaceae 335
Sterculia apetala (Jacq.) Karst.
 var. elata (Ducke) E. Taylor, Sterculiaceae 324
Syagrus romanzoffiana
 (Cham.) Glassman, Arecaceae 45
Tagetes erecta L., Asteraceae 67
Tradescantia spathacea Sw., Commelinaceae 129
Vitex montevidensis Cham., Verbenaceae 337
Wissadula periplocifolia Presl., Malvaceae 223
Peru Balsam Substitute
Humiria balsamifera
 (Aubl.) St.-Hil., Humiriaceae 183
Phagedenic Ulcers
Euphorbia tirucalli L., Euphorbiaceae 153
Pharyngitis
Bixa orellana L., Bixaceae 85
Canna gigantea Desf., Cannaceae 110
Genipa americana L., Rubiaceae 298
Psidium guajava L., Myrtaceae 256
Phlebitis. See also Circulatory Problems
Davilla rugosa Poir., Dilleniaceae 145
Piles. See Hemorrhoids
Pityriasis
Annona spinescens Mart., Annonaceae 13
Ocotea cymbarum H.B.K., Lauraceae 200
Placenta Expulsion.
See also Childbirth, Foetus Expulsion
Chenopodium ambrosioides L., Chenopodiaceae ... 118
Crescentia cujete L., Bignoniaceae 80
Pneumonia. See also Pulmonary Disorders
Copaifera officinalis (Jacq.) L., Caesalpiniaceae 102
Poison. See also Poison Antidote, Toxic
–arrow
Dieffenbachia seguine (Jacq.) Schott, Araceae 35
–dart
Naucleopsis amara Ducke, Moraceae 249
–fish
Clibadium surinamense L., Asteraceae 58
Gustavia hexapetala
 (Aubl.) J.E. Smith, Lecythidaceae 205
Ichthyothere terminalis
 (Spr.) S.F. Blake, Asteraceae 61
–snake
Mikania officinalis Mart., Asteraceae 62
Poison Antidote. See also Cassava
Poison Antidote, Snake Poison Antidote
Aristolochia gigantea
 Mart. & Zucc., Aristolochiaceae 48
Cayaponia espelina
 (Manso) Cogn., Cucurbitaceae 135
Cocos nucifera L., Arecaceae 40

POISON ANTIDOTE – PURGATIVE: MEDICINAL INDEX

Eclipta prostrata (L.) L., Asteraceae 59
Fevillea trilobata L., Cucurbitaceae 136
Flaveria bidentis (L.) Ktze., Asteraceae 60
Gomphrena leucocephala Mart., Amaranthaceae 4
Hypericum brasiliense Choisy, Clusiaceae 122
Leopoldinia major Wallace, Arecaceae 43
Mikania officinalis Mart., Asteraceae 62
Piper geniculatum Sw., Piperaceae 275
Senna occidentalis (L.) Link, Caesalpiniaceae 105
Senna quinqueangulata
   (Rich.) Ir. & Barn., Caesalpiniaceae 106
Senna uniflora
   (P. Miller) Ir. & Barn., Caesalpiniaceae 106
–cassava
Bixa orellana L., Bixaceae 85
Fevillea trilobata L., Cucurbitaceae 136
Tabebuia leucoxylon (L.) DC., Bignoniaceae 83
–plant
Cayaponia espelina (Manso) Cogn., Cucurbitaceae 135
–snake
Aristolochia spp., all, Aristolochiaceae 49
Aristolochia birostris Duch., Aristolochiaceae 46
Aristolochia triangularis Cham., Aristolochiaceae ... 48
Mikania officinalis Mart., Asteraceae 62
Thevetia ahouai (L.) DC., Apocynaceae 28

Poisonous. See Toxic

Poultice. See also Sinapism
Wissadula periplocifolia Presl., Malvaceae 223

Pregnancy. See also Childbirth
Bixa orellana L., Bixaceae 85
Cocos nucifera L., Arecaceae 40

Prolapsed Rectum. See Rectal Prolapse
Prolapsed Uterus. See Uterine Prolapse
Prostatitis
Gallesia gorazema (Vell.) Moq., Phytolaccaceae ... 271
Hymenaea courbaril L., Caesalpiniaceae 103

Proteolytic
Jacaratia spinosa
   (Aubl.) A. DC., Caricaceae (CHEM.) 113

Prurigo
Aristolochia cymbifera
   Mart. & Zucc., Aristolochiaceae 46

Pruritus. See also Itch
Caraipa grandifolia Mart., Clusiaceae 121
Dieffenbachia seguine (Jacq.) Schott, Araceae 35
Solanum nigrum L., Solanaceae 321

Psoriasis
Copaifera officinalis (Jacq.) L., Caesalpiniaceae 102
Himatanthus phagedaenica
   (Mart.) Woods., Apocynaceae 26
Solanum mammosum L., Solanaceae 321
Solanum nigrum L., Solanaceae 321

Pterygium Remover
Cyperus ligularis L., Cyperaceae 142
Marsdenia amylacea
   (Barb.-Rodr.) Malme, Asclepiadaceae 51

Puerperal Fever. See also Childbirth
Guettarda angelica Mart., Rubiaceae 298

Pulmonary Conditions.
See also Pneumonia, Tuberculosis
Anadenanthera falcata

   (Benth.) Brenan, Mimosaceae 236
Chaptalia nutans (L.) Polak., Asteraceae 57
Cunila microcephala Benth., Lamiaceae 192
Guettarda angelica Mart., Rubiaceae 298
Hylocereus undatus (Haw.) Br. & Rose, Cactaceae .. 95
Lucuma rivicoa Gaertn., Sapotaceae 309
Myracroduon urundeuva
   Fr. All., Anacardiaceae 9
Prunus subcoriacea
   (Chod. & Hassl.) Hoehne, Rosaceae 294
Sauvagesia erecta L., Ochnaceae 262
Urera subpeltata Miq., Urticaceae 331
Waltheria viscosissima St.-Hil., Sterculiaceae 325

Pungent
Cinnamodendron axillare
   (Nees & Mart.) Endl., Canellaceae 110
Piper tuberculatum Jacq., Piperaceae 276

Purgative. See also Carthatic, Hydragogue
Allamanda cathartica L., Apocynaceae 20
Allamanda doniana M. Arg., Apocynaceae 20
Anacardium occidentale L., Anacardiaceae 7
Anchietea pyrifolia (Mart.) G. Don, Violaceae 338
Andira inermis (Sw.) H.B.K., Fabaceae 162
Anisolobus cururu (Mart.) M. Arg., Apocynaceae 21
Anisosperma passiflora Manso, Cucurbitaceae 135
Boerhavia erecta L., Nyctaginaceae 258
Boerhavia paniculata Rich., Nyctaginaceae 258
Borreria tenella Cham. & Schl., Rubiaceae 296
Bromelia antiacantha Bertol., Bromeliaceae 91
Brunfelsia uniflora (Pohl) D. Don, also
   B. grandiflora D. Don, Solanaceae 316
Caladium bicolor (Aiton) Vent., Araceae 34
Calonyction aculeatum
   (L.) House, Convolvulaceae 129
Carapa guianensis Aubl., Meliaceae 227
Cayaponia cabocla (Vell.) Mart., Cucurbitaceae ... 135
Cayaponia espelina
   (Manso) Cogn., Cucurbitaceae 135
Cayaponia martiana
   (Cogn.) Cogn., Cucurbitaceae 135
Cayaponia pilosa Cogn., Cucurbitaceae 135
Chamaecrista fasciculata
   (Michx.) Greene, Caesalpiniaceae 102
Chiococca alba (L.) Hitch., Rubiaceae 297
Clematis dioica L., Ranunculaceae 290
Clusia rosea Jacq., Clusiaceae 122
Crescentia cujete L., Bignoniaceae 80
Croton floribundus Spreng., Euphorbiaceae 150
Cuscuta racemosa Mart., Convolvulaceae 130
Cypella herbertii Herb., Iridaceae 186
Davilla rugosa Poir., Dilleniaceae 145
Desmoncus orthacanthos Mart., Arecaceae 40
Dipladenia illustris M. Arg., Apocynaceae 23
Dodonaea viscosa Jacq., Sapindaceae 305
Dorstenia brasiliensis Lam., Moraceae 247
Erythrina corallodendron L., Fabaceae 166
Erythrina fusca Lour., Fabaceae 166
Erythroxylum campestre St.-Hil., Erythroxylaceae . 149
Euphorbia cotinoides Miq., Euphorbiaceae 152
Euphorbia hirta L., Euphorbiaceae 152
Euphorbia papillosa St.-Hil., Euphorbiaceae 152
Fevillea trilobata L., Cucurbitaceae 136
Fevillea uncipetala Kuhlm., Cucurbitaceae 138

MEDICINAL INDEX: PURGATIVE – RABIES

Ficus gomelleira Kunth & Bouché, Moraceae 248
Ficus insipida Willd., Moraceae 248
Galphimia brasiliensis Juss., Malpighiaceae 220
Genipa americana L., Rubiaceae 298
Griffinia hyacinthina Ker-Gawl., Amaryllidaceae 6
Guarea trichilioides L., Meliaceae 227
Guarea tuberculata Vell., Meliaceae 229
Gurania multiflora Cogn., Cucurbitaceae 138
Gurania paulista Cogn., Cucurbitaceae 138
Heimia salicifolia
  (H.B.K.) Link & Otto, Lythraceae 214
Himatanthus alba (L.) Woods., Apocynaceae 24
Himatanthus lancifolia
  (M. Arg.) Woods., Apocynaceae 26
Himatanthus sucuuba (Spr.) Woods., Apocynaceae . 26
Hippeastrum puniceum (Lam.) Kuntze
  [includes Hippeastrum equestre
  (L.) Hebert], Amaryllidaceae 6
Hura crepitans L., Euphorbiaceae 153
Hybanthus atropurpureus Taub., Violaceae 338
Ipomoea acetosifolia (Vahl)
  Roem. & Schult., Convolvulaceae 130
Ipomoea pes-caprae (L.) R. Br., see also
  CHEM & PHARM: Ipomoea spp: I batatoides Meissn., I.
  capparpides Choisy, I. echioides Choisy, I. igantea
  Choisy, I. longicuspis Meissn., I. silvana Choisy, & I.
  sinuata Ortega, Convolvulaceae 130
Isostigma megapotamicum
  (Spr.) Sherff, Asteraceae 61
Jatropha curcas L., Euphorbiaceae 154
Jatropha elliptica (Pohl) M. Arg., Euphorbiaceae .. 154
Jatropha gossypiifolia L., Euphorbiaceae 154
Jatropha multifida L., Euphorbiaceae 154
Jatropha urens L., Euphorbiaceae 155
Jessenia bataua (Mart.) Burret, Arecaceae 43
Joannesia heveoides Ducke, Euphorbiaceae 155
Laetia apetala Jacq., Flacourtiaceae 178
Lagenaria siceraria
  (Molina) Standl., Cucurbitaceae 138
Lindernia diffusa Wettst., Scrophulariaceae 311
Lithraea molleoides (Vell.) Engl., Anacardiaceae 9
Luffa operculata (L.) Cogn., Cucurbitaceae 138
Macrosiphonia longiflora
  (Desf.) M. Arg., Apocynaceae 26
Matayba purgans Radlk.., Sapindaceae 306
Maytenus boaria Mol., Celastraceae 115
Melothria fluminensis Gardn., Cucurbitaceae 139
Mesechites sulphurea (Vell.) M. Arg., Apocynaceae 27
Mimosa pudica L., Mimosaceae 240
Mimosa velloziana Mart., Mimosaceae 240
Momordica charantia L., Cucurbitaceae 139
Omphalea diandra M. Arg., Euphorbiaceae 156
Operculina alata (Ham.) Urb., Convolvulaceae 131
Operculina macrocarpa Urb., Convolvulaceae 131
Philodendron bipinnatifidum Schott, Araceae 36
Philodendron imbe Schott, Araceae 36
Philodendron ochrostemon Schott, Araceae 37
Philodendron selloum Koch, Araceae 37
Pisonia aculeata L., Nyctaginaceae 258
Pisonia alcalina Fr. All., also
  P. subcordata Sw., Nyctaginaceae 258
Plumbago scandens L., Plumbaginaceae 279
Plumeria alba L., Apocynaceae 28

Polygala paniculata L., Polygalaceae 284
Rauwolfia ligustrina
  Willd. ex Roem. & Schult., Apocynaceae 28
Rollinia exalbida (Vell.) Mart., Annonaceae 15
Ruellia tuberosa L., Acanthaceae 1
Schinus molle L., Anacardiaceae 9
Sebastiania macrocarpa M. Arg., Euphorbiaceae .. 157
Senna affinis (Benth.) Ir. & Barn., Caesalpiniaceae 104
Senna alata (L.) Roxb., Caesalpiniaceae 104
Senna bicapsularis (L.) Roxb., Caesalpiniaceae 104
Senna oblongifolia
  (Vog.) Ir. & Barn., Caesalpiniaceae 105
Senna obtusifolia
  (L.) Ir. & Barn., Caesalpiniaceae 105
Senna occidentalis (L.) Link, Caesalpiniaceae 105
Senna quinqueangulata
  (Rich.) Ir. & Barn., Caesalpiniaceae 106
Senna rugosa
  (G. Don) Ir. & Barn., Caesalpiniaceae 106
Senna septentrionalis
  (Viv.) Ir. & Barn., Caesalpiniaceae 106
Senna spp.: S. alexandrina Miller
  & S. italica Miller, Caesalpiniaceae 107
Sicyos polyacanthus Cogn., Cucurbitaceae 139
Smilax oblongifolia Pohl, Liliaceae 208
Sophora tomentosa L., Fabaceae 172
Tabebuia aurea (Manso) Moore, Bignoniaceae 82
Tabernaemontana citrifolia L., Apocynaceae 28
Terminalia argentea Mart., Combretaceae 126
Thevetia ahouai (L.) DC., Apocynaceae 28
Trianosperma glandulosa Mart., Cucurbitaceae 140
Trianosperma trilobata Cogn., Cucurbitaceae 140
Trichilia cathartica Mart., Meliaceae 229
Trichilia catigua Juss., Meliaceae 229
Trichilia hirta L., Meliaceae 229
Vataireopsis araroba (Aguiar) Ducke, Fabaceae 172
Vismia acuminata (L.) Pers., Clusiaceae 123
Wilbrandia ebracteata Cogn., Cucurbitaceae 140
Wilbrandia verticillata
  (Vell.) Cogn., Cucurbitaceae 140
Ximenia americana L., Olacaceae 263
Ximenia coriacea Engl., Olacaceae 263

Q

Quassia Substitute
Tachia guianenesis Aubl., Gentianaceae 180
Quinine Substitute
Cestrum pseudoquina Mart., Solanaceae 317
Coutarea hexandra (Jacq.) K. Sch., Rubiaceae 297
Esenbeckia intermedia Mart., Rutaceae 301
Tachia guianenesis Aubl., Gentianaceae 180

R

Rabies (Hydrophobia)
Cayaponia martiana
  (Cogn.) Cogn., Cucurbitaceae 135
Cayaponia tayuya (Mart.) Cogn., Cucurbitaceae 135
Clematis denticulata Vell., Ranunculaceae 290

Echinodorus macrophyllus
   (Kunth) Mich., Alismataceae 2
Mikania parviflora (Aubl.) Karst., Asteraceae 62
Rachitism (Rickets). *See also* Scurvy
Lophophytum mirabile
   Schott & Endl., Balanophoraceae 73
Radiation Burns
Stryphnodendron adstringens
   (Mart.) Cov., Mimosaceae 242
Recovery after illness
Bathysa cuspidata Hook., Rubiaceae 296
Rectal Prolapse
Blepharocalyx salicifolius
   (H.B.K.) Berg, Myrtaceae 253
Oxalis corniculata L., Oxalidaceae 266
Simaba ferruginea St.-Hil., Simaroubaceae 314
Refreshant
Attalea spectabilis Mart., Arecaceae 39
Craniolaria annua L., Martyniaceae 224
Hedyosmum brasiliense Mart., Chloranthaceae 119
Ilex paraguariensis St.-Hil., Aquifoliaceae 31
Mauritiella aculeata (Kunth) Burret, Arecaceae 43
Regeneration of Tissue
Mabea fistulifera Mart., Euphorbiaceae 155
Renal Disorders. *See* Colic (Renal),
Kidney Disease, Kidney Stones,
Lithiasis, Urinary Problems
Resolvent
Amaranthus viridis L., Amaranthaceae 3
Anisolobus cururu (Mart.) M. Arg., Apocynaceae 21
Annona dioica St.-Hil., Annonaceae 12
Annona reticulata L., Annonaceae 13
Bidens cynapiifolia H.B.K., Asteraceae 56
Cissampelos ovalifolia DC., Menispermaceae 233
Cissampelos sympodialis Eichl., Menispermaceae . 233
Clusia rosea Jacq., Clusiaceae 122
Cochlospermum regium
   (Mart. & Schl.) Pilg., Cochlospermaceae 125
Costus spiralis (Jacq.) Roscoe, Costaceae 132
Cydista aequinoctialis Miers, Bignoniaceae 80
Echites macrocalyx M. Arg., Apocynaceae 23
Elephantopus mollis H.B.K., Asteraceae 59
Ficus gomelleira Kunth & Bouché, Moraceae 248
Heliotropium elongatum Willd., Boraginaceae 88
Heliotropium indicum L., Boraginaceae 89
Imperata brasiliensis Trin., also
   Imperata contracta Hitch., Poaceae 281
Kielmeyera coriacea Mart., Clusiaceae 122
Mabea fistulifera Mart., Euphorbiaceae 155
Machaerium ferox (Mart.) Ducke, Fabaceae 168
Mammea americana L., Clusiaceae 123
Momordica charantia L., Cucurbitaceae 139
Monnieria trifolia Loefl., Rutaceae 302
Ocotea opifera Mart., Lauraceae 201
Parahancornia amapa (Hub.) Ducke, Apocynaceae 27
Parthenium hysterophorus L., Asteraceae 64
Periandra mediterranea (Vell.) Taub., Fabaceae 170
Philodendron speciosum Schott, Araceae 209
Physalis angulata L., Solanaceae 318
Piper angustifolium R. & Pav., Piperaceae 274
Piper mollicomum Kunth, Piperaceae 276
Rumex brasiliensis Link, Polygonaceae 287

Schrankia leptocarpa DC., Mimosaceae 242
Senna latifolia
   (Meyer) Ir. & Barn., Caesalpiniaceae 105
Sicyos polyacanthus Cogn., Cucurbitaceae 139
Sterculia chicha St.-Hil., Sterculiaceae 324
Urera baccifera Gaud., Urticaceae 331
Virola surinamensis (Rol.) Warb., Myristicaceae 252
Vismia guianensis (Aubl.) Choisy, Clusiaceae 124
Xanthium orientale L., *X. spinosum* L.
   & *X. strumarium* L., Asteraceae 67
Respiratory Problems. *See also* Asthma
Anadenanthera colubrina
   (Vell.) Brenan, Mimosaceae 236
Bidens pilosa L., Asteraceae 57
Cecropia hololeuca Miq., Moraceae 247
Crescentia cujete L., Bignoniaceae 80
Dorstenia asaroides Gardn., Moraceae 247
Hyptis fasciculata Benth., Lamiaceae 192
Mikania periplocifolia Hook. & Arn., Asteraceae ... 62
Myrocarpus frondosus Fr. All., Fabaceae 170
Operculina alata (Ham.) Urb., Convolvulaceae 131
Operculina macrocarpa Urb., Convolvulaceae 131
Passiflora edulis Sims, Passifloraceae 269
Phlebodium aureum
   (L.) J.E. Smith, Polypodiaceae 288
Vochysia thyrsoidea Pohl, Vochysiaceae 340
Restorative
Heterothalamus alienus (Spr.) O. Ktze., Asteraceae 60
Parkinsonia aculeata L., Caesalpiniaceae 104
Revulsant
Cleome aculeata L., Capparaceae 112
Rhatany Substitute
Krameria argentea Mart., Krameriaceae 191
Krameria spartioides Berg, Krameriaceae 191
Krameria tomentosa St.-Hil., Krameriaceae 191
Rheumatism
Acacia paniculata Willd., Mimosaceae 236
Ageratum conyzoides L., Asteraceae 53
Agonandra brasiliensis Miers, Opiliaceae 265
Aiovea meissneri Mez, Lauraceae 197
Andradea floribunda Fr. All., Nyctaginaceae 257
Aniba permollis (Nees) Mez, Lauraceae 197
Annona dioica St.-Hil., Annonaceae 12
Annona foetida Mart., Annonaceae 12
Annona glabra L., Annonaceae 13
Annona spinescens Mart., Annonaceae 13
Annona squamosa L., Annonaceae 13
Attalea spectabilis Mart., Arecaceae 39
Baccharis dentata (Vell.) G.M. Barroso, Asteraceae 54
Baccharis notosergila Gris., Asteraceae 54
Baccharis trimera (Less.) DC., Asteraceae 54
Bactris insignis (Mart.) Baill., Arecaceae 39
Bauhinia rutilans Spr. ex Benth., Caesalpiniaceae ... 99
Bignonia exoleta Vell., Bignoniaceae 79
Bowdichia virgilioides H.B.K., Fabaceae 163
Brunfelsia uniflora (Pohl) D. Don, also
   B. grandiflora D. Don, Solanaceae 316
Buchnera aquatica Aubl., Scrophulariaceae 310
Bulbostylis capillaris Clarke, Cyperaceae 142
Calolisianthus pendulus
   (Mart.) Gilg, Gentianaceae 179
Calonyction aculeatum
   (L.) House, Convolvulaceae 129

MEDICINAL INDEX: RHEUMATISM

Calophyllum brasiliense Camb., Clusiaceae 120
Calotropis procera (Ait.) Ait. f., Asclepiadaceae 50
Canna gigantea Desf., Cannaceae 110
Canna glauca L., Cannaceae 110
Canna indica L., Cannaceae 111
Capparis urens B. Rodr., Capparaceae 111
Caraipa grandifolia Mart., Clusiaceae 121
Caraipa minor Huber, Clusiaceae 121
Carapa guianensis Aubl., Meliaceae 217
Casearia sylvestris Sw., Flacourtiaceae 178
Cayaponia tayuya (Mart.) Cogn., Cucurbitaceae 135
Cestrum calycinum Willd., Solanaceae 317
Cestrum parqui L'Herit., Solanaceae 317
Cissus palmata Poir., Vitaceae 339
Clematis denticulata Vell., Ranunculaceae 290
Cleome gigantea L., Capparaceae 112
Clusia rosea Jacq., Clusiaceae 122
Cochlospermum regium
   (Mart. & Schl.) Pilg., Cochlospermaceae 125
Commelina nudiflora L., Commelinaceae 126
Commelina vestita Seub., Commelinaceae 128
Copaifera cearensis
   Huber ex Ducke, Caesalpiniaceae 102
Copernicia prunifera (Mill.) H. Moore, Arecaceae .. 40
Cordia coffeoides Warm., Boraginaceae 87
Cordyline dracaenoides Kunth, Liliaceae 207
Crataeva benthamii Eichl., Capparaceae 112
Cyrtocymura scorpioides
   (Lam.) H. Robinson, Asteraceae 58
Dodonaea viscosa Jacq., Sapindaceae 305
Dorstenia brasiliensis Lam., Moraceae 247
Dorstenia cayapia Vell., Moraceae 248
Duguetia riparia Hub., Annonaceae 14
Echinodorus macrophyllus
   (Kunth) Mich., Alismataceae 2
Elaeis oleifera (H.B.K.) Cortez, Arecaceae 40
Elephantopus mollis H.B.K., Asteraceae 59
Elionurus bilinguis (Trin.) Hack., Poaceae 281
Ephedra triandra Tul., Ephedraceae 148
Erythrina crista-galli L., Fabaceae 166
Erythrina fusca Lour., Fabaceae 166
Eugenia brasiliensis Lam., Myrtaceae 253
Eugenia uniflora L., Myrtaceae 254
Fevillea trilobata L., Cucurbitaceae 136
Ficus gomelleira Kunth & Bouché, Moraceae 248
Gallesia gorazema (Vell.) Moq., Phytolaccaceae ... 271
Guarea trichilioides L., Meliaceae 227
Hancornia speciosa Gomes, Apocynaceae 24
Herreria salsaparilha Mart., Liliaceae 207
Himatanthus sucuuba (Spr.) Woods., Apocynaceae . 26
Hura crepitans L., Euphorbiaceae 153
Hydrocotyle bonariensis Lam., Apiaceae 19
Hydrocotyle leucocephala
   Cham. & Schlecht., Apiaceae 20
Ipomoea pes-caprae (L.) R. Br., Convolvulaceae .. 130
Jatropha elliptica (Pohl) M. Arg., Euphorbiaceae .. 154
Jatropha gossypiifolia L., Euphorbiaceae 154
Lantana camara L., Verbenaceae 33
Lantana microphylla Cham., also L. mixta L.,
   L. pseudothea (St.-Hil.) Schauer, Verbenaceae 335
Leonotis nepetaefolia R. Br., Lamiaceae 194
Licaria canella (Meissn.) Kosterm., Lauraceae 199

Limonium brasiliense
   (Boiss.) O. Ktze., Plumbaginaceae 278
Lithraea molleoides (Vell.) Engl., Anacardiaceae 9
Macfadyena unguis-cati (L.) Gentry, Bignoniaceae . 81
Marsypianthes chamaedrys
   (Vahl) O. Ktze., Lamiaceae 194
Maytenus laevis Reiss., Celastraceae 115
Melothrianthus smilacifolius
   (Cogn.) M. Crovetto, Cucurbitaceae 139
Mikania cordifolia (L. f.) Willd., Asteraceae 61
Mikania hirsutissima DC., Asteraceae 62
Mikania parviflora (Aubl.) Karst., Asteraceae 62
Mimosa malacocentra Mart., Mimosaceae 239
Mimosa pudica L., Mimosaceae 240
Mimosa velloziana Mart., Mimosaceae 240
Momordica charantia L., Cucurbitaceae 139
Monstera adansonii Schott, Araceae 36
Montrichardia linifera (Arruda) Schott, Araceae 36
Ocimum fluminensis Vell., Lamiaceae 195
Ocotea guianensis Aubl., Lauraceae 201
Ocotea opifera Mart., Lauraceae 201
Ocotea pretiosa
   (Nees & Mart.) Benth. & Hook., Lauraceae 201
Ouratea jabotapita Engl., Ochnaceae 261
Ouratea parviflora (DC.) Baill., Ochnaceae 261
Peperomia hederacea Miq., Piperaceae 273
Petiveria alliacea L., Phytolaccaceae 271
Philodendron bipinnatifidum Schott, Araceae 36
Philodendron hederaceum
   (Jacq.) Schott var. hederaceum, Araceae 36
Philodendron imbe Schott, Araceae 36
Philodendron ochrostemon Schott, Araceae 37
Philodendron pedatum (Hook.) Kunth, Araceae 37
Philodendron speciosum Schott, Araceae 37
Physalis angulata L., Solanaceae 318
Piper arboreum Aubl., Piperaceae 274
Piper callosum R. & Pav., Piperaceae 274
Piper colubrinum Link, Piperaceae 275
Pisonia aculeata L., Nyctaginaceae 258
Polygonum hydropiperoides
   Michx., Polygonaceae 286
Polygonum spectabile Mart., Polygonaceae 287
Protium icicariba (DC.) March., Burseraceae 94
Pteridium aquilinum (L.) Kuhn, Dennstaedtiaceae . 144
Pterodon apparicioi Peders., Fabaceae 170
Pterodon pubescens Benth., Fabaceae 171
Ptychopetalum olacoides Benth., Olacaceae 262
Raphia taedigera (Mart.) Mart., Arecaceae 45
Saccoglottis guianensis Benth., Humiriaceae 185
Salacia impressifolia
   (Miers) A.C. Sm., Hippocrateaceae 183
Salpichroa origanifolia (Lam.) Thell., Solanaceae 319
Schinus lentiscifolius March., Anacardiaceae 9
Schinus molle L., Anacardiaceae 9
Seguieria americana L., Phytolaccaceae 272
Senna alata (L.) Roxb., Caesalpiniaceae 104
Siparuna laurifolia (H.B.K.) DC., Monimiaceae ... 246
Smilax campestris Gris., Liliaceae 208
Smilax longifolia Rich. (includes S. brasiliensis
   Spreng.), Liliaceae 208
Sparattosperma leucanthum
   (Vell.) K. Sch., Bignoniaceae 82

RHEUMATISM – SCURVY: MEDICINAL INDEX

Symphonia globulifera L. f., Clusiaceae 123
Tabebuia serratifolia (Vahl) Nichol., Bignoniaceae .. 83
Tagetes erecta L., Asteraceae 67
Tagetes minuta L., Asteraceae 67
Tillandsia usneoides L., Bromeliaceae 91
Torrubia olfersiana
 (Link, Klotzsch & Otto) Standl., Nyctaginaceae ... 258
Tournefortia elegans Cham., Boraginaceae 89
Tovomita brasiliensis (Mart.) Walp., Clusiaceae 123
Tradescantia effusa Mart., Commelinaceae 129
Trichilia catigua Juss., Meliaceae 229
Virola macrophylla
 (Spr. ex Benth.) Warb., Myristicaceae 250
Virola oleifera (Schott) A.C. Smith, Myristicaceae . 250
Vismia guianensis (Aubl.) Choisy, Clusiaceae 124
Vitex agnus-castus L., Verbenaceae 336
Vitex gardneriana Schauer, Verbenaceae 336
Wilbrandia ebracteata Cogn., Cucurbitaceae 140
Wilbrandia verticillata
 (Vell.) Cogn.,Cucurbitaceae 140
Xylopia frutescens Aubl., Annonaceae 16

Rickets. See Rachitism, Scurvy

Ringworm
Arrabidaea chica (H.B.K.) Bur., Bignoniaceae 78
Caraipa grandifolia Mart., Clusiaceae 121
Carapa guianensis Aubl., Meliaceae 227
Crotalaria verrucosa L., Fabaceae 163
Fevillea trilobata L., Cucurbitaceae 136
Fevillea uncipetala Kuhlm., Cucurbitaceae 138
Himatanthus lancifolia
 (M. Arg.) Woods., Apocynaceae 26
Porophyllum ruderale (Jacq.) Cass., Asteraceae 64
Rauwolfia blanchetii DC., Apocynaceae 28
Seguieria americana L., Phytolaccaceae 272
Sorocea bonplandii (Baill.) Burger, Moraceae 249
Tabebuia impetiginosa
 (Mart.) Standl., Bignoniaceae 83
Urospatha caudata
 (Poepp. & Endl.) Schott, Araceae 37
Vatairea guianensis Aubl., Fabaceae 172
Vismia latifolia (Aubl.) Choisy, Clusiaceae 124
Xyris laxifolia Mart., Xyridaceae 342
Xyris pallida Mart., Xyridaceae 342

Rosemary Substitute
Heterothalamus alienus (Spr.) O. Ktze., Asteraceae 60

Rubefacient
Buchnera aquatica Aubl., Scrophulariaceae 310
Clematis denticulata Vell., Ranunculaceae 290
Clematis dioica L., Ranunculaceae 290
Cleome spinosa Jacq., Capparaceae 112
Hura crepitans L., Euphorbiaceae 153
Jatropha multifida L., Euphorbiaceae 154
Mikania lindleyana DC., Asteraceae 62
Monstera adansonii Schott, Araceae 36

S

Salivation
Canna glauca L., Cannaceae 110
Crotalaria verrucosa L., Fabaceae 163

Scabies
Allamanda cathartica L., Apocynaceae 20

Aristolochia esperanzae
 O. Kuntze, Aristolochiaceae 48
Caraipa densifolia Mart., Clusiaceae 121
Caraipa grandifolia Mart., Clusiaceae 121
Dracontium asperum K. Koch, Araceae 35
Lantana camara L., Verbenaceae 334
Leiothrix flavescens (Bong.) Ruhl., Eriocaulaceae .. 148
Macairea radula (Bonpl.) DC., Melastomataceae .. 225
Momordica charantia L., Cucurbitaceae 139
Pisonia cordifolia Mart., Nyctaginaceae 258
Rauwolfia blanchetii DC., Apocynaceae 28
Tabebuia impetiginosa
 (Mart.) Standl., Bignoniaceae 83

Scalp Conditions. See also Dandruff
Dipteryx odorata (Aubl.) Willd., Fabaceae 166
Ludwigia repens (L.) Hara, Onagraceae 264
Senna septentrionalis
 (Viv.) Ir. & Barn., Caesalpiniaceae 106
Zanthoxylum pterota H.B.K., Rutaceae 303

Schistosomiasis (Bilharzia).
See also Anthelmintic
Pterodon apparicioi
 Peders., Fabaceae (CHEM. & PHARM.) 170
Pterodon pubescens Benth., Fabaceae
 (CHEM. & PHARM.) 171

Sciatica
Brasilopuntia brasiliensis
 (Willd.) Berg., Cactaceae 95

Scrofula
Albizzia lebbeck (L.) Benth., Mimosaceae 236
Calolisianthus pendulus
 (Mart.) Gilg, Gentianaceae 179
Clematis dioica L., Ranunculaceae 290
Mimosa pudica L., Mimosaceae 240
Mimosa velloziana Mart., Mimosaceae 240
Pradosia lactescens (Vell.) Radlk., Sapotaceae 310
Smilax longifolia Rich. (includes S. brasiliensis
 Spreng.), Liliaceae 208
Xanthium orientale L., X. spinosum L.
 & X. strumarium L., Asteraceae 67

Scurvy. See also Rachitism
Anacardium occidentale L., Anacardiaceae 7
Begonia acida Mart., Begoniaceae 75
Berberis laurina Thunb., Berberidaceae 76
Bidens graveolens Mart., Asteraceae 56
Bidens pilosa L., Asteraceae 57
Cereus jamacaru DC., Cactaceae 95
Cereus peruvianus (L.) Mill., Cactaceae 95
Croton floribundus Spreng., Euphorbiaceae 150
Cinnamodendron axillare
 (Nees & Mart.) Endl., Canellaceae 110
Cleome polygama L., Capparaceae 112
Drimys winteri Forst., Winteraceae 340
Hylocereus undatus (Haw.) Br. & Rose, Cactaceae .. 95
Lophophytum mirabile
 Schott & Endl., Balanophoraceae 73
Melocactus melocactoides (Hoffm.) DC., Cactaceae . 97
Oxalis cordata St.-Hil., Oxalidaceae 266
Rollinia orthopetala DC., Annonaceae 15
Samolus valerandi L., Primulaceae 290
Sesuvium portulacastrum L., Aizoaceae 1
Tetracera aspera Willd., Dilleniaceae 146

MEDICINAL INDEX: SCURVY – SKIN DISEASE

Trianosperma glandulosa Mart., Cucurbitaceae 140
Trianosperma trilobata Cogn., Cucurbitaceae 140
Tropaeolum pentaphyllum Lam., Tropaeolaceae 327

Sedative, including Nerve Sedative
Acosmium dasycarpum (Vog.) Yakovl., Fabaceae .. 162
Acosmium subelegans
  (Mohlenb.) Yakovl., Fabaceae 162
Carica papaya L., Caricaceae 113
Cestrum calycinum Willd., Solanaceae 317
Datura suaveolens Humb. & Bonpl., Solanaceae ... 318
Erythrina corallodendron L., Fabaceae 166
Euphorbia hirta
  L., Euphorbiaceae (CHEM. & PHARM.) 152
Ficus trigona L. f., Moraceae 249
Hylocereus undatus (Haw.) Br. & Rose, Cactaceae .. 95
Indigofera suffruticosa Mill., Fabaceae 168
Kalanchoe pinnata (Lam.) Pers., Crassulaceae 133
Lepismium myosurus Pfeiff., Cactaceae 96
Mimosa verrucosa Benth., Mimosaceae 240
Nicandra physaloides (L.) Gaertn., Solanaceae 318
Opuntia vulgaris Mill., Cactaceae 97
Passiflora alata Dryand., Passifloraceae 267
Passiflora edulis Sims, Passifloraceae 269
Peltodon radicans Pohl, Lamiaceae 195
Piper tuberculatum Jacq., Piperaceae 276
Porophyllum ruderale (Jacq.) Cass., Asteraceae 64
Rhipsalis macrocarpa Miq., Cactaceae 97
Solanum nigrum L., Solanaceae 321
Tagetes erecta L., Asteraceae 67
Tibouchina aspera Aubl., Melastomataceae 226
Torresea cearensis Fr. All., Fabaceae 172

Senna Substitute
Chamaecrista fasciculata
  (Michx.) Greene, Caesalpiniaceae 102
Senna alata (L.) Roxb., Caesalpiniaceae 104
Senna uniflora
  (P. Miller) Ir. & Barn., Caesalpiniaceae 106

Sexual Impotence
Eryngium foetidum L., Apiaceae 19

Sexually Transmitted Disease. *See* Blennorrhagia, Gonorrhoea, HIV-1, Syphilis, Venereal Disease, Shingles

Shingles
Caraipa excelsa Ducke, Clusiaceae 121

Sialagogue
Anchietea pyrifolia (Mart.) G. Don, Violaceae 338
Bidens pilosa L., Asteraceae 57
Ottonia jaborandi (Vell.) Kunth, Piperaceae 272
Pilocarpus pinnatifolius Lem., Rutaceae 302
Piper ceanothifolium H.B.K., Piperaceae 275
Piper marginatum Jacq., Piperaceae 275
Piper reticulatum L., Piperaceae 276

Sinapism (Mustard Plaster). *See also* Poultice
Capparis urens B. Rodr., Capparaceae 111
Polygonum hydropiperoides
  Michx., Polygonaceae 26

Sinusitis
Jatropha curcas L., Euphorbiaceae 154
Luffa operculata (L.) Cogn., Cucurbitaceae 138

Skin Disease. *See also* Dartre, Eczema, Erysipelas, Exanthema,

Leishmaniasis, Pityriasis, Prurigo, Psoriasis, Ringworm, Scabies, Tinea, Ulcers, Vitiligo, Yaws
Albizzia lebbeck (L.) Benth., Mimosaceae 236
Alternanthera achyrantha R. Br., Amaranthaceae 3
Anacardium humile St.-Hil., Anacardiaceae 7
Anacardium nanum St.-Hil., Anacardiaceae 7
Anacardium occidentale L., Anacardiaceae 7
Anchietea pyrifolia (Mart.) G. Don, Violaceae 338
Anemone decapetala L., Ranunculaceae 290
Apium sellowianum Wolf, Apiaceae 18
Aristolochia triangularis Cham., Aristolochiaceae ... 48
Arrabidaea chica (H.B.K.) Bur., Bignoniaceae 78
Baccharidastrum triplinerve
  (Less.) Cabr., Asteraceae 53
Bowdichia virgilioides H.B.K., Fabaceae 163
Bredemeyera floribunda Willd., Polygalaceae 283
Cabralea canjerana (Vell.) Mart., Meliaceae 227
Caraipa densifolia Mart., Clusiaceae 121
Caraipa insidiosa B. Rodr., Clusiaceae 121
Caraipa silvatica B. Rodr., Clusiaceae 121
Casearia inaequilatera Camb., Flacourtiaceae 178
Cassia grandis L., Caesalpiniaceae 101
Cayaponia tayuya (Mart.) Cogn., Cucurbitaceae 135
Cereus jamacaru DC., Cactaceae 95
Cestrum calycinum Willd., Solanaceae 317
Cestrum parqui L'Herit., Solanaceae 317
Chaptalia nutans (L.) Polak., Asteraceae 57
Clarisia racemosa Ruiz & Pav., Moraceae 247
Clematis dioica L., Ranunculaceae 290
Clibadium surinamense L., Asteraceae 58
Commelina nudiflora L., Commelinaceae 126
Copaifera officinalis (Jacq.) L., Caesalpiniaceae 102
Copernicia prunifera (Mill.) H. Moore, Arecaceae . 40
Crescentia cujete L., Bignoniaceae 80
Crotalaria verrucosa L., Fabaceae 163
Cybianthus detergens Mart., Myrsinaceae 253
Desmoncus orthacanthos Mart., Arecaceae 40
Dorstenia brasiliensis Lam., Moraceae 247
Dorstenia cayapia Vell., Moraceae 248
Echinodorus grandiflorus
  (Cham. & Schl.) Mich., Alismataceae 2
Echinodorus macrophyllus
  (Kunth) Mich., Alismataceae 2
Echinodorus pubescens Mart., Alismataceae 2
Guarea spiciflora Juss., Meliaceae 227
Guazuma ulmifolia Lam. var. *tomentella* Schum.,
  var. *ulmifolia*, Sterculiaceae 323
Heliotropium indicum L., Boraginaceae 89
Herreria salsaparilha Mart., Liliaceae 207
Himatanthus lancifolia
  (M. Arg.) Woods., Apocynaceae 26
Hymenaea courbaril L., Caesalpiniaceae 103
Ipomoea acetosifolia
  (Vahl) Roem. & Schult., Convolvulaceae 130
Jacaranda brasiliana (Lam.) Pers., Bignoniaceae ... 80
Jacaranda caroba (Vell.) DC., Bignoniaceae 80
Jacaranda copaia (Aubl.) D. Don, Bignoniaceae 80
Julocroton stipularis M. Arg., Euphorbiaceae 155
Macairea radula (Bonpl.) DC., Melastomataceae .. 225
Mammea americana L., Clusiaceae 123
Maytenus ilicifolia Mart., Celastraceae 115

Echinodorus macrophyllus
  (Kunth) Mich., Alismataceae 2
Mikania parviflora (Aubl.) Karst., Asteraceae 62
Rachitism (Rickets). *See also* **Scurvy**
Lophophytum mirabile
  Schott & Endl., Balanophoraceae 73
Radiation Burns
Stryphnodendron adstringens
  (Mart.) Cov., Mimosaceae 242
Recovery after illness
Bathysa cuspidata Hook., Rubiaceae 296
Rectal Prolapse
Blepharocalyx salicifolius
  (H.B.K.) Berg, Myrtaceae 253
Oxalis corniculata L., Oxalidaceae 266
Simaba ferruginea St.-Hil., Simaroubaceae 314
Refreshant
Attalea spectabilis Mart., Arecaceae 39
Craniolaria annua L., Martyniaceae 224
Hedyosmum brasiliense Mart., Chloranthaceae 119
Ilex paraguariensis St.-Hil., Aquifoliaceae 31
Mauritiella aculeata (Kunth) Burret, Arecaceae 43
Regeneration of Tissue
Mabea fistulifera Mart., Euphorbiaceae 155
Renal Disorders. *See* **Colic (Renal),**
  Kidney Disease, Kidney Stones,
  Lithiasis, Urinary Problems
Resolvent
Amaranthus viridis L., Amaranthaceae 3
Anisolobus cururu (Mart.) M. Arg., Apocynaceae 21
Annona dioica St.-Hil., Annonaceae 12
Annona reticulata L., Annonaceae 13
Bidens cynapiifolia H.B.K., Asteraceae 56
Cissampelos ovalifolia DC., Menispermaceae 233
Cissampelos sympodialis Eichl., Menispermaceae . 233
Clusia rosea Jacq., Clusiaceae 122
Cochlospermum regium
  (Mart. & Schl.) Pilg., Cochlospermaceae 125
Costus spiralis (Jacq.) Roscoe, Costaceae 132
Cydista aequinoctialis Miers, Bignoniaceae 80
Echites macrocalyx M. Arg., Apocynaceae 23
Elephantopus mollis H.B.K., Asteraceae 59
Ficus gomelleira Kunth & Bouché, Moraceae 248
Heliotropium elongatum Willd., Boraginaceae 88
Heliotropium indicum L., Boraginaceae 89
Imperata brasiliensis Trin., also
  Imperata contracta Hitch., Poaceae 281
Kielmeyera coriacea Mart., Clusiaceae 122
Mabea fistulifera Mart., Euphorbiaceae 155
Machaerium ferox (Mart.) Ducke, Fabaceae 168
Mammea americana L., Clusiaceae 123
Momordica charantia L., Cucurbitaceae 139
Monnieria trifolia Loefl., Rutaceae 302
Ocotea opifera Mart., Lauraceae 201
Parahancornia amapa (Hub.) Ducke, Apocynaceae 27
Parthenium hysterophorus L., Asteraceae 64
Periandra mediterranea (Vell.) Taub., Fabaceae ... 170
Philodendron speciosum Schott, Araceae 37
Physalis angulata L., Solanaceae 318
Piper angustifolium R. & Pav., Piperaceae 274
Piper mollicomum Kunth, Piperaceae 276
Rumex brasiliensis Link, Polygonaceae 287

Schrankia leptocarpa DC., Mimosaceae 242
Senna latifolia
  (Meyer) Ir. & Barn., Caesalpiniaceae 105
Sicyos polyacanthus Cogn., Cucurbitaceae 139
Sterculia chicha St.-Hil., Sterculiaceae 324
Urera baccifera Gaud., Urticaceae 331
Virola surinamensis (Rol.) Warb., Myristicaceae 252
Vismia guianensis (Aubl.) Choisy, Clusiaceae 124
Xanthium orientale L., *X. spinosum* L.
  & *X. strumarium* L., Asteraceae 67
Respiratory Problems. *See also* **Asthma**
Anadenanthera colubrina
  (Vell.) Brenan, Mimosaceae 236
Bidens pilosa L., Asteraceae 57
Cecropia hololeuca Miq., Moraceae 247
Crescentia cujete L., Bignoniaceae 80
Dorstenia asaroides Gardn., Moraceae 247
Hyptis fasciculata Benth., Lamiaceae 192
Mikania periplocifolia Hook. & Arn., Asteraceae 62
Myrocarpus frondosus Fr. All., Fabaceae 170
Operculina alata (Ham.) Urb., Convolvulaceae 131
Operculina macrocarpa Urb., Convolvulaceae 131
Passiflora edulis Sims, Passifloraceae 269
Phlebodium aureum
  (L.) J.E. Smith, Polypodiaceae 288
Vochysia thyrsoidea Pohl, Vochysiaceae 340
Restorative
Heterothalamus alienus (Spr.) O. Ktze., Asteraceae 60
Parkinsonia aculeata L., Caesalpiniaceae 104
Revulsant
Cleome aculeata L., Capparaceae 112
Rhatany Substitute
Krameria argentea Mart., Krameriaceae 191
Krameria spartioides Berg, Krameriaceae 191
Krameria tomentosa St.-Hil., Krameriaceae 191
Rheumatism
Acacia paniculata Willd., Mimosaceae 236
Ageratum conyzoides L., Asteraceae 53
Agonandra brasiliensis Miers, Opiliaceae 265
Aiovea meissneri Mez, Lauraceae 197
Andradea floribunda Fr. All., Nyctaginaceae 257
Aniba permollis (Nees) Mez, Lauraceae 197
Annona dioica St.-Hil., Annonaceae 12
Annona foetida Mart., Annonaceae 12
Annona glabra L., Annonaceae 13
Annona spinescens Mart., Annonaceae 13
Annona squamosa L., Annonaceae 13
Attalea spectabilis Mart., Arecaceae 39
Baccharis dentata (Vell.) G.M. Barroso, Asteraceae 54
Baccharis notosergila Gris., Asteraceae 54
Baccharis trimera (Less.) DC., Asteraceae 54
Bactris insignis (Mart.) Baill., Arecaceae 39
Bauhinia rutilans Spr. ex Benth., Caesalpiniaceae ... 99
Bignonia exoleta Vell., Bignoniaceae 79
Bowdichia virgilioides H.B.K., Fabaceae 163
Brunfelsia uniflora (Pohl) D. Don, also
  B. grandiflora D. Don, Solanaceae 316
Buchnera aquatica Aubl., Scrophulariaceae 310
Bulbostylis capillaris Clarke, Cyperaceae 142
Calolisianthus pendulus
  (Mart.) Gilg, Gentianaceae 179
Calonyction aculeatum
  (L.) House, Convolvulaceae 129

MEDICINAL INDEX: RHEUMATISM

Calophyllum brasiliense Camb., Clusiaceae 120
Calotropis procera (Ait.) Ait. f., Asclepiadaceae 50
Canna gigantea Desf., Cannaceae 110
Canna glauca L., Cannaceae 110
Canna indica L., Cannaceae 111
Capparis urens B. Rodr., Capparaceae 111
Caraipa grandifolia Mart., Clusiaceae 121
Caraipa minor Huber, Clusiaceae 121
Carapa guianensis Aubl., Meliaceae 217
Casearia sylvestris Sw., Flacourtiaceae 178
Cayaponia tayuya (Mart.) Cogn., Cucurbitaceae 135
Cestrum calycinum Willd., Solanaceae 317
Cestrum parqui L'Herit., Solanaceae 317
Cissus palmata Poir., Vitaceae 339
Clematis denticulata Vell., Ranunculaceae 290
Cleome gigantea L., Capparaceae 112
Clusia rosea Jacq., Clusiaceae 122
Cochlospermum regium
  (Mart. & Schl.) Pilg., Cochlospermaceae 125
Commelina nudiflora L., Commelinaceae 126
Commelina vestita Seub., Commelinaceae 128
Copaifera cearensis
  Huber ex Ducke, Caesalpiniaceae 102
Copernicia prunifera (Mill.) H. Moore, Arecaceae .. 40
Cordia coffeoides Warm., Boraginaceae 87
Cordyline dracaenoides Kunth, Liliaceae 207
Crataeva benthamii Eichl., Capparaceae 112
Cyrtocymura scorpioides
  (Lam.) H. Robinson, Asteraceae 58
Dodonaea viscosa Jacq., Sapindaceae 305
Dorstenia brasiliensis Lam., Moraceae 247
Dorstenia cayapia Vell., Moraceae 248
Duguetia riparia Hub., Annonaceae 14
Echinodorus macrophyllus
  (Kunth) Mich., Alismataceae 2
Elaeis oleifera (H.B.K.) Cortez, Arecaceae 40
Elephantopus mollis H.B.K., Asteraceae 59
Elionurus bilinguis (Trin.) Hack., Poaceae 281
Ephedra triandra Tul., Ephedraceae 148
Erythrina crista-galli L., Fabaceae 166
Erythrina fusca Lour., Fabaceae 166
Eugenia brasiliensis Lam., Myrtaceae 253
Eugenia uniflora L., Myrtaceae 254
Fevillea trilobata L., Cucurbitaceae 136
Ficus gomelleira Kunth & Bouché, Moraceae 248
Gallesia gorazema (Vell.) Moq., Phytolaccaceae ... 271
Guarea trichilioides L., Meliaceae 227
Hancornia speciosa Gomes, Apocynaceae 24
Herreria salsaparilha Mart., Liliaceae 207
Himatanthus sucuuba (Spr.) Woods., Apocynaceae . 26
Hura crepitans L., Euphorbiaceae 153
Hydrocotyle bonariensis Lam., Apiaceae 19
Hydrocotyle leucocephala
  Cham. & Schlecht., Apiaceae 20
Ipomoea pes-caprae (L.) R. Br., Convolvulaceae .. 130
Jatropha elliptica (Pohl) M. Arg., Euphorbiaceae .. 154
Jatropha gossypiifolia L., Euphorbiaceae 154
Lantana camara L., Verbenaceae 33
Lantana microphylla Cham., also *L. mixta* L.,
  L. pseudothea (St.-Hil.) Schauer, Verbenaceae 335
Leonotis nepetaefolia R. Br., Lamiaceae 194
Licaria canella (Meissn.) Kosterm., Lauraceae 199

Limonium brasiliense
  (Boiss.) O. Ktze., Plumbaginaceae 278
Lithraea molleoides (Vell.) Engl., Anacardiaceae 9
Macfadyena unguis-cati (L.) Gentry, Bignoniaceae . 81
Marsypianthes chamaedrys
  (Vahl) O. Ktze., Lamiaceae 194
Maytenus laevis Reiss., Celastraceae 115
Melothrianthus smilacifolius
  (Cogn.) M. Crovetto, Cucurbitaceae 139
Mikania cordifolia (L. f.) Willd., Asteraceae 61
Mikania hirsutissima DC., Asteraceae 62
Mikania parviflora (Aubl.) Karst., Asteraceae 62
Mimosa malacocentra Mart., Mimosaceae 239
Mimosa pudica L., Mimosaceae 240
Mimosa velloziana Mart., Mimosaceae 240
Momordica charantia L., Cucurbitaceae 139
Monstera adansonii Schott, Araceae 36
Montrichardia linifera (Arruda) Schott, Araceae 36
Ocimum fluminensis Vell., Lamiaceae 195
Ocotea guianensis Aubl., Lauraceae 201
Ocotea opifera Mart., Lauraceae 201
Ocotea pretiosa
  (Nees & Mart.) Benth. & Hook., Lauraceae 201
Ouratea jabotapita Engl., Ochnaceae 261
Ouratea parviflora (DC.) Baill., Ochnaceae 261
Peperomia hederacea Miq., Piperaceae 273
Petiveria alliacea L., Phytolaccaceae 271
Philodendron bipinnatifidum Schott, Araceae 36
Philodendron hederaceum
  (Jacq.) Schott var. *hederaceum*, Araceae 36
Philodendron imbe Schott, Araceae 36
Philodendron ochrostemon Schott, Araceae 37
Philodendron pedatum (Hook.) Kunth, Araceae 37
Philodendron speciosum Schott, Araceae 37
Physalis angulata L., Solanaceae 318
Piper arboreum Aubl., Piperaceae 274
Piper callosum R. & Pav., Piperaceae 274
Piper colubrinum Link, Piperaceae 275
Pisonia aculeata L., Nyctaginaceae 258
Polygonum hydropiperoides
  Michx., Polygonaceae 286
Polygonum spectabile Mart., Polygonaceae 287
Protium icicariba (DC.) March., Burseraceae 94
Pteridium aquilinum (L.) Kuhn, Dennstaedtiaceae . 144
Pterodon apparicioi Peders., Fabaceae 170
Pterodon pubescens Benth., Fabaceae 171
Ptychopetalum olacoides Benth., Olacaceae 262
Raphia taedigera (Mart.) Mart., Arecaceae 45
Saccoglottis guianensis Benth., Humiriaceae 185
Salacia impressifolia
  (Miers) A.C. Sm., Hippocrateaceae 183
Salpichroa origanifolia (Lam.) Thell., Solanaceae 319
Schinus lentiscifolius March., Anacardiaceae 9
Schinus molle L., Anacardiaceae 9
Seguieria americana L., Phytolaccaceae 272
Senna alata (L.) Roxb., Caesalpiniaceae 104
Siparuna laurifolia (H.B.K.) DC., Monimiaceae ... 246
Smilax campestris Gris., Liliaceae 208
Smilax longifolia Rich. (includes *S. brasiliensis*
  Spreng.), Liliaceae 208
Sparattosperma leucanthum
  (Vell.) K. Sch., Bignoniaceae 82

Symphonia globulifera L. f., Clusiaceae 123
Tabebuia serratifolia (Vahl) Nichol., Bignoniaceae .. 83
Tagetes erecta L., Asteraceae 67
Tagetes minuta L., Asteraceae 67
Tillandsia usneoides L., Bromeliaceae 91
Torrubia olfersiana
  (Link, Klotzsch & Otto) Standl., Nyctaginaceae ... 258
Tournefortia elegans Cham., Boraginaceae 89
Tovomita brasiliensis (Mart.) Walp., Clusiaceae 123
Tradescantia effusa Mart., Commelinaceae 129
Trichilia catigua Juss., Meliaceae 229
Virola macrophylla
  (Spr. ex Benth.) Warb., Myristicaceae 250
Virola oleifera (Schott) A.C. Smith, Myristicaceae .. 250
Vismia guianensis (Aubl.) Choisy, Clusiaceae 124
Vitex agnus-castus L., Verbenaceae 336
Vitex gardneriana Schauer, Verbenaceae 336
Wilbrandia ebracteata Cogn., Cucurbitaceae 140
Wilbrandia verticillata
  (Vell.) Cogn.,Cucurbitaceae 140
Xylopia frutescens Aubl., Annonaceae 16

Rickets. *See* **Rachitism, Scurvy**

Ringworm
Arrabidaea chica (H.B.K.) Bur., Bignoniaceae 78
Caraipa grandifolia Mart., Clusiaceae 121
Carapa guianensis Aubl., Meliaceae 227
Crotalaria verrucosa L., Fabaceae 163
Fevillea trilobata L., Cucurbitaceae 136
Fevillea uncipetala Kuhlm., Cucurbitaceae 138
Himatanthus lancifolia
  (M. Arg.) Woods., Apocynaceae 26
Porophyllum ruderale (Jacq.) Cass., Asteraceae 64
Rauwolfia blanchetii DC., Apocynaceae 28
Seguieria americana L., Phytolaccaceae 272
Sorocea bonplandii (Baill.) Burger, Moraceae 249
Tabebuia impetiginosa
  (Mart.) Standl., Bignoniaceae 83
Urospatha caudata
  (Poepp. & Endl.) Schott, Araceae 37
Vatairea guianensis Aubl., Fabaceae 172
Vismia latifolia (Aubl.) Choisy, Clusiaceae 124
Xyris laxifolia Mart., Xyridaceae 342
Xyris pallida Mart., Xyridaceae 342

Rosemary Substitute
Heterothalamus alienus (Spr.) O. Ktze., Asteraceae 60

Rubefacient
Buchnera aquatica Aubl., Scrophulariaceae 310
Clematis denticulata Vell., Ranunculaceae 290
Clematis dioica L., Ranunculaceae 290
Cleome spinosa Jacq., Capparaceae 112
Hura crepitans L., Euphorbiaceae 153
Jatropha multifida L., Euphorbiaceae 154
Mikania lindleyana DC., Asteraceae 62
Monstera adansonii Schott, Araceae 36

S

Salivation
Canna glauca L., Cannaceae 110
Crotalaria verrucosa L., Fabaceae 163

Scabies
Allamanda cathartica L., Apocynaceae 20

Aristolochia esperanzae
  O. Kuntze, Aristolochiaceae 48
Caraipa densifolia Mart., Clusiaceae 121
Caraipa grandifolia Mart., Clusiaceae 121
Dracontium asperum K. Koch, Araceae 35
Lantana camara L., Verbenaceae 334
Leiothrix flavescens (Bong.) Ruhl., Eriocaulaceae .. 148
Macairea radula (Bonpl.) DC., Melastomataceae .. 225
Momordica charantia L., Cucurbitaceae 139
Pisonia cordifolia Mart., Nyctaginaceae 258
Rauwolfia blanchetii DC., Apocynaceae 28
Tabebuia impetiginosa
  (Mart.) Standl., Bignoniaceae 83

Scalp Conditions. *See also* **Dandruff**
Dipteryx odorata (Aubl.) Willd., Fabaceae 166
Ludwigia repens (L.) Hara, Onagraceae 264
Senna septentrionalis
  (Viv.) Ir. & Barn., Caesalpiniaceae 106
Zanthoxylum pterota H.B.K., Rutaceae 303

Schistosomiasis (Bilharzia).
See also **Anthelmintic**
Pterodon apparicioi
  Peders., Fabaceae (CHEM. & PHARM.) 170
Pterodon pubescens Benth., Fabaceae
  (CHEM. & PHARM.) 171

Sciatica
Brasilopuntia brasiliensis
  (Willd.) Berg., Cactaceae 95

Scrofula
Albizzia lebbeck (L.) Benth., Mimosaceae 236
Calolisianthus pendulus
  (Mart.) Gilg, Gentianaceae 179
Clematis dioica L., Ranunculaceae 290
Mimosa pudica L., Mimosaceae 240
Mimosa velloziana Mart., Mimosaceae 240
Pradosia lactescens (Vell.) Radlk., Sapotaceae 310
Smilax longifolia Rich. (includes *S. brasiliensis*
  Spreng.), Liliaceae 208
Xanthium orientale L., *X. spinosum* L.
  & *X. strumarium* L., Asteraceae 67

Scurvy. *See also* **Rachitism**
Anacardium occidentale L., Anacardiaceae 7
Begonia acida Mart., Begoniaceae 75
Berberis laurina Thunb., Berberidaceae 76
Bidens graveolens Mart., Asteraceae 56
Bidens pilosa L., Asteraceae 57
Cereus jamacaru DC., Cactaceae 95
Cereus peruvianus (L.) Mill., Cactaceae 95
Croton floribundus Spreng., Euphorbiaceae 150
Cinnamodendron axillare
  (Nees & Mart.) Endl., Canellaceae 110
Cleome polygama L., Capparaceae 112
Drimys winteri Forst., Winteraceae 340
Hylocereus undatus (Haw.) Br. & Rose, Cactaceae .. 95
Lophophytum mirabile
  Schott & Endl., Balanophoraceae 73
Melocactus melocactoides (Hoffm.) DC., Cactaceae . 97
Oxalis cordata St.-Hil., Oxalidaceae 266
Rollinia orthopetala DC., Annonaceae 15
Samolus valerandi L., Primulaceae 290
Sesuvium portulacastrum L., Aizoaceae 1
Tetracera aspera Willd., Dilleniaceae 146

MEDICINAL INDEX: SCURVY – SKIN DISEASE

Trianosperma glandulosa Mart., Cucurbitaceae 140
Trianosperma trilobata Cogn., Cucurbitaceae 140
Tropaeolum pentaphyllum Lam., Tropaeolaceae 327

Sedative, including Nerve Sedative
Acosmium dasycarpum (Vog.) Yakovl., Fabaceae .. 162
Acosmium subelegans
  (Mohlenb.) Yakovl., Fabaceae 162
Carica papaya L., Caricaceae 113
Cestrum calycinum Willd., Solanaceae 317
Datura suaveolens Humb. & Bonpl., Solanaceae ... 318
Erythrina corallodendron L., Fabaceae 166
Euphorbia hirta
  L., Euphorbiaceae (CHEM. & PHARM.) 152
Ficus trigona L. f., Moraceae 249
Hylocereus undatus (Haw.) Br. & Rose, Cactaceae .. 95
Indigofera suffruticosa Mill., Fabaceae 168
Kalanchoe pinnata (Lam.) Pers., Crassulaceae 133
Lepismium myosurus Pfeiff., Cactaceae 96
Mimosa verrucosa Benth., Mimosaceae 240
Nicandra physaloides (L.) Gaertn., Solanaceae 318
Opuntia vulgaris Mill., Cactaceae 97
Passiflora alata Dryand., Passifloraceae 267
Passiflora edulis Sims, Passifloraceae 269
Peltodon radicans Pohl, Lamiaceae 195
Piper tuberculatum Jacq., Piperaceae 276
Porophyllum ruderale (Jacq.) Cass., Asteraceae 64
Rhipsalis macrocarpa Miq., Cactaceae 97
Solanum nigrum L., Solanaceae 321
Tagetes erecta L., Asteraceae 67
Tibouchina aspera Aubl., Melastomataceae 226
Torresea cearensis Fr. All., Fabaceae 172

Senna Substitute
Chamaecrista fasciculata
  (Michx.) Greene, Caesalpiniaceae 102
Senna alata (L.) Roxb., Caesalpiniaceae 104
Senna uniflora
  (P. Miller) Ir. & Barn., Caesalpiniaceae 106

Sexual Impotence
Eryngium foetidum L., Apiaceae 19

Sexually Transmitted Disease. *See* Blennorrhagia, Gonorrhoea, HIV-1, Syphilis, Venereal Disease, Shingles

Shingles
Caraipa excelsa Ducke, Clusiaceae 121

Sialagogue
Anchietea pyrifolia (Mart.) G. Don, Violaceae 338
Bidens pilosa L., Asteraceae 57
Ottonia jaborandi (Vell.) Kunth, Piperaceae 272
Pilocarpus pinnatifolius Lem., Rutaceae 302
Piper ceanothifolium H.B.K., Piperaceae 275
Piper marginatum Jacq., Piperaceae 275
Piper reticulatum L., Piperaceae 276

Sinapism (Mustard Plaster). *See also* Poultice
Capparis urens B. Rodr., Capparaceae 111
Polygonum hydropiperoides
  Michx., Polygonaceae 26

Sinusitis
Jatropha curcas L., Euphorbiaceae 154
Luffa operculata (L.) Cogn., Cucurbitaceae 138

Skin Disease. *See also* Dartre, Eczema, Erysipelas, Exanthema,

Leishmaniasis, Pityriasis, Prurigo, Psoriasis, Ringworm, Scabies, Tinea, Ulcers, Vitiligo, Yaws
Albizzia lebbeck (L.) Benth., Mimosaceae 236
Alternanthera achyrantha R. Br., Amaranthaceae 3
Anacardium humile St.-Hil., Anacardiaceae 7
Anacardium nanum St.-Hil., Anacardiaceae 7
Anacardium occidentale L., Anacardiaceae 7
Anchietea pyrifolia (Mart.) G. Don, Violaceae 338
Anemone decapetala L., Ranunculaceae 290
Apium sellowianum Wolf, Apiaceae 18
Aristolochia triangularis Cham., Aristolochiaceae ... 48
Arrabidaea chica (H.B.K.) Bur., Bignoniaceae 78
Baccharidastrum triplinerve
  (Less.) Cabr., Asteraceae 53
Bowdichia virgilioides H.B.K., Fabaceae 163
Bredemeyera floribunda Willd., Polygalaceae 283
Cabralea canjerana (Vell.) Mart., Meliaceae 227
Caraipa densifolia Mart., Clusiaceae 121
Caraipa insidiosa B. Rodr., Clusiaceae 121
Caraipa silvatica B. Rodr., Clusiaceae 121
Casearia inaequilatera Camb., Flacourtiaceae 178
Cassia grandis L., Caesalpiniaceae 101
Cayaponia tayuya (Mart.) Cogn., Cucurbitaceae ... 135
Cereus jamacaru DC., Cactaceae 95
Cestrum calycinum Willd., Solanaceae 317
Cestrum parqui L'Herit., Solanaceae 317
Chaptalia nutans (L.) Polak., Asteraceae 57
Clarisia racemosa Ruiz & Pav., Moraceae 247
Clematis dioica L., Ranunculaceae 290
Clibadium surinamense L., Asteraceae 58
Commelina nudiflora L., Commelinaceae 126
Copaifera officinalis (Jacq.) L., Caesalpiniaceae 102
Copernicia prunifera (Mill.) H. Moore, Arecaceae . 40
Crescentia cujete L., Bignoniaceae 80
Crotalaria verrucosa L., Fabaceae 163
Cybianthus detergens Mart., Myrsinaceae 253
Desmoncus orthacanthos Mart., Arecaceae 40
Dorstenia brasiliensis Lam., Moraceae 247
Dorstenia cayapia Vell., Moraceae 248
Echinodorus grandiflorus
  (Cham. & Schl.) Mich., Alismataceae 2
Echinodorus macrophyllus
  (Kunth) Mich., Alismataceae 2
Echinodorus pubescens Mart., Alismataceae 2
Guarea spiciflora Juss., Meliaceae 227
Guazuma ulmifolia Lam. var. *tomentella* Schum.,
  var. *ulmifolia*, Sterculiaceae 323
Heliotropium indicum L., Boraginaceae 89
Herreria salsaparilha Mart., Liliaceae 207
Himatanthus lancifolia
  (M. Arg.) Woods., Apocynaceae 26
Hymenaea courbaril L., Caesalpiniaceae 103
Ipomoea acetosifolia
  (Vahl) Roem. & Schult., Convolvulaceae 130
Jacaranda brasiliana (Lam.) Pers., Bignoniaceae ... 80
Jacaranda caroba (Vell.) DC., Bignoniaceae 80
Jacaranda copaia (Aubl.) D. Don, Bignoniaceae 80
Julocroton stipularis M. Arg., Euphorbiaceae 155
Macairea radula (Bonpl.) DC., Melastomataceae .. 225
Mammea americana L., Clusiaceae 123
Maytenus ilicifolia Mart., Celastraceae 115

Melothrianthus smilacifolius
  (Cogn.) M. Crovetto, Cucurbitaceae 139
Mikania lindleyana DC., Asteraceae 62
Ocotea cymbarum H.B.K., Lauraceae 200
Operculina alata (Ham.) Urb., Convolvulaceae 131
Operculina macrocarpa Urb., Convolvulaceae 131
Paspalum extenuatum Nees, Poaceae 282
Passiflora amethystina Mikan, Passifloraceae 269
Passiflora caerulea L., Passifloraceae 269
Peltodon radicans Pohl, Lamiaceae 195
Pisonia cordifolia Mart., Nyctaginaceae 258
Platonia insignis Mart., Clusiaceae 123
Pontederia cordifolia Mart., Pontederiaceae 288
Portulaca grandiflora Hook., Portulacaceae 288
Ranunculus apiifolius Pers., Ranunculaceae 290
Ruellia tuberosa L., Acanthaceae 1
Schinus molle L., Anacardiaceae 9
Sebastiania macrocarpa M. Arg., Euphorbiaceae .. 157
Senna occidentalis (L.) Link, Caesalpiniaceae 105
Senna quinqueangulata
  (Rich.) Ir. & Barn.,Caesalpiniaceae 106
Smilax longifolia Rich. (includes
  S. brasiliensis Spreng.), Liliaceae 208
Solanum aculeatissimum Jacq., Solanaceae 319
Solanum cernuum Vell., Solanaceae 319
Stromanthe sanguinea Sond., Marantaceae 224
Tragia volubilis L., Euphorbiaceae 158
Vataireopsis araroba (Aguiar) Ducke, Fabaceae 172
Virola oleifera (Schott) A.C. Smith, Myristicaceae . 250
Vismia guianensis (Aubl.) Choisy, Clusiaceae 124
Vismia japurensis Reich., Clusiaceae 124
Vismia reichardtiana
  (O. Ktze.) Ewan, Clusiaceae 124
Zanthoxylum pterota H.B.K., Rutaceae 303
Zeyheria digitalis (Vell.) Hoehne, Bignoniaceae 84

Skin Eruptions
Hancornia speciosa Gomes, Apocynaceae 24

Skin Spot Remover
Caraipa excelsa Ducke, Clusiaceae 121
Caraipa grandifolia Mart., Clusiaceae 121
Clematis dioica L., Ranunculaceae 290
Vatairea guianensis Aubl., Fabaceae 172

Sleep Disorders. *See* Insomnia

Slimming (Weight Reduction)
Baccharis trimera (Less.) DC., Asteraceae 54
Cordia ecalyculata Vell., Boraginaceae 87
Cordia obscura Cham., Boraginaceae 88
Cordia salicifolia Cham., Boraginaceae 88
Ilex paraguariensis St.-Hil., Aquifoliaceae 31

Smallpox
Cocos nucifera L., Arecaceae 40

Snake Poison Antidote
Aristolochia birostris Duch., Aristolochiaceae 46
Mikania officinalis Mart., Asteraceae 62
Thevetia ahouai (L.) DC., Apocynaceae 28

Snakebite
Abuta rufescens Aubl., Menispermaceae 231
Alisma palaefolium Kunth, Alismataceae 2
Amaranthus spinosus L., Amaranthaceae 3
Anacampta riedellii (M. Arg.) Mgf., Apocynaceae ... 21
Annona crassifolia Mart., Annonaceae 12
Aristolochia elegans Mast., Aristolochiaceae 48

Ayapana triplinerve
  (Vahl) King & Robinson, Asteraceae 53
Boerhavia coccinea Mill., Nyctaginaceae 257
Bredemeyera floribunda Willd., Polygalaceae 283
Buddleja brasiliensis Jacq. ex Spr., Buddlejaceae 93
Byrsonima crassifolia H.B.K., Malpighiaceae 219
Caesalpinia bonduc (L.) Roxb., Caesalpiniaceae 99
Casearia cambessedesii Eichl., Flacourtiaceae 176
Casearia sylvestris Sw., Flacourtiaceae 178
Cereus peruvianus (L.) Mill., Cactaceae 94
Chiococca alba (L.) Hitch., Rubiaceae 297
Cissampelos glaberrima St.-Hil., Menispermaceae 233
Conocliniopsis prasiifolia
  (DC.) King & Robinson, Asteraceae 58
Craniolaria integrifolia Cham., Martyniaceae 224
Crataeva benthamii Eichl., Capparaceae 112
Cyperus gracilescens
  Roem. & Schult., Cyperaceae 142
Dieffenbachia seguine (Jacq.) Schott, Araceae 35
Dipladenia illustris M. Arg., Apocynaceae 23
Dorstenia asaroides Gardn., Moraceae 247
Dorstenia brasiliensis Lam., Moraceae 247
Dorstenia cayapia Vell., Moraceae 248
Dracontium asperum K. Koch, Araceae 35
Elephantopus mollis H.B.K., Asteraceae 59
Erythroxylum anguifugum Mart., Erythroxylaceae . 148
Euphorbia hirta L., Euphorbiaceae 152
Fevillea trilobata L., Cucurbitaceae 136
Heterothalamus psiadioides Less., Asteraceae 60
Himatanthus alba (L.) Woods., Apocynaceae 24
Indigofera suffruticosa Mill., Fabaceae 168
Isoetes martii A. Braun, Isoetaceae 189
Jatropha curcas L., Euphorbiaceae 154
Jatropha elliptica (Pohl) M. Arg., Euphorbiaceae .. 154
Lafoensia densiflora Pohl, Lythraceae 214
Macfadyena unguis-cati (L.) Gentry, Bignoniaceae . 81
Mandevilla velutina (Mart. ex Stadelm.) Woods.
  var. *velutina*, Apocynaceae 27
Maranta arundinacea L., Marantaceae 223
Marsypianthes chamaedrys
  (Vahl) O. Ktze., Lamiaceae 194
Mikania cordifolia (L. f.) Willd., Asteraceae 61
Mikania glomerata Spreng., Asteraceae 61
Mikania parviflora (Aubl.) Karst., Asteraceae 62
Monnieria trifolia Loefl., Rutaceae 302
Peltodon radicans Pohl, Lamiaceae 195
Pentaclethra macroloba
  (Willd.) O. Ktze., Mimosaceae 242
Pfaffia jubata Mart., Amaranthaceae 5
Piper ceanothifolium H.B.K., Piperaceae 275
Piper marginatum Jacq., Piperaceae 275
Plumeria alba L., Apocynaceae 28
Polygala paniculata L., Polygalaceae 284
Potalia amara Aubl., Loganiaceae 209
Selaginella stellata Spring, Selaginellaceae 313
Senna rugosa
  (G. Don) Ir. & Barn., Caesalpiniaceae 106
Triplaris macrocalyx Casar., Polygonaceae 286
Virola oleifera (Schott) A.C. Smith, Myristicaceae . 250
Xylopia frutescens Aubl., Annonaceae 16

Soothing
Buddleja brasiliensis Jacq. ex Spr., Buddlejaceae 93
Protium icicariba (DC.) March., Burseraceae 94

Soporific

Acosmium dasycarpum (Vog.) Yakovl., Fabaceae .. 162
Acosmium subelegans
  (Mohlenb.) Yakovl., Fabaceae 162
Aloysia triphylla (L'Her.) Britt., Verbenaceae 332
Brunfelsia uniflora (Pohl) D. Don, also
  B. grandiflora D. Don, Solanaceae 316
Buchnera virgata H.B.K., Scrophulariaceae 310
Croton zehntneri Pax & Hoffm., Euphorbiaceae 151
Cymbopogon schoenanthus (L.) Spreng., Poaceae 280
Erythrina crista-galli L., Fabaceae 166
Erythrina fusca Lour., Fabaceae 166
Passiflora alata Dryand., Passifloraceae 267

Sore Throat. *See* Throat Conditions

Sores. *See also* Breast Sores, Ulcers

Amasonia arborea H.B.K., Verbenaceae 333
Bidens pilosa L., Asteraceae 57
Bromelia arenaria Ule, Bromeliaceae 91
Caesalpinia ferrea Mart. ex Tul., Caesalpiniaceae . 100
Campsiandra comosa Benth.
  var. *laurifolia* (Benth.) Cowan, Caesalpiniaceae ... 100
Cedrela fissilis Vell., Meliaceae 227
Chaptalia nutans (L.) Polak., Asteraceae 57
Costus spiralis (Jacq.) Roscoe, Costaceae 132
Curatella americana L., Dilleniaceae 144
Cuscuta racemosa Mart., Convolvulaceae 130
Dipteryx odorata (Aubl.) Willd., Fabaceae 166
Dracontium asperum K. Koch, Araceae 35
Genipa americana L., Rubiaceae 298
Hibiscus tiliaceus L., Malvaceae 221
Humiria balsamifera (Aubl.) St.-Hil., Humiriaceae 183
Inga lateriflora Miq., Mimosaceae 237
Lagenaria siceraria
  (Molina) Standl., Cucurbitaceae 138
Phthirusa adunca
  (Meyer) Maguire, Loranthaceae 211
Piper angustifolium R. & Pav., Piperaceae 274
Pithecellobium unguis-cati
  (L.) Benth., Mimosaceae 242
Portulaca pilosa L., Portulacaceae 289
Pothomorphe umbellata (L.) Miq., Piperaceae 277
Senna latifolia
  (Meyer) Ir. & Barn., Caesalpiniaceae 105
Stryphnodendron adstringens
  (Mart.) Cov., Mimosaceae 242
Thalia geniculata L., Marantaceae 224
Virola oleifera (Schott) A.C. Smith, Myristicaceae . 250
Xanthium orientale L., *X. spinosum* L.
  & *X. strumarium* L., Asteraceae 67
Zizyphus joazeiro Mart., Rhamnaceae 293

Sour

Bidens graveolens Mart., Asteraceae 56
Bromelia antiacantha Bertol., Bromeliaceae 91
Clematis campestris St.-Hil., Ranunculaceae 290
Renealmia occidentalis Sweet, also
  R. sylvestris Horan., Zingiberaceae 342

Spasmodic (Spasms). *See also* Angina

Aloysia triphylla (L'Her.) Britt., Verbenaceae 332
Angelonia integerrima Spreng., Scrophulariaceae .. 310
Aniba canelilla (H.B.K.) Mez, Lauraceae 197
Annona muricata L., Annonaceae 13
Arrabidaea chica (H.B.K.) Bur., Bignoniaceae 78

Bauhinia rutilans Spr. ex Benth., Caesalpiniaceae ... 99
Calyptranthes aromatica St.-Hil., Myrtaceae 253
Carica papaya L., Caricaceae (CHEM. & PHARM.) ... 113
Cestrum calycinum Willd., Solanaceae 317
Cunila microcephala Benth., Lamiaceae 192
Cyperus sesquiflorus
  (Torrey) Mattf. & Kükent., Cyperaceae 142
Dipladenia fragrans DC., Apocynaceae 23
Dipteryx odorata (Aubl.) Willd., Fabaceae 166
Dracontium polyphyllum L., Araceae 36
Drimys winteri Forst., Winteraceae 340
Eryngium foetidum L., Apiaceae 19
Erythrina verna Vell., Fabaceae 168
Euphorbia hirta
  L., Euphorbiaceae (CHEM. & PHARM.) 152
Gallesia gorazema (Vell.) Moq., Phytolaccaceae ... 271
Hypericum brasiliense Choisy, Clusiaceae 122
Hyptis atrorubens Poit., Lamiaceae 192
Hyptis fasciculata Benth., Lamiaceae 192
Hyptis suaveolens Poit., Lamiaceae 193
Indigofera suffruticosa Mill., Fabaceae 168
Lantana brasiliensis Link, Verbenaceae 334
Leonotis nepetaefolia R. Br., Lamiaceae 194
Leucas martinicensis (Jacq.) R. Br., Lamiaceae 194
Licaria camara (Schomb.) Kosterm., Lauraceae 198
Lippia alba (Mill.) N.E. Brown, Verbenaceae 335
Lithraea molleoides (Vell.) Engl., Anacardiaceae 9
Marsypianthes chamaedrys
  (Vahl) O. Ktze., Lamiaceae 194
Mollinedia schottiana (Spr.) Perk., Monimiaceae .. 245
Muntingia calabura L., Tiliaceae 327
Nectandra turbacensis Nees, Lauraceae 200
Ocimum micranthum Willd., Lamiaceae 195
Passiflora gardneri Mast., Passifloraceae 270
Passiflora macrocarpa Mast., Passifloraceae 270
Petiveria alliacea L., Phytolaccaceae 271
Piper marginatum Jacq., Piperaceae 275
Rollinia sylvatica (St.-Hil.) Mart., Annonaceae 15
Rumohra adiantiformis
  (G. Forst.) Ching, Dryopteridaceae 147
Schinus molle L., Anacardiaceae 9
Silybum marianum Gaertn., Asteraceae 65
Siparuna brasiliensis (Spr.) DC., Monimiaceae 245
Siparuna guianensis Aubl., Monimiaceae 245
Solanum nigrum L., Solanaceae 321
Spondias macrocarpa Engl., Anacardiaceae 10
Spondias mombin L., Anacardiaceae 10
Torresea cearensis Fr. All., Fabaceae 172
Virola oleifera (Schott) A.C. Smith, Myristicaceae . 250
Zanthoxylum rhoifolium Lam., Rutaceae 303

Spleen Conditions

Anisolobus cururu (Mart.) M. Arg., Apocynaceae 21
Ficus gomelleira Kunth & Bouché, Moraceae 248
Genipa americana L., Rubiaceae 298
Hackelochloa granularis (L.) O. Ktze., Poaceae ... 281
Pothomorphe umbellata (L.) Miq., Piperaceae 277
Strychnos pseudoquina St.-Hil., Loganiaceae 209

Sprains

Clusia rosea Jacq., Clusiaceae 122
Solidago chilensis Meyen, Asteraceae 65

Stimulant. *See also* Excitant

Acmella oleracea (L.) R.K. Jansen, Asteraceae 52

Acmella repens (Walt.) L.C. Rich., Asteraceae 52
Anacardium occidentale L., Anacardiaceae 7
Aristolochia triangularis Cham., Aristolochiaceae ... 48
Aristolochia trilobata L., Aristolochiaceae 48
Ayapana triplinerve
   (Vahl) King & Robinson, Asteraceae 53
Bidens pilosa L., Asteraceae 57
Calotropis procera (Ait.) Ait. f., Asclepiadaceae 50
Cecropia palmata Willd., Moraceae 247
Chaptalia nutans (L.) Polak., Asteraceae 57
Citronella congonha (Mart.) Howard, Icacinaceae . 185
Citronella mucronata
   (R. & Pav.) Don, Icacinaceae 186
Conyza blakei (Cabr.) Cabr., Asteraceae 58
Copaifera officinalis (Jacq.) L., Caesalpiniaceae 102
Cunila microcephala Benth., Lamiaceae 192
Cusparia febrifuga Humb., Rutaceae 300
Cyperus rotundus L., Cyperaceae 142
Cyperus sesquiflorus
   (Torrey) Mattf. & Kükent., Cyperaceae 142
Davilla rugosa Poir., Dilleniaceae 145
Dicypellium caryophyllatum
   Nees & Mart., Lauraceae 198
Dorstenia asaroides Gardn., Moraceae 247
Dorstenia brasiliensis Lam., Moraceae 247
Erythroxylum cataractarum
   Spruce, Erythroxylaceae 149
Erythroxylum coca Lam., Erythroxylaceae 149
Glandularia peruviana (L.) Small, Verbenaceae ... 334
Glechon spathulata Benth., Lamiaceae 192
Hedyosmum brasiliense Mart., Chloranthaceae 119
Hypericum teretiusculum St.-Hil., Clusiaceae 122
Hyptis crenata Pohl, Lamiaceae 192
Ilex paraguariensis St.-Hil., Aquifoliaceae 31
Lantana microphylla Cham., also *L. mixta* L.,
   L. pseudothea (St.-Hil.) Schauer, Verbenaceae 335
Licaria puchury-major
   (Mart.) Kosterm., Lauraceae 199
Mammea americana L., Clusiaceae 123
Maquira sclerophylla
   (Ducke) C. C. Berg, Moraceae 249
Maytenus gonoclada Mart., Celastraceae 115
Maytenus laevis Reiss., Celastraceae 115
Paullinia cupana Kunth, Sapindaceae 306
Peltodon longipes St.-Hil., Lamiaceae 195
Petiveria alliacea L., Phytolaccaceae 271
Phyllanthus nobilis M. Arg., Euphorbiaceae 157
Physalis pubescens L., Solanaceae 314
Piper aduncum L., Piperaceae 274
Piper tuberculatum Jacq., Piperaceae 276
Polygonum punctatum Elliot, Polygonaceae 287
Polygonum spectabile Mart., Polygonaceae 287
Protium icicariba (DC.) March., Burseraceae 94
Psoralea glandulosa L., Fabaceae 170
Schinus molle L., Anacardiaceae 9
Siparuna guianensis Aubl., Monimiaceae 245
Stachytarpheta cayennensis
   (Rich.) Vahl, Verbenaceae 335
Stachytarpheta jamaicensis
   (L.) Vahl, Verbenaceae 336
Tanacetum vulgare L., Asteraceae 67
Turnera diffusa Willd., Turneraceae 327
Turnera opifera Mart., Turneraceae 328

Vernonanthura brasiliana
   (L.) H. Robinson, Asteraceae 67
Waltheria communis St.-Hil., Sterculiaceae 325
Zanthoxylum hyemale St.-Hil., Rutaceae 302

Stings
Annona ambotay Aubl., Annonaceae 12
Arrabidaea foetida Bur. & K. Sch., Bignoniaceae 79
Bixa orellana L., Bixaceae 85
Bredemeyera floribunda Willd., Polygalaceae 283
Carapa guianensis Aubl., Meliaceae 227
Dieffenbachia seguine (Jacq.) Schott, Araceae 35
Heliotropium indicum L., Boraginaceae 89
Hyptis mutabilis (Rich.) Briq., Lamiaceae 193
Kalanchoe brasiliensis Camb., Crassulaceae 133
Mammea americana L., Clusiaceae 123
Marsypianthes chamaedrys
   (Vahl) O. Ktze., Lamiaceae 194
Ocimum micranthum Willd., Lamiaceae 195
Peltodon radicans Pohl, Lamiaceae 195
Selaginella stellata Spring, Selaginellaceae 313
Sida rhombifolia L., Malvaceae 222
Syagrus coronata (Mart.) Becc., Arecaceae 45

–ant
Arrabidaea foetida Bur. & K. Sch., Bignoniaceae 79

–scorpion
Arrabidaea foetida Bur. & K. Sch., Bignoniaceae 79
Mikania parviflora (Aubl.) Karst., Asteraceae 62

Stomach Problems.
***See also* Hyperacidity, Nausea**
Calea pinnatifida (R. Br.) Less., Asteraceae 57
Cayaponia tayuya (Mart.) Cogn., Cucurbitaceae ... 135
Cecropia leucocoma Miq., Moraceae 247
Chaptalia nutans (L.) Polak., Asteraceae 57
Chondodendron platyphyllum
   (Mart.) Miers, Menispermaceae 231
Croton hemiargyreus M. Arg., Euphorbiaceae 151
Croton sincorensis Mart., Euphorbiaceae 151
Croton spp., including *C. cascarilla*
   (L.) Bennet, *C. glabellus* L. & *C. paniculatus*
   M. Arg., Euphorbiaceae 152
Evolvulus alsinoides L., Convolvulaceae 130
Hyptis incana Briq., Lamiaceae 192
Jacaratia spinosa (Aubl.) A. DC., Caricaceae 113
Jodina rhombifolia Hook. & Arn., Santalaceae 304
Ludwigia suffruticosa (L.) Gomes, Onagraceae 264
Machaerium lunatum (L.) Ducke, Fabaceae 168
Mariscus jacquinii H.B.K., Cyperaceae 143
Mikania officinalis Mart., Asteraceae 62
Monopteryx uacu Spruce ex Benth., Fabaceae 169
Nectandra pichurim (H.B.K.) Mez, Lauraceae 200
Pfaffia jubata Mart., Amaranthaceae 5
Strychnos pseudoquina St.-Hil., Loganiaceae 209
Strychnos trinervis (Vell.) Mart., Loganiaceae 210
Tanaecium nocturnum
   (B. Rodr.) Bur. & K. Sch., Bignoniaceae 84
Turnera rupestris Aubl., Turneraceae 328
Virola surinamensis (Rol.) Warb., Myristicaceae 252

Stomachache (Gastralgia)
Achyrocline satureioides (Lam.) DC., Asteraceae 52
Andira retusa (Poir.) H.B.K., Fabaceae 162
Aristolochia trilobata L., Aristolochiaceae 48

Bertholletia excelsa
  Humb. & Bonpl., Lecythidaceae 204
Calolisianthus pendulus
  (Mart.) Gilg, Gentianaceae 179
Capraria biflora L., Scrophulariaceae 311
Carapa guianensis Aubl., Meliaceae 227
Chondodendron platyphyllum
  (Mart.) Miers, Menispermaceae 231
Coleus barbatus Benth., Lamiaceae 191
Dipteryx odorata (Aubl.) Willd., Fabaceae 166
Elephantopus mollis H.B.K., Asteraceae 59
Eleutherine plicata Herb., Iridaceae 186
Guatteria ouregon (Aubl.) Dun., Annonaceae 14
Hyptis incana Briq., Lamiaceae 192
Ilex paraguariensis St.-Hil., Aquifoliaceae 31
Leonurus sibiricus L., Lamiaceae 194
Maytenus obtusifolia Mart., Celastraceae 116
Myrcia lanceolata Camb., Myrtaceae 255
Peperomia elongata Miq., Piperaceae 273
Picrolemma pseudocoffea Ducke, Simaroubaceae . 314
Piper callosum R. & Pav., Piperaceae 274
Piper cavalcantei Yunck., Piperaceae 275
Scleria pratensis L., Cyperaceae 143
Solanum nigrum L., Solanaceae 321
Spondias macrocarpa Engl., Anacardiaceae 10
Spondias mombin L., Anacardiaceae 10
Stachytarpheta cayennensis
  (Rich.) Vahl, Verbenaceae 335
Vitex agnus-castus L., Verbenaceae 336
Xylopia benthamiana Fries, Annonaceae 16

Stomachic
Abuta rufescens Aubl., Menispermaceae 231
Achyrocline satureioides (Lam.) DC., Asteraceae 52
Aiovea meissneri Mez, Lauraceae 197
Angelonia integerrima Spreng., Scrophulariaceae .. 310
Aniba permollis (Nees) Mez, Lauraceae 197
Annona squamosa L., Annonaceae 13
Aristolochia trilobata L., Aristolochiaceae 48
Aspidosperma excelsum Benth., Apocynaceae 21
Baccharis trimera (Less.) DC., Asteraceae 54
Carica papaya L., Caricaceae 113
Chenopodium ambrosioides L., Chenopodiaceae ... 118
Cinnamodendron axillare
  (Nees & Mart.) Endl., Canellaceae 110
Cissampelos glaberrima St.-Hil., Menispermaceae 233
Clusia panapanari Choisy, Clusiaceae 122
Copaifera officinalis (Jacq.) L., Caesalpiniaceae 102
Coutoubea ramosa Aubl., Gentianaceae 179
Coutoubea spicata Aubl., Gentianaceae 179
Crataeva benthamii Eichl., Capparaceae 112
Croton salutaris Casar., Euphorbiaceae 151
Croton sonderianus M. Arg., Euphorbiaceae 151
Cuscuta racemosa Mart., Convolvulaceae 130
Cyperus sesquiflorus
  (Torrey) Mattf. & Kükent., Cyperaceae 142
Deianira pallescens Cham. & Schl., Gentianaceae . 180
Drimys winteri Forst., Winteraceae 340
Egletes viscosa (L.) Less., Asteraceae 59
Fevillea trilobata L., Cucurbitaceae 136
Fevillea unicipetala Kuhlm., Cucurbitaceae 138
Geissospermum laeve (Vell.) Baill., Apocynaceae 23
Genipa americana L., Rubiaceae 298
Grindelia buphthalmoides DC., Asteraceae 60

Guettarda angelica Mart., Rubiaceae 298
Hedyosmum brasiliense Mart., Chloranthaceae 119
Hibiscus sabdariffa L., Malvaceae 221
Hortia brasiliensis Vand., Rutaceae 301
Hymenaea courbaril L., Caesalpiniaceae 103
Hypolytrum laxum Schrad., Cyperaceae 143
Hyptis mutabilis (Rich.) Briq., Lamiaceae 193
Hyptis umbrosa Salzm., Lamiaceae 193
Lantana brasiliensis Link, Verbenaceae 334
Leonotis nepetaefolia R. Br., Lamiaceae 194
Lippia alba (Mill.) N.E. Brown, Verbenaceae 335
Lippia gratissima
  (Gill. & Hook.) Troncoso, Verbenaceae 335
Mentha crispa L., Lamiaceae 194
Nectandra puberula Nees, Lauraceae 200
Ocotea pulchella Mart., Lauraceae 201
Oldenlandia corymbosa L., Rubiaceae 299
Ottonia corcovadensis Miq., Piperaceae 272
Ouratea guianensis Aubl., Ochnaceae 261
Peperomia rotundifolia H.B.K., Piperaceae 274
Piper ceanothifolium H.B.K., Piperaceae 275
Piper geniculatum Sw., Piperaceae 275
Piper gigantifolium Jacq., Piperaceae 275
Piper marginatum Jacq., Piperaceae 275
Piper mollicomum Kunth, Piperaceae 276
Piper reticulatum L., Piperaceae 276
Pluchea suaveolens (Vell.) O. Ktze., Asteraceae 64
Raputia aromatica Aubl., Rutaceae 302
Raputia magnifica Engl., Rutaceae 302
Raulinoreitzia tremula
  (Hook. & Arn.) King & Robinson, Asteraceae 64
Renealmia exaltata L. f., Zingiberaceae 342
Renealmia occidentalis Sweet, also
  R. sylvestris Horan., Zingiberaceae 342
Sauvagesia erecta L., Ochnaceae 262
Sida acuta Burm., Malvaceae 221
Siparuna brasiliensis (Spr.) DC., Monimiaceae 245
Siparuna camporum (Tul.) DC., Monimiaceae 245
Solidago chilensis Meyen, Asteraceae 65
Spondias macrocarpa Engl., Anacardiaceae 10
Spondias mombin L., Anacardiaceae 10
Strychnos subcordata Spr. ex Benth., Loganiaceae 209
Syagrus comosa Mart., Arecaceae 45
Syagrus oleracea (Mart.) Becc., Arecaceae 45
Tontelea brachypoda Miers, Hippocrateaceae 183
Virola oleifera (Schott) A.C. Smith, Myristicaceae . 250
Zanthoxylum rhoifolium Lam., Rutaceae 303
Zizyphus joazeiro Mart., Rhamnaceae 293

Stomatitis
Begonia luxurians Scheidw., Begoniaceae 76
Buchnera aquatica Aubl., Scrophulariaceae 310
Hypericum connatum Lam., Clusiaceae 122
Krameria tomentosa St.-Hil., Krameriaceae 191
Sparattosperma leucanthum
  (Vell.) K. Sch., Bignoniaceae 82

Storax Substitute
Styrax ferrugineum Nees & Mart., Styracaceae 325

Strengthener. *See also* Fortifier
Brosimum parinarioides Ducke, Moraceae 246
Connarus patrisii Planch., Connaraceae 129
Rhabdodendron amazonicum
  (Spr. ex Benth.) Hub., Rhamnaceae 291

STUPEFACIENT – SUDORIFIC: MEDICINAL INDEX

Stupefacient
Datura arborea L., Solanaceae 317
Datura stramonium L., Solanaceae 318
Styptic. *See* **Astringent**
Subcutaneous Manifestations
Sapium hamatum Pax & Hoffm., Euphorbiaceae ... 157
Sudorific (Diaphoretic)
Acanthospermum australe
  (Loefl.) O. Ktze., Asteraceae 51
Acanthospermum hispidum DC., Asteraceae 52
Adiantum trapeziforme L., Adiantaceae 1
Anacardium occidentale L., Anacardiaceae 7
Andradea floribunda Fr. All., Nyctaginaceae 257
Andropogon bicornis L., Poaceae 279
Andropogon condensatus H.B.K., Poaceae 279
Annona squamosa L., Annonaceae 13
Aristolochia birostris Duch., Aristolochiaceae 46
Aristolochia cordigera Willd., Aristolochiaceae 46
Aristolochia trilobata L., Aristolochiaceae 53
Ayapana triplinerve
  (Vahl) King & Robinson, Asteraceae 53
Blanchetia heterotricha DC., Asteraceae 57
Bomarea salsilloides Roem., Amaryllidaceae 6
Borreria asclepiadea Cham. & Schl., substitute
  for Cephaelis ipecacuanha Rich., Rubiaceae 296
Buddleja brasiliensis Jacq. ex Spr., Buddlejaceae 93
Canna gigantea Desf., Cannaceae 110
Canna glauca L., Cannaceae 110
Canna indica L., Cannaceae 111
Canna lutea Roscoe, Cannaceae 111
Caryocar villosum (Aubl.) Pers., Caryocaraceae 114
Cephaelis ipecacuanha Rich., Rubiaceae 296
Chenopodium ambrosioides L., Chenopodiaceae ... 118
Cissampelos glaberrima St.-Hil., Menispermaceae 233
Cissampelos ovalifolia DC., Menispermaceae 233
Combretum leprosum Mart., Combretaceae 126
Cordia coffeoides Warm., Boraginaceae 87
Costus spicatus (Jacq.) Sw., Costaceae 132
Cunila spicata L., Lamiaceae 192
Cuphea balsamona Cham., Lythraceae 213
Cuphea carthagenensis
  (Jacq.) MacBride, Lythraceae 213
Cuphea ingrata Cham. & Schl., Lythraceae 214
Cyperus rotundus L., Cyperaceae 142
Cyperus sesquiflorus
  (Torrey) Mattf. & Kükent., Cyperaceae 142
Diodia polymorpha Cham. & Schl., substitute for
  Cephaelis ipecacuanha Rich., Rubiaceae 297
Dipteryx alata Vog., Fabaceae 165
Dodonaea viscosa Jacq., Sapindaceae 305
Dorstenia asaroides Gardn., Moraceae 247
Dorstenia brasiliensis Lam., Moraceae 247
Drimys winteri Forst., Winteraceae 340
Elephantopus micropappus Less., Asteraceae 59
Elephantopus mollis H.B.K., Asteraceae 59
Ephedra triandra Tul., Ephedraceae 148
Erythrina velutina Willd., Fabaceae 166
Erythroxylum cataractarum
  Spruce, Erythroxylaceae 149
Erythroxylum coca Lam., Erythroxylaceae 149
Glechon ciliata Benth., Lamiaceae 192
Glechon spathulata Benth., Lamiaceae 192

Heimia salicifolia
  (H.B.K.) Link & Otto, Lythraceae 214
Herreria salsaparilha Mart., Liliaceae 207
Hybanthus ipecacuanha (L.) Baill., Violaceae, same
  use as Cephaelis ipecacuanha Rich., Rubiaceae .. 339
Hyptis atrorubens Poit., Lamiaceae 192
Hyptis crenata Pohl, Lamiaceae 192
Hyptis suaveolens Poit., Lamiaceae 193
Hyptis umbrosa Salzm., Lamiaceae 193
Ionidium poaya St.-Hil., Violaceae, same use as
  Cephaelis ipecacuanha Rich., Rubiaceae 339
Jacaranda copaia (Aubl.) D. Don, Bignoniaceae 80
Jacaranda subrhombea DC., Bignoniaceae 81
Keithia denudata Benth., Lamiaceae 193
Lantana camara L., Verbenaceae 334
Leucas martinicensis (Jacq.) R. Br., Lamiaceae 194
Lipostoma campanuliflorum D. Don, also
  L. capitata D. Don, substitutes for
  Cephaelis ipecacuanha Rich., Rubiaceae 299
Lippia alba (Mill.) N.E. Brown, Verbenaceae 335
Luxemburgia glazioviana Gilg, Ochnaceae 260
Luxemburgia polyandra St.-Hil., Ochnaceae 261
Machaonia brasiliensis Cham. & Schl., Rubiaceae 299
Manettia ignita (Vell.) K. Sch., substitute
  for Cephaelis ipecacuanha Rich., Rubiaceae 299
Melampodium divaricatum (Rich.) DC., Asteraceae 61
Monnieria trifolia Loefl., Rutaceae 302
Ocimum fluminensis Vell., Lamiaceae 195
Ocimum micranthum Willd., Lamiaceae 195
Ocotea pretiosa
  (Nees & Mart.) Benth.& Hook., Lauraceae 201
Ocotea teleiandra (Messn.) Mez, Lauraceae 203
Ottonia jaborandi (Vell.) Kunth, Piperaceae 272
Parkinsonia aculeata L., Caesalpiniaceae 104
Petiveria alliacea L., Phytolaccaceae 271
Phyllanthus niruri L., Euphorbiaceae 156
Pilocarpus pinnatifolius Lem., Rutaceae 302
Piper elongatum Vahl, Piperaceae 275
Piper geniculatum Sw., Piperaceae 275
Polygala angulata DC., Polygalaceae 284
Polygala klotzschii Chodat, Polygalaceae 284
Porophyllum ruderale (Jacq.) Cass., Asteraceae 64
Psoralea glandulosa L., Fabaceae 170
Remirea maritima Aubl., Cyperaceae 143
Ruellia tuberosa L., Acanthaceae 1
Schinus molle L., Anacardiaceae 9
Senna occidentalis (L.) Link, Caesalpiniaceae 105
Senna quinqueangulata
  (Rich.) Ir. & Barn., Caesalpiniaceae 106
Senna uniflora
  (P. Miller) Ir. & Barn.,Caesalpiniaceae 106
Sisyrinchium vaginatum Spreng., Iridaceae 186
Solanum cernuum Vell., Solanaceae 319
Sophora tomentosa L., Fabaceae 172
Spigelia flemingiana Cham. & Schl., Loganiaceae . 209
Spigelia glabrata Mart., Loganiaceae 209
Stachytarpheta cayennensis
  (Rich.) Vahl, Verbenaceae 335
Stachytarpheta jamaicensis
  (L.) Vahl, Verbenaceae 336
Swartzia panacoco (Aubl.) Cowan
  var. panacoco, Caesalpiniaceae 107
Tetracera aspera Willd., Dilleniaceae 146

Tetracera volubilis L., Dilleniaceae 146	Cybistax antisyphilitica
Tragia volubilis L., Euphorbiaceae 158	(Mart.) Mart., Bignoniaceae 80
Verbena erinoides Lam., Verbenaceae 336	Echinodorus grandiflorus
Waltheria communis St.-Hil., Sterculiaceae 325	(Cham. & Schl.) Mich., Alismataceae 2
Zanthoxylum pterota H.B.K., Rutaceae 303	Echinodorus macrophyllus

Suppuration
Chromolaena hirsuta
(Hook. & Arn.) King & Robinson, Asteraceae 58
Elaeis guineensis Jacq., Arecaceae 40
Ipomoea acetosifolia
(Vahl) Roem. & Schult., Convolvulaceae 130
Maclura brasiliensis Endl., Moraceae 249
Patagonula americana L., Boraginaceae 89
Psidium arboreum Vell., Myrtaceae 256

Sweating. See Sudorific

Swelling
Piper marginatum Jacq., Piperaceae 275
Pothomorphe umbellata (L.) Miq., Piperaceae 277

–arthritic
Guarea trichilioides L., Meliaceae 227

–legs
Davilla rugosa Poir., Dilleniaceae 145
Elaeis guineensis Jacq., Arecaceae 40
Phoradendron crassifolium
(Pohl) Eichl., Loranthaceae 211
Tetracera breyniana Schl., Dilleniaceae 146

Syphilis
Alternanthera achyrantha R. Br., Amaranthaceae 3
Anacardium humile St.-Hil., Anacardiaceae 7
Anacardium nanum St.-Hil., Anacardiaceae 7
Anacardium occidentale L., Anacardiaceae 7
Anchietea pyrifolia (Mart.) G. Don, Violaceae 338
Anemopaegma arvense (Vell.) Stapf, Bignoniaceae . 78
Aniba canelilla (H.B.K.) Mez, Lauraceae 197
Apuleia leiocarpa
(Vog.) MacBride, Caesalpiniaceae 98
Bauhinia rutilans Spr. ex Benth., Caesalpiniaceae ... 99
Bowdichia nitida Spruce ex Benth., Fabaceae 163
Bowdichia virgilioides H.B.K., Fabaceae 163
Byrsonima verbascifolia
(L.) Rich., Malpighiaceae 220
Cayaponia espelina
(Manso) Cogn., Cucurbitaceae 135
Cayaponia martiana
(Cogn.) Cogn., Cucurbitaceae 135
Cayaponia pilosa Cogn., Cucurbitaceae 135
Cayaponia tayuya (Mart.) Cogn., Cucurbitaceae ... 135
Chaptalia nutans (L.) Polak., Asteraceae 57
Clematis dioica L., Ranunculaceae 290
Conocarpus erecta L., Combretaceae 126
Copernicia prunifera (Mill.) H. Moore, Arecaceae .. 40
Costus cuspidatus
(Nees & Mart.) Maas, Costaceae 132
Costus spiralis (Jacq.) Roscoe, Costaceae 132
Cremastus sceptrum Bur. & K. Sch., Bignoniaceae .. 79
Croton floribundus Spreng., Euphorbiaceae 150
Croton triqueter Lam., Euphorbiaceae 151
Cuphea balsamona Cham., Lythraceae 213
Cuphea carthagenensis
(Jacq.) MacBride, Lythraceae 213
Cuphea ingrata Cham. & Schl., Lythraceae 214

Echinodorus grandiflorus
(Cham. & Schl.) Mich., Alismataceae 2
Echinodorus macrophyllus
(Kunth) Mich., Alismataceae 2
Echinodorus pubescens Mart., Alismataceae 2
Elephantopus mollis H.B.K., Asteraceae 59
Euphorbia cotinoides Miq., Euphorbiaceae 152
Euphorbia papillosa St.-Hil., Euphorbiaceae 152
Evolvulus holosericeus H.B.K., Convolvulaceae 130
Ficus gomelleira Kunth & Bouché, Moraceae 248
Genipa americana L., Rubiaceae 298
Guarea spiciflora Juss., Meliaceae 227
Guarea tuberculata Vell., Meliaceae 229
Guazuma ulmifolia Lam.,
var. ulmifolia, Sterculiaceae 323
Heliotropium elongatum Willd., Boraginaceae 88
Herreria salsaparilha Mart., Liliaceae 207
Himatanthus lancifolia
(M. Arg.) Woods., Apocynaceae 26
Hippobroma longiflora (L.) G. Don [including
Lobelia longiflora L.], Campanulaceae 109
Jacaranda brasiliana (Lam.) Pers., Bignoniaceae ... 80
Jacaranda caroba (Vell.) DC., Bignoniaceae 80
Jacaranda copaia (Aubl.) D. Don, Bignoniaceae 80
Jacaranda micrantha Cham., Bignoniaceae 81
Jacaranda mimosifolia D. Don, Bignoniaceae 81
Jacaranda spp., including J. clausseniana Casar.,
J. decurrens Cham., J. elegans Mart.,
J. heterophylla Bur. & Pet., J. oxyphylla Cham.,
J. paucifoliata Mart., J. puberula Cham.,
J. rufa Manso, J. semiserrata Cham.,
& J. tomentosa R.Br., Bignoniaceae 81
Jatropha elliptica (Pohl) M. Arg., Euphorbiaceae .. 154
Jatropha multifida L., Euphorbiaceae 154
Macrosiphonia velame
(St.-Hil.) M. Arg., Apocynaceae 26
Marcgravia rectiflora
Tr. & Planch., Marcgraviaceae 224
Martinella obovata
(H.B.K.) Bur. & K. Sch., Bignoniaceae 82
Melothrianthus smilacifolius
(Cogn.) M. Crovetto, Cucurbitaceae 139
Mikania parviflora (Aubl.) Karst., Asteraceae 62
Modiolastrum pinnatipartitum
(St.-Hil.& Naudin) Krapovickas, Malvaceae 221
Muehlenbeckia sagittifolia
(Ort.) Meissn., Polygonaceae 285
Operculina alata (Ham.) Urb., Convolvulaceae 131
Operculina macrocarpa Urb., Convolvulaceae 131
Parahancornia amapa (Hub.) Ducke, Apocynaceae . 27
Patagonula americana L., Boraginaceae 89
Peperomia hederacea Miq., Piperaceae 273
Pereskia aculeata Mill., Cactaceae 97
Pereskia bleo H.B.K., Cactaceae 97
Piptocarpha rotundifolia (Less.) Bak., Asteraceae .. 64
Potalia amara Aubl., Loganiaceae 209
Protium icicariba (DC.) March., Burseraceae 94
Reisseckia smilacina (Sm.) Steud., Rhamnaceae 293
Renealmia occidentalis Sweet, also
Renealmia sylvestris Horan., Zingiberaceae 342

Rumex brasiliensis Link, Polygonaceae 287
Sapium hamatum Pax & Hoffm., Euphorbiaceae ... 157
Sebastiania macrocarpa M. Arg., Euphorbiaceae .. 157
Senna hirsuta (L.) Ir. & Barn.
    var. *puberula* Ir. & Barn., Caesalpiniaceae 105
Senna macranthera
    (Collad.) Ir. & Barn., Caesalpiniaceae 105
Sida macrodon DC., Malvaceae 222
Simarouba versicolor St.-Hil., Simaroubaceae 315
Smilax campestris Gris., Liliaceae 208
Smilax longifolia Rich. (includes
    S. brasiliensis Spreng.), Liliaceae 208
Sparattosperma leucanthum
    (Vell.) K. Sch., Bignoniaceae 82
Stachytarpheta jamaicensis
    (L.) Vahl, Verbenaceae 336
Tabebuia caraiba (Mart.) Bur., Bignoniaceae 82
Tabebuia chrysotricha
    (Mart.) Standl., Bignoniaceae 82
Tabebuia ipe (Mart.) Standl., Bignoniaceae 83
Tabebuia serratifolia (Vahl) Nichol., Bignoniaceae .. 83
Tetracera aspera Willd., Dilleniaceae 146
Tetracera volubilis L., Dilleniaceae 146
Tournefortia laevigata Lam., Boraginaceae 89
Turnera diffusa Willd., Turneraceae 327
Turnera opifera Mart., Turneraceae 328
Urera caracasana Jacq., Urticaceae 331
Waltheria indica L., Sterculiaceae 325
Wilbrandia ebracteata Cogn., Cucurbitaceae 140
Wilbrandia verticillata
    (Vell.) Cogn., Cucurbitaceae 140
Zeyheria digitalis (Vell.) Hoehne, Bignoniaceae 84

T

Tachycardia
Cissus sicyoides L., Vitaceae 339
Taenifuge. *See also* Anthelmintic, Vermifuge
Astrocaryum aculeatissimum
    (Schott) Burret, Arecaceae 39
Cocos nucifera L., Arecaceae 40
Cucurbita pepo L., Cucurbitaceae 136
Phlebodium aureum
    (L.) J.E. Smith, Polypodiaceae 288
Tanniferous
Terminalia tanibouca Smith, Combretaceae 126
Tart. *See* Sour
Tea (Thea) Substitute
Tournefortia volubilis L., Boraginaceae 90
Teeth. *See* Toothache
Teething
Operculina alata (Ham.) Urb., Convolvulaceae 131
Operculina macrocarpa Urb., Convolvulaceae 131
Ruellia tuberosa L., Acanthaceae 1
Tendonitis (Animal)
Calophyllum brasiliense Camb., Clusiaceae 120
Testicular Problems.
    ***See also* Hydrocele, Orchitis**
Leandra lacunosa Cogn., Melastomataceae 225
Marcgravia rectiflora
    Tr. & Planch., Marcgraviaceae 224

Tetanus
Copaifera officinalis (Jacq.) L., Caesalpiniaceae 102
Tetterworm
Fevillea uncipetala Kuhlm., Cucurbitaceae 138
Thermetic
Pilea microphylla (L.) Liebm., Urticaceae 331
Thorn Remover
Turnera ulmifolia L., Turneraceae 328
Throat Conditions. *See also* Catarrh
Acmella oleracea (L.) R.K. Jansen, Asteraceae 52
Acmella repens (Walt.) L.C. Rich., Asteraceae 52
Anacardium occidentale L., Anacardiaceae 7
Ananas comosus (L.) Merrill, Bromeliaceae 90
Ayapana triplinerve
    (Vahl) King & Robinson, Asteraceae 53
Berberis laurina Thunb., Berberidaceae 76
Cariniana legalis (Mart.) O. Ktze., Lecythidaceae . 204
Chromolaena hirsuta
    (Hook. & Arn.) King & Robinson, Asteraceae 58
Coccoloba marginata Benth., Polygonaceae 285
Commelina vestita Seub., Commelinaceae 128
Commelina virginica L., Commelinaceae 128
Copaifera officinalis (Jacq.) L., Caesalpiniaceae 102
Cuscuta racemosa Mart., Convolvulaceae 130
Deianira pallescens Cham. & Schl., Gentianaceae . 180
Dichorisandra affinis Mart., Commelinaceae 128
Dichorisandra leucophthalmos
    Hook., Commelinaceae 128
Echinodorus macrophyllus
    (Kunth) Mich., Alismataceae 2
Eryngium pristis Cham. & Schlecht., Apiaceae 19
Erythrina crista-galli L., Fabaceae 166
Hyptis crenata Pohl, Lamiaceae 192
Jacaranda copaia (Aubl.) D. Don, Bignoniaceae 80
Maclura brasiliensis Endl., Moraceae 249
Oxalis amara St.-Hil., Oxalidaceae 266
Oxalis cordata St.-Hil., Oxalidaceae 266
Oxalis martiana Zucc., also other
    Oxalis spp., Oxalidaceae 267
Peperomia pellucida H.B.K., Piperaceae 273
Plantago brasiliensis Sims, Plantaginaceae 278
Rollinia sylvatica (St.-Hil.) Mart., Annonaceae 15
Siparuna brasiliensis (Spr.) DC., Monimiaceae 245
Sparattosperma leucanthum
    (Vell.) K. Sch., Bignoniaceae 83
Tabebuia umbellata (Sond.) Sandw., Bignoniaceae .. 83
Tibouchina clavata
    (Pers.) Wurdack, Melastomataceae 226
Tradescantia effusa Mart., Commelinaceae 129
Xanthosoma striatipes
    (Kunth & Bouché) Madison, Arecaceae 37
Throat, Sore
Bidens pilosa L., Asteraceae 57
Coccoloba marginata Benth., Polygonaceae 285
Commelina vestita Seub., Commelinaceae 128
Commelina virginica L., Commelinaceae 128
Deianira pallescens Cham. & Schl., Gentianaceae . 180
Dichorisandra affinis Mart., Commelinaceae 128
Dichorisandra leucophthalmos
    Hook., Commelinaceae 128
Erythrina crista-galli L., Fabaceae 166
Hyptis crenata Pohl, Lamiaceae 192

MEDICINAL INDEX: THROAT, SORE – TONIC

Oxalis amara St.-Hil., Oxalidaceae 266
Oxalis cordata St.-Hil., Oxalidaceae 266
Oxalis martiana Zucc., also many other
   Oxalis spp., Oxalidaceae 267
Peperomia pellucida H.B.K., Piperaceae 273
Plantago guilleminiana Dcne., Plantaginaceae 278
Siparuna brasiliensis (Spr.) DC., Monimiaceae 245
Tradescantia effusa Mart., Commelinaceae 129

Thrush
Manilkara zapota (L.) Van Royen, Sapotaceae 309

Tick Eliminator
Carpotroche longifolia Benth., Flacourtiaceae 176

Tinea. See also **Ringworm**
Commelina nudiflora L., Commelinaceae 126
Cybianthus detergens Mart., Myrsinaceae 253

Tonic
Abuta candicans Rich., Menispermaceae 231
Abuta rufescens Aubl., Menispermaceae 231
Abuta selloana Eichl., Menispermaceae 231
Acanthospermum australe
   (Loefl.) O. Ktze., Asteraceae 51
Acanthospermum hispidum DC., Asteraceae 52
Ageratum conyzoides L., Asteraceae 53
Ambrosia artemisiifolia L., Asteraceae 53
Anacardium occidentale L., Anacardiaceae 7
Aristolochia triangularis Cham., Aristolochiaceae ... 48
Aristolochia trilobata L., Aristolochiaceae 48
Ayapana triplinerve
   (Vahl) King & Robinson, Asteraceae 53
Baccharis articulata (Lam.) Pers., Asteraceae 54
Baccharis dracunculifolia DC., Asteraceae 54
Baccharis spp., Asteraceae 56
Baccharis trimera (Less.) DC., Asteraceae 54
Bathysa cuspidata Hook., Rubiaceae 296
Brosimum potabile Ducke, Moraceae 246
Bumelia sartorum Mart., Sapotaceae 308
Caesalpinia echinata Lam., Caesalpiniaceae 100
Calolisianthus pendulus
   (Mart.) Gilg, Gentianaceae 179
Calotropis procera (Ait.) Ait. f., Asclepiadaceae 50
Campsiandra comosa Benth. var.
   laurifolia (Benth.) Cowan, Caesalpiniaceae 100
Canna indica L., Cannaceae 111
Carapa guianensis Aubl., Meliaceae 227
Casearia ovata Willd., Flacourtiaceae 178
Casearia sylvestris Sw., Flacourtiaceae 178
Cayaponia espelina
   (Manso) Cogn., Cucurbitaceae 135
Cecropia hololeuca Miq., Moraceae 247
Cestrum pseudoquina Mart., Solanaceae 317
Chaptalia nutans (L.) Polak., Asteraceae 57
Cinnamodendron axillare
   (Nees & Mart.) Endl., Canellaceae 110
Cissampelos fasciculata Benth., Menispermaceae . 231
Cissampelos glaberrima St.-Hil., Menispermaceae 233
Cissampelos ovalifolia DC., Menispermaceae 233
Cissampelos pareira L., Menispermaceae 233
Cissampelos sympodialis Eichl., Menispermaceae . 233
Clibadium surinamense L., Asteraceae 58
Colletia paradoxa (Spr.) Escalante, Rhamnaceae ... 291
Copaifera cearensis
   Huber ex Ducke, Caesalpiniaceae 102

Copaifera multijuga Hayne, Caesalpiniaceae 102
Cordia multispicata Cham., Boraginaceae 88
Cordia salicifolia Cham., Boraginaceae 88
Costus spicatus (Jacq.) Sw., Costaceae 132
Coutarea hexandra (Jacq.) K. Sch., Rubiaceae 297
Coutoubea spicata Aubl., Gentianaceae 179
Crataeva benthamii Eichl., Capparaceae 112
Crataeva tapia L., Capparaceae 112
Cryptocarya minima Mez, Lauraceae 198
Curtia tenuifolia (Aubl.) Knobl., Gentianaceae 180
Cusparia febrifuga Humb., Rutaceae 300
Cymbopogon schoenanthus (L.) Spreng., Poaceae 280
Dalechampia ficifolia Lam., Euphorbiaceae 152
Davilla rugosa Poir., Dilleniaceae 145
Deianira pallescens Cham. & Schl., Gentianaceae . 180
Dicypellium caryophyllatum
   Nees & Mart., Lauraceae 198
Discaria americana Gill. & Hook., Rhamnaceae ... 291
Dorstenia asaroides Gardn., Moraceae 247
Dorstenia brasiliensis Lam., Moraceae 247
Drimys winteri Forst., Winteraceae 340
Echinodorus grandiflorus
   (Cham. & Schl.) Mich., Alismataceae 2
Echinodorus pubescens Mart., Alismataceae 2
Elephantopus mollis H.B.K., Asteraceae 59
Esenbeckia febrifuga Juss., Rutaceae 301
Esenbeckia intermedia Mart., Rutaceae 301
Evolvulus alsinoides L., Convolvulaceae 130
Exostemma australe St.-Hil., Rubiaceae 298
Fevillea trilobata L., Cucurbitaceae 136
Fevillea uncipetala Kuhlm., Cucurbitaceae 138
Ficus gomelleira Kunth & Bouché, Moraceae 248
Galipea multiflora Schult., Rutaceae 301
Geissospermum laeve (Vell.) Baill., Apocynaceae ... 24
Gomphrena mollis Mart., Amaranthaceae 4
Gomphrena officinalis Mart., Amaranthaceae 4
Guettarda angelica Mart., Rubiaceae 298
Guettarda argentea Lam., Rubiaceae 298
Guettarda uruguayensis
   Cham. & Schl., Rubiaceae 298
Gustavia hexapetala
   (Aubl.) J.E. Smith, Lecythidaceae 205
Hedyosmum brasiliense Mart., Chloranthaceae 119
Heliotropium lanceolatum Loefgr., Boraginaceae ... 89
Hibiscus sabdariffa L., Malvaceae 221
Himatanthus drastica
   (Mart.) Woods., Apocynaceae 24
Hortia brasiliensis Vand., Rutaceae 301
Hymenaea courbaril L., Caesalpiniaceae 103
Hyptis crenata Pohl, Lamiaceae 192
Hyptis multiflora Pohl, Lamiaceae 193
Hyptis mutabilis (Rich.) Briq., Lamiaceae 193
Hyptis umbrosa Salzm., Lamiaceae 193
Ilex acrodonta Reiss., Aquifoliaceae 31
Ilex paraguariensis St.-Hil., Aquifoliaceae 31
Jacaranda caroba (Vell.) DC., Bignoniaceae 80
Jatropha urens L., Euphorbiaceae 155
Kielmeyera coriacea Mart., Clusiaceae 122
Kielmeyera speciosa St.-Hil., Clusiaceae 123
Ladenbergia hexandra Klotz., Rubiaceae 299
Ladenbergia lambertiana Klotz., Rubiaceae 299
Lafoensia pacari St.-Hil., Lythraceae 215
Lantana camara L., Verbenaceae 334

Lantana microphylla Cham., also *L. mixta* L.,
  L. pseudothea (St.-Hil.) Schauer, Verbenaceae 335
Leiphaimos aphylla (Jacq.) Gilg, Gentianaceae 180
Leonotis nepetaefolia R. Br., Lamiaceae 194
Leucas martinicensis (Jacq.) R. Br., Lamiaceae 194
Licaria puchury-major
  (Mart.) Kosterm., Lauraceae 199
Lithraea molleoides (Vell.) Engl., Anacardiaceae 9
Mabea fistulifera Mart., Euphorbiaceae 155
Margyricarpus setosus Ruiz & Pav., Rosaceae 294
Mariscus jacquinii H.B.K., Cyperaceae 143
Marupa francoana Miers, Simaroubaceae 313
Mauritia flexuosa L. f., Arecaceae 43
Mauritiella aculeata (Kunth) Burret, Arecaceae 43
Maytenus gonoclada Mart., Celastraceae 115
Maytenus ilicifolia Mart., Celastraceae 115
Metrodorea pubescens St.-Hil. & Tul., Rutaceae ... 301
Mikania officinalis Mart., Asteraceae 62
Mimosa pudica L., Mimosaceae 240
Mimosa velloziana Mart., Mimosaceae 240
Monnieria trifolia Loefl., Rutaceae 302
Myracroduon urundeuva
  Fr. All., Anacardiaceae 9
Nectandra globosa (Aubl.) Mez, Lauraceae 199
Nectandra leucantha Nees, Lauraceae 199
Nymphoides indica (L.) O. Ktze., Menyanthaceae . 235
Ocotea cujumary Mart., Lauraceae 200
Ocotea cymbarum H.B.K., Lauraceae 200
Ocotea rodiei (Schomb.) Mez, Lauraceae 201
Ocotea spectabilis (Meissn.) Mez, Lauraceae 201
Ocotea squarrosa Mart. ex Nees, Lauraceae 203
Ouratea jabotapita Engl., Ochnaceae 261
Ouratea parviflora (DC.) Baill., Ochnaceae 261
Parahancornia amapa (Hub.) Ducke, Apocynaceae 27
Passiflora foetida L., Passifloraceae 269
Paullinia cupana Kunth, Sapindaceae 306
Peperomia hederacea Miq., Piperaceae 273
Peperomia rotundifolia H.B.K., Piperaceae 274
Peschiera affinis (M. Arg.) Miers, Apocynaceae 27
Peschiera laeta (Mart.) Miers, Apocynaceae 27
Pfaffia jubata Mart., Amaranthaceae 5
Pfaffia paniculata (Mart.) Kuntze, Amaranthaceae 5
Phyllanthus conami Sw., Euphorbiaceae 156
Phyllanthus niruri L., Euphorbiaceae 156
Phyllanthus nobilis M. Arg, Euphorbiaceae 157
Picramnia bahiensis Turcz., Simaroubaceae 313
Picramnia camboita Engl., Simaroubaceae 314
Picramnia ciliata Mart., Simaroubaceae 314
Piper geniculatum Sw., Piperaceae 275
Piper marginatum Jacq., Piperaceae 275
Plantago guilleminiana Dcne., Plantaginaceae 278
Pyrostegia ignea (Vell.) Pres., Bignoniaceae 82
Raulinoreitzia tremula
  (Hook. & Arn.) King & Robinson, Asteraceae 64
Rauwolfia bahiensis DC., Apocynaceae 28
Renealmia exaltata L. f., Zingiberaceae 342
Renealmia occidentalis Sweet, also
  R. sylvestris Horan., Zingiberaceae 342
Rollinia salicifolia Schl., Annonaceae 15
Rumex brasiliensis Link, Polygonaceae 287
Sapindus saponaria L., Sapindaceae 306
Schinus molle L., Anacardiaceae 9
Schultesia stenophylla Mart., Gentianaceae 180

Senna affinis (Benth.) Ir. & Barn., Caesalpiniaceae 104
Senna hirsuta (L.) Ir. & Barn.
  var. *puberula* Ir. & Barn., Caesalpiniaceae 105
Senna multijuga Rich. var. *verrucosa*
  (Vog.) Ir. & Barn., Caesalpiniaceae 105
Senna occidentalis (L.) Link, Caesalpiniaceae 105
Senna quinqueangulata
  (Rich.) Ir. & Barn., Caesalpiniaceae 106
Senna uniflora
  (P. Miller) Ir. & Barn., Caesalpiniaceae 106
Sida acuta Burm., Malvaceae 221
Simaba ferruginea St.-Hil., Simaroubaceae 314
Simarouba versicolor St.-Hil., Simaroubaceae 315
Sinningia allagophylla
  (Mart.) Wiehl., Gesneriaceae 181
Smilax oblongifolia Pohl, Liliaceae 208
Solanum variabile Mart., Solanaceae 322
Spondias macrocarpa Engl., Anacardiaceae 10
Spondias mombin L., Anacardiaceae 10
Stachytarpheta cayennensis
  (Rich.) Vahl, Verbenaceae 335
Stachytarpheta jamaicensis (L.) Vahl, Verbenaceae 336
Strychnos pseudoquina St.-Hil., Loganiaceae 209
Syagrus oleracea (Mart.) Becc., Arecaceae 45
Symplocos platyphylla
  (Pohl) Benth., Symplocaceae 326
Symplocos pubescens Klotzsch, Symplocaceae 326
Tabebuia leucoxylon (L.) DC., Bignoniaceae 83
Tabernaemontana citrifolia L., Apocynaceae 28
Tanacetum vulgare L., Asteraceae 67
Trichilia catigua Juss., Meliaceae 229
Turnera diffusa Willd., Turneraceae 327
Turnera opifera Mart., Turneraceae 328
Turnera ulmifolia L., Turneraceae 328
Verbena erinoides Lam., Verbenaceae 336
Vismia latifolia (Aubl.) Choisy, Clusiaceae 124
Xylopia frutescens Aubl., Annonaceae 16
Zanthoxylum hyemale St.-Hil., Rutaceae 302

Tonka Bean Substitute
Torresea cearensis Fr. All., Fabaceae 172

Tonsillitis (Amygdalitis)
Begonia luxurians Scheidw., Begoniaceae 76
Cinnamodendron axillare
  (Nees & Mart.) Endl., Canellaceae 110
Commelina nudiflora L., Commelinaceae 126
Hypericum connatum Lam., Clusiaceae 122
Kalanchoe pinnata (Lam.) Pers., Crassulaceae 133
Plantago myosurus Lam., Plantaginaceae 278
Senna occidentalis (L.) Link, Caesalpiniaceae 105

Tooth Extraction
Quassia amara L., Simaroubaceae 314

Toothache (Antiodontalgic, Odontalgic)
Acmella oleracea (L.) R.K. Jansen, Asteraceae 52
Acmella repens (Walt.) L.C. Rich., Asteraceae 52
Aniba rosaeodora Ducke, Lauraceae 197
Astronium fraxinifolium Schott, Anacardiaceae 9
Avicennia germinans (L.) L., Verbenaceae 334
Bidens pilosa L., Asteraceae 57
Caesalpinia echinata Lam., Caesalpiniaceae 100
Calotropis procera (Ait.) Ait. f., Asclepiadaceae 52
Canna gigantea Desf., Cannaceae 110
Centropogon cornutus (L.) Druce, Campanulaceae 109

Erythrina corallodendron L., Fabaceae 166
Kielmeyera speciosa St.-Hil., Clusiaceae 123
Maclura tinctoria (L.) D. Don, Moraceae 249
Ottonia corcovadensis Miq., Piperaceae 272
Ottonia jaborandi (Vell.) Kunth, Piperaceae 272
Oxalis corniculata L., Oxalidaceae 266
Petiveria alliacea L., Phytolaccaceae 271
Piper geniculatum Sw., Piperaceae 275
Plumbago scandens L., Plumbaginaceae 279
Protium icicariba (DC.) March., Burseraceae 94
Thevetia ahouai (L.) DC., Apocynaceae 28
Zanthoxylum rhoifolium Lam., Rutaceae 303
Zizyphus joazeiro Mart., Rhamnaceae 293

Toxic *(includes toxic in large doses)*
Abrus precatorius L., Fabaceae 160
Abuta candicans Rich., Menispermaceae 231
Acnistus arborescens (L.) Schl., Solanaceae 316
Allamanda doniana M. Arg., Apocynaceae 20
Andira retusa (Poir.) H.B.K., Fabaceae 162
Andira vermifuga Mart. ex Benth., Fabaceae 162
Araujia sericifera Brot., Asclepiadaceae 50
Brosimum acutifolium Huber, also
  B. obovata Ducke, Moraceae 246
Brunfelsia uniflora (Pohl) D. Don, also
  B. grandiflora D. Don, Solanaceae 316
Carica papaya L., Caricaceae 113
Cestrum calycinum Willd., Solanaceae 317
Chiococca alba (L.) Hitch., Rubiaceae 297
Chondodendron platyphyllum
  (Mart.) Miers, Menispermaceae 231
Clematis campestris St.-Hil., Ranunculaceae 290
Clematis dioica L., Ranunculaceae 290
Cocculus filipendula Mart., Menispermaceae 234
Cusparia toxicaria Spr. ex Engl., Rutaceae 301
Datura arborea L., Solanaceae 317
Datura suaveolens Humb. & Bonpl., Solanaceae ... 318
Davilla rugosa Poir., Dilleniaceae 145
Dipladenia fragrans DC., Apocynaceae 23
Dipladenia illustris M. Arg., Apocynaceae 23
Dracontium polyphyllum L., Araceae 36
Euphorbia tirucalli L., Euphorbiaceae 153
Fevillea uncipetala Kuhlm., Cucurbitaceae 138
Ficus maxima P. Mill., Moraceae 249
Haynaldia exaltata
  (Pohl) Kanitz, Campanulaceae 109
Heliotropium spp., Boraginaceae 89
Himatanthus fallax
  (M. Arg.) Woods., Apocynaceae 25
Hippobroma longiflora
  (L.) G. Don, Campanulaceae 109
Hura crepitans L., Euphorbiaceae 153
Hybanthus atropurpureus Taub., Violaceae 338
Hydrocotyle bonariensis Lam., Apiaceae 19
Hydrocotyle leucocephala
  Cham. & Schlecht., Apiaceae 20
Joannesia princeps Vell., Euphorbiaceae 155
Lagenaria siceraria
  (Molina) Standl., Cucurbitaceae 138
Maprounea brasiliensis L., Euphorbiaceae 155
Mesechites sulphurea (Vell.) M. Arg., Apocynaceae .. 27
Montrichardia linifera (Arruda) Schott, Araceae 36
Mucuna pruriens (L.) DC., Fabaceae 169
Passiflora macrocarpa Mast., Passifloraceae 270

Petiveria alliacea L., Phytolaccaceae 271
Pteridium aquilinum
  (L.) Kuhn, Dennstaedtiaceae 144
Salpichroa origanifolia (Lam.) Thell., Solanaceae .. 319
Samolus valerandi L., Primulaceae 290
Sapium hamatum Pax & Hoffm., Euphorbiaceae ... 157
Schultesia stenophylla Mart., Gentianaceae 180
Senecio brasiliensis Less., Asteraceae 65
Simarouba versicolor St.-Hil., Simaroubaceae 315
Solanum aculeatissimum Jacq., Solanaceae 319
Solanum ciliatum Lam., Solanaceae 319
Spigelia anthelmia L., Loganiaceae 209
Stryphnodendron coriaceum Benth., Mimosaceae . 243
Tachia guianensis Aubl., Gentianaceae 180
Tanaecium nocturnum
  (B. Rodr.) Bur. & K. Sch., Bignoniaceae 84
Thevetia ahouai (L.) DC., Apocynaceae 28

Trachoma
Abrus precatorius L., Fabaceae (PHARM.) 160

Trance Inducer
Datura insignis B. Rodr., Solanaceae 318

Tranquilizer
Calotropis procera (Ait.) Ait. f., Asclepiadaceae 50

Tremor Inducer
Brunfelsia uniflora (Pohl) D. Don, also
  B. grandiflora D. Don, Solanaceae 316

Tuberculosis (Consumption).
See also Scrofula
Acmella oleracea (L.) R.K. Jansen, Asteraceae 52
Acmella repens (Walt.) L.C. Rich., Asteraceae 52
Astronium fraxinifolium Schott, Anacardiaceae 9
Brasilopuntia brasiliensis (Willd.) Berg., Cactaceae 95
Byrsonima coccolobifolia H.B.K., Malpighiaceae .. 218
Jessenia bataua (Mart.) Burret, Arecaceae 43
Microgramma vaccinifolia
  (Langsd. & Fisch.) Copel., Polypodiaceae 288
Pteridium aquilinum
  (L.) Kuhn, Dennstaedtiaceae 144
Solanum aculeatissimum Jacq., Solanaceae 319
Xylopia frutescens Aubl., Annonaceae 16

Tumors
Caladium bicolor (Aiton) Vent.
  var. poecile (Schott) Engler, Araceae 35
Calophyllum brasiliense Camb., Clusiaceae 120
Canna glauca L., Cannaceae 110
Costus spicatus (Jacq.) Sw., Costaceae 132
Costus spiralis (Jacq.) Roscoe, Costaceae 132
Dodonaea viscosa Jacq., Sapindaceae 305
Gallesia gorazema
  (Vell.) Moq., Phytolaccaceae 271
Ipomoea pes-caprae (L.) R. Br., Convolvulaceae .. 130
Jatropha elliptica (Pohl) M. Arg., Euphorbiaceae .. 154
Jatropha urens L., Euphorbiaceae 155
Lemna minor L., Lemnaceae 207
Leucas martinicensis (Jacq.) R. Br., Lamiaceae 194
Lithraea molleoides (Vell.) Engl., Anacardiaceae 9
Ludwigia peruviana (L.) Hara, Onagraceae 264
Maytenus spp., Celastraceae (CHEM. & PHARM.) 116
Mimosa pudica L., Mimosaceae 240
Mimosa velloziana Mart., Mimosaceae 240
Sapium hamatum Pax & Hoffm., Euphorbiaceae ... 157
Schinus molle L., Anacardiaceae 9

TUMORS – ULCERS: MEDICINAL INDEX

Schinus terebinthifolius Raddi, Anacardiaceae 10
Sida rhombea L., Malvaceae 222
Tabebuia spp., Bignoniaceae 83
Turnera ulmifolia L., Turneraceae 328
Wissadula periplocifolia Presl., Malvaceae 223

Typhoid Fever. See also Fever
Aristolochia cordigera Willd., Aristolochiaceae 46
Dorstenia asaroides Gardn., Moraceae 247

U

Ulcers (External & Internal). See also Aphthae, Phagedenic Ulcers, Skin Ulcers
Abrus precatorius L., Fabaceae 160
Acanthosyris spinescens
  (Mart. & Endl.) Gris., Santalaceae 304
Aiovea brasiliensis Meissn., Lauraceae 196
Anacardium occidentale L., Anacardiaceae 7
Andira vermifuga Mart. ex Benth., Fabaceae 162
Annona cornifolia St.-Hil., Annonaceae 12
Annona foetida Mart., Annonaceae 12
Annona spinescens Mart., Annonaceae 13
Annona squamosa L., Annonaceae 13
Aristolochia cymbifera
  Mart. & Zucc., Aristolochiaceae 46
Aristolochia triangularis Cham., Aristolochiaceae ... 48
Aristolochia trilobata L., Aristolochiaceae 48
Auxemma oncocalyx
  (Fr. All.) Taub., Boraginaceae 87
Baccharidastrum triplinerve
  (Less.) Cabr., Asteraceae 53
Baccharis lundii DC., Asteraceae 54
Baccharis trimera (Less.) DC., Asteraceae 54
Bidens graveolens Mart., Asteraceae 56
Bowdichia nitida Spruce ex Benth., Fabaceae 163
Caladium sororium Schott, Araceae 35
Calophyllum brasiliense Camb., Clusiaceae 120
Canna indica L., Cannaceae 111
Carapa guianensis Aubl., Meliaceae 227
Casearia adstringens Mart., Flacourtiaceae 176
Casearia cambessedesii Eichl., Flacourtiaceae 176
Cedrela fissilis Vell., Meliaceae 227
Cereus jamacaru DC., Cactaceae 95
Cereus peruvianus (L.) Mill., Cactaceae 94
Cestrum bracteatum Link & Otto, Solanaceae 317
Chaptalia nutans (L.) Polak., Asteraceae 57
Chromolaena laevigata
  (Lam.) King & Robinson, Asteraceae 58
Clidemia blepharoides DC., Melastomataceae 225
Cordia verbenacea DC., Boraginaceae 88
Coussapoa asperifolia Tréc., Moraceae 247
Croton floribundus Spreng., Euphorbiaceae 150
Cryptocarya minima Mez, Lauraceae 198
Curatella americana L., Dilleniaceae 144
Dracontium polyphyllum L., Araceae 36
Echinodorus macrophyllus
  (Kunth) Mich., Alismataceae 2
Echites peltata Vell., Apocynaceae 23
Eryngium pristis Cham. & Schlecht., Apiaceae 19
Erythrina corallodendron L., Fabaceae 166
Euphorbia phosphorea Mart., Euphorbiaceae 153
Euphorbia tirucalli L., Euphorbiaceae 153

Euterpe oleracea Mart., Arecaceae 42
Ficus gomelleira Kunth & Bouché, Moraceae 248
Gustavia hexapetala
  (Aubl.) J.E. Smith, Lecythidaceae 205
Heliotropium elongatum Willd., Boraginaceae 88
Heliotropium indicum L., Boraginaceae 89
Hibiscus tiliaceus L., Malvaceae 221
Himatanthus drastica
  (Mart.) Woods., Apocynaceae 24
Himatanthus phagedaenica
  (Mart.) Woods., Apocynaceae 26
Hura crepitans L., Euphorbiaceae 153
Hylocereus undatus (Haw.) Br. & Rose, Cactaceae .. 95
Ichthyothere terminalis
  (Spr.) S.F. Blake, Asteraceae 61
Ilex paraguariensis St.-Hil., Aquifoliaceae 31
Ipomoea pes-caprae (L.) R. Br., Convolvulaceae .. 130
Jacaranda brasiliana (Lam.) Pers., Bignoniaceae ... 80
Jacaranda subrhombea DC., Bignoniaceae 81
Jatropha multifida L., Euphorbiaceae 154
Jodina rhombifolia Hook. & Arn., Santalaceae 304
Lafoensia densiflora Pohl, Lythraceae 214
Leonotis nepetaefolia R. Br., Lamiaceae 194
Mabea fistulifera Mart., Euphorbiaceae 155
Magonia pubescens St.-Hil., Sapindaceae 305
Marsdenia amylacea
  (Barb.-Rodr.) Malme, Asclepiadaceae 51
Maytenus boaria Mol., Celastraceae 115
Maytenus ilicifolia Mart., Celastraceae 115
Maytenus obtusifolia Mart., Celastraceae 116
Maytenus spp., Celastraceae (CHEM. & PHARM.) 116
Mikania lindleyana DC., Asteraceae 62
Mikania parviflora (Aubl.) Karst., Asteraceae 62
Monstera adansonii Schott, Araceae 36
Montrichardia linifera (Arruda) Schott, Araceae 36
Myracroduon urundeuva
  Fr. All., Anacardiaceae 9
Myrcia tingens Berg, Myrtaceae 255
Nectandra leucothyrsus Meissn., Lauraceae 199
Nymphaea rudgeana G. Meyer, Nymphaeaceae 259
Omphalea diandra M. Arg., Euphorbiaceae 156
Orbignya phalerata Mart., Arecaceae 43
Ouratea jabotapita Engl., Ochnaceae 261
Ouratea parviflora (DC.) Baill., Ochnaceae 261
Parapiptadenia rigida
  (Benth.) Brenan, Mimosaceae 240
Parkia oppositifolia (Spruce) Benth., Mimosaceae 240
Parkia pectinata Benth., Mimosaceae 240
Pentaclethra macroloba
  (Willd.) O. Ktze., Mimosaceae 242
Philodendron bipinnatifidum Schott, Araceae 36
Pisonia cordifolia Mart., Nyctaginaceae 258
Pithecellobium avaremotemo Mart., Mimosaceae .. 242
Polygonum punctatum Elliot, Polygonaceae 287
Polygonum spectabile Mart., Polygonaceae 287
Portulaca oleracea L., Portulacaceae 289
Portulaca pilosa L., Portulacaceae 289
Protium heptaphyllum (Aubl.) March., Burseraceae 93
Protium icicariba (DC.) March., Burseraceae 94
Renealmia exaltata L.f., Zingiberaceae 342
Renealmia occidentalis Sweet, also
  R. sylvestris Horan., Zingiberaceae 342
Scoparia dulcis L., Scrophulariaceae 312

MEDICINAL INDEX: ULCERS – VENEREAL DISEASE

Senna hirsuta (L.) Ir. & Barn.
  var. puberula Ir. & Barn., Caesalpiniaceae 105
Sida macrodon DC., Malvaceae 222
Solanum cernuum Vell., Solanaceae 319
Solanum insidiosum Mart., Solanaceae 320
Solanum nigrum L., Solanaceae 321
Solanum paniculatum L., Solanaceae 321
Solanum verbascifolium L., Solanaceae 322
Sparattosperma leucanthum
  (Vell.) K. Sch., Bignoniaceae 82
Stachytarpheta cayennensis
  (Rich.) Vahl, Verbenaceae 335
Stryphnodendron coriaceum Benth., Mimosaceae . 243
Tabebuia ipe (Mart.) Standl., Bignoniaceae 83
Terminalia tanibouca Smith, Combretaceae 126
Thevetia ahouai (L.) DC., Apocynaceae 28
Trianosperma glandulosa Mart., Cucurbitaceae 140
Trianosperma trilobata Cogn., Cucurbitaceae 140
Turnera diffusa Willd., Turneraceae 327
Turnera opifera Mart., Turneraceae 328
Virola sebifera Aubl., Myristicaceae 250
Virola surinamensis (Rol.) Warb., Myristicaceae ... 252
Vouacapoua americana Aubl., Caesalpiniaceae 108
Waltheria viscosissima St.-Hil., Sterculiaceae 325
Zschokkea arborescens M. Arg., Apocynaceae 29

Ulcers (Animal)
Magonia pubescens St.-Hil., Sapindaceae 305
Plumbago scandens L., Plumbaginaceae 279

Urethritis
Blepharocalyx salicifolius
  (H.B.K.) Berg, Myrtaceae 253
Campomanesia aurea Berg, also
  C. xanthocarpa Berg, Myrtaceae 253
Canna glauca L., Cannaceae 110
Casearia guyanensis (Aubl.) Urb., Flacourtiaceae ... 177
Clitoria guianensis (Aubl.) Benth., Fabaceae 163
Costus spicatus (Jacq.) Sw., Costaceae 132
Jacaranda copaia (Aubl.) D. Don, Bignoniaceae 80
Krameria tomentosa St.-Hil., Krameriaceae 191
Myrocarpus frondosus Fr. All., Fabaceae 170
Spondias macrocarpa Engl., Anacardiaceae 10
Spondias mombin L., Anacardiaceae 10

Uric Acid Excess
Mikania hirsutissima DC., Asteraceae 62
Stryphnodendron adstringens
  (Mart.) Cov., Mimosaceae 242

Urinary Antiseptic, Antiblennorrhagic, Antileucorrhoea
Copaifera officinalis (Jacq.) L., Caesalpiniaceae 102

Urinary Problems. *See also* Albuminuria, Anuria, Bladder Disease, Cystitis, Diuretic, Hematuria, Kidney Disease, Urethritis
Acanthospermum australe
  (Loefl.) O. Ktze., Asteraceae 51
Amasonia arborea H.B.K., Verbenaceae 333
Bassovia lucida Dunal, Solanaceae 316
Borreria verbenoides Cham. & Schl., Rubiaceae ... 296
Cissampelos glaberrima St.-Hil., Menispermaceae 233
Jacaranda brasiliana (Lam.) Pers., Bignoniaceae ... 80
Jatropha urens L., Euphorbiaceae 155

Mikania hirsutissima DC., Asteraceae 62
Periandra mediterranea (Vell.) Taub., Fabaceae ... 170
Phyllanthus conami Sw., Euphorbiaceae 156
Phyllanthus niruri L., Euphorbiaceae 156
Scoparia dulcis L., Scrophulariaceae 312
Silybum marianum Gaertn., Asteraceae 65

Urine Retention
Calathea grandiflora Lindl., Marantaceae 223
Eryngium foetidum L., Apiaceae 19
Hymenaea courbaril L., Caesalpiniaceae 103
Microtea debilis Sw., Phytolaccaceae 271
Pilea microphylla (L.) Liebm., Urticaceae 331
Sida rhombea L., Malvaceae 222

Urogenital Problems. *See also* Urethritis
Jatropha urens L., Euphorbiaceae 155
Turnera opifera Mart., Turneraceae 328

Uterine Disorders (Metritis). *See also* Leucorrhoea, Metrorrhagia
Chloris polydactyla Sw., Poaceae 280
Phthirusa adunca
  (Meyer) Maguire, Loranthaceae 211
Piper aduncum L., Piperaceae 274
Schinus terebinthifolius Raddi, Anacardiaceae 10
Sicana odorifera Naud., Cucurbitaceae 139
Silybum marianum Gaertn., Asteraceae 65
Trixis antimenorrhoea (Schrank) Mart., Asteraceae . 67

Uterine Prolapse. *See also* Childbirth
Piper aduncum L., Piperaceae 274

V

Vaginal Conditions. *See also* Leucorrhoea
Casearia guyanensis (Aubl.) Urb., Flacourtiaceae . 177
Krameria tomentosa St.-Hil., Krameriaceae 191
Parkia pendula Benth. ex Walp., Mimosaceae 240
Phthirusa adunca (Meyer) Maguire, Loranthaceae 211
Pithecellobium avaremotemo Mart., Mimosaceae .. 242
Stryphnodendron coriaceum Benth., Mimosaceae . 243
Stryphnodendron polyphyllum
  Mart., Mimosaceae 244
Triumfetta semitriloba Jacq., Tiliaceae 327

Varicose Veins
Davilla rugosa Poir., Dilleniaceae 145
Lafoensia densiflora Pohl, Lythraceae 214
Orbignya phalerata Mart., Arecaceae 43

Vasoconstrictor
Carica papaya L., Caricaceae (CHEM. & PHARM.) 113
Xylopia sericea St.-Hil., Annonaceae 16

Veins. *See* Circulatory Problems, Phlebitis, Varicose Veins, Vasoconstrictor

Venereal Disease. *See* Blennorrhagia, Gonorrhoea, Herpes, HIV-1, Syphilis, Venereal Disease (Unspecified)

Venereal Disease (Unspecified)
Dodonaea viscosa Jacq., Sapindaceae 305
Entada polystachya (Jacq.) DC., Mimosaceae 237
Himatanthus fallax (M. Arg.) Woods., Apocynaceae 25
Macfadyena unguis-cati (L.) Gentry, Bignoniaceae . 81
Pisonia aculeata L., Nyctaginaceae 258
Tragia volubilis L., Euphorbiaceae 158

Vitex montevidensis Cham., Verbenaceae 337
Vermifuge.
  See **Anthelmintic, Taenifuge**
Vesicant
  Anacardium humile St.-Hil., Anacardiaceae 7
  Anacardium nanum St.-Hil., Anacardiaceae 7
  Anacardium occidentale L., Anacardiaceae 7
  Clematis dioica L., Ranunculaceae 290
  Monstera adansonii Schott, Araceae 36
Veterinary Use (note: *= Toxic in Animals)
  Anisosperma passiflora Manso, Cucurbitaceae 135
  Baccharis articulata (Lam.) Pers., Asteraceae 54
  Calophyllum brasiliense Camb., Clusiaceae 120
  Caryocar coriaceum Wittm., Caryocaraceae 114
  Magonia pubescens St.-Hil., Sapindaceae 305
  Plumbago scandens L., Plumbaginaceae 279
  **Pteridium aquilinum*
    (L.) Kuhn, Dennstaedtiaceae 144
  **Solanum ciliatum* Lam., Solanaceae 319
  –**cattle**
  Cayaponia pilosa Cogn., Cucurbitaceae 135
  **Clematis dioica* L., Ranunculaceae 290
  Clusia rosea Jacq., Clusiaceae 122
  Hyptis mutabilis (Rich.) Briq., Lamiaceae 193
  Macrosiphonia longiflora
    (Desf.) M. Arg., Apocynaceae 26
  Macrosiphonia velame
    (St.-Hil.) M. Arg., Apocynaceae 26
  **Schultesia stenophylla* Mart., Gentianaceae 180
  **Senecio brasiliensis* Less., Asteraceae 65
  –**glanders**
  Solidago chilensis Meyen, Asteraceae 65
  –**horses.** *See also* **Veterinary Use**–**glanders**
  Imperata brasiliensis Trin., also
    Imperata contracta Hitch., Poaceae 281
  Magonia pubescens St.-Hil., Sapindaceae 305
  Plumbago scandens L., Plumbaginaceae 279
  –**mules**
  Buddleja cambara Arech., Buddlejaceae 93
  –**poultry**
  Momordica charantia L., Cucurbitaceae 139
  –**rabbits**
  Zizyphus joazeiro Mart., Rhamnaceae (PHARM.) 293
  –**rats**
  Stryphnodendron polyphyllum
    Mart., Mimosaceae (PHARM.) 244
Virus. *See* **HIV-1**
Vitiligo
  Brosimum gaudichaudii Tréc., Moraceae 246
Vomitive. *See* **Emetic**
Vulnerary. *See* **Wounds**

W

Warts
  Anacardium occidentale L., Anacardiaceae 7
  Carica papaya L., Caricaceae 113
  Commelina nudiflora L., Commelinaceae 126
  Euphorbia phosphorea Mart., Euphorbiaceae 153
  Himatanthus alba (L.) Woods., Apocynaceae 24

Himatanthus phagedaenica
  (Mart.) Woods., Apocynaceae 26
Oxalis corniculata L., Oxalidaceae 266
Plumbago scandens L., Plumbaginaceae 279
Plumeria alba L., Apocynaceae 28
Sapium hamatum Pax & Hoffm., Euphorbiaceae ... 157
Solanum lycocarpum St.-Hil., Solanaceae 321
Weakness
  Baccharis articulata (Lam.) Pers., Asteraceae 54
Weight Reduction. *See* **Slimming**
Whitlow
  Crataeva tapia L., Capparaceae 112
  Elaeis guineensis Jacq., Arecaceae 40
  Plumbago scandens L., Plumbaginaceae 279
Whooping Cough
  Anchietea pyrifolia (Mart.) G. Don, Violaceae 338
  Bauhinia radiata Vell., Caesalpiniaceae 99
  Cardiospermum grandiflorum Sw., Sapindaceae ... 305
  Cayaponia espelina
    (Manso) Cogn., Cucurbitaceae 135
  Cecropia hololeuca Miq., Moraceae 247
  Cupania racemosa Radlk., Sapindaceae 305
  Dioscorea silvestris Vell., Dioscoreaceae 147
  Dracontium asperum K. Koch, Araceae 35
  Erythrina corallodendron L., Fabaceae 166
  Leonurus sibiricus L., Lamiaceae 194
  Mikania parviflora (Aubl.) Karst., Asteraceae 62
  Ocimum micranthum Willd., Lamiaceae 195
Womb Strengthener.
  See also **Uterine Prolapse**
  Ocotea pulchella Mart., Lauraceae 201
  Piper aduncum L., Piperaceae 274
Worms
  Ambrosia artemisiifolia L., Asteraceae 53
  Anacardium occidentale L., Anacardiaceae 7
  Andira vermifuga Mart. ex Benth., Fabaceae 162
  Annona squamosa L., Annonaceae 13
  Aristolochia triangularis Cham., Aristolochiaceae ... 48
  Bellucia grossularioides (L.) Tr., Melastomataceae 225
  Caesalpinia bonduc (L.) Roxb., Caesalpiniaceae 99
  Calyptranthes aromatica St.-Hil., Myrtaceae 253
  Caraipa grandifolia Mart., Clusiaceae 121
  Carica papaya L., Caricaceae 113
  Couma utilis (Mart.) M. Arg., Apocynaceae 23
  Duguetia riparia Hub., Annonaceae 14
  Himatanthus phagedaenica
    (Mart.) Woods., Apocynaceae 26
  Mikania parviflora (Aubl.) Karst., Asteraceae 62
  Polygonum acuminatum H.B.K., Polygonaceae 286
  Polygonum spectabile Mart., Polygonaceae 286
  Spigelia anthelmia L., Loganiaceae 209
  –*tapeworms*
  Calyptranthes aromatica St.-Hil., Myrtaceae 253
Wounds (Vulnerary)
  Ageratum conyzoides L., Asteraceae 53
  Annona squamosa L., Annonaceae 13
  Arrabidaea chica (H.B.K.) Bur., Bignoniaceae 78
  Auxemma oncocalyx (Fr. All.) Taub., Boraginaceae . 87
  Bidens pilosa L., Asteraceae 57
  Blanchetia heterotricha DC., Asteraceae 57
  Caesalpinia ferrea Mart. ex Tul., Caesalpiniaceae . 100
  Caladium bicolor (Aiton) Vent., Araceae 34

MEDICINAL INDEX: WOUNDS – YELLOW FEVER

Casearia cambessedesii Eichl., Flacourtiaceae 176
Casearia sylvestris Sw., Flacourtiaceae 178
Cecropia palmata Willd., Moraceae 247
Ceiba pentandra (L.) Gaertn., Bombacaceae 86
Cereus peruvianus (L.) Mill., Cactaceae 94
Cestrum bracteatum Link & Otto, Solanaceae 317
Cissampelos ovalifolia DC., Menispermaceae 233
Cleome polygama L., Capparaceae 112
Cleome spinosa Jacq., Capparaceae 112
Copaifera cearensis
   Huber ex Ducke, Caesalpiniaceae 102
Copaifera officinalis (Jacq.) L., Caesalpiniaceae 102
Cordia ecalyculata Vell., Boraginaceae 87
Cordia verbenacea DC., Boraginaceae 88
Croton floribundus Spreng., Euphorbiaceae 150
Croton salutaris Casar., Euphorbiaceae 151
Cuscuta racemosa Mart., Convolvulaceae 130
Cyrtopodium andersoni R. Br., Orchidaceae 266
Erigeron tweediei Hook. & Arn., Asteraceae 60
Euphorbia hirta L., Euphorbiaceae 152
Euterpe edulis Mart., Arecaceae 41
Galinsoga parviflora Cav., Asteraceae 60
Grindelia scorzonerifolia Hook. & Arn., Asteraceae 60
Heimia salicifolia
   (H.B.K.) Link & Otto, Lythraceae 214
Heliotropium indicum L., Boraginaceae 89
Hibiscus tiliaceus L., Malvaceae 21
Himatanthus sucuuba (Spr.) Woods., Apocynaceae . 26
Hymenaea courbaril L., Caesalpiniaceae 103
Hypericum brasiliense Choisy, Clusiaceae 122
Hyptis spicigera Lam., Lamiaceae 193
Ipomoea acetosifolia
   (Vahl) Roem. & Schult., Convolvulaceae 130
Ipomoea pes-caprae (L.) R. Br., Convolvulaceae .. 130
Ischnosiphon arouma Koern., Marantaceae 223
Jacaranda brasiliana (Lam.) Pers., Bignoniaceae ... 80
Jodina rhombifolia Hook. & Arn., Santalaceae 304
Jungia floribunda Less., Asteraceae 61
Lithraea molleoides (Vell.) Engl., Anacardiaceae 9
Ludwigia natans (H.B.K.) Ell., Onagraceae 264
Maclura tinctoria (L.) D. Don, Moraceae 249
Macrosiphonia longiflora
   (Desf.) M. Arg., Apocynaceae 26
Macrosiphonia velame
   (St.-Hil.) M. Arg., Apocynaceae 26
Mammea americana L., Clusiaceae 123
Marsdenia amylacea
   (Barb.-Rodr.) Malme, Asclepiadaceae 51
Maytenus boaria Mol., Celastraceae 115
Maytenus communis Reiss., Celastraceae 115
Maytenus ilicifolia Mart., Celastraceae 115
Mikania parviflora (Aubl.) Karst., Asteraceae 62
Mouriri apiranga Spruce, Melastomataceae 225
Nymphaea ampla DC., Nymphaeaceae 259
Nymphaea rudgeana G. Meyer, Nymphaeaceae ... 259
Oenothera catharinensis Camb., Onagraceae 264
Ouratea hexasperma (St.-Hil.) Baill., Ochnaceae .. 261
Parahancornia amapa
   (Hub.) Ducke, Apocynaceae 27
Parkia oppositifolia (Spruce) Benth., Mimosaceae 240
Parkia pectinata Benth., Mimosaceae 240
Patagonula americana L., Boraginaceae 89

Peschiera affinis (M. Arg.) Miers, Apocynaceae 27
Peschiera laeta (Mart.) Miers, Apocynaceae 27
Piper angustifolium R. & Pav., Piperaceae 274
Pothomorphe peltata L., Piperaceae 277
Protium aracouchini (Aubl.) March., Burseraceae ... 93
Psidium guajava L., Myrtaceae 256
Psoralea glandulosa L., Fabaceae 170
Schinus molle L., Anacardiaceae 9
Senecio brasiliensis Less., Asteraceae 65
Sida rhombea L., Malvaceae 222
Simaba ferruginea St.-Hil., Simaroubaceae 314
Solidago chilensis Meyen, Asteraceae 65
Stryphnodendron adstringens
   (Mart.) Cov., Mimosaceae 242
Syagrus coronata (Mart.) Becc., Arecaceae 45
Virola surinamensis (Rol.) Warb., Myristicaceae 252
Wissadula periplocifolia Presl., Malvaceae 223
Ximenia americana L., Olacaceae 263
Ximenia coriacea Engl., Olacaceae 263

Y

Yaws (Pian)
Himatanthus lancifolia
   (M. Arg.) Woods., Apocynaceae 26
Yellow Fever
Cordia coffeoides Warm., Boraginaceae 87
Senna occidentalis (L.) Link, Caesalpiniaceae 105
Senna quinqueangulata
   (Rich.) Ir. & Barn., Caesalpiniaceae 106
Stachytarpheta jamaicensis
   (L.) Vahl, Verbenaceae 336

Common Names Index

A

Abacate-do-mato
　Tontelea brachypoda Miers, Hippocrateaceae 183
Abacaterana
　Pleurothyrium cuneifolium Nees, Lauraceae 203
Abacaxi
　Ananas comosus (L.) Merrill, Bromeliaceae 90
Abagerú *(abajeru)*
　Chrysobalanus icaco L., Chrysobalanaceae 119
Abajeru *(abagerú)*
　Chrysobalanus icaco L., Chrysobalanaceae 119
Abecedária
　Acmella repens (Walt.) L.C. Rich., Asteraceae 52
Abiu
　Lucuma caimito Roem. & Schult., Sapotaceae 309
Abóbora
　Cucurbita pepo L., Cucurbitaceae 136
Abóbora-do-mato
　Melothria fluminensis Gardn., Cucurbitaceae 139
Abobreira-do-mato
　Cayaponia cabocla (Vell.) Mart., also
　　Cayaponia spp., Cucurbitaceae 135
Abobrinha
　Cayaponia martiana (Cogn.) Cogn., also
　　Cayaponia spp., Cucurbitaceae 135
Abobrinha-do-mato
　Cayaponia martiana (Cogn.) Cogn., also
　　Cayaponia spp., Cucurbitaceae 135
　Cayaponia pilosa Cogn., Cucurbitaceae 135
　Cayaponia tayuya (Mart.) Cogn., Cucurbitaceae 135
　Trianosperma diversifolia Cogn., Cucurbitaceae 139
　Trianosperma glandulosa Mart., Cucurbitaceae 140
　Wilbrandia verticillata (Vell.)
　　Cogn., Cucurbitaceae 140
Abre-sol
　Heimia salicifolia (H.B.K.)
　　Link & Otto, Lythraceae 214
Abricó
　Mammea americana L., Clusiaceae 123
Abricó-do-pará
　Mammea americana L., Clusiaceae 123
Abroco
　Xanthium orientale L., *X. spinosum* L.
　　and *X. strumarium* L., Asteraceae 68
Abuta
　Abuta concolor Poepp. & Endl., Menispermaceae . 231
Abutinha
　Cissampelos glaberrima St.-Hil., Menispermaceae 233
Abútua
　Abuta candicans Rich., Menispermaceae 231
　Abuta concolor Poepp. & Endl., Menispermaceae . 231
　Abuta rufescens Aubl., Menispermaceae 231
　Abuta selloana Eichl., Menispermaceae 231

Cissampelos fasciculata Benth., Menispermaceae . 231
Cissampelos glaberrima St.-Hil., Menispermaceae 233
Cissampelos pareira L., Menispermaceae 233
Sciadotenia paraensis
　(Eichl.) Diels, Menispermaceae 234
Abútua-da-terra
　Chondodendron platyphyllum
　　(Mart.) Miers, Menispermaceae 231
Abútua-do-rio
　Cissampelos fluminensis Eichl., Menispermaceae .. 233
Abútua-grande
　Chondodendron platyphyllum
　　(Mart.) Miers, Menispermaceae 231
Abútua-miúda
　Cocculus filipendula Mart., Menispermaceae 234
Abútua-pequena
　Cissampelos ovalifolia DC., Menispermaceae 233
Abútua-preta
　Chondodendron platyphyllum
　　(Mart.) Miers, Menispermaceae 231
Açacu *(assacu)*
　Hura crepitans L., Euphorbiaceae 153
Açacu-i
　Euphorbia cotinoides Miq., Euphorbiaceae 152
Açacurana
　Erythrina fusca Lour., Fabaceae 166
Açafroa
　Bixa orellana L., Bixaceae 85
　Guarea trichilioides L., Meliaceae 228
Açafroeira-da-terra
　Bixa orellana L., Bixaceae 85
Açaí
　Euterpe oleracea Mart., Arecaceae 42
　also Uses: *Physalis angulata* L., Solanaceae 318
Acaíba
　Spondias mombin L., Anacardiaceae 10
Açaizeiro
　Euterpe oleracea Mart., Arecaceae 42
Acapociba
　Allamanda doniana M. Arg., Apocynaceae 20
Acapu
　Vouacapoua americana Aubl., Caesalpiniaceae 108
Acapu-do-igapó
　Campsiandra comosa Benth. var.
　　laurifolia (Benth.) Cowan, Caesalpiniaceae 100
Acapurana
　Campsiandra comosa Benth. var.
　　laurifolia (Benth.) Cowan, Caesalpiniaceae 100
Acariçoba
　Hydrocotyle bonariensis Lam., Apiaceae 19
　Hydrocotyle leucocephala
　　Cham. & Schlecht., Apiaceae 20
Acariquara-branca
　Geissospermum sericeum
　　Benth. & Hook., Apocynaceae 24

Acarirana
Geissospermum sericeum
Benth. & Hook., Apocynaceae 24
Acoara-muru
Cordia grandiflora DC., Boraginaceae 87
Cordia magnolifolia Cham., Boraginaceae 87
Açoita-cavalo
Luehea divaricata Mart. & Zucc., Tiliaceae 326
Luehea rufescens St.-Hil., Tiliaceae 327
Acuá
Saccoglottis guianensis Benth., Humiriaceae 185
Açucena
Hedychium coronarium Koenig, Zingiberaceae 342
Hippeastrum puniceum
(Lam.) Kuntze, Amaryllidaceae 6
Açucena-d'água
Hymenocallis tubiflora Salisb., Amaryllidaceae 7
Açucena-do-brejo
Datura arborea L., Solanaceae 317
Açucena-do-campo
Hippeastrum psittacinum Herb., Amaryllidaceae 6
Açucena-do-jardim
Hippeastrum vittatum (L'Hérit.)
Herb., Amaryllidaceae 6
Acuralzinho
Euphorbia thymifolia L., Euphorbiaceae 153
Acurí
Scheelea phalerata (Mart. ex Spreng.)
Burret, Arecaceae 45
Adima
Sauvagesia erecta L., Ochnaceae 262
Agaí
Thevetia ahouai (L.) DC., Apocynaceae 28
Agoniada
Himatanthus lancifolia
(M. Arg.) Woods., Apocynaceae 26
Agreste
Imperata brasiliensis Trin., Poaceae 281
Agrião
Sphagneticola trilobata (L.) Pruski, Asteraceae 65
Agrião-bravo
Acmella repens (Walt.) L.C. Rich., Asteraceae 52
Agrião-do-Brasil
Acmella repens (Walt.) L.C. Rich., Asteraceae 52
Agrião-do-brejo
Eclipta prostrata (L.) L., Asteraceae 59
Agrião-do-pará
Acmella oleracea (L.) R.K. Jansen, Asteraceae 52
Acmella repens (Walt.) L.C. Rich., Asteraceae 52
Aguaçu
Orbignya phalerata Mart., Arecaceae 43
Aguapé
Azolla caroliniana Willd., Salviniaceae 304
Echinodorus grandiflorus
(Cham. & Schl.) Mich., Alistmataceae 2
Eichhornia crassipes Solms, Pontederiaceae 288
Pontederia cordifolia Mart., Pontederiaceae 288
Aguapé-da-flor-amarela
Nymphaea rudgeana G. Meyer, Nymphaeaceae 259

Aguapé-da-flor-branca
Nymphaea ampla DC., Nymphaeaceae 259
Aguapé-da-meia-noite
Nymphaea rudgeana G. Meyer, Nymphaeaceae 259
Aguapé-de-flor-miúda
Nymphoides indica (L.) O. Ktze., Menyanthaceae . 235
Aguapé-de-flor-roxa
Eichhornia crassipes Solms, Pontederiaceae 288
Aguapé-do-grande
Nymphaea ampla DC., Nymphaeaceae 259
Aguaraquinhá
Heliotropium elongatum Willd., Boraginaceae 88
Agutiguepe
Maranta arundinacea L., Marantaceae 223
Aiapana
Ayapana triplinerve
(Vahl) King & H. Robinson, Asteraceae 53
Aipo
Apium sellowianum Wolf, Apiaceae 18
Aipo-bravo
Apium sellowianum Wolf, Apiaceae 18
Airi
Astrocaryum aculeatissimum
(Schott) Burret, Arecaceae 39
Aiúba
Aniba permollis (Nees) Mez, Lauraceae 197
Ajuba
Aniba permollis (Nees) Mez, Lauraceae 197
Alafavaca-de-caboclo
Hyptis mutabilis (Rich.) Briq., Lamiaceae 193
Alamanda
Allamanda cathartica L., Apocynaceae 20
Alamanda-cheirosa
Dipladenia fragrans DC., Apocynaceae 23
Alamanda-de-flor-grande
Allamanda cathartica L., Apocynaceae 20
Alamanda-de-jacobina
Allamanda blanchetii M. Arg., Apocynaceae 20
Albará
Canna glauca L., Cannaceae 110
Albina
Turnera ulmifolia L., Turneraceae 328
Alcaçuz-bravo
Senna rugosa
(G. Don) Ir. & Barn., Caesalpiniaceae 106
Alcaçuz-da-terra
Periandra mediterranea (Vell.) Taub., Fabaceae ... 170
Alcaçuz-do-cerrado
Periandra mediterranea (Vell.) Taub., Fabaceae ... 170
Alecrim-bravo
Hypericum brasiliense Choisy, Clusiaceae 122
Lantana microphylla Cham., Verbenaceae 335
Alecrim-da-praia
Bulbostylis capillaris Clarke, Cyperaceae 142
Alecrim-das-paredes
Pterocaulon virgatum DC., Asteraceae 64
Alecrim-de-angola
Piper arboreum Aubl., Piperaceae 274
Vitex agnus-castus L., Verbenaceae 336

Alecrim-do-campo
Baccharis dentata (Vell.) G.M. Barroso, Asteraceae 54
Baccharis dracunculifolia DC., Asteraceae 54
Baccharis ramosissima Gardn., Asteraceae 54
Heterothalamus alienus (Spr.) O. Ktze., Asteraceae 60
Heterothalamus psiadioides Less., Asteraceae 60
Lantana microphylla Cham., Verbenaceae 335
Lippia alba (Mill.) N.E. Brown, Verbenaceae 335

Alecrim-do-mato
Baccharis dentata
(Vell.) G.M. Barroso, Asteraceae 54

Alecrim-do-norte
Vitex agnus-castus L., Verbenaceae 336

Aleluia
Senna macranthera
(Collad.) Ir. & Barn., Caesalpiniaceae 105
Senna multijuga Rich. var.
verrucosa (Vog.) Ir. & Barn., Caesalpiniaceae 105

Alfavaca
Ocimum fluminensis Vell., Lamiaceae 195
Ocimum micranthum Willd., Lamiaceae 195

Alfavaca-brava
Monnieria trifolia Loefl., Rutaceae 302

Alfavaca-de-cheiro
Marsypianthes chamaedrys
(Vahl) O. Ktze., Lamiaceae 194
Ocimum fluminensis Vell., Lamiaceae 195
Peltodon longipes St.-Hil., Lamiaceae 195

Alfavaca-de-cobra
Monnieria trifolia Loefl., Rutaceae 302
Peperomia pellucida H.B.K., Piperaceae 273
Piper eucalyptifolium (Miq.) Rudge, Piperaceae 275

Alfavaca-do-campo
Ocimum micranthum Willd., Lamiaceae 195

Alfavacão
Hyptis mutabilis (Rich.) Briq., Lamiaceae 193

Algodão-bravo
Cochlospermum orinocense
(H.B.K.) Steud., Cochlospermaceae 125
Cochlospermum regium
(Mart. & Schl.) Pilg., Cochlospermaceae 125

Algodão-o-brejo
Hibiscus bifurcatus Cav., Malvaceae 221

Algodoeiro-bravo
Hibiscus bifurcatus Cav., Malvaceae 221

Algodoeiro-da-praia
Hibiscus tiliaceus L., Malvaceae 221

Algodoeiro-do-campo
Cochlospermum regium
(Mart. & Schl.) Pilg., Cochlospermaceae 125

Alho-da-campina
Cipura paludosa Aubl., Iridaceae 186

Alho-do-campo
Cipura paludosa Aubl., Iridaceae 186

Alho-do-mato
Cipura paludosa Aubl., Iridaceae 186

Alho-silvestre
Nothoscordum striatum Kunth, Iridaceae 186

Alicuri
Syagrus schizophylla (Mart.) Glassman, Arecaceae . 46

Almecegueira
Protium icicariba (DC.) March., Burseraceae 94
Protium heptaphyllum (Aubl.) March., Burseraceae 93

Almíscar
Styrax glabratum Schott, Styracaceae 325

Amajouva
Aiovea brasiliensis Meissn., Lauraceae 197

Amandurana
Hibiscus bifurcatus Cav., Malvaceae 221

Amapá
Brosimum parinarioides Ducke, Moraceae 246
Parahancornia amapa (Hub.) Ducke, Apocynaceae 27

Amapá-de-várzea
Brosimum potabile Ducke, Moraceae 246

Amapá-doce
Brosimum potabile Ducke, Moraceae 246

Amarelinho
Raputia magnifica Engl., Rutaceae 302

Amarelinho-da-serra
Cusparia febrifuga Humb., Rutaceae 300

Amarelo
Cusparia febrifuga Humb., Rutaceae 300

Ambaia-caá
Aristolochia cymbifera
Mart. & Zucc., Aristolochiaceae 46

Ambaia-embo
Aristolochia cymbifera
Mart. & Zucc., Aristolochiaceae 46

Ambrosia, Ambrósia
Ambrosia artemisiifolia L., Asteraceae 53
Chenopodium ambrosioides L., Chenopodiaceae ... 118

Ambrósia-do-méxico
Chenopodium ambrosioides L., Chenopodiaceae ... 118

Amburana
Torresea cearensis Fr. All., Fabaceae 172

Amburana-brava
Dipteryx alata Vog., Fabaceae 165

Ameixa
Ximenia americana L., Olacaceae 263
Ximenia coriacea Engl., Olacaceae 263

Ameixa-brava
Ximenia coriacea Engl., Olacaceae 263

Ameixa-de-espinho
Ximenia americana L., Olacaceae 263

Ameixa-do-brasil
Ximenia americana L., Olacaceae 263

Amêndoa-de-espinho
Caryocar villosum (Aubl.) Pers., Caryocaraceae 114

Amendoeirana
Desmodium axillare (Sw.) DC., Fabaceae 164
Senna rugosa (G. Don) Ir.
& Barn., Caesalpiniaceae 106

Amonjeaba
Sacciolepis myuros (Lam.) Chase, Poaceae 282

Amor-crescido
Portulaca grandiflora Hook., Portulacaceae 289
Portulaca pilosa L., Portulacaceae 289

Amor-de-negro
Acanthospermum australe
(Loefl.) O. Ktze., Asteraceae 51

Acanthospermum hispidum DC., Asteraceae 52
Xanthium orientale L., *X. spinosum* L.
and *X. strumarium* L., Asteraceae 68
Amor-do-campo
Desmodium triflorum DC., Fabaceae 164
Triumfetta rhomboidea Jacq., Tiliaceae 327
Amora-branca
Rubus brasiliensis Mart., Rosaceae 294
Amora-brava
Rubus brasiliensis Mart., Rosaceae 294
Amora-do-mato
Coutarea hexandra (Jacq.) K. Sch., Rubiaceae 297
Amora-preta
Rubus brasiliensis Mart., Rosaceae 294
Amora-verde
Rubus brasiliensis Mart., Rosaceae 294
Amoreira-do-brasil
Rubus brasiliensis Mart., Rosaceae 294
Amoreira-do-mato
Brosimum gaudichaudii Tréc., Moraceae 246
Rubus brasiliensis Mart., Rosaceae 294
Amores-o-campo
Desmodium axillare (Sw.) DC., Fabaceae 164
Amorzinho-seco
Desmodium triflorum DC., Fabaceae 164
Ana-da-costa
Leonurus sibiricus L., Lamiaceae 194
Anabi
Potalia amara Aubl., Loganiaceae 209
Anacuri
Scheelea phalerata
  (Mart. ex Spreng.) Burret, Arecaceae 45
Ananás
Ananas comosus (L.) Merrill, Bromeliaceae 90
Anapinta
Cayaponia cabocla (Vell.) Mart., also
  Cayaponia spp., Cucurbitaceae 135
Cayaponia tayuya (Mart.) Cogn., Cucurbitaceae 135
Wilbrandia verticillata
  (Vell.) Cogn., Cucurbitaceae 140
Anauerá
Licania macrophylla Benth., Chrysobalanaceae 120
Anavinga
Casearia ovata Willd., Flacourtiaceae 178
Andá-açu
Joannesia princeps Vell., Euphorbiaceae 155
Andacá, Andacaá
Commelina virginica L., Commelinaceae 128
Panicum brevifolium L., Poaceae 282
Panicum trichanthum Nees, Poaceae 282
Andira-da-várzea
Vatairea guianensis Aubl., Fabaceae 172
Andirá-poampé
Bignonia exoleta Vell., Bignoniaceae 79
Andirá-uxi
Andira inermis (Sw.) H.B.K., Fabaceae 162
Andira retusa (Poir.) H.B.K., Fabaceae 162
Andiroba
Anisosperma passiflora Manso, Cucurbitaceae 135
Carapa guianensis Aubl., Meliaceae 227

Anêmone
Anemone decapetala L., Ranunculaceae 290
Anêmone-de-dez-folhas
Anemone decapetala L., Ranunculaceae 290
Angélica
Guettarda angelica Mart., Rubiaceae 298
Guettarda argentea Lam., Rubiaceae 298
Angélica-brava
Guettarda angelica Mart., Rubiaceae 298
Angélica-de-rama
Araujia sericifera Brot., Asclepiadaceae 50
Angélica-do-mato
Guettarda angelica Mart., Rubiaceae 298
Angélica-mansa
Guettarda angelica Mart., Rubiaceae 298
Angelicó
Aristolochia cordigera Willd., Aristolochiaceae 46
Aristolochia trilobata L., Aristolochiaceae 48
Angelim
Sweetia fruticosa Spreng., Fabaceae 172
Angelim-amargoso
Andira vermifuga Mart. ex Benth., Fabaceae 162
Vataireopsis araroba (Aguiar) Ducke, Fabaceae 172
Angelim-araroba
Vataireopsis araroba (Aguiar) Ducke, Fabaceae 172
Angelim-coco
Andira legalis (Vell.) Tol., and Andira spp.,
  under Andira vermifuga, Fabaceae 162
Angelim-da-várzea
Andira inermis (Sw.) H.B.K., Fabaceae 162
Angelim-do-campo
Andira vermifuga Mart. ex Benth., Fabaceae 162
Angelim-pedra
Sweetia fruticosa Spreng., Fabaceae 172
Angelônia
Angelonia integerrima Spreng., Scrophulariaceae .. 310
Angico
Anadenanthera colubrina
  (Vell.) Brenan, Mimosaceae 236
Anadenanthera falcata
  (Benth.) Brenan, Mimosaceae 236
Anadenanthera macrocarpa
  (Benth.) Brenan, Mimosaceae 236
Anadenanthera peregrina
  (L.) Speg., Mimosaceae 236
Pithecellobium avaremotemo Mart., Mimosaceae .. 242
Angico-branco
Anadenanthera colubrina
  (Vell.) Brenan, Mimosaceae 236
Parapiptadenia rigida
  (Benth.) Brenan, Mimosaceae 240
Angico-bravo
Anadenanthera macrocarpa
  (Benth.) Brenan, Mimosaceae 236
Angico-cedro
Parapiptadenia rigida
  (Benth.) Brenan, Mimosaceae 240
Angico-de-curtume
Parapiptadenia rigida
  (Benth.) Brenan, Mimosaceae 240

ANGICO-DO-BANHADO – ARAPABACA: COMMON NAMES INDEX

Angico-do-banhado
Parapiptadenia rigida
(Benth.) Brenan, Mimosaceae 240
Angico-do-cerrado
Anadenanthera macrocarpa
(Benth.) Brenan, Mimosaceae 236
Angico-dos-montes
Parapiptadenia rigida
(Benth.) Brenan, Mimosaceae 240
Angico-preto
Anadenanthera macrocarpa
(Benth.) Brenan, Mimosaceae 236
Angico-rosa
Parapiptadenia rigida
(Benth.) Brenan, Mimosaceae 240
Angico-verdadeiro
Parapiptadenia rigida
(Benth.) Brenan, Mimosaceae 240
Angico-vermelho
Anadenanthera peregrina
(L.) Speg., Mimosaceae 236
Angustura
Cusparia febrifuga Humb., Rutaceae 300
Esenbeckia febrifuga Juss., Rutaceae 301
Esenbeckia intermedia Mart., Rutaceae 301
Galipea multiflora Schult., Rutaceae 301
Angustura-venenosa
Cusparia toxicaria Spr. ex Engl., Rutaceae 301
Anhanga-piri
Clidemia blepharoides DC., Melastomataceae 225
Anhuiba-do-brejo
Nectandra leucothyrsus Meissn., Lauraceae 200
Anil
Indigofera suffruticosa Mill., Fabaceae 168
Anil-trepador
Cissus sicyoides L., Vitaceae 339
Anileira
Indigofera suffruticosa Mill., Fabaceae 168
Anima-membeca
Calathea grandiflora Lindl., Marantaceae 223
Aninga
Montrichardia linifera (Arruda) Schott, Araceae 36
Philodendron speciosum Schott, Araceae 37
Aninga-açu
Montrichardia linifera (Arruda) Schott, Araceae 36
Aninga-da-água
Caladium sororium Schott, Araceae 35
Aninga-para
Dieffenbachia seguine (Jacq.) Schott, Araceae 35
Aninga-pari
Clidemia blepharoides DC., Melastomataceae 225
Aninga-piri
Clidemia blepharoides DC., Melastomataceae 225
Aninga-uba
Dieffenbachia seguine (Jacq.) Schott, Araceae 35
Aniúba
Aniba permollis (Nees) Mez, Lauraceae 197
Anserina-vermífuga
Chenopodium ambrosioides L., Chenopodiaceae ... 118

Anzol-de-lontra
Strychnos subcordata Spr. ex Benth., Loganiaceae 210
Apanha-saia
Hybanthus atropurpureus Taub., Violaceae 338
Apé
Nymphaea rudgeana G. Meyer, Nymphaeaceae 259
Apê
Urospatha caudata
(Poepp. & Endl.) Schott, Araceae 37
Apê-do-sertão
Brosimum gaudichaudii Tréc., Moraceae 246
Apeí
Dorstenia reniformis Pohl, Moraceae 248
Aperana
Nymphoides indica (L.) O. Ktze., Menyanthaceae . 235
Aperta-ruão
Leandra lacunosa Cogn., Melastomataceae 225
Piper aduncum L., Piperaceae 274
Piper angustifolium R. & Pav., Piperaceae 274
Aperta-ruão-do-ceará
Piper elongatum Vahl, Piperaceae 275
Apii
Dorstenia asaroides Gardn., Moraceae 247
Apiranga
Mouriri apiranga Spruce, Melastomataceae 225
Apogitaguará
Esenbeckia intermedia Mart., Rutaceae 301
Apuí
Clusia grandiflora Splitg., Clusiaceae 121
Ficus trigona L. f., Moraceae 249
Apuí-açu
Ficus insipida Willd., Moraceae 248
Ará
Caladium bicolor (Aiton) Vent., Araceae 34
Araçá
Psidium cattleyanum Sabine, Myrtaceae 256
Araçá-cinzento
Psidium cinereum Mart., Myrtaceae 256
Araçá-de-anta
Bellucia grossularioides (L.) Tr., Melastomataceae 225
Araçá-de-pedra
Psidium cattleyanum Sabine, Myrtaceae 256
Araçá-do-campo
Psidium cattleyanum Sabine, Myrtaceae 256
Araçá-iba
Psidium cattleyanum Sabine, Myrtaceae 256
Araçá-pelea
Psidium arboreum Vell., Myrtaceae 256
Araçá-rasteiro
Campomanesia aurea Berg, Myrtaceae 253
Araçazeiro-grande
Psidium arboreum Vell., Myrtaceae 256
Araçazeiro
Psidium cattleyanum Sabine, Myrtaceae 256
Aracuchini
Protium aracouchini (Aubl.) March., Burseraceae ... 93
Arapabaca
Spigelia anthelmia L., Loganiaceae 209
Spigelia flemingiana Cham. & Schl., Loganiaceae . 209

Spigelia glabrata Mart., Loganiaceae 209
Arapoca
Raputia magnifica Engl., Rutaceae 302
Arapoca-amarela
Galipea dichotoma Sald., Rutaceae 301
Arapoca-branca
Raputia alba (Nees & Mart.) Engl., Rutaceae 302
Arapoca-de-cheiro
Raputia aromatica Aubl., Rutaceae 302
Arara-tucupé
Parkia oppositifolia (Spruce) Benth., Mimosaceae 240
Araracanga
Aspidosperma desmanthum M. Arg., Apocynaceae . 21
Araraúba-da-terra-firme
Aspidosperma desmanthum M. Arg., Apocynaceae . 21
Araroba
Vataireopsis araroba (Aguiar) Ducke, Fabaceae 172
Araruta
Maranta arundinacea L., Marantaceae 223
Araruta-bastarda
Canna edulis Ker-Gawl., Cannaceae 110
Araruta-de-porco
Canna edulis Ker-Gawl., Cannaceae 110
Araruta-do-campo
Connarus suberosus Planch., Connaraceae 129
Aratanha
Astronium fraxinifolium Schott, Anacardiaceae 9
Araticu-grande
Rollinia sylvatica (St.-Hil.) Mart., Annonaceae 15
Araticum
Annona crassifolia Mart., Annonaceae 12
Annona glabra L., Annonaceae 13
Annona marcgravii Mart., Annonaceae 13
Annona reticulata L., Annonaceae 13
Bocagea alba St.-Hil., Annonaceae 14
Bocagea viridis St.-Hil., Annonaceae 14
Araticum-alvadio
Rollinia exalbida (Vell.) Mart., Annonaceae 15
Araticum-bravo
Annona glabra L., Annonaceae 13
Araticum-cagão
Annona marcgravii Mart., Annonaceae 13
Araticum-cortiça
Annona glabra L., Annonaceae 13
Araticum-da-água
Annona glabra L., Annonaceae 13
Araticum-da-caatinga
Annona foetida Mart., Annonaceae 12
Araticum-da-mata
Rollinia sylvatica (St.-Hil.) Mart., Annonaceae 15
Araticum-das-catingas
Annona cornifolia St.-Hil., Annonaceae 12
Araticum-de-comer
Annona muricata L., Annonaceae 13
Araticum-de-espinho
Annona spinescens Mart., Annonaceae 13
Araticum-de-paca
Annona marcgravii Mart., Annonaceae 13

Araticum-de-santa-catarina
Rollinia salicifolia Schl., Annonaceae 15
Araticum-do-brejo
Annona glabra L., Annonaceae 13
Annona spinescens Mart., Annonaceae 13
Araticum-do-campo
Annona coriacea Mart., Annonaceae 12
Annona cornifolia St.-Hil., Annonaceae 12
Annona dioica St.-Hil., Annonaceae 12
Duguetia furfuracea
  (St.-Hil.) Benth. & Hook., Annonaceae 14
Araticum-do-cerrado
Annona crassifolia Mart., Annonaceae 12
Araticum-do-grande
Annona muricata L., Annonaceae 13
Araticum-do-mangue
Annona glabra L., Annonaceae 13
Araticum-do-mato
Rollinia sylvatica (St.-Hil.) Mart., Annonaceae 15
Araticum-do-morro
Rollinia sylvatica (St.-Hil.) Mart., Annonaceae 15
Araticum-do-pará
Annona cornifolia St.-Hil., Annonaceae 12
Araticum-do-rio
Annona spinescens Mart., Annonaceae 13
Araticum-do-tabuleiro
Annona coriacea Mart., Annonaceae 12
Araticum-folha-de-salgueiro
Rollinia salicifolia Schl., Annonaceae 15
Araticum-fruta-de-pau
Talauma ovata St.-Hil., Magnoliaceae 216
Araticum-grande
Annona dioica St.-Hil., Annonaceae 12
Duguetia furfuracea
  (St.-Hil.) Benth. & Hook., Annonaceae 14
Araticum-mirim
Annona cornifolia St.-Hil., Annonaceae 12
Araticum-pana
Annona marcgravii Mart., Annonaceae 13
Araticum-panã
Annona crassifolia Mart., Annonaceae 12
Araticum-ponhé
Annona marcgravii Mart., Annonaceae 13
Areeiro
Hura crepitans L., Euphorbiaceae 153
Aricurí
Syagrus coronata (Mart.) Becc., Arecaceae 45
Syagrus schizophylla (Mart.) Glassman, Arecaceae . 46
Ariri
Allagoptera campestris (Mart.) Kuntze, Arecaceae .. 39
Syagrus schizophylla (Mart.) Glassman, Arecaceae . 46
Ariu
Chrysobalanus icaco L., Chrysobalanaceae 119
Arnica
Jungia floribunda Less., Asteraceae 61
Solidago chilensis Meyen, Asteraceae 65
Arnica-da-serra
Heterothalamus alienus (Spr.) O. Ktze., Asteraceae 60

Arnica-do-campo
Chionolaena latifolia (Benth.) Baker, Asteraceae 57
Arnica-silvestre
Solidago chilensis Meyen, Asteraceae 65
Aroeira
Astronium fraxinifolium Schott, Anacardiaceae 9
Myracroduon urundeuva
Fr. All., Anacardiaceae 9
Schinus molle L., Anacardiaceae 9
Aroeira-branca
Lithraea molleoides (Vell.) Engl., Anacardiaceae 9
Aroeira-brava
Lithraea molleoides (Vell.) Engl., Anacardiaceae 9
Aroeira-do-campo
Astronium fraxinifolium Schott, Anacardiaceae 9
Schinus lentiscifolius March., Anacardiaceae 9
Aroeira-do-sertão
Myracroduon urundeuva
Fr. All., Anacardiaceae 9
Aroeira-folha-de-salsa
Schinus molle L., Anacardiaceae 9
Aroeira-mansa
Schinus molle L., Anacardiaceae 9
Schinus terebinthifolius Raddi, Anacardiaceae 10
Aroeira-preta
Astronium fraxinifolium Schott, Anacardiaceae 9
Myracroduon urundeuva
Fr. All., Anacardiaceae 9
Aroeira-vermelha
Astronium fraxinifolium Schott, Anacardiaceae 9
Schinus terebinthifolius Raddi, Anacardiaceae 10
Aroeirinha
Lithraea molleoides (Vell.) Engl., Anacardiaceae 9
Schinus molle L., Anacardiaceae 9
Arranca-pedras
Phyllanthus niruri L., Euphorbiaceae 156
Arre-diabo
Jatropha urens L., Euphorbiaceae 155
Arrebenta-boi
Hippobroma longiflora
(L.) G. Don, Campanulaceae 109
Solanum aculeatissimum Jacq., Solanaceae 319
Arrebenta-cavalo
Solanum aculeatissimum Jacq., Solanaceae 319
Solanum ciliatum Lam., Solanaceae 319
Arrebenta-cavalos
Haynaldia exaltata (Pohl) Kanitz, Campanulaceae 109
Arrebenta-pedras
Phyllanthus acutifolius Spreng., Euphorbiaceae 156
Phyllanthus niruri L., Euphorbiaceae 156
Phyllanthus tenellus Roxb., Euphorbiaceae 157
Arriózes
Caesalpinia bonduc (L.) Roxb., Caesalpiniaceae 99
Arroz-das-águas
Luziola peruviana Pers., Poaceae 281
Arroz-do-brejo
Luziola peruviana Pers., Poaceae 281
Arroz-silvestre
Luziola peruviana Pers., Poaceae 281

Arruda-do-campo
Hypericum teretiusculum St.-Hil., Clusiaceae 122
Aruaaca
Lindernia diffusa Wettst., Scrophulariaceae 312
Aruca
Calea pinnatifida (R. Br.) Less., Asteraceae 57
Arumá
Ischnosiphon arouma Koern., Marantaceae 223
Arumã-membeca
Ischnosiphon arouma Koern., Marantaceae 223
Arumarana
Thalia geniculata L., Marantaceae 224
Arumbeva
Opuntia vulgaris Mill., Cactaceae 97
Aruru
Protium schomburgkianum Engl., Burseraceae 94
Árvore do bálsamo
Styrax pohlii DC., Styracaceae 325
Árvore-da-preguiça
Cecropia palmata Willd., Moraceae 247
Árvore-de-bálsamo
Jatropha multifida L., Euphorbiaceae 154
Árvore-de-chocalho
Sorocea bonplandii (Baill.) Burger, Moraceae 249
Árvore-de-coral
Euphorbia tirucalli L., Euphorbiaceae 153
Árvore-de-coral
Jatropha multifida L., Euphorbiaceae 154
Árvore-de-lã
Ceiba pentandra (L.) Gaertn., Bombacaceae 86
Árvore-de-leite
Sapium hamatum Pax & Hoffm., Euphorbiaceae ... 157
Árvore-de-são-sebastião
Euphorbia tirucalli L., Euphorbiaceae 153
Árvore-de-seda
Ceiba pentandra (L.) Gaertn., Bombacaceae 86
Árvore-de-umbela
Cordia umbraculifera DC., Boraginaceae 88
Árvore-do-sebo
Virola surinamensis (Rol.) Warb., Myristicaceae 252
Árvore-dos-feiticeiros
Connarus patrisii Planch., Connaraceae 129
Assa-peixe
Boehmeria caudata Sw., Urticaceae 330
Cyrtocymura scorpioides
(Lam.) H. Robinson, Asteraceae 59
Vernonanthura brasiliana
(L.) H. Robinson, Asteraceae 67
Assacu *(açacu)*
Hura crepitans L., Euphorbiaceae 153
Assapeixe
Magonia pubescens St.-Hil., Sapindaceae 305
Ata
Annona muricata L., Annonaceae 13
Annona reticulata L., Annonaceae 13
Annona squamosa L., Annonaceae 13
Ataúba
Guarea tuberculata Vell., Meliaceae 229

Atepele
Marcgravia rectiflora
  Tr. & Planch., Marcgraviaceae 224
Atitara
Desmoncus orthacanthos Mart., Arecaceae 40
Aturiá
Machaerium lunatum (L.) Ducke, Fabaceae 168
Au-uva
Aniba permollis (Nees) Mez, Lauraceae 197
Auaçu
Orbignya phalerata Mart., Arecaceae 43
Auaí
Thevetia ahouai (L.) DC., Apocynaceae 28
Avaramo
Pithecellobium unguis-cati
  (L.) Benth., Mimosaceae 242
Avaremotemo
Pithecellobium avaremotemo Mart., Mimosaceae .. 242
Aveia-da-terra
Avena quadridentata Doell, Poaceae 280
Aveia-do-campo
Avena quadridentata Doell, Poaceae 280
Aveia-do-mato
Avena quadridentata Doell, Poaceae 280
Avelós
Euphorbia tirucalli L., Euphorbiaceae 153
Avenca-da-terra
Adiantopsis chlorophylla (Sw.) Fée, Adiantaceae 1
Avenca-de-espiga
Anemia phyllitidis (L.) Sw., Schizaeaceae 310
Avenca-de-folha-miúda
Adiantum cuneatum Langsd. & Fisch., Adiantaceae ... 1
Avenca-dos-córregos
Adiantum trapeziforme L., Adiantaceae 1
Avenca-dourada
Phlebodium aureum
  (L.) J.E. Smith, Polypodiaceae 288
Avenca-grande
Cyathea microdonta (Desv.) Domin, Cyatheaceae . 141
Avenca-paulista
Adiantum trapeziforme L., Adiantaceae 1
Avencão
Adiantum cuneatum Langsd. & Fisch., Adiantaceae ... 1
Adiantum trapeziforme L., Adiantaceae 1
Avineira
Andira inermis (Sw.) H.B.K., Fabaceae 162
Avoadeira
Porophyllum ruderale (Jacq.) Cass., Asteraceae 64
Avoador
Mimosa malacocentra Mart., Mimosaceae 239
Axuá
Saccoglottis guianensis Benth., Humiriaceae 185
Azeda-de-ourives
Begonia acida Mart., Begoniaceae 75
Azeda-de-são-paulo
Begonia paulensis DC., Begoniaceae 76
Azeda-graúda
Rumex brasiliensis Link, Polygonaceae 287

Azedinha
Begonia acida Mart., Begoniaceae 75
Hibiscus sabdariffa L., Malvaceae 221
Oxalis amara St.-Hil., Oxalidaceae 266
Oxalis cordata St.-Hil., Oxalidaceae 266
Oxalis corniculata L., Oxalidaceae 266
Azedinha-amargosa
Oxalis amara St.-Hil., Oxalidaceae 266
Azedinha-do-brejo
Begonia acida Mart., Begoniaceae 75
Azedinha-do-campo
Oxalis cordata St.-Hil., Oxalidaceae 266
Azeitona-brava
Vitex montevidensis Cham., Verbenaceae 337
Azeitona-do-mato
Vitex montevidensis Cham., Verbenaceae 337
Azougue
Wilbrandia verticillata
  (Vell.) Cogn., Cucurbitaceae 140
Azougue-do-brasil
Cayaponia tayuya (Mart.) Cogn., also
  Cayaponia spp., Cucurbitaceae 135
Wilbrandia verticillata
  (Vell.) Cogn., Cucurbitaceae 140
Azougue-dos-pobres
Melothrianthus smilacifolius
  (Cogn.) M. Crovetto, Cucurbitaceae 139
Wilbrandia verticillata
  (Vell.) Cogn., Cucurbitaceae 140

B

Babá
Solanum aculeatissimum Jacq., Solanaceae 319
Solanum agrarium Sendt., Solanaceae 319
Baba-de-boi
Syagrus romanzoffiana
  (Cham.) Glassman, Arecaceae 45
Babaçu *(babassu)*
Orbignya phalerata Mart., Arecaceae 43
Babado-de-nossa-senhora
Macrosiphonia longiflora
  (Desf.) M. Arg., Apocynaceae 26
Babão
Solanum agrarium Sendt., Solanaceae 319
Syagrus comosa Mart., Arecaceae 45
Babassu *(babaçu)*
Orbignya phalerata Mart., Arecaceae 43
Babosa-de-árvore
Anthurium affine Schott, Araceae 33
Babosa-do-mato
Anthurium affine Schott, Araceae 33
Bacabá
Oenocarpus distichus Mart., Arecaceae 43
Bacaba-de-azeite
Oenocarpus distichus Mart., Arecaceae 43
Bacaba-de-óleo
Oenocarpus distichus Mart., Arecaceae 43
Bacopá
Buchnera aquatica Aubl., Scrophulariaceae 310

Bacupari-cipó
Peritassa calypsoides
(Camb.) A.C. Sm., Hippocrateaceae 183
Bacuralzinho
Euphorbia thymifolia L., Euphorbiaceae 153
Bacuri
Platonia insignis Mart., Clusiaceae 123
Scheelea phalerata
(Mart. ex Spreng.) Burret, Arecaceae 45
Baga-da-praia
Chondodendron platyphyllum
(Mart.) Miers, Menispermaceae 231
Coccoloba laevis Casar., Polygonaceae 285
Baga-de-caboclo
Abuta selloana Eichl., Menispermaceae 231
Baguaçu
Orbignya phalerata Mart., Arecaceae 43
Talauma ovata St.-Hil., Magnoliaceae 216
Baicuri-açu
Samolus valerandi L., Primulaceae 290
Baicuru
Limonium brasiliense
(Boiss.) O. Ktze., Plumbaginaceae 278
Bainha-de-espada
Sorocea bonplandii (Baill.) Burger, Moraceae 249
Balãozinho
Cardiospermum grandiflorum Sw., Sapindaceae ... 305
Physalis angulata L., Solanaceae 318
Balata
Manilkara bidentata (A. DC.) Chev., Sapotaceae .. 309
Balata-verdadeira
Manilkara bidentata (A. DC.) Chev., Sapotaceae .. 309
Baleeira
Cordia monosperma (Jacq.) Roem. & Schult.,
Boraginaceae 87
Balsa
Ochroma pyramidale (Cav.) Urb., Bombacaceae 86
Balsaminha
Capraria biflora L., Scrophulariaceae 311
Bálsamo
Naucleopsis amara Ducke, Moraceae 249
Bálsamo-de-jacareúba
Calophyllum brasiliense Camb., Clusiaceae: Uses . 120
Bálsamo-de-landim
Calophyllum brasiliense Camb., Clusiaceae: Uses .. 120
Bálsamo-de-tolu
Myroxylon balsamum (L.) Harms, Fabaceae 170
Bálsamo-de-umiri
Humiria balsamifera
(Aubl.) St.-Hil., Humiriaceae: Uses 183
Bálsamo-do-peru
Myroxylon balsamum (L.) Harms, Fabaceae 170
Balsamona
Cuphea balsamona Cham., Lythraceae 213
Bamburral
Hyptis suaveolens Poit., Lamiaceae 193
Hyptis umbrosa Salzm., Lamiaceae 193
Banana-do-brejo
Philodendron bipinnatifidum Schott, Araceae 36

Xanthosoma striatipes
(Kunth & Bouché) Madison, Araceae 37
Banana-do-mato
Bromelia antiacantha Bertol., Bromeliaceae 91
Banana-imbê
Philodendron bipinnatifidum Schott, Araceae 36
Bananeira-brava
Canna gigantea Desf., Cannaceae 110
Heliconia bihai L., Heliconiaceae 181
Bananeira-d'água
Dieffenbachia seguine (Jacq.) Schott, Araceae 35
Bananeira-do-mato
Canna glauca L., Cannaceae 110
Bananeirinha
Canna glauca L., Cannaceae 110
Bananeirinha-da-índia
Canna indica L., Cannaceae 111
Bananeirinha-de-flor-amarela
Canna lutea Roscoe, Cannaceae 111
Bananeirinha-do-mato
Calathea grandiflora Lindl., Marantaceae 223
Heliconia angusta Vell., Heliconiaceae 181
Heliconia bihai L., Heliconiaceae 181
Bananeirinha-roxa
Canna warszewiczii Dietr., Cannaceae 111
Barariçô
Trimezia lurida Salisb., Iridaceae 186
Baratinha
Caraipa minor Huber, Clusiaceae 121
Baraúna
Schinopsis brasiliensis Engl., Anacardiaceae 9
Barba-branca
Clematis denticulata Vell., Ranunculaceae 290
Barba-de-bode
Aristida pallens Cav., Poaceae 280
Elionurus candidus (Trin.) Hack., Poaceae 281
Panicum petrosum Trin., Poaceae 282
Barba-de-boi
Remirea maritima Aubl., Cyperaceae 143
Triumfetta rhomboidea Jacq., Tiliaceae 327
Barba-de-paca
Nepsera aquatica Naud., Melastomataceae 226
Barba-de-pau
Tillandsia usneoides L., Bromeliaceae 91
Barba-de-são-pedro
Polygala paniculata L., Polygalaceae 284
Barba-de-timão
Stryphnodendron adstringens
(Mart.) Cov., Mimosaceae 242
Barba-de-velho
Clematis campestris St.-Hil., Ranunculaceae 290
Clematis denticulata Vell., Ranunculaceae 290
Clematis dioica L., Ranunculaceae 290
Tillandsia usneoides L., Bromeliaceae 91
Barbadinho
Acacia paniculata Willd., Mimosaceae 236
Barbasco
Buddleja brasiliensis Jacq. ex Spr., Buddlejaceae 93
Clibadium leiocarpum Mart., Asteraceae 58
Pterocaulon virgatum DC., Asteraceae 64

Barbasco-do-brasil
Buddleja brasiliensis Jacq. ex Spr., Buddlejaceae 93
Barbatimão
Jacaranda brasiliana (Lam.) Pers., Bignoniaceae ... 80
Stryphnodendron adstringens
(Mart.) Cov., Mimosaceae 242
Stryphnodendron coriaceum Benth., Mimosaceae . 243
Stryphnodendron polyphyllum
Mart., Mimosaceae 244
Baririçô
Trimezia juncifolia Benth. & Hook., Iridaceae 186
Baronesa
Eichhornia crassipes Solms, Pontederiaceae 288
Barriguda
Chorisia crispiflora H.B.K., Bombacaceae 86
Barriguda-de-espinho
Ceiba pentandra (L.) Gaertn., Bombacaceae 86
Barrigudo
Jacaratia spinosa (Aubl.) A. DC., Caricaceae 113
Baru
Dipteryx alata Vog., Fabaceae 165
Batão
Andradea floribunda Fr. All., Nyctaginaceae 257
Astronium fraxinifolium Schott, Anacardiaceae 9
Batata-brava
Cissampelos fasciculata Benth., Menispermaceae . 231
Batata-caapeba
Cissampelos fasciculata Benth., Menispermaceae . 231
Batata-cogumelo
Leiphaimos aphylla (Jacq.) Gilg, Gentianaceae 180
Batata-da-praia
Ipomoea pes-caprae (L.) R. Br., Convolvulaceae .. 130
Batata-da-uva-do-mato
Cissampelos fasciculata Benth., Menispermaceae . 231
Batata-de-caboclo
Bignonia exoleta Vell., Bignoniaceae 79
Batata-de-escamas
Lophophytum mirabile
Schott & Endl., Balanophoraceae 73
Batata-de-porco
Boerhavia coccinea Mill., Nyctaginaceae 257
Batata-de-purga
Operculina alata (Ham.) Urb., Convolvulaceae 131
Operculina macrocarpa Urb., Convolvulaceae 131
Batata-de-sucupira
Pterodon pubescens Benth., Fabaceae: Uses 171
Batata-do-campo
Sinningia allagophylla
(Mart.) Wiehl., Gesneriaceae 181
Batata-do-mar
Ipomoea pes-caprae (L.) R. Br., Convolvulaceae .. 130
Batata-miúda
Bignonia exoleta Vell., Bignoniaceae 79
Batata-ovo
Commelina robusta Kunth, Commelinaceae 128
Batatão
Operculina alata (Ham.) Urb., Convolvulaceae 131
Batatão-roxo
Ipomoea pentaphylla Jacq., Convolvulaceae 130

Batatinha-amarela
Trimezia lurida Salisb., Iridaceae 186
Batatinha-d'água
Isoetes martii A. Braun, Isoetaceae 189
Batatinha-de-purga
Trimezia juncifolia Benth. & Hook., Iridaceae 186
Batatinha-do-campo
Sinningia allagophylla
(Mart.) Wiehl., Gesneriaceae 181
Batatinha-purgative
Cypella herbertii Herb., Iridaceae 186
Bate-testa
Physalis pubescens L., Solanaceae 318
Batiputá
Ouratea jabotapita Engl., Ochnaceae 261
Ouratea parviflora (DC.) Baill., Ochnaceae 261
Bebiri
Ocotea rodiei (Schomb.) Mez, Lauraceae 201
Bebiru
Ocotea rodiei (Schomb.) Mez, Lauraceae 201
Begônia
Begonia luxurians Scheidw., Begoniaceae 76
Belas
Pyrostegia ignea (Vell.) Pres., Bignoniaceae 82
Beldroega
Portulaca oleracea L., Portulacaceae 289
Beldroega-da-praia
Sesuvium portulacastrum L., Aizoaceae 1
Beldroega-de-flor-grande
Portulaca grandiflora Hook., Portulacaceae 289
Beldroega-grande
Talinum racemosum (L.) Rohr., Portulacaceae 289
Beldroega-miúda
Sesuvium portulacastrum L., Aizoaceae 1
Beldroega-pequena
Portulaca oleracea L., Portulacaceae 289
Benjoeiro
Styrax ferrugineum Nees & Mart., Styracaceae 325
Styrax pohlii DC., Styracaceae 325
Berberiz
Berberis laurina Thunb., Berberidaceae 76
Berberis spinulosa St.-Hil., Berberidaceae 76
Berberiz-da-terra
Berberis laurina Thunb., Berberidaceae 76
Beri
Canna edulis Ker-Gawl., Cannaceae 110
Betis
Piper eucalyptifolium (Miq.) Rudge, Piperaceae 275
Betônica-brava
Hyptis multiflora Pohl, Lamiaceae 193
Bico-de-arara
Erythrina fusca Lour., Fabaceae 166
Bico-de-papagaio
Centropogon cornutus
(L.) Druce, Campanulaceae 109
Bico-de-pato
Deianira pallescens Cham. & Schl., Gentianaceae . 180
Bicuíba
Virola oleifera (Schott) A.C. Smith, Myristicaceae . 250

Virola surinamensis (Rol.) Warb., Myristicaceae 252
Bicuíba-vermelha
Virola oleifera (Schott) A.C. Smith, Myristicaceae . 250
Bilreiro
Guarea trichilioides L., Meliaceae 228
Biribá
Rollinia orthopetala DC., Annonaceae 15
Biru-manso
Canna edulis Ker-Gawl., Cannaceae 110
Bisturi-do-mato
Cyrtopodium andersoni R. Br., Orchidaceae 266
Cyrtopodium punctatum Lindl., Orchidaceae 266
Bisturi-vegetal
Cyrtopodium andersoni R. Br., Orchidaceae 266
Cyrtopodium punctatum Lindl., Orchidaceae 266
Bitre
Piper marginatum Jacq., Piperaceae 276
Boa-noite
Calonyction aculeatum
(L.) House, Convolvulaceae 129
Lophophytum mirabile
Schott & Endl., Balanophoraceae 73
Boaria
Maytenus boaria Mol., Celastraceae 115
Bobó
Solanum aculeatissimum Jacq., Solanaceae 319
Boca-de-sapo
Deianira pallescens Cham. & Schl., Gentianaceae . 180
Boca-de-velha
Salacia impressifolia
(Miers) A.C. Sm., Hippocrateaceae 183
Bocuba
Virola oleifera
(Schott) A.C. Smith, Myristicaceae 250
Boi-gordo
Senna rugosa
(G. Don) Ir. & Barn., Caesalpiniaceae 106
Boia-caá
Marsypianthes chamaedrys
(Vahl) O. Ktze., Lamiaceae 194
Boizinho
Kielmeyera speciosa St.-Hil., Clusiaceae 123
Boldo
Coleus barbatus Benth., Lamiaceae 191
Boleira
Joannesia princeps Vell., Euphorbiaceae 155
Bolsa-de-pastor
Solanum cernuum Vell., Solanaceae 319
Bordão-de-velho
Pithecellobium avaremotemo Mart., Mimosaceae .. 242
Borragem-brava
Heliotropium indicum L., Boraginaceae 89
Botão-de-ouro
Acmella repens (Walt.) L.C. Rich., Asteraceae 52
Ranunculus apiifolius Pers., Ranunculaceae 290
Xyris laxifolia Mart., Xyridaceae 342
Xyris pallida Mart., Xyridaceae 342
Botica-inteira
Bredemeyera floribunda Willd., Polygalaceae 283

Botuto
Cochlospermum orinocense
(H.B.K.) Steud., Cochlospermaceae 125
Bracken fern
Pteridium aquilinum
(L.) Kuhn, Dennstaedtiaceae 144
Braço-de-mono
Solanum martii Sendt., Solanaceae 321
Braço-de-preguiça
Solanum cernuum Vell., Solanaceae 319
Brandão
Sebastiania macrocarpa M. Arg., Euphorbiaceae .. 157
Branquilho
Sebastiania klotzschiana M. Arg., Euphorbiaceae .. 157
Braúna
Schinopsis brasiliensis Engl., Anacardiaceae 9
Brazil nut
Bertholletia excelsa
Humb. & Bonpl., Lecythidaceae 204
Brazil wood
Caesalpinia echinata Lam., Caesalpiniaceae 100
Brazilian copal
Caesalpinia echinata Lam., Caesalpiniaceae: USES 100
Brazilian ginseng
Pfaffia iresinoides Spreng., under Chem. & Pharm.:
Pfaffia paniculata (Mart.) Kuntze, Amaranthaceae .. 6
Brazilian nutmeg
Cryptocarya moschata
Nees & Mart. ex Nees, Lauraceae 198
Brazilian sassafras
Ocotea pretiosa
(Nees & Mart.) Benth. & Hook., Lauraceae 201
Bredinho
Iresine polymorpha Mart., Amaranthaceae 4
Bredo
Amaranthus blitum L., Amaranthaceae 3
Amaranthus viridis L., Amaranthaceae 3
Bredo-branco
Amaranthus spinosus L., Amaranthaceae 3
Bredo-da-praia
Philoxerus portulacoides St.-Hil., Amaranthaceae 5
Sesuvium portulacastrum L., Aizoaceae 1
Bredo-de-espinho
Amaranthus spinosus L., Amaranthaceae 3
Bredo-de-porco
Boerhavia coccinea Mill., Nyctaginaceae 257
Boerhavia paniculata Rich., Nyctaginaceae 258
Bredo-de-santo-antonio
Amaranthus spinosus L., Amaranthaceae 3
Bredo-fedorento
Cleome polygama L., Capparaceae 112
Bredo-macho
Amaranthus blitum L., Amaranthaceae 3
Bredo-malabar
Amaranthus blitum L., Amaranthaceae 3
Bredo-rabaça
Amaranthus blitum L., Amaranthaceae 3
Bredo-vermelho
Amaranthus spinosus L., Amaranthaceae 3

Brejaúva
Astrocaryum aculeatissimum
(Schott) Burret, Arecacae 39
Breu
Protium heptaphyllum (Aubl.) March., Burseraceae 93
Breu-branco
Protium heptaphyllum (Aubl.) March., Burseraceae 93
Protium icicariba (DC.) March., Burseraceae 94
Breu-jauaricica
Protium heptaphyllum (Aubl.) March., Burseraceae 93
Brilhantina
Pilea microphylla (L.) Liebm., Urticaceae 331
Brusca
Discaria americana Gill. & Hook., Rhamnaceae ... 293
Bucha-dos-paulistas
Gurania paulista Cogn., Cucurbitaceae 138
Buchinha
Luffa operculata (L.) Cogn., Cucurbitaceae 138
Bucho-de-rã
Physalis angulata L., Solanaceae 318
Bugrinho
Cordia salicifolia Cham., Boraginaceae 88
Buranhém
Pradosia lactescens (Vell.) Radlk., Sapotaceae 310
Buri-do-campo
Allagoptera campestris (Mart.) Kuntze, Arecaceae 39
Buriti
Mauritia flexuosa L. f., Arecaceae 43
Buritirana
Mauritiella aculeata (Kunth) Burret, Arecaceae 43
Burra-leitera
Euphorbia hyssopifolia L., Euphorbiaceae 153
Butiá
Butia yatay (Mart.) Becc., Arecaceae 39
Butinha
Cissampelos glaberrima St.-Hil., Menispermaceae 233
Bútua
Abuta concolor Poepp. & Endl., Menispermaceae . 231
Abuta rufescens Aubl., Menispermaceae 231
Abuta selloana Eichl., Menispermaceae 231
Cissampelos fasciculata Benth., Menispermaceae . 231
Butuá-de-corvo
Cochlospermum regium
(Mart. & Schl.) Pilg., Cochlospermaceae 125

C

Caá-açu
Byrsonima spicata Rich., Malpighiaceae 219
Caá-ataia
Lindernia diffusa Wettst., Scrophulariaceae 312
Caá-cambuí
Euphorbia hirta L., Euphorbiaceae 152
Caá-chira
Oldenlandia corymbosa L., Rubiaceae 299
Caá-cica
Euphorbia hirta L., Euphorbiaceae 152
Caá-membeca
Polygala spectabilis DC., Polygalaceae 284

Caa-opiá
Vismia guianensis (Aubl.) Choisy, Clusiaceae 124
Caá-peuá
Pothomorphe peltata L., Piperaceae 277
Caacapoc
Campsiandra comosa Benth. var.
laurifolia (Benth.) Cowan, Caesalpiniaceae 100
Caapeba
Abuta concolor Poepp. & Endl., Menispermaceae . 231
Cissampelos glaberrima St.-Hil., Menispermaceae 233
Piper rohrii C. DC., Piperaceae 276
Pothomorphe peltata L., Piperaceae 277
Pothomorphe umbellata (L.) Miq., Piperaceae 277
Caapeba-cheirosa
Piper marginatum Jacq., Piperaceae 276
Caapeba-do-norte
Pothomorphe peltata L., Piperaceae 277
Caapi
Banisteriopsis caapi (Spr.) Morton, Malpighiaceae 217
Caapiá
Dorstenia asaroides Gardn., Moraceae 247
Dorstenia brasiliensis Lam., Moraceae 247
Dorstenia cayapia Vell., Moraceae 248
Caapiá-açu
Dorstenia brasiliensis Lam., Moraceae 247
Caaponga
Alternanthera brasiliana
(L.) O. Ktze., Amaranthaceae 3
Portulaca oleracea L., Portulacaceae 289
Caapononga
Plumbago scandens L., Plumbaginaceae 279
Caapuçara
Dalechampia ficifolia Lam., Euphorbiaceae 152
Caapuera-branca
Solanum cernuum Vell., Solanaceae 319
Caataia
Plumbago scandens L., Plumbaginaceae 279
Caatiguá
Trichilia catigua Juss., Meliaceae 229
Caatinga
Costus spicatus (Jacq.) Sw., also
Costus spiralis (Jacq.) Roscoe, Costaceae 132
Caavitinga
Solanum mauritianum Scop., Solanaceae 321
Caavurana
Solanum caavurana Vell., Solanaceae 319
Cabaça
Lagenaria siceraria
(Molina) Standl., Cucurbitaceae 138
Cabaça-amargosa
Lagenaria siceraria
(Molina) Standl., Cucurbitaceae 138
Cabacinha
Luffa operculata (L.) Cogn., Cucurbitaceae 138
Wilbrandia verticillata
(Vell.) Cogn., Cucurbitaceae 140
Cabão-de-bugre
Bredemeyera floribunda Willd., Polygalaceae 283
Cabeça-de-frade
Melocactus melocactoides
(Hoffm.) DC., Cactaceae 97

Cabeça-de-negro
 Annona coriacea Mart., Annonaceae 12
 Annona crassifolia Mart., Annonaceae 12
 Cayaponia tayuya (Mart.) Cogn., also
  Cayaponia spp., Cucurbitaceae 135
 Trianosperma glandulosa Mart., Cucurbitaceae 140
 Wilbrandia verticillata (Vell.)
  Cogn., Cucurbitaceae 140
Cabeleira
 Caryocar glabrum (Aubl.) Pers., Caryocaraceae 114
Cabelo-de-negro
 Connarus suberosus Planch., Connaraceae 129
 Erythroxylum campestre St.-Hil., Erythroxylaceae . 149
Cabo-de-formão
 Sweetia fruticosa Spreng., Fabaceae 172
Cabo-de-machado
 Aspidosperma discolor Benth., Apocynaceae 21
Cabo-verde
 Senna affinis (Benth.) Ir. & Barn., Caesalpiniaceae 104
 Senna macranthera
  (Collad.) Ir. & Barn., Caesalpiniaceae 105
Caboreíba
 Myroxylon balsamum (L.) Harms, Fabaceae 170
Caboriba
 Myroxylon balsamum (L.) Harms, Fabaceae 170
Cabriuva
 Myrocarpus frondosus Fr. All., Fabaceae 170
Cabriuva-parda
 Myrocarpus frondosus Fr. All., Fabaceae 170
Cabuçu
 Coccoloba marginata Benth., Polygonaceae 285
Cacaba
 Oenocarpus distichus Mart., Arecaceae 43
Cacália-amarga
 Baccharis trimera (Less.) DC., Asteraceae 54
Caçaú
 Aristolochia cymbifera
  Mart. & Zucc., Aristolochiaceae 46
 Aristolochia elegans Mast., Aristolochiaceae 48
 Aristolochia triangularis Cham., Aristolochiaceae ... 48
Cacau-branco
 Carpotroche longifolia Benth., Flacourtiaceae 176
Caçaui
 Aristolochia cymbifera
  Mart. & Zucc., Aristolochiaceae 46
Cachaceiro
 Rhabdodendron amazonicum
  (Spr. ex Benth.) Hub., Rhabdodendraceae 291
Cacto-rosa
 Pereskia bleo H.B.K., Cactaceae 97
Caculucage
 Pluchea suaveolens (Vell.) O. Ktze., Asteraceae 64
Caeté-açu
 Calathea grandiflora Lindl., Marantaceae 223
 Canna gigantea Desf., Cannaceae 110
Caeté-bravo
 Stromanthe sanguinea Sond., Marantaceae 224
Caeté-de-talo-roxo
 Canna warszewiczii Dietr., Cannaceae 111

Caeté-do-mato
 Canna gigantea Desf., Cannaceae 110
Caeté-imbiri
 Canna glauca L., Cannaceae 110
Caeté-mirim
 Canna warszewiczii Dietr., Cannaceae 111
Caeté-roxo
 Canna warszewiczii Dietr., Cannaceae 111
Café-açu
 Renealmia exaltata L. f., Zingiberaceae 342
Café-bravo
 Casearia guyanensis (Aubl.) Urb., Flacourtiaceae . 177
 Casearia sylvestris Sw., Flacourtiaceae 178
Café-do-diabo
 Casearia guyanensis (Aubl.) Urb., Flacourtiaceae . 177
Café-do-mato
 Canna lanuginosa Roscoe, Cannaceae 111
 Casearia guyanensis (Aubl.) Urb., Flacourtiaceae . 177
 Cordia coffeoides Warm., Boraginaceae 87
 Cordia ecalyculata Vell., Boraginaceae 87
 Cordia salicifolia Cham., Boraginaceae 88
 Peschiera laeta (Mart.) Miers, Apocynaceae 27
Caferana
 Picrolemma pseudocoffea Ducke, Simaroubaceae . 314
 Tachia guianensis Aubl., Gentianaceae 181
Cafezinho
 Cordia ecalyculata Vell., Boraginaceae 87
Cagaiteira
 Eugenia dysenterica DC., Myrtaceae 253
Caiapiá
 Dorstenia brasiliensis Lam., Moraceae 247
 Dorstenia cayapia Vell., Moraceae 248
Caiaté
 Omphalea diandra M. Arg., Euphorbiaceae 156
Caiauá
 Elaeis oleifera (H.B.K.) Cortez, Arecaceae 40
Caiaué
 Elaeis oleifera (H.B.K.) Cortez, Arecaceae 40
Caiauê
 Elaeis oleifera (H.B.K.) Cortez, Arecaceae 40
Caiçara
 Sweetia fruticosa Spreng., Fabaceae 172
Caimbé
 Coussapoa asperifolia Tréc., Moraceae 247
 Curatella americana L., Dilleniaceae 144
Cainana
 Chiococca alba (L.) Hitch., Rubiaceae 297
Cainca
 Chiococca alba (L.) Hitch., Rubiaceae 297
Caixão
 Cariniana legalis (Mart.) O. Ktze., Lecythidaceae . 205
Cajá
 Spondias mombin L., Anacardiaceae 10
Cajá-mirim
 Spondias mombin L., Anacardiaceae 10
Cajati
 Cryptocarya mandioccana Meissn., Lauraceae 198
Cajazeira
 Spondias mombin L., Anacardiaceae 10

Cajiru
 Arrabidaea chica (H.B.K.) Bur., Bignoniaceae 78
Cajueiro
 Anacardium occidentale L., Anacardiaceae 7
Cajueiro-anão
 Anacardium humile St.-Hil. and
 Anacardium nanum St.-Hil., Anacardiaceae 7
Cajueiro-branco
 Curatella americana L., Dilleniaceae 144
Cajueiro-do-campo
 Anacardium humile St.-Hil. and
 Anacardium nanum St.-Hil., Anacardiaceae 7
Cajuí
 Anacardium humile St.-Hil. and
 Anacardium nanum St.-Hil., Anacardiaceae 7
Calabura
 Muntingia calabura L., Tiliaceae 327
Caládio
 Caladium bicolor (Aiton) Vent., Araceae 34
Calaguala
 Rumohra adiantiformis
 (G. Forst.) Ching, Dryopteridaceae 147
Cálamo-branco
 Mariscus jacquinii H.B.K., Cyperaceae 143
Calcanhar-de-cotia
 Guarea tuberculata Vell., Meliaceae 229
Calção-de-velho
 Buddleja brasiliensis Jacq. ex Spr., Buddlejaceae 93
Calças-de-velho
 Buddleja brasiliensis Jacq. ex Spr., Buddlejaceae 93
Calumba
 Simaba salubris Engl., Simaroubaceae 315
Calumbi
 Mimosa malacocentra Mart., Mimosaceae 239
Calunga
 Aristolochia trilobata L., Aristolochiaceae 48
 Simaba ferruginea St.-Hil., Simaroubaceae 314
 Simaba glandulifera Gardn., Simaroubaceae 315
 Simaba salubris Engl., Simaroubaceae 315
Camacã
 Guazuma ulmifolia
 Lam. var. tomentella Schum., Sterculiaceae 323
Camapu
 Physalis angulata L., Solanaceae 318
 Physalis pubescens L., Solanaceae 318
Camará
 Chromolaena laevigata
 (Lam.) King & H. Robinson, Asteraceae 58
 Lantana camara L., Verbenaceae 334
Camará-de-bilro
 Geissospermum laeve (Vell.) Baill., Apocynaceae 24
Cambaibinha
 Davilla rugosa Poir., Dilleniaceae 145
Cambará
 Buddleja cambara Arech., Buddlejaceae 93
 Chromolaena laevigata
 (Lam.) King & H. Robinson, Asteraceae 58
 Lantana camara L., Verbenaceae 334
Cambará-branco
 Lantana brasiliensis Link, Verbenaceae 334

Cambará-de-capoeira
 Verbena bonariensis L., Verbenaceae 336
Cambará-de-cheiro
 Lantana camara L., Verbenaceae 334
 Licaria camara (Schomb.) Kosterm., Lauraceae 199
Cambará-de-chumbo
 Lantana camara L., Verbenaceae 334
Cambará-de-espinho
 Lantana camara L., Verbenaceae 334
Cambará-de-folha-grande
 Gochnatia polymorpha (Less.) Cabr., Asteraceae 60
 Lantana macrophylla Schauer, Verbenaceae 335
Cambará-do-mato
 Gochnatia polymorpha (Less.) Cabr., Asteraceae 60
Cambará-juba
 Lantana camara L., Verbenaceae 334
Cambará-rosa
 Lantana lilacina Desf., Verbenaceae 335
Camboatá
 Cupania racemosa Radlk., Sapindaceae 305
 Guarea trichilioides L., Meliaceae 228
 Guarea tuberculata Vell., Meliaceae 229
 Jacaranda caroba (Vell.) DC., Bignoniaceae 80
Camboatá
 Picramnia camboita Engl., Simaroubaceae 314
Camboatã-da-baía
 Picramnia bahiensis Turcz., Simaroubaceae 314
Camboatá-pequeno
 Jacaranda caroba (Vell.) DC., Bignoniaceae 80
Camboita
 Picramnia camboita Engl., Simaroubaceae 314
Cambraia
 Croton salutaris Casar., Euphorbiaceae 151
Cambuí
 Schinus terebinthifolius Raddi, Anacardiaceae 10
Cambuí-branco
 Anadenanthera colubrina
 (Vell.) Brenan, Mimosaceae 236
Cambuí-da-restinga
 Sophora tomentosa L., Fabaceae 172
Cambuí-fero
 Anadenanthera macrocarpa
 (Benth.) Brenan, Mimosaceae 236
Campainha-branca
 Ipomoea acetosifolia
 (Vahl) Roem. & Schult., Convolvulaceae 130
Campainha-dos-tintureiros
 Ipomoea pentaphylla Jacq., Convolvulaceae 130
Camucá
 Marsdenia amylacea
 (Barb.-Rodr.) Malme, Asclepiadaceae 51
Cana
 Canna indica L., Cannaceae 111
Cana-branca
 Costus spicatus (Jacq.) Sw. also
 Costus spiralis (Jacq.) Roscoe, Costaceae 132
 Renealmia occidentalis Sweet, Zingiberaceae 343
Cana-brava
 Gynerium parviflorum Nees, Poaceae 281

Cana-da-índia
Canna indica L., Cannaceae 111
Cana-da-terra
Costus cuspidatus
  (Nees & Mart.) Maas, Costaceae 132
Cana-de-imbé
Dieffenbachia seguine (Jacq.) Schott, Araceae 35
Cana-de-macaco
Costus spicatus (Jacq.) Sw., also
  Costus spiralis (Jacq.) Roscoe, Costaceae 132
Cana-do-brejo
Costus spicatus (Jacq.) Sw., also
  Costus spiralis (Jacq.) Roscoe, Costaceae 132
Renealmia exaltata L. f., Zingiberaceae 342
Xanthosoma striatipes
  (Kunth & Bouché) Madison, Araceae 37
Cana-do-mato
Costus cuspidatus
  (Nees & Mart.) Maas, Costaceae 132
Renealmia occidentalis Sweet, Zingiberaceae 343
Cana-do-rio
Costus cuspidatus
  (Nees & Mart.) Maas, Costaceae 132
Gynerium parviflorum Nees, Poaceae 281
Cana-ubá
Gynerium parviflorum Nees, Poaceae 281
Canafístula
Cassia ferruginea
  (Schrad.) Schrad. ex DC., Caesalpiniaceae 100
Canafístula-da-mata
Senna corymbosa
  (Lam.) Ir. & Barn., Caesalpiniaceae 104
Canaiá
Mauritiella aculeata (Kunth) Burret, Arecaceae 43
Cananã
Euphorbia phosphorea Mart., Euphorbiaceae 153
Cananga
Virola macrophylla
  (Spr. ex Benth.) Warb., Myristicaceae 250
Canarana
Costus spicatus (Jacq.) Sw., also
  Costus spiralis (Jacq.) Roscoe, Costaceae 132
Canaru-caá
Cordia multispicata Cham., Boraginaceae 88
Cancerosa
Jodina rhombifolia Hook. & Arn., Santalaceae 304
Maytenus ilicifolia Mart., Celastraceae 115
Canchalágua
Sisyrinchium vaginatum Spreng., Iridaceae 186
Cancorosa-de-três-pontas
Jodina rhombifolia Hook. & Arn., Santalaceae 304
Candeia
Piptocarpha rotundifolia (Less.) Bak., Asteraceae .. 64
Candeiá
Cladonia pyxidata (L.) Ach., Cladoniaceae 120
Canduá
Cladonia miniata Mey., Cladoniaceae 120
Cladonia pyxidata (L.) Ach., Cladoniaceae 120
Canela-abacate
Cryptocarya minima Mez, Lauraceae 198

Canela-amarela
Nectandra leucantha Nees, Lauraceae 199
Canela-amarela-de-cheiro
Aiovea meissneri Mez, Lauraceae 197
Canela-amarga
Drimys winteri Forst., Winteraceae 340
Nectandra puberula Nees, Lauraceae 200
Canela-amargosa
Ocotea squarrosa Mart. ex Nees, Lauraceae 203
Canela-bebiru
Ocotea rodiei (Schomb.) Mez, Lauraceae 201
Canela-branca
Cinnamodendron axillare
  (Nees & Mart.) Endl., Canellaceae 110
Nectandra leucothyrsus Meissn., Lauraceae 200
Canela-braúna
Ocotea spectabilis (Meissn.) Mez, Lauraceae 201
Canela-caixeta
Licaria canella (Meissn.) Kosterm., Lauraceae 199
Canela-cheirosa
Ocotea pretiosa (Nees & Mart.)
  Benth. & Hook., Lauraceae 201
Canela-da-capoeira
Nectandra leucantha Nees, Lauraceae 199
Canela-da-vargem
Nectandra leucothyrsus Meissn., Lauraceae 200
Canela-de-catarro
Nectandra leucothyrsus Meissn., Lauraceae 200
Canela-de-cheiro
Ocotea opifera Mart., Lauraceae 201
Canela-de-cunhã
Croton zehntneri Pax & Hoffm., Euphorbiaceae 152
Canela-de-espinho
Scutia buxifolia Reiss., Rhamnaceae 293
Canela-de-goiás
Mezilaurus crassiramea
  (Meissn.) Taub. ex Mez, Lauraceae 199
Canela-de-velha
Miconia albicans (Sw.) Tr., Melastomataceae 225
Canela-de-velho
Croton zehntneri Pax & Hoffm., Euphorbiaceae 152
Canela-do-brejo
Cryptocarya minima Mez, Lauraceae 198
Ocotea pulchella Mart., Lauraceae 201
Canela-funcho
Ocotea pretiosa (Nees & Mart.)
  Benth. & Hook., Lauraceae 201
Canela-iacuá
Ocotea teleiandra (Messn.) Mez, Lauraceae 203
Canela-lageana
Ocotea pulchella Mart., Lauraceae 201
Canela-limão
Ocotea rodiei (Schomb.) Mez, Lauraceae 201
Ocotea teleiandra (Messn.) Mez, Lauraceae 203
Canela-mescla
Ocotea spectabilis (Meissn.) Mez, Lauraceae 201
Canela-mirim
Nectandra leucantha Nees, Lauraceae 199

Canela-parda
  Nectandra puberula Nees, Lauraceae 200
Canela-preta
  Nectandra globosa (Aubl.) Mez, Lauraceae 199
  Ocotea pulchella Mart., Lauraceae 201
  Ocotea spectabilis (Meissn.) Mez, Lauraceae 201
Canela-sassafrás
  Ocotea pretiosa (Nees & Mart.)
    Benth. & Hook., Lauraceae 201
Canela-sassafrás-preta
  Ocotea cymbarum H.B.K., Lauraceae 200
Canela-seca
  Nectandra leucantha Nees, Lauraceae 199
Caneleira
  Ocotea pulchella Mart., Lauraceae 201
Caneleira-cravo
  Dicypellium caryophyllatum
    Nees & Mart., Lauraceae 198
Caneleira-de-cheiro
  Ocotea opifera Mart., Lauraceae 201
Caneleira-do-mato
  Nectandra canescens Nees, Lauraceae 199
Canelinha
  Croton zehntneri Pax & Hoffm., Euphorbiaceae 152
  Ocotea pretiosa (Nees & Mart.)
    Benth. & Hook., Lauraceae 201
  Ocotea pulchella Mart., Lauraceae 201
Cangerana
  Cabralea canjerana (Vell.) Mart., Meliaceae 227
Canguçu
  Buchnera virgata H.B.K., Scrophulariaceae 310
Canguçu-preto
  Buchnera virgata H.B.K., Scrophulariaceae 310
Cânhamo-brasileiro
  Hibiscus cannabinus L., Malvaceae 221
Canjerana
  Guarea trichilioides L., Meliaceae 228
Canjica
  Sweetia fruticosa Spreng., Fabaceae 172
Cansanção
  Jatropha urens L., Euphorbiaceae 155
  Laportea aestuans (L.) Chew, Urticaceae 330
  Urera baccifera Gaud., Urticaceae 331
  Urera caracasana Jacq., Urticaceae 331
  Urera subpeltata Miq., Urticaceae 331
Cansanção-de-leite
  Jatropha urens L., Euphorbiaceae 155
Cansanção-verdadeiro
  Urera aurantiaca Wedd., Urticaceae 331
Canudeiro
  Mabea fistulifera Mart., Euphorbiaceae 155
Canudo-amargoso
  Geissospermum laeve (Vell.) Baill., Apocynaceae 24
Canudo-de-pito
  Carpotroche brasiliensis
    (Raddi) Endl., Flacourtiaceae 176
  Mabea fistulifera Mart., Euphorbiaceae 155
  Senna multijuga Rich. var.
    verrucosa (Vog.) Ir. & Barn., Caesalpiniaceae 105
  Senna septentrionalis

  (Viv.) Ir. & Barn., Caesalpiniaceae 106
Canudo-de-purga
  Rauwolfia blanchetii DC., Apocynaceae 28
Caopiá
  Vismia guianensis (Aubl.) Choisy, Clusiaceae 124
Capa-homem
  Aristolochia cymbifera Mart.
    & Zucc., Aristolochiaceae 46
  Aristolochia trilobata L., Aristolochiaceae 48
  Davilla rugosa Poir., Dilleniaceae 145
  Echites peltata Vell., Apocynaceae 23
Caparosa
  Neea theifera Oersted, Nyctaginaceae 258
  Oenothera catharinensis Camb., Onagraceae 264
  Vismia acuminata (L.) Pers., Clusiaceae 123
Caparosa-do-campo
  Neea theifera Oersted, Nyctaginaceae 258
Capeba
  Pothomorphe umbellata (L.) Miq., Piperaceae 277
Caperiçoba-branc
  Chenopodium hircinum Schrad., Chenopodiaceae . 119
Capetiraguá
  Philoxerus portulacoides St.-Hil., Amaranthaceae 5
Capiçaba
  Polygonum acuminatum H.B.K., Polygonaceae 286
Capilário
  Adiantum cuneatum Langsd. & Fisch., Adiantaceae ... 1
Capim-açu
  Andropogon minarum Kunth, Poaceae 280
  Cyperus ligularis L., Cyperaceae 142
  Mariscus flavus Vahl, Cyperaceae 143
  Panicum megiston Schult., Poaceae 282
Capim-agreste
  Imperata brasiliensis Trin., Poaceae 281
Capim-amargoso
  Andropogon bicornis L., Poaceae 279
  Elionurus candidus (Trin.) Hack., Poaceae 281
  Pappophorum mucronulatum Nees, Poaceae 282
Capim-amonjeaba
  Sacciolepis myuros (Lam.) Chase, Poaceae 282
Capim-andacaá
  Panicum trichanthum Nees, Poaceae 282
Capim-arroz
  Luziola peruviana Pers., Poaceae 281
Capim-barba-de-bode
  Aristida pallens Cav., Poaceae 280
Capim-batatal
  Chloris distichophylla (Nees) Lag., Poaceae 280
Capim-branco
  Chloris polydactyla Sw., Poaceae 280
Capim-catinguento
  Melinis minutiflora Beauv., Poaceae 281
Capim-cebola
  Chloris distichophylla (Nees) Lag., Poaceae 280
Capim-cheiroso
  Cyperus sesquiflorus
    (Torrey) Mattf. & Kükent., Cyperaceae 142
Capim-chuvisco
  Panicum brevifolium L., Poaceae 282

Capim-cidreira
Cymbopogon schoenanthus (L.) Spreng., Poaceae 280
Cyperus sesquiflorus (Torrey)
Mattf. & Kükent., Cyperaceae 142
Capim-d'agua
Andropogon bicornis L., Poaceae 279
Capim-da-praia-açu
Panicum megiston Schult., Poaceae 282
Capim-de-bezerro
Andropogon bicornis L., Poacea 279
Capim-de-bode
Aristida pallens Cav., Poaceae 280
Capim-de-cheiro
Cyperus sesquiflorus
(Torrey) Mattf. & Kükent., Cyperaceae 142
Capim-de-sapo
Paspalum extenuatum Nees, Poaceae 282
Capim-de-um-só-botão
Kyllinga pungens Link, Cyperaceae 143
Capim-gigante
Panicum megiston Schult., Poaceae 282
Capim-gomoso
Commelina nudiflora L., Commelinaceae 126
Capim-gordo
Melinis minutiflora Beauv., Poaceae 281
Capim-gordura
Melinis minutiflora Beauv., Poaceae 281
Capim-guiamum
Chloris polydactyla Sw., Poaceae 280
Capim-jasmin-da-serra
Elionurus bilinguis (Trin.) Hack., Poaceae 281
Capim-limão
Cymbopogon schoenanthus (L.) Spreng., Poaceae 280
Cyperus sesquiflorus (Torrey)
Mattf. & Kükent., Cyperaceae 142
Elionurus candidus (Trin.) Hack., Poaceae 281
Capim-lixa
Panicum megiston Schult., Poaceae 282
Capim-mão-de-sapo
Paspalum extenuatum Nees, Poaceae 282
Capim-massapê
Imperata brasiliensis Trin., Poaceae 281
Capim-melado
Melinis minutiflora Beauv., Poaceae 281
Capim-mimoso
Hackelochloa granularis (L.) O. Ktze., Poaceae ... 281
Panicum brevifolium L., Poaceae 282
Panicum trichanthum Nees, Poaceae 282
Capim-mimoso-de-cacho
Setaria scandens Schrad., Poaceae 282
Capim-mole
Andropogon bicornis L., Poaceae 279
Capim-navalha-mole
Hypolytrum laxum Schrad., Cyperaceae 143
Capim-peba
Andropogon bicornis L., Poaceae 279
Capim-rabo-de-raposa
Andropogon bicornis L., Poaceae 279
Setaria scandens Schrad., Poaceae 282

Capim-rabo-de-rato
Setaria scandens Schrad., Poaceae 282
Capim-rei
Abolboda poarchon Seub., Xyridaceae 342
Trimezia lurida Salisb., Iridaceae 186
Capim-santo
Cymbopogon schoenanthus (L.) Spreng., Poaceae 280
Capim-sapê
Andropogon bicornis L., Poaceae 279
Imperata brasiliensis Trin., Poaceae 281
Capim-taboquinha
Panicum megiston Schult., Poaceae 282
Capim-vassoura
Andropogon bicornis L., Poaceae 279
Capim-vindecaá
Panicum trichanthum Nees, Poaceae 282
Capiscaba-mirim
Cyperus gracilescens
Roem. & Schult., Cyperaceae 142
Capitão-do-campo
Cordia obscura Cham., Boraginaceae 88
Terminalia argentea Mart., Combretaceae 126
Capitão-do-mato
Cayaponia cabocla (Vell.) Mart. also
Cayaponia spp., Cucurbitaceae 135
Capitão-preto
Strychnos trinervis (Vell.) Mart., Loganiaceae 210
Capitiçova
Polygonum punctatum Elliot, Polygonaceae 287
Polygonum spectabile Mart., Polygonaceae 287
Capitiú
Renealmia occidentalis Sweet, Zingiberaceae 343
Siparuna guianensis Aubl., Monimiaceae 245
Capitiú-do-amazonas
Siparuna laurifolia (H.B.K.) DC., Monimiaceae ... 246
Capivara
Aristolochia birostris Duch., Aristolochiaceae 46
Capixingui
Croton floribundus Spreng., Euphorbiaceae 150
Capoeira-branca
Solanum mauritianum Scop., Solanaceae 321
Capororoca-picante
Drimys winteri Forst., Winteraceae 340
Capuchinha
Macairea radula (Bonpl.) DC., Melastomataceae .. 225
Tropaeolum pentaphyllum Lam., Tropaeolaceae ... 327
Caputuna
Metrodorea pubescens St.-Hil. & Tul., Rutaceae ... 301
Caputuva
Metrodorea pubescens St.-Hil. & Tul., Rutaceae ... 301
Caquera
Senna bicapsularis (L.) Roxb., Caesalpiniaceae 104
Senna uniflora (P. Miller)
Ir. & Barn., Caesalpiniaceae 106
Cará-de-caboclo
Bomarea salsilloides Roem., Amaryllidaceae 6
Cará-de-folha-colorida
Dioscorea glandulosa Klotz., Dioscoreaceae 147
Cará-de-pedra
Dioscorea silvestris Vell., Dioscoreaceae 147

Cará-de-sapo
   Dioscorea laxiflora Mart., Dioscoreaceae 147
Cará-do-mato
   Bomarea spectabilis Schrenk, Amaryllidaceae 6
Cará-liso
   Dioscorea glandulosa Klotz., Dioscoreaceae 147
Cará-sem-barba
   Dioscorea glandulosa Klotz., Dioscoreaceae 147
Caracasana
   Urera caracasana Jacq., Urticaceae 331
Caraguatá
   Bromelia pinguin L., Bromeliaceae 91
   Eryngium elegans Cham. & Schlecht., Apiaceae 19
   Eryngium pandanifolium
      Cham. & Schlecht., Apiaceae 19
   Eryngium pristis Cham. & Schlecht., Apiaceae 19
Caraguatá-branco
   Eryngium pandanifolium
      Cham. & Schlecht., Apiaceae 19
Caraguatá-do-banhado
   Eryngium pandanifolium
      Cham. & Schlecht., Apiaceae 19
Caraguatá-elegante
   Eryngium elegans Cham. & Schlecht., Apiaceae 19
Caraguatá-falso
   Eryngium paniculatum Cav. & Domb.
      ex Delar., Apiaceae 19
Caraíba
   Cordia insignis Cham., Boraginaceae 87
   Tabebuia caraiba (Mart.) Bur., Bignoniaceae 82
Carajuru
   Arrabidaea chica (H.B.K.) Bur., Bignoniaceae 78
Caraná
   Mauritiella aculeata (Kunth) Burret, Arecaceae 43
Caranaí
   Mauritiella aculeata (Kunth) Burret, Arecaceae 43
Carango
   Pfaffia paniculata (Mart.) Kuntze, Amaranthaceae 5
Carapanaúba
   Aspidosperma excelsum Benth., Apocynaceae 21
   Aspidosperma nitidum Benth., Apocynaceae 21
Carapiá
   Dorstenia brasiliensis Lam., Moraceae 247
   Dorstenia cayapia Vell., Moraceae 248
   Sida macrodon DC., Malvaceae 222
Caratinga
   Dioscorea glandulosa Klotz., Dioscoreaceae 147
Caratinga-brava
   Dioscorea laxiflora Mart., Dioscoreaceae 147
Caratinga-do-mato
   Dioscorea laxiflora Mart., Dioscoreaceae 147
Carauá
   Bromelia pinguin L., Bromeliaceae 91
Carauatá
   Bromelia antiacantha Bertol., Bromeliaceae 91
Caraúba
   Jacaranda copaia (Aubl.) D. Don, Bignoniaceae 80
Caraúba-do-campo
   Tabebuia caraiba (Mart.) Bur., Bignoniaceae 82

Caraxixi
   Solanum nigrum L., Solanaceae 321
Cardamom
   Renealmia occidentalis Sweet, Zingiberaceae 343
Cardamomo-da-terra
   Renealmia occidentalis Sweet, Zingiberaceae 342
Cardamomo-do-brasil
   Renealmia exaltata L. f., Zingiberaceae 342
Cardieiro
   Cereus jamacaru DC., Cactaceae 95
Cardo-ananás
   Hylocereus undatus (Haw.) Br. & Rose, Cactaceae .. 95
Cardo-asnal
   Silybum marianum Gaertn., Asteraceae 65
Cardo-limão
   Hylocereus undatus (Haw.) Br. & Rose, Cactaceae .. 95
Cardo-melão
   Melocactus melocactoides (Hoffm.) DC., Cactaceae 97
   Notocactus ottonis (Lem.) Berg., Cactaceae 97
Cardo-santo
   Silybum marianum Gaertn., Asteraceae 65
Carijó
   Cayaponia espelina (Manso) Cogn.,
      also *Cayaponia* spp., Cucurbitaceae 135
   Davilla rugosa Poir., Dilleniaceae 145
Carnaúba
   Copernicia prunifera (Mill.) H. Moore, Arecaceae .. 40
Carnaubeira
   Copernicia prunifera (Mill.) H. Moore, Arecaceae .. 40
Carne-de-anta
   Maytenus obtusifolia Mart., Celastraceae 116
Caroá-caá
   Peperomia hederacea Miq., Piperaceae 273
Caroatá
   Bromelia pinguin L., Bromeliaceae 91
Caroba
   Jacaranda brasiliana (Lam.) Pers., Bignoniaceae ... 80
   Jacaranda caroba (Vell.) DC., Bignoniaceae 80
   Jacaranda cuspidifolia Mart., Bignoniaceae 81
   Jacaranda micrantha Cham., Bignoniaceae 81
   Schinus lentiscifolius March., Anacardiaceae 9
Caroba-branca
   Sparattosperma leucanthum
      (Vell.) K. Sch., Bignoniaceae 82
Caroba-de-flor-branca
   Sparattosperma leucanthum
      (Vell.) K. Sch., Bignoniaceae 82
Caroba-de-flor-verde
   Cybistax antisyphilitica
      (Mart.) Mart., Bignoniaceae 80
Caroba-do-campo
   Cremastus sceptrum Bur. & K. Sch., Bignoniaceae .. 79
   Cybistax antisyphilitica
      (Mart.) Mart., Bignoniaceae 80
   Jacaranda caroba (Vell.) DC., Bignoniaceae 80
Caroba-do-carrasco
   Jacaranda caroba (Vell.) DC., Bignoniaceae 80
Caroba-do-mato
   Jacaranda copaia (Aubl.) D. Don, Bignoniaceae 80

CAROBA-GUAÇU – CASCA-DOCE: COMMON NAMES INDEX

Caroba-guaçu
  Jacaranda mimosifolia D. Don, Bignoniaceae 81
Caroba-miúda
  Jacaranda caroba (Vell.) DC., Bignoniaceae 80
Caroba-preta
  Jacaranda subrhombea DC., Bignoniaceae 81
Caroba-roxa
  Jacaranda subrhombea DC., Bignoniaceae 81
Carobão
  Jacaranda micrantha Cham., Bignoniaceae 81
Carobeira
  Tabebuia caraiba (Mart.) Bur., Bignoniaceae 82
Carobinha
  Jacaranda caroba (Vell.) DC., Bignoniaceae 80
Carobinha-do-campo
  Jacaranda subrhombea DC., Bignoniaceae 81
Carobinha-verde
  Cybistax antisyphilitica (Mart.)
    Mart., Bignoniaceae 80
Carobuçu
  Jacaranda copaia (Aubl.) D. Don, Bignoniaceae 80
Carqueja
  Baccharis articulata (Lam.) Pers., Asteraceae 54
  Baccharis lundii DC., Asteraceae 54
  Baccharis notosergila Gris., Asteraceae 54
  Baccharis spp., Asteraceae 54
  Baccharis trimera (Less.) DC., Asteraceae 54
Carqueja-amargosa
  Baccharis trimera (Less.) DC., Asteraceae 54
Carqueja-do-morro
  Baccharis articulata (Lam.) Pers., Asteraceae 54
Carqueja-doce
  Baccharis articulata (Lam.) Pers., Asteraceae 54
Carqueja-miúda
  Baccharis articulata (Lam.) Pers., Asteraceae 54
Carquejinha
  Baccharis articulata (Lam.) Pers., Asteraceae 54
Carrancudo
  Maytenus obtusifolia Mart., Celastraceae 116
Carrapeta
  Guarea trichilioides L., Meliaceae 228
  Trichilia hirta L., Meliaceae 229
Carrapichinho
  Triumfetta semitriloba Jacq., Tiliaceae 327
Carrapicho
  Acanthospermum hispidum DC., Asteraceae 52
  Achyranthes indica L., Amaranthaceae 3
  Bidens pilosa L., Asteraceae 57
  Desmodium triflorum DC., Fabaceae 164
  Tropaeolum pentaphyllum Lam., Tropaeolaceae ... 327
Carrapicho-da-calçada
  Triumfetta rhomboidea Jacq., Tiliaceae 327
Carrapicho-de-agulha
  Bidens cynapiifolia H.B.K., Asteraceae 56
  Bidens pilosa L., Asteraceae 57
Carrapicho-de-calçada
  Triumfetta semitriloba Jacq., Tiliaceae 327
Carrapicho-de-carneiro
  Xanthium orientale L., *X. spinosum* L.
    and *X. strumarium* L., Asteraceae 68

Carrapicho-de-cavalo
  Krameria tomentosa St.-Hil., Krameriaceae 191
  Remirea maritima Aubl., Cyperaceae 143
Carrapicho-de-duas-pontas
  Bidens pilosa L., Asteraceae 57
Carrapicho-de-linho
  Triumfetta semitriloba Jacq., Tiliaceae 327
Carrapicho-do-ceará
  Krameria argentea Mart., Krameriaceae 191
Carrapicho-grande
  Xanthium orientale L., *X. spinosum* L.
    and *X. strumarium* L., Asteraceae 68
Carrapicho-rasteiro
  Acanthospermum australe
    (Loefl.) O. Ktze., Asteraceae 51
  Desmodium axillare (Sw.) DC., Fabaceae 164
Caru-caá
  Cordia multispicata Cham., Boraginaceae 88
Carúa-piranga
  Attalea spectabilis Mart., Arecaceae 39
Caruru
  Amaranthus spinosus L., Amaranthaceae 3
  Amaranthus viridis L., Amaranthaceae 3
Caruru-azedo
  Hibiscus sabdariffa L., Malvaceae 221
Caruru-bravo
  Amaranthus viridis L., Amaranthaceae 3
Caruru-da-guiné
  Hibiscus sabdariffa L., Malvaceae 221
Caruru-de-espinho
  Amaranthus spinosus L., Amaranthaceae 3
  Solanum juciri Mart., Solanaceae 321
Caruru-de-porco
  Amaranthus blitum L., Amaranthaceae 3
Caruru-de-sapo
  Oxalis martiana Zucc., Oxalidaceae 267
Caruru-de-soldado
  Amaranthus viridis L., Amaranthaceae 3
Caruru-de-veado
  Tournefortia elegans Cham., Boraginaceae 89
Caruru-miúdo
  Amaranthus blitum L., Amaranthaceae 3
  Amaranthus viridis L., Amaranthaceae 3
Caruru-verdadeiro
  Amaranthus blitum L., Amaranthaceae 3
Caruru-verde
  Amaranthus viridis L., Amaranthaceae 3
Carvoeira
  Callisthene major Mart., Vochysiaceae 340
Casca-cheirosa
  Ocotea pretiosa (Nees & Mart.)
    Benth. & Hook., Lauraceae 201
Casca-d'anta
  Drimys winteri Forst., Winteraceae 340
Casca-de-anta-brava
  Rauwolfia bahiensis DC., Apocynaceae 28
Casca-do-maranhão
  Aniba canelilla (H.B.K.) Mez, Lauraceae 197
Casca-doce
  Andradea floribunda Fr. All., Nyctaginaceae 257

Casca-paratudo
Cinnamodendron axillare
(Nees & Mart.) Endl., Cannaceae 110
Casca-preciosa
Aniba canelilla (H.B.K.) Mez, Lauraceae 197
Ocotea pretiosa (Nees & Mart.)
Benth. & Hook., Lauraceae 201
Casca-sacaca
Croton cajucara Benth., Euphorbiaceae 150
Cascaveleira
Thevetia ahouai (L.) DC., Apocynaceae 28
Cascos
Dioscorea laxiflora Mart., Dioscoreaceae 147
Cashew apple
USES: *Anacardium occidentale* L., Anacardiaceae 7
Casinga
Chiococca alba (L.) Hitch., Rubiaceae 297
Cássia-das-antilhas
Chamaecrista fasciculata
(Michx.) Greene, Caesalpiniaceae 102
Cássia-de-empingem
Chamaecrista mimosoides
(L.) Ir. & Barn., Caesalpiniaceae 102
Cássia-murici
Senna multijuga Rich. var.
verrucosa (Vog.) Ir. & Barn., Caesalpiniaceae 105
Castanha
Omphalea diandra M. Arg., Euphorbiaceae 156
Castanha-caetá
Omphalea diandra M. Arg., Euphorbiaceae 156
Castanha-comadre-de-azeite
Omphalea diandra M. Arg., Euphorbiaceae 156
Castanha-de-arara
Joannesia heveoides Ducke, Euphorbiaceae 155
Castanha-de-bugre
Anisosperma passiflora Manso, Cucurbitaceae 135
Castanha-de-cotia
Omphalea diandra M. Arg., Euphorbiaceae 156
Castanha-de-jatobá
Anisosperma passiflora Manso, Cucurbitaceae 135
Castanha-de-peixe
Omphalea diandra M. Arg., Euphorbiaceae 156
Castanha-do-pará
Bertholletia excelsa
Humb. & Bonpl., Lecythidaceae 204
Castanha-mineira
Anisosperma passiflora Manso, Cucurbitaceae 135
Tontelea brachypoda Miers, Hippocrateaceae 183
Castanha-sapucaia
Lecythis pisonis Camb., Lecythidaceae 207
Castanheira-do-pará *(Brazil nut)*
Bertholletia excelsa
Humb. & Bonpl., Lecythidaceae 204
Castanna-de-azeite
Omphalea diandra M. Arg., Euphorbiaceae 156
Cataguá
Metrodorea pubescens St.-Hil. & Tul., Rutaceae ... 301
Cataí-guaçu
Pilocarpus pinnatifolius Lem., Rutaceae 302

Cataia
Drimys winteri Forst., Winteraceae 340
Polygonum acuminatum H.B.K., Polygonaceae 286
Catajé
Pothomorphe peltata L., Piperaceae 277
Catauari
Crataeva benthamii Eichl., Capparaceae 112
Catauré
Crataeva benthamii Eichl., Capparaceae 112
Catiguá
Trichilia catigua Juss., Meliaceae 229
Catinga-de-barrão
Ageratum conyzoides L., Asteraceae 53
Catinga-de-bode
Ageratum conyzoides L., Asteraceae 53
Catinga-de-mulata
Croton zehntneri Pax & Hoffm., Euphorbiaceae 152
Leucas martinicensis (Jacq.) R. Br., Lamiaceae 194
Tanacetum vulgare L., Asteraceae 67
Catinga-de-negro
Cleome gigantea L., Capparaceae 112
Cleome speciosa H.B.K., Capparaceae 112
Catinga-de-porco
Caesalpinia microphylla Mart., Caesalpiniaceae ... 100
Catinga-de-tatu
Cleome gigantea L., Capparaceae 112
Catinga-preta
Cordia verbenacea DC., Boraginaceae 88
Catingueira
Caesalpinia bracteosa Tul., Caesalpiniaceae 100
Caesalpinia pyramidalis Tul., Caesalpiniaceae 100
Catingueiro-da-folha-miúda
Caesalpinia microphylla Mart., Caesalpiniaceae ... 100
Catingueiro-de-porco
Caesalpinia microphylla Mart., Caesalpiniaceae ... 100
Catojé
Cissampelos glaberrima
St.-Hil., Menispermaceae 233
Catolé
Syagrus comosa Mart., Arecaceae 45
Syagrus oleracea (Mart.) Becc., Arecaceae 45
Catoré
Crataeva benthamii Eichl., Capparaceae 112
Cattail
Typha domingensis Pers., Typhaceae 328
Catuaba
Anemopaegma arvense (Vell.) Stapf, Bignoniaceae . 78
Phyllanthus nobilis M. Arg., Euphorbiaceae 157
Trichilia catuaba (Silva) Rizz., Meliaceae 229
Catuaba-cipó
Secondatia floribunda DC., Apocynaceae 28
Catuaba-verdadeira
Anemopaegma arvense (Vell.) Stapf, Bignoniaceae . 78
Cauaçu
Coccoloba mollis Casar., Polygonaceae 285
Exostemma australe St.-Hil., Rubiaceae 298
Caúna
Ilex brevicuspis Reiss., Aquifoliaceae 31
Caúna-da-serra
Ilex brevicuspis Reiss., Aquifoliaceae 31

Cavalheiro-das-onze-horas
Portulaca grandiflora Hook., Portulacaceae 289
Cavalinha
Equisetum giganteum L., Equisetaceae 148
Cavalinho
Equisetum giganteum L., Equisetaceae 148
Caxapora-do-gentio
Terminalia argentea Mart., Combretaceae 126
Caxinguba
Ficus insipida Willd., Moraceae 248
Ficus maxima P. Mill., Moraceae 248
Cebola berrante
Hippeastrum puniceum
  (Lam.) Kuntze, Amaryllidaceae 6
Cebola-barrão
Hippeastrum vittatum
  (L'Hérit.) Herb., Amaryllidaceae 6
Cebola-branca
Hymenocallis tubiflora Salisb., Amaryllidaceae 7
Cebola-brava
Clusia rosea Jacq., Clusiaceae 122
Crinum scabrum Sims, Amaryllidaceae 6
Griffinia hyacinthina Ker.-Gawl., Amaryllidaceae 6
Hymenocallis tubiflora Salisb., Amaryllidaceae 7
Cebola-cecem
Hippeastrum vittatum
  (L'Hérit.) Herb., Amaryllidaceae 6
Cebola-do-mato
Griffinia hyacinthina Ker.-Gawl., Amaryllidaceae 6
Hippeastrum vittatum
  (L'Hérit.) Herb., Amaryllidaceae 6
Cebola-grande-da-mata
Clusia grandiflora Splitg., Clusiaceae 121
Cebolinha-do-campo
Cipura paludosa Aubl., Iridaceae 186
Cedrão
Guarea trichilioides L., Meliaceae 228
Cedro
Cedrela fissilis Vell., Meliaceae 227
Cedrela odorata L., Meliaceae 227
Cedro-batata
Cedrela fissilis Vell., Meliaceae 227
Cedro-branco
Cedrela fissilis Vell., Meliaceae 227
Cedro-do-amazonas
Cedrela odorata L., Meliaceae 227
Cedro-preto
Nectandra globosa (Aubl.) Mez, Lauraceae 199
Cedro-rosa
Cedrela fissilis Vell., Meliaceae 227
Cedro-vermelho
Cedrela fissilis Vell., Meliaceae 227
Cega-olho
Hippobroma longiflora
  (L.) G. Don, Campanulaceae 109
Celidônia
Boerhavia coccinea Mill., Nyctaginaceae 257
Trixis antimenorrhoea (Schrank) Mart., Asteraceae . 67
Cengolo-de-porco
Cariniana legalis (Mart.) O. Ktze., Lecythidaceae . 205

Centáurea-do-brasil
Deianira nervosa Cham. & Schl., Gentianaceae 180
Centáurea-menor
Curtia tenuifolia (Aubl.) Knobl., Gentianaceae 180
Cerebuna
Avicennia germinans (L.) L., Verbenaceae 334
Cereja-de-purga
Melothria fluminensis Gardn., Cucurbitaceae 139
Ceriba
Bactris insignis (Mart.) Baill., Arecaceae 39
Cerveja-de-índio
Ampelozizyphus amazonicus Ducke, Rhamnaceae . 291
Cerveja-de-pobre
Agonandra brasiliensis Miers, Opiliaceae 265
Chà-bravo
Ottonia corcovadensis Miq., Piperaceae 272
Chá-cravo
Capraria biflora L., Scrophulariaceae 311
Chá-da-américa
Capraria biflora L., Scrophulariaceae 311
Chá-da-campanha
Echinodorus grandiflorus
  (Cham. & Schl.) Mich., Alismataceae 2
Echinodorus macrophyllus
  (Kunth) Mich., Alismataceae 2
Chá-da-terra
Capraria biflora L., Scrophulariaceae 311
Turnera rupestris Aubl., Turneraceae 328
Chá-de-boi
Capraria biflora L., Scrophulariaceae 311
Chá-de-bugre
Cordia ecalyculata Vell., Boraginaceae 87
Cordia salicifolia Cham., Boraginaceae 88
Hedyosmum brasiliense Mart., Chloranthaceae 119
Chá-de-frade
Cordia ecalyculata Vell., Boraginaceae 87
Leonurus sibiricus L., Lamiaceae 194
Chá-de-marajó
Capraria biflora L., Scrophulariaceae 311
Chá-de-negro-mina
Cordia salicifolia Cham., Boraginaceae 88
Chá-de-soldado
Hedyosmum brasiliense Mart., Chloranthaceae 119
Chá-do-tabuleiro
Lippia alba (Mill.) N.E. Brown, Verbenaceae 335
Chá-mate
Ilex paraguariensis St.-Hil., Aquifoliaceae 31
Chá-mineiro
Echinodorus pubescens Mart., Alismataceae 2
Chá-mineiro-verdadeiro
Tournefortia volubilis L., Boraginaceae 90
Chá-preto
Capraria biflora L., Scrophulariaceae 311
Chagari
Cuphea balsamona Cham., Lythraceae 213
Chagas
Tropaeolum pentaphyllum Lam., Tropaeolaceae 327
Chagas-miúdas
Tropaeolum pentaphyllum Lam., Tropaeolaceae 327

Chanana
Turnera opifera Mart., Turneraceae 328
Turnera ulmifolia L., Turneraceae 328
Chapada
Acosmium dasycarpum (Vog.) Yakovl., Fabaceae .. 161
Chapadinha
Acosmium dasycarpum (Vog.) Yakovl., Fabaceae .. 161
Chaparro
Byrsonima coccolobifolia H.B.K., Malpighiaceae .. 218
Chapéu-de-couro
Echinodorus macrophyllus
  (Kunth) Mich., Alismataceae 2
Chapéu-de-napoleão
Thevetia ahouai (L.) DC., Apocynaceae 28
Charrua
Chromolaena hirsuta (Hook. & Arn.)
  King & H. Robinson, Asteraceae 58
Chibatã
Astronium fraxinifolium Schott, Anacardiaceae 9
Chica
Arrabidaea chica (H.B.K.) Bur., Bignoniaceae 78
Chica red
CHEM.: Arrabidaea chica
  (H.B.K.) Bur., Bignoniaceae 78
Chichá
Sterculia apetala (Jacq.) Karst.
  var. elata Ducke E. Taylor, Sterculiaceae 325
Sterculia chicha St.-Hil., Sterculiaceae 325
Chifre-de-veado
Ibicella lutea (Lindl.) Van Eselt., Martyniaceae 224
Chilca
Raulinoreitzia tremula (Hook. & Arn.)
  King & H. Robinson, Asteraceae 65
Chocalho-de-cascavel
Crotalaria verrucosa L., Fabaceae 163
Chonta
Bactris insignis (Mart.) Baill., Arecaceae 39
Chuchuguacha
Maytenus laevis Reiss., Celastraceae 115
Chuchuhuasca
Maytenus laevis Reiss., Celastraceae 115
Chumbinho
Lantana camara L., Verbenaceae 334
Chupa-ferro
Galipea multiflora Schult., Rutaceae 301
Cicuta-falsa
Hydrocotyle leucocephala
  Cham. & Schlecht., Apiaceae 20
Cidrão
Aloysia triphylla (L'Her.) Britt., Verbenaceae 332
Lippia gratissima (Gill. & Hook.)
  Troncoso, Verbenaceae 335
Cidreira
Siparuna brasiliensis (Spr.) DC., Monimiaceae 245
Cidrilha
Aloysia triphylla (L'Her.) Britt., Verbenaceae 332
Lippia alba (Mill.) N.E. Brown, Verbenaceae 335
Siparuna brasiliensis (Spr.) DC., Monimiaceae 245
Cidró
Aloysia triphylla (L'Her.) Britt., Verbenaceae 332

Cigua
Nectandra turbacensis Nees, Lauraceae 200
Cila
Hymenocallis tubiflora Salisb., Amaryllidaceae 7
Cila-da-terra
Hymenocallis tubiflora Salisb., Amaryllidaceae 7
Cincho
Sorocea bonplandii (Baill.) Burger, Moraceae 249
Cinco-chagas
Cybistax antisyphilitica
  (Mart.) Mart., Bignoniaceae 80
Sparattosperma leucanthum
  (Vell.) K. Sch., Bignoniaceae 82
Cinco-folhas
Cybistax antisyphilitica
  (Mart.) Mart., Bignoniaceae 80
Sparattosperma leucanthum
  (Vell.) K. Sch., Bignoniaceae 82
Cinzeiro
Terminalia tanibouca Smith, Combretaceae 126
Cinzeiro-do-mato
Symplocos pubescens Klotzsch, Symplocaceae 326
Cioula
Mouriri guianensis Aubl., Melastomataceae 226
Ciparoba
Cissampelos glaberrima St.-Hil., Menispermaceae 233
Cipó
Tetracera volubilis L., Dilleniaceae 146
Cipó-amargoso
Abuta candicans Rich., Menispermaceae 231
Cipó-azougue
Melothrianthus smilacifolius
  (Cogn.) M. Crovetto, Cucurbitaceae 139
Wilbrandia verticillata
  (Vell.) Cogn., Cucurbitaceae 140
Cipó-barba-branca
Clematis campestris St.-Hil., Ranunculaceae 290
Cipó-bela-flor
Pyrostegia ignea (Vell.) Pres., Bignoniaceae 82
Cipó-cabeludo
Mikania hirsutissima DC., Asteraceae 62
Mikania setigera Schultz-Bip.
  ex Baker, Asteraceae 62
Cipó-caboclo
Davilla rugosa Poir., Dilleniaceae 145
Cipó-caboclo-venenoso
Doliocarpus rolandri Gmel., Dilleniaceae 146
Cipó-camarão
Arrabidaea agnus-castus
  (Cham.) DC., Bignoniaceae 78
Cipó-capa-homem
Davilla rugosa Poir., Dilleniaceae 145
Cipó-capador
Echites peltata Vell., Apocynaceae 23
Cipó-catinga
Mikania parviflora (Aubl.) Karst., Asteraceae 62
Cipó-chumbo
Cassytha filiformis L., Lauraceae 198
Cuscuta racemosa Mart., Convolvulaceae 130

Cipó-corimbó
Tanaecium nocturnum
  (B. Rodr.) Bur. & K. Sch., Bignoniaceae 84
Cipó-cravo
Tynanthus cognatus (Cham.) Miers, also
  T. elegans (Cham.) Miers, and *T. fasciculatus*
  (Vell.) Miers, Bignoniaceae 84
Cipó-cruz
Arrabidaea chica (H.B.K.) Bur., Bignoniaceae 78
Chiocócca alba (L.) Hitch., Rubiaceae 297
Clematis dioica L., Ranunculaceae 290
Cipó-cruzeiro
Strychnos trinervis (Vell.) Mart., Loganiaceae 210
Cipó-curimbo
Tanaecium nocturnum
  (B. Rodr.) Bur. & K. Sch., Bignoniaceae 84
Cipó-cururu
Anisolobus cururu (Mart.) M. Arg., Apocynaceae 21
Odontadenia speciosa Benth., Apocynaceae 27
Cipó-da-areia
Ephedra triandra Tul., Ephedraceae 148
Cipó-da-beira-mar
Entada polystachya (Jacq.) DC., Mimosaceae 237
Cipó-da-praia
Ipomoea acetosifolia (Vahl) Roem.
  & Schult., Convolvulaceae 130
Ipomoea pes-caprae (L.) R. Br., Convolvulaceae .. 130
Remirea maritima Aubl., Cyperaceae 143
Cipó-d'agua
Doliocarpus rolandri Gmel., Dilleniaceae 146
Cipó-d'alho
Adenocalymma alliacea
  (Lam.) Miers, Bignoniaceae 78
Cipó-de-alho
Seguieria americana L., Phytolaccaceae 272
Cipó-de-caboclo
Davilla rugosa Poir., Dilleniaceae 145
Tetracera volubilis L., Dilleniaceae 146
Cipó-de-cabras
Cissampelos pareira L., Menispermaceae 233
Cipó-de-carijá
Davilla rugosa Poir., Dilleniaceae 145
Cipó-de-carneiro
Haemadyction gaudichaudii DC., Apocynaceae 24
Cipó-de-cesto
Cydista aequinoctialis Miers, Bignoniaceae 80
Cipó-de-cobra
Cissampelos glaberrima St.-Hil., Menispermaceae 233
Cipó-de-copacabana
Peritassa calypsoides
  (Camb.) A.C. Sm., Hippocrateaceae 183
Cipó-de-corda
Cydista aequinoctialis Miers, Bignoniaceae 80
Cipó-de-fogo
Euphorbia phosphorea Mart., Euphorbiaceae 153
Pyrostegia ignea (Vell.) Pres., Bignoniaceae 82
Cipó-de-gato
Macfadyena unguis-cati (L.) Gentry, Bignoniaceae . 81
Cipó-de-gota
Cissampelos pareira L., Menispermaceae 233

Cipó-de-imbê
Philodendron imbe Schott, Araceae 36
Philodendron ochrostemon Schott, Araceae 37
Philodendron selloum Koch, Araceae 37
Cipó-de-jaboti
Fevillea trilobata L., Cucurbitaceae 136
Cipó-de-lagartixa
Pyrostegia ignea (Vell.) Pres., Bignoniaceae 82
Cipó-de-lagarto
Pyrostegia ignea (Vell.) Pres., Bignoniaceae 82
Cipó-de-lavadeira
Reisseckia smilacina (Sm.) Steud., Rhamnaceae 293
Cipó-de-leite
Mesechites sulphurea (Vell.) M. Arg., Apocynaceae 27
Tragia volubilis L., Euphorbiaceae 158
Cipó-de-paina
Echites peltata Vell., Apocynaceae 23
Cipó-de-parque
Araujia sericifera Brot., Asclepiadaceae 50
Cipó-de-rama
Araujia sericifera Brot., Asclepiadaceae 50
Cipó-de-rego
Arrabidaea agnus-castus
  (Cham.) DC., Bignoniaceae 78
Cipó-de-são-joão
Pyrostegia ignea (Vell.) Pres., Bignoniaceae 82
Cipó-de-sapo
Araujia sericifera Brot., Asclepiadaceae 50
Cipó-de-seda
Araujia sericifera Brot., Asclepiadaceae 50
Cipó-do-banhado
Ranunculus apiifolius Pers., Ranunculaceae 290
Cipó-do-coração
Aristolochia cordigera Willd., Aristolochiaceae 46
Cipó-do-reino
Clematis campestris St.-Hil., Ranunculaceae 290
Clematis dioica L., Ranunculaceae 290
Cipó-em
Smilax longifolia Rich., Liliaceae 208
Cipó-escada
Bauhinia langsdorffiana Bong., Caesalpiniaceae 99
Bauhinia radiata Vell., Caesalpiniaceae 99
Fevillea trilobata L., Cucurbitaceae 136
Cipó-gimbé
Philodendron bipinnatifidum Schott, Araceae 36
Cipó-imbé, Cipó-imbê
Philodendron bipinnatifidum Schott, Araceae 36
Philodendron imbe Schott, Araceae 36
Cipó-ira
Guatteria scandens Ducke, Annonaceae 15
Cipó-jarrinha
Aristolochia triangularis Cham., Aristolochiaceae ... 48
Cipó-jatobá
Fevillea uncipetala Kuhlm., Cucurbitaceae 138
Cipó-mata-cobras
Aristolochia cymbifera
  Mart. & Zucc., Aristolochiaceae 46
Cipó-mil-homens
Aristolochia triangularis Cham., Aristolochiaceae ... 48

Cipó-milhomens
 Aristolochia elegans Mast., Aristolochiaceae 48
Cipó-mole
 Pisonia aculeata L., Nyctaginaceae 258
Cipó-paratudo
 Aristolochia cymbifera
  Mart. & Zucc., Aristolochiaceae 47
Cipó-paré
 Tanaecium nocturnum
  (B. Rodr.) Bur. & K. Sch., Bignoniaceae 84
Cipó-peludo
 Micrograma vaccinifolia
  (Langsd. & Fisch.) Copel., Polypodiaceae 288
Cipó-prata
 Clematis dioica L., Ranunculaceae 290
Cipó-preto
 Hippocratea volubilis L., Hippocrateaceae 183
Cipó-pucá
 Cissus sicyoides L., Vitaceae 339
Cipó-puci
 Cissus sicyoides L., Vitaceae 339
Cipó-quina
 Smilax oblongifolia Pohl, Liliaceae 208
Cipó-ramo
 Araujia sericifera Brot., Asclepiadaceae 50
Cipó-rego
 Arrabidaea agnus-castus
  (Cham.) DC., Bignoniaceae 78
Cipó-santo
 Echites peltata Vell., Apocynaceae 23
Cipó-seda
 Araujia sericifera Brot., Asclepiadaceae 50
Cipó-suma
 Anchietea pyrifolia (Mart.) G. Don, Violaceae 338
Cipó-três-quinas
 Arrabidaea agnus-castus
  (Cham.) DC., Bignoniaceae 78
Cipó-tripa-de-galinha
 Dalechampia ficifolia Lam., Euphorbiaceae 152
Cipó-urtiguinha
 Tragia volubilis L., Euphorbiaceae 158
Cipó-vermelho
 Davilla rugosa Poir., Dilleniaceae 145
 Doliocarpus rolandri Gmel., Dilleniaceae 146
 Tetracera aspera Willd., Dilleniaceae 146
 Tetracera breyniana Schl., Dilleniaceae 146
Cipotaí
 Capparis lineata Pers., Capparaceae 111
 Capparis urens B. Rodr., Capparaceae 111
Cipozinho-do-campo
 Araujia sericifera Brot., Asclepiadaceae 50
Ciúme
 Calotropis procera (Ait.) Ait. f., Asclepiadaceae 50
Coagerucu
 Xylopia frutescens Aubl., Annonaceae 16
Coapiranga
 Arrabidaea chica (H.B.K.) Bur., Bignoniaceae 78
Coari-bravo
 Tagetes minuta L., Asteraceae 67

Coatindiba
 Celtis brasiliensis Planch., Ulmaceae 330
 Celtis morifolia Planch., Ulmaceae 330
Coaxicó
 Cryptocarya guyanensis Meissn., Lauraceae 198
Coaxinguba
 Ficus insipida Willd., Moraceae 248
 Ficus maxima P. Mill., Moraceae 248
Coca
 Erythroxylum coca Lam., Erythroxylaceae 150
Cocão
 Raputia magnifica Engl., Rutaceae 302
Cocklebur
 Xanthium orientale L., *X. spinosum* L.
  and *X. strumarium* L., Asteraceae 68
Coco-amargoso
 Syagrus pseudococos
  (Raddi) Glassman, Arecaceae 45
Coco-babão
 Syagrus oleracea (Mart.) Becc., Arecaceae 45
Coco-de-airi
 Astrocaryum aculeatissimum
  (Schott) Burret, Arecaceae 39
Coco-de-cachorro
 Syagrus romanzoffiana
  (Cham.) Glassman, Arecaceae 45
Coco-de-purga
 Joannesia princeps Vell., Euphorbiaceae 155
Coco-de-quaresma
 Syagrus oleracea (Mart.) Becc., Arecaceae 45
Coco-de-sapo
 Syagrus romanzoffiana
  (Cham.) Glassman, Arecaceae 45
Coco-de-vassoura
 Allagoptera campestris (Mart.) Kuntze, Arecaceae .. 39
Coco-feijão
 Dipteryx alata Vog., Fabaceae 165
Coco-guariroba
 Syagrus oleracea (Mart.) Becc., Arecaceae 45
Coco-naiá
 Orbignya phalerata Mart., Arecaceae 43
Coco-pindo-ba
 Orbignya phalerata Mart., Arecaceae 43
Coco-verde
 Syagrus pseudococos
  (Raddi) Glassman, Arecaceae 45
Cocorobó
 Chloris distichophylla (Nees) Lag., Poaceae 280
Coentrilho
 Zanthoxylum hyemale St.-Hil., Rutaceae 302
Coentro-bravo
 Eryngium foetidum L., Apiaceae 19
Coentro-da-colônia
 Eryngium foetidum L., Apiaceae 19
Coentro-de-caboclo
 Eryngium foetidum L., Apiaceae 19
Coerana
 Bassovia lucida Dunal, Solanaceae 316
 Cestrum amictum Schl., Solanaceae 317

Cestrum bracteatum Link & Otto, Solanaceae 317
Cestrum calycinum Willd., Solanaceae 317
Cestrum parqui L'Herit., Solanaceae 317
Cogumelo-de-caboclo
 Scybalium fungiforme
  Schott & Endl., Balanophoraceae 74
Cogumelo-de-sangue
 Scybalium fungiforme
  Schott & Endl., Balanophoraceae 74
Coifa-do-diabo
 Aristolochia cymbifera
  Mart. & Zucc., Aristolochiaceae 47
Coirama
 Kalanchoe brasiliensis Camb., Crassulaceae 133
 Kalanchoe pinnata (Lam.) Pers., Crassulaceae ... 133
Coirama-branca
 Kalanchoe brasiliensis Camb., Crassulaceae 133
Coité
 Crescentia cujete L., Bignoniaceae 80
Cola-de-cavalo
 Equisetum giganteum L., Equisetaceae 148
Cola-de-sapateiro
 Cyrtopodium andersoni R. Br., Orchidaceae 266
Comadre-de-azeite
 Omphalea diandra M. Arg., Euphorbiaceae 156
Comaí
 Zschokkea arborescens M. Arg., Apocynaceae 29
Comandaíba
 Sophora tomentosa L., Fabaceae 172
Comida-de-jaboti
 Peperomia pellucida H.B.K., Piperaceae 273
Comigo-ninguém-pode
 Dieffenbachia seguine (Jacq.) Schott, Araceae ... 35
Conabi
 Clibadium surinamense L., Asteraceae 58
 Ichthyothere terminalis
  (Spr.) S.F. Blake, Asteraceae 61
 Phyllanthus conami Sw., Euphorbiaceae 156
Conambi
 Clibadium surinamense L., Asteraceae 58
 Phyllanthus conami Sw., Euphorbiaceae 156
Conami
 Phyllanthus conami Sw., Euphorbiaceae 156
Condessa
 Annona reticulata L., Annonaceae 13
Conduru
 Brosimum gaudichaudii Tréc., Moraceae 246
Congonha
 Citronella congonha (Mart.) Howard, Icacinaceae . 185
 Ilex brevicuspis Reiss., Aquifoliaceae 31
 Ilex paraguariensis St.-Hil., Aquifoliaceae 31
 Psoralea glandulosa L., Fabaceae 170
 Salpichroa origanifolia (Lam.) Thell., Solanaceae 319
Congonha-brava
 Maytenus communis Reiss., Celastraceae 115
Congonha-brava-de-folha-miúda
 Maytenus obtusifolia Mart., Celastraceae 116
Congonha-de-bugre
 Citronella congonha (Mart.) Howard, Icacinaceae . 185

Congonha-do-brejo
 Echinodorus grandiflorus
  (Cham. & Schl.) Mich., Alismataceae 2
Congonha-do-campo
 Luxemburgia glazioviana Gilg., Ochnaceae 260
 Luxemburgia polyandra St.-Hil., Ochnaceae 260
Congonha-do-mato
 Luxemburgia glazioviana Gilg., Ochnaceae 260
 Luxemburgia polyandra St.-Hil., Ochnaceae 260
Congonha-do-sertão
 Citronella congonha (Mart.) Howard, Icacinaceae . 185
 Citronella mucronata
  (R. & Pav.) Don, Icacinaceae 186
Congonha-falsa
 Citronella congonha (Mart.) Howard, Icacinaceae . 185
Congonha-grande
 Maytenus communis Reiss., Celastraceae 115
Congonha-verdadeira
 Citronella mucronata
  (R. & Pav.) Don, Icacinaceae 186
Conta-de-cobra
 Dorstenia brasiliensis Lam., Moraceae 247
Contra-erva-do-Peru
 Flaveria bidentis (L.) Ktze., Asteraceae 60
Contraerva
 Dorstenia brasiliensis Lam., Moraceae 247
Convetinga
 Solanum mauritianum Scop., Solanaceae 321
Copaíba
 Copaifera multijuga Hayne, Caesalpiniaceae 102
Copaíba-verdadeira
 Copaifera officinalis (Jacq.) L., Caesalpiniaceae 102
Copaíva
 Copaifera officinalis (Jacq.) L., Caesalpiniaceae 102
Copo-de-leite
 Datura suaveolens Humb. & Bonpl., Solanaceae ... 318
Coqueiro-amargoso
 Syagrus oleracea (Mart.) Becc., Arecaceae 45
Coqueiro-catolé
 Syagrus comosa Mart., Arecaceae 45
Coqueiro-da-bahia
 Cocos nucifera L., Arecaceae 40
Coqueiro-de-santa-catarina
 Syagrus romanzoffiana
  (Cham.) Glassman, Arecaceae 45
Coqueiro-de-venus
 Cordyline dracaenoides Kunth, Liliaceae 207
Coqueiro-jataí
 Butia yatay (Mart.) Becc., Arecaceae 39
Coqueiro-juvena
 Syagrus romanzoffiana
  (Cham.) Glassman, Arecaceae 45
Coqueiro-naiá
 Scheelea phalerata
  (Mart. ex Spreng.) Burret, Arecaceae 45
Coqueiro-pissandó
 Allagoptera campestris (Mart.) Kuntze, Arecaceae .. 39
Coquidá
 Swartzia chrysantha B. Rodr., Caesalpiniaceae ... 107

Coquilho
Canna glauca L., Cannaceae 110
Coração
Piper gigantifolium Jacq., Piperaceae 275
Coração-de-estudante
Begonia luxurians Scheidw., Begoniaceae 76
Coração-de-Jesus
Mikania cordifolia (L. f.) Willd., Asteraceae 61
Mikania officinalis Mart., Asteraceae 62
Coração-de-negro
Albizzia lebbeck (L.) Benth., Mimosaceae 236
Coração-verde
Ocotea rodiei (Schomb.) Mez, Lauraceae 201
Coral
Jatropha multifida L., Euphorbiaceae 154
Machaonia brasiliensis Cham. & Schl., Rubiaceae 299
Manettia ignita (Vell.) K. Sch., Rubiaceae 299
Coral-dos-jardins
Jatropha multifida L., Euphorbiaceae 154
Coralina
Heterothalamus psiadioides Less., Asteraceae 60
Corango
Gomphrena leucocephala Mart., Amaranthaceae 4
Cordão-de-frade
Borreria verticillata (L.) Meyer, Rubiaceae 296
Leonotis nepetaefolia R. Br., Lamiaceae 194
Leucas martinicensis (Jacq.) R. Br., Lamiaceae 194
Cordão-de-são-francisco
Leonotis nepetaefolia R. Br., Lamiaceae 194
Leonurus sibiricus L., Lamiaceae 194
Leucas martinicensis (Jacq.) R. Br., Lamiaceae 194
Parkia pendula Benth. ex Walp., Mimosaceae 240
Cordobá
Tradescantia spathacea Sw., Commelinaceae 129
Corimbó
Tanaecium nocturnum
(B. Rodr.) Bur. & K. Sch., Bignoniaceae 84
Corimbó-da-mata
Tanaecium nocturnum
(B. Rodr.) Bur. & K. Sch., Bignoniaceae 84
Corindiba
Celtis brasiliensis Planch., Ulmaceae 330
Corindiúba
Celtis brasiliensis Planch., Ulmaceae 330
Cornos-do-diabo
Ibicella lutea (Lindl.) Van Eselt., Martyniaceae 224
Coroá
Sicana odorifera Naud., Cucurbitaceae 139
Coroa-de-cristo
Colletia paradoxa (Spr.) Escalante, Rhamnaceae ... 291
Euphorbia tirucalli L., Euphorbiaceae 153
Coroa-de-frade
Melocactus melocactoides
(Hoffm.) DC., Cactaceae 97
Corongo
Gomphrena leucocephala Mart., Amaranthaceae 4
Coronilha
Scutia buxifolia Reiss., Rhamnaceae 293
Corre-corre
Evolvulus alsinoides L., Convolvulaceae 130

Corrente
Achyranthes ficoidea Lam., Amaranthaceae 3
Pfaffia glomerata (Spreng.) Peders., Amaranthaceae .. 4
Corticeira
Annona glabra L., Annonaceae 13
Erythrina crista-galli L., Fabaceae 166
Cortina-de-pobre
Cissus sicyoides L., Vitaceae 339
Corubá
Celtis morifolia Planch., Ulmaceae 330
Costa-branca
Chaptalia nutans (L.) Polak., Asteraceae 57
Cotieira
Joannesia princeps Vell., Euphorbiaceae 155
Couve-cravinho
Porophyllum ruderale (Jacq.) Cass., Asteraceae 64
Couve-de-vedado
Porophyllum ruderale (Jacq.) Cass., Asteraceae 64
Couvinha
Porophyllum ruderale (Jacq.) Cass., Asteraceae 64
Craveiro-da-terra
Calyptranthes aromatica St.-Hil., Myrtaceae 253
Pseudocaryophyllus sericeus Berg, Myrtaceae 256
Craveiro-do-campo
Calyptranthes variabilis Berg, Myrtaceae 253
Craveiro-do-maranhão
Dicypellium caryophyllatum
Nees & Mart., Lauraceae 198
Cravinho
Croton zehntneri Pax & Hoffm., Euphorbiaceae 152
Dicypellium caryophyllatum
Nees & Mart., Lauraceae 198
Cravo-de-defunto
Tagetes erecta L., Asteraceae 67
Tagetes minuta L., Asteraceae 67
Cravo-de-defunto-miúdo
Tagetes minuta L., Asteraceae 67
Cravo-de-urubu
Porophyllum ruderale (Jacq.) Cass., Asteraceae 64
Cravo-do-campo
Calyptranthes variabilis Berg, Myrtaceae 253
Isostigma megapotamicum (Spr.)
Sherff, Asteraceae 61
Cravo-do-mato
Dicypellium caryophyllatum
Nees & Mart., Lauraceae 198
Tillandsia aeranthos
(Loisel.) L.B. Smith, Bromeliaceae 91
Crindiúva
Celtis brasiliensis Planch., Ulmaceae 330
Crista-de-galo
Amaranthus spinosus L., Amaranthaceae 3
Heliotropium curassavicum L., Boraginaceae 88
Heliotropium elongatum Willd., Boraginaceae 88
Heliotropium indicum L., Boraginaceae 89
Crista-de-peru
Centropogon cornutus (L.) Druce, Campanulaceae 109
Croatá-falso
Eryngium paniculatum
Cav. & Domb. ex Delar., Apiaceae 19

Cruá – Cutiti: Common Names Index

Cruá
Sicana odorifera Naud., Cucurbitaceae 139
Cruili
Mouriri guianensis Aubl., Melastomataceae 226
Crumbamba
Desmoncus polyacanthos Mart., Arecaceae 40
Cruz-de-malta
Ludwigia peruviana (L.) Hara, Onagraceae 264
Ludwigia repens (L.) Hara, Onagraceae 264
Ludwigia suffruticosa (L.) Gomes, Onagraceae 264
Cruzeirinha
Chiococca alba (L.) Hitch., Rubiaceae 297
Cruzeiro
Declieuxia cordigera Mart. & Zucc., Rubiaceae 297
Cuambu
Bidens pilosa L., Asteraceae 57
Cubatã-vermelho
Astronium fraxinifolium Schott, Anacardiaceae 9
Cuia
Lagenaria siceraria
   (Molina) Standl., Cucurbitaceae 138
Cuia-rana
Terminalia tanibouca Smith, Combretaceae 126
Cuieira
Crescentia cujete L., Bignoniaceae 80
Cuieté
Crescentia cujete L., Bignoniaceae 80
Lagenaria siceraria
   (Molina) Standl., Cucurbitaceae 138
Cuimari
Ocotea cujumary Mart., Lauraceae 200
Cuipuna
Myrcia tingens Berg, Myrtaceae 255
Cuité-açu
Renealmia occidentalis Sweet, Zingiberaceae 343
Cuiumaru
Ocotea cujumary Mart., Lauraceae 200
Cujumari-da-guiana
Ocotea guianensis Aubl., Lauraceae 201
Cujumari-mirim
Ocotea guianensis Aubl., Lauraceae 201
Cujumari-rana
Ocotea guianensis Aubl., Lauraceae 201
Cujumaru
Ocotea cujumary Mart., Lauraceae 200
Culantrilho
Adiantum concinnum Humb. & Bonp., Adiantaceae .. 1
Cumã
Couma utilis (Mart.) M. Arg., Apocynaceae 23
Cumacá
Marsdenia amylacea
   (Barb.-Rodr.) Malme, Asclepiadaceae 51
Cumacaá
Marsdenia amylacea
   (Barb.-Rodr.) Malme, Asclepiadaceae 51
Cumaí
Couma utilis (Mart.) M. Arg., Apocynaceae 23
Zschokkea arborescens M. Arg., Apocynaceae 29

Cumaná
Marsdenia amylacea
   (Barb.-Rodr.) Malme, Asclepiadaceae 51
Cumandá
Campsiandra comosa Benth. var.
   laurifolia (Benth.) Cowan, Caesalpiniaceae 100
Cumapé
Anisolobus cururu (Mart.) M. Arg., Apocynaceae 21
Cumaru
Dipteryx odorata (Aubl.) Willd., Fabaceae 166
Torresea cearensis Fr. All., Fabaceae 172
Cumaru-amarelo
Dipteryx odorata (Aubl.) Willd., Fabaceae 166
Cumaru-das-caatingas
Torresea cearensis Fr. All., Fabaceae 172
Cumaru-do-amazonas
Dipteryx odorata (Aubl.) Willd., Fabaceae 166
Cumaru-do-ceará
Torresea cearensis Fr. All., Fabaceae 172
Cumaru-do-nordeste
Torresea cearensis Fr. All., Fabaceae 172
Cumaru-verdadeiro
Dipteryx odorata (Aubl.) Willd., Fabaceae 166
Cumarurana
Andira inermis (Sw.) H.B.K., Fabaceae 162
Andira retusa (Poir.) H.B.K., Fabaceae 162
Dipteryx alata Vog., Fabaceae 165
Cumba
Craniolaria annua L., Martyniaceae 224
Craniolaria integrifolia Cham., Martyniaceae 224
Philodendron imbe Schott, Araceae 36
Cumbaru
Dipteryx alata Vog., Fabaceae 165
Cumichá
Pisonia cordifolia Mart., Nyctaginaceae 258
Cunabi
Ichthyothere terminalis
   (Spr.) S.F. Blake, Asteraceae 61
Cunambi
Ichthyothere terminalis
   (Spr.) S.F. Blake, Asteraceae 61
Cupaí
Clusia rosea Jacq., Clusiaceae 122
Curatá
Coccoloba laevis Casar., Polygonaceae 285
Curro
Colletia paradoxa (Spr.) Escalante, Rhamnaceae ... 291
Curuá
Sicana odorifera Naud., Cucurbitaceae 139
Curubá
Celtis morifolia Planch., Ulmaceae 330
Curumi
Muntingia calabura L., Tiliaceae 327
Curupitá
Sapium hamatum Pax & Hoffm., Euphorbiaceae ... 157
Cururu
Anisolobus cururu (Mart.) M. Arg., Apocynaceae 21
Cutiti
Lucuma rivicoa Gaertn., Sapotaceae 309

Cutitiribá
Lucuma rivicoa Gaertn., Sapotaceae 309
Cutiuba
Bowdichia virgilioides H.B.K., Fabaceae 163
Cutúbeo-brasileira
Coutoubea spicata Aubl., Gentianaceae 179
Cuvitinga
Solanum mauritianum Scop., Solanaceae 321
Solanum verbascifolium L., Solanaceae 322

D

Daião
Kalanchoe pinnata (Lam.) Pers., Crassulaceae 133
Dama-da-noite
Calonyction aculeatum
(L.) House, Convolvulaceae 129
Dambê
Chiococca alba (L.) Hitch., Rubiaceae 297
Damiana
Turnera diffusa Willd., Turneraceae 327
Turnera guianensis Aubl., Turneraceae 328
Turnera opifera Mart., Turneraceae 328
Dartrial
Senna alata (L.) Roxb., Caesalpiniaceae 104
Dedal
Lafoensia pacari St.-Hil., Lythraceae 215
Dedal-de-dama
Allamanda cathartica L., Apocynaceae 20
Dedaleira-amarela
Lafoensia pacari St.-Hil., Lythraceae 215
Dendezeiro
Elaeis guineensis Jacq., Arecaceae 40
Dendezeiro-do-pará
Elaeis oleifera (H.B.K.) Cortez, Arecaceae 40
Diambarana
Coutoubea ramosa Aubl., Gentianaceae 179
Diamburu
Jacaratia spinosa (Aubl.) A. DC., Caricaceae 113
Didi-da-porteira
Commelina nudiflora L., Commelinaceae 126
Commelina pohliana Seub., Commelinaceae 127
Disciplina
Cayaponia espelina (Manso) Cogn., also
Cayaponia spp., Cucurbitaceae 135
Dichorisandra affinis Mart., Commelinaceae 128
Dorme-maria
Mimosa velloziana Mart., Mimosaceae 240
Dormideira
Mimosa pudica L., Mimosaceae 240
Mimosa velloziana Mart., Mimosaceae 240
Dormideira-grande
Mimosa velloziana Mart., Mimosaceae 240
Douradinha
Lindernia diffusa Wettst., Scrophulariaceae 312
Waltheria communis St.-Hil., Sterculiaceae 325
Douradinha-do-campo
Lindernia crustacea F. Muell., Scrophulariaceae ... 311
Waltheria communis St.-Hil., Sterculiaceae 325

Douradinha-do-pará
Lindernia crustacea F. Muell., Scrophulariaceae ... 311
Douradinha-falsa
Byrsonima verbascifolia
(L.) Rich., Malpighiaceae 220
Dracena
Cordyline dracaenoides Kunth, Liliaceae 207
Dragão-fedorento
Monstera adansonii Schott, Araceae 36
Duckweed
Lemna minor L., Lemnaceae 207
Dumb cane
CHEM. & PHARM.:*Dieffenbachia seguine*
(Jacq.) Schott, Araceae 35
Dumiringama
Vallesia cymbifolia Ortega, Apocynaceae 29
Dyer's mulberry
Maclura tinctoria (L.) D. Don, Moraceae 249

E

Ébano-amarelo
Tabebuia leucoxylon (L.) DC., Bignoniaceae 83
Ébano-oriental
Albizzia lebbeck (L.) Benth., Mimosaceae 236
Elemi
Protium icicariba (DC.) March., Burseraceae 94
Elixir-paregórico
Peperomia elongata Miq., Piperaceae 273
Piper callosum R. & Pav., Piperaceae 274
Piper cavalcantei Yunck., Piperaceae 275
Embaúba
Cecropia hololeuca Miq., Moraceae 247
Cecropia palmata Willd., Moraceae 247
Embaúba-branca
Cecropia leucocoma Miq., Moraceae 247
Cecropia palmata Willd., Moraceae 247
Embaúba-prateada
Cecropia hololeuca Miq., Moraceae 247
Embira
Guazuma ulmifolia
Lam. var. *ulmifolia*, Sterculiaceae 323
Rollinia exalbida (Vell.) Mart., Annonaceae 15
Urena lobata L., Malvaceae 223
Xylopia aromatica (Lam.) Mart., Annonaceae 15
Embira-brava
Helicteres ovata Lam., Sterculiaceae 324
Embira-do-mato
Helicteres ovata Lam., Sterculiaceae 324
Embira-vermelha
Rollinia salicifolia Schl., Annonaceae 15
Embirataia
Duguetia riparia Hub., Annonaceae 14
Embiriba
Xylopia benthamiana Fries, Annonaceae 16
Embiriba-pacovi
Xylopia benthamiana Fries, Annonaceae 16
Embiru
Guazuma ulmifolia Lam.
var. *ulmifolia*, Sterculiaceae 323

Emburi
Allagoptera campestris (Mart.) Kuntze, Arecaceae .. 39
Enfira-bobó
Annona cornifolia St.-Hil., Annonaceae 12
Ensacadinha
Cardiospermum grandiflorum Sw., Sapindaceae ... 305
Envira
Guatteria ouregon (Aubl.) Dun., Annonaceae 14
Xylopia aromatica (Lam.) Mart., Annonaceae 15
Xylopia frutescens Aubl., Annonaceae 16
Envira-amarela
Xylopia benthamiana Fries, Annonaceae 16
Envirataí
Duguetia riparia Hub., Annonaceae 14
Envirataia
Annona ambotay Aubl., Annonaceae 12
Envireira
Annona cornifolia St.-Hil., Annonaceae 12
Xylopia aromatica (Lam.) Mart., Annonaceae 15
Erva-almíscar
Hedyosmum brasiliense Mart., Chloranthaceae 119
Erva-andorinha
Euphorbia hirta L., Euphorbiaceae 152
Euphorbia hyssopifolia L., Euphorbiaceae 153
Trixis antimenorrhoea (Schrank) Mart., Asteraceae . 67
Erva-azeda
Begonia acida Mart., Begoniaceae 75
Erva-baleeira
Cordia monosperma
(Jacq.) Roem. & Schult., Boraginaceae 87
Cordia verbenacea DC., Boraginaceae 88
Erva-botão
Borreria verticillata (L.) Meyer, Rubiaceae 296
Eclipta prostrata (L.) L., Asteraceae 59
Erva-cancerosa
Jodina rhombifolia Hook. & Arn., Santalaceae 304
Maytenus ilicifolia Mart., Celastraceae 115
Erva-cancorosa
Jodina rhombifolia Hook. & Arn., Santalaceae 304
Erva-capitão
Hydrocotyle bonariensis Lam., Apiaceae 19
Hydrocotyle leucocephala
Cham. & Schlecht., Apiaceae 20
Erva-capitão-miúda
Hydrocotyle leucocephala
Cham. & Schlecht., Apiaceae 20
Erva-chumbo
Cassytha filiformis L., Lauraceae 198
Erva-cidreira
Aloysia triphylla (L'Her.) Britt., Verbenaceae 332
Lippia alba (Mill.) N.E. Brown, Verbenaceae 335
Erva-cidreira-do-mato
Siparuna brasiliensis (Spr.) DC., Monimiaceae 245
Erva-cidreira-dos-campos
Siparuna camporum (Tul.) DC., Monimiaceae 245
Erva-cigana
Cremastus sceptrum Bur. & K. Sch., Bignoniaceae .. 79
Erva-colégio
Elephantopus mollis H.B.K., Asteraceae 59

Erva-couvinha
Porophyllum ruderale (Jacq.) Cass., Asteraceae 64
Erva-da-costa
Kalanchoe brasiliensis Camb., Crassulaceae 133
Erva-da-vida
Heimia salicifolia
(H.B.K.) Link & Otto, Lythraceae 214
Erva-d'alho
Petiveria alliacea L., Phytolaccaceae 271
Erva-de-andorinha
Euphorbia caecorum Mart., Euphorbiaceae 152
Erva-de-anta
Citronella congonha (Mart.) Howard, Icacinaceae . 185
Erva-de-anta-com-espinho
Citronella mucronata
(R. & Pav.) Don, Icacinaceae 186
Erva-de-bicho
Cuphea melvilla Lindl., Lythraceae 214
Polygonum acuminatum H.B.K., Polygonaceae 286
Polygonum punctatum Elliot, Polygonaceae 287
Polygonum spectabile Mart., Polygonaceae 287
Erva-de-botão
Eclipta prostrata (L.) L., Asteraceae 59
Erva-de-charrua
Chromolaena hirsuta
(Hook. & Arn.) King & H. Robinson, Asteraceae ... 58
Erva-de-chumbo
Cassytha filiformis L., Lauraceae 198
Erva-de-cigana
Cremastus sceptrum Bur. & K. Sch., Bignoniaceae .. 79
Erva-de-cobra
Marsypianthes chamaedrys
(Vahl) O. Ktze., Lamiaceae 194
Mikania cordifolia (L. f.) Willd., Asteraceae 61
Erva-de-colégio
Elephantopus mollis H.B.K., Asteraceae 59
Erva-de-empigem
Xyris laxifolia Mart., Xyridaceae 342
Erva-de-gato
Clematis dioica L., Ranunculaceae 290
Erva-de-guiné
Petiveria alliacea L., Phytolaccaceae 271
Erva-de-jaboti
Peperomia pellucida H.B.K., Piperaceae 273
Piper aduncum L., Piperaceae 274
Erva-de-lagarto
Calea pinnatifida (R. Br.) Less., Asteraceae 57
Microgramma vaccinifolia
(Langsd. & Fisch.) Copel., Polypodiaceae 288
Stomatanthes oblongifolius
(Spr.) H. Robinson, Asteraceae 65
Tournefortia laevigata Lam., Boraginaceae 89
Erva-de-leite
Euphorbia hyssopifolia L., Euphorbiaceae 153
Erva-de-macaé
Leonurus sibiricus L., Lamiaceae 194
Erva-de-morcego
Macfadyena unguis-cati (L.) Gentry, Bignoniaceae . 81

Erva-de-mulher
Trixis antimenorrhoea (Schrank) Mart., Asteraceae . 67
Erva-de-nossa-senhora
Cissampelos glaberrima St.-Hil., Menispermaceae 233
Cissampelos pareira L., Menispermaceae 233
Erva-de-paracari
Marsypianthes chamaedrys
(Vahl) O. Ktze., Lamiaceae 194
Erva-de-parida
Declieuxia aristolochia M. Arg., Rubiaceae 297
Erva-de-passarinho
Phoradendron crassifolium
(Pohl) Eichl., Loranthaceae 211
Phthirusa adunca (Meyer) Maguire, Loranthaceae 211
Struthanthus marginatus
(Desf.) Bl., Loranthaceae 213
Erva-de-passarinho-de-folha-grande
Phoradendron crassifolium
(Pohl) Eichl., Loranthaceae 211
Erva-de-pinto
Alternanthera achyrantha R. Br., Amaranthaceae 3
Erva-de-rato
Caesalpinia microphylla Mart., Caesalpiniaceae ... 100
Erva-de-sangue
Cuphea balsamona Cham., Lythraceae 213
Erva-de-santa-luzia
Commelina sulcata Willd., Commelinaceae 128
Commelina virginica L., Commelinaceae 128
Euphorbia caecorum Mart., Euphorbiaceae 152
Euphorbia hirta L., Euphorbiaceae 152
Euphorbia hyssopifolia L., Euphorbiaceae 153
Euphorbia thymifolia L., Euphorbiaceae 153
Erva-de-santa-maria
Chenopodium ambrosioides L., Chenopodiaceae ... 118
Dracontium polyphyllum L., Araceae 36
Erva-de-santo-antônio
Baccharidastrum triplinerve
(Less.) Cabr., Asteraceae 53
Erva-de-são martinho
Sauvagesia erecta L., Ochnaceae 262
Erva-de-são-caetano
Momordica charantia L., Cucurbitaceae 139
Erva-de-são-domingos
Macfadyena unguis-cati (L.) Gentry, Bignoniaceae . 81
Erva-de-são-joão
Ageratum conyzoides L., Asteraceae 53
Erva-de-sapo
Begonia acida Mart., Begoniaceae 75
Begonia hirtella Link, Begoniaceae 76
Mikania cordifolia (L. f.) Willd., Asteraceae 61
Erva-de-saracura
Begonia acida Mart., Begoniaceae 75
Begonia hirtella Link, Begoniaceae 76
Erva-de-soldado
Hedyosmum brasiliense Mart., Chloranthaceae 119
Peperomia elongata Miq., Piperaceae 273
Piper angustifolium R. & Pav., Piperaceae 274
Piper elongatum Vahl, Piperaceae 275
Erva-de-teiú
Casearia sylvestris Sw., Flacourtiaceae 178

Erva-de-veado
Dodonaea viscosa Jacq., Sapindaceae 305
Erva-de-vidro
Peperomia transparens Miq., Piperaceae 274
Erva-do-brejo
Alisma palaefolium Kunth, Alismataceae 2
Echinodorus grandiflorus
(Cham. & Schl.) Mich., Alismataceae 2
Echinodorus macrophyllus
(Kunth) Mich., Alismataceae 2
Erva-do-diabo
Plumbago scandens L., Plumbaginaceae 279
Erva-do-pântano
Alisma palaefolium Kunth, Alismataceae 2
Echinodorus grandiflorus
(Cham. & Schl.) Mich., Alismataceae 2
Echinodorus macrophyllus
(Kunth) Mich., Alismataceae 2
Erva-do-santo-filho
Leonurus sibiricus L., Lamiaceae 194
Erva-dos-feridos
Canna gigantea Desf., Cannaceae 110
Canna glauca L., Cannaceae 110
Erva-dos-zangões
Leonurus sibiricus L., Lamiaceae 194
Erva-dutra
Mikania hirsutissima DC., Asteraceae 62
Erva-ferro
Heliotropium elongatum Willd., Boraginaceae 88
Erva-formiga
Heterothalamus psiadioides Less., Asteraceae 60
Erva-galega
Evolvulus holosericeus H.B.K., Convolvulaceae 130
Erva-gorda
Pilea microphylla (L.) Liebm., Urticaceae 331
Erva-grossa
Elephantopus mollis H.B.K., Asteraceae 59
Erva-jararaca
Dracontium asperum K. Koch, Araceae 35
Erva-lanceta
Conyza blakei (Cabr.) Cabr., Asteraceae 58
Senecio brasiliensis Less., Asteraceae 65
Solidago chilensis Meyen, Asteraceae 65
Erva-lombrigueira
Spigelia anthelmia L., Loganiaceae 209
Spigelia glabrata Mart., Loganiaceae 209
Erva-macaé
Leonurus sibiricus L., Lamiaceae 194
Erva-mate
Ilex brevicuspis Reiss., Aquifoliaceae 31
Ilex paraguariensis St.-Hil., Aquifoliaceae 31
Erva-mijona
Acanthospermum australe
(Loefl.) O. Ktze., Asteraceae 51
Commelina virginica L., Commelinaceae 128
Microtea debilis Sw., Phytolaccaceae 271
Erva-mineira
Acanthospermum australe
(Loefl.) O. Ktze., Asteraceae 51

Erva-mole
 Gomphrena mollis Mart., Amaranthaceae 4
Erva-mole-falsa
 Gomphrena mollis Mart., Amaranthaceae 4
Erva-moura
 Solanum nigrum L., Solanaceae 321
Erva-moura-do-peru
 Physalis pubescens L., Solanaceae 318
Erva-moura-do-sertão
 Cinnamodendron axillare
  (Nees & Mart.) Endl., Canellaceae 110
Erva-picão
 Bidens pilosa L., Asteraceae 57
Erva-pipi
 Petiveria alliacea L., Phytolaccaceae 271
Erva-pombinha
 Phyllanthus acutifolius Spreng., Euphorbiaceae 156
 Phyllanthus diffusus Klotz., Euphorbiaceae 156
 Phyllanthus niruri L., Euphorbiaceae 156
 Phyllanthus tenellus Roxb., Euphorbiaceae 157
Erva-preá
 Blanchetia heterotricha DC., Asteraceae 57
 Cyrtocymura scorpioides (Lam.)
  H. Robinson, Asteraceae 59
 Vernonanthura brasiliana (L.)
  H. Robinson, Asteraceae 67
Erva-purgante
 Jatropha gossypiifolia L., Euphorbiaceae 154
Erva-santa
 Baccharidastrum triplinerve
  (Less.) Cabr., Asteraceae 53
 Echites peltata Vell., Apocynaceae 23
 Mollinedia schottiana (Spr.) Perk., Monimiaceae .. 245
 Siparuna guianensis Aubl., Monimiaceae 245
 Stachytarpheta elatior Schrad., Verbenaceae 336
Erva-silveira
 Microgramma vaccinifolia
  (Langsd. & Fisch.) Copel., Polypodiaceae 288
Erva-silvina
 Microgramma vaccinifolia
  (Langsd. & Fisch.) Copel., Polypodiaceae 288
Erva-teresa
 Microgramma vaccinifolia
  (Langsd. & Fisch.) Copel., Polypodiaceae 288
Erva-tostão
 Boerhavia coccinea Mill., Nyctaginaceae 257
 Boerhavia hirsuta, Nyctaginaceae under Uses:
  Acanthospermum hispidum DC., Asteraceae 52
 Boerhavia paniculata Rich., Nyctaginaceae 258
Erva-tostão-de-minas
 Boerhavia erecta L., Nyctaginaceae 258
Erva-venenosa
 Dipladenia illustris M. Arg., Apocynaceae 23
Ervanço
 Alternanthera brasiliana
  (L.) O. Ktze., Amaranthaceae 3
Ervinha-de-parida
 Declieuxia aristolochia M. Arg., Rubiaceae 297
Escada-de-jabuti
 Bauhinia guianensis Aubl., Caesalpiniaceae 99

Bauhinia rutilans Spr. ex Benth., Caesalpiniaceae ... 99
Esfola-bainha
 Xylopia aromatica (Lam.) Mart., Annonaceae 15
Espadana
 Typha domingensis Pers., Typhaceae 328
Espelina-falsa
 Clitoria guianensis (Aubl.) Benth., Fabaceae 163
Esperta
 Peschiera laeta (Mart.) Miers, Apocynaceae 27
Espiga-da-terra
 Lophophytum mirabile
  Schott & Endl., Balanophoraceae 73
Espiga-de-ouro
 Solidago chilensis Meyen, Asteraceae 65
Espiga-de-sangue
 Helosis cayennensis
  (Swartz) Spreng., Balanophoraceae 73
Espinheira
 Mimosa bimucronata (DC.) O. Ktze., Mimosaceae 238
Espinheira-santa
 Maytenus ilicifolia Mart., Celastraceae 115
Espinheiro
 Mimosa hostilis Benth., Mimosaceae 238
 Zanthoxylum pterota H.B.K., Rutaceae 303
Espinheiro-amarelo
 Maclura brasiliensis Endl., Moraceae 249
Espinheiro-branco
 Maclura brasiliensis Endl., Moraceae 249
Espinheiro-bravo
 Maclura brasiliensis Endl., Moraceae 249
Espinheiro-de-cerca
 Mimosa bimucronata (DC.) O. Ktze., Mimosaceae 238
Espinheiro-preto
 Mimosa hostilis Benth., Mimosaceae 238
Espinho-branco
 Maclura tinctoria (L.) D. Don, Moraceae 249
Espinho-de-agulha
 Acanthospermum australe
  (Loefl.) O. Ktze., Asteraceae 51
Espinho-de-carneiro
 Xanthium orientale L., *X. spinosum* L.
  and *X. strumarium* L., Asteraceae 68
Espinho-de-cerca
 Mimosa bimucronata (DC.) O. Ktze., Mimosaceae 238
 Mimosa malacocentra Mart., Mimosaceae 239
Espinho-de-deus
 Maytenus ilicifolia Mart., Celastraceae 115
Espinho-de-maricá
 Mimosa bimucronata (DC.) O. Ktze., Mimosaceae 238
Espinho-de-são-joão
 Berberis laurina Thunb., Berberidaceae 76
Espinho-de-touro
 Scutia buxifolia Reiss., Rhamnaceae 293
Espinho-de-vintém
 Zanthoxylum rhoifolium Lam., Rutaceae 303
Espinho-decarneiro
 Acanthospermum australe
  (Loefl.) O. Ktze., Asteraceae 51

Espinho-roxo
  Mimosa bimucronata (DC.) O. Ktze., Mimosaceae 238
  Piptadenia polyptera Benth., Mimosaceae 242
Esponja-de-raiz
  Scybalium fungiforme
    Schott & Endl., Balanophoraceae 74
Espora-de-galo
  Pisonia aculeata L., Nyctaginaceae 258
Esporão-de-galo-falso
  Acnistus arborescens (L.) Schl., Solanaceae 316
Estopeira
  Cariniana legalis (Mart.) O. Ktze., Lecythidaceae . 205
Estoraque
  Pluchea suaveolens (Vell.) O. Ktze., Asteraceae 64
Estramônio
  Datura stramonium L., Solanaceae 318
Estrela
  Leonurus sibiricus L., Lamiaceae 194

F

Facheiro
  Cereus jamacaru DC., Cactaceae 95
Falsa-ipeca
  Ruellia tuberosa L., Acanthaceae 1
Falsa-quina
  Strychnos pseudoquina St.-Hil., Loganiaceae 209
Falsa-tiririca
  Hypoxis decumbens L., Hypoxidaceae 185
False poaias
  Uses: *Ionidium poaya* St.-Hil., Violaceae 339
Falso-boldo
  Coleus barbatus Benth., Lamiaceae 191
Falso-café
  Tachia guianensis Aubl., Gentianaceae 181
Falso-guaco
  Mikania periplocifolia Hook. & Arn., Asteraceae 62
Falso-jaborandi
  Ottonia corcovadensis Miq., Piperaceae 272
Falso-mate
  Citronella congonha (Mart.) Howard, Icacinaceae . 185
Farinha-seca
  Cybianthus detergens Mart., Myrsinaceae 253
Fava-café
  Mucuna pruriens (L.) DC., Fabaceae 169
Fava-de-santo-inácio-falsa
  Fevillea trilobata L., Cucurbitaceae 136
Fava-de-empingem
  Vatairea guianensis Aubl., Fabaceae 172
Fava-tonca
  Dipteryx odorata (Aubl.) Willd., Fabaceae 166
Faveira
  Vatairea guianensis Aubl., Fabaceae 172
Faveira-amarela
  Vatairea guianensis Aubl., Fabaceae 172
Faveiro
  Pterodon pubescens Benth., Fabaceae 171
Faxina-vermelha
  Dodonaea viscosa Jacq., Sapindaceae 305

Fazendaeiro
  Galinsoga parviflora Cav., Asteraceae 60
Fedegoso
  Heliotropium indicum L., Boraginaceae 89
  Senna alata (L.) Roxb., Caesalpiniaceae 104
  Senna corymbosa
    (Lam.) Ir. & Barn., Caesalpiniaceae 104
  Senna latifolia
    (Meyer) Ir. & Barn., Caesalpiniaceae 105
  Senna leiophylla
    (Vog.) Ir. & Barn., Caesalpiniaceae 105
  Senna oblongifolia
    (Vog.) Ir. & Barn., Caesalpiniaceae 105
  Senna occidentalis (L.) Link, Caesalpiniaceae 105
Fedegoso-de-folha-torta
  Senna corymbosa
    (Lam.) Ir. & Barn., Caesalpiniaceae 104
Fedegoso-do-mato
  Heliotropium elongatum Willd., Boraginaceae 88
  Senna hirsuta (L.) Ir. & Barn.
    var. *puberula* Ir. & Barn., Caesalpiniaceae 105
Fedegoso-do-pará
  Senna uniflora (P. Miller)
    Ir. & Barn., Caesalpiniaceae 106
Fedegoso-dormideira
  Chamaecrista fasciculata
    (Michx.) Greene, Caesalpiniaceae 102
Fedegoso-grande
  Senna quinqueangulata
    (Rich.) Ir. & Barn., Caesalpiniaceae 106
Fedegoso-legítimo
  Senna affinis
    (Benth.) Ir. & Barn., Caesalpiniaceae 104
Fedorento
  Siparuna guianensis Aubl., Monimiaceae 245
Feijão
  Dipteryx alata Vog., Fabaceae 165
Feijão-bravo
  Erythrina fusca Lour., Fabaceae 166
  Galactia neesii DC., Fabaceae 168
Feijão-café
  Mucuna pruriens (L.) DC., Fabaceae 169
Feijão-coco
  Dipteryx alata Vog., Fabaceae 165
Feijão-da-praia
  Sophora tomentosa L., Fabaceae 172
Fel-da-terra
  Deianira erubescens
    Cham. & Schl., Gentianaceae 179
  Schultesia stenophylla Mart., Gentianaceae 180
  Scybalium fungiforme
    Schott & Endl., Balanophoraceae 74
  Tachia guianensis Aubl., Gentianaceae 181
Fel-de-gentio
  Cayaponia espelina (Manso) Cogn., also
    Cayaponia spp., Cucurbitaceae 135
Feto-águia
  Pteridium aquilinum
    (L.) Kuhn, Dennstaedtiaceae 144

Figo-do-inferno
Jatropha curcas L., Euphorbiaceae 154
Figueira
Brasilopuntia brasiliensis
(Willd.) Berg., Cactaceae 95
Figueira-brava
Ficus maxima P. Mill., Moraceae 248
Figueira-de-lombrigueiro
Ficus maxima P. Mill., Moraceae 248
Figueira-do-inferno
Datura stramonium L., Solanaceae 318
Figueira-do-mato
Ficus insipida Willd., Moraceae 248
Figueirinha
Dorstenia brasiliensis Lam., Moraceae 247
Fios-de-ovos
Cuscuta racemosa Mart., Convolvulaceae 130
Flecha-de-urubu
Cyperus ligularis L., Cyperaceae 142
Flexa
Gynerium parviflorum Nees, Poaceae 281
Flor-da-paixão
Passiflora alata Dryand., Passifloraceae 267
Passiflora amethystina Mikan, Passifloraceae 269
Passiflora caerulea L., Passifloraceae 269
Passiflora edulis Sims, Passifloraceae 269
Passiflora mucronata Lam., Passifloraceae 270
Flor-das-almas
Senecio brasiliensis Less., Asteraceae 65
Flor-das-lavadeiras
Commelina virginica L., Commelinaceae 128
Flor-de-babado
Dipladenia illustris M. Arg., Apocynaceae 23
Macrosiphonia longiflora
(Desf.) M. Arg., Apocynaceae 26
Macrosiphonia velame
(St.-Hil.) M. Arg., Apocynaceae 26
Flor-de-coral
Erythrina corallodendron L., Fabaceae 166
Erythrina crista-galli L., Fabaceae 166
Jatropha multifida L., Euphorbiaceae 154
Flor-de-onze-horas
Portulaca grandiflora Hook., Portulacaceae 289
Flor-de-pérolas
Torrubia olfersiana
(Link, Klotzsch & Otto) Standl., Nyctaginaceae ... 258
Flor-de-santa-cruz
Declieuxia cordigera Mart. & Zucc., Rubiaceae 297
Flor-de-sapo
Holostylis reniformis Duch., Aristolochiaceae ... 50
Flor-de-seda
Calotropis procera (Ait.) Ait. f., Asclepiadaceae 50
Folha-cheirosa
Anthurium oxycarpum Poepp., Araceae 33
Folha-da-costa
Kalanchoe brasiliensis Camb., Crassulaceae 133
Kalanchoe pinnata (Lam.) Pers., Crassulaceae 133
Folha-da-fonte
Philodendron bipinnatifidum Schott, Araceae 36

Philodendron hederaceum (Jacq.) Schott
var. *hederaceum*, Araceae 36
Folha-da-fortuna
Kalanchoe brasiliensis Camb., Crassulaceae 133
Kalanchoe pinnata (Lam.) Pers., Crassulaceae 133
Folha-de-lixa
Davilla rugosa Poir., Dilleniaceae 145
Folha-de-louro
Plumbago scandens L., Plumbaginaceae 279
Folha-de-santana
Boehmeria caudata Sw., Urticaceae 330
Folha-de-uruba
Philodendron pedatum (Hook.) Kunth, Araceae 37
Folha-furada
Monstera adansonii Schott, Araceae 36
Folha-gorda
Pilea microphylla (L.) Liebm., Urticaceae 331
Folha-grossa
Kalanchoe brasiliensis Camb., Crassulaceae 133
Folha-preciosa
Aniba canelilla (H.B.K.) Mez, Lauraceae 197
Folha-rota
Monstera adansonii Schott, Araceae 36
Monstera obliqua Miquel, Araceae 36
Folha-santa
Echites macrocalyx M. Arg., Apocynaceae 23
Kielmeyera coriacea Mart., Clusiaceae 122
Kielmeyera speciosa St.-Hil., Clusiaceae 123
Formigueira
Triplaris noli-tangere Wedd., Polygonaceae 287
Forno-do-jacaré
Victoria amazonica
(Poepp.) Sower., Nymphaeaceae 260
Forquilha
Euphorbia tirucalli L., Euphorbiaceae 153
Fruta-de-arara
Joannesia princeps Vell., Euphorbiaceae 155
Fruta-de-conde
Annona squamosa L., Annonaceae 13
Fruta-de-conde pequena
Rollinia exalbida (Vell.) Mart., Annonaceae 15
Fruta-de-condessa
Annona reticulata L., Annonaceae 13
Fruta-de-cotia
Carpotroche brasiliensis
(Raddi) Endl., Flacourtiaceae 176
Carpotroche longifolia Benth., Flacourtiaceae 176
Fruta-de-gentio
Cayaponia pilosa Cogn., also
Cayaponia spp., Cucurbitaceae 135
Fruta-de-guará
Solanum mauritianum Scop., Solanaceae 321
Fruta-de-lobo
Solanum grandiflorum Ruiz & Pav., Solanaceae ... 320
Solanum lycocarpum St.-Hil., Solanaceae 321
Solanum mauritianum Scop., Solanaceae 321
Solanum verbascifolium L., Solanaceae 322
Fruta-de-morcego
Piper geniculatum Sw., Piperaceae 275

Fruta-de-perdiz
  Margyricarpus setosus Ruiz & Pav., Rosaceae 294
Fruta-de-pomba
  Erythroxylum anguifugum Mart., Erythroxylaceae . 148
Fruta-de-sabiá
  Acnistus arborescens (L.) Schl., Solanaceae 316
  Schinus terebinthifolius Raddi, Anacardiaceae 10
Fruta-de-tatu
  Eugenia supra-axillaris Spring, Myrtaceae 254
Fruta-de-tucano
  Erythroxylum campestre St.-Hil., Erythroxylaceae . 149
Fruto de imbé
  Philodendron sellowum Koch, Araceae 37
Fruto-de-babado
  Carpotroche brasiliensis
  (Raddi) Endl., Flacourtiaceae 176
Fruto-de-macaco
  Carpotroche brasiliensis
  (Raddi) Endl., Flacourtiaceae 176
Fumo-bravo
  Chamissoa altissima H.B.K., Amaranthaceae 4
  Chamissoa macrocarpa H.B.K., Amaranthaceae 4
  Elephantopus mollis H.B.K., Asteraceae 59
  Solanum grandiflorum Ruiz & Pav., Solanaceae ... 320
  Solanum mauritianum Scop., Solanaceae 321
Fumo-bravo-do-ceará
  Chamissoa macrocarpa H.B.K., Amaranthaceae 4
Fumo-da-mata
  Elephantopus mollis H.B.K., Asteraceae 59
Funcho-brabo
  Solanum verbascifolium L., Solanaceae 322
Fura-capa
  Bidens pilosa L., Asteraceae 57

G

Gameleira
  Ficus gomelleira Kunth & Bouché, Moraceae 248
Gameleira-branca
  Ficus gomelleira Kunth & Bouché, Moraceae 248
  Ficus insipida Willd., Moraceae 248
Gameleira-roxa
  Ficus insipida Willd., Moraceae 248
  Ficus maxima P. Mill., Moraceae 248
Ganha-saia
  Centropogon cornutus (L.) Druce, Campanulaceae 109
  Hybanthus atropurpureus Taub., Violaceae 338
Gapuí
  Martinella obovata
  (H.B.K.) Bur. & K. Sch., Bignoniaceae 82
Gapuí-cipó
  Martinella obovata
  (H.B.K.) Bur. & K. Sch., Bignoniaceae 82
Garanhoto
  Jatropha elliptica (Pohl) M. Arg., Euphorbiaceae .. 154
Garapa
  Apuleia leiocarpa
  (Vog.) MacBride, Caesalpiniaceae 98

Garapuvira
  Patagonula americana L., Boraginaceae 89
Gema-de-ovo
  Apuleia leiocarpa
  (Vog.) MacBride, Caesalpiniaceae 98
  Raputia magnifica Engl., Rutaceae 302
Genciana
  Coutoubea spicata Aubl., Gentianaceae 179
Genciana-brasileira
  Calolisianthus pendulus
  (Mart.) Gilg, Gentianaceae 179
Genciana-da-terra
  Microcolea quadrangularis
  (Lam.) Gris., Gentianaceae 180
  Lisianthus spp., Gentianaceae 179
Genciana-do-brasil
  Calolisianthus pendulus
  (Mart.) Gilg, Gentianaceae 179
  Coutoubea spicata Aubl., Gentianaceae 179
Genciana-sem-folhas
  Leiphaimos aphylla (Jacq.) Gilg, Gentianaceae 180
Genipapo *(jenipapo)*
  Genipa americana L., Rubiaceae 298
Gentiana-da-terra
  Zygostigma australe
  (Cham. & Schl.) Gris., Gentianaceae 181
Gerimataia
  Vitex gardneriana Schauer, Verbenaceae 336
Gerimato
  Vitex gardneriana Schauer, Verbenaceae 336
Gerimum
  Cucurbita pepo L., Cucurbitaceae 136
Gervão
  Stachytarpheta dichotoma Vahl, Verbenaceae 336
Gervão-bastardo
  Bouchea laetevirens Schauer, Verbenaceae 334
Gervão-cheiroso
  Verbena erinoides Lam., Verbenaceae 336
Gervão-das-taperas
  Stachytarpheta cayennensis
  (Rich.) Vahl, Verbenaceae 336
Gervão-de-folha-grande
  Bouchea pseudogervao
  (St.-Hil.) Cham., Verbenaceae 334
Gervão-de-folha-larga
  Bouchea pseudogervao
  (St.-Hil.) Cham., Verbenaceae 334
Gervão-do-alagadiço
  Stachytarpheta elatior Schrad., Verbenaceae 336
Gervão-falso
  Bouchea laetevirens Schauer, Verbenaceae 334
  Bouchea pseudogervao
  (St.-Hil.) Cham., Verbenaceae 334
Gervão-roxo
  Stachytarpheta cayennensis
  (Rich.) Vahl, Verbenaceae 336
Gervão-verdadeiro
  Stachytarpheta jamaicensis
  (L.) Vahl, Verbenaceae 336

Gipico *(jipico)*
  Entada paranaguana B. Rodr., Mimosaceae 237
  Entada polyphylla Benth., Mimosaceae 237
Gipoca *(jipoca)*
  Entada paranaguana B. Rodr., Mimosaceae 237
  Entada polyphylla Benth., Mimosaceae 237
Gipooca *(jipooca)*
  Entada paranaguana B. Rodr., Mimosaceae 237
  Entada polyphylla Benth., Mimosaceae 237
Girassol-do-mato
  Grindelia buphthalmoides DC., Asteraceae 60
Gitó
  Guarea trichilioides L., Meliaceae 228
Goa powder
  Vataireopsis araroba (Aguiar) Ducke, Fabaceae 173
Goambu
  Bidens pilosa L., Asteraceae 57
Goiabeira
  Psidium guajava L., Myrtaceae 256
Goiabeira-brava
  Psidium arboreum Vell., Myrtaceae 256
Goiabeira-do-mato
  Psidium arboreum Vell., Myrtaceae 256
Goldenrod
  Solidago chilensis Meyen, Asteraceae 65
Golfo
  Nymphoides indica (L.) O. Ktze., Menyanthaceae . 235
  Nymphaea rudgeana G. Meyer, Nymphaeaceae 259
Goma-arábica
  Vochysia thyrsoidea Pohl, Vochysiaceae 340
Gomável
  Astronium fraxinifolium Schott, Anacardiaceae 9
Gomeira
  Vochysia thyrsoidea Pohl, Vochysiaceae 340
Gonçalo-alves
  Astronium fraxinifolium Schott, Anacardiaceae 9
Goraná-timbó
  Dahlstedtia pinnata (Benth.) Malme, Fabaceae 163
Gracuí
  Sweetia fruticosa Spreng., Fabaceae 172
Grama-da-terra
  Commelina nudiflora L., Commelinaceae 126
Graminha-de-araraquara
  Chloris distichophylla (Nees) Lag., Poaceae 280
Grão-de-cavalo
  Caryocar villosum (Aubl.) Pers., Caryocaraceae 114
Grão-de-galo
  Celtis iguanaea Sarg., Ulmaceae 330
  Cordia grandiflora DC., Boraginaceae 87
  Cordia insignis Cham., Boraginaceae 87
  Cordia magnolifolia Cham., Boraginaceae 87
  Peschiera laeta (Mart.) Miers, Apocynaceae 27
  Salpichroa origanifolia (Lam.) Thell., Solanaceae 319
Grão-de-galo-miúdo
  Celtis spinosissima Miq., Ulmaceae 330
Grão-de-porco
  Cordia grandiflora DC., Boraginaceae 87
Grãozinho-de-galo
  Celtis spinosissima Miq., Ulmaceae 330

Grapiá
  Apuleia leiocarpa
    (Vog.) MacBride, Caesalpiniaceae 98
Grapiapunha
  Apuleia leiocarpa
    (Vog.) MacBride, Caesalpiniaceae 98
Gravatá
  Bromelia antiacantha Bertol., Bromeliaceae 91
Gravatá-da-praia
  Bromelia antiacantha Bertol., Bromeliaceae 91
Gravatá-de-raposa
  Bromelia antiacantha Bertol., Bromeliaceae 91
Gravatá-do-mato
  Bromelia antiacantha Bertol., Bromeliaceae 91
Gravatá-falso
  Eryngium elegans Cham. & Schlecht., Apiaceae 19
Graviola
  Annona muricata L., Annonaceae 13
Groselha-da-américa
  Pereskia aculeata Mill., Cactaceae 97
Grumarim
  Esenbeckia febrifuga Juss., Rutaceae 301
Grumixaba
  Eugenia brasiliensis Lam., Myrtaceae 253
Grumixama
  Eugenia brasiliensis Lam., Myrtaceae 253
Guabiroba
  Blepharocalyx salicifolius
    (H.B.K.) Berg, Myrtaceae 253
  Campomanesia aurea Berg, Myrtaceae 253
Guabiroba-do-campo
  Campomanesia aurea Berg, Myrtaceae 253
Guabiroba-do-rio-grande-do-sul
  Blepharocalyx salicifolius
    (H.B.K.) Berg, Myrtaceae 253
Guaçatonga, Guaçatunga
  Calea pinnatifida (R. Br.) Less., Asteraceae 57
  Casearia cambessedesii Eichl., Flacourtiaceae 176
  Casearia inaequilatera Camb., Flacourtiaceae 178
  Casearia sylvestris Sw., Flacourtiaceae 178
Guaco
  Galphimia brasiliensis Juss., Malpighiaceae 220
  Mikania cordifolia (L. f.) Willd., Asteraceae 61
  Mikania glomerata Spreng., Asteraceae 61
  Mikania hirsutissima DC., Asteraceae 62
  Mikania parviflora (Aubl.) Karst., Asteraceae 62
  Mikania periplocifolia Hook. & Arn., Asteraceae ... 62
  Mikania setigera Schultz-Bip. ex Baker, Asteraceae 62
Guaco-bravo
  Aristolochia cordigera Willd., Aristolochiaceae 46
Guaco-da-serra
  Mikania officinalis Mart., Asteraceae 62
Guaco-de-quintal
  Mikania periplocifolia Hook. & Arn., Asteraceae ... 62
Guaco-verdadeiro
  Mikania periplocifolia Hook. & Arn., Asteraceae ... 62
Guacurí
  Scheelea phalerata
    (Mart. ex Spreng.) Burret, Arecaceae 45

Guagiru
  Arrabidaea chica (H.B.K.) Bur., Bignoniaceae 78
Guaicuru
  Borreria verbenoides Cham. & Schl., Rubiaceae ... 296
  Limonium brasiliense
    (Boiss.) O. Ktze., Plumbaginaceae 278
Guaipipocaíba
  Pithecellobium avaremotemo Mart., Mimosaceae .. 242
Guaiuvira
  Patagonula americana L., Boraginaceae 89
Guajabara
  Coccoloba laevis Casar., Polygonaceae 285
  Coccoloba marginata Benth., Polygonaceae 285
Guajaraí
  Zschokkea arborescens M. Arg., Apocynaceae 29
Guajeru
  Chrysobalanus icaco L., Chrysobalanaceae 119
Guajuriva
  Coccoloba marginata Benth., Polygonaceae 285
Guajuru
  Chrysobalanus icaco L., Chrysobalanaceae 119
Guajuvira
  Patagonula americana L., Boraginaceae 89
Guambé
  Philodendron selloum Koch, Araceae 37
Guanandi
  Calophyllum brasiliense Camb., Clusiaceae 120
  Symphonia globulifera L. f., Clusiaceae 123
Guanandi-cedro
  Calophyllum brasiliense Camb., Clusiaceae 120
Guandi
  Calophyllum brasiliense Camb., Clusiaceae 120
Guandi-carvalho
  Calophyllum brasiliense Camb., Clusiaceae 120
Guaparonga
  Marlierea tomentosa Camb., Myrtaceae 255
Guapeba
  Pouteria laurifolia Radlk., Sapotaceae 309
Guapebeira
  Pouteria laurifolia Radlk., Sapotaceae 309
Guapeva
  Fevillea trilobata L., Cucurbitaceae 136
Guapoí
  Protium icicariba (DC.) March., Burseraceae 94
Guaporanga
  Marlierea tomentosa Camb., Myrtaceae 255
Guapuí
  Clusia grandiflora Splitg., Clusiaceae 121
Guarabu
  Astronium fraxinifolium Schott, Anacardiaceae 9
Guaraiúva
  Patagonula americana L., Boraginaceae 89
Guarajuru-piranga
  Arrabidaea chica (H.B.K.) Bur., Bignoniaceae 78
Guaraná
  Paullinia cupana Kunth, Sapindaceae 306
Guarapiraca
  Anadenanthera macrocarpa
    (Benth.) Brenan, Mimosaceae 236

Guararema
  Agonandra brasiliensis Miers, Opiliaceae 265
  Gallesia gorazema (Vell.) Moq., Phytolaccaceae ... 271
Guardião
  Cayaponia tayuya (Mart.) Cogn., also
    Cayaponia spp., Cucurbitaceae 135
  Melothria fluminensis Gardn., Cucurbitaceae 139
Guaririnha
  Phlebodium decumanum
    (Willd.) J. Smith, Polypodiaceae 288
Guariroba
  Syagrus comosa Mart., Arecaceae 45
  Syagrus oleracea (Mart.) Becc., Arecaceae 45
  Syagrus pseudococos (Raddi) Glassman, Arecaceae 45
Guariroba-do-campo
  Syagrus comosa Mart., Arecaceae 45
Guaritá
  Zanthoxylum rhoifolium Lam., Rutaceae 303
Guariuba
  Clarisia racemosa Ruiz & Pav., Moraceae 247
Guarucaia
  Parapiptadenia rigida
    (Benth.) Brenan, Mimosaceae 240
Guaruga
  Galipea multiflora Schult., Rutaceae 301
Guava
  Psidium guajava L., Myrtaceae 256
Guaxima
  Helicteres ovata Lam., Sterculiaceae 324
  Sida micrantha St.-Hil., Malvaceae 222
  Sida rhombea L., Malvaceae 222
Guaxima-roxa
  Urena lobata L., Malvaceae 223
Guaximinga
  Galipea multiflora Schult., Rutaceae 301
Guaxinduba-preta
  Ficus maxima P. Mill., Moraceae 248
Guaxuma
  Sida acuta Burm., Malvaceae 221
  Sida rhombea L., Malvaceae 222
  Sida rhombifolia L., Malvaceae 222
  Triumfetta semitriloba Jacq., Tiliaceae 327
Guembé
  Philodendron pedatum (Hook.) Kunth, Araceae 37
Guimbê
  Philodendron bipinnatifidum Schott, Araceae 36
Guimberana
  Philodendron hederaceum
    (Jacq.) Schott var. *hederaceum*, Araceae 36
Guiné
  Petiveria alliacea L., Phytolaccaceae 271
Guitó
  Sapindus saponaria L., Sapindaceae 306
Guriri-do-campo
  Allagoptera campestris (Mart.) Kuntze, Arecaceae .. 39

H

Hamuí
  Ocotea cymbarum H.B.K., Lauraceae 200

Hortelã-brava
Hyptis atrorubens Poit., Lamiaceae 192
Hortelã-de-folha-miúda
Mentha crispa L., Lamiaceae 195
Hortelã-de-panela
Mentha crispa L., Lamiaceae 195
Hortelã-do-brasil
Marsypianthes chamaedrys
(Vahl) O. Ktze., Lamiaceae 194
Hortelã-do-brejo
Hedyosmum brasiliense Mart., Chloranthaceae 119
Hortelã-do-campo
Marsypianthes chamaedrys
(Vahl) O. Ktze., Lamiaceae 194
Peltodon longipes St.-Hil., Lamiaceae 195
Hortelã-do-mato
Peltodon radicans Pohl, Lamiaceae 195
Hortelã-rasteira
Mentha crispa L., Lamiaceae 195
Hortênsia
Calotropis procera (Ait.) Ait. f., Asclepiadaceae 50

I

Iagê
Banisteriopsis caapi (Spr.) Morton, Malpighiaceae 217
Iapana
Ayapana triplinerve
(Vahl) King & H. Robinson, Asteraceae 53
Iará-açu
Leopoldinia major Wallace, Arecaceae 43
Ibaporoiti
Eugenia brasiliensis Lam., Myrtaceae 253
Ibatimó
Stryphnodendron adstringens
(Mart.) Cov., Mimosaceae 242
Ibipitanga
Eugenia uniflora L., Myrtaceae 255
Ibirapitanga
Caesalpinia echinata Lam., Caesalpiniaceae 100
Ibirarema
Seguieria americana L., Phytolaccaceae 272
Ibirataí
Pilocarpus pinnatifolius Lem., Rutaceae 302
Ibita-obi
Caesalpinia ferrea Mart. ex Tul., Caesalpiniaceae . 100
Ieuri-cumajé
Anthurium oxycarpum Poepp., Araceae 33
Imbé
Philodendron imbe Schott, Araceae 36
Imbê
Monstera adansonii Schott, Araceae 36
Philodendron bipinnatifidum Schott, Araceae 36
Imbé-de-comer
Philodendron selloum Koch, Araceae 37
Imbê-furado
Monstera adansonii Schott, Araceae 36
Imbê-miúdo
Philodendron ochrostemon Schott, Araceae 37

Imbê-são-pedro
Monstera adansonii Schott, Araceae 36
Imbiri
Canna glauca L., Cannaceae 110
Imburana
Torresea cearensis Fr. All., Fabaceae 172
Imburana-de-cheiro
Torresea cearensis Fr. All., Fabaceae 172
Imburi
Allagoptera campestris (Mart.) Kuntze, Arecaceae .. 39
Indigo
Indigofera suffruticosa Mill., Fabaceae 168
Infalível
Alternanthera brasiliana
(L.) O. Ktze., Amaranthaceae 3
Piptocarpha rotundifolia (Less.) Bak., Asteraceae .. 64
Ingá-de-flor-amarela
Inga setigera DC., Mimosaceae 237
Ingá-xixi
Inga alba (Sw.) Willd., Mimosaceae 237
Inga lateriflora Miq., Mimosaceae 237
Inhambuquiçaua
Caraipa insidiosa B. Rodr., Clusiaceae 121
Inimbó
Caesalpinia bonduc (L.) Roxb., Caesalpiniaceae 99
Inimboja
Caesalpinia bonduc (L.) Roxb., Caesalpiniaceae 99
Invirataí
Duguetia riparia Hub., Annonaceae 14
Ipadu
Erythroxylum coca Lam., Erythroxylaceae 150
Ipadu-mirim
Erythroxylum cataractarum
Spruce, Erythroxylaceae 149
Ipê
Tabebuia chrysotricha
(Mart.) Standl., Bignoniaceae 82
Tabebuia serratifolia (Vahl) Nichol., Bignoniaceae .. 83
Ipê-açu
Tabebuia leucoxylon (L.) DC., Bignoniaceae 83
Ipê-amarelo
Tabebuia chrysotricha
(Mart.) Standl., Bignoniaceae 82
Tabebuia serratifolia (Vahl) Nichol., Bignoniaceae .. 83
Tabebuia umbellata (Sond.) Sandw., Bignoniaceae .. 83
Ipê-batata
Sparattosperma leucanthum
(Vell.) K. Sch., Bignoniaceae 82
Ipê-branco
Patagonula americana L., Boraginaceae 89
Sparattosperma leucanthum
(Vell.) K. Sch., Bignoniaceae 82
Ipê-caboclo
Tabebuia leucoxylon (L.) DC., Bignoniaceae 83
Ipê-contra-sarna
Tabebuia impetiginosa
(Mart.) Standl., Bignoniaceae 83
Ipê-da-várzea
Cybistax antisyphilitica (Mart.)
Mart., Bignoniaceae 80

Ipê-de-flor-verde
 Cybistax antisyphilitica (Mart.)
   Mart., Bignoniaceae 80
Ipê-do-brejo
 Tabebuia chrysotricha (Mart.)
   Standl., Bignoniaceae 82
 Tabebuia umbellata (Sond.) Sandw., Bignoniaceae .. 83
Ipê-do-campo
 Tabebuia serratifolia (Vahl) Nichol., Bignoniaceae .. 83
Ipê-falso
 Senna macranthera
   (Collad.) Ir. & Barn., Caesalpiniaceae 105
Ipê-mirim
 Tabebuia ipe (Mart.) Standl., Bignoniaceae 83
Ipê-preto
 Tabebuia ipe (Mart.) Standl., Bignoniaceae 83
Ipê-rosa
 Tabebuia ipe (Mart.) Standl., Bignoniaceae 83
Ipê-roxo
 Tabebuia impetiginosa
   (Mart.) Standl., Bignoniaceae 83
 Tabebuia ipe (Mart.) Standl., Bignoniaceae 83
Ipê-tabaco
 Tabebuia chrysotricha
   (Mart.) Standl., Bignoniaceae 82
 Tabebuia ipe (Mart.) Standl., Bignoniaceae 83
 Tabebuia leucoxylon (L.) DC., Bignoniaceae 83
Ipê-verde
 Cybistax antisyphilitica
   (Mart.) Mart., Bignoniaceae 80
Ipeca
 Cephaelis ipecacuanha Rich., Rubiaceae 296
Ipecac *(poaia)*
 Cephaelis ipecacuanha Rich., Rubiaceae 296
Ipecacuanha
 Cephaelis ipecacuanha Rich., Rubiaceae 296
   also under Uses: *Ionidium poaya*
   St.-Hil., Violaceae 339
 Corynostylis hybanthus
   (L.) Mart. & Zucc., Violaceae 338
 Polygala angulata DC., Polygalaceae 283
Ipecacuanha-branca
 Hybanthus ipecacuanha (L.) Baill., Violaceae 339
Ipecacuanha-de-flor-roxa
 Ruellia geminiflora H.B.K., Acanthaceae 1
Ipecacuanha-falsa
 Boerhavia coccinea Mill., Nyctaginaceae 257
Ipês-boia
 Sparattosperma leucanthum
   (Vell.) K. Sch., Bignoniaceae 82
Ipeúva
 Tabebuia ipe (Mart.) Standl., Bignoniaceae 83
 Tabebuia serratifolia (Vahl) Nichol., Bignoniaceae .. 83
Iride-branca
 Clematis campestris St.-Hil., Ranunculaceae 290
Irurapia
 Celtis iguanaea Sarg., Ulmaceae 330
Itabocaba
 Allamanda doniana M. Arg., Apocynaceae 20

Itapicuru
 Callisthene major Mart., Vochysiaceae 340
Itapiúva
 Callisthene major Mart., Vochysiaceae 340
Itaúba-camará
 Licaria camara (Schomb.) Kosterm., Lauraceae 199
Ituá
 Matayba purgans Radlk., Sapindaceae 306
Iuçara
 Euterpe edulis Mart., Arecaceae 41
Ivitinga
 Luehea rufescens St.-Hil., Tiliaceae 327

J

Jaborandi
 Ottonia corcovadensis Miq., Piperaceae 272
 Pilocarpus pinnatifolius Lem., Rutaceae 302
 Piper eucalyptifolium (Miq.) Rudge, Piperaceae 275
Jaborandi-da-mata-virgem
 Ottonia jaborandi (Vell.) Kunth, Piperaceae 272
Jaborandi-de-três-folhas
 Monnieria trifolia Loefl., Rutaceae 302
Jaborandi-do-mato
 Ottonia jaborandi (Vell.) Kunth, Piperaceae 272
 Piper aduncum L., Piperaceae 274
Jaborandi-do-norte
 Pilocarpus pinnatifolius Lem., Rutaceae 302
Jaborandi-do-pará
 Monnieria trifolia Loefl., Rutaceae 302
Jaborandi-do-rio
 Piper geniculatum Sw., Piperaceae 275
Jaborandi-falso
 Piper ceanothifolium H.B.K., Piperaceae 275
 Piper geniculatum Sw., Piperaceae 275
 Piper reticulatum L., Piperaceae 276
Jaborandi-manso
 Piper colubrinum Link, Piperaceae 275
 Piper mollicomum Kunth, Piperaceae 276
Jabotapitá
 Ouratea guianensis Aubl., Ochnaceae 261
 Ouratea jabotapita Engl., Ochnaceae 261
 Ouratea parviflora (DC.) Baill., Ochnaceae 261
Jabuticaba-de-cipó
 Chondodendron platyphyllum
   (Mart.) Miers, Menispermaceae 231
Jacamim-renepeá
 Alsodeia flavescens (Aubl.) Spreng., Violaceae 338
Jaçapé
 Cyperus sesquiflorus
   (Torrey) Mattf. & Kükent., Cyperaceae 142
Jacará-mirim
 Callisthene major Mart., Vochysiaceae 340
Jacarandá
 Jacaranda brasiliana (Lam.) Pers., Bignoniaceae ... 80
Jacarandá-caroba
 Jacaranda mimosifolia D. Don, Bignoniaceae 81
Jacarandá-mimoso
 Jacaranda mimosifolia D. Don, Bignoniaceae 81

Jacarandá-preto
Jacaranda brasiliana (Lam.) Pers., Bignoniaceae ... 80
Jacaratiá
Jacaratia spinosa (Aubl.) A. DC., Caricaceae 113
Jacaré-açu
Tachia guianensis Aubl., Gentianaceae 181
Jacaré-aru
Tachia guianensis Aubl., Gentianaceae 181
Jacaré-do-mato
Cybianthus detergens Mart., Myrsinaceae 253
Jacareúba
Calophyllum brasiliense Camb., Clusiaceae 120
Jacitara
Desmoncus orthacanthos Mart., Arecaceae 40
Desmoncus polyacanthos Mart., Arecaceae 40
Jacuacanga
Costus spicatus (Jacq.) Sw., also
Costus spiralis (Jacq.) Roscoe, Costaceae 132
Jacuruaru
Tachia guianensis Aubl., Gentianaceae 181
Jaguara-muru
Cordia magnolifolia Cham., Boraginaceae 87
Jalapa
Ipomoea pes-caprae (L.) R. Br., Chem. & Pharm.,
re: *Ipomoea* spp., Convolvulaceae 130
Mandevilla velutina (Mart. ex Stadelm.) Woods.
var. *velutina*, Apocynaceae 27
Operculina alata (Ham.) Urb., Convolvulaceae 131
Operculina macrocarpa Urb., Convolvulaceae 131
Jalapa-vermelha
Dipladenia illustris M. Arg., Apocynaceae 23
Jalapão
Jatropha elliptica (Pohl) M. Arg., Euphorbiaceae .. 154
Jatropha gossypiifolia L., Euphorbiaceae 154
Jamacaru
Cereus jamacaru DC., Cactaceae 95
Jamaru
Lagenaria siceraria
(Molina) Standl., Cucurbitaceae 138
Jambu
Acmella repens (Walt.) L.C. Rich., Asteraceae 53
Janaguba
Himatanthus sucuuba (Spr.) Woods., Apocynaceae . 26
Janaúba
Himatanthus drastica
(Mart.) Woods., Apocynaceae 24
Japana
Ayapana triplinerve
(Vahl) King & H. Robinson, Asteraceae 53
Japana-branca
Ayapana triplinerve
(Vahl) King & H. Robinson, Asteraceae 53
Japecanga
Dioscorea basiclavicaulis
Rizz. & Mattos, Dioscoreaceae 146
Herreria salsaparilha Mart., Liliaceae 207
Smilax campestris Gris., Liliaceae 208
Japecanga-vermelha
Smilax longifolia Rich., Liliaceae 208

Japim-caá
Amasonia arborea H.B.K., Verbenaceae 333
Jará-açu
Leopoldinia major Wallace, Arecaceae 43
Jararaca
Dracontium asperum K. Koch, Araceae 35
Dracontium polyphyllum L., Araceae 36
Jararaca-mirim
Dracontium polyphyllum L., Araceae 36
Jararaca-taia
Dracontium asperum K. Koch, Araceae 35
Jararaca-tajá
Dracontium asperum K. Koch, Araceae 35
Jaraugaúba
Bomarea salsilloides Roem., Amaryllidaceae 6
Jarra-do-diabo
Aristolochia cymbifera
Mart. & Zucc., Aristolochiaceae 47
Jarrinha
Aristolochia birostris Duch., Aristolochiaceae 46
Aristolochia cymbifera
Mart. & Zucc., Aristolochiaceae 47
Aristolochia elegans Mast., Aristolochiaceae 48
Aristolochia esperanzae
O. Kuntze, Aristolochiaceae 48
Aristolochia trilobata L., Aristolochiaceae 48
Jarrinha-concha
Aristolochia triangularis Cham., Aristolochiaceae ... 48
Jarrinha-monstro
Aristolochia gigantea
Mart. & Zucc., Aristolochiaceae 48
Jarrinha-pintada
Aristolochia elegans Mast., Aristolochiaceae 48
Jarrinha-triangular
Aristolochia triangularis Cham., Aristolochiaceae ... 48
Jasmim-amarelo
Galphimia brasiliensis Juss., Malpighiaceae 220
Jasmim-azul
Plumbago scandens L., Plumbaginaceae 279
Jasmim-da-itália
Hippobroma longiflora
(L.) G. Don, Campanulaceae 109
Jasmim-da-mata
Tabernaemontana citrifolia L., Apocynaceae 28
Jasmim-de-cachorro
Hippobroma longiflora
(L.) G. Don, Campanulaceae 109
Jasmim-de-caiena
Himatanthus alba (L.) Woods., Apocynaceae 24
Plumeria alba L., Apocynaceae 28
Jasmim-de-leita
Plumeria alba L., Apocynaceae 28
Jasmim-de-leite
Himatanthus alba (L.) Woods., Apocynaceae 24
Peschiera laeta (Mart.) Miers, Apocynaceae 27
Jasmim-do-mato
Calea pinnatifida (R. Br.) Less., Asteraceae 57
Jasmim-do-pará
Himatanthus alba (L.) Woods., Apocynaceae 24

Plumeria alba L., Apocynaceae 28
Jasmim-manga
Himatanthus drastica
(Mart.) Woods., Apocynaceae 24
Jasmim-mango-falso
Himatanthus phagedaenica
(Mart.) Woods., Apocynaceae 26
Jasmin-de-cachorro
Peschiera laeta (Mart.) Miers, Apocynaceae 27
Jataí
Hymenaea courbaril L., Caesalpiniaceae 103
Jataíba
Guarea trichilioides L., Meliaceae 228
Jatobá
Apuleia leiocarpa
(Vog.) MacBride, Caesalpiniaceae 98
Fevillea uncipetala Kuhlm., Cucurbitaceae 138
Hymenaea courbaril L., Caesalpiniaceae 103
Jatobá-mirim
Copaifera officinalis (Jacq.) L., Caesalpiniaceae 102
Jauaricica
Protium heptaphyllum (Aubl.) March., Burseraceae 93
Jejerecu
Xylopia aromatica (Lam.) Mart., Annonaceae 15
Jenipá
Genipa americana L., Rubiaceae 298
Jenipapeirol
Genipa americana L., Rubiaceae 298
Jenipapinho
Conocarpus erecta L., Combretaceae 126
Jenipapo *(genipapo)*
Genipa americana L., Rubiaceae 298
Jeniparana
Gustavia hexapetala
(Aubl.) J.E. Smith, Lecythidaceae 205
Jequiriti
Abrus precatorius L., Fabaceae 160
Jequitá
Desmoncus orthacanthos Mart., Arecaceae 40
Jequitibá-branco
Cariniana legalis (Mart.) O. Ktze., Lecythidaceae . 205
Jequitibá-cedro
Cariniana legalis (Mart.) O. Ktze., Lecythidaceae . 205
Jequitibá-rosa
Cariniana legalis (Mart.) O. Ktze., Lecythidaceae . 205
Jererecu
Xylopia frutescens Aubl., Annonaceae 16
Jericó
Selaginella convoluta Spring, Selaginellaceae 313
Jerivá
Syagrus romanzoffiana
(Cham.) Glassman, Arecaceae 45
Jiçara
Euterpe edulis Mart., Arecaceae 41
Jinja
Eugenia uniflora L., Myrtaceae 255
Jipico *(gipico)*
Entada paranaguana B. Rodr., Mimosaceae 237
Entada polyphylla Benth., Mimosaceae 237

Jipoca *(gipoca)*
Entada paranaguana B. Rodr., Mimosaceae 237
Entada polyphylla Benth., Mimosaceae 237
Jipooca *(gipooca)*
Entada paranaguana B. Rodr., Mimosaceae 237
Entada polyphylla Benth., Mimosaceae 237
Jiquirioba
Solanum juciri Mart., Solanaceae 321
Jiraraca
Dracontium polyphyllum L., Araceae 36
Jitaí
Apuleia leiocarpa
(Vog.) MacBride, Caesalpiniaceae 98
Jitó
Guarea spiciflora Juss., Meliaceae 227
Guarea tuberculata Vell., Meliaceae 229
Trichilia cathartica Mart., Meliaceae 229
Joá-miúdo
Celtis iguanaea Sarg., Ulmaceae 330
João-da-costa
Echites peltata Vell., Apocynaceae 23
Joazeiro
Zizyphus joazeiro Mart., Rhamnaceae 293
Jorro-jorro
Thevetia ahouai (L.) DC., Apocynaceae 28
Juá
Solanum aculeatissimum Jacq., Solanaceae 319
Solanum ciliatum Lam., Solanaceae 319
Solanum juciri Mart., Solanaceae 321
Zizyphus joazeiro Mart., Rhamnaceae 293
Juá-bravo
Solanum insidiosum Mart., Solanaceae 320
Solanum mammosum L., Solanaceae 321
Juá-de-capote
Physalis angulata L., Solanaceae 318
Juá-poca
Physalis pubescens L., Solanaceae 318
Juá-vermelho
Solanum ciliatum Lam., Solanaceae 319
Juazeiro
Zizyphus joazeiro Mart., Rhamnaceae 293
Jubeba
Solanum paniculatum L., Solanaceae 321
Jucá
Caesalpinia ferrea Mart. ex Tul., Caesalpiniaceae . 100
Jucapê
Imperata brasiliensis Trin., Poaceae 281
Juçara
Euterpe edulis Mart., Arecaceae 41
Euterpe oleracea Mart., Arecaceae 42
Juciri
Solanum juciri Mart., Solanaceae 321
Jujuíra
Astronium fraxinifolium Schott, Anacardiaceae 9
Jumbeba
Brasilopuntia brasiliensis
(Willd.) Berg., Cactaceae 95
Pereskia bleo H.B.K., Cactaceae 97

Junça-miúda
Cyperus gracilescens
Roem. & Schult., Cyperaceae 142
Junco
Mariscus jacquinii H.B.K., Cyperaceae 143
Junco-miúdo
Cyperus gracilescens
Roem. & Schult., Cyperaceae 142
Jupati
Raphia taedigera (Mart.) Mart., Arecaceae 45
Jupicaí
Xyris laxifolia Mart., Xyridaceae 342
Jupicanga
Solanum variabile Mart., Solanaceae 322
Juqueri
Solanum juciri Mart., Solanaceae 321
Juqueri-grande
Machaerium ferox (Mart.) Ducke, Fabaceae 168
Juquiri
Mimosa pudica L., Mimosaceae 240
Juquirirana
Caesalpinia bonduc (L.) Roxb., Caesalpiniaceae 99
Jurema
Mimosa acutistipula Benth., Mimosaceae 237
Mimosa hostilis Benth., Mimosaceae 238
Mimosa malacocentra Mart., Mimosaceae 239
Mimosa verrucosa Benth., Mimosaceae 240
Jurema-preta
Mimosa acutistipula Benth., Mimosaceae 237
Mimosa hostilis Benth., Mimosaceae 238
Jureminha
Mimosa malacocentra Mart., Mimosaceae 239
Juripeba
Solanum paniculatum L., Solanaceae 321
Jurubeba
Pereskia bleo H.B.K., Cactaceae 97
Solanum paniculatum L., Solanaceae 321
Jurubeba-branca
Solanum albidum Dun., Solanaceae 319
Jurubeba-de-espinho
Solanum insidiosum Mart., Solanaceae 320
Jurubeba-do-pará
Solanum mammosum L., Solanaceae 321
Jurubeba-grande
Solanum grandiflorum Ruiz & Pav., Solanaceae ... 320
Jurubeba-verdadeira
Solanum paniculatum L., Solanaceae 321
Jurubebinha
Solanum paniculatum L., Solanaceae 321
Jurumbeba
Brasilopuntia brasiliensis (Willd.) Berg., Cactaceae 95
Jurutê
Cordia obscura Cham., Boraginaceae 88
Juta-nacional
Triumfetta semitriloba Jacq., Tiliaceae 327
Jutaí
Apuleia leiocarpa
(Vog.) MacBride, Caesalpiniaceae 98
Hymenaea courbaril L., Caesalpiniaceae 103

Jutaí-açu
Hymenaea courbaril L., Caesalpiniaceae 103
Juuna
Solanum paniculatum L., Solanaceae 321
Juva
Zanthoxylum rhoifolium Lam., Rutaceae 303
Juvena
Solanum paniculatum L., Solanaceae 321
Juvevê
Zanthoxylum rhoifolium Lam., Rutaceae 303

L

Labaça
Rumex brasiliensis Link, Polygonaceae 287
Lacrão
Vismia japurensis Reich., Clusiaceae 124
Lacre
Vismia acuminata (L.) Pers., Clusiaceae 123
Vismia guianensis (Aubl.) Choisy, Clusiaceae 124
Vismia latifolia (Aubl.) Choisy, Clusiaceae 124
Vismia reichardtiana (O. Ktze.) Ewan, Clusiaceae . 124
Lacre-branco
Miconia albicans (Sw.) Tr., Melastomataceae 225
Vismia guianensis (Aubl.) Choisy, Clusiaceae 124
Lágrima-de-nossa-senhora
Pithecellobium cochleatum
(Willd.) Mart., Mimosaceae 242
Landim
Calophyllum brasiliense Camb., Clusiaceae 120
Symphonia globulifera L. f., Clusiaceae 123
Typha domingensis Pers., Typhaceae 328
Laranja-brava
Esenbeckia febrifuga Juss., Rutaceae 301
Polygala klotzschii Chodat, Polygalaceae 284
Laranjeira-do-mato
Cordia coffeoides Warm., Boraginaceae 87
Cordia salicifolia Cham., Boraginaceae 88
Esenbeckia febrifuga Juss., Rutaceae 301
Metrodorea pubescens St.-Hil. & Tul., Rutaceae ... 301
Laranjeiro-da-terra
Esenbeckia febrifuga Juss., Rutaceae 301
Laranjinha
Polygala klotzschii Chodat, Polygalaceae 284
Zanthoxylum rhoifolium Lam., Rutaceae 303
Laranjinha-de-vaqueiro
Zizyphus joazeiro Mart., Rhamnaceae 293
Laranjinha-do-mato
Zanthoxylum tingoassuiba, Rutaceae 303
Lava-prato
Senna occidentalis (L.) Link, Caesalpiniaceae 105
Lava-pratos
Senna latifolia (Meyer)
Ir. & Barn., Caesalpiniaceae 105
Lavadeira
Leonurus sibiricus L., Lamiaceae 194
Leiteira
Brosimum potabile Ducke, Moraceae 246
Euphorbia cotinoides Miq., Euphorbiaceae 152

Peschiera affinis (M. Arg.) Miers, Apocynaceae 27
Lemon grass
Cymbopogon schoenanthus (L.) Spreng., Poaceae 280
Lençol-de-santa-bárbara
Pothomorphe umbellata (L.) Miq., Piperaceae 277
Lenha-branca
Maytenus obtusifolia Mart., Celastraceae 116
Lentilha-d'água
Lemna minor L., Lemnaceae 207
Lentilha-d'água-caparosa
Lemna minor L., Lemnaceae 207
Levantina
Leonurus sibiricus L., Lamiaceae 194
Licuri
Syagrus coronata (Mart.) Becc., Arecaceae 45
Licurizeiro
Syagrus coronata (Mart.) Becc., Arecaceae 45
Liga-liga
Dorstenia brasiliensis Lam., Moraceae 247
Liga-osso
Dorstenia brasiliensis Lam., Moraceae 247
Limão-bravo
Siparuna brasiliensis (Spr.) DC., Monimiaceae 245
Limão-do-mato
Cordia coffeoides Warm., Boraginaceae 87
Siparuna brasiliensis (Spr.) DC., Monimiaceae 245
Limãozinho
Maytenus obtusifolia Mart., Celastraceae 116
Polygala klotzschii Chodat, Polygalaceae 284
Siparuna brasiliensis (Spr.) DC., Monimiaceae 245
Zanthoxylum rhoifolium Lam., Rutaceae 303
Limoeiro-bravo
Siparuna cujabana (Mart.) DC., Monimiaceae 245
Limoeiro-do-campo
Styrax ferrugineum Nees & Mart., Styracaceae 325
Limoeiro-do-mato
Metrodorea pubescens St.-Hil. & Tul., Rutaceae ... 301
Limpa-viola
Clibadium rotundifolium DC., Asteraceae 58
Língua-de-araçari
Eryngium pristis Cham. & Schlecht., Apiaceae 19
Língua-de-sapo
Peperomia transparens Miq., Piperaceae 274
Língua-de-teiú
Casearia sylvestris Sw., Flacourtiaceae 178
Língua-de-tucano
Eryngium pristis Cham. & Schlecht., Apiaceae 19
Lingua-de-vaca
Chaptalia nutans (L.) Polak., Asteraceae 57
Elephantopus mollis H.B.K., Asteraceae 59
Lírio rajado
Crinum scabrum Sims, Amaryllidaceae 6
Lírio-do-brejo
Hedychium coronarium Koenig, Zingiberaceae 342
Lírio-folha-de-palmeira
Eleutherine plicata Herb., Iridaceae 186
Lírio-roxo-do-campo
Trimezia juncifolia Benth. & Hook., Iridaceae 186

Lixa-vegetal
Equisetum giganteum L., Equisetaceae 148
Lixeira
Curatella americana L., Dilleniaceae 144
Lobeira
Solanum grandiflorum Ruiz & Pav., Solanaceae ... 320
Solanum lycocarpum St.-Hil., Solanaceae 321
Lombrigueira
Ficus insipida Willd., Moraceae 248
Spigelia anthelmia L., Loganiaceae 209
Losna
Artemisia absinthium, see *Baccharis articulata*
 (Lam.) Pers., Asteraceae: USES 54
Losna-do-mato
Egletes viscosa (L.) Less., Asteraceae 59
Louco
Plumbago scandens L., Plumbaginaceae 279
Louro
Ocotea opifera Mart., Lauraceae 201
Ocotea teleiandra (Messn.) Mez, Lauraceae 203
Louro-abacate
Cryptocarya minima Mez, Lauraceae 198
Pleurothyrium cuneifolium Nees, Lauraceae 203
Louro-amarelo-de-cheiro
Aiovea meissneri Mez, Lauraceae 197
Louro-amargoso
Nectandra puberula Nees, Lauraceae 200
Louro-anhuiba
Nectandra leucothyrsus Meissn., Lauraceae 200
Louro-branco
Ocotea guianensis Aubl., Lauraceae 201
Louro-bravo
Nectandra canescens Nees, Lauraceae 199
Louro-cheiroso
Dicypellium caryophyllatum
 Nees & Mart., Lauraceae 198
Ocotea pretiosa (Nees & Mart.)
 Benth. & Hook., Lauraceae 201
Louro-cravo
Dicypellium caryophyllatum
 Nees & Mart., Lauraceae 198
Louro-cujumari
Ocotea cujumary Mart., Lauraceae 200
Louro-das-guianas
Ocotea guianensis Aubl., Lauraceae 201
Louro-inhamuí
Ocotea cymbarum H.B.K., Lauraceae 200
Louro-mamori
Ocotea cymbarum H.B.K., Lauraceae 200
Louro-mole
Cordia ecalyculata Vell., Boraginaceae 87
Louro-pixurim
Nectandra pichurim (H.B.K.) Mez, Lauraceae 200
Louro-preto
Nectandra puberula Nees, Lauraceae 200
Ocotea spectabilis (Meissn.) Mez, Lauraceae 201
Louro-puxuri
Licaria puchury-major
 (Mart.) Kosterm., Lauraceae 199

LOURO-SALGUEIRO – MAMONINHA: COMMON NAMES INDEX

Louro-salgueiro
   Cordia ecalyculata Vell., Boraginaceae 87
Louro-tamancão
   Ocotea guianensis Aubl., Lauraceae 201
Louro-vermelho
   Nectandra globosa (Aubl.) Mez, Lauraceae 199
Lupiticha
   Sida carpinifolia (L. f.) K. Sch., Malvaceae 222

M

Macaqueiro
   Guarea trichilioides L., Meliaceae 228
Macela
   Achyrocline satureioides (Lam.) DC., Asteraceae 52
Macela-da-terra
   Egletes viscosa (L.) Less., Asteraceae 59
Macela-do-campo
   Achyrocline satureioides (Lam.) DC., Asteraceae 52
   Bidens pilosa L., Asteraceae 57
Macela-do-sertão
   Egletes viscosa (L.) Less., Asteraceae 59
Macela-miúda
   Solidago chilensis Meyen, Asteraceae 65
Macieira
   Piptocarpha rotundifolia (Less.) Bak., Asteraceae .. 64
Macucu
   Caraipa densifolia Mart., Clusiaceae 121
Madacaru-de-leite
   Euphorbia phosphorea Mart., Euphorbiaceae 153
Magabeira-brava
   Lafoensia pacari St.-Hil., Lythraceae 215
Magerioba
   Senna occidentalis (L.) Link, Caesalpiniaceae 105
Magnólia-da-mata
   Talauma ovata St.-Hil., Magnoliaceae 216
Magnólia-do-brejo
   Talauma ovata St.-Hil., Magnoliaceae 216
Maiaca
   Xyris pallida Mart., Xyridaceae 342
Maioba
   Senna occidentalis (L.) Link, Caesalpiniaceae 105
Majorana
   Hibiscus bifurcatus Cav., Malvaceae 221
Mal-me-quer
   Noticastrum diffusum (Pers.) Cabr., Asteraceae 62
Mal-me-quer-do-pântano
   Erigeron tweediei Hook. & Arn., Asteraceae 60
Maleiteira
   Euphorbia cotinoides Miq., Euphorbiaceae 152
Malícia
   Schrankia leptocarpa DC., Mimosaceae 242
Malícia-das-mulheres
   Mimosa velloziana Mart., Mimosaceae 240
Malícia-de-mulher
   Mimosa invisa Mart., Mimosaceae 239
   Mimosa pudica L., Mimosaceae 240
Malícia-roxa
   Schrankia leptocarpa DC., Mimosaceae 242

Malmequer
   Grindelia buphthalmoides DC., Asteraceae 60
   Grindelia scorzonerifolia
     Hook. & Am., Asteraceae 60
Malva-branca
   Waltheria indica L., Sterculiaceae 325
   Waltheria viscosissima St.-Hil., Sterculiaceae 325
Malva-de-marajó
   Hyptis crenata Pohl, Lamiaceae 192
Malva-do-campo
   Kielmeyera speciosa St.-Hil., Clusiaceae 123
   Sida macrodon DC., Malvaceae 222
Malva-pedra
   Phyllanthus niruri L., Euphorbiaceae 156
Malva-preta
   Sida micrantha St.-Hil., Malvaceae 222
   Sida rhombifolia L., Malvaceae 222
Malva-roxa
   Urena lobata L., Malvaceae 223
Malva-santa
   Coleus barbatus Benth., Lamiaceae 191
Malva-veludo
   Waltheria indica L., Sterculiaceae 325
Malvaísco
   Pothomorphe umbellata (L.) Miq., Piperaceae 277
   Sida micrantha St.-Hil., Malvaceae 222
   Urena lobata L., Malvaceae 223
   Wissadula periplocifolia Presl., Malvaceae 223
Malvarisco
   Piper marginatum Jacq., Piperaceae 276
   Pothomorphe peltata L., Piperaceae 277
Malvavisco
   Pothomorphe umbellata (L.) Miq., Piperaceae 277
Mama-cadela
   Brosimum gaudichaudii Tréc., Moraceae 246
Mamangá
   Senna occidentalis (L.) Link, Caesalpiniaceae 105
Mamão
   Carica papaya L., Caricaceae 113
Mamão-de-veado
   Jacaratia spinosa (Aubl.) A. DC., Caricaceae 113
Mamão-do-mato
   Jacaratia spinosa (Aubl.) A. DC., Caricaceae 113
Mamão-rana
   Jacaratia spinosa (Aubl.) A. DC., Caricaceae 113
Mambu-açu
   Acmella repens (Walt.) L.C. Rich., Asteraceae 53
Mamica-de-cadela
   Zanthoxylum rhoifolium Lam., Rutaceae 303
Maminha-de-porca
   Zanthoxylum rhoifolium Lam., Rutaceae 303
Mamoeiro
   Carica papaya L., Caricaceae 113
Mamoiero bravo
   Jacaratia spinosa (Aubl.) A. DC., Caricaceae 113
Mamona-do-mato
   Mabea fistulifera Mart., Euphorbiaceae 155
Mamoninha
   Jatropha gossypiifolia L., Euphorbiaceae 154

Mamuí
Jacaratia spinosa (Aubl.) A. DC., Caricaceae 113
Maná-de-raposa
Bromelia antiacantha Bertol., Bromeliaceae 91
Manacá
Brunfelsia uniflora (Pohl) D. Don, Solanaceae 316
Manacá-cheiroso
Brunfelsia uniflora (Pohl) D. Don, Solanaceae 316
Mandacaru
Cereus jamacaru DC., Cactaceae 95
Cereus peruvianus (L.) Mill., Cactaceae 95
Mandacaru-de-boi
Cereus jamacaru DC., Cactaceae 95
Mandecravo
Pluchea suaveolens (Vell.) O. Ktze., Asteraceae 64
Mandobi-guaçu
Jatropha curcas L., Euphorbiaceae 154
Mandubirana
Desmodium axillare (Sw.) DC., Fabaceae 164
Manduirana
Senna macranthera (Collad.)
  Ir. & Barn., Caesalpiniaceae 105
Mangabinha-do-norte
Hancornia speciosa Gomes, Apocynaceae 24
Mangabeira
Hancornia speciosa Gomes, Apocynaceae 24
Mangará
Caladium bicolor (Aiton) Vent., Araceae 34
Xanthosoma violaceum Schott, Araceae 37
Mangarito-grande
Xanthosoma violaceum Schott, Araceae 37
Mangarito-roxo
Xanthosoma violaceum Schott, Araceae 37
Mangericão
Hyptis mutabilis (Rich.) Briq., Lamiaceae 193
Mangericão-grande
Ocimum micranthum Willd., Lamiaceae 195
Mangerioba
Senna corymbosa
  (Lam.) Ir. & Barn., Caesalpiniaceae 104
Mangerona
Glechon ciliata Benth., Lamiaceae 192
Mangerona-do-campo
Glechon spathulata Benth., Lamiaceae 192
Mangue
Conocarpus erecta L., Combretaceae 126
Rhizophora mangle L., Rhizophoraceae 294
Mangue-amarelo
Avicennia germinans (L.) L., Verbenaceae 334
Mangue-branco
Avicennia germinans (L.) L., Verbenaceae 334
Pisonia alcalina Fr. All., Nyctaginaceae 258
Mangue-de-botão
Conocarpus erecta L., Combretaceae 126
Mangue-manso
Avicennia germinans (L.) L., Verbenaceae 334
Mangue-vermelho
Rhizophora mangle L., Rhizophoraceae 294

Manguerana
Tovomita brasiliensis (Mart.) Walp., Clusiaceae 123
Manibu
Cyperus ligularis L., Cyperaceae 142
Manobi-açu
Commelina robusta Kunth, Commelinaceae 128
Mão-aberta
Caladium bicolor (Aiton) Vent.
  var. *poecile* (Schott) Engler, Araceae 35
Mão-de-calango
Macfadyena unguis-cati
  (L.) Gentry, Bignoniaceae 81
Mãos-de-sapo
Ludwigia suffruticosa (L.) Gomes, Onagraceae 264
Maquiné-do-mato
Mesechites sulphurea (Vell.) M. Arg., Apocynaceae 27
Maracá
Canna glauca L., Cannaceae 110
Maracujá
Passiflora alata Dryand., Passifloraceae 267
Passiflora caerulea L., Passifloraceae 269
Passiflora edulis Sims, Passifloraceae 269
Passiflora laurifolia L., Passifloraceae 270
Passiflora macrocarpa Mast., Passifloraceae 270
Maracujá-açu
Passiflora macrocarpa Mast., Passifloraceae 270
Maracujá-azul
Passiflora caerulea L., Passifloraceae 269
Maracujá-catinga
Passiflora foetida L., Passifloraceae 269
Maracujá-comum
Passiflora edulis Sims, Passifloraceae 269
Passiflora laurifolia L., Passifloraceae 270
Maracujá-de-cobra
Passiflora caerulea L., Passifloraceae 269
Maracujá-de-estalo
Passiflora foetida L., Passifloraceae 269
Maracujá-de-ponche
Passiflora edulis Sims, Passifloraceae 269
Maracujá-do-mato
Passiflora coccinea Aubl., Passifloraceae 269
Maracujá-do-piauí
Passiflora gardneri Mast., Passifloraceae 270
Maracujá-doce
Passiflora edulis Sims, Passifloraceae 269
Maracujá-fedorento
Passiflora foetida L., Passifloraceae 269
Maracujá-mamão
Passiflora macrocarpa Mast., Passifloraceae 270
Maracujá-melão
Passiflora macrocarpa Mast., Passifloraceae 270
Maracujá-mirim
Passiflora edulis Sims, Passifloraceae 269
Maracujá-peroba
Passiflora edulis Sims, Passifloraceae 269
Maracujá-poranga
Passiflora coccinea Aubl., Passifloraceae 269
Maracujá-roxo
Passiflora edulis Sims, Passifloraceae 269

Marapuama
 Ptychopetalum olacoides Benth., Olacaceae 262
 Ptychopetalum uncinatum Anselm., Olacaceae 263
Marcela
 Achyrocline satureioides (Lam.) DC., Asteraceae 52
 Pfaffia jubata Mart., Amaranthaceae 5
Marcela-da-mata
 Achyrocline satureioides (Lam.) DC., Asteraceae 52
Marcela-do-campo
 Pfaffia jubata Mart., Amaranthaceae 5
Marcela-do-cerrado
 Pfaffia jubata Mart., Amaranthaceae 5
Marfim-de-ramá
 Bredemeyera floribunda Willd., Polygalaceae 283
Margarita
 Tibouchina aspera Aubl., Melastomataceae 226
Mari
 Geoffroea striata (Willd.) Morong, Fabaceae 168
Mari-mari
 Geoffroea striata (Willd.) Morong, Fabaceae 168
Maria-mole
 Commelina nudiflora L., Commelinaceae 126
 Commelina virginica L., Commelinaceae 128
 Peperomia pellucida H.B.K., Piperaceae 273
 Senecio brasiliensis Less., Asteraceae 65
Maria-preta
 Ageratum conyzoides L., Asteraceae 53
 Blanchetia heterotricha DC., Asteraceae 57
 Conocliniopsis prasiifolia (DC.) King &
  H. Robinson, Asteraceae 58
 Cordia verbenacea DC., Boraginaceae 88
 Senna alata (L.) Roxb., Caesalpiniaceae 104
 Solanum nigrum L., Solanaceae 321
Maria-preta-verdadeira
 Conocliniopsis prasiifolia
  (DC.) King & H. Robinson, Asteraceae 58
Maria-rezadeira
 Cordia verbenacea DC., Boraginaceae 88
Mariana
 Acnistus arborescens (L.) Schl., Solanaceae 316
Marianeira
 Acnistus arborescens (L.) Schl., Solanaceae 316
 Bassovia lucida Dunal, Solanaceae 316
Marianinha
 Commelina nudiflora L., Commelinaceae 126
 Commelina virginica L., Commelinaceae 128
Maricá
 Mimosa bimucronata (DC.) O. Ktze., Mimosaceae 238
Maricaua
 Datura insignis B. Rodr., Solanaceae 318
Maricotinha
 Monnieria trifolia Loefl., Rutaceae 302
Marigeriona-grande
 Senna alata (L.) Roxb., Caesalpiniaceae 104
Marinheiro
 Geoffroea striata (Willd.) Morong, Fabaceae 168
 Guarea trichilioides L., Meliaceae 228
 Trichilia cathartica Mart., Meliaceae 229
Marinheiro-de-folha-larga
 Guarea spiciflora Juss., Meliaceae 227

Marizeiro
 Geoffroea striata (Willd.) Morong, Fabaceae 168
Marmelada
 Alibertia edulis (Rich.) Rich., Rubiaceae 295
Marmelada-de-cachorro
 Alibertia edulis (Rich.) Rich., Rubiaceae 295
Marmeleiro
 Croton hemiargyreus M. Arg., Euphorbiaceae 151
 Croton sonderianus M. Arg., Euphorbiaceae 151
Marmeleiro-branco
 Croton sincorensis Mart., Euphorbiaceae 151
Marmeleiro-do-campo
 Casearia cambessedesii Eichl., Flacourtiaceae 176
 Maprounea brasiliensis L., Euphorbiaceae 155
Marmeleiro-do-mato
 Casearia cambessedesii Eichl., Flacourtiaceae 176
Marmeleiro-preto
 Croton hemiargyreus M. Arg., Euphorbiaceae 151
 Croton sonderianus M. Arg., Euphorbiaceae 151
Marmelinho
 Tournefortia paniculata Cham., Boraginaceae 90
Marolinho
 Annona coriacea Mart., Annonaceae 12
Marolo
 Annona coriacea Mart., Annonaceae 12
 Annona crassifolia Mart., Annonaceae 12
Maroto
 Acanthospermum hispidum DC., Asteraceae 52
Marqueza-de-belas
 Pyrostegia ignea (Vell.) Pres., Bignoniaceae 82
Marroio
 Hyptis fasciculata Benth., Lamiaceae 192
 Leonurus sibiricus L., Lamiaceae 194
Marsh mallow substitute
 Uses: *Sida rhombea* L., Malvaceae 222
Marubá
 Quassia amara L., Simaroubaceae 314
Marupá
 Jacaranda copaia (Aubl.) D. Don, Bignoniaceae 80
 Marupa francoana Miers, Simaroubaceae 313
 Quassia amara L., Simaroubaceae 314
 Simarouba amara Aubl., Simaroubaceae 315
Marupá-falso
 Jacaranda copaia (Aubl.) D. Don, Bignoniaceae 80
Marupá-piranga
 Eleutherine plicata Herb., Iridaceae 186
Marupaís
 Simarouba versicolor St.-Hil., Simaroubaceae 315
Maruparaíba
 Simarouba amara Aubl., Simaroubaceae 315
Marupazinho
 Eleutherine plicata Herb., Iridaceae 186
Marupitá
 Sapium hamatum Pax & Hoffm., Euphorbiaceae ... 157
Massapê
 Imperata brasiliensis Trin., Poaceae 281
Mastruço
 Acmella repens (Walt.) L.C. Rich., Asteraceae 53
 Chenopodium ambrosioides L., Chenopodiaceae ... 118

Mastruz
Chenopodium ambrosioides L., Chenopodiaceae ... 118
Mata-barata
Andira humilis Benth., see *Andira vermifuga*, USES:
Andira spp., Fabaceae 162
Simarouba versicolor St.-Hil., Simaroubaceae 315
Mata-cana
Cuphea ingrata Cham. & Schl., Lythraceae 214
Mata-cavalo
Solanum ciliatum Lam., Solanaceae 319
Mata-olho
Pouteria salicifolia Hook. & Arn., Sapotaceae 310
Mata-paca
Calea pinnatifida (R. Br.) Less., Asteraceae 57
Mata-pasto
Acanthospermum australe
(Loefl.) O. Ktze., Asteraceae 51
Senna obtusifolia (L.) Ir. & Barn., Caesalpiniaceae 105
Mata-piolho
Carpotroche brasiliensis
(Raddi) Endl., Flacourtiaceae 176
Mata-zombando
Datura stramonium L., Solanaceae 318
Schultesia stenophylla Mart., Gentianaceae 180
Matacana
Lindernia crustacea F. Muell., Scrophulariaceae ... 311
Matafome
Physalis angulata L., Solanaceae 318
Matapasto
Senna alata (L.) Roxb., Caesalpiniaceae 104
Senna occidentalis (L.) Link, Caesalpiniaceae 105
Senna uniflora
(P. Miller) Ir. & Barn., Caesalpiniaceae 106
Matapau
Clusia rosea Jacq., Clusiaceae 122
Mate
Citronella congonha (Mart.) Howard, Icacinaceae . 185
Ilex paraguariensis St.-Hil., Aquifoliaceae 31
Mate-do-campo
Luxemburgia glazioviana Gilg., Ochnaceae 260
Luxemburgia polyandra St.-Hil., Ochnaceae 260
Matega
Byrsonima coccolobifolia H.B.K., Malpighiaceae .. 218
Matias
Vernonanthura brasiliana
(L.) H. Robinson, Asteraceae 67
Matico
Piper angustifolium R. & Pav., Piperaceae 274
Piper elongatum Vahl, Piperaceae 275
Matico-falso
Piper aduncum L., Piperaceae 274
Matucan
Lindernia crustacea F. Muell., Scrophulariaceae ... 311
Medicineiro
Jatropha elliptica (Pohl) M. Arg., Euphorbiaceae .. 154
Melancia-da-praia
Solanum agrarium Sendt., Solanaceae 319
Melão-de-caboclo
Sicana odorifera Naud., Cucurbitaceae 139

Melão-de-morcego
Melothria fluminensis Gardn., Cucurbitaceae 139
Melão-de-são-caetano
Momordica charantia L., Cucurbitaceae 139
Melindre
Glandularia peruviana (L.) Small, Verbenaceae ... 334
Mendanha
Esenbeckia febrifuga Juss., Rutaceae 301
Mentrasto
Ageratum conyzoides L., Asteraceae 53
Hyptis spicigera Lam., Lamiaceae 193
Mentrasto-grande
Hyptis suaveolens Poit., Lamiaceae 193
Mercurial
Modiolastrum pinnatipartitum
(St.-Hil. & Naudin) Krapovickas, Malvaceae 221
Mercúrio-da-terra-firme
Brosimum acutifolium Huber, Moraceae 246
Mercúrio-vegetal
Brosimum acutifolium Huber, Moraceae 246
Meru
Canna edulis Ker-Gawl., Cannaceae 110
Mescla
Protium icicariba (DC.) March., Burseraceae 94
Mil-homens
Aristolochia birostris Duch., Aristolochiaceae 46
Aristolochia esperanzae
O. Kuntze, Aristolochiaceae 48
Aristolochia trilobata L., Aristolochiaceae 48
Mil-homens-do-rio-grande-do-sul
Aristolochia triangularis Cham., Aristolochiaceae ... 48
Milfacadas
Hypericum brasiliense Choisy, Clusiaceae 122
Milfuradas
Hypericum brasiliense Choisy, Clusiaceae 122
Milho-de-cobra
Dracontium asperum K. Koch, Araceae 35
Lophophytum mirabile Schott &
Endl., Balanophoraceae 73
Milhome
Aristolochia cymbifera
Mart. & Zucc., Aristolochiaceae 47
Aristolochia gigantea
Mart. & Zucc., Aristolochiaceae 48
Milhome-de-babado
Aristolochia elegans Mast., Aristolochiaceae 48
Milhomens
Aristolochia cymbifera
Mart. & Zucc., Aristolochiaceae 47
Aristolochia gigantea
Mart. & Zucc., Aristolochiaceae 48
Miloló
Annona reticulata L., Annonaceae 13
Mimosinho
Hackelochloa granularis (L.) O. Ktze., Poaceae ... 281
Minuana
Oenothera catharinensis Camb., Onagraceae 264
Miri
Dipholis nigra Gr., Sapotaceae 309

Miriti
Mauritia flexuosa L. f., Arecaceae 43
Mititoroba
Lucuma rivicoa Gaertn., Sapotaceae 309
Mofumbo
Combretum leprosum Mart., Combretaceae 126
Molongó
Ambelania tenuifolia Aubl., Apocynaceae 21
Zschokkea arborescens M. Arg., Apocynaceae 29
Morango-do-acre
Ephedra americana Willd., Ephedraceae 147
Morcegueira
Andira retusa (Poir.) H.B.K., Fabaceae 162
Moreira
Maclura tinctoria (L.) D. Don, Moraceae 249
Mororó
Bauhinia forficata Link, Caesalpiniaceae 99
Morrão-de-candeia
Croton triqueter Lam., Euphorbiaceae 151
Morrião-d'água
Samolus valerandi L., Primulaceae 290
Muçambê
Cleome spinosa Jacq., Capparaceae 112
Muçambê-catinga
Cleome gigantea L., Capparaceae 112
Muçambê-de-espinhos
Cleome spinosa Jacq., Capparaceae 112
Muçambê-de-três-folhas
Cleome polygama L., Capparaceae 112
Muçambê-fedorento
Cleome aculeata L., Capparaceae 112
Mucataia
Nectandra canescens Nees, Lauraceae 199
Mucuna
Mucuna pruriens (L.) DC., Fabaceae 169
Muira-itá
Caesalpinia ferrea Mart. ex Tul., Caesalpiniaceae . 100
Muira-piranga
Brosimum acutifolium Huber, Moraceae 246
Muirá-tinga
Maquira sclerophylla
 (Ducke) C. C. Berg, Moraceae 249
Muiracutua
Doliocarpus rolandri Gmel., Dilleniaceae 146
Muirapuama
Ptychopetalum olacoides Benth., Olacaceae 262
Ptychopetalum uncinatum Anselm., Olacaceae 263
Rhabdodendron amazonicum
 (Spr. ex Benth.) Hub., Rhabdodendraceae 291
Muiraqueteca
Davilla rugosa Poir., Dilleniaceae 145
Doliocarpus rolandri Gmel., Dilleniaceae 146
Muiratã
Ptychopetalum olacoides Benth., Olacaceae 262
Ptychopetalum uncinatum Anselm., Olacaceae 263
Muiratetec
Davilla rugosa Poir., Dilleniaceae 145
Mulateiro
Pentaclethra macroloba
 (Willd.) O. Ktze., Mimosaceae 242

Mulher-pobre
Jacaranda cuspidifolia Mart., Bignoniaceae 81
Mulungu
Erythrina corallodendron L., Fabaceae 166
Erythrina crista-galli L., Fabaceae 166
Erythrina falcata Benth., Fabaceae 166
Erythrina fusca Lour., Fabaceae 166
Erythrina velutina Willd., Fabaceae 166
Erythrina verna Vell., Fabaceae 168
Muraré
Nymphoides indica (L.) O. Ktze., Menyanthaceae . 235
Mureci
Byrsonima coccolobifolia H.B.K., Malpighiaceae .. 218
Murici
Byrsonima chrysophylla H.B.K., Malpighiaceae 218
Murici-açu
Byrsonima verbascifolia (L.) Rich., Malpighiaceae 220
Murici-amarelo
Senna multijuga Rich. var.
 verrucosa (Vog.) Ir. & Barn., Caesalpiniaceae 105
Murici-da-mata
Byrsonima verbascifolia (L.) Rich., Malpighiaceae 220
Murici-do-campo
Byrsonima crassifolia H.B.K., Malpighiaceae 219
Murici-guaçu
Byrsonima verbascifolia (L.) Rich., Malpighiaceae 220
Murici-penima
Byrsonima chrysophylla H.B.K., Malpighiaceae 218
Muriri
Mouriri guianensis Aubl., Melastomataceae 226
Murta
Mouriri guianensis Aubl., Melastomataceae 226
Murta-de-parida
Mouriri guianensis Aubl., Melastomataceae 226
Murta-do-mato
Coutarea hexandra (Jacq.) K. Sch., Rubiaceae 297
Murta-parida
Myrcia lanceolata Camb., Myrtaceae 255
Muru
Canna lutea Roscoe, Cannaceae 111
Muruchi
Byrsonima chrysophylla H.B.K., Malpighiaceae 218
Muruchi-rasteiro
Byrsonima verbascifolia (L.) Rich., Malpighiaceae 220
Murumuru
Astrocaryum murumuru Mart., Arecaceae 39
Mururé
Brosimum acutifolium Huber, Moraceae 246
Brosimum utile (H.B.K.) Pittier, Moraceae 246
Cabomba piauhyensis Gard., Nymphaeaceae 259
Eichhornia crassipes Solms, Pontederiaceae 288
Ludwigia natans (H.B.K.) Ell., Onagraceae 264
Ludwigia repens (L.) Hara, Onagraceae 264
Nymphaea rudgeana G. Meyer, Nymphaeaceae 259
Mururé-rendado
Azolla caroliniana Willd., Salviniaceae 304
Mutamba
Guazuma ulmifolia
 Lam. var. *ulmifolia*, Sterculiaceae 323

Muuba
  Bellucia grossularioides (L.) Tr., Melastomataceae 225

N

Naiá
  Scheelea phalerata
    (Mart. ex Spreng.) Burret, Arecaceae 45
Navalha-miúda
  Hypolytrum laxum Schrad., Cyperaceae 143
Negramina
  Siparuna brasiliensis (Spr.) DC., Monimiaceae 245
  Siparuna guianensis Aubl., Monimiaceae 245
Nhaborandi
  Piper geniculatum Sw., Piperaceae 275
Nhandi
  Piper marginatum Jacq., Piperaceae 276
Nhandiroba
  Fevillea trilobata L., Cucurbitaceae 136
Nhandu
  Piper marginatum Jacq., Piperaceae 276
Nó-de-porco
  Heteropteris aphrodisiaca
    O. Mach., Malpighiaceae 220
Noz-de-serpente
  Fevillea trilobata L., Cucurbitaceae 136
Noz-moscada-do-brasil
  Cryptocarya moschata
    Nees & Mart. ex Nees, Lauraceae 198
Noz-moscada-do-pará
  Nectandra pichurim (H.B.K.) Mez, Lauraceae 200
Noz-vômica
  Strychnos trinervis (Vell.) Mart., Loganiaceae 210
Nú-de-cachorro
  Heteropteris aphrodisiaca
    O. Mach., Malpighiaceae 220

O

Oajuru
  Arrabidaea chica (H.B.K.) Bur., Bignoniaceae 78
Oanani
  Symphonia globulifera L. f., Clusiaceae 123
Oiti-tereba
  Lucuma rivicoa Gaertn., Sapotaceae 309
Oiticica
  Clarisia racemosa Ruiz & Pav., Moraceae 247
Oiticica-cica
  Clarisia racemosa Ruiz & Pav., Moraceae 247
Oiticica-vermelha
  Clarisia racemosa Ruiz & Pav., Moraceae 247
Oiticicia
  Maclura tinctoria (L.) D. Don, Moraceae 249
Olandi
  Calophyllum brasiliense Camb., Clusiaceae 120
Óleo-elétrico
  Piper callosum R. & Pav., Piperaceae 274
Óleo-pardo
  Myrocarpus frondosus Fr. All., Fabaceae 170

Óleo-vermelho
  Myroxylon balsamum (L.) Harms, Fabaceae 170
Olho-de-burro
  Mucuna pruriens (L.) DC., Fabaceae 169
Olho-de-gato
  Caesalpinia bonduc (L.) Roxb., Caesalpiniaceae 99
Olhos de porco
  Miconia albicans (Sw.) Tr., Melastomataceae 225
Onze-horas
  Portulaca grandiflora Hook., Portulacaceae 289
Ora-pro-nobis
  Pereskia aculeata Mill., Cactaceae 97
  Pereskia bleo H.B.K., Cactaceae 97
  Portulaca oleracea L., Portulacaceae 289
Orango-do-campo
  Ephedra triandra Tul., Ephedraceae 148
Orelha-de-gato
  Hypericum brasiliense Choisy, Clusiaceae 122
  Hypericum connatum Lam., Clusiaceae 122
  Tibouchina clavata
    (Pers.) Wurdack, Melastomataceae 226
Orelha-de-mico
  Ilex brevicuspis Reiss., Aquifoliaceae 31
Orelha-de-monge
  Kalanchoe brasiliensis Camb., Crassulaceae 133
Orelha-de-onça
  Chondodendron platyphyllum
    (Mart.) Miers, Menispermaceae 231
  Cissampelos ovalifolia DC., Menispermaceae 233
  Cissampelos pareira L., Menispermaceae 233
  Cissampelos sympodialis Eichl., Menispermaceae . 233
  Lindernia crustacea F. Muell., Scrophulariaceae ... 311
  Tibouchina clavata
    (Pers.) Wurdack, Melastomataceae 226
Orelha-de-onça-rasteira
  Hydrocotyle leucocephala
    Cham. & Schlecht., Apiaceae 20
Orelha-de-rato
  Lindernia diffusa Wettst., Scrophulariaceae 312
Orélia
  Allamanda cathartica L., Apocynaceae 20
Ouregon
  Guatteria ouregon (Aubl.) Dun., Annonaceae 14
Ovo-de-galo
  Salpichroa origanifolia (Lam.) Thell., Solanaceae 319

P

Pacapiá
  Fevillea uncipetala Kuhlm., Cucurbitaceae 138
Pacaratepê
  Anacampta riedellii (M. Arg.) Mgf., Apocynaceae ... 21
Pacari
  Lafoensia densiflora Pohl, Lythraceae 214
  Lafoensia pacari St.-Hil., Lythraceae 215
Pachinhos
  Xylopia aromatica (Lam.) Mart., Annonaceae 15
Paco-caatinga
  Costus spicatus (Jacq.) Sw., also
    Costus spiralis (Jacq.) Roscoe, Costaceae 132

Paco-seroca

Renealmia occidentalis Sweet, Zingiberaceae 343

Pacoté

Cochlospermum orinocense
(H.B.K.) Steud., Cochlospermaceae 125

Pacová

Costus spicatus (Jacq.) Sw., also
Costus spiralis (Jacq.) Roscoe, Costaceae 132
Renealmia exaltata L. f., Zingiberaceae 342
Renealmia occidentalis Sweet, Zingiberaceae 343

Pacová-catinga

Renealmia exaltata L. f., Zingiberaceae 342

Pacovi

Xylopia aromatica (Lam.) Mart., Annonaceae 15
Xylopia frutescens Aubl., Annonaceae 16

Pacuarana

Canna lanuginosa Roscoe, Cannaceae 111

Pacuri

Lafoensia pacari St.-Hil., Lythraceae 215

Paia-marioba

Polygonum acuminatum H.B.K., Polygonaceae 286

Paina-de-penas

Echites peltata Vell., Apocynaceae 23

Paina-de-seda

Araujia sericifera Brot., Asclepiadaceae 50

Paina-do-campo

Araujia sericifera Brot., Asclepiadaceae 50

Paina-lisa

Ceiba pentandra (L.) Gaertn., Bombacaceae 86

Paineira

Chorisia crispiflora H.B.K., Bombacaceae 86

Paipuna

Myrcia tingens Berg, Myrtaceae 255

Pajamarioba

Senna occidentalis (L.) Link, Caesalpiniaceae 106

Pali

Piper geniculatum Sw., Piperaceae 275

Palim

Piper geniculatum Sw., Piperaceae 275

Palissandra

Jacaranda mimosifolia D. Don, Bignoniaceae 81

Palma-santa

Opuntia vulgaris Mill., Cactaceae 97

Palmatória

Opuntia vulgaris Mill., Cactaceae 97

Palmatória-grande

Brasilopuntia brasiliensis
(Willd.) Berg., Cactaceae 95

Palmeira

Attalea oleifera Barb. Rodr., Arecaceae 39

Palmeira-do-brejo

Desmoncus orthacanthos Mart., Arecaceae 40

Palmeira-real

Bactris insignis (Mart.) Baill., Arecaceae 39

Palminha-das-pedras

Selaginella erythropus Spring, Selaginellaceae 313

Palmiteiro

Euterpe oleracea Mart., Arecaceae 42

Palmito

Euterpe edulis Mart., Arecaceae 41

Palmito amargoso

Syagrus comosa Mart., Arecaceae 45

Palmito-amargoso

Syagrus pseudococos
(Raddi) Glassman, Arecaceae 45

Palmito-doce

Euterpe edulis Mart., Arecaceae 41

Palmito-juçara

Euterpe edulis Mart., Arecaceae 41

Panacéia

Gomphrena officinalis Mart., Amaranthaceae 4
Solanum cernuum Vell., Solanaceae 319
Solanum martii Sendt., Solanaceae 321

Panapanari

Clusia panapanari Choisy, Clusiaceae 122

Panduarana

Canna lanuginosa Roscoe, Cannaceae 111

Pané

Abuta rufescens Aubl., Menispermaceae 231

Pao-de-peru

Aristolochia elegans Mast., Aristolochiaceae 48

Papaterra

Lindernia diffusa Wettst., Scrophulariaceae 312

Papaya

Carica papaya L., Caricaceae 113

Papo-de-galo

Aristolochia cymbifera
Mart. & Zucc., Aristolochiaceae 47

Papo-de-peru

Aristolochia cymbifera
Mart. & Zucc., Aristolochiaceae 47
Aristolochia gigantea
Mart. & Zucc., Aristolochiaceae 48
Aristolochia trilobata L., Aristolochiaceae 48

Papo-de-peru-de-babado

Aristolochia gigantea
Mart. & Zucc., Aristolochiaceae 48

Papo-de-peru-do-grande

Aristolochia gigantea
Mart. & Zucc., Aristolochiaceae 48

Papo-de-peru-do-miudo

Aristolochia esperanzae
O. Kuntze, Aristolochiaceae 48

Papoula-de-são-francisco

Hibiscus cannabinus L., Malvaceae 221

Paqueretê

Anacampta riedellii (M. Arg.) Mgf., Apocynaceae ... 21

Pará-pará

Cordia umbraculifera DC., Boraginaceae 88

Paracari

Marsypianthes chamaedrys
(Vahl) O. Ktze., Lamiaceae 194
Peltodon radicans Pohl, Lamiaceae 195
Tetralacrium veroniciforme
Turcz., Scrophulariaceae 312

Paraci

Eichhornia crassipes Solms, Pontederiaceae 288

Paracuru

Marsypianthes chamaedrys
(Vahl) O. Ktze., Lamiaceae 194

Paraguaia
    Anchietea pyrifolia (Mart.) G. Don, Violaceae 338
Paraíba
    Simarouba amara Aubl., Simaroubaceae 315
    Simarouba versicolor St.-Hil., Simaroubaceae 315
Paraíba-mirim
    Simaba glandulifera Gardn., Simaroubaceae 315
Parala
    Diospyros paralea Steud., Ebenaceae 147
Paramarioba
    Senna hirsuta (L.) Ir. & Barn. var.
        puberula Ir. & Barn., Caesalpiniaceae 105
    Senna occidentalis (L.) Link, Caesalpiniaceae 106
Parapará
    Jacaranda copaia (Aubl.) D. Don, Bignoniaceae 80
Paratucu
    Tabernaemontana citrifolia L., Apocynaceae 28
Paratudinho
    Gomphrena officinalis Mart., Amaranthaceae 4
Paratudo
    Drimys winteri Forst., Winteraceae 340
    Gomphrena leucocephala Mart., Amaranthaceae 4
    Gomphrena officinalis Mart., Amaranthaceae 4
    Pfaffia paniculata (Mart.) Kuntze, Amaranthaceae 5
    Piptocarpha rotundifolia (Less.) Bak., Asteraceae .. 64
    Tabebuia aurea (Manso) Moore, Bignoniaceae 82
Paratudo-aromatico
    Cinnamodendron axillare
        (Nees & Mart.) Endl., Canellaceae 110
Paratudo-do-campo
    Gomphrena macrocephala St.-Hil., Amaranthaceae .. 4
Paraturá
    Remirea maritima Aubl., Cyperaceae 143
Paricá
    Anadenanthera peregrina (L.) Speg., Mimosaceae 236
    Parkia oppositifolia (Spruce) Benth., Mimosaceae 240
    Parkia pectinata Benth., Mimosaceae 240
Paricá-da-terra-firme
    Anadenanthera peregrina (L.) Speg., Mimosaceae 236
Paricarana
    Bowdichia virgilioides H.B.K., Fabaceae 163
Parietária
    Parietaria boehmerioides Mart., Urticaceae 331
Parimá
    Gynerium parviflorum Nees, Poaceae 281
Pariparoba
    Piper mikanianum (Kunth) Steud., Piperaceae 276
    Piper rohrii C. DC., Piperaceae 276
    Pothomorphe peltata L., Piperaceae 277
    Pothomorphe umbellata (L.) Miq., Piperaceae 277
Pariparoba-do-rio-grande
    Piper parthenium Mart., Piperaceae 276
Pariri piranga
    Arrabidaea chica (H.B.K.) Bur., Bignoniaceae 78
Parreira-brava
    Abuta concolor Poepp. & Endl., Menispermaceae . 231
    Abuta rufescens Aubl., Menispermaceae 231
    Chondodendron platyphyllum
        (Mart.) Miers, Menispermaceae 231
    Cissampelos pareira L., Menispermaceae 233

Parreira-brava-do-rio
    Cissampelos fluminensis Eichl., Menispermaceae .. 233
Parreira-brava-lisa
    Cissampelos glaberrima St.-Hil., Menispermaceae 233
Parreira-caapeba
    Cissampelos glaberrima St.-Hil., Menispermaceae 233
Parreirinha
    Cremastus sceptrum Bur. & K. Sch., Bignoniaceae .. 79
Partasana
    Typha domingensis Pers., Typhaceae 328
Pasta-miúda *(duckweed)*
    Lemna minor L., Lemnaceae 207
Pata-de-boi
    Bauhinia candicans Benth., Caesalpiniaceae 99
Pata-de-vaca
    Bauhinia candicans Benth., Caesalpiniaceae 99
    Bauhinia forficata Link, Caesalpiniaceae 99
Pataquera
    Conobea aquatica Aubl., Scrophulariaceae 311
    Conobea scoparioides Benth., Scrophulariaceae 311
Pataquira
    Conobea scoparioides Benth., Scrophulariaceae 311
Patauá
    Jessenia bataua (Mart.) Burret, Arecaceae 43
Pati
    Syagrus oleracea (Mart.) Becc., Arecaceae 45
Pati-amargosa
    Syagrus oleracea (Mart.) Becc., Arecaceae 45
Pati-amargoso
    Syagrus pseudococos (Raddi) Glassman, Arecaceae 45
Pau-amarante
    Caesalpinia bracteosa Tul., Caesalpiniaceae 100
Pau-bálsamo
    Myrocarpus frondosus Fr. All., Fabaceae 170
Pau-branco
    Auxemma oncocalyx (Fr. All.) Taub., Boraginaceae . 87
Pau-brasil
    Caesalpinia echinata Lam., Caesalpiniaceae 100
Pau-breu
    Symphonia globulifera L. f., Clusiaceae 123
Pau-caixão
    Bredemeyera floribunda Willd., Polygalaceae 283
Pau-cardoso
    Cyathea armata (Sw.) Domin, Cyatheaceae 141
Pau-cravo
    Dicypellium caryophyllatum
        Nees & Mart., Lauraceae 198
Pau-cumaru
    Dipteryx alata Vog., Fabaceae 165
Pau-d'alho
    Crataeva tapia L., Capparaceae 112
    Gallesia gorazema (Vell.) Moq., Phytolaccaceae .. 271
    Seguieria americana L., Phytolaccaceae 272
Pau-d'alho-do-campo
    Agonandra brasiliensis Miers, Opiliaceae 265
Pau-d'arco
    Patagonula americana L., Boraginaceae 89
    Tabebuia aurea (Manso) Moore, Bignoniaceae 82
    Tabebuia serratifolia (Vahl) Nichol., Bignoniaceae .. 83

Pau-d'arco-amarelo
Tabebuia chrysotricha
(Mart.) Standl., Bignoniaceae 82
Pau-d'arco-da-beira
Tabebuia barbata (May) Sandw., Bignoniaceae 82
Pau-d'arco-roxo
Tabebuia impetiginosa
(Mart.) Standl., Bignoniaceae 83
Pau-de-angola, Pau-d'angola
Piper arboreum Aubl., Piperaceae 274
Piper marginatum Jacq., Piperaceae 276
Vitex agnus-castus L., Verbenaceae 336
Pau-de-anjo
Carpotroche brasiliensis
(Raddi) Endl., Flacourtiaceae 176
Pau-de-azeite
Ilex acrodonta Reiss., Aquifoliaceae 31
Pau-de-balsa
Ochroma pyramidale (Cav.) Urb., Bombacaceae 86
Pau-de-boaz
Anadenanthera falcata (Benth.)
Brenan, Mimosaceae 236
Pau-de-cangalha
Symplocos parviflora Benth., Symplocaceae 326
Pau-de-cinza
Symplocos pubescens Klotzsch, Symplocaceae 326
Pau-de-cobra
Potalia amara Aubl., Loganiaceae 209
Pau-de-colher
Peschiera laeta (Mart.) Miers, Apocynaceae 27
Zschokkea arborescens M. Arg., Apocynaceae 29
Pau-de-cortiça
Kielmeyera speciosa St.-Hil., Clusiaceae 123
Pau-de-cotia
Carpotroche brasiliensis
(Raddi) Endl., Flacourtiaceae 176
Pau-de-curtume
Byrsonima spicata Rich., Malpighiaceae 219
Pau-de-gasolina
Ocotea cymbarum H.B.K., Lauraceae 200
Pau-de-lacre
Vismia guianensis (Aubl.) Choisy, Clusiaceae 124
Vismia japurensis Reich., Clusiaceae 124
Vismia latifolia (Aubl.) Choisy, Clusiaceae 124
Pau-de-lagarto
Calea pinnatifida (R. Br.) Less., Asteraceae 57
Casearia sylvestris Sw., Flacourtiaceae 178
Pau-de-leite
Euphorbia hyssopifolia L., Euphorbiaceae 153
Euphorbia phosphorea Mart., Euphorbiaceae 153
Himatanthus alba (L.) Woods., Apocynaceae 24
Plumeria alba L., Apocynaceae 28
Rauwolfia ligustrina Willd. ex
Roem. & Schult., Apocynaceae 28
Pau-de-lepra
Carpotroche brasiliensis
(Raddi) Endl., Flacourtiaceae 176
Pau-de-moquem
Vernonanthura brasiliana (L.) H.
Robinson, Asteraceae 67

Pau-de-mutamba
Guazuma ulmifolia Lam. var.
tomentella Schum., Sterculiaceae 323
Pau-de-novato
Triplaris weigeltiana (Reichb.)
O. Ktze., Polygonaceae 287
Pau-de-óleo
Copaifera officinalis (Jacq.) L., Caesalpiniaceae 102
Pau-de-piranha
Laetia apetala Jacq., Flacourtiaceae 178
Pau-de-praga
Leonotis nepetaefolia R. Br., Lamiaceae 194
Leucas martinicensis (Jacq.) R. Br., Lamiaceae 194
Pau-de-querosene
Ocotea cymbarum H.B.K., Lauraceae 200
Pau-de-rato
Caesalpinia microphylla Mart., Caesalpiniaceae ... 100
Caesalpinia pyramidalis Tul., Caesalpiniaceae 100
Pau-de-remo
Aspidosperma nitidum Benth., Apocynaceae 21
Pradosia lactescens (Vell.) Radlk., Sapotaceae 310
Pau-de-sangue
Vismia latifolia (Aubl.) Choisy, Clusiaceae 124
Pau-de-santa-ana
Nectandra puberula Nees, Lauraceae 200
Pau-de-santo
Cabralea canjerana (Vell.) Mart., Meliaceae 227
Pau-de-são-josé
Kielmeyera coriacea Mart., Clusiaceae 122
Pau-de-sebo
Sapindus saponaria L., Sapindaceae 306
Pau-de-seda
Muntingia calabura L., Tiliaceae 327
Pau-de-vassoura
Coccoloba mollis Casar., Polygonaceae 285
Pau-de-vinho
Vochysia thyrsoidea Pohl, Vochysiaceae 340
Pau-doce
Pradosia lactescens (Vell.) Radlk., Sapotaceae 310
Pau-d'óleo
Copaifera cearensis Huber
ex Ducke, Caesalpiniaceae 102
Pau-fava
Senna macranthera (Collad.) Ir.
& Barn., Caesalpiniaceae 105
Pau-ferro
Caesalpinia ferrea Mart. ex Tul., Caesalpiniaceae . 100
Connarus suberosus Planch., Connaraceae 129
Swartzia panacoco (Aubl.) Cowan
var. *panacoco*, Caesalpiniaceae 107
Pau-forquilha
Geissospermum laeve (Vell.) Baill., Apocynaceae 24
Pau-marfim
Agonandra brasiliensis Miers, Opiliaceae 265
Pau-mulato
Pentaclethra macroloba (Willd.)
O. Ktze., Mimosaceae 242
Pau-para-tudo
Drimys winteri Forst., Winteraceae 340

Leonurus sibiricus L., Lamiaceae 194
Pau-paraíba
  Simarouba versicolor St.-Hil., Simaroubaceae 315
  Triplaris macrocalyx Casar., Polygonaceae 287
Pau-pereira
  Geissospermum laeve (Vell.) Baill., Apocynaceae 24
Pau-pereira-falso
  Picramnia ciliata Mart., Simaroubaceae 314
Pau-pernambuco
  Caesalpinia echinata Lam., Caesalpiniaceae 100
Pau-pimenta
  Cinnamodendron axillare (Nees &
  Mart.) Endl., Canellaceae 110
Pau-pombo
  Marupa francoana Miers, Simaroubaceae 313
Pau-rendoso
  Bredemeyera floribunda Willd., Polygalaceae 283
Pau-rosa *(rosewood)*
  Aniba rosaeodora Ducke, Lauraceae 197
Pau-santo
  Kielmeyera coriacea Mart., Clusiaceae 122
  Kielmeyera petiolaris Mart., Clusiaceae 122
  Kielmeyera speciosa St.-Hil., Clusiaceae 123
  Swartzia panacoco
    (Aubl.) Cowan var. *panacoco,* Caesalpiniaceae 107
Pau-sassafrás
  Ocotea cymbarum H.B.K., Lauraceae 200
Pau-terra-do-mato
  Callisthene major Mart., Vochysiaceae 340
Pau-violeta
  Dalbergia gracilis Benth., Fabaceae 163
Paud'arco
  Tabebuia leucoxylon (L.) DC., Bignoniaceae 83
Pavoá
  Eichhornia crassipes Solms, Pontederiaceae 288
Pawpaw
  Carica papaya L., Caricaceae 113
Paxiubarana-miúda
  Tovomita brasiliensis (Mart.) Walp., Clusiaceae 123
Pé-de-cabra
  Ipomoea pes-caprae (L.) R. Br., Convolvulaceae .. 130
Pé-de-elefante
  Elephantopus mollis H.B.K., Asteraceae 59
Pé-de-galinha
  Chloris distichophylla (Nees) Lag., Poaceae 280
  Chloris polydactyla Sw., Poaceae 280
Pé-de-papagaio
  Selaginella convoluta Spring, Selaginellaceae 313
Pé-de-perdiz
  Simarouba versicolor St.-Hil., Simaroubaceae 315
Pé-de-pombo
  Oxalis corniculata L., Oxalidaceae 266
Pedra-ume-caá
  Myrcia amazonica DC., Myrtaceae 255
  Myrcia sphaerocarpa DC., Myrtaceae 255
Pega-pinto
  Boerhavia coccinea Mill., Nyctaginaceae 257
Peito-de-moça
  Solanum mammosum L., Solanaceae 321

Peito-de-vaca
  Solanum mammosum L., Solanaceae 321
Pente-de-macaco
  Calliandra tweedii Benth., Mimosaceae 237
Pepino-de-papagaio
  Gurania multiflora Cogn., Cucurbitaceae 138
Pepino-do-mato
  Ambelania tenuifolia Aubl., Apocynaceae 21
Pequi
  Caryocar brasiliense Camb., Caryocaraceae 114
  Caryocar coriaceum Wittm., Caryocaraceae 114
  Caryocar villosum (Aubl.) Pers., Caryocaraceae 114
Pequi-da-areia
  Caryocar glabrum (Aubl.) Pers., Caryocaraceae 114
Pequiá
  Caryocar brasiliense Camb., Caryocaraceae 114
  Caryocar coriaceum Wittm., Caryocaraceae 114
Pequiá-verdadeiro
  Caryocar villosum (Aubl.) Pers., Caryocaraceae 114
Pequiarana
  Caryocar glabrum (Aubl.) Pers., Caryocaraceae 114
Pequiarana-da-terra-firme
  Caryocar glabrum (Aubl.) Pers., Caryocaraceae 114
Pequiarana-vermelha
  Caryocar glabrum (Aubl.) Pers., Caryocaraceae 114
Pere-siriúba
  Avicennia germinans (L.) L., Verbenaceae 334
Pereira
  Geissospermum sericeum
    Benth. & Hook., Apocynaceae 24
Pereira-das-ilhas
  Tabebuia leucoxylon (L.) DC., Bignoniaceae 83
Pereiro
  Geissospermum laeve (Vell.) Baill., Apocynaceae 24
Pereiro-amarelo
  Aspidosperma nigricans Handro, Apocynaceae 21
Perexi
  Portulaca grandiflora Hook., Portulacaceae 289
Periná
  Costus spicatus (Jacq.) Sw., also
  Costus spiralis (Jacq.) Roscoe, Costaceae 132
Periquiteira
  Cochlospermum regium
    (Mart. & Schl.) Pilg., Cochlospermaceae 125
Periquiteira-da-mata
  Cochlospermum orinocense
    (H.B.K.) Steud., Cochlospermaceae 125
Periquiteira-do-campo
  Cochlospermum regium
    (Mart. & Schl.) Pilg., Cochlospermaceae 125
Periquiteira-grande-da-terra-firme
  Cochlospermum orinocense
    (H.B.K.) Steud., Cochlospermaceae 125
Periquito
  Alternanthera achyrantha R. Br., Amaranthaceae 3
Perna-de-saracura
  Raulinoreitzia tremula
    (Hook. & Arn.) King & H. Robinson, Asteraceae ... 65

Peroba
Aspidosperma discolor Benth., Apocynaceae 21
Peroba-amargosa
Aspidosperma polyneuron M. Arg., Apocynaceae 21
Peroba-rosa
Aspidosperma polyneuron M. Arg., Apocynaceae 21
Perobinha
Acosmium subelegans
(Mohlenb.) Yakovl., Fabaceae 162
Perobinha-branca
Acosmium subelegans
(Mohlenb.) Yakovl., Fabaceae 162
Perobinha-do-campo
Acosmium subelegans
(Mohlenb.) Yakovl., Fabaceae 162
Pérola-vegetal
Phyllanthus nobilis M. Arg., Euphorbiaceae 157
Perpétua-da-mata
Alternanthera brasiliana
(L.) O. Ktze., Amaranthaceae 3
Perpétua-do-brasil
Alternanthera brasiliana
(L.) O. Ktze., Amaranthaceae 3
Perpétua-do-mato
Gomphrena officinalis Mart., Amaranthaceae 4
Persicária-do-brasil
Polygonum punctatum Elliot, Polygonaceae 287
Polygonum spectabile Mart., Polygonaceae 287
Peru balsam
Myroxylon balsamum (L.) Harms, Fabaceae 170
Peruvian rhatany substitute
Krameria argentea, Krameriaceae 191
Krameria spartioides, Krameriaceae 191
USES: *Krameria tomentosa* St.-Hil., Krameriaceae . 191
Pessegueiro-bravo
Prunus subcoriacea
(Chod. & Hassl.) Hoehne, Rosaceae 294
Pessegueiro-de-curtume
Byrsonima spicata Rich., Malpighiaceae 219
Pessegueiro-do-mato
Prunus subcoriacea
(Chod. & Hassl.) Hoehne, Rosaceae 294
Petiá
Caryocar villosum (Aubl.) Pers., Caryocaraceae 114
Peúva
Tabebuia ipe (Mart.) Standl., Bignoniaceae 83
Peúva-roxa
Tabebuia ipe (Mart.) Standl., Bignoniaceae 83
Pião-branco
Jatropha curcas L., Euphorbiaceae 154
Picão
Bidens graveolens Mart., Asteraceae 56
Bidens pilosa L., Asteraceae 57
Picão-branco
Galinsoga parviflora Cav., Asteraceae 60
Picão-da-praia
Acanthospermum australe
(Loefl.) O. Ktze., Asteraceae 51
Melampodium divaricatum (Rich.) DC., Asteraceae 61

Picão-do-campo
Bidens pilosa L., Asteraceae 57
Picão-preto
Bidens pilosa L., Asteraceae 57
Pimenta-da-costa
Xylopia aromatica (Lam.) Mart., Annonaceae 15
Pimenta-d'agua, Pimenta d'água
Acmella repens (Walt.) L.C. Rich., Asteraceae 52
Polygonum acuminatum H.B.K., Polygonaceae 286
Pimenta-darta
Piper tuberculatum Jacq., Piperaceae 276
Pimenta-de-árvore
Xylopia aromatica (Lam.) Mart., Annonaceae 15
Pimenta-de-bugre
Xylopia aromatica (Lam.) Mart., Annonaceae 15
Pimenta-de-cachorro
Pilocarpus pinnatifolius Lem., Rutaceae 302
Pimenta-de-cobra
Monnieria trifolia Loefl., Rutaceae 302
Pimenta-de-folha-grande
Xylopia aromatica (Lam.) Mart., Annonaceae 15
Pimenta-de-folha-larga
Piper elongatum Vahl, Piperaceae 275
Pimenta-de-gentio
Xylopia aromatica (Lam.) Mart., Annonaceae 15
Xylopia frutescens Aubl., Annonaceae 16
Pimenta-de-lagarta
Monnieria trifolia Loefl., Rutaceae 302
Pimenta-de-macaco
Cleome polygama L., Capparaceae 112
Piper aduncum L., Piperaceae 274
Xylopia aromatica (Lam.) Mart., Annonaceae 15
Xylopia frutescens Aubl., Annonaceae 16
Pimenta-de-negro
Xylopia aromatica (Lam.) Mart., Annonaceae 15
Pimenta-do-campo
Xylopia aromatica (Lam.) Mart., Annonaceae 15
Pimenta-do-mato
Piper marginatum Jacq., Piperaceae 276
Xylopia frutescens Aubl., Annonaceae 16
Pimenta-do-sertão
Xylopia aromatica (Lam.) Mart., Annonaceae 15
Xylopia frutescens Aubl., Annonaceae 16
Pimenta-dos-índios
Piper marginatum Jacq., Piperaceae 276
Pimenta-dos-negros
Xylopia aromatica (Lam.) Mart., Annonaceae 15
Pimenta-longa
Piper aduncum L., Piperaceae 274
Piper tuberculatum Jacq., Piperaceae 276
Pimenta-matico
Piper elongatum Vahl, Piperaceae 275
Pindaíba
Styrax ferrugineum Nees & Mart., Styracaceae 325
Xylopia frutescens Aubl., Annonaceae 16
Pindaíba-preta
Guatteria nigrescens Mart., Annonaceae 14
Pindaíba-vermelha
Xylopia sericea St.-Hil., Annonaceae 16

Pindaibuna
Styrax ferrugineum Nees & Mart., Styracaceae 325
Pindó
Syagrus romanzoffiana
(Cham.) Glassman, Arecaceae 45
Pindoba
Attalea oleifera Barb. Rodr., Arecaceae 39
Pingo-pingo
Ephedra americana Willd., Ephedraceae 147
Pinguaciba
Geissospermum laeve (Vell.) Baill., Apocynaceae 24
Pinha
Annona muricata L., Annonaceae 13
Annona reticulata L., Annonaceae 13
Annona squamosa L., Annonaceae 13
Pinha-de-raiz
Lophophytum mirabile
Schott & Endl., Balanophoraceae 73
Pinha-do-brejo
Talauma ovata St.-Hil., Magnoliaceae 216
Pinha-queimadeira
Jatropha urens L., Euphorbiaceae 155
Pinhão
Jatropha curcas L., Euphorbiaceae 154
Kielmeyera speciosa St.-Hil., Clusiaceae 123
Pinhão-de-purga
Jatropha curcas L., Euphorbiaceae 154
Pinhão-do-inferno
Jatropha curcas L., Euphorbiaceae 154
Pinhão-do-paraguai
Jatropha curcas L., Euphorbiaceae 154
Pinhão-manso
Jatropha curcas L., Euphorbiaceae 154
Pinhão-roxo
Jatropha gossypiifolia L., Euphorbiaceae 154
Piolho-de-padre
Bidens pilosa L., Asteraceae 57
Pipi
Petiveria alliacea L., Phytolaccaceae 271
Piqui
Caryocar brasiliense Camb., Caryocaraceae 114
Caryocar coriaceum Wittm., Caryocaraceae 114
Caryocar villosum (Aubl.) Pers., Caryocaraceae 114
Piquiá
Caryocar villosum (Aubl.) Pers., Caryocaraceae 114
Piraguaia
Anchietea pyrifolia (Mart.) G. Don, Violaceae 338
Corynostylis hybanthus
(L.) Mart. & Zucc., Violaceae 338
Piranha
Laetia apetala Jacq., Flacourtiaceae 178
Pirarucu
Kalanchoe pinnata (Lam.) Pers., Crassulaceae 133
Piriá
Euterpe oleracea Mart., Arecaceae 42
Piriguáo
Bactris insignis (Mart.) Baill., Arecaceae 39
Piriguara
Anchietea pyrifolia (Mart.) G. Don, Violaceae 338

Piripirioca
Cyperus corymbosus Rottb., Cyperaceae 142
Pirixi
Philoxerus portulacoides St.-Hil., Amaranthaceae 5
Pissandu
Allagoptera campestris (Mart.) Kuntze, Arecaceae .. 39
Pitacaiá
Hylocereus undatus (Haw.) Br. & Rose, Cactaceae .. 95
Pitaguará
Esenbeckia intermedia Mart., Rutaceae 301
Pitanga
Eugenia sulcata Spring, Myrtaceae 254
Eugenia uniflora L., Myrtaceae 255
Pitanga-vermelha
Eugenia uniflora L., Myrtaceae 255
Pitangatuba
Eugenia uniflora L., Myrtaceae 255
Pitangueira
Eugenia uniflora L., Myrtaceae 255
Pitangueira-selvagem
Eugenia sulcata Spring, Myrtaceae 254
Pitangui
Eugenia sulcata Spring, Myrtaceae 254
Pitomba-grande-da-mata
Talisia esculenta Radlk., Sapindaceae 306
Piúva
Tabebuia serratifolia (Vahl) Nichol., Bignoniaceae .. 83
Piúva-do-charco
Tabebuia serratifolia (Vahl) Nichol., Bignoniaceae .. 83
Pixurim
Licaria puchury-major
(Mart.) Kosterm., Lauraceae 199
Pluma
Polypodium brasiliense Poir., Polypodiaceae 288
Pteridium aquilinum (L.) Kuhn, Dennstaedtiaceae . 144
Pluma-grande
Pteridium aquilinum (L.) Kuhn, Dennstaedtiaceae . 144
Pó-da bahia
Vataireopsis araroba (Aguiar) Ducke, Fabaceae 173
Pó-de-mico
Mucuna pruriens (L.) DC., Fabaceae 169
Sicyos polyacanthus Cogn., Cucurbitaceae 139
Poaia
Borreria verticillata (L.) Meyer, Rubiaceae 296
Cephaelis ipecacuanha Rich., Rubiaceae 296
Chiococca alba (L.) Hitch., Rubiaceae 297
Ionidium poaya St.-Hil., Violaceae 339
Polygala angulata DC., Polygalaceae 283
Polygala comata Mart., Polygalaceae 284
Poaia-branca
Hybanthus ipecacuanha (L.) Baill., Violaceae 339
Poaia-comprida
Borreria verticillata (L.) Meyer, Rubiaceae 296
Poaia-da-areia
Lipostoma campanuliflorum D. Don, Rubiaceae ... 299
Poaia-da-praia
Hybanthus ipecacuanha (L.) Baill., Violaceae 339
Machaonia brasiliensis Cham. & Schl., Rubiaceae 299
Manettia ignita (Vell.) K. Sch., Rubiaceae 299

Poaia-de-cipó
Machaonia brasiliensis Cham. & Schl., Rubiaceae 299
Manettia ignita (Vell.) K. Sch., Rubiaceae 299
Poaia-de-haste-comprida
Borreria verbenoides Cham. & Schl., Rubiaceae ... 296
Poaia-de-minas
Manettia ignita (Vell.) K. Sch., Rubiaceae 299
Poaia-do-arador
Borreria poaya (St.-Hil.) DC., Rubiaceae 296
Poaia-do-campo
Borreria asclepiadea Cham. & Schl., Rubiaceae ... 296
Diodia polymorpha Cham. & Schl., Rubiaceae 297
Polygala angulata DC., Polygalaceae 283
Poaia-do-cerrado
Borreria tenella Cham. & Schl., Rubiaceae 296
Poaia-do-mato
Machaonia brasiliensis Cham. & Schl., Rubiaceae 299
Manettia ignita (Vell.) K. Sch., Rubiaceae 299
Poaia-do-rio
Machaonia brasiliensis Cham. & Schl., Rubiaceae 299
Manettia ignita (Vell.) K. Sch., Rubiaceae 299
Poaia-rasteira
Borreria asclepiadea Cham. & Schl., Rubiaceae ... 296
Borreria poaya (St.-Hil.) DC., Rubiaceae 296
Poaia-rosário
Borreria verticillata (L.) Meyer, Rubiaceae 296
Pobre-velha
Costus spicatus (Jacq.) Sw., also
  Costus spiralis (Jacq.) Roscoe, Costaceae 132
Poejo
Cunila microcephala Benth., Lamiaceae 192
Cunila spicata L., Lamiaceae 192
Poejo-da-praia
Acanthospermum australe
  (Loefl.) O. Ktze., Asteraceae 51
Poejo-do-campo
Keithia denudata Benth., Lamiaceae 193
Poejo-do-mato
Manettia ignita (Vell.) K. Sch., Rubiaceae 299
Porangaba
Cordia ecalyculata Vell., Boraginaceae 87
Cordia salicifolia Cham., Boraginaceae 88
Porongo
Lagenaria siceraria
  (Molina) Standl., Cucurbitaceae 138
Potincoba
Polygonum hydropiperoides
  Michx., Polygonaceae 286
Pracajá-nambi
Tibouchina clavata
  (Pers.) Wurdack, Melastomataceae 226
Pracaxi
Pentaclethra macroloba
  (Willd.) O. Ktze., Mimosaceae 242
Praguá
Heteropteris syringifolia Gris., Malpighiaceae 220
Preciosa
Aniba canelilla (H.B.K.) Mez, Lauraceae 197
Ocotea pretiosa
  (Nees & Mart.) Benth. & Hook., Lauraceae 201

Priprioca
Cyperus corymbosus Rottb., Cyperaceae 142
Pucá
Cissus sicyoides L., Vitaceae 339
Puçá
Rauwolfia bahiensis DC., Apocynaceae 28
Pumpkin *(gerimum)*
Cucurbita pepo L., Cucurbitaceae 136
Purga-de-caboclo
Cayaponia martiana (Cogn.) Cogn., Cucurbitaceae 135
Cayaponia pilosa Cogn., Cucurbitaceae 135
Purga-de-caiapó
Cayaponia cabocla (Vell.) Mart., also
  Cayaponia spp., Cucurbitaceae 135
Cayaponia pilosa Cogn., Cucurbitaceae 135
Purga-de-campo
Hybanthus ipecacuanha (L.) Baill., Violaceae 339
Purga-de-carijó
Cayaponia espelina (Manso) Cogn., also
  Cayaponia spp., Cucurbitaceae 135
Purga-de-gentio
Cayaponia cabocla (Vell.) Mart., also
  Cayaponia spp., Cucurbitaceae 135
Cayaponia martiana
  (Cogn.) Cogn., Cucurbitaceae 135
Cayaponia pilosa Cogn., Cucurbitaceae 135
Joannesia princeps Vell., Euphorbiaceae 155
Purga-de-joão-paes
Lindernia diffusa Wettst., Scrophulariaceae 312
Purga-de-leite
Sebastiania macrocarpa M. Arg., Euphorbiaceae .. 157
Purga-de-veado
Hybanthus atropurpureus Taub., Violaceae 338
Purga-de-vento
Hybanthus atropurpureus Taub., Violaceae 338
Purga-do-campo
Dipladenia illustris M. Arg., Apocynaceae 23
Ionidium poaya St.-Hil., Violaceae 339
Purga-do-joão-paes
Luffa operculata (L.) Cogn., Cucurbitaceae 138
Purga-do-mato
Cayaponia pilosa Cogn., also
  Cayaponia spp., Cucurbitaceae 135
Purga-dos-paulistas
Joannesia princeps Vell., Euphorbiaceae 155
Luffa operculata (L.) Cogn., Cucurbitaceae 138
Purga-preta
Chiococca alba (L.) Hitch., Rubiaceae 297
Purslane
Portulaca oleracea L., Portulacaceae 289
Puru
Urera aurantiaca Wedd., Urticaceae 331
Purui
Alibertia edulis (Rich.) Rich., Rubiaceae 295
Purunara
Anchietea pyrifolia (Mart.) G. Don, Violaceae 338
Purunga
Lagenaria siceraria
  (Molina) Standl., Cucurbitaceae 138

Puxuri
Licaria puchury-major
 (Mart.) Kosterm., Lauraceae 199
Nectandra pichurim (H.B.K.) Mez, Lauraceae 200
Puxuri-bravo
Aniba puchury-minor (Mart.) Mez, Lauraceae 197
Puxuri-do-maranhão
Aniba puchury-minor (Mart.) Mez, Lauraceae 197
Puxuri-mirim
Aniba puchury-minor (Mart.) Mez, Lauraceae 197
Puxuri-pequeno
Aniba puchury-minor (Mart.) Mez, Lauraceae 197
Puxurim
Licaria puchury-major
 (Mart.) Kosterm., Lauraceae 199

Q

Quaró
Galphimia brasiliensis Juss., Malpighiaceae 220
Quassia
Quassia amara L., Simaroubaceae 314
Quássia-do-pará
Tachia guianensis Aubl., Gentianaceae 181
Quatro-patacas
Allamanda cathartica L., Apocynaceae 20
Quebra-arado
Heimia salicifolia
 (H.B.K.) Link & Otto, Lythraceae 214
Quebra-foice
Calliandra tweedii Benth., Mimosaceae 237
Quebra-pedra, Quebra-pedras
Phyllanthus acutifolius Spreng., Euphorbiaceae 156
Phyllanthus niruri L., Euphorbiaceae 156
Phyllanthus sellowianus M. Arg., Euphorbiaceae .. 157
Phyllanthus tenellus Roxb., Euphorbiaceae 157
Queimadura
Plumbago scandens L., Plumbaginaceae 279
Quenopódio
Chenopodium ambrosioides L., Chenopodiaceae ... 118
Quiabo-azedo
Hibiscus sabdariffa L., Malvaceae 221
Quiabo-de-angola
Hibiscus sabdariffa L., Malvaceae 221
Quiabo-róseo
Hibiscus sabdariffa L., Malvaceae 221
Quiabo-roxo
Hibiscus sabdariffa L., Malvaceae 221
Quina
Cestrum pseudoquina Mart., Solanaceae 317
Colletia paradoxa (Spr.) Escalante, Rhamnaceae ... 291
Naucleopsis amara Ducke, Moraceae 249
Quassia amara L., Simaroubaceae 314
Quina-amargosa
Tachia guianensis Aubl., Gentianaceae 181
Quina-branca
Strychnos pseudoquina St.-Hil., Loganiaceae 209
Quina-brava
Coutarea hexandra (Jacq.) K. Sch., Rubiaceae 297

Quina-cruzeiro
Berberis laurina Thunb., Berberidaceae 76
Strychnos pseudoquina St.-Hil., Loganiaceae 209
Strychnos trinervis (Vell.) Mart., Loganiaceae 210
Tachia guianensis Aubl., Gentianaceae 181
Quina-da-terra
Cestrum pseudoquina Mart., Solanaceae 317
Quina-de-camamu
Dipladenia illustris M. Arg., Apocynaceae 23
Quina-de-cipó
Strychnos trinervis (Vell.) Mart., Loganiaceae 210
Quina-de-folha-larga
Ladenbergia hexandra Klotz., Rubiaceae 299
Quina-de-pernambuco
Coutarea hexandra (Jacq.) K. Sch., Rubiaceae 297
Quina-de-raiz-preta
Chiococca alba (L.) Hitch., Rubiaceae 297
Quina-de-rego
Aspidosperma discolor Benth., Apocynaceae 21
Quina-de-santa-catarina
Exostemma australe St.-Hil., Rubiaceae 298
Quina-de-são-paulo
Solanum pseudoquina St.-Hil., Solanaceae 322
Quina-do-campo
Discaria americana Gill. & Hook., Rhamnaceae ... 293
Hortia brasiliensis Vand., Rutaceae 301
Quina-do-mato
Bathysa cuspidata Hook., Rubiaceae 296
Cestrum pseudoquina Mart., Solanaceae 317
Esenbeckia febrifuga Juss., Rutaceae 301
Exostemma australe St.-Hil., Rubiaceae 298
Quina-do-pará
Casearia adstringens Mart., Flacourtiaceae 176
Cestrum pseudoquina Mart., Solanaceae 317
Coutarea hexandra (Jacq.) K. Sch., Rubiaceae 297
Quina-do-paraná
Exostemma australe St.-Hil., Rubiaceae 298
Quina-do-piauí
Coutarea hexandra (Jacq.) K. Sch., Rubiaceae 297
Quina-do-rio-de-janeiro
Ladenbergia hexandra Klotz., Rubiaceae 299
Quina-do-rio-grande
Discaria americana Gill. & Hook., Rhamnaceae ... 293
Quina-do-rio-negro
Ladenbergia lambertiana Klotz., Rubiaceae 299
Quina-laranjeira
Esenbeckia febrifuga Juss., Rutaceae 301
Quina-mole
Himatanthus lancifolia
 (M. Arg.) Woods., Apocynaceae 26
Quina-quina
Ladenbergia hexandra Klotz., Rubiaceae 299
Quinarana
Geissospermum sericeum
 Benth. & Hook., Apocynaceae 24
Quingombô-de-espinho
Ibicella lutea (Lindl.) Van Eselt., Martyniaceae 224
Quinino-dos-pobres
Leonurus sibiricus L., Lamiaceae 194

Quinôa – Rosa-curandeira: Common Names Index

Quinôa
Chenopodium hircinum Schrad., Chenopodiaceae . 119
Quintilho
Nicandra physaloides (L.) Gaertn., Solanaceae 318
Quitoco
Pluchea laxiflora Hook. & Arn., Asteraceae 64
Pluchea suaveolens (Vell.) O. Ktze., Asteraceae 64
Quixaba
Bumelia sartorum Mart., Sapotaceae 308
Quixabeira
Bumelia sartorum Mart., Sapotaceae 308

R

Rabo-de-bugio
Cyathea armata (Sw.) Domin, Cyatheaceae 141
Cyathea microdonta (Desv.) Domin, Cyatheaceae . 141
Rabo-de-jacaré
Rhipsalis macrocarpa Miq., Cactaceae 97
Rabo-de-macaco
Cyathea armata (Sw.) Domin, Cyatheaceae 141
Rabo-de-rato
Lepismium myosurus Pfeiff., Cactaceae 96
Rabo-de-rojão
Solidago chilensis Meyen, Asteraceae 65
Rabo-de-tatu
Cyrtopodium andersoni R. Br., Orchidaceae 266
Rabugem-de-cachorro
Marsypianthes chamaedrys
  (Vahl) O. Ktze., Lamiaceae 194
Peltodon radicans Pohl, Lamiaceae 195
Rainha-dos-lagos
Pontederia cordifolia Mart., Pontederiaceae 288
Raivosa
Himatanthus drastica
  (Mart.) Woods., Apocynaceae 24
Raiz-amarga
Calolisianthus pendulus
  (Mart.) Gilg, Gentianaceae 179
Raiz-amargosa
Coutoubea spicata Aubl., Gentianaceae 179
Deianira nervosa Cham. & Schl., Gentianaceae 180
Raiz-de-bugre
Cayaponia tayuya (Mart.) Cogn., also
  Cayaponia spp., Cucurbitaceae 135
Raiz-de-cobra
Jatropha elliptica (Pohl) M. Arg., Euphorbiaceae .. 154
Raiz-de-frade
Chiococca alba (L.) Hitch., Rubiaceae 297
Raiz-de-joão-da-coasta
Bredemeyera floribunda Willd., Polygalaceae 283
Raiz-de-josé-domingues
Aristolochia cymbifera
  Mart. & Zucc., Aristolochiaceae 47
Raiz-de-lagarto
Jatropha elliptica (Pohl) M. Arg., Euphorbiaceae .. 154
Raiz-de-laranja
Jatropha elliptica (Pohl) M. Arg., Euphorbiaceae .. 154

Raiz-de-quina
Chiococca alba (L.) Hitch., Rubiaceae 297
Raiz-de-são-joão
Berberis laurina Thunb., Berberidaceae 76
Raiz-de-serpentária
Chiococca alba (L.) Hitch., Rubiaceae 297
Raiz-de-teiú
Jatropha elliptica (Pohl) M. Arg., Euphorbiaceae .. 154
Jatropha gossypiifolia L., Euphorbiaceae 154
Mabea fistulifera Mart., Euphorbiaceae 155
Raiz-do-padre
Gomphrena officinalis Mart., Amaranthaceae 4
Raiz-doce
Periandra mediterranea (Vell.) Taub., Fabaceae ... 170
Ranúnculo
Ranunculus bonariensis Poir., Ranunculaceae 291
Ranúnculo-aipo
Ranunculus apiifolius Pers., Ranunculaceae 290
Rapé-dos-índios
Maquira sclerophylla
  (Ducke) C. C. Berg, Moraceae 249
Ratanhia
Krameria argentea Mart., Krameriaceae 191
Krameria spartioides Berg, Krameriaceae 191
Ratanhia-da-terra
Krameria argentea Mart., Krameriaceae 191
Krameria tomentosa St.-Hil., Krameriaceae 191
Ratanhia-do-ceará
Krameria argentea Mart., Krameriaceae 191
Ratânia
Krameria spartioides Berg, Krameriaceae 191
Red mangrove
Rhizophora mangle L., Rhizophoraceae 294
Redondinho
Cabomba piauhyensis Gard., Nymphaeaceae 259
Relógio
Sida angustifolia Lam., Malvaceae 222
Sida rhombea L., Malvaceae 222
Sida rhombifolia L., Malvaceae 222
Relógio-de-vaqueiro
Sida acuta Burm., Malvaceae 221
Relógio-vassoura
Sida acuta Burm., Malvaceae 221
Resedá-amarelo
Galphimia brasiliensis Juss., Malpighiaceae 220
Ressurreição
Selaginella convoluta Spring, Selaginellaceae 313
Retirante
Acanthospermum hispidum DC., Asteraceae 52
Rinchão
Stachytarpheta cayennensis
  (Rich.) Vahl, Verbenaceae 336
Stachytarpheta dichotoma Vahl, Verbenaceae 336
Rompe-gibão
Bumelia sartorum Mart., Sapotaceae 308
Mimosa malacocentra Mart., Mimosaceae 239
Rosa-curandeira
Pereskia bleo H.B.K., Cactaceae 97

Rosa-da-turquia
Parkinsonia aculeata L., Caesalpiniaceae 104
Rosa-do-campo
Dipladenia fragrans DC., Apocynaceae 23
Dipladenia illustris M. Arg., Apocynaceae 23
Rosa-infalível
Dipladenia illustris M. Arg., Apocynaceae 23
Rosa-mole
Pereskia bleo H.B.K., Cactaceae 97
Rosca
Helicteres ovata Lam., Sterculiaceae 324
Rosela
Hibiscus sabdariffa L., Malvaceae 221
Rosewood oil
Aniba rosaeodora Ducke, Lauraceae 197
Rubim
Borreria tenella Cham. & Schl., Rubiaceae 296
Leonotis nepetaefolia R. Br., Lamiaceae 194
Leonurus sibiricus L., Lamiaceae 194
Rucurí
Scheelea phalerata
  (Mart. ex Spreng.) Burret, Arecaceae 45
Ruibarbo-do-campo
Cypella herbertii Herb., Iridaceae 186
Rutim
Desmoncus polyacanthos Mart., Arecaceae 40

S

Sabão-de-soldado
Sapindus saponaria L., Sapindaceae 306
Sabeú-una
Himatanthus drastica
  (Mart.) Woods., Apocynaceae 24
Sabiá
Mimosa caesalpiniaefolia Benth., Mimosaceae 238
Sabiá-una
Himatanthus phagedaenica
  (Mart.) Woods., Apocynaceae 26
Saboeiro
Sapindus saponaria L., Sapindaceae 306
Symplocos pubescens Klotzsch, Symplocaceae 326
Sabonete
Sapindus saponaria L., Sapindaceae 306
Saboneteira
Sapindus saponaria L., Sapindaceae 306
Sabugueiro-do-mato
Borreria verbenoides Cham. & Schl., Rubiaceae ... 296
Sacaca
Croton cajucara Benth., Euphorbiaceae 150
Saca-estrepe
Turnera ulmifolia L., Turneraceae 328
Sacarrolha
Helicteres ovata Lam., Sterculiaceae 324
Saia-branca
Datura arborea L., Solanaceae 317
Datura suaveolens Humb. & Bonpl., Solanaceae ... 318
Saião
Kalanchoe brasiliensis Camb., Crassulaceae 133

Salerma
Gomphrena officinalis Mart., Amaranthaceae 4
Salsa
Muehlenbeckia sagittifolia
  (Ort.) Meissn., Polygonaceae 285
Salsa-branca
Lippia alba (Mill.) N.E. Brown, Verbenaceae 335
Salsa-da-praia
Ipomoea acetosifolia
  (Vahl) Roem. & Schult., Convolvulaceae 130
Ipomoea pes-caprae (L.) R. Br., Convolvulaceae .. 130
Salsa-de-espinho
Herreria salsaparilha Mart., Liliaceae 207
Salsa-de-marajó
Hyptis crenata Pohl, Lamiaceae 192
Salsa-do-campo
Herreria salsaparilha Mart., Liliaceae 207
Salsa-do-rio-grande
Muehlenbeckia sagittifolia
  (Ort.) Meissn., Polygonaceae 285
Salsa-do-rio-novo
Smilax longifolia Rich., Liliaceae 208
Salsa-limão
Lippia alba (Mill.) N.E. Brown, Verbenaceae 335
Salsa-moura
Cissus palmata Poir., Vitaceae 339
Salsaparrilha
Herreria salsaparilha Mart., Liliaceae 207
Muehlenbeckia sagittifolia
  (Ort.) Meissn., Polygonaceae 285
Smilax longifolia Rich., Liliaceae 208
Salva
Hyptis crenata Pohl, Lamiaceae 192
Salva-branca
Lippia alba (Mill.) N.E. Brown, Verbenaceae 335
Salva-de-marajó
Hyptis crenata Pohl, Lamiaceae 192
Hyptis incana Briq., Lamiaceae 192
Salva-limão
Aloysia triphylla (L'Her.) Britt., Verbenaceae 332
Lippia alba (Mill.) N.E. Brown, Verbenaceae 335
Salvavidas
Maytenus ilicifolia Mart., Celastraceae 115
Peperomia rotundifolia H.B.K., Piperaceae 274
Samambaia
Pteridium aquilinum (L.) Kuhn, Dennstaedtiaceae . 144
Selaginella stellata Spring, Selaginellaceae 313
Samambaia-açu
Cyathea armata (Sw.) Domin, Cyatheaceae 141
Cyathea microdonta (Desv.) Domin, Cyatheaceae . 141
Samambaia-das-queimadas
Pteridium aquilinum (L.) Kuhn, Dennstaedtiaceae . 144
Samambaia-das-roças
Pteridium aquilinum (L.) Kuhn, Dennstaedtiaceae . 144
Samambaia-das-taperas
Pteridium aquilinum (L.) Kuhn, Dennstaedtiaceae . 144
Sambacaitá
Hyptis mutabilis (Rich.) Briq., Lamiaceae 193
Sambacão
Hyptis mutabilis (Rich.) Briq., Lamiaceae 193

Sambacuité
  Hyptis mutabilis (Rich.) Briq., Lamiaceae 193
Sambaíba
  Curatella americana L., Dilleniaceae 144
  Doliocarpus rolandri Gmel., Dilleniaceae 146
Sambaibinha
  Davilla rugosa Poir., Dilleniaceae 145
Sambaité
  Hyptis mutabilis (Rich.) Briq., Lamiaceae 193
Sanandu
  Erythrina corallodendron L., Fabaceae 166
  Erythrina falcata Benth., Fabaceae 166
Sananduva
  Erythrina corallodendron L., Fabaceae 166
  Erythrina crista-galli L., Fabaceae 166
Sangue-de-drago
  Croton salutaris Casar., Euphorbiaceae 151
  Croton urucurana Baill., Euphorbiaceae 151
Santa-maria
  Allamanda cathartica L., Apocynaceae 20
  Ocimum fluminensis Vell., Lamiaceae 195
  Peltodon longipes St.-Hil., Lamiaceae 195
Santa-rita
  Laplacea fruticosa (Schr.) Kobuski, Theaceae 326
São-joão
  Senna bicapsularis (L.) Roxb., Caesalpiniaceae 104
São-joão-caá
  Unxia camphorata L. f., Asteraceae 67
São-raimundo
  Kalanchoe pinnata (Lam.) Pers., Crassulaceae 133
Sapatinho-de-iaiá
  Tropaeolum pentaphyllum Lam., Tropaeolaceae 327
Sapatinho-do-diabo
  Tropaeolum pentaphyllum Lam., Tropaeolaceae 327
Sapê
  Andropogon bicornis L., Poaceae 279
  Imperata brasiliensis Trin., Poaceae 281
Sapê-macho
  Solidago chilensis Meyen, Asteraceae 65
Sapo-taia
  Capparis cynophallophora L., Capparaceae 111
Sapopema
  Aspidosperma nitidum Benth., Apocynaceae 21
Sapoti
  Manilkara zapota (L.) Van Royen, Sapotaceae 309
Sapotizeiro
  Manilkara zapota (L.) Van Royen, Sapotaceae 309
Sapucaia
  Lecythis amara Aubl., Lecythidaceae 206
Sapucaia-amargosa
  Lecythis amara Aubl., Lecythidaceae 206
Sapucainha
  Carpotroche brasiliensis
    (Raddi) Endl., Flacourtiaceae 176
Sapupira
  Bowdichia nitida Spruce ex Benth., Fabaceae 163
Saputá
  Peritassa calypsoides
    (Camb.) A.C. Sm., Hippocrateaceae 183

Salacia impressifolia
  (Miers) A.C. Sm., Hippocrateaceae 183
Saracura
  Ludwigia natans (H.B.K.) Ell., Onagraceae 264
Saracura-muirá
  Ampelozizyphus amazonicus Ducke, Rhamnaceae . 291
Sarandi
  Phyllanthus sellowianus M. Arg., Euphorbiaceae .. 157
  Pouteria salicifolia Hook. & Arn., Sapotaceae 310
Sarandi-branco
  Phyllanthus sellowianus M. Arg., Euphorbiaceae .. 157
Sarandi-vermelho
  Phyllanthus sellowianus M. Arg., Euphorbiaceae .. 157
Sarsaparilla
  Smilax longifolia Rich., Liliaceae 208
Sassafrás
  Ocotea pretiosa
    (Nees & Mart.) Benth. & Hook., Lauraceae 201
Sassafrás-do-amazonas
  Ocotea cymbarum H.B.K., Lauraceae 200
Sassafrás-do-pará
  Ocotea cymbarum H.B.K., Lauraceae 200
Sebepira
  Bowdichia nitida Spruce ex Benth., Fabaceae 163
Seda-vegetal
  Araujia sericifera Brot., Asclepiadaceae 50
Segurelha-brava
  Seguieria americana L., Phytolaccaceae 272
Selidônia
  Boerhavia coccinea Mill., Nyctaginaceae 257
Sem-vergonha
  Pereskia bleo H.B.K., Cactaceae 97
Sempreviva
  Leiothrix flavescens (Bong.) Ruhl., Eriocaulaceae .. 148
Sene-do-campo
  Chamaecrista cathartica
    (Mart.) Ir. & Barn., Caesalpiniaceae 101
Senna
  Senna affinis (Benth.) Ir.
    & Barn., CHEM., Caesalpiniaceae 104
Sensitiva
  Chamaecrista mimosoides
    (L.) Ir. & Barn., Caesalpiniaceae 102
  Mimosa pudica L., Mimosaceae 240
  Mimosa velloziana Mart., Mimosaceae 240
Sereíba-tinga
  Avicennia germinans (L.) L., Verbenaceae 334
Sertão
  Leonurus sibiricus L., Lamiaceae 194
Sessenta-feridas
  Acacia paniculata Willd., Mimosaceae 236
Sete-marias
  Cleome spinosa Jacq., Capparaceae 112
Sete-sangrias
  Cuphea aperta Koehne, Lythraceae 213
  Cuphea balsamona Cham., Lythraceae 213
  Cuphea carthagenensis
    (Jacq.) MacBride, Lythraceae 213
  Cuphea ingrata Cham. & Schl., Lythraceae 214

Declieuxia cordigera Mart. & Zucc., Rubiaceae 297
Heliotropium lanceolatum Loefgr., Boraginaceae 89
Polycarpaea corymbosa
   (L.) Lam., Caryophyllaceae 115
Symplocos parviflora Benth., Symplocaceae 326
Symplocos platyphylla
   (Pohl) Benth., Symplocaceae 326
Symplocos pubescens Klotzsch, Symplocaceae 326
Sete-sangrias-do-campo
Cuphea carthagenensis
   (Jacq.) MacBride, Lythraceae 214
Silva-da-praia
Caesalpinia bonduc (L.) Roxb., Caesalpiniaceae 99
Simaruba
Simarouba amara Aubl., Simaroubaceae 315
Simaruba-copaia
Jacaranda copaia (Aubl.) D. Don, Bignoniaceae 80
Simaruba-falsa
Jacaranda copaia (Aubl.) D. Don, Bignoniaceae 80
Siriúba
Avicennia germinans (L.) L., Verbenaceae 334
Sobro
Aspidosperma polyneuron M. Arg., Apocynaceae 21
Soldanela
Nymphoides indica (L.) O. Ktze., Menyanthaceae . 235
Soldanela-d'água
Nymphoides indica (L.) O. Ktze., Menyanthaceae . 235
Solidônia
Boerhavia coccinea Mill., Nyctaginaceae 257
Boerhavia paniculata Rich., Nyctaginaceae 258
Trixis antimenorrhoea (Schrank) Mart., Asteraceae . 67
Sombra-de-touro
Acanthosyris spinescens
   (Mart. & Endl.) Gris., Santalaceae 304
Jodina rhombifolia Hook. & Arn., Santalaceae 304
Maytenus ilicifolia Mart., Celastraceae 115
Vitex montevidensis Cham., Verbenaceae 337
Sorva
Couma macrocarpa B. Rodr., Apocynaceae 23
Couma utilis (Mart.) M. Arg., Apocynaceae 23
Sorva-da-mata
Couma macrocarpa B. Rodr., Apocynaceae 23
Sorva-do-pará
Couma utilis (Mart.) M. Arg., Apocynaceae 23
Sorva-pequena
Couma utilis (Mart.) M. Arg., Apocynaceae 23
Sorveira
Couma macrocarpa B. Rodr., Apocynaceae 23
Couma utilis (Mart.) M. Arg., Apocynaceae 23
Sorvinha
Couma utilis (Mart.) M. Arg., Apocynaceae 23
Zschokkea arborescens M. Arg., Apocynaceae 29
Suaçucaá
Elephantopus mollis H.B.K., Asteraceae 59
Suçuaiá
Elephantopus micropappus Less., Asteraceae 59
Elephantopus mollis H.B.K., Asteraceae 59
Sucuba
Himatanthus sucuuba (Spr.) Woods., Apocynaceae . 26

Sucuíba
Himatanthus phagedaenica
   (Mart.) Woods., Apocynaceae 26
Sucupira
Bowdichia nitida Spruce ex Benth., Fabaceae 163
Bowdichia virgilioides H.B.K., Fabaceae 163
Ouratea hexasperma (St.-Hil.) Baill., Ochnaceae .. 261
Sucupira-açu
Bowdichia virgilioides H.B.K., Fabaceae 163
Sucupira-amarela
Bowdichia virgilioides H.B.K., Fabaceae 163
Sweetia fruticosa Spreng., Fabaceae 172
Sucupira-branca
Bowdichia virgilioides H.B.K., Fabaceae 163
Pterodon apparicioi Peders., Fabaceae 170
Pterodon pubescens Benth., Fabaceae 171
Sucupira-do-campo
Bowdichia virgilioides H.B.K., Fabaceae 163
Sucupira-do-cerrado
Bowdichia virgilioides H.B.K., Fabaceae 163
Sucuriju
Mikania lindleyana DC., Asteraceae 62
Sucuuba
Himatanthus drastica
   (Mart.) Woods., Apocynaceae 24
Himatanthus fallax
   (M. Arg.) Woods., Apocynaceae 25
Himatanthus phagedaenica
   (Mart.) Woods., Apocynaceae 26
Himatanthus sucuuba (Spr.) Woods., Apocynaceae . 26
Suê
Solanum nigrum L., Solanaceae 321
Suinã
Erythrina corallodendron L., Fabaceae 166
Erythrina crista-galli L., Fabaceae 166
Erythrina falcata Benth., Fabaceae 166
Erythrina fusca Lour., Fabaceae 166
Sumaré
Cyrtopodium andersoni R. Br., Orchidaceae 266
Sumaré-da-mata
Cyrtopodium punctatum Lindl., Orchidaceae 266
Sumaré-da-pedra
Cyrtopodium andersoni R. Br., Orchidaceae 266
Sumaré-do-pau
Cyrtopodium punctatum Lindl., Orchidaceae 266
Sumaúma
Ceiba pentandra (L.) Gaertn., Bombacaceae 86
Sumaumeira
Ceiba pentandra (L.) Gaertn., Bombacaceae 86
Sumaumeira-da-várzea
Ceiba pentandra (L.) Gaertn., Bombacaceae 86
Surineia
Nectandra puberula Nees, Lauraceae 200
Surucuina
Eclipta prostrata (L.) L., Asteraceae 59
Sururu
Passiflora mucronata Lam., Passifloraceae 270

T

Tabacarana
  Pluchea suaveolens (Vell.) O. Ktze., Asteraceae 64
Tabua
  Typha domingensis Pers., Typhaceae 328
Tachi
  Triplaris weigeltiana
    (Reichb.) O. Ktze., Polygonaceae 287
Tachi-preto-da-várzea
  Triplaris weigeltiana
    (Reichb.) O. Ktze., Polygonaceae 287
Tachizeiro
  Triplaris weigeltiana
    (Reichb.) O. Ktze., Polygonaceae 287
Tahebo
  Tabebuia umbellata (Sond.) Sandw.,
    Uses, Bignoniaceae 83
Taiá-açu
  Xanthosoma violaceum Schott, Araceae 37
Taiarana
  Xanthosoma violaceum Schott, Araceae 37
Taioba
  Xanthosoma violaceum Schott, Araceae 37
Taioba-verdadeira
  Xanthosoma violaceum Schott, Araceae 37
Taiuiá
  Cayaponia spp., see *Cayaponia tayuya*
    (Mart.) Cogn., Chem., Cucurbitaceae 135
  Trianosperma glandulosa Mart., Cucurbitaceae 140
  Wilbrandia ebracteata Cogn., Cucurbitaceae 140
Taiuiá-de-pimenta
  Cayaponia martiana (Cogn.) Cogn., also
    Cayaponia spp., Cucurbitaceae 135
Taiuiá-grande
  Cayaponia martiana (Cogn.) Cogn., also
    Cayaponia spp., Cucurbitaceae 135
Taiuiá-miúdo
  Melothria fluminensis Gardn., Cucurbitaceae 139
Taiyiá
  Cayaponia martiana (Cogn.) Cogn., also
    Cayaponia spp., Cucurbitaceae 135
Tajá
  Caladium bicolor (Aiton) Vent., Araceae 34
Tajá-de-cobra
  Dracontium asperum K. Koch, Araceae 35
Tajuba
  Maclura tinctoria (L.) D. Don, Moraceae 249
Talaúma
  Talauma ovata St.-Hil., Magnoliaceae 216
Tamacoaré
  Caraipa insidiosa B. Rodr., Clusiaceae 121
Tamacoari
  Caraipa densifolia Mart., Clusiaceae 121
Tamacuari
  Caraipa densifolia Mart., Clusiaceae 121
Tamanqueira
  Ocotea guianensis Aubl., Lauraceae 201

Zanthoxylum rhoifolium Lam., Rutaceae 303
Tamanqueira-da-terra-firme
  Zanthoxylum rhoifolium Lam., Rutaceae 303
Tamaquaré
  Caraipa excelsa Ducke, Clusiaceae 121
  Caraipa insidiosa B. Rodr., Clusiaceae 121
Tamaquaré-brando
  Caraipa densifolia Mart., Clusiaceae 121
Tamaquaré-do-cerrado
  Caraipa densifolia Mart., Clusiaceae 121
Tamaquaré-grande
  Caraipa grandifolia Mart., Clusiaceae 121
Tamaquaré-miudo
  Caraipa minor Huber, Clusiaceae 121
Tamaquari
  Caraipa densifolia Mart., Clusiaceae 121
Tamiarana
  Dalechampia ficifolia Lam., Euphorbiaceae 152
  Tragia volubilis L., Euphorbiaceae 158
Tamaquari-miudo
  Caraipa minor Huber, Clusiaceae 121
Tamurá-tuira
  Tabebuia serratifolia (Vahl) Nichol., Bignoniaceae .. 83
Tanchagem
  Plantago brasiliensis Sims, Plantaginaceae 278
  Plantago guilleminiana Dcne., Plantaginaceae 278
Tanchagem-miúda
  Plantago myosurus Lam., Plantaginaceae 278
Tangará
  Boerhavia coccinea Mill., Nyctaginaceae 257
Tangaraca
  Boerhavia coccinea Mill., Nyctaginaceae 257
Tangaraca-açu
  Coccoloba arborescens
    (Vell.) How., Polygonaceae 285
Tangarana
  Triplaris weigeltiana
    (Reichb.) O. Ktze., Polygonaceae 287
Tanibouca
  Terminalia tanibouca Smith, Combretaceae 126
Tanrigudinho
  Boerhavia paniculata Rich., Nyctaginaceae 258
Tansy
  Tanacetum vulgare L., Asteraceae 67
Tapaciriba
  Andradea floribunda Fr. All., Nyctaginaceae 257
  Pisonia aculeata L., Nyctaginaceae 258
Tapaciriba-amarela
  Andradea floribunda Fr. All., Nyctaginaceae 257
Tapaciriba-branca
  Pisonia alcalina Fr. All., Nyctaginaceae 258
Taperebá
  Spondias mombin L., Anacardiaceae 10
Taperebá-açu
  Spondias macrocarpa Engl., Anacardiaceae 10
Taperibá
  Spondias mombin L., Anacardiaceae 10
Tapiá
  Crataeva tapia L., Capparaceae 112

Tapicuru
Peritassa calypsoides
 (Camb.) A.C. Sm., Hippocrateaceae 183
Tapinhoã-amarelo
Pouteria laurifolia Radlk., Sapotaceae 309
Tapirapecu
Elephantopus mollis H.B.K., Asteraceae 59
Tapixava
Scoparia dulcis L., Scrophulariaceae 312
Tapuoca
Himatanthus lancifolia
 (M. Arg.) Woods., Apocynaceae 26
Taquari-do-mato
Panicum brevifolium L., Poaceae 282
Taquera
Lagenaria siceraria
 (Molina) Standl., Cucurbitaceae 138
Tariri
Picramnia ciliata Mart., Simaroubaceae 314
Taropé
Dorstenia brasiliensis Lam., Moraceae 247
Tarumã
Vitex montevidensis Cham., Verbenaceae 337
Tarumã-romã
Vitex montevidensis Cham., Verbenaceae 337
Tasneira
Tanacetum vulgare L., Asteraceae 67
Tasneirinha
Senecio brasiliensis Less., Asteraceae 65
Tataíba
Maclura brasiliensis Endl., Moraceae 249
Tatajuba
Maclura tinctoria (L.) D. Don, Moraceae 249
Tatajuba-do-brejo
Maclura brasiliensis Endl., Moraceae 249
Tatu
Agonandra brasiliensis Miers, Opiliaceae 265
Tatu-cáa
Eugenia supra-axillaris Spring, Myrtaceae 254
Taúba
Maclura tinctoria (L.) D. Don, Moraceae 249
Teim
Jatropha elliptica (Pohl) M. Arg., Euphorbiaceae .. 154
Teiú-iba
Jatropha elliptica (Pohl) M. Arg., Euphorbiaceae .. 154
Tejuíba
Jatropha elliptica (Pohl) M. Arg., Euphorbiaceae .. 154
Tembetari
Zanthoxylum hyemale St.-Hil., Rutaceae 302
Tembetaru
Zanthoxylum hyemale St.-Hil., Rutaceae 302
Zanthoxylum rhoifolium Lam., Rutaceae 303
Zanthoxylum tingoassuiba St.-Hil., Rutaceae 303
Thorn-apple
Datura stramonium L., Solanaceae 318
Tiborna
Himatanthus drastica
 (Mart.) Woods., Apocynaceae 24
Himatanthus phagedaenica
 (Mart.) Woods., Apocynaceae 26
Tiborna-traiçoeira
Himatanthus fallax
 (M. Arg.) Woods., Apocynaceae 25
Tigarea
Tetracera aspera Willd., Dilleniaceae 146
Timbó
Araujia sericifera Brot., Asclepiadaceae 50
Timbó-açu
Magonia pubescens St.-Hil., Sapindaceae 305
Timbó-de-raiz
Dahlstedtia pinnata (Benth.) Malme, Fabaceae 163
Timbó-manso
Monstera adansonii Schott, Araceae 36
Timbó-mirim
Indigofera suffruticosa Mill., Fabaceae 168
Timbopeba
Magonia pubescens St.-Hil., Sapindaceae 305
Timborana
Arrabidaea foetida Bur. & K. Sch., Bignoniaceae 79
Timutu
Polygala timoutou Aubl., Polygalaceae 284
Tinguá-ab
Tachia guianensis Aubl., Gentianaceae 181
Tinguaciba
Zanthoxylum rhoifolium Lam., Rutaceae 303
Zanthoxylum tingoassuiba St.-Hil., Rutaceae 303
Tinguaciba-do-pará
Tachia guianensis Aubl., Gentianaceae 181
Tinguciba
Zanthoxylum rhoifolium Lam., Rutaceae 303
Tinguí
Magonia pubescens St.-Hil., Sapindaceae 305
Tinguí-açu
Magonia pubescens St.-Hil., Sapindaceae 305
Tinguí-da-praia
Buddleja brasiliensis Jacq. ex Spr., Buddlejaceae 93
Tinguí-de-cola
Magonia pubescens St.-Hil., Sapindaceae 305
Tinguí-de-leite
Thevetia ahouai (L.) DC., Apocynaceae 28
Tinguí-do-cerrado
Magonia pubescens St.-Hil., Sapindaceae 305
Tinhorão
Caladium bicolor (Aiton) Vent., Araceae 34
Tipi
Petiveria alliacea L., Phytolaccaceae 271
Tiriba
Callisthene major Mart., Vochysiaceae 340
Tiririca
Cyperus gracilescens
 Roem. & Schult., Cyperaceae 142
Cyperus rotundus L., Cyperaceae 142
Hypolytrum laxum Schrad., Cyperaceae 143
Scleria pratensis L., Cyperaceae 143
Tiú
Dorstenia brasiliensis Lam., Moraceae 247
Jatropha elliptica (Pohl) M. Arg., Euphorbiaceae .. 154

Toé
Datura insignis B. Rodr., Solanaceae 318
Tolu balsam
Myroxylon balsamum (L.) Harms, Fabaceae 170
Tomba
Cayaponia tayuya (Mart.) Cogn., also
Cayaponia spp., Cucurbitaceae 135
Tonka bean
Dipteryx odorata (Aubl.) Willd., Fabaceae 166
Topa
Ochroma pyramidale (Cav.) Urb., Bombacaceae 86
Topete-de-cardeal
Calliandra tweedii Benth., Mimosaceae 237
Torém
Cecropia palmata Willd., Moraceae 247
Touca-do-diabo
Aristolochia cymbifera
Mart. & Zucc., Aristolochiaceae 47
Tracuá
Philodendron imbe Schott, Araceae 36
Tramanhem
Vernonanthura brasiliana
(L.) H. Robinson, Asteraceae 67
Trapiá
Crataeva benthamii Eichl., Capparaceae 112
Crataeva tapia L., Capparaceae 112
Trapoeraba
Commelina nudiflora L., Commelinaceae 126
Commelina platyphylla
Klotz. ex Seub., Commelinaceae 127
Commelina virginica L., Commelinaceae 128
Dichorisandra affinis Mart., Commelinaceae 128
Tradescantia diuretica Mart., Commelinaceae 128
Trapoeraba-açu
Commelina robusta Kunth, Commelinaceae 128
Tradescantia spathacea Sw., Commelinaceae 129
Trapoeraba-azul
Commelina nudiflora L., Commelinaceae 126
Commelina pohliana Seub., Commelinaceae 127
Commelina vestita Seub., Commelinaceae 128
Commelina virginica L., Commelinaceae 128
Dichorisandra leucophthalmos
Hook., Commelinaceae 128
Trapoeraba-rana
Commelina nudiflora L., Commelinaceae 126
Trapoeraba-verdadeira
Tradescantia diuretica Mart., Commelinaceae 128
Trapoerba-branca
Tradescantia effusa Mart., Commelinaceae 129
Três-corações
Oxalis corniculata L., Oxalidaceae 266
Três-folhas
Esenbeckia febrifuga Juss., Rutaceae 301
Três-folhas-vermelha
Esenbeckia febrifuga Juss., Rutaceae 301
Trevo
Oxalis corniculata L., Oxalidaceae 266
Trevo-do-campo
Desmodium triflorum DC., Fabaceae 164

Tripa-de-galinha
Dalbergia gracilis Benth., Fabaceae 163
Trombeta
Datura stramonium L., Solanaceae 318
Trombeta-branca
Datura arborea L., Solanaceae 317
Trombeta-cheirosa
Datura suaveolens Humb. & Bonpl., Solanaceae ... 318
Trombeteira
Datura arborea L., Solanaceae 317
Tuampoca
Trichilia barraensis DC., Meliaceae 229
Tuapoca
Trichilia barraensis DC., Meliaceae 229
Tucujá
Zschokkea arborescens M. Arg., Apocynaceae 29
Tuia
Smilax oblongifolia Pohl, Liliaceae 208
Tuna
Cereus peruvianus (L.) Mill., Cactaceae 95
Tuparapo
Tachia guianensis Aubl., Gentianaceae 181
Tuparobá
Tachia guianensis Aubl., Gentianaceae 181
Tuparubo
Tachia guianensis Aubl., Gentianaceae 181
Tupeiçaba
Buddleja stachioides Cham., Buddlejaceae 93
Tupeiçava
Scoparia dulcis L., Scrophulariaceae 312
Tupiçaba
Scoparia dulcis L., Scrophulariaceae 312
Tupitixa
Sida rhombea L., Malvaceae 222
Sida rhombifolia L., Malvaceae 222
Tupitixá
Sida acuta Burm., Malvaceae 221
Tupixaba
Scoparia dulcis L., Scrophulariaceae 312
Turco
Parkinsonia aculeata L., Caesalpiniaceae 104
Turubi
Julocroton stipularis M. Arg., Euphorbiaceae 155
Tutiriba
Lucuma rivicoa Gaertn., Sapotaceae 309

U

Uá-iandi
Calophyllum brasiliense Camb., Clusiaceae 120
Uaçacu
Hura crepitans L., Euphorbiaceae 153
Uachuá
Saccoglottis guianensis Benth., Humiriaceae 185
Uaco
Mikania cordifolia (L. f.) Willd., Asteraceae 61
Uacu
Monopteryx uacu Spruce ex Benth., Fabaceae 169

Uacurí
Scheelea phalerata
(Mart. ex Spreng.) Burret, Arecaceae 45
Uafé
Urera subpeltata Miq., Urticaceae 331
Uaimiuru
Salacia impressifolia
(Miers) A.C. Sm., Hippocrateaceae 183
Uanani
Symphonia globulifera L. f., Clusiaceae 123
Uapé
Nymphaea rudgeana G. Meyer, Nymphaeaceae 259
Uauaçu
Attalea spectabilis Mart., Arecaceae 39
Uaxuá
Saccoglottis guianensis Benth., Humiriaceae 185
Ubá
Gynerium parviflorum Nees, Poaceae 281
Ubacaia, Ubá-caiá
Costus cuspidatus
(Nees & Mart.) Maas, Costaceae 132
Costus spicatus (Jacq.) Sw., also
Costus spiralis (Jacq.) Roscoe, Costaceae 132
Ubatã
Astronium fraxinifolium Schott, Anacardiaceae 9
Ubirarema
Seguieria americana L., Phytolaccaceae 272
Ucansanção
Jatropha urens L., Euphorbiaceae 155
Ucuhuba *(ucuuba)*
Virola macrophylla
(Spr. ex Benth.) Warb., Myristicaceae 250
Ucuuba
Virola macrophylla
(Spr. ex Benth.) Warb., Myristicaceae 250
Virola sebifera Aubl., Myristicaceae 250
Virola surinamensis (Rol.) Warb., Myristicaceae 252
Ucuuba-branca
Virola surinamensis (Rol.) Warb., Myristicaceae 252
Ucuuba-cheirosa
Virola surinamensis (Rol.) Warb., Myristicaceae 252
Ucuuba-da-terra-firme
Virola sebifera Aubl., Myristicaceae 250
Ucuuba-vermelha
Virola sebifera Aubl., Myristicaceae 250
Uirarí-terém
Strychnos subcordata Spr. ex Benth., Loganiaceae 210
Umari
Geoffroea striata (Willd.) Morong, Fabaceae 168
Umbamba
Desmoncus polyacanthos Mart., Arecaceae 40
Umbaru
Hibiscus cannabinus L., Malvaceae 221
Umbu-caá
Aristolochia cymbifera
Mart. & Zucc., Aristolochiaceae 47
Aristolochia trilobata L., Aristolochiaceae 48
Umiri
Humiria balsamifera (Aubl.) St.-Hil., Humiriaceae 183

Umiri-de-cheiro
Humiria balsamifera (Aubl.) St.-Hil., Humiriaceae 183
Umiri-do-pará
Humiria balsamifera (Aubl.) St.-Hil., Humiriaceae 183
Umirizeiro
Humiria balsamifera (Aubl.) St.-Hil., Humiriaceae 183
Unha-de-boi
Bauhinia candicans Benth., Caesalpiniaceae 99
Bauhinia langsdorffiana Bong., Caesalpiniaceae 99
Unha-de-gato
Acacia paniculata Willd., Mimosaceae 236
Macfadyena unguis-cati (L.) Gentry, Bignoniaceae . 81
Mimosa bimucronata (DC.) O. Ktze., Mimosaceae 238
Mimosa malacocentra Mart., Mimosaceae 239
Unha-de-vaca
Bauhinia candicans Benth., Caesalpiniaceae 99
Bauhinia forficata Link, Caesalpiniaceae 99
Urtiga
Dalechampia scandens L., Euphorbiaceae 152
Jatropha urens L., Euphorbiaceae 155
Pilea microphylla (L.) Liebm., Urticaceae 331
Urtiga-branca
Urera aurantiaca Wedd., Urticaceae 331
Urtiga-brava
Urera baccifera Gaud., Urticaceae 331
Urera caracasana Jacq., Urticaceae 331
Urtiga-de-folha-grande
Laportea aestuans (L.) Chew, Urticaceae 330
Urtiga-fogo
Urera baccifera Gaud., Urticaceae 331
Urtiga-grande
Laportea aestuans (L.) Chew, Urticaceae 330
Urera baccifera Gaud., Urticaceae 331
Urera subpeltata Miq., Urticaceae 331
Urtiga-mansa
Boehmeria caudata Sw., Urticaceae 330
Urtiga-vermelha
Laportea aestuans (L.) Chew, Urticaceae 330
Urera baccifera Gaud., Urticaceae 331
Urtigão
Urera baccifera Gaud., Urticaceae 331
Urera subpeltata Miq., Urticaceae 331
Urtiguinha-de-cipó
Tragia volubilis L., Euphorbiaceae 158
Uru-de-pobre
Tradescantia spathacea Sw., Commelinaceae 129
Urubamba
Desmoncus orthacanthos Mart., Arecaceae 40
Urubu-caá
Aristolochia gigantea
Mart. & Zucc., Aristolochiaceae 48
Urucu
Bixa orellana L., Bixaceae 85
Urucum
Bixa orellana L., Bixaceae 85
also see *B. orellana* under USES:
Physalis angulata L., Solanaceae 318
Urucurana
Croton urucurana Baill., Euphorbiaceae 151

Urucuri – Vilanova: Common Names Index

Urucuri
Syagrus coronata (Mart.) Becc., Arecaceae 45
Syagrus schizophylla (Mart.) Glassman, Arecaceae . 46
Urum
Desmoncus orthacanthos Mart., Arecaceae 40
Urumbeba
Brasilopuntia brasiliensis (Willd.) Berg., Cactaceae 95
Hylocereus undatus (Haw.) Br. & Rose, Cactaceae .. 95
Urumbeva
Cereus peruvianus (L.) Mill., Cactaceae 95
Opuntia vulgaris Mill., Cactaceae 97
Urundeúva
Myracroduon urundeuva
Fr. All., Anacardiaceae 9
Uruparaíba
Tabebuia leucoxylon (L.) DC., Bignoniaceae 83
Utuapoca
Guarea spiciflora Juss., Meliaceae 227
Trichilia barraensis DC., Meliaceae 229
Uva-de-espinho
Berberis laurina Thunb., Berberidaceae 76
Uva-de-gentio
Abuta selloana Eichl., Menispermaceae 231
Uva-do-campo
Cissus salutaris H.B.K., Vitaceae 339
Uva-do-mato
Chondodendron platyphyllum
(Mart.) Miers, Menispermaceae 231
Uva-espim-do-brasil
Berberis laurina Thunb., Berberidaceae 76
Uxi-de-morcego
Andira retusa (Poir.) H.B.K., Fabaceae 162
Uxirana
Andira retusa (Poir.) H.B.K., Fabaceae 162

V

Vapuronga
Marlierea tomentosa Camb., Myrtaceae 255
Vassoura
Baccharis dracunculifolia DC., Asteraceae 54
Baccharis trimera (Less.) DC., Asteraceae 54
Buddleja brasiliensis Jacq. ex Spr., Buddlejaceae 93
Buddleja stachioides Cham., Buddlejaceae 93
Diodia polymorpha Cham. & Schl., Rubiaceae 297
Sida carpinifolia (L. f.) K. Sch., Malvaceae 222
Sida rhombea L., Malvaceae 222
Vassoura-de-ferro
Raulinoreitzia tremula (Hook. & Arn.)
King & H. Robinson, Asteraceae 65
Vassoura-do-campo
Dodonaea viscosa Jacq., Sapindaceae 305
Vassoura-preta
Sida acuta Burm., Malvaceae 221
Vassoura-vermelha
Dodonaea viscosa Jacq., Sapindaceae 305
Vassourinha
Baccharis dracunculifolia DC., Asteraceae 54
Buddleja stachioides Cham., Buddlejaceae 93

Diodia polymorpha Cham. & Schl., Rubiaceae 297
Heimia salicifolia
(H.B.K.) Link & Otto, Lythraceae 214
Scoparia dulcis L., Scrophulariaceae 312
Sida acuta Burm., Malvaceae 221
Sida carpinifolia (L. f.) K. Sch., Malvaceae 222
Sida rhombea L., Malvaceae 222
Sida rhombifolia L., Malvaceae 222
Vassourinha-de-botão
Scoparia dulcis L., Scrophulariaceae 312
Vassourinha-de-relógio
Sida angustifolia Lam., Malvaceae 222
Vassourinha-do-campo
Conobea scoparioides Benth., Scrophulariaceae 311
Vassourinha-doce
Hyptis plectranthoides Benth., Lamiaceae 193
Vassourinha-miuda
Sida micrantha St.-Hil., Malvaceae 222
Velame
Croton triqueter Lam., Euphorbiaceae 151
Croton urucurana Baill., Euphorbiaceae 151
Velame-branco
Macrosiphonia longiflora
(Desf.) M. Arg., Apocynaceae 26
Macrosiphonia velame
(St.-Hil.) M. Arg., Apocynaceae 26
Velame-de-cheiro
Croton floribundus Spreng., Euphorbiaceae 150
Velame-do-campo
Julocroton humilis Diedr., Euphorbiaceae 155
Velame-do-mato
Solanum cernuum Vell., Solanaceae 319
Velame-do-rio-grande-do-sul
Macrosiphonia longiflora
(Desf.) M. Arg., Apocynaceae 26
Macrosiphonia velame
(St.-Hil.) M. Arg., Apocynaceae 26
Veludinha
Guettarda uruguayensis
Cham. & Schl., Rubiaceae 298
Ventre-livre
Piper callosum R. & Pav., Piperaceae 274
Verbasco
Buddleja brasiliensis Jacq. ex Spr., Buddlejaceae 93
Verbena-falsa
Stachytarpheta cayennensis
(Rich.) Vahl, Verbenaceae 336
Stachytarpheta dichotoma Vahl, Verbenaceae 336
Verbena-melindre
Glandularia peruviana (L.) Small, Verbenaceae ... 334
Verga-tesa
Galactia peduncularis (Benth.) Taub., Fabaceae ... 168
Vergonha
Mimosa pudica L., Mimosaceae 240
Vermelho
Tetracera volubilis L., Dilleniaceae 146
Verônica
Dalbergia subcymosa Ducke, Fabaceae 164
Vilanova
Parthenium hysterophorus L., Asteraceae 64

Vinagreira
  Hibiscus sabdariffa L., Malvaceae 221
Vindecaá
  Panicum brevifolium L., Poaceae 282
Vinheiro-do-campo
  Vochysia thyrsoidea Pohl, Vochysiaceae 340
Vinho de coco
  Cocos nucifera L., USES, Arecaceae 45
Vinho de jurema
  Mimosa hostilis Benth.: USES, Mimosaceae 238
Violeta-de-petrópolis
  Angelonia integerrima Spreng., Scrophulariaceae .. 310
Violeta-do-campo
  Angelonia integerrima Spreng., Scrophulariaceae .. 310
Vira-vira
  Lucilia nitens Less., Asteraceae 61
Visgueiro
  Parkia oppositifolia (Spruce) Benth., Mimosaceae 240
Visguero
  Parkia pectinata Benth., Mimosaceae 240
Vitória-régia
  Victoria amazonica
  (Poepp.) Sower., Nymphaeaceae 260
Voandeira
  Ilex brevicuspis Reiss., Aquifoliaceae 31

W

Water hyacinth
  Eichhornia crassipes Solms, Pontederiaceae 288
West Indian arrowroot
  Maranta arundinacea L., Marantaceae 223
Wormwood
  Artemisia absinthium: see USES *Bacchaaris articulata*
  (Lam.) Pers., Asteraceae 54

X

Ximbuí
  Peperomia pellucida H.B.K., Piperaceae 273

Z

Zabumba
  Datura stramonium L., Solanaceae 318
Zabumba-branca
  Datura arborea L., Solanaceae 317
  Datura suaveolens Humb. & Bonpl., Solanaceae ... 318
Zangatempo
  Anthurium affine Schott, Araceae 33
Zanzo
  Sida rhombea L., Malvaceae 222
Zebradim
  Ottonia corcovadensis Miq., Piperaceae 272

Species Index

Abolboda poarchon Seub., Xyridaceae 342
Abrus precatorius L., Fabaceae 160
Abuta candicans Rich., Menispermaceae 231
Abuta concolor Poepp. & Endl., Menispermaceae ... 231
Abuta rufescens Aubl., Menispermaceae 231
    Abuta rufescens: illustration, 232
Abuta selloana Eichl., Menispermaceae 231
Acacia paniculata Willd., Mimosaceae 236
Acanthaceae 1
Acanthospermum australe
    (Loefl.) O. Ktze., Asteraceae 52
Acanthospermum hispidum DC. 52
Acanthosyris spinescens
    (Mart. & Endl.) Gris., Santalaceae 304
Achyranthes ficoidea Lam., Amaranthaceae 3
Achyranthes indica L., Amaranthaceae 3
Achyrocline satureioides (Lam.) DC., Asteraceae 52
Acmella oleracea (L.) R.K. Jansen, Asteraceae 52
Acmella repens (Walt.) L.C. Rich., Asteraceae 52
Acnistus arborescens (L.) Schl., Solanaceae 316
Acosmium dasycarpum (Vog.) Yakovl., Fabaceae 161
    Acosmium dasycarpum: illustration, 161
Acosmium subelegans
    (Mohlenb.) Yakovl., Fabaceae 162
Adenocalymma alliacea (Lam.) Miers, Bignoniaceae 78
Adiantaceae 1
Adiantopsis chlorophylla (Sw.) Fée, Adiantaceae 1
Adiantum concinnum Humb. & Bonp., Adiantaceae ... 1
Adiantum cuneatum Langsd. & Fisch., Adiantaceae ... 1
Adiantum trapeziforme L., Adiantaceae 1
Ageratum conyzoides L., Asteraceae 53
Agonandra brasiliensis Miers, Opiliaceae 265
    Agonandra brasiliensis: illustration, 265
Aiovea brasiliensis Meissn., Lauraceae 196
Aiovea meissneri Mez, Lauraceae 197
Aizoaceae 2
Alibertia edulis (Rich.) Rich., Rubiaceae 294
Albizzia lebbeck (L.) Benth., Mimosaceae 236
Alisma palaefolium Kunth, Alismataceae 2
Alismataceae 2
Allagoptera campestris (Mart.) Kuntze, Arecaceae 39
Allamanda blanchetii M. Arg., Apocynaceae 20
Allamanda cathartica L., Apocynaceae 20
Allamanda doniana M. Arg., Apocynaceae 20
Aloysia triphylla (L'Her.) Britt., Verbenaceae 332
    Aloysia triphylla: illustration, 333
Alsodeia flavescens (Aubl.) Spreng., Violaceae 337
Alternanthera achyrantha R. Br., Amaranthaceae 3
Alternanthera brasiliana (L.) O. Ktze., Amaranthaceae 3
Amaranthaceae 3
Amaranthus blitum L., Amaranthaceae 3
Amaranthus spinosus L., Amaranthaceae 3
Amaranthus viridis L., Amaranthaceae 3
Amaryllidaceae 6
Amasonia arborea H.B.K., Verbenaceae 333
Ambelania tenuifolia Aubl., Apocynaceae 20
Ambrosia artemisiifolia L., Asteraceae 53
Ampelozizyphus amazonicus Ducke, Rhamnaceae ... 291

Anacampta riedellii (M. Arg.) Mgf., Apocynaceae 21
Anacardiaceae 7
Anacardium humile St.-Hil., Anacardiaceae 7
Anacardium nanum St.-Hil., Anacardiaceae 7
Anacardium occidentale L., Anacardiaceae 7
    Anacardium occidentale: illustration, 8
Anadenanthera colubrina
    (Vell.) Brenan, Mimosaceae 236
Anadenanthera falcata
    (Benth.) Brenan, Mimosaceae 236
Anadenanthera macrocarpa
    (Benth.) Brenan, Mimosaceae 236
Anadenanthera peregrina (L.) Speg., Mimosaceae .. 236
Ananas comosus (L.) Merrill, Bromeliaceae 90
Anchietea pyrifolia (Mart.) G. Don, Violaceae 338
    Anchietea pyrifolia: illustration, 338
Andira anthelmia (Vell.) MacBride, Fabaceae 162
    Andira anthelmia: illustration, 162
Andira fraxinifolia Benth., Fabaceae 162
Andira humilis Benth., Fabaceae 162
Andira inermis (Sw.) H.B.K., Fabaceae 162
Andira legalis (Vell.) Tol., Fabaceae 162
Andira retusa (Poir.) H.B.K., Fabaceae 162
Andira spp., Fabaceae 162
Andira vermifuga Mart. ex Benth., Fabaceae 162
Andradea floribunda Fr. All., Nyctaginaceae 257
Andropogon bicornis L., Poaceae 279
Andropogon condensatus H.B.K., Poaceae 279
Andropogon minarum Kunth, Poaceae 280
Anemia phyllitidis (L.) Sw., Schizaeaceae 310
Anemone decapetala L., Ranunculaceae 290
Anemopaegma album Mart., Bignoniaceae 78
Anemopaegma arvense (Vell.) Stapf, Bignoniaceae 78
    Anemopaegma arvense: illustration, 79
Anemopaegma glaucum Mart., Bignoniaceae 78
Anemopaegma scabriusculum Mart., Bignoniaceae ... 78
Anemopaegma spp., Bignoniaceae 78
Angelonia integerrima Spreng., Scrophulariaceae ... 310
Aniba canelilla (H.B.K.) Mez, Lauraceae 197
Aniba duckei Kosterm., Lauraceae 197
Aniba permollis (Nees) Mez, Lauraceae 197
Aniba puchury-minor (Mart.) Mez, Lauraceae 197
Aniba rosaeodora Ducke, Lauraceae 197
Aniba spp., Lauraceae 197
Anisolobus cururu (Mart.) M. Arg., Apocynaceae 21
Anisosperma passiflora Manso, Cucurbitaceae 135
Annona ambotay Aubl., Annonaceae 12
Annona coriacea Mart., Annonaceae 12
Annona cornifolia St.-Hil., Annonaceae 12
Annona crassifolia Mart., Annonaceae 12
Annona dioica St.-Hil., Annonaceae 12
Annona foetida Mart., Annonaceae 12
Annona glabra L., Annonaceae 13
Annona marcgravii Mart., Annonaceae 13
Annona muricata L., Annonaceae 13
Annona reticulata L., Annonaceae 13
Annona spinescens Mart., Annonaceae 13
Annona squamosa L., Annonaceae 13

Annonaceae 11
Anthurium affine Schott, Araceae 33
Anthurium oxycarpum Poepp., Araceae 33
Apiaceae 18
Apium sellowianum Wolf, Apiaceae 18
Apocynaceae 20
Apuleia leiocarpa (Vog.) MacBride, Caesalpiniaceae . 98
Aquifoliaceae 31
Araceae 33
Araujia sericifera Brot., Asclepiadaceae 50
Arecaceae 39
Aristida pallens Cav., Poaceae 280
Aristolochia allemani Hoehne, Aristolochiaceae 49
Aristolochia amazonica Ule, Aristolochiaceae 49
Aristolochia arcuata Mast., Aristolochiaceae 49
Aristolochia barbata Jacq., Aristolochiaceae 49
Aristolochia birostris Duch., Aristolochiaceae 46
Aristolochia burchellii Mast., Aristolochiaceae 50
Aristolochia cordigera Willd., Aristolochiaceae 46
Aristolochia cymbifera
    Mart. & Zucc., Aristolochiaceae 46
    Aristolochia cymbifera: illustration, 47
Aristolochia elegans Mast., Aristolochiaceae 48
Aristolochia esperanzae
    O. Kuntze, Aristolochiaceae 48
Aristolochia gigantea
    Mart. & Zucc., Aristolochiaceae 48
Aristolochia maxima Jacq., Aristolochiaceae 50
Aristolochia sipho L'Her., Aristolochiaceae 50
Aristolochia spp., Aristolochiaceae 46
Aristolochia triangularis Cham., Aristolochiaceae 48
Aristolochia trilobata L., Aristolochiaceae 48
    Aristolochia trilobata: illustration, 49
Aristolochiaceae 46
Arnica montana L. 65
Arrabidaea agnus-castus (Cham.) DC., Bignoniaceae 78
Arrabidaea chica (H.B.K.) Bur., Bignoniaceae 78
Arrabidaea foetida Bur. & K. Sch., Bignoniaceae 79
Artemisia absinthium L., Asteraceae 54
Asclepiadaceae 50
Aspidosperma desmanthum M. Arg., Apocynaceae 21
Aspidosperma discolor Benth., Apocynaceae 21
Aspidosperma excelsum Benth., Apocynaceae 21
Aspidosperma nigricans Handro, Apocynaceae 21
Aspidosperma nitidum Benth., Apocynaceae 21
Aspidosperma polyneuron M. Arg., Apocynaceae 21
Aspidosperma spp., Apocynaceae 22
Asteraceae 52
Astrocaryum aculeatissimum
    (Schott) Burret, Arecaceae 39
Astrocaryum murumuru Mart., Arecaceae 39
Astronium fraxinifolium Schott, Anacardiaceae 9
Attalea oleifera Barb. Rodr., Arecaceae 39
Attalea spectabilis Mart., Arecaceae 39
Auxemma oncocalyx (Fr. All.) Taub., Boraginaceae 87
Avena quadridentata Doell, Poaceae 280
Avicennia germinans (L.) L., Verbenaceae 334
Ayapana triplinerve (Vahl)
    King & H. Robinson, Asteraceae 53
Azolla caroliniana Willd., Salviniaceae 304
Baccharidastrum triplinerve
    (Less.) Cabr., Asteraceae 53
Baccharis articulata (Lam.) Pers., Asteraceae 54

Baccharis cordifolia DC., Asteraceae 56
Baccharis dentata (Vell.) G.M. Barroso, Asteraceae .. 54
Baccharis dracunculifolia DC., Asteraceae 54
Baccharis gaudichaudii DC., Asteraceae 56
Baccharis lundii DC., Asteraceae 54
Baccharis megapotamica Spreng., Asteraceae 56
Baccharis notosergila Gris., Asteraceae 54
Baccharis ochracea Spr., Asteraceae 56
Baccharis ramosissima Gardn., Asteraceae 54
Baccharis spp., Asteraceae 56
Baccharis stenocephala Baker, Asteraceae 56
Baccharis tarchonanthoides DC., Asteraceae 56
Baccharis trimera (Less.) DC., Asteraceae 54
    Baccharis trimera: illustration, 55
Bactris insignis (Mart.) Baill., Arecaceae 39
Balanophoraceae 73
Banisteriopsis caapi (Spr.) Morton, Malpighiaceae .. 217
    Banisteriopsis caapi: illustration, 218
Bassovia lucida Dunal, Solanaceae 316
Bathysa cuspidata Hook., Rubiaceae 296
Bauhinia candicans Benth., Caesalpiniaceae 99
Bauhinia forficata Link, Caesalpiniaceae 99
    Bauhinia forficata: illustration, 98
Bauhinia guianensis Aubl., Caesalpiniaceae 99
Bauhinia langsdorffiana Bong., Caesalpiniaceae 99
Bauhinia radiata Vell., Caesalpiniaceae 99
Bauhinia rutilans Spr. ex Benth., Caesalpiniaceae 99
Begonia acida Mart., Begoniaceae 75
Begonia hirtella Link, Begoniaceae 76
Begonia luxurians Scheidw., Begoniaceae 76
Begonia paulensis DC., Begoniaceae 76
    Begonia paulensis: illustration, 75
Begoniaceae 75
Bellucia grossularioides (L.) Tr., Melastomataceae .. 225
Berberidaceae 76
Berberis laurina Thunb., Berberidaceae 76
    Berberis laurina: illustration, 77
Berberis spinulosa St.-Hil., Berberidaceae 76
Bertholletia excelsa Humb. & Bonpl., Lecythidaceae 204
    Bertholletia excelsa: illustration, 205
Bidens cynapiifolia H.B.K., Asteraceae 56
Bidens graveolens Mart., Asteraceae 56
Bidens pilosa L., Asteraceae 57
Bignonia exoleta Vell., Bignoniaceae 79
Bignoniaceae 78
Bixa orellana L., Bixaceae .... 85 & 306, 318
Bixaceae 85
Blanchetia heterotricha DC., Asteraceae 57
Blepharocalyx saliciifolius
    (H.B.K.) Berg, Myrtaceae 253
Bocagea alba St.-Hil., Annonaceae 14
Bocagea viridis St.-Hil., Annonaceae 14
Boehmeria caudata Sw., Urticaceae 330
Boerhavia coccinea Mill., Nyctaginaceae 257
Boerhavia erecta L., Nyctaginaceae 258
Boerhavia hirsuta, Nyctaginaceae 52
Boerhavia paniculata Rich., Nyctaginaceae 258
Bomarea salsilloides Roem., Amaryllidaceae 6
Bomarea spectabilis Schrenk, Amaryllidaceae 6
Bombacaceae 86
Boraginaceae 87
Borreria asclepiadea Cham. & Schl., Rubiaceae 296
Borreria capitata (Ruiz & Pav.), Rubiaceae 296
Borreria latifolia K. Sch., Rubiaceae 296

Borreria poaya (St.-Hil.) DC., Rubiaceae 296
Borreria tenella Cham. & Schl., Rubiaceae 296
Borreria verbenoides Cham. & Schl., Rubiaceae 296
Borreria verticillata (L.) Meyer, Rubiaceae 296
Bouchea laetevirens Schauer, Verbenaceae 334
Bouchea pseudogervao
    (St.-Hil.) Cham., Verbenaceae 334
Bowdichia nitida Spruce ex Benth., Fabaceae 163
Bowdichia virgilioides H.B.K., Fabaceae 163
Brasilopuntia brasiliensis (Willd.) Berg, Cactaceae ... 95
    Brasilopuntia brasiliensis: illustration, 96
Bredemeyera floribunda Willd., Polygalaceae 283
Bromelia antiacantha Bertol., Bromeliaceae 91
Bromelia arenaria Ule, Bromeliaceae 91
Bromelia pinguin L., Bromeliaceae 91
Bromeliaceae 90
Brosimum acutifolium Huber, Moraceae 246
Brosimum gaudichaudii Tréc., Moraceae 246
Brosimum obovata Ducke, Moraceae 246
Brosimum parinarioides Ducke, Moraceae 246
Brosimum potabile Ducke, Moraceae 246
Brosimum utile (H.B.K.) Pittier, Moraceae 246
Brunfelsia grandiflora D. Don, Solanaceae 316
    Brunfelsia grandiflora: illustration, 316
Brunfelsia spp., Solanaceae 316
Brunfelsia uniflora (Pohl) D. Don, Solanaceae 316
Buchnera aquatica Aubl., Scrophulariaceae 310
Buchnera virgata H.B.K., Scrophulariaceae 310
Buddleja brasiliensis Jacq. ex Spr., Buddlejaceae 93
Buddleja cambara Arech., Buddlejaceae 93
Buddleja stachioides Cham., Buddlejaceae 93
Buddlejaceae 93
Bulbostylis capillaris Clarke, Cyperaceae 142
Bumelia sartorum Mart., Sapotaceae 308
Burseraceae 93
Butia yatay (Mart.) Becc., Arecaceae 39
Byrsonima chrysophylla H.B.K., Malpighiaceae 218
Byrsonima coccolobifolia H.B.K., Malpighiaceae 218
    Byrsonima coccolobifolia: illustration, 219
Byrsonima crassifolia H.B.K., Malpighiaceae 219
Byrsonima spicata Rich., Malpighiaceae 219
Byrsonima verbascifolia (L.) Rich., Malpighiaceae .. 220
Cabomba piauhyensis Gard., Nymphaeaceae 259
Cabralea canjerana (Vell.) Mart., Meliaceae 227
Cactaceae 95
Caesalpinia bonduc (L.) Roxb., Caesalpiniaceae 99
Caesalpinia bracteosa Tul., Caesalpiniaceae 100
Caesalpinia echinata Lam., Caesalpiniaceae 100
    Caesalpinia echinata: illustration, 101
Caesalpinia ferrea Mart. ex Tul., Caesalpiniaceae 100
Caesalpinia microphylla Mart., Caesalpiniaceae 100
Caesalpinia pyramidalis Tul., Caesalpiniaceae 100
Caesalpiniaceae 98
Caladium bicolor (Aiton) Vent., Araceae 34
Caladium bicolor (Aiton) Vent.
    var. *poecile* (Schott) Engler, Araceae 35
    Caladium bicolor: illustration, 34
Caladium sororium Schott, Araceae 35
Calathea grandiflora Lindl., Marantaceae 223
Calea pinnatifida (R. Br.) Less., Asteraceae 57
Calliandra tweediei Benth., Mimosaceae 237
Callisthene major Mart., Vochysiaceae 340
Calolisianthus amplissimus
    (Mart.) Gilg, Gentianaceae 179

Calolisianthus pendulus (Mart.) Gilg, Gentianaceae 179
Calolisianthus spp., Gentianaceae 179
Calonyction aculeatum (L.) House, Convolvulaceae 129
Calophyllum brasiliense Camb., Clusiaceae 120
Calotropis procera (Ait.) Ait. f., Asclepiadaceae 50
Calyptranthes aromatica St.-Hil., Myrtaceae 253
Calyptranthes variabilis Berg, Myrtaceae 253
Campanulaceae 109
Campomanesia aurea Berg, Myrtaceae 253
Campomanesia xanthocarpa Berg, Myrtaceae 253
Campsiandra comosa Benth.
    var. *laurifolia* (Benth.) Cowan, Caesalpiniaceae ... 100
Canellaceae 110
Canna edulis Ker-Gawl., Cannaceae 110
Canna gigantea Desf., Cannaceae 110
Canna glauca L., Cannaceae 110
Canna indica L., Cannaceae 111
Canna lanuginosa Roscoe, Cannaceae 111
Canna lutea Roscoe, Cannaceae 111
Canna warszewiczii Dietr., Cannaceae 111
Cannaceae 110
Capparaceae 111
Capparis cynophallophora L., Capparaceae 111
Capparis lineata Pers., Capparaceae 111
Capparis urens B. Rodr., Capparaceae 111
Capraria biflora L., Scrophulariaceae 311
    Capraria biflora: illustration, 311
Caraipa densifolia Mart., Clusiaceae 121
Caraipa excelsa Ducke, Clusiaceae 121
Caraipa grandifolia Mart., Clusiaceae 121
Caraipa insidiosa B. Rodr., Clusiaceae 121
Caraipa minor Huber, Clusiaceae 121
Caraipa silvatica B. Rodr., Clusiaceae 121
Carapa guianensis Aubl., Meliaceae 227
Cardiospermum grandiflorum Sw., Sapindaceae 305
Carica papaya L., Caricaceae 113
Caricaceae 113
Cariniana legalis (Mart.) O. Ktze., Lecythidaceae ... 204
    Cariniana legalis: illustration, 206
Carpotroche brasiliensis
    (Raddi) Endl., Flacourtiaceae 176
    Carpotroche brasiliensis: illustration, 177
Carpotroche longifolia Benth., Flacourtiaceae 176
Caryocar brasiliense Camb., Caryocaraceae 114
Caryocar coriaceum Wittm., Caryocaraceae 114
Caryocar glabrum (Aubl.) Pers., Caryocaraceae 114
Caryocar villosum (Aubl.) Pers., Caryocaraceae 114
Caryocaraceae 114
Caryophyllaceae 115
Casearia adstringens Mart., Flacourtiaceae 176
Casearia cambessedesii Eichl., Flacourtiaceae 176
Casearia guyanensis (Aubl.) Urb., Flacourtiaceae 177
Casearia inaequilatera Camb., Flacourtiaceae 178
Casearia ovata Willd., Flacourtiaceae 178
Casearia sylvestris Sw., Flacourtiaceae 178
Cassia see also *Senna*, Caesalpiniaceae 106
Cassia ferruginea (Schrad.)
    Schrad. ex DC., Caesalpiniaceae 100
Cassia grandis L., Caesalpiniaceae 101
Cassytha filiformis L., Lauraceae 198
Cayaponia cabocla (Vell.) Mart., Cucurbitaceae 135
Cayaponia cordifolia Cogn., Cucurbitaceae 136
Cayaponia espelina (Manso) Cogn., Cucurbitaceae . 135

Cayaponia martiana (Cogn.) Cogn., Cucurbitaceae . 135
Cayaponia pedata Cogn., Cucurbitaceae 136
Cayaponia pilosa Cogn., Cucurbitaceae 135
Cayaponia spp., Cucurbitaceae 136
Cayaponia tayuya (Mart.) Cogn., Cucurbitaceae 135
Cayaponia triangularis Cogn., Cucurbitaceae 136
Cecropia hololeuca Miq., Moraceae 247
Cecropia leucocoma Miq., Moraceae 247
Cecropia palmata Willd., Moraceae 247
Cedrela fissilis Vell., Meliaceae 227
    Cedrela fissilis: illustration, 228
Cedrela odorata L., Meliaceae 227
Ceiba pentandra (L.) Gaertn., Bombacaceae 86
Celastraceae 115
Celtis brasiliensis Planch., Ulmaceae 330
Celtis iguanaea Sarg., Ulmaceae 330
Celtis morifolia Planch., Ulmaceae 330
Celtis spinosissima Miq., Ulmaceae 330
Centropogon cornutus (L.) Druce, Campanulaceae .. 109
Cephaelis ipecacuanha Rich., Rubiaceae .... 296 &
    284, 297, 299, 339
Cereus jamacaru DC., Cactaceae 95
Cereus peruvianus (L.) Mill., Cactaceae 95
Cestrum amictum Schl., Solanaceae 317
Cestrum bracteatum Link & Otto, Solanaceae 317
Cestrum calycinum Willd., Solanaceae 317
Cestrum parqui L'Herit., Solanaceae 317
Cestrum pseudoquina Mart., Solanaceae 317
Chamaecrista cathartica
    (Mart.) Ir. & Barn., Caesalpiniaceae 101
Chamaecrista fasciculata
    (Michx.) Greene, Caesalpiniaceae 102
Chamaecrista mimosoides
    (L.) Ir. & Barn., Caesalpiniaceae 102
Chamissoa altissima H.B.K., Amaranthaceae 4
Chamissoa macrocarpa H.B.K., Amaranthaceae 4
Chaptalia nutans (L.) Polak., Asteraceae 57
Chenopodiaceae 118
Chenopodium ambrosioides L., Chenopodiaceae 118
Chenopodium hircinum Schrad., Chenopodiaceae ... 119
Chiococca alba (L.) Hitch., Rubiaceae 297
Chionolaena latifolia (Benth.) Baker, Asteraceae 57
Chloranthaceae 119
Chloris distichophylla (Nees) Lag., Poaceae 280
Chloris polydactyla Sw., Poaceae 280
Chondodendron platyphyllum
    (Mart.) Miers, Menispermaceae 231
Chondodendron tomentosum, Menispermaceae 231
Chorisia crispiflora H.B.K., Bombacaceae 86
Chromolaena hirsuta (Hook. & Arn.)
    King & H. Robinson, Asteraceae 58
Chromolaena laevigata
    (Lam.) King & H. Robinson, Asteraceae 58
Chrysobalanaceae 119
Chrysobalanus icaco L., Chrysobalanaceae 119
Cinnamodendron axillare
    (Nees & Mart.) Endl., Canellaceae 110
Cipura paludosa Aubl., Iridaceae 186
    Cipura paludosa: illustration, 187
Cissampelos fasciculata Benth., Menispermaceae 231
Cissampelos fluminensis Eichl., Menispermaceae ... 233
Cissampelos glaberrima St.-Hil., Menispermaceae .. 233
Cissampelos ovalifolia DC., Menispermaceae 233

Cissampelos pareira L., Menispermaceae 233
Cissampelos sympodialis Eichl., Menispermaceae ... 233
Cissus palmata Poir., Vitaceae 339
Cissus salutaris H.B.K., Vitaceae 339
Cissus sicyoides L., Vitaceae 339
Citronella congonha (Mart.) Howard, Icacinaceae ... 185
Citronella mucronata (R. & Pav.) Don, Icacinaceae . 186
Cladonia miniata Mey., Cladoniaceae 120
Cladonia pyxidata (L.) Ach., Cladoniaceae 120
Cladoniaceae 120
Clarisia racemosa Ruiz & Pav., Moraceae 247
Clematis denticulata Vell., Ranunculaceae 290
Clematis dioica L., Ranunculaceae 290
Cleome aculeata L., Capparaceae 112
Cleome gigantea L., Capparaceae 112
Cleome polygama L., Capparaceae 112
Cleome speciosa H.B.K., Capparaceae 112
Cleome spinosa Jacq., Capparaceae 112
Clibadium leiocarpum Mart., Asteraceae 58
Clibadium rotundifolium DC., Asteraceae 58
Clibadium surinamense L., Asteraceae 58
Clidemia blepharoides DC., Melastomataceae 225
Clitoria guianensis (Aubl.) Benth., Fabaceae 163
Clusia grandiflora Splitg., Clusiaceae 121
Clusia insignis Mart., Clusiaceae 121
Clusia panapanari Choisy, Clusiaceae 122
Clusia rosea Jacq., Clusiaceae 122
Clusiaceae 120
Coccoloba arborescens (Vell.) How., Polygonaceae . 285
Coccoloba laevis Casar., Polygonaceae 285
Coccoloba marginata Benth., Polygonaceae 285
Coccoloba mollis Casar., Polygonaceae 285
Cocculus filipendula Mart., Menispermaceae 234
Cochlospermaceae 125
Cochlospermum orinocense
    (H.B.K.) Steud., Cochlospermaceae 125
Cochlospermum regium
    (Mart. & Schl.) Pilg., Cochlospermaceae 125
Cocos nucifera L., Arecaceae 40
Coleus barbatus Benth., Lamiaceae 191
Coleus forskohlii (Willd.) Briq., Lamiaceae 191
Colletia paradoxa (Spr.) Escalante, Rhamnaceae 291
Combretaceae 126
Combretum leprosum Mart., Combretaceae 126
Commelina nudiflora L., Commelinaceae 126
Commelina platyphylla
    Klotz. ex Seub., Commelinaceae 126
Commelina pohliana Seub., Commelinaceae 127
Commelina robusta Kunth, Commelinaceae 128
Commelina sulcata Willd., Commelinaceae 128
Commelina vestita Seub., Commelinaceae 128
Commelina virginica L., Commelinaceae 128
Commelinaceae 126
Connarus patrisii Planch., Connaraceae 129
Connarus suberosus Planch., Connaraceae 129
Connaraceae 129
Conobea aquatica Aubl., Scrophulariaceae 311
Conobea scoparioides Benth., Scrophulariaceae 311
Conocarpus erecta L., Combretaceae 126
Conocliniopsis prasiifolia
    (DC.) King & H. Robinson, Asteraceae 58
Convolvulaceae 129
Conyza blakei (Cabr.) Cabr., Asteraceae 58

Copaifera cearensis – Dichorisandra affinis: Species Index

Copaifera cearensis
   Huber ex Ducke, Caesalpiniaceae 102
Copaifera langsdorffii Desf., Caesalpiniaceae 102
Copaifera multijuga Hayne, Caesalpiniaceae 102
Copaifera officinalis (Jacq.) L., Caesalpiniaceae 102
Copaifera reticulata Ducke, Caesalpiniaceae 102
Copernicia prunifera (Mill.) H. Moore, Arecaceae 40
   Copernicia prunifera: illustration, 41
Cordia coffeoides Warm., Boraginaceae 87
Cordia ecalyculata Vell., Boraginaceae 87
Cordia grandiflora DC., Boraginaceae 87
Cordia insignis Cham., Boraginaceae 87
Cordia magnolifolia Cham., Boraginaceae 87
Cordia monosperma (Jacq.)
   Roem. & Schult., Boraginaceae 87
Cordia multispicata Cham., Boraginaceae 88
Cordia obscura Cham., Boraginaceae 88
Cordia salicifolia Cham., Boraginaceae 88
Cordia umbraculifera DC., Boraginaceae 88
Cordia verbenacea DC., Boraginaceae 88
Cordyline dracaenoides Kunth, Liliaceae 207
Corynostylis hybanthus
   (L.) Mart. & Zucc., Violaceae 338
Costaceae 132
Costus cuspidatus (Nees & Mart.) Maas, Costaceae . 132
Costus spicatus (Jacq.) Sw., Costaceae 132
Costus spiralis (Jacq.) Roscoe, Costaceae 132
Couma macrocarpa B. Rodr., Apocynaceae 23
Couma utilis (Mart.) M. Arg., Apocynaceae 23
Coussapoa asperifolia Tréc., Moraceae 247
Coutarea hexandra (Jacq.) K. Sch., Rubiaceae 297
Coutoubea ramosa Aubl., Gentianaceae 179
Coutoubea spicata Aubl., Gentianaceae 179
Craniolaria annua L., Martyniaceae 224
Craniolaria integrifolia Cham., Martyniaceae 224
Crassulaceae 133
Crataeva benthamii Eichl., Capparaceae 112
Crataeva tapia L., Capparaceae 112
Cremastus sceptrum Bur. & K. Sch., Bignoniaceae 79
Crescentia cujete L., Bignoniaceae 80
Crinum scabrum Sims, Amaryllidaceae 6
Crotalaria verrucosa L., Fabaceae 163
Croton cajucara Benth., Euphorbiaceae 150
Croton cascarilla (L.) Bennet, Euphorbiaceae 152
Croton floribundus Spreng., Euphorbiaceae 150
Croton glabellus L., Euphorbiaceae 152
Croton hemiargyreus M. Arg., Euphorbiaceae 151
Croton moritibensis Baill., Euphorbiaceae 150
Croton paniculatus M. Arg., Euphorbiaceae 152
Croton salutaris Casar., Euphorbiaceae 151
Croton sincorensis Mart., Euphorbiaceae 151
Croton sonderianus M. Arg., Euphorbiaceae 151
Croton spp., Euphorbiaceae 152
Croton triqueter Lam., Euphorbiaceae 151
Croton urucurana Baill., Euphorbiaceae 151
Croton zehntneri Pax & Hoffm., Euphorbiaceae 151
Cryptocarya guyanensis Meissn., Lauraceae 198
Cryptocarya mandioccana Meissn., Lauraceae 198
Cryptocarya minima Mez, Lauraceae 198
Cryptocarya moschata
   Nees & Mart. ex Nees, Lauraceae 198
Cucurbita pepo L., Cucurbitaceae 136
Cucurbitaceae 135

Cunila microcephala Benth., Lamiaceae 192
Cunila spicata L., Lamiaceae 192
Cupania racemosa Radlk., Sapindaceae 305
Cuphea aperta Koehne, Lythraceae 213
Cuphea balsamona Cham., Lythraceae 213
Cuphea carthagenensis
   (Jacq.) MacBride, Lythraceae 213
Cuphea ingrata Cham. & Schl., Lythraceae 214
   Cuphea ingrata: illustration, 213
Cuphea melvilla Lindl., Lythraceae 214
Cuphea spp., Lythraceae 214
Curatella americana L., Dilleniaceae 144
   Curatella americana: illustration, 145
Curtia tenuifolia (Aubl.) Knobl., Gentianaceae 180
Cuscuta racemosa Mart., Convolvulaceae 130
Cuscuta spp., Convolvulaceae 130
Cuscuta umbellata H.B.K., Convolvulaceae 130
Cusparia febrifuga Humb., Rutaceae 300
Cusparia toxicaria Spr. ex Engl., Rutaceae 301
Cyathea armata (Sw.) Domin, Cyatheaceae 141
Cyathea microdonta (Desv.) Domin, Cyatheaceae ... 141
Cyatheaceae 141
Cybianthus detergens Mart., Myrsinaceae 253
Cybistax antisyphilitica (Mart.) Mart., Bignoniaceae .. 80
Cydista aequinoctialis Miers, Bignoniaceae 80
Cymbopogon schoenanthus (L.) Spreng., Poaceae ... 280
Cypella herbertii Herb., Iridaceae 186
   Cypella herbertii: illustration, 188
Cyperaceae 142
Cyperus corymbosus Rottb., Cyperaceae 142
Cyperus gracilescens Roem. & Schult., Cyperaceae . 142
Cyperus ligularis L., Cyperaceae 142
Cyperus rotundus L., Cyperaceae 142
Cyperus sesquiflorus (Torrey)
   Mattf. & Kükent., Cyperaceae 142
Cyrtocymura scorpioides
   (Lam.) H. Robinson, Asteraceae 58
Cyrtopodium andersoni R. Br., Orchidaceae 266
Cyrtopodium punctatum Lindl., Orchidaceae 266
Dahlstedtia pentaphylla (Taub.) Burk., Fabaceae 163
Dahlstedtia pinnata (Benth.) Malme, Fabaceae 163
Dalbergia gracilis Benth., Fabaceae 163
Dalbergia subcymosa Ducke, Fabaceae 164
   Dalbergia subcymosa: illustration, 164
Dalechampia ficifolia Lam., Euphorbiaceae 152
Dalechampia scandens L., Euphorbiaceae 152
Datura arborea L., Solanaceae 317
Datura insignis B. Rodr., Solanaceae 317, 318
Datura stramonium L., Solanaceae 318
Datura suaveolens Humb. & Bonpl., Solanaceae 318
Davilla rugosa Poir., Dilleniaceae 145
Declieuxia aristolochia M. Arg., Rubiaceae 297
Declieuxia cordigera Mart. & Zucc., Rubiaceae 297
Deianira erubescens
   Cham. & Schl., Gentianaceae 180
Deianira nervosa Cham. & Schl., Gentianaceae 180
Deianira pallescens Cham. & Schl., Gentianaceae ... 180
Dennstaedtiaceae 144
Desmodium axillare (Sw.) DC. 164
Desmodium triflorum DC., Fabaceae 164
Desmoncus orthacanthos Mart., Arecaceae 40
Desmoncus polyacanthos Mart., Arecaceae 40
Dichorisandra affinis Mart., Commelinaceae 128

Dichorisandra leucophthalmos
  Hook., Commelinaceae 128
Dichorisandra luschnathiana
  Kunth, Commelinaceae 128
Dichorisandra picta Hook., Commelinaceae 128
Dichorisandra spp., Commelinaceae 128
Dichorisandra thyrsiflora Mikan, Commelinaceae .. 128
Dichorisandra villosula Mart., Commelinaceae 128
Dicypellium caryophyllatum
  Nees & Mart., Lauraceae 198
Dieffenbachia seguine (Jacq.) Schott, Araceae 35
Dilleniaceae 144
Diodia polymorpha Cham. & Schl., Rubiaceae 297
Dioscorea basiclavicaulis
  Rizz. & Mattos, Dioscoreaceae 146
Dioscorea glandulosa Klotz., Dioscoreaceae 147
Dioscorea laxiflora Mart., Dioscoreaceae 147
Dioscorea silvestris Vell., Dioscoreaceae 147
Dioscoreaceae 146
Diospyros paralea Steud., Ebenaceae 147
Dipholis nigra Gr., Sapotaceae 309
Dipladenia amabilis Hort., Apocynaceae 23
Dipladenia atropurpurea
  (Lindl.) DC., Apocynaceae 23
Dipladenia atroviolacea (Lem.) DC., Apocynaceae ... 23
Dipladenia fragrans DC., Apocynaceae 23
  Dipladenia fragrans: illustration, 22
Dipladenia gentianoides M. Arg., Apocynaceae 23
Dipladenia illustris M. Arg., Apocynaceae 23
Dipladenia riedelii M. Arg., Apocynaceae 23
Dipladenia spigeliifolia M. Arg., Apocynaceae 23
Dipladenia splendens (Hook.) DC., Apocynaceae 23
Dipladenia spp., Apocynaceae 23
Dipteryx alata Vog., Fabaceae 165
  Dipteryx alata: illustration, 165
Dipteryx odorata (Aubl.) Willd., Fabaceae 166
Discaria americana Gill. & Hook., Rhamnaceae 291
Discaria febrifuga Mart., Rhamnaceae 293
Dodonaea viscosa Jacq., Sapindaceae 305
Doliocarpus rolandri Gmel., Dilleniaceae 146
Dorstenia asaroides Gardn., Moraceae 247
Dorstenia brasiliensis Lam., Moraceae 247
Dorstenia cayapia Vell., Moraceae 248
Dorstenia reniformis Pohl, Moraceae 248
Dracontium asperum K. Koch, Araceae 35
Dracontium polyphyllum L., Araceae 36
Drimys winteri Forst., Winteraceae 340
  Drimys winteri: illustration, 341
Dryopteridaceae 147
Duguetia furfuracea (St.-Hil.)
  Benth. & Hook., Annonaceae 14
Duguetia riparia Hub., Annonaceae 14
Ebenaceae 147
Echinodorus grandiflorus
  (Cham. & Schl.) Mich., Alismataceae 2
Echinodorus macrophyllus
  (Kunth) Mich., Alismataceae 2
Echinodorus pubescens Mart., Alismataceae 2
Echites macrocalyx M. Arg., Apocynaceae 23
Echites peltata Vell., Apocynaceae 23
Eclipta prostrata (L.) L., Asteraceae 59
Egletes viscosa (L.) Less., Asteraceae 59
Eichhornia crassipes Solms, Pontederiaceae 288

Elephantopus micropappus Less., Asteraceae 59
Elephantopus mollis H.B.K., Asteraceae 59
Elaeis guineensis Jacq., Arecaceae 40
Elaeis oleifera (H.B.K.) Cortez, Arecaceae 40
Eleutherine plicata Herb., Iridaceae 186
Elionurus bilinguis (Trin.) Hack., Poaceae 281
Elionurus candidus (Trin.) Hack., Poaceae 281
Elionurus latiflorus Nees, Poaceae 281
Entada paranaguana B. Rodr., Mimosaceae 237
Entada polyphylla Benth., Mimosaceae 237
Entada polystachya (Jacq.) DC., Mimosaceae 237
Ephedra americana Willd., Ephedraceae 147
Ephedra triandra Tul., Ephedraceae 148
Ephedraceae 147
Equisetaceae 148
Equisetum giganteum L., Equisetaceae 148
Equisetum martii Milde, Equisetaceae 148
Equisetum ramosissimum Desf., Equisetaceae 148
Erigeron tweediei Hook. & Arn., Asteraceae 60
Eriocaulaceae 148
Eryngium elegans Cham. & Schlecht., Apiaceae 19
Eryngium foetidum L., Apiaceae 19
Eryngium pandanifolium
  Cham. & Schlecht., Apiaceae 19
Eryngium paniculatum Cav.
  & Domb. ex Delar., Apiaceae 19
Eryngium pristis Cham. & Schlecht., Apiaceae 19
Erythrina corallodendron L., Fabaceae 166
Erythrina crista-galli L., Fabaceae 166
Erythrina falcata Benth., Fabaceae 166
Erythrina fusca Lour., Fabaceae 166
Erythrina velutina Willd., Fabaceae 166
Erythrina verna Vell., Fabaceae 168
Erythroxylaceae 148
Erythroxylum anguifugum Mart., Erythroxylaceae ... 148
Erythroxylum campestre St.-Hil., Erythroxylaceae 149
Erythroxylum cataractarum Spruce, Erythroxylaceae 149
Erythroxylum coca Lam., Erythroxylaceae 149
  Erythroxylum coca: illustration, 149
Erythroxylum coca
  var. *ipadu* Plowman, Erythroxylaceae 149
Esenbeckia febrifuga Juss., Rutaceae 301
Esenbeckia intermedia Mart., Rutaceae 301
Eugenia brasiliensis Lam., Myrtaceae 253
Eugenia dysenterica DC., Myrtaceae 253
  Eugenia dysenterica: illustration, 254
Eugenia sulcata Spring, Myrtaceae 254
Eugenia supra-axillaris Spring, Myrtaceae 254
Eugenia uniflora L., Myrtaceae 254
Euphorbia caecorum Mart., Euphorbiaceae 152
Euphorbia cotinoides Miq., Euphorbiaceae 152
Euphorbia hirta L., Euphorbiaceae 152
Euphorbia hyssopifolia L., Euphorbiaceae 153
Euphorbia papillosa St-Hil., Euphorbiaceae 152
Euphorbia phosphorea Mart., Euphorbiaceae 153
Euphorbia prostrata Ait., Euphorbiaceae 153
Euphorbia thymifolia L., Euphorbiaceae 153
Euphorbia tirucalli L., Euphorbiaceae 153
Euphorbiaceae 150
Euterpe edulis Mart., Arecaceae 41
Euterpe oleracea Mart., Arecaceae .... 42 & *318, 306*
  Euterpe oleracea: illustration, 42
Evolvulus alsinoides L., Convolvulaceae 130

Evolvulus holosericeus – Hypoxidaceae: Species Index

Evolvulus holosericeus H.B.K., Convolvulaceae 130
Exostemma australe St.-Hil., Rubiaceae 298
Fabaceae 160
Fevillea trilobata L., Cucurbitaceae 136
Fevillea uncipetala Kuhlm., Cucurbitaceae 138
Ficus gomelleira Kunth & Bouché, Moraceae 248
Ficus insipida Willd., Moraceae 248
Ficus maxima P. Mill., Moraceae 248
Ficus trigona L.f., Moraceae 249
Flacourtiaceae 176
Flaveria bidentis (L.) Ktze., Asteraceae 60
Galactia neesii DC., Fabaceae 168
   Galactia neesii: illustration, 167
Galactia peduncularis (Benth.) Taub., Fabaceae. 168
Galinsoga parviflora Cav., Asteraceae 60
Galipea dichotoma Sald., Rutaceae 301
Galipea multiflora Schult., Rutaceae 301
Gallesia gorazema (Vell.) Moq., Phytolaccaceae 271
Galphimia brasiliensis Juss., Malpighiaceae 220
Geissospermum laeve (Vell.) Baill., Apocynaceae 23
Geissospermum sericeum
   Benth. & Hook., Apocynaceae 24
Geissospermum spp., Apocynaceae 24
Genipa americana L., Rubiaceae 298
Gentianaceae 179
Geoffroea striata (Willd.) Morong, Fabaceae 168
Gesneriaceae 181
Glandularia peruviana (L.) Small, Verbenaceae 334
Glechon ciliata Benth., Lamiaceae 192
Glechon spathulata Benth., Lamiaceae 192
Gochnatia polymorpha (Less.) Cabr., Asteraceae 60
Gomphrena leucocephala Mart., Amaranthaceae 4
Gomphrena macrocephala St.-Hil., Amaranthaceae 4
Gomphrena mollis Mart., Amaranthaceae 4
Gomphrena officinalis Mart., Amaranthaceae 4
Griffinia hyacinthina Ker.-Gawl., Amaryllidaceae 6
Grindelia buphthalmoides DC., Asteraceae 60
Grindelia scorzonerifolia Hook. & Arn., Asteraceae .. 60
Guarea spiciflora Juss., Meliaceae 227
Guarea trichilioides L., Meliaceae 227
Guarea tuberculata Vell., Meliaceae 229
Guatteria nigrescens Mart., Annonaceae 14
Guatteria ouregon (Aubl.) Dun., Annonaceae 14
Guatteria scandens Ducke, Annonaceae 15
Guazuma ulmifolia Lam.
   var. tomentella Schum., Sterculiaceae 323
Guazuma ulmifolia Lam.
   var. ulmifolia, Sterculiaceae 323
Guettarda angelica Mart., Rubiaceae 298
Guettarda argentea Lam., Rubiaceae 298
Guettarda uruguayensis Cham. & Schl., Rubiaceae . 298
Gurania multiflora Cogn., Cucurbitaceae 138
Gurania paulista Cogn., Cucurbitaceae 138
Gustavia hexapetala (Aubl.)
   J.E. Smith, Lecythidaceae 205
Gynerium parviflorum Nees, Poaceae 281
Gynerium sagittatum (Pers.) Beauv., Poaceae 281
Hackelochloa granularis (L.) O. Ktze., Poaceae 281
Haemadyction gaudichaudii DC., Apocynaceae 24
Hancornia speciosa Gomes, Apocynaceae 24
   Hancornia speciosa: illustration, 25
Haynaldia exaltata (Pohl) Kanitz, Campanulaceae ... 109
Hedychium coronarium Koenig, Zingiberaceae 342

Hedyosmum brasiliense Mart., Chloranthaceae 119
Heimia salicifolia (H.B.K.)
   Link & Otto, Lythraceae 214
Heliconia angusta Vell., Heliconiaceae 181
   Heliconia angusta: illustration, 182
Heliconia bihai L., Heliconiaceae 181
Heliconiaceae 181
Helicteres ovata Lam., Sterculiaceae 324
   Helicteres ovata: illustration, 324
Heliotropium curassavicum L., Boraginaceae 88
Heliotropium elongatum Willd., Boraginaceae 88
Heliotropium indicum L., Boraginaceae 89
Heliotropium lanceolatum Loefgr., Boraginaceae 89
Helosis cayennensis
   (Swartz) Spreng., Balanophoraceae 73
   Helosis cayennensis: illustration, 74
Herreria salsaparilha Mart., Liliaceae 207
Heteropteris aphrodisiaca O. Mach., Malpighiaceae 220
Heteropteris syringifolia Gris., Malpighiaceae 220
Heterothalamus alienus (Spr.) O. Ktze., Asteraceae .. 60
Heterothalamus psiadioides Less., Asteraceae 60
Hibiscus bifurcatus Cav., Malvaceae 221
Hibiscus cannabinus L., Malvaceae 221
Hibiscus sabdariffa L., Malvaceae 221
Hibiscus tiliaceus L., Malvaceae 221
Himatanthus alba (L.) Woods., Apocynaceae 24
Himatanthus drastica (Mart.) Woods., Apocynaceae .. 24
Himatanthus fallax (M. Arg.) Woods., Apocynaceae .. 25
Himatanthus lancifolia
   (M. Arg.) Woods., Apocynaceae 26
Himatanthus phagedaenica
   (Mart.) Woods., Apocynaceae 26
Himatanthus sucuuba (Spr.) Woods., Apocynaceae 26
Hippeastrum psittacinum Herb., Amaryllidaceae 6
Hippeastrum puniceum
   (Lam.) Kuntze, Amaryllidaceae 6
Hippeastrum vittatum (L'Hérit.) Herb., Amaryllidaceae 6
Hippobroma longiflora (L.) G. Don, Campanulaceae 109
Hippocratea volubilis L., Hippocrateaceae 183
Hippocrateaceae 183
Holostylis reniformis Duch., Aristolochiaceae 50
Hortia brasiliensis Vand., Rutaceae 301
Humiria balsamifera (Aubl.) St.-Hil., Humiriaceae .. 183
Humiriaceae 183
Hura crepitans L., Euphorbiaceae 153
Hybanthus atropurpureus Taub., Violaceae 338
Hybanthus ipecacuanha (L.) Baill., Violaceae 339
Hydrastis canadensis, Ranunculaceae 76
Hydrocotyle bonariensis Lam., Apiaceae 19
Hydrocotyle leucocephala
   Cham. & Schlecht., Apiaceae 19
Hylocereus undatus (Haw.) Br. & Rose, Cactaceae 95
Hymenaea courbaril L., Caesalpiniaceae 103
   Hymenaea courbaril, illustration, 103
Hymenaea spp., Caesalpiniaceae 104
Hymenaea stigonocarpa Mart., Caesalpiniaceae 104
Hymenaea stilbocarpa Hayne, Caesalpiniaceae 104
Hymenocallis tubiflora Salisb., Amaryllidaceae 7
Hypericum brasiliense Choisy, Clusiaceae 122
Hypericum connatum Lam., Clusiaceae 122
Hypericum teretiusculum St.-Hil., Clusiaceae 122
Hypolytrum laxum Schrad., Cyperaceae 143
Hypoxidaceae 185

Hypoxis decumbens L., Hypoxidaceae 185	*Jacaratia spinosa* (Aubl.) A. DC., Caricaceae 113
Hyptis atrorubens Poit., Lamiaceae 192	*Jatropha curcas* L., Euphorbiaceae 154
Hyptis crenata Pohl, Lamiaceae 192	*Jatropha elliptica* (Pohl) M. Arg., Euphorbiaceae 154
Hyptis fasciculata Benth., Lamiaceae 192	*Jatropha gossypiifolia* L., Euphorbiaceae 154
Hyptis incana Briq., Lamiaceae 192	*Jatropha multifida* L., Euphorbiaceae 154
Hyptis multiflora Pohl, Lamiaceae 193	*Jatropha pohliana* M. Arg., Euphorbiaceae 154
Hyptis mutabilis (Rich.) Briq., Lamiaceae 193	*Jatropha urens* L., Euphorbiaceae 155
Hyptis plectranthoides Benth., Lamiaceae 193	*Jessenia bataua* (Mart.) Burret, Arecaceae 43
Hyptis spicigera Lam., Lamiaceae 193	*Joannesia heveoides* Ducke, Euphorbiaceae 155
Hyptis suaveolens Poit., Lamiaceae 193	*Joannesia princeps* Vell., Euphorbiaceae 155
Hyptis umbrosa Salzm., Lamiaceae 193	*Jodina rhombifolia* Hook. & Arn., Santalaceae 304
Ibicella lutea (Lindl.) Van Eselt., Martyniaceae 224	*Julocroton humilis* Diedr., Euphorbiaceae 155
Icacinaceae 185	*Julocroton stipularis* M. Arg., Euphorbiaceae 155
Ichthyothere terminalis (Spr.) S.F. Blake, Asteraceae . 61	*Jungia floribunda* Less., Asteraceae 61
Ilex acrodonta Reiss., Aquifoliaceae 31	*Kalanchoe brasiliensis* Camb., Crassulaceae 133
Ilex brevicuspis Reiss., Aquifoliaceae 31	*Kalanchoe pinnata* (Lam.) Pers., Crassulaceae 133
Ilex paraguariensis St.-Hil., Aquifoliaceae ...... 31 & *185*	*Kalanchoe* spp., Crassulaceae 134
Ilex paraguariensis: illustration, 32	*Keithia denudata* Benth., Lamiaceae 193
Imperata brasiliensis Trin., Poaceae 281	*Kielmeyera coriacea* Mart., Clusiaceae 122
Imperata contracta Hitch., Poaceae 281	*Kielmeyera petiolaris* Mart., Clusiaceae 122
Indigofera suffruticosa Mill., Fabaceae 168	*Kielmeyera rosea* Mart., Clusiaceae 122
Inga alba (Sw.) Willd., Mimosaceae 237	*Kielmeyera speciosa* St.-Hil., Clusiaceae 123
Inga lateriflora Miq., Mimosaceae 237	*Krameria argentea* Mart., Krameriaceae 191
Inga setigera DC., Mimosaceae 237	*Krameria argentea:* illustration, 190
Ionidium poaya St.-Hil., Violaceae 339	*Krameria spartioides* Berg, Krameriaceae 191
Ipomoea acetosifolia (Vahl)	*Krameria tomentosa* St.-Hil., Krameriaceae 191
Roem. & Schult., Convolvulaceae 130	*Krameria triandra* R. & Pav., Krameriaceae 191
Ipomoea batatoides Meissn., Convolvulaceae 131	Krameriaceae 191
Ipomoea capparoides Choisy, Convolvulaceae 131	*Kyllinga pungens* Link, Cyperaceae 143
Ipomoea echioides Choisy, Convolvulaceae 131	*Ladenbergia hexandra* Klotz., Rubiaceae 299
Ipomoea gigantea Choisy, Convolvulaceae 131	*Ladenbergia lambertiana* Klotz., Rubiaceae 299
Ipomoea longicuspis Meissn., Convolvulaceae 131	*Laetia apetala* Jacq., Flacourtiaceae 178
Ipomoea pentaphylla Jacq., Convolvulaceae 130	*Lafoensia densiflora* Pohl, Lythraceae 214
Ipomoea pes-caprae (L.) R. Br., Convolvulaceae 130	*Lafoensia densiflora:* illustration, 215
Ipomoea silvana Choisy, Convolvulaceae 131	*Lafoensia pacari* St.-Hil., Lythraceae 215
Ipomoea sinuata Ortega, Convolvulaceae 131	*Lagenaria siceraria* (Molina) Standl., Cucurbitaceae 138
Ipomoea spp., Convolvulaceae 131	Lamiaceae 191
Iresine polymorpha Mart., Amaranthaceae 4	*Lantana brasiliensis* Link, Verbenaceae 334
Iridaceae 186	*Lantana camara* L., Verbenaceae 334
Ischnosiphon arouma Koern., Marantaceae 223	*Lantana lilacina* Desf., Verbenaceae 335
Isoetaceae 189	*Lantana macrophylla* Schauer, Verbenaceae 335
Isoetes martii A. Braun, Isoetaceae 189	*Lantana microphylla* Cham., Verbenaceae 335
Isoetes martii: illustration, 189	*Lantana mixta* L., Verbenaceae 335
Isostigma megapotamicum (Spr.) Sherff, Asteraceae .. 61	*Lantana pseudothea*
Jacaranda brasiliana (Lam.) Pers., Bignoniaceae 80	(St.-Hil.) Schauer, Verbenaceae 335
Jacaranda caroba (Vell.) DC., Bignoniaceae 80	*Lantana* spp., Verbenaceae 335
Jacaranda claussenia na Casar., Bignoniaceae 81	*Laplacea fruticosa* (Schr.) Kobuski, Theaceae 326
Jacaranda copaia (Aubl.) D. Don, Bignoniaceae 80	*Laportea aestuans* (L.) Chew, Urticaceae 330
Jacaranda cuspidifolia Mart., Bignoniaceae 81	Lauraceae 196
Jacaranda decurrens Cham., Bignoniaceae 81	*Leandra lacunosa* Cogn., Melastomataceae 225
Jacaranda elegans Mart., Bignoniaceae 81	Lecythidaceae 204
Jacaranda heterophylla	*Lecythis amara* Aubl., Lecythidaceae 205
Bur. & Pet., Bignoniaceae 81	*Lecythis pisonis* Camb., Lecythidaceae 206
Jacaranda micrantha Cham., Bignoniaceae 81	*Leiothrix flavescens* (Bong.) Ruhl., Eriocaulaceae 148
Jacaranda mimosifolia D. Don, Bignoniaceae 81	*Leiphaimos aphylla* (Jacq.) Gilg, Gentianaceae 180
Jacaranda oxyphylla Cham., Bignoniaceae 81	*Lemna minor* L., Lemnaceae 207
Jacaranda paucifoliata Mart., Bignoniaceae 81	Lemnaceae 207
Jacaranda puberula Cham., Bignoniaceae 81	*Leonotis nepetaefolia* R. Br., Lamiaceae 194
Jacaranda rufa Manso, Bignoniaceae 81	*Leonurus sibiricus* L., Lamiaceae 194
Jacaranda semiserrata Cham., Bignoniaceae 81	*Leopoldinia major* Wallace, Arecaceae 43
Jacaranda subrhombea DC., Bignoniaceae 81	*Lepismium myosurus* Pfeiff., Cactaceae 96
Jacaranda spp., Bignoniaceae 81	*Leucas martinicensis* (Jacq.) R. Br., Lamiaceae 194
Jacaranda tomentosa R. Br., Bignoniaceae 81	*Licania macrophylla* Benth., Chrysobalanaceae 120

Licaria camara (Schomb.) Kosterm., Lauraceae 198
Licaria canella (Meissn.) Kosterm., Lauraceae 199
Licaria puchury-major
  (Mart.) Kosterm., Lauraceae 199
Liliaceae 207
Limonium brasiliense
  (Boiss.) O. Ktze., Plantaginaceae 278
Lindernia crustacea F. Muell., Scrophulariaceae 311
Lindernia diffusa Wettst., Scrophulariaceae 311
Lipostoma campanuliflorum D. Don, Rubiaceae 299
Lipostoma capitata D. Don, Rubiaceae 299
Lippia alba (Mill.) N.E. Brown, Verbenaceae 335
Lippia gratissima (Gill. & Hook.)
  Troncoso, Verbenaceae 335
Lisianthus alpestris Mart., Gentianaceae 179
Lisianthus amplissimus Mart., Gentianaceae 179
Lisianthus brevifolius Gris., Gentianaceae 179
Lisianthus campanuloides Spruce, Gentianaceae 179
Lisianthus coerulescens Aubl., Gentianaceae 179
Lisianthus obtusifolius Gris., Gentianaceae 179
Lisianthus purpurascens Aubl., Gentianaceae 179
Lisianthus spp., Gentianaceae 179
Lisianthus uliginosus Gris., Gentianaceae 179
Lisianthus vividiflorus Mart., Gentianaceae 179
Lithraea molleoides (Vell.) Engl., Anacardiaceae 9
Loganiaceae 209
Lophophytum mirabile
  Schott & Endl., Balanophoraceae 73
Loranthaceae 211
Lucilia nitens Less., Asteraceae 61
Lucuma caimito Roem. & Schult., Sapotaceae 309
Lucuma rivicoa Gaertn., Sapotaceae 309
Ludwigia natans (H.B.K.) Ell., Onagraceae 264
Ludwigia peruviana (L.) Hara, Onagraceae 264
Ludwigia repens (L.) Hara, Onagraceae 264
Ludwigia suffruticosa (L.) Gomes, Onagraceae 264
Luehea divaricata Mart. & Zucc., Tiliaceae 326
Luehea rufescens St.-Hil., Tiliaceae 327
Luffa operculata (L.) Cogn., Cucurbitaceae 138
  Luffa operculata: illustration, 137
Luxemburgia glazioviana Gilg, Ochnaceae 260
Luxemburgia polyandra St.-Hil., Ochnaceae 261
Luziola peruviana Pers., Poaceae 281
Lythraceae 213
Mabea fistulifera Mart., Euphorbiaceae 155
Macairea radula (Bonpl.) DC., Melastomataceae 225
Macfadyena unguis-cati (L.) Gentry, Bignoniaceae 81
Machaerium ferox (Mart.) Ducke, Fabaceae 168
Machaerium lunatum (L.) Ducke, Fabaceae 168
Machaonia brasiliensis Cham. & Schl., Rubiaceae .. 299
Maclura brasiliensis Endl., Moraceae 249
Maclura tinctoria (L.) D. Don, Moraceae 249
Macrosiphonia longiflora
  (Desf.) M. Arg., Apocynaceae 26
Macrosiphonia velame
  (St.-Hil.) M. Arg., Apocynaceae 26
Magnoliaceae 216
Magonia pubescens St.-Hil., Sapindaceae 305
Malpighiaceae 217
Malvaceae 221
Mammea americana L., Clusiaceae 123
Mandevilla velutina (Mart. ex Stadelm.) Woods.
  var. *velutina*, Apocynaceae 27

Manettia ignita (Vell.) K. Sch., Rubiaceae 299
Manilkara bidentata (A. DC.) Chev., Sapotaceae 309
Manilkara zapota (L.) Van Royen, Sapotaceae 309
Maprounea brasiliensis L., Euphorbiaceae 155
Maquira sclerophylla
  (Ducke) C. C. Berg, Moraceae 249
Maranta arundinacea L., Marantaceae 223
Marantaceae 223
Marcgravia rectiflora
  Tr. & Planch., Marcgraviaceae 224
Marcgraviaceae 224
Margyricarpus setosus Ruiz & Pav., Rosaceae 294
Mariscus flavus Vahl, Cyperaceae 143
Mariscus jacquinii H.B.K., Cyperaceae 143
Marlierea tomentosa Camb., Myrtaceae 255
Marsdenia amylacea
  (Barb.-Rodr.) Malme, Asclepiadaceae 51
Marsypianthes chamaedrys
  (Vahl) O. Ktze., Lamiaceae 194
Martinella obovata (H.B.K.)
  Bur. & K. Sch., Bignoniaceae 82
Martyniaceae 224
Marupa francoana Miers, Simaroubaceae 313
Mauritia flexuosa L. f., Arecaceae 43
  Mauritia flexuosa: illustration, 44
Mauritiella aculeata (Kunth) Burret, Arecaceae 43
Matayba purgans Radlk., Sapindaceae 306
Maytenus boaria Mol., Celastraceae 115
Maytenus communis Reiss., Celastraceae 115
Maytenus gonoclada Mart., Celastraceae 115
Maytenus ilicifolia Mart., Celastraceae . 115 & *133, 249*
Maytenus laevis Reiss., Celastraceae 115
Maytenus obtusifolia Mart., Celastraceae 116
Maytenus spp., Celastraceae .... 116 & *183*
Melampodium divaricatum (Rich.) DC., Asteraceae .. 61
Melastomataceae 225
Meliaceae 227
Melinis minutiflora Beauv., Poaceae 281
Melocactus melocactoides (Hoffm.) DC., Cactaceae .. 97
Melothria fluminensis Gardn., Cucurbitaceae 139
Melothrianthus smilacifolius
  (Cogn.) M. Crovetto, Cucurbitaceae 139
Menispermaceae 231
Mentha crispa L., Lamiaceae 194
Menyanthaceae 235
Mesechites sulphurea (Vell.) M. Arg., Apocynaceae ... 27
Metrodorea pubescens St.-Hil. & Tul., Rutaceae 301
Mezilaurus crassiramea (Meissn.)
  Taub. ex Mez, Lauraceae 199
Miconia albicans (Sw.) Tr., Melastomataceae 225
Miconia spp., Melastomataceae 225
Microcolea quadrangularis
  (Lam.) Gris., Gentianaceae 180
Microgramma vaccinifolia
  (Langsd. & Fisch.) Copel., Polypodiaceae 288
Microtea debilis Sw., Phytolaccaceae 271
Mikania cordifolia (L. f.) Willd., Asteraceae 61
Mikania glomerata Spreng., Asteraceae 61
  Mikania glomerata: illustration, 63
Mikania hirsutissima DC., Asteraceae 62
Mikania lindleyana DC., Asteraceae 62
Mikania officinalis Mart., Asteraceae 62
Mikania parviflora (Aubl.) Karst., Asteraceae 62

Mikania periplocifolia Hook. & Arn., Asteraceae 62
Mikania setigera Schultz-Bip. ex Baker, Asteraceae ... 62
Mimosa acutistipula Benth., Mimosaceae 237
Mimosa bimucronata (DC.) O. Ktze., Mimosaceae .. 238
Mimosa caesalpiniaefolia Benth., Mimosaceae 238
Mimosa hostilis Benth., Mimosaceae .... 238 & 240
  Mimosa hostilis: illustration, 238
Mimosa invisa Mart., Mimosaceae 239
Mimosa malacocentra Mart., Mimosaceae 239
Mimosa pudica L., Mimosaceae 240
Mimosa velloziana Mart., Mimosaceae 240
Mimosa verrucosa Benth., Mimosaceae 240
  Mimosa verrucosa: illustration, 239
Mimosaceae 236
Modiolastrum pinnatipartitum
  (St.-Hil. & Naudin) Krapovickas, Malvaceae 221
Mollinedia schottiana (Spr.) Perk., Monimiaceae 245
Momordica charantia L., Cucurbitaceae 139
Monimiaceae 245
Monnieria trifolia Loefl., Rutaceae 302
Monopteryx uacu Spruce ex Benth., Fabaceae 169
Monstera adansonii Schott, Araceae 36
Monstera obliqua Miquel, Araceae 36
Montrichardia linifera (Arruda) Schott, Araceae 36
Moraceae 246
Mouriri apiranga Spruce, Melastomataceae 225
Mouriri guianensis Aubl., Melastomataceae 225
Mucuna pruriens (L.) DC., Fabaceae 169
Muehlenbeckia sagittifolia
  (Ort.) Meissn., Polygonaceae 285
Muntingia calabura L., Tiliaceae 327
Myracroduon urundeuva
  Fr. All., Anacardiaceae 9
Myrcia amazonica DC., Myrtaceae 255
Myrcia lanceolata Camb., Myrtaceae 255
Myrcia sphaerocarpa DC., Myrtaceae 255
Myrcia tingens Berg, Myrtaceae 255
Myrocarpus fastigiatus Fr. All., Fabaceae 170
Myrocarpus frondosus Fr. All., Fabaceae 170
Myroxylon balsamum (L.) Harms, Fabaceae 170
  Myroxylon balsamum: illustration, 169
Myristicaceae 250
Myrsinaceae 253
Myrtaceae 253
Naucleopsis amara Ducke, Moraceae 249
Nectandra canescens Nees, Lauraceae 199
Nectandra globosa (Aubl.) Mez, Lauraceae 199
Nectandra leucantha Nees, Lauraceae 199
Nectandra leucothyrsus Meissn., Lauraceae 199
Nectandra pichurim (H.B.K.) Mez, Lauraceae 200
Nectandra puberula Nees, Lauraceae 200
Nectandra turbacensis Nees, Lauraceae 200
Neea theifera Oersted, Nyctaginaceae 258
Nepsera aquatica Naud., Melastomataceae 226
Nicandra physaloides (L.) Gaertn., Solanaceae 318
Nothoscordum striatum Kunth, Iridaceae 186
Noticastrum diffusum (Pers.) Cabr., Asteraceae 62
Notocactus ottonis (Lem.) Berg., Cactaceae 97
Nyctaginaceae 257
Nymphaea ampla DC., Nymphaeaceae 259
Nymphaea rudgeana G. Meyer, Nymphaeaceae 259
  Nymphaea rudgeana: illustration, 260
Nymphaeaceae 259

Nymphoides indica (L.) O. Ktze., Menyanthaceae 235
  Nymphoides indica: illustration, 235
Ochnaceae 260
Ochroma pyramidale (Cav.) Urb., Bombacaceae 86
Ocimum fluminensis Vell., Lamiaceae 195
Ocimum micranthum Willd., Lamiaceae 195
Ocimum nudicaule Benth., Lamiaceae 195
Ocimum sellowii Benth., Lamiaceae 195
Ocotea cujumary Mart., Lauraceae 200
Ocotea cymbarum H.B.K., Lauraceae 200
Ocotea guianensis Aubl., Lauraceae 201
Ocotea opifera Mart., Lauraceae 201
Ocotea pretiosa (Nees & Mart.)
  Benth. & Hook., Lauraceae 201
  Ocotea pretiosa: illustration, 202
Ocotea pulchella Mart., Lauraceae 201
Ocotea rodiei (Schomb.) Mez, Lauraceae 201
Ocotea spectabilis (Meissn.) Mez, Lauraceae 201
Ocotea squarrosa Mart. ex Nees, Lauraceae 203
Ocotea teleiandra (Messn.) Mez, Lauraceae 203
Odontadenia speciosa Benth., Apocynaceae 27
Oenocarpus distichus Mart., Arecaceae 43
Oenothera catharinensis Camb., Onagraceae 264
Olacaceae 262
Oldenlandia corymbosa L., Rubiaceae 299
Omphalea diandra M. Arg., Euphorbiaceae 156
Onagraceae 264
Operculina alata (Ham.) Urb., Convolvulaceae 131
Operculina macrocarpa Urb., Convolvulaceae 131
Operculina spp., Convolvulaceae 131
Opiliaceae 265
Opuntia vulgaris Mill., Cactaceae 97
Orbignya phalerata Mart., Arecaceae 43
Orchidaceae 266
Ottonia corcovadensis Miq., Piperaceae 272
Ottonia jaborandi (Vell.) Kunth, Piperaceae 272
Ouratea guianensis Aubl., Ochnaceae 261
Ouratea hexasperma (St.-Hil.) Baill., Ochnaceae 261
Ouratea jabotapita Engl., Ochnaceae 261
Ouratea parviflora (DC.) Baill., Ochnaceae 261
Ouratea spp., Ochnaceae 262
Oxalidaceae 266
Oxalis amara St.-Hil., Oxalidaceae 266
Oxalis articulata Sav., Oxalidaceae 267
Oxalis bahiensis Prog., Oxalidaceae 267
Oxalis bipartita St.-Hil., Oxalidaceae 267
Oxalis chrysantha Prog., Oxalidaceae 267
Oxalis cordata St.-Hil., Oxalidaceae 266
Oxalis corniculata L., Oxalidaceae 266
  Oxalis corniculata: illustration, 267
Oxalis eriocarpa DC., Oxalidaceae 267
Oxalis martiana Zucc., Oxalidaceae 267
  Oxalis martiana: illustration, 268
Oxalis oxyptera Prog., Oxalidaceae 267
Oxalis spp., Oxalidaceae 267
Oxalis triangularis St.-Hil., Oxalidaceae 267
Panicum brevifolium L., Poaceae 282
Panicum megiston Schult., Poaceae 282
Panicum petrosum Trin., Poaceae 282
Panicum trichanthum Nees, Poaceae 282
Pappophorum mucronulatum Nees, Poaceae 282
Parahancornia amapa (Hub.) Ducke, Apocynaceae .. 27
  Parahancornia amapa: illustration, 25

Parapiptadenia rigida
   (Benth.) Brenan, Mimosaceae 240
Parietaria boehmerioides Mart., Urticaceae 331
Parkia oppositifolia (Spruce) Benth., Mimosaceae ... 240
   Parkia oppositifolia: illustration, 241
Parkia pectinata Benth., Mimosaceae 240
Parkia pendula Benth. ex Walp., Mimosaceae 240
Parkinsonia aculeata L., Caesalpiniaceae 104
Parthenium hysterophorus L., Asteraceae 64
Paspalum extenuatum Nees, Poaceae 282
Passiflora alata Dryand., Passifloraceae 267
Passiflora amethystina Mikan, Passifloraceae 269
Passiflora caerulea L., Passifloraceae 269
Passiflora coccinea Aubl., Passifloraceae 269
Passiflora edulis Sims, Passifloraceae 269
Passiflora foetida L., Passifloraceae 269
Passiflora gardneri Mast., Passifloraceae 270
Passiflora incarnata L., Passifloraceae. 270
Passiflora laurifolia L., Passifloraceae 270
Passiflora macrocarpa Mast., Passifloraceae 270
Passiflora mucronata Lam, Passifloraceae. 270
Passiflora spp., Passifloraceae 270
Passifloraceae 267
Patagonula americana L., Boraginaceae 89
Paullinia cupana Kunth, Sapindaceae 306
   Paullinia cupana: illustration, 307
Peltodon longipes St.-Hil., Lamiaceae 195
Peltodon radicans Pohl, Lamiaceae 195
Pentaclethra macroloba
   (Willd.) O. Ktze., Mimosaceae 242
Peperomia elongata Miq., Piperaceae 273
Peperomia hederacea Miq., Piperaceae 273
Peperomia pellucida H.B.K., Piperaceae 273
   Peperomia pellucida: illustration, 273
Peperomia rotundifolia H.B.K., Piperaceae 274
Peperomia transparens Miq., Piperaceae 274
Pereskia aculeata Mill., Cactaceae 97
Pereskia bleo H.B.K., Cactaceae 97
Periandra mediterranea (Vell.) Taub., Fabaceae 170
Peritassa calypsoides
   (Camb.) A.C. Sm., Hippocrateaceae 183
Peschiera affinis (M. Arg.) Miers, Apocynaceae 27
Peschiera laeta (Mart.) Miers, Apocynaceae 27
Petiveria alliacea L., Phytolaccaceae 271
Pfaffia glomerata (Spreng.) Peders., Amaranthaceae 4
Pfaffia iresinoides Spreng., Amaranthaceae 5
Pfaffia jubata Mart., Amaranthaceae 5
Pfaffia paniculata (Mart.) Kuntze, Amaranthaceae 5
Philodendron bipinnatifidum Schott, Araceae 36
Philodendron hederaceum (Jacq.) Schott
   var. *hederaceum*, Araceae 36
Philodendron imbe Schott, Araceae 36
Philodendron ochrostemon Schott, Araceae 37
Philodendron pedatum (Hook.) Kunth, Araceae 37
   Philodendron pedatum: illustration, 38
Philodendron selloum Koch, Araceae 37
Philodendron speciosum Schott, Araceae 37
Philoxerus portulacoides St.-Hil., Amaranthaceae 5
Phlebodium aureum (L.) J.E. Smith, Polypodiaceae . 288
Phlebodium decumanum
   (Willd.) J. Smith, Polypodiaceae 288
Phoradendron crassifolium
   (Pohl) Eichl., Loranthaceae 211

Phthirusa adunca (Meyer) Maguire, Loranthaceae ... 211
Phyllanthus acutifolius Spreng., Euphorbiaceae 156
Phyllanthus amarus
   Thonn. & Schum., Euphorbiaceae 156
Phyllanthus conami Sw., Euphorbiaceae 156
Phyllanthus diffusus Klotz., Euphorbiaceae 156
Phyllanthus lathyroides M. Arg., Euphorbiaceae 157
Phyllanthus niruri L., Euphorbiaceae 156
Phyllanthus nobilis M. Arg., Euphorbiaceae 157
Phyllanthus sellowianus M. Arg., Euphorbiaceae 157
Phyllanthus tenellus Roxb., Euphorbiaceae 157
Physalis angulata L., Solanaceae 318
Physalis pubescens L., Solanaceae 318
Phytolaccaceae 271
Picramnia bahiensis Turcz., Simaroubaceae 313
Picramnia camboita Engl., Simaroubaceae 314
Picramnia ciliata Mart., Simaroubaceae 314
Picrolemma pseudocoffea Ducke, Simaroubaceae ... 314
Pilea microphylla (L.) Liebm., Urticaceae 331
Pilocarpus pinnatifolius Lem., Rutaceae 302
Piper aduncum L., Piperaceae 274
Piper angustifolium R. & Pav., Piperaceae 274
Piper arboreum Aubl., Piperaceae 274
Piper callosum R. & Pav., Piperaceae 274
Piper cavalcantei Yunck., Piperaceae 275
Piper ceanothifolium H.B.K., Piperaceae 275
Piper colubrinum Link, Piperaceae 275
Piper elongatum Vahl, Piperaceae 275
Piper eucalyptifolium (Miq.) Rudge, Piperaceae 275
Piper geniculatum Sw., Piperaceae 275
Piper gigantifolium Jacq., Piperaceae 275
Piper marginatum Jacq., Piperaceae 275
Piper mikanianum (Kunth) Steud., Piperaceae 276
Piper mollicomum Kunth, Piperaceae 276
Piper parthenium Mart., Piperaceae 276
Piper reticulatum L., Piperaceae 276
Piper rohrii C. DC., Piperaceae 276
Piper tuberculatum Jacq., Piperaceae 276
Piperaceae 272
Piptadenia polyptera Benth., Mimosaceae 242
Piptocarpha rotundifolia (Less.) Bak., Asteraceae 64
Pisonia aculeata L., Nyctaginaceae 258
Pisonia alcalina Fr. All., Nyctaginaceae 258
Pisonia cordifolia Mart., Nyctaginaceae 258
Pisonia subcordata Sw., Nyctaginaceae 258
Pithecellobium avaremotemo Mart., Mimosaceae 242
Pithecellobium cochleatum
   (Willd.) Mart., Mimosaceae 242
Pithecellobium spp., Mimosaceae 242
Pithecellobium unguis-cati (L.) Benth., Mimosaceae 242
Plantaginaceae 278
Plantago brasiliensis Sims, Plantaginaceae 278
Plantago guilleminiana Dcne., Plantaginaceae 278
Plantago myosurus Lam., Plantaginaceae 278
Platonia insignis Mart., Clusiaceae 123
Pleurothyrium cuneifolium Nees, Lauraceae 203
Pluchea laxiflora Hook. & Arn., Asteraceae 64
Pluchea suaveolens (Vell.) O. Ktze., Asteraceae 64
Plumbaginaceae 278
Plumbago scandens L., Plumbaginaceae 279
Plumeria alba L., Apocynaceae 28
Poaceae 279
Polycarpaea corymbosa (L.) Lam., Caryophyllaceae 115

SPECIES INDEX: POLYGALA ANGULATA – SCHULTESIA STENOPHYLLA

Polygala angulata DC., Polygalaceae 283
Polygala comata Mart., Polygalaceae 284
Polygala klotzschii Chodat, Polygalaceae 284
Polygala paniculata L., Polygalaceae 284
Polygala senega L., Polygalaceae 284
Polygala spectabilis DC., Polygalaceae 284
Polygala timoutou Aubl., Polygalaceae 284
Polygalaceae 283
Polygonaceae 285
Polygonum acuminatum H.B.K., Polygonaceae 286
Polygonum hydropiperoides Michx., Polygonaceae . 286
 Polygonum hydropiperoides: illustration, 286
Polygonum punctatum Elliot, Polygonaceae 287
Polygonum spectabile Mart., Polygonaceae 287
Polypodiaceae 288
Polypodium brasiliense Poir., Polypodiaceae 288
Pontederia cordifolia Mart., Pontederiaceae 288
Pontederiaceae 288
Porophyllum ruderale (Jacq.) Cass., Asteraceae 64
Portulaca grandiflora Hook., Portulacaceae 288
Portulaca oleracea L., Portulacaceae 289
Portulaca pilosa L., Portulacaceae 289
Portulacaceae 288
Potalia amara Aubl., Loganiaceae 209
Pothomorphe peltata L., Piperaceae 277
Pothomorphe umbellata (L.) Miq., Piperaceae 277
Pouteria laurifolia Radlk., Sapotaceae 309
Pouteria obtusifolia Baehni, Sapotaceae 310
Pouteria salicifolia Hook. & Arn., Sapotaceae 310
Pradosia lactescens (Vell.) Radlk., Sapotaceae 310
Primulaceae 290
Protium aracouchini (Aubl.) March., Burseraceae 93
Protium brasiliense Engl., Burseraceae 94
 Protium brasiliense: illustration, 94
Protium cordatum Hub., Burseraceae 94
Protium elegans Engl., Burseraceae 94
Protium heptaphyllum (Aubl.) March., Burseraceae ... 93
Protium icicariba (DC.) March., Burseraceae 94
Protium insigne Engl., Burseraceae 94
Protium opacum Swart., Burseraceae 95
Protium sagotianum March., Burseraceae 94
Protium schomburgkianum Engl., Burseraceae 94
Protium spp., Burseraceae 94
Protium spruceanum (Benth.) Engl., Burseraceae ... 94
Protium unifoliolatum Engl., Burseraceae 94
Prunus subcoriacea
 (Chod. & Hassl.) Hoehne, Rosaceae 294
Pseudocaryophyllus sericeus Berg, Myrtaceae 256
Psidium arboreum Vell., Myrtaceae 256
Psidium cattleyanum Sabine, Myrtaceae 256
Psidium cinereum Mart., Myrtaceae 256
Psidium guajava L., Myrtaceae 256
Psoralea glandulosa L., Fabaceae 170
 Psoralea glandulosa: illustration, 171
Pteridium aquilinum (L.) Kuhn, Dennstaedtiaceae ... 144
Pterocaulon virgatum DC., Asteraceae 64
Pterodon apparicioi Peders., Fabaceae 170
 Pterodon apparicioi: illustration, 171
Pterodon pubescens Benth., Fabaceae 171
Ptychopetalum olacoides Benth., Olacaceae 262
Ptychopetalum uncinatum Anselm., Olacaceae 262
Pyrostegia ignea (Vell.) Pres., Bignoniaceae 82
Quassia amara L., Simaroubaceae 314

Ranunculaceae 290
Ranunculus apiifolius Pers., Ranunculaceae 290
Ranunculus bonariensis Poir., Ranunculaceae 291
Raphia taedigera (Mart.) Mart., Arecaceae 45
Raputia alba (Nees & Mart.) Engl., Rutaceae 302
Raputia aromatica Aubl., Rutaceae 302
Raputia magnifica Engl., Rutaceae 302
Raulinoreitzia tremula (Hook.
 & Arn.) King & H. Robinson, Asteraceae 64
Rauwolfia bahiensis DC., Apocynaceae 28
Rauwolfia blanchetii DC., Apocynaceae 28
Rauwolfia ligustrina Willd. ex
 Roem. & Schult., Apocynaceae 28
Reisseckia smilacina (Sm.) Steud., Rhamnaceae 293
Remirea maritima Aubl., Cyperaceae 143
Renealmia exaltata L.f., Zingiberaceae 342
Renealmia occidentalis Sweet, Zingiberaceae 342
Renealmia sylvestris Horan., Zingiberaceae 342
Rhabdodendraceae 291
Rhabdodendron amazonicum
 (Spr. ex Benth.) Hub., Rhabdodendraceae 291
Rhamnaceae 291
Rhipsalis macrocarpa Miq., Cactaceae 97
Rhizophora mangle L., Rhizophoraceae 294
 Rhizophora mangle: illustration, 295
Rhizophoraceae 294
Rollinia exalbida (Vell.) Mart., Annonaceae 15
Rollinia orthopetala DC., Annonaceae 15
Rollinia salicifolia Schl., Annonaceae 15
Rollinia sylvatica (St.-Hil.) Mart., Annonaceae 15
Rosaceae 294
Rubus brasiliensis Mart., Rosaceae 294
Ruellia geminiflora H.B.K., Acanthaceae 1
Ruellia tuberosa L., Acanthaceae 1
Rubiaceae 294
Rumex brasiliensis Link, Polygonaceae 287
Rumohra adiantiformis
 (G. Forst.) Ching, Dryopteridaceae 147
Rutaceae 300
Sacciolepis myuros (Lam.) Chase, Poaceae 282
Saccoglottis guianensis Benth., Humiriaceae 185
 Saccoglottis guianensis: illustration, 184
Salacia impressifolia
 (Miers) A.C. Sm., Hippocrateaceae 183
Salacia spp., Hippocrateaceae 183
Salpichroa origanifolia (Lam.) Thell., Solanaceae ... 319
Salviniaceae 304
Samolus valerandi L., Primulaceae 290
Santalaceae 305
Sapindaceae 305
Sapindus saponaria L., Sapindaceae 306
Sapium hamatum Pax & Hoffm., Euphorbiaceae ... 157
Sapotaceae 308
Sauvagesia erecta L., Ochnaceae 262
Scheelea phalerata
 (Mart. ex Spreng.) Burret, Arecaceae 45
Schinopsis brasiliensis Engl., Anacardiaceae 9
Schinus lentiscifolius March., Anacardiaceae 9
Schinus molle L., Anacardiaceae 9
Schinus terebinthifolius Raddi, Anacardiaceae 10
Schizaeaceae 310
Schrankia leptocarpa DC., Mimosaceae 242
Schultesia stenophylla Mart., Gentianaceae 180

Sciadotenia paraensis
  (Eichl.) Diels, Menispermaceae 234
Scleria pratensis L., Cyperaceae 143
Scoparia dulcis L., Scrophulariaceae 312
Scrophulariaceae 310
Scutia buxifolia Reiss., Rhamnaceae 293
Scybalium fungiforme
  Schott & Endl., Balanophoraceae 74
Sebastiania klotzschiana M. Arg., Euphorbiaceae 157
Sebastiania macrocarpa M. Arg., Euphorbiaceae 157
Sebastiania potamophila Pax, Euphorbiaceae 157
Secondatia floribunda DC., Apocynaceae 28
Sedum sp. 133
Seguieria americana L., Phytolaccaceae 272
Selaginella convoluta Spring, Selaginellaceae 313
Selaginella erythropus Spring, Selaginellaceae 313
Selaginella stellata Spring, Selaginellaceae 313
Selaginellaceae 313
Senecio brasiliensis Less., Asteraceae 65
  Senecio brasiliensis: illustration, 66
Senna affinis (Benth.) Ir. & Barn., Caesalpiniaceae ... 104
Senna alata (L.) Roxb., Caesalpiniaceae 104
Senna alexandrina Miller, Caesalpiniaceae 107
Senna bicapsularis (L.) Roxb., Caesalpiniaceae 104
Senna corymbosa
  (Lam.) Ir. & Barn., Caesalpiniaceae 104
Senna hirsuta (L.) Ir. & Barn.
  var. *puberula* Ir. & Barn., Caesalpiniaceae 105
Senna italicus Miller, Caesalpiniaceae 107
Senna latifolia (Meyer) Ir. & Barn., Caesalpiniaceae 105
Senna leiophylla (Vog.) Ir. & Barn., Caesalpiniaceae 105
Senna macranthera
  (Collad.) Ir. & Barn., Caesalpiniaceae 105
Senna multijuga Rich. var.
  verrucosa (Vog.) Ir. & Barn., Caesalpiniaceae 105
Senna oblongifolia
  (Vog.) Ir. & Barn., Caesalpiniaceae 105
Senna obtusifolia (L.) Ir. & Barn., Caesalpiniaceae .. 105
Senna occidentalis (L.) Link, Caesalpiniaceae 105
Senna quinqueangulata
  (Rich.) Ir. & Barn., Caesalpiniaceae 106
Senna rugosa (G. Don) Ir. & Barn., Caesalpiniaceae 106
  Senna rugosa: illustration, 107
Senna septentrionalis
  (Viv.) Ir. & Barn., Caesalpiniaceae 106
Senna spp., Caesalpiniaceae 106
Senna uniflora
  (P. Miller) Ir. & Barn., Caesalpiniaceae 106
Sesuvium portulacastrum L., Aizoaceae 1
Setaria scandens Schrad., Poaceae 282
Sicana odorifera Naud., Cucurbitaceae 139
Sicyos polyacanthus Cogn., Cucurbitaceae 139
Sida acuta Burm., Malvaceae 221
Sida angustifolia Lam., Malvaceae 222
Sida carpinifolia (L. f.) K. Sch., Malvaceae 222
Sida macrodon DC., Malvaceae 222
Sida micrantha St.-Hil., Malvaceae 222
Sida rhombea L., Malvaceae 222
Sida rhombifolia L., Malvaceae 222
Silybum marianum Gaertn., Asteraceae 65
Simaba ferruginea St.-Hil., Simaroubaceae 314
Simaba glandulifera Gardn., Simaroubaceae 314
Simaba salubris Engl., Simaroubaceae 315

Simarouba amara Aubl., Simaroubaceae 315
Simarouba versicolor St.-Hil., Simaroubaceae 315
Simaroubaceae 313
Sinningia allagophylla (Mart.) Wiehl., Gesneriaceae 181
Siparuna brasiliensis (Spr.) DC., Monimiaceae 245
Siparuna camporum (Tul.) DC., Monimiaceae 245
Siparuna cujabana (Mart.) DC., Monimiaceae 245
Siparuna guianensis Aubl., Monimiaceae 245
Siparuna laurifolia (H.B.K.) DC., Monimiaceae 246
Sisyrinchium vaginatum Spreng., Iridaceae 186
Smilax brasiliensis Spreng., Liliaceae 208
Smilax campestris Gris., Liliaceae 208
  Smilax campestris: illustration, 208
Smilax longifolia Rich., Liliaceae 208
Smilax oblongifolia Pohl, Liliaceae 208
Solanaceae 316
Solanum aculeatissimum Jacq., Solanaceae 319
Solanum agrarium Sendt., Solanaceae 319
Solanum albidum Dun., Solanaceae 319
Solanum ambrosiacum Vell., Solanaceae 319
Solanum caavurana Vell., Solanaceae 319
Solanum cernuum Vell., Solanaceae 319
Solanum ciliatum Lam., Solanaceae 319
Solanum grandiflorum Ruiz & Pav., Solanaceae 320
Solanum insidiosum Mart., Solanaceae 320
  Solanum insidiosum: illustration, 320
Solanum juciri Mart., Solanaceae 321
Solanum juripeba Rich., Solanaceae 321
Solanum lycocarpum St.-Hil., Solanaceae 321
Solanum mammosum L., Solanaceae 321
Solanum martii Sendt. 321
Solanum mauritianum Scop., Solanaceae 321
Solanum nigrum L., Solanaceae 321
Solanum paniculatum L., Solanaceae 321
  Solanum paniculatum: illustration, 320
Solanum pseudoquina St.-Hil., Solanaceae 322
Solanum spp. [Solanaceae] alkaloids, chemistry of 322
Solanum variabile Mart., Solanaceae 322
Solanum verbascifolium L., Solanaceae 322
Solidago chilensis Meyen, Asteraceae 65
Sophora tomentosa L., Fabaceae 172
Sorocea bonplandii (Baill.) Burger, Moraceae 249
Sparattosperma leucanthum
  (Vell.) K. Sch., Bignoniaceae 82
Sphagneticola trilobata (L.) Pruski, Asteraceae 65
Spigelia anthelmia L., Loganiaceae 209
Spigelia flemingiana Cham. & Schl., Loganiaceae ... 209
Spigelia glabrata Mart., Loganiaceae 209
Spondias macrocarpa Engl., Anacardiaceae 10
Spondias mombin L., Anacardiaceae 10
Stachytarpheta cayennensis
  (Rich.) Vahl, Verbenaceae 335
Stachytarpheta dichotoma Vahl, Verbenaceae 336
Stachytarpheta elatior Schrad., Verbenaceae 336
Stachytarpheta jamaicensis (L.) Vahl, Verbenaceae . 336
Sterculia apetala (Jacq.) Karst.
  var. *elata* (Ducke) E. Taylor, Sterculiaceae 324
Sterculia chicha St.-Hil., Sterculiaceae 325
Sterculiaceae 323
Stomatanthes oblongifolius
  (Spr.) H. Robinson, Asteraceae 65
Stromanthe sanguinea Sond., Marantaceae 224
Struthanthus marginatus (Desf.) Bl., Loranthaceae .. 213
  Struthanthus marginatus: illustration, 212

SPECIES INDEX: STRYCHNOS PSEUDOQUINA – UROSPATHA CAUDATA

Strychnos pseudoquina St.-Hil., Loganiaceae 209
   Strychnos pseudoquina: illustration, 210
Strychnos subcordata Spr. ex Benth, Loganiaceae. ... 209
Strychnos spp., Loganiaceae .... 209 & 211, 231
Strychnos torresiana
   Krukoff & Monachino, Loganiaceae 210
Strychnos trinervis (Vell.) Mart., Loganiaceae 210
   Strychnos trinervis: illustration, 210
Stryphnodendron adstringens
   (Mart.) Cov., Mimosaceae 242
Stryphnodendron coriaceum Benth., Mimosaceae ... 243
   Stryphnodendron coriaceum: illustration, 243
Stryphnodendron polyphyllum Mart., Mimosaceae .. 244
Styracaceae 325
Styrax ferrugineum Nees & Mart., Styracaceae 325
Styrax glabratum Schott, Styracaceae 325
Styrax pohlii DC., Styracaceae 325
Swartzia chrysantha B. Rodr., Caesalpiniaceae 107
Swartzia panacoco (Aubl.) Cowan
   var. panacoco, Caesalpiniaceae 107
Sweetia fruticosa Spreng., Fabaceae 172
Syagrus comosa Mart., Arecaceae 45
Syagrus coronata (Mart.) Becc., Arecaceae 45
Syagrus oleracea (Mart.) Becc., Arecaceae 45
Syagrus pseudococos (Raddi) Glassman, Arecaceae .. 45
Syagrus romanzoffiana (Cham.) Glassman, Arecaceae 45
Syagrus schizophylla (Mart.) Glassman, Arecaceae 46
Symphonia globulifera L.f., Clusiaceae 123
Symplocaceae 326
Symplocos parviflora Benth., Symplocaceae 326
Symplocos platyphylla (Pohl) Benth., Symplocaceae 326
Symplocos pubescens Klotzsch, Symplocaceae 326
Tabebuia aurea (Manso) Moore, Bignoniaceae 82
Tabebuia barbata (May) Sandw., Bignoniaceae 82
Tabebuia caraiba (Mart.) Bur., Bignoniaceae 82
Tabebuia chrysotricha (Mart.) Standl., Bignoniaceae . 82
Tabebuia impetiginosa (Mart.) Standl., Bignoniaceae . 83
Tabebuia ipe (Mart.) Standl., Bignoniaceae 83
Tabebuia leucoxylon (L.) DC., Bignoniaceae 83
Tabebuia serratifolia (Vahl) Nichol., Bignoniaceae ... 83
Tabebuia spp., Bignoniaceae 83
Tabebuia umbellata (Sond.) Sandw., Bignoniaceae 83
Tabernaemontana citrifolia L., Apocynaceae 28
Tachia guianensis Aubl., Gentianaceae 180
Tagetes erecta L., Asteraceae 67
Tagetes minuta L., Asteraceae 67
Talauma ovata St.-Hil., Magnoliaceae 216
   Talauma ovata: illustration, 217
Talinum racemosum (L.) Rohr., Portulacaceae 289
Talisia esculenta Radlk., Sapindaceae 306
Tanacetum vulgare L., Asteraceae 67
Tanaecium nocturnum (B. Rodr.)
   Bur. & K. Sch., Bignoniaceae 84
Terminalia argentea Mart., Combretaceae 126
Terminalia tanibouca Smith, Combretaceae 126
Ternstroemia brasiliensis Camb., Theaceae 326
Tetracera aspera Willd., Dilleniaceae 146
Tetracera breyniana Schl., Dilleniaceae 146
Tetracera volubilis L., Dilleniaceae 146
Tetralacrium veroniciforme
   Turcz., Scrophulariaceae 312
Thalia geniculata L., Marantaceae 224
Theaceae 326
Thevetia ahouai (L.) DC., Apocynaceae 28

Tibouchina aspera Aubl., Melastomataceae 226
Tibouchina clavata
   (Pers.) Wurdack, Melastomataceae 226
Tiliaceae 326
Tillandsia aeranthos
   (Loisel.) L.B. Smith, Bromeliaceae 91
   Tillandsia aeranthos: illustration, 92
Tillandsia usneoides L., Bromeliaceae 91
Tontelea brachypoda Miers, Hippocrateaceae 183
Torresea cearensis Fr. All., Fabaceae 172
Torrubia olfersiana
   (Link, Klotzsch & Otto) Standl., Nyctaginaceae ... 258
Tournefortia elegans Cham., Boraginaceae 89
Tournefortia laevigata Lam., Boraginaceae 89
Tournefortia paniculata Cham., Boraginaceae 89
Tournefortia volubilis L., Boraginaceae 90
Tovomita brasiliensis (Mart.) Walp., Clusiaceae 123
Tradescantia diuretica Mart., Commelinaceae 128
Tradescantia effusa Mart., Commelinaceae 129
Tradescantia spathacea Sw., Commelinaceae 129
   Tradescantia spathacea: illustration, 127
Tragia volubilis L., Euphorbiaceae 158
Trianosperma diversifolia Cogn., Cucurbitaceae 139
Trianosperma glandulosa Mart., Cucurbitaceae 140
Trichilia barraensis DC., Meliaceae 229
Trichilia cathartica Mart., Meliaceae 229
Trichilia catigua Juss., Meliaceae 229
Trichilia catuaba (Silva) Rizz., Meliaceae 229
   Trichilia catuaba: illustration, 230
Trichilia hirta L., Meliaceae 229
Trimezia juncifolia Benth. & Hook., Iridaceae 186
Trimezia lurida Salisb., Iridaceae 186
Triplaris macrocalyx Casar., Polygonaceae 287
Triplaris noli-tangere Wedd., Polygonaceae 287
Triplaris weigeltiana
   (Reichb.) O. Ktze., Polygonaceae 287
Triumfetta rhomboidea Jacq., Tiliaceae 327
Triumfetta semitriloba Jacq., Tiliaceae 327
Trixis antimenorrhoea (Schrank) Mart., Asteraceae 67
Tropaeolaceae 327
Tropaeolum pentaphyllum Lam., Tropaeolaceae 327
Turnera diffusa Willd., Turneraceae .... 327 & 328
Turnera guianensis Aubl., Turneraceae 328
Turnera opifera Mart., Turneraceae 328
Turnera rupestris Aubl., Turneraceae 328
Turnera ulmifolia L., Turneraceae 328
Turneraceae 327
Tynanthus cognatus (Cham.) Miers, Bignoniaceae 84
Tynanthus elegans (Cham.), Bignoniaceae 84
Tynanthus fasciculatus
   (Vell.) Miers, Bignoniaceae 84
Typha domingensis Pers., Typhaceae 329
Typhaceae 328
Ulmaceae 330
Unxia camphorata L. f., Asteraceae 67
Urena lobata L., Malvaceae 223
Urera aurantiaca Wedd., Urticaceae 331
Urera baccifera Gaud., Urticaceae 331
Urera caracasana Jacq., Urticaceae 331
Urera subpeltata Miq., Urticaceae 331
   Urera subpeltata: illustration, 332
Urticaceae 330
Urospatha caudata (Poepp.
   & Endl.) Schott, Araceae 37

Vallesia cymbifolia Ortega, Apocynaceae 29
Vatairea guianensis Aubl., Fabaceae 172
Vataireopsis araroba (Aguiar) Ducke, Fabaceae 172
   Vataireopsis araroba: illustration, 171
Verbena bonariensis L., Verbenaceae 336
Verbena erinoides Lam., Verbenaceae 336
Verbenaceae 332
Vernonanthura brasiliana
   (L.) H. Robinson, Asteraceae 67
Victoria amazonica (Poepp.) Sower., Nymphaeaceae 259
   Victoria amazonica: illustration, 261
Violaceae 337
Virola macrophylla
   (Spr. ex Benth.) Warb., Myristicaceae 250
Virola oleifera (Schott) A.C. Smith, Myristicaceae ... 250
Virola sebifera Aubl., Myristicaceae 250
Virola spp., Myristicaceae 252
Virola surinamensis (Rol.) Warb., Myristicaceae 252
   Virola surinamensis: illustration, 251
Vismia acuminata (L.) Pers., Clusiaceae 123
Vismia guianensis (Aubl.) Choisy, Clusiaceae 124
Vismia japurensis Reich., Clusiaceae 124
Vismia latifolia (Aubl.) Choisy, Clusiaceae 124
Vismia reichardtiana (O. Ktze.) Ewan, Clusiaceae ... 124
Vitaceae 339
Vitex agnus-castus L., Verbenaceae 336
Vitex gardneriana Schauer, Verbenaceae 336
Vitex montevidensis Cham., Verbenaceae 337
Vochysia thyrsoidea Pohl, Vochysiaceae 340
Vochysiaceae 340
Vouacapoua americana Aubl., Caesalpiniaceae 107
Waltheria communis St.-Hil., Sterculiaceae 325
Waltheria indica L., Sterculiaceae 325
Waltheria viscosissima St.-Hil., Sterculiaceae 325
Wilbrandia ebracteata Cogn., Cucurbitaceae 140
Wilbrandia spp., Cucurbitaceae 140
Wilbrandia verticillata (Vell.) Cogn., Cucurbitaceae 140
Winteraceae 340
Wissadula periplocifolia Presl., Malvaceae 223
Xanthium orientale L., Asteraceae 67
Xanthium spinosum L., Asteraceae 67
Xanthium strumarium L., Asteraceae 67
Xanthosoma striatipes
   (Kunth & Bouché) Madison, Araceae 37
Xanthosoma violaceum Schott, Araceae 37
Ximenia americana L., Olacaceae 263
Ximenia coriacea Engl., Olacaceae 263
Xylopia aromatica (Lam.) Mart., Annonaceae . 15 & *180*
   Xylopia aromatica: illustration, 17
Xylopia benthamiana Fries, Annonaceae 16
Xylopia frutescens Aubl., Annonaceae 16
Xylopia sericea St.-Hil., Annonaceae 16
Xyridaceae 342
Xyris laxifolia Mart., Xyridaceae 342
Xyris pallida Mart., Xyridaceae 342
Zanthoxylum hyemale St.-Hil., Rutaceae 302
Zanthoxylum pterota H.B.K., Rutaceae 303
Zanthoxylum rhoifolium Lam., Rutaceae 303
Zanthoxylum tingoassuiba St.-Hil., Rutaceae 303
Zeyheria digitalis (Vell.) Hoehne, Bignoniaceae 84
Zingiberaceae 342
Zizyphus joazeiro Mart., Rhamnaceae 293
   Zizyphus joazeiro: illustration, 292

Zschokkea arborescens M. Arg., Apocynaceae 29
Zygostigma australe
   (Cham. & Schl.) Gris., Gentianaceae 181

Vallesia cymbifolia – Zygostigma australe: Species Index

Vallesia cymbifolia Ortega, Apocynaceae 29
Vatairea guianensis Aubl., Fabaceae 172
Vataireopsis araroba (Aguiar) Ducke, Fabaceae 172
   Vataireopsis araroba: illustration, 171
Verbena bonariensis L., Verbenaceae 336
Verbena erinoides Lam., Verbenaceae 336
Verbenaceae 332
Vernonanthura brasiliana
   (L.) H. Robinson, Asteraceae 67
Victoria amazonica (Poepp.) Sower., Nymphaeaceae 259
   Victoria amazonica: illustration, 261
Violaceae 337
Virola macrophylla
   (Spr. ex Benth.) Warb., Myristicaceae 250
Virola oleifera (Schott) A.C. Smith, Myristicaceae ... 250
Virola sebifera Aubl., Myristicaceae 250
Virola spp., Myristicaceae 252
Virola surinamensis (Rol.) Warb., Myristicaceae 252
   Virola surinamensis: illustration, 251
Vismia acuminata (L.) Pers., Clusiaceae 123
Vismia guianensis (Aubl.) Choisy, Clusiaceae 124
Vismia japurensis Reich., Clusiaceae 124
Vismia latifolia (Aubl.) Choisy, Clusiaceae 124
Vismia reichardtiana (O. Ktze.) Ewan, Clusiaceae ... 124
Vitaceae 339
Vitex agnus-castus L., Verbenaceae 336
Vitex gardneriana Schauer, Verbenaceae 336
Vitex montevidensis Cham., Verbenaceae 337
Vochysia thyrsoidea Pohl, Vochysiaceae 340
Vochysiaceae 340
Vouacapoua americana Aubl., Caesalpiniaceae 107
Waltheria communis St.-Hil., Sterculiaceae 325
Waltheria indica L., Sterculiaceae 325
Waltheria viscosissima St.-Hil., Sterculiaceae 325
Wilbrandia ebracteata Cogn., Cucurbitaceae 140
Wilbrandia spp., Cucurbitaceae 140
Wilbrandia verticillata (Vell.) Cogn., Cucurbitaceae 140
Winteraceae 340
Wissadula periplocifolia Presl., Malvaceae 223
Xanthium orientale L., Asteraceae 67
Xanthium spinosum L., Asteraceae 67
Xanthium strumarium L., Asteraceae 67
Xanthosoma striatipes
   (Kunth & Bouché) Madison, Araceae 37
Xanthosoma violaceum Schott, Araceae 37
Ximenia americana L., Olacaceae 263
Ximenia coriacea Engl., Olacaceae 263
Xylopia aromatica (Lam.) Mart., Annonaceae . 15 & *180*
   Xylopia aromatica: illustration, 17
Xylopia benthamiana Fries, Annonaceae 16
Xylopia frutescens Aubl., Annonaceae 16
Xylopia sericea St.-Hil., Annonaceae 16
Xyridaceae 342
Xyris laxifolia Mart., Xyridaceae 342
Xyris pallida Mart., Xyridaceae 342
Zanthoxylum hyemale St.-Hil., Rutaceae 302
Zanthoxylum pterota H.B.K., Rutaceae 303
Zanthoxylum rhoifolium Lam., Rutaceae 303
Zanthoxylum tingoassuiba St.-Hil., Rutaceae 303
Zeyheria digitalis (Vell.) Hoehne, Bignoniaceae 84
Zingiberaceae 342
Zizyphus joazeiro Mart., Rhamnaceae 293
   Zizyphus joazeiro: illustration, 292

Zschokkea arborescens M. Arg., Apocynaceae 29
Zygostigma australe
   (Cham. & Schl.) Gris., Gentianaceae 181